1 MONTH OF
FREE
READING

at
www.ForgottenBooks.com

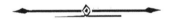

By purchasing this book you are
eligible for one month membership to
ForgottenBooks.com, giving you
unlimited access to our entire
collection of over 1,000,000 titles via
our web site and mobile apps.

To claim your free month visit:
www.forgottenbooks.com/free47307

ISBN 978-0-428-98865-4
PIBN 10047307

MEDICAL NEWS

AND

ABSTRACT.

VOLUME XXXIX.

EDITED BY

I. MINIS HAYS, A.M., M.D.

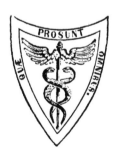

PHILADELPHIA:
HENRY C. LEA'S SON & CO.
1881.

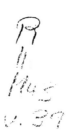

COLLINS, PRINTER.

CONTENTS OF NUMBER 457.

JANUARY, 1881.

CLINICS.

CLINICAL LECTURES.

HOSPITAL NOTES.

MONTHLY ABSTRACT.

ANATOMY AND PHYSIOLOGY.

MATERIA MEDICA AND THERAPEUTICS.

MEDICINE.

MEDICAL NEWS.

THE

MEDICAL NEWS AND ABSTRACT.

VOL. XXXIX. No. 1.   JANUARY, 1881.   WHOLE No. 457.

CLINICS.

Clinical Lectures.

GALVANISM, OR FARADISM? WHICH IS TO BE USED, AND WHEN?

A CLINICAL LECTURE DELIVERED AT JEFFERSON COLLEGE HOSPITAL,

By ROBERTS BARTHOLOW, M.D., LL.D.,

PROFESSOR OF THERAPEUTICS AND MATERIA MEDICA IN JEFFERSON MEDICAL COLLEGE, PHILADELPHIA.

GENTLEMEN: We have had before us many cases in which the applications of electricity have been directed. Sometimes it is the galvanic. sometimes the faradic current which we employ for diagnosis or for treatment. A little inquiry will easily demonstrate, that, if we use electricity as it should be used, both kinds of batteries are necessary. In the purchase of an instrument, the buyer is sometimes misled by the statement that a particular battery furnishes all the currents—a primary or galvanic current, and the various secondary currents. A faradic instrument, of course, furnishes an induced current, and the induction exerted between the coils of the primary wire may be utilized, as well as that from the secondary wire, so that various modifications of the induced currents are available. But no one should be deluded into believing that a faradic battery can also furnish a galvanic current. Pray, do not understand me as saying that the two forms of batteries cannot be combined in the same apparatus. These may, of course, be put in one box, both faradic and galvanic combinations, and the dealers now make very beautiful and perfect instruments of this kind.

I am thus minute in stating these elementary facts, because I am frequently interrogated by students and physicians in regard to these points. I start out with the declaration, then, that if you expect to use electricity in a truly scientific way, you must be provided with both kinds of apparatus, either separately, or combined in one box. Much may be done by faradic application alone ; but in its own sphere, and if employed merely to affect the imagination of the patient, it will be quite as successful as both. I hope none here present, however, will descend to electricity quackery, whether openly or under the guise of its scientific use. As I proceed with the subject, I will indicate in passing the form of current used in particular cases. I wish also to address myself more especially to current delusions about the use of electricity. Let us take for illustration a common form of paralysis—hemiplegia. No spectacle is more often seen than the tinkering of an old hemiplegia with a faradic battery. The muscles are daily shaken up, and physician and patient are finally at their wits' end, for no improvement follows. No one, at all acquainted with the subject, would expect to benefit an ordinary hemiplegia by faradizing the muscles of the paralyzed members, unless two conditions existed: 1, wasting, degeneration, and impaired electro-contractility; 2, late rigidity. In many cases of hemiplegia, the muscles are of their normal size and firmness, and readily respond to faradic stimulation; then no good can be done by applying electricity. When late rigidity exists, the faradic and galvanic currents are useful if rightly applied. Observe the conditions present. On one side the flexors rigidly contracted, and drawing in the fingers on the palm. The nails cannot be cut, and the cast-off epidermis accumulating decomposes; ulcerations occur, and a horrible fetor is given forth. On the other side, the extensors of the fingers, relatively less powerful in the normal state, also, are now relatively weaker, and are unable to oppose the over-action of the extensors. As the galvanic current, when continuously applied, allays spasm and over-action, the flexors should have proper galvanic applications. As the extensors are weak and need stimulating, the faradic current should be applied to them. The same method of management is applicable to *torticollis*, or wry neck. On one side are the rigid, over-acting muscles; on the other, a group of weak or paretic muscles, quite unequal to maintain the contest with their antagonists. To galvanize and relax the one, and faradize and strengthen the other, are the obvious indications, and the successful method of treatment.

In paralyses due to disease of the spinal cord both forms of currents are applicable to diagnosis and to treatment. Thus, we meet with cases in which the muscles react differently to the faradic and galvanic currents—cases in which the muscles will not respond to faradic, but will respond to galvanic stimulation. There are other examples of paralysis in which the muscular contractility to both currents is retained; and still other cases present themselves in which the response to current stimulation is impaired merely and not lost.

I have already stated a fact, of which you have repeatedly seen the verification in this amphitheatre, that in ordinary hemiplegias the electrocontractility is preserved. When paraplegia, for example, is produced by disease of the dorso-lumbar enlargement of the cord, which is the centre for the nerves proceeding to the lower extremities, the power of the muscles to respond to the faradic current is presently entirely lost, but these paralyzed muscles are then found to contract to a slowly interrupted galvanic current. Further, when a paraplegia is due to disease of the cord, *above* the dorso-lumbar enlargement, leaving that untouched, the muscles of the lower extremities respond readily to the faradic and galvanic currents. In still other cases, say, disseminated myelitis, with lesions all along the cord, leaving tracts of healthy tissue, the muscles connected by nerve filaments to the diseased part of the cord lose their power to contract, and those muscles connected with the healthy parts of the cord retain their power to contract, on faradic stimulation. In fact, the diagnostic point is, that paralyzed members receiving their innervation from a diseased part of the spinal cord lose their electro-contractility to the faradic current, and preserve it when that part of the cord from which the nerves are given off is in a healthy state, although elsewhere the cord may be diseased. The importance, then, of using both currents is very obvious. But there are other examples, not less striking. In cases of disease and injury of motor nerve trunks, the contractility of the muscles receiving filaments from them is variously affected. When the initial hyperæmia occurs in neuritis, the irritability of the nerve, for a brief period is heightened, and the muscular contraction occurs with abnormal readiness on faradic and galvanic stimu- lation; but soon the electro-contractility declines, and is then extinguished as to the faradic current, but is retained as to the galvanic current. Not only do the muscles fail to respond to the faradic current, but they respond with more than usual readiness to the galvanic current—to a less strength of current than indeed suffices to move the healthy muscles. There are differences as to anodal and cathodal opening and closing of the circuit, which are expressed in definite formula, but not to distract your attention from the fundamental proposition, I merely mention this fact. The mus- cles degenerate as the injuries to the nerve proceed, and finally they cease to respond to the galvanic current. If the nerve recovers from the effects of the inflammation, the contractility of the muscles to the faradic current is finally restored, and the response to galvanic excitation lessens in readi- ness until it becomes normal.

It has been observed that in these cases of neuritis, the response to the will, as recovery takes place, precedes by many days the response to the faradic current, reversing the order in which the loss of contrae- tility occurred. These changes in the muscular reaction to galvanism and faradism, are entitled by Erb "the reactions of degeneration," an expressive phrase coming into general use, and with which you should be familiar. These reactions of degeneration take place when the spinal cord or the nerve trunks are diseased. They are typically exhibited in the cases of facial paralysis. A current of cold air directed against the seventh nerve in front of the external auditory foramen—the *pes anserinus*—produces, sometimes, a paralysis of all the muscles to which the nerve filaments are distributed. You have had various examples of this malady brought before you, and its peculiarities pointed out. In a short time after the muscles are paralyzed, it is found that no move- ments can be induced by a faradic current, never so strong, and that a gal- vanic current barely strong enough to cause contractions on the healthy side will act energetically on the paralyzed muscles. These facts have been exhibited in cases in your presence. If we compare such a facial paralysis with that which accompanies hemiplegia, we observe great dif- ferences in the reactions: in the latter both faradic and galvanic currents act energetically ; in the former, only the galvanic produces responses.

Galvanism and faradism are much more important in the treatment of paralyses characterized by the reactions of degeneration than in hemiple- gias. Both currents are required. As the galvanic current only can cause movements of the muscles, in certain cases, this must be applied until the contractility to faradism is restored—for it is found that persist- ent use of the former has this result. When the faradic current causes movements, it can then be continued until the cure is effected. If the degenerating muscles do not respond to either currents, then it may be concluded that the muscular elements have disappeared, being replaced by connective tissue and fat. Certain paralyses from disease of the anterior cornua of the spinal cord—infantile paralysis, for example—are characterized by the rapidity with which the muscles waste. These affections are designated by Charcot amyotrophic, to express this peculiarity. Electricity is our special resource to arrest these trophic degenerations. In these affections the reactions of degenerations are perfectly characteristic, and hence the galvanic current must be used until the contractility to the faradic current is restored. If the wasting of the muscles proceeds unchecked and the anatomical elements are destroyed, no electrical applications will be of any service. They must be undertaken, therefore, before the muscles are too far gone to be restored. When, by systematic excitation, the muscles have recovered their normal volume and contractility, electricity can accomplish nothing more, for the centric disease on which all depends may not be remediable.

In morbid states involving *sensibility* the faradic current is of little service. A very high tension current, with excessively rapid interruptions applied along the trajectory of a nerve, is sometimes serviceable in a neuralgia. The power to relieve pain is the property of the galvanic current. A descending stabile current is, theoretically, the best form of application to relieve the irritability of a sensory nerve, but in practice it is found that the direction of the current is of little moment, the relief being the same in what direction soever the electricity may be flowing. It follows then, of course, that the galvanic and not the faradic current is to be used in the treatment of neuralgia. The use of the faradic current in such cases is one of the medical delusions against which we must protest.

In the treatment of internal maladies the galvanic current is chiefly used. It has been abundantly proved that this form of electricity penetrates to the deepest organs and tissues, whilst faradism does not so penetrate. Galvanism affects the calibre of the vessels, and thus has an influence on the nutrition of the tissues. If the faradic current is applied directly to the sympathetic nerves, the vessels innervated by these nerves are thrown into a condition of tetanic spasm, and the blood stream is arrested. Applied on the surface, however, such effects do not follow, because the current does not penetrate sufficiently. The galvanic current does penetrate to the vessels when applied to the surface, and hence the important results which may follow its proper administration. It is important to understand the mode in which galvanism affects the circulation. We owe, I think, chiefly to the labours of Onimus and Legros the facts which I am now about to submit. The normal movement of a healthy arteriole is that known as vermicular. An impulse beginning at one point is transmitted by a succession of waves to a distant point, and as one part contracts, another dilates. Now Onimus and Legros have shown that whilst the faradic current tetanizes and stops the distribution of blood, the galvanic promotes and enlarges the vermicular movements, and thus increases the quantity of blood passing in a given time. The nutrition of organs and tissues must, necessarily, be promoted by the galvanic current. In this, probably, we have an explanation of Remak's " catalytic effects." The practical application of these principles is of much importance. If we wish to arrest hemorrhage from an organ, such as the uterus, to which we can apply the electrodes directly, which form of electricity ought we to use? the faradic or galvanic? The former unquestionably, for it not only causes strong uterine contractions, tetanizes, but it also affects the vessels in the same way. I need hardly stop to say that faradism is an excellent expedient in uterine inertia with hemorrhage.

On the other hand, suppose our object be to improve the condition of an enlarged, flabby, and congested uterus, the vessels being dilated, the blood-streams sluggish—then the galvanic current should be applied, for under its use the tone of the vessels would be restored, and the blood-streams would be propelled with more force and rapidity. In any attempts to improve the nutrition of the deeper parts of the body beyond the reach of direct applications, the galvanic current only can be used, since the faradic does not diffuse to the necessary depth. In the treatment of those neuroses of the skin, due to changes in the condition of the sympathetic ganglia, remarkable results are often obtained from the form of galvanization known as centric. The tonic and reconstituent effects which follow the application of galvanism to the cervical sympathetic, to the pneumogastric, and to the spinal cord, are doubtless due to the increased action of the vessels and to the stimulation of the nervous apparatus presiding over the movements of the chylopoietic viscera. Also, doubtless, something is due to the action of the current on the trophic system. What explanation, soever, may be adopted, the fact remains that stimulation by galvanism of the important apparatus of animal and organic life, mentioned just now, has remarkably good effects in some disorders of nutrition. I may mention, in illustration, the curative influence of galvanism in exophthalmic goitre. I mean, of course, this malady as it does exist, free from any structural lesions of the heart and of the thyroid gland. Under the persistent use of galvanism the rapid action of the heart, the dilatation and increased pulsation of the vessels of the neck and of the thyroid, the enlargement of the thyroid due to enlargement of its vessels, and the protrusion of the eyes cease, and permanently cease in favourable cases.

There is a form of faradic application, which is alleged to promote nutrition—the general electrization of Beard and Rockwell—in which the whole surface is in turn stimulated by faradic applications to the skin. This acts on the cutaneous nerves and vessels, and does generally promote the activity of the nutritive functions, but it is slow and not efficient. Weir Mitchell applies the faradic current in another way. He throws all the muscles of the body in turn into action by a faradic current of sufficient strength. This acts by increasing the circulation and the oxidation processes in the muscles, for muscular contraction can no more take place than any force can be evolved without the consumption of material. As the most of the heat production of the body occurs in the muscular tissue, the increase of muscular contraction means increased temperature and consequent greater activity in the nutritive functions generally. Indeed, making all the muscles contract by a faradic current is exercising them, and thus Mitchell succeeds in exercising his patients without voluntary efforts on their part.

In further exemplification of the power of galvanism to affect the function of nutrition may be mentioned the solution of cataract, which, it is alleged, has been accomplished by application of a galvanic current to the affected eye. An additional case, lately published in Virchow's *Archiv*, by Dr. Neftel, of New York, has been warmly disputed by Knapp, Agnew, and Loring, who have shown that Dr. Neftel was over-sanguine.

Galvanism can alone be used to affect the condition of the brain and spinal cord. Faradism does not pass the barrier of the bony envelope to these parts, but galvanism has been experimentally shown to do so. That galvanism, and not faradism, should be used when it is proposed to reach these parts, seems, therefore, conclusive. There can be little question that galvanism is highly serviceable in certain vascular states of the intracranial organs. We must bear in mind how galvanism affects the vessels, in order to apply it correctly. I have already stated that Onimus and Legros have shown how galvanism promotes the normal vermicular motions of the vessels, and is, therefore, indicated when the circulation is languid from paresis of the vessel walls. That state of the intracranial circulation which exists when atheromatous changes have occurred in the vessels, and the walls of the arterioles are yielding, and miliary aneurisms forming, and characterized objectively by failing memory, weakened power of attention, vertiginous sensations, etc., is much improved by the daily application of a weak galvanic current to the head, kept up for some weeks or months; the individual applications, however, being less than five minutes in duration.

The propriety and utility of applying galvanism to the brain, in cases of embolism and cerebral hemorrhage, are much disputed. The rule is to apply galvanism, only, after all acute symptoms have subsided. As, however, the collateral hyperæmia and œdema do much mischief, it is surely desirable to prevent or limit them. We possess no agents which can act on the contractility of the vessels with the promptness and efficiency of galvanism. If rightly applied, the current being weak, substantial good may be done in the direction I have indicated. Sudden, strong applications, shocks, may do serious harm. The relaxed state of the vessels following acute meningitis, or cerebro-spinal meningitis may be toned up, and soft, unorganized exudations remaining after the acute inflammation, absorbed, under the stimulation of galvanism, but only currents of moderate strength are at all proper. I need hardly add that faradic applications are useless under these circumstances, and could only do injury if persisted in.

As a general rule, in the neuroses of the respiratory organs galvanism is used rather than faradism, but there are some exceptions. Remarkably good results are obtained in some cases of asthma by galvanization of the pneumogastric, sympathetic, and phrenic. A very successful case has lately been reported in which faradism was alone used. I have seen hiccough promptly arrested by a strong faradic current, when galvanism was used in vain; but this success of the faradic application was due to the action of inhibition. The reflex hiccough was arrested by the simultaneons arrival at the centre of another impression. The method of treating hiccough by faradism consists in sending through the walls of the thorax a strong current, just as the spasm is about to occur. The result is—the hiccough is inhibited. Neuralgia of the cardiac plexus, of the solar plexus, and of the stomach, or gastralgia, are most effectively treated by galvanism. Torpor of the muscular layer of the large intestine may be successfully overcome by both currents, but they differ in action; faradism affects the bowel rather at the point of contact, and induces strong tetanic contractions; galvanism originates movements, which are propagated in a vermicular manner much more widely. The best results are obtained by a combination of the two agents.

No systematic attempts have been made to promote the functional activity of the chylopoietic viscera by galvanic treatment, but it is highly probable that this remedy might be used with good results. The state of functional depression, diseases characterized by impaired nutrition, etc., are those which might be much improved by systematic galvanic treatment.

Both currents are used in the maladies of the sexual system, male and female. I have already indicated the principles regulating the employment of faradism and galvanism in uterine diseases. Probably faradism is more effective as a stimulant in amenorrhœa, as it is in uterine inertia, whilst galvanism is more serviceable in the vascular states characterized by relaxation. In the treatment of impotence in the male both forms of currents are useful, but their action is not the same. When the erections are wanting in force, due to imperfect filling of the veins of the erectile tissue, galvanism is more effective because of its power to increase the vermicnlar movements of the vessel's walls. When anæsthesia of the external organs exists, generally or in part, the faradic brush is serviceable.

In the treatment of affections of the chylopoietic system, one electrode properly insulated should rest in the rectum, and the other should be applied over the abdomen, all parts being brought successively within the circuit. A properly insulated electrode, flexible, and of the right length, could be readily introduced into the stomach. From such a position of the electrode, the current could be diverted to the various organs, and especially to the semi-lunar ganglion and solar plexus. The recent observations of Da Costa and Longstreth on the changes in the renal ganglion in Bright's disease, furnish an additional motive for further extension of galvanic applications by intra-stomachal electrodes.

Finally, gentlemen, as the manner of applying electrodes is important, I must say something of the details concerned. In faradic applications well-moistened sponge electrodes are used when it is desired to reach the muscles, for the conductivity of the tissues is determined by the amount of water present in them. When single muscles are to be stimulated, the olive-pointed electrodes of Duchenne are best, and they must be covered by soft leather, and not by sponge. When muscular groups of large size are to be acted on, large sponge electrodes may be used. The larger the electrode, and the more thoroughly moistened, the less the pain. When the skin alone is to be faradized, all moisture should be carefully wiped off, and some drying powder dusted over the surface. When galvanic applications are to be made, the form and size of the electrodes will depend on the object in view ; for single muscles, and separate nerve trunks, small electrodes are employed ; for large muscular groups, and for pain in many nerve filaments, large, well-moistened sponge electrodes are best.

The injunction, in systematic works, to add a little salt to the water with which the sponge electrodes are moistened, is proper only in the case of galvanic applications to the face and head. In neuralgias of the extremities, especially of long standing, I am convinced that we should use powerful currents, and, therefore, make the applications with large electrodes, moistened, but not with salt water. Not sufficient attention is paid to the duration and number of the *séances*. In galvanic applications about the head the sittings should not exceed five minutes, but they may be repeated several—say three—times a day. In neuralgias the applications should be more prolonged, and should be repeated at short intervals. Much better results would be obtained in these affections, sciatica, for example, if the applications of galvanism were fifteen minutes long, and repeated every three or four hours. These statements are based on some experience with these frequent applications, and are not merely speculative theories. In the treatment of muscular paralysis by faradism, it should be remembered that the muscles are readily fatigued, and that no benefit results from treatment which has this effect. As a rule, the smallest strength of current which will induce muscular contractions, is only necessary. The individual muscles will bear exercise in this way from five to fifteen minutes, and the applications may be repeated about twice daily.

Every physician employing electricity as a remedy should give the necessary time and attention to the applications, and should resist the inclination to get through with them as quickly as possible, when numerous and fatiguing. Provided with suitable apparatus, and an adequate knowledge of the subject, the physician will find himself possessed of a most valuable remedy, capable of results which none other can achieve in its own province.

ON THE INTERDIAGNOSIS OF INSENSIBILITY FROM VARIOUS CAUSES.

By REGINALD SOUTHEY, M.D. Oxon., F.R.C.P.,
Physician and Lecturer at St. Bartholomew's Hospital.

GENTLEMEN: Questions somewhat of the following kind are likely to be put to you one day, and are full alike of clinical interest and medico-legal importance: What is the matter with an individual who has been picked up on the road insensible, irrational, or inarticulate, and about whom no antecedents whatever are known? Is he ill, drunk, drugged, suffering from brain concussion, or from coma after an apoplectic or epileptic fit?

Syncope, trance, catalepsy, and coma are names severally used by medical writers to designate states of insensibility which the lay public group vaguely under fits.

Syncope is fainting; it may be otherwise described as a condition of body in which there is a death-like pallor, with loss of muscular power and of consciousness. Trance is a state of death-like faintness in which, however, some consciousness is retained, although the person is unable to move or speak. A faint is ordinarily (when an individual has not lost a very large amount of blood) an exceedingly transitory affair. A person collapses rather than falls to the ground in a faint; his knees bend under him, he subsides into the sitting posture, his head drops forward, and by the time the head has thus sunk to the level of the heart, or below it, the circulation through the brain becomes sufficiently restored for consciousness to return. In a faint a person seldom bruises his face. Upon waking up he may feel sick or giddy, or alarmed, but his brain resumes its thinking function usually at once and entirely.

In states of trance—of which I possess no personal experience, but may refer you to accounts to be read in Smith's "Forensic Medicine," pp. 540–542, and Forsyth's "Medical Jurisprudence," pp. 125–130, 155, and pp. 165–188—it appears that the body is to all appearance inanimate, and there is no power to move a muscle, the limbs meanwhile remaining perfectly flexible. The peculiarity attached to this condition is that the individual may hear, see, and remember all that goes on about him. There is no perceptible pulse or respiration, and hence trance has been mistaken for death, but we possess no recent or philosophical observations upon this form of faint. The recorded cases do not tell us of the temperature, or whether or not the muscles react to galvanic stimulus. Burial alive in this condition, except at sea, is highly improbable, but in no case would you be justified in making a post-mortem or consigning a body to burial unless you were satisfied from the presence of rigor mortis or appearances of putrefaction that death was actual.   Catalepsy, again, is a rare inanimate condition; still I once had a case under my care which accorded well with the descriptions that have been given of it.

A young man of nineteen was picked up in Fleet Street insensible, not fallen, but standing stiffly, unable to move or to articulate.   Here are the features that distinguish this state, all which he presented in other similar seizures which he had for several days afterwards while in the hospital.   Thus while carrying something about, or sitting up in bed, or attempting to poke the fire, his eyes would suddenly acquire a fixed gaze, and he would remain arrested as it were in his act.   We could set his limbs in any posture we pleased, and there he remained like a mesmerized cock, to the amusement of the nurses and other patients.   I watched him on several occasions.   There was not the slightest twitching or spasm of any of his muscles.   His pulse was slow, and so were his respirations, his extremities cold and flabby, the axillary temperature remained natural.   He would bear pinching or pricking without flinching, and took no account of our bawling his name close by his ear.   There was no reason to think that he was feigning, and it would be difficult, I fancy, to feign and act a disease so well as he did.   To quote from Dr. Copland's Dictionary, vol. i. p. 292: "The statue-like appearance and muteness of the cataleptic alone suffices to distinguish this disease.   There is neither the lividity of asphyxia, the pallor and general flexibility of syncope, the stertor of coma, the paralysis of apoplexy, nor the movement and dreamy mental automatism of somnambulism."

Coma, however, because arising from very various causes, is the single one of the several states mentioned by them as likely to offer much difficulty in diagnosis.   Coma may be due—1. To *pressure* exercised on the brain, arising (a) from within the ventricles, effusion therein; (b) from depressed fracture; (c) from effusions outside the brain between hair and membranes.   2. To *alteration* in molecular state of brain from some concussion, contusion, bruising, œdema, apoplectic extravasation.   3. To brain poisoning by insufficiently oxidized blood, uræmic blood, narcotics, anæsthetics, inebriants.

I cannot give you certain symptoms for diagnosing each of these causes of coma, but I may aid you in excluding some of them, and thus help you to arrive at a correct diagnosis in particular instances.   The profound coma produced by serous effusion into the ventricles of the brain, to judge from what I have seen in dropsy, renal or cardiac, and by what happens in tubercular meningitis, is gradually reached through a stage of sopor.   The individual at first is sleepy, then dreamy and slow of apprehension, difficult to awake, and finally incapable of being aroused at all.   Reflex movements may be excited for a while, later the face is pale, the temperature falls.   The breath is either Cheyne-Stokes or principally diaphragmatic and stertorous.   At first there is power to swallow, afterwards acts of deglutition fail to be coördinated.   The pupils are non-characteristic, but more often dilated than contracted.   (a) The coma due to depressed fractures, or to effusion of blood or pus or fluid between the brain and the membranes, is as sudden in its advent as its cause may have been.   Usually the breath is stertorous, the pupils are contracted, and the temperature is normal or above normal, the skin perspires profusely.   No or only slight reflex response is made to galvanic or cutaneous stimulation.

You will be guided to the diagnosis of fractured skull by bleeding or oozing of bloody serum from the ear or nose or by ecchymosis of the eye, and towards large apoplectic effusion of blood upon the surface of the brain by the stertor of the breathing and complete absence of reflex irritability.   (b) When the coma is due to alteration in the molecular state of the brain, local contusion, or apoplectic extravasations, the face is usually pale, the temperature fallen below normal;

the reflex irritability, although variable, is apt to be greater on one side of the body than on the other; the pupils may be unequal, and evidence of some hemiplegia is generally discoverable in the muscles of the face or eye.

It seems like hair-splitting in diagnosis to dwell upon what may aid you to distinguish between coma due to general compression of the brain substance and coma due to more localized brain injury, with general circulatory and nutritional disturbance, but I give you the best clues I can, such as have served me sometimes well; the evidence of any hemiplegia in a case of profound coma is always in favour of localized injury of brain rather than of general pressure.

The coma may, however, be due to some brain-poisoning, the sources of which I have grouped under heading 3. Now, deficiency of oxygen and excess of carbonic acid in blood produces coma—as, for example, in the inhalation of laughing-gas or nitrous oxide, when the face is black, the veins turgid, the skin hot, the muscles irritable, and reflex spinal irritability is heightened.

Again, the blood-poisoning may be due to the action of some gas inhaled which interferes with or arrests the oxygen-carrying properties of the blood-cells. Sulphuretted hydrogen and carbonic oxide both appear to act in this way. The circumstances of the accident, the conditions under which the person was found, as well as some significant clinical appearances, already discussed by me, should facilitate the recognition of this source of coma. This blood change, if profound, is not recovered from.

Brain-poisoning and coma by anæsthetics and inebriants are usually detectable by the odour of the breath of the comatose poison.

You may occasionally feel a little uncertain as between apoplexy and dead drunkenness. We had an illustrative case the other day in our wards. A man who had been intoxicated by rum was admitted, and very profoundly comatose he was. No reflex movements were excitable; his face was cyanotic; there were gurgling râles in his throat, and I believe he might have died suffocated if I had left him in the position in which the nurse had placed him in bed, for he had a large tongue and uvula, with somewhat swollen and œdematous fauces; and as he lay on a flat bolster, with his head back, his tongue slipped back in his mouth, and nearly closed the opening of the glottis. Propping him up with a bed rest, and pulling his tongue forwards, his breathing quickly improved, and his face assumed a less blue colour. Still for some ten minutes I was unable to get any movement of either leg by tickling the soles of the feet, and the pupils were unequal, one rather smaller than the other, and both quite irresponsive to the stimulus of light. It was true he smelt of liquor, but he was quite properly admitted by the house-physician, since treatment and lapse of time alone could decide whether his coma was due to alcohol alone, or to disease *plus* alcohol. You may remember what I ordered in that case, as a piece of practice which is prompt, rational, and attended by no possible risks—the throwing up the rectum of a pint and a half of cold water, with a tablespoonful of common salt dissolved in it. It brought him out of his profound coma at once, for he asked for a night-stool almost directly afterwards. The stomach-pumping and belabouring with a galvanic battery of a comatose person, who may be the subject of gravescent apoplexy, belong to the surgery of the past, when active practice corresponded too closely with lynch-law-like punishment.

In every case of coma count the respiration, observe the quality of the breathing, and its ordinary effect upon the blood by the colour of the lips. Examine the pulse carefully for quality, frequency, regularity. Touch the eyeballs, examine the pupils for reaction to light, their condition—dilated, contracted, unequal, irregular; tickle the soles of the feet, to test what amount of reflex muscular action can be co-ordinated. The breathing in most states of coma is heavy and slow; notice if it be stertorous, Cheyne-Stokes-like, wholly diaphragmatic, or if the intercostals act.   Next take temperature in the axilla or rectum. A remarkably low temperature, four degrees or more below normal, betokens usually uræmic coma, acetonæmia, or grave concussion of the brain.   After epilepsy, apoplexy, intoxication, the temperature is more often normal, or even slightly above normal.

Uræmic coma will again be separately distinguished most often by some slight œdema of eyelids or extremities, wax-like pallor, bronchitic sounds, very foul breath, smelling of beef-tea ; a brown furred tongue, pearly conjunctivæ, and dilated pupils bespeak urea poisoning.   Diabetic coma is indicated by oppressed noisy breathing, effected by abundant muscular effort, but attended by some lividity in evidence of impaired oxidizing changes at the pulmonary capillaries, of which we at present do not understand the exact cause.

In the coma that has succeeded an epileptic fit you may expect to find bruises, torn or dirtied clothes, indications of the tongue having been bitten.

Finally, the mode of recovering consciousness after intoxication differs much from what is observed in persons recovering from the coma that succeeds an epileptic fit.   After intoxication I have noticed that while the sense of hearing is recovered soon, the lower attributes of mind, the sensorial instincts, reappear early, the individual who was comatosely drunk hears correctly before he sees correctly, and sometimes before he can stand.   It is curious to notice the manner in which he repeats a word of your question over and over again, like a parrot, and perceive how some grotesque idea grows out of the jingle or jangle of a phrase mumbled over more or less thickly.

How differently do the mental faculties recover after brain concussion and commotion as after epilepsy.   How the intellectually reduced "egomet" is in a dreamy state and staggers in his gait, hears questions put to him correctly, answers them articulately, apparently rationally, but having done so straightway forgets what he has said, cannot tell where he is or what he is or was doing.   He is conscious of some confusion in his own memory, and shows often some high measure of judgment in his distrust of himself, and says, "I cannot recollect where I was going." ·

Intellectual wholeness or sanity lies outside to-day's lecture, and I mention this merely as a clue to past coma, whether from drink or cerebral commotion.

It remains for me to point out the distinctive features of opium coma.   There is profound stupor, with closed eyelids, contracted pupils, upturned eyeballs; the face is pale, the skin cool, clammy ; the forehead beaded with heavy perspiration; the limbs are lax, but, for a while, reflex motions are readily excited. The respiration now slackens, falls in frequency, perhaps, as I have seen it do, to as low an ebb as 6 per minute, the pulse remaining fair at 80.   The coma now is very profound; you may prick, stimulate by galvanism, call, flick, stimulate by what means you please, little or no further purposive response. is returned by co-ordinated muscular movements.   The body will not walk; it is only dragged about, if the advice given has been to walk the man about.   Next the lips get livid ; the surface of the body colder ; the breath is sobbing, and at long irregular intervals ; the pulse hardly to be felt at the wrist, and death is imminent by asthenia or sudden failure of the heart's action.   Now for what may you mistake this coma, and what may be most easily confounded with it ?   Apoplexy into the pons Varolii, since, as was pointed out long since by Dr. Wilks, who illustrated the fact by several examples of cases that had fallen under his observation, apoplexy into the pons is attended by great contraction of the pupils.

If, then, in any case of profound coma, with extremely contracted pupils, you suspect opium to be its cause, but have no corroborative fact, no laudanum bottle, no opium-smelling substance, or mark of subcutaneous morphia syringing upon the body, or soot of opium-smoking inside the nostril to aid you, remember that the case may still be apoplexy into the pons, a source of coma not likely to be benefited either by bastinado, beating with towels, walking about, or all the ex-tracts of coffee which can be pumped into the body at either extremity.—*Lancet*, Dec. 4, 1880.

Hospital Notes.

Galactocele; Incision; Cure.

Mrs. T——, aged eighteen, first came under Mr. PEARCE GOULD's care in the out-patient room of the Westminster Hospital, on August 19th, 1878. She was a robust, healthy-looking young woman, who stated that two years before she struck her right breast against a chair, and three months afterwards noticed a small lump in the breast close to the nipple. She had been married fifteen months, and was confined of her first child in February. "Just a little milk came" in the right breast, but not enough to enable her to suckle with it. There was no pain in it, but as it felt different from the other, and did not secrete milk, she sought advice.

The left breast was well developed, with a good nipple, and secreted freely. The right gland was almost the same size as the left, but was almost completely occupied by a tense, rounded, fluctuating swelling, a little involuted mammary tissue being felt at the lower part; the nipple was flattened out by the swelling; the skin was not reddened, and there was no enlargement of the axillary glands. She was seen again on Aug. 23d, when the swelling was distinctly larger and "pointing," the contained milk being visible as a white spot in the centre of a red area. A small incision, radiating from the nipple, evacuated about half a pint of creamy fluid, and the sac completely collapsed; a horsehair drain was inserted, and the breast supported by a bandage of cotton-wool. A thick, milky discharge continued to flow from the wound for several weeks, and then gradually became thinner and less, and finally ceased in March, 1879. Extract of bella-donna was applied over the breast at first, and later on pressure was employed. The fluid was examined microscopically, and found to be a clear liquid containing colostrum corpuscles, oil globules, and fine granules.

Remarks.—Lacteal cysts are not common. The history and appearance of this case left no room for doubt as to its nature. These cysts have been stated to arise from dilatation of the sinuses or large ducts, or from rupture of a duct and extra-vasation of milk, in which case they have been found to increase "rapidly and distinctly every time the infant sucks" Here this feature was not noticed, and the history of a previous injury and inability to suckle with the breast render it probable that there was obstruction to one, or perhaps more, of the lacteal ducts. Out of seventeen cases of galactocele recorded by Gross there had been a pre-vious blow in two. It has been stated that such cysts never burst; this one "pointed" most distinctly, and at least threatened to burst.—*Lancet*, Nov. 27, 1880.

MONTHLY ABSTRACT.

Anatomy and Physiology.

The Cortical Centre for Movements of the Face.

In a recent issue of the *Progrès Médical*, M. BALLET records a case at La Salpêtrière confirmatory of the views of Charcot and Pitres as to the centre for the movements of the facial muscles being seated in the lower third of the parietal and ascending frontal convolutions. It is certainly very rare to meet with cases of facial paralysis arising from limited central lesions. The patient in this case was a woman seventy-one years of age, who for some time had been the subject of senile tremors. She was admitted to the hospital with well-marked left facial paralysis, but with no impairment of motility of the limbs beyond a very slight degree of weakness in the left arm. Sensibility was unaffected. During the same day there appeared conjugate deviation of the eyes to the right, and the face became more strongly drawn to this side. The following day coma supervened, the eye and head being strongly deviated to the right, and death took place three days later. Post-mortem examination showed a recent clot weighing five grammes in the cortex of the right cerebral hemisphere, occupying the lower part of the ascending frontal convolution and bounding the fissure of Sylvius. On section it was found to have destroyed the inferior frontal fasciculus, and to have encroached upon the corresponding parietal fasciculus, without, however, reaching deeply enough to involve the central gray nuclei. M. Ballet remarks that few cases hitherto published so clearly establish the seat of the psycho-motor centre of the face, the majority of such cases being those of facial paralysis associated with brachial monoplegia, with lesions extending beyond the limit assigned to the face centre. In this case, however, the hemorrhage and surrounding softening were limited almost entirely to the lower third of the ascending frontal gyrus, and had led to a facial "monoplegia" of the opposite side. The paresis of the arm, which increased slightly as the case advanced, was probably due to a slight extension of the hemorrhage, and to the pressure produced by this lesion upon the centre for the upper limb, which is in close contiguity to the facial centre.—*Lancet*, October 2, 1880.

Materia Medica and Therapeutics.

Indications of Anæsthesia by the Application of Chloroform to the Skin.

M. ALBERT HENOCQUE observes (*Gazette Hebdom.*, Nov. 10) that the Biological Society was deeply interested, at its meeting on the 13th inst., by a communication from Prof. BROWN-SÉQUARD, concerning certain profound modifications rapidly produced in the great organic functions and the properties of the nervous and muscular tissues, by the application of chloroform to the skin. The distinctness of the phenomena observed, their constancy, their absolute novelty, and the facility of their demonstration, are so many reasons for their successful reproduction in any physiological laboratory.

"Up to the present time Prof. Brown-Séquard has been able to expound the results of more than sixty experiments, which I have assisted him in performing. The origin of these investigations was an unexpected fact which occurred during laboratory work. In order that a guinea-pig should be killed, upon which an experiment was performed some months before, it was placed under a bell into which ether had been poured. Anæsthesia taking place too slowly, a strong dose of chloroform was poured into the tube of the bell furnished with a sponge, so that the drops fell between the shoulder and the neck of the animal, *i. e.*, the epileptogenous region. It was immediately seized with a violent attack of epilepsy—a phenomenon never before observed in this guinea-pig, although it had had some epileptic predecessors. Prof. Brown-Séquard, wishing to at once investigate this fact, poured some chloroform on the same region of another guinea-pig, with the effect of inducing not epilepsy, but profound anæsthesia, together with a series of phenomena which have been many times verified since, and the most general type of which may be summed up in the following manner:—

"If we pour chloroform rapidly on the shoulder of a guinea-pig, a reflex contraction of the platysma myoides and subjacent muscles immediately appears; the animal at first tries to escape, but in a short time its respiration diminishes, its temperature descends, it staggers, and becomes torpid. It allows itself to be placed on the side or the back without attempting to re-assume a normal attitude; and then it falls almost suddenly into a state of anæsthesia, which may last for several hours, during which sensibility may disappear absolutely—the animal remaining inert, in a state of the most complete resolution, resembling that of anæsthetic sleep. If we operate on a young cat, the result is quite striking. It is well known that this animal is difficult to anæsthetize by chloroform, and that in a few minutes after the cessation of the inspirations it wakes up during a period of agitation somewhat alarming to those exposed to the attacks of the claws of the now furious animal. We can readily understand, therefore, the natural astonishment produced at the Biological Society, where any one might handle a young cat which the local application of chloroform practised an hour previously had plunged in such a sleep that the most vigorous pinching did not elicit any movement demonstrating the existence of sensibility. This condition, resembling shock, or the state of syncope following severe injuries or profound drunkenness, persisted in this animal for several hours, there being scarcely observable, from time to time, some automatic movements of the paws, seeming to announce an approaching awakening.

" Such are the most immediately striking phenomena which the local application of chloroform produces. We may add that certain differences are observed, according to the animal employed; but the capital result—the production of the most profound resolution of general anæsthesia—is obtained in the guinea-pig, the rabbit, the cat, and the dog. This fact already in itself is of great interest; but the investigation of other phenomena has exhibited results of considerable importance in physiology, some of these being so singular, or rather so novel, that it requires that they should be seen in order to be admitted. It will be readily understood that the series of phenomena produced by the local application of chloroform offers variations, but we shall not mention these in detail, it sufficing to trace their principal features; and, as will be seen, the facts observed are already rather numerous. Thus, the guinea-pig or cat, which we have left inert on our table, begins to show signs of muscular or nervous activity in the shape of tremors of the four paws. It raises itself in a staggering manner, taking the attitude of paraplegia or hemiplegia which it had presented prior to the anæsthesia; and two cats exhibited manifest signs of delirium. The animal gradually becomes conscious and recovers its activity. Sometimes there remains a state of hyperæsthesia, which may be very considerable, the skin becoming the seat of a more or less active state of inflammation, if the dose of chloroform was considerable, and especially if the experiment had been repeated several times. The experiment may also prove fatal. Death may either supervene suddenly, as by sideration, or it may come on more slowly after a series of very characteristic symptoms have been observed, such as convulsions, epilepsy, diminution of the reflex faculty on the side on which the application had been made, pupillary contraction in the cat, or considerable dilatation in the dog. The respiration then becomes slower, being sometimes confined to the upper portion of the thorax; the diaphragm seems paralyzed, or at all events contracts no longer on one side; and, finally, the temperature becomes lower and lower; and the animal, if it be not sacrificed by opening the thorax, dies suddenly, generally without convulsions.

" It is then that the physiologist may verify a series of ultimate manifestations which accompany or follow death, and which trench upon most important problems in the investigation of the organic functions. The animal having been opened immediately after death, or just when this seemed imminent, the predominant characters in the aspect of the organs are found to be turgescence of the vessels of the intestines, of the spleen, and of the other viscera, and the red colour of the vascular arborescences; the aorta contains blood; the two ventricles are gorged with blood, and the blood of the vena cava is of a much less black colour than in the normal condition. In a word, we here find the characteristics of death in a state of syncope. The study of the excitability of the nerves and muscles presents results which are even far more interesting for the physiologist, and which may be thus summed up: 'The excitability of the muscles and nerves of the limbs and trunk, as well as the excitability of the nerves to mechanical action and galvanic currents, are modified.' Not only is a relatively very feeble galvanic current sufficient, Prof. Brown-Séquard observes, to bring these parts into play, but we find that the persistence of this irritability after death is much greater than in healthy animals killed by opening the thorax. In the guinea-pig especially, the persistence of excitability in the sciatic and brachial nerves has been met with three or four times greater than in guinea-pigs not submitted to the action of chloroform—the excitability lasting an hour and a quarter instead of from twenty to twenty-five minutes, as is habitually observed. Phenomena of not less importance than the preceding have been discovered from observation of the galvanic excitability of the phrenic nerves and various portions of the diaphragm. To use Prof. Brown-Séquard's own words, 'In two dogs and in several guinea-pigs, after opening the thorax, the phrenic nerve of one side was found to have lost its excitability, completely in one case, and almost completely in others. The corresponding half of the diaphragm also underwent a notable diminution of irritability, which only continued the fourth or the third of the ordinary period of persistence of this property of the muscle after the thorax has been opened. It is the phrenic nerve and half of the diaphragm of the opposite side to that of the application of the chloroform that thus become inhibited and paralyzed, not only as regards their action which depends on nerve-cells, but also their property of tissue.' In other words, the phrenic nerve of the opposite side to the application of chloroform, in certain cases, presents a diminution, or even a cessation, of its galvanic irritability. Excited by strong, medium, or feeble induced currents, the phrenic nerve no longer causes the contraction of the half of the diaphragm which corresponds to it, or a comparatively very strong current is required to produce contractions. Finally, in one case, which we can never forget, the lateral half of the diaphragm, situated on the opposite side to that of the application of the chloroform, was unexcitable by the strongest galvanic current that we are in the habit of using—the muscular excitability having disappeared. Truly a singular phenomenon, since it is the first occasion in which the loss of muscular excitability resulting from a remote irritation has been observed.

"We will not insist upon the peculiarity of this crossed action on the phrenic nerve and the diaphragm, because we are not about to put forth on this occasion a complete theory of these phenomena. Can such a theory, indeed, be advanced already? I should feel greatly disposed to answer in the affirmative, and to indicate the fundamental conclusions flowing from it, did I not fear trenching on the reserve necessary with regard to Prof. Brown-Séquard, in a matter still the subject of daily investigation, and which will shortly form the subject of his public lectures. Still, even at present, I may sum up the theoretical outlines characterizing these phenomena. We have here to do with one of the phenomena connected with inhibition; that is, the arrest of function. A remote action takes place, through the skin, on the nervous system. Such inhibition may go on to simple syncope, syncope with asphyxia, or finally to syncope with arrest of the exchanges. And, in fact, the diminution of temperature, the modifications in muscular and nervous excitability, the presence of red blood in the veins, of blood in the aorta—this condition of syncope, resembling at the same time anæsthetic sleep, the coma of drunkenness, sideration, or the state of shock, presents all the characteristics assigned by Prof. Brown-Séquard to the group of inhibitory phenomena which he has described under the name of 'arrest of the exchanges.' We shall have occasion to return to these theoretical considerations and their development. At present it suffices to have exhibited a series of facts possessing an importance of the first order. These facts can be reproduced, for their verification is easy; nothing but an animal and a bottle of chloroform being requisite for the principal features. But it is of importance to avoid a cause of error arising from the absorption of the chloroform by the lungs. Such a complication may be avoided by applying to the mouth of the animal the muzzle which is generally employed in chloroforming, but on this occasion terminating it with a caoutchouc tube sufficiently long to avoid the respiration of the vapour of the chloroform. I may add, however, that this precaution is not indispensable, for Prof. Brown-Séquard has frequently found that the respiration of the vapours of chloroform, which may take place during these experiments, does not induce any sensible modification of the symptoms. More than this, it has been observed that the injection of chloroform as an enema produced in a dog no phenomena analogous to those described, and which yet were later manifested in this same dog as a consequence of the application of chloroform to the skin."—*Med. Times and Gazette,* Nov. 27, 1880.

———

The Use of Martin's Elastic Bandage.

Dr. PAUL BRUNS, of Tübingen, is a warm advocate of the employment of the India-rubber bandage, and asserts unhesitatingly that Martin's method of treating ulcers of the leg is the best and most effectual that has hitherto been practised. Seventeen cases of ulcer thus treated are reported by this surgeon (*Berliner Klinische Wochenschrift,* Nos. 25, 26, 1880), in order to prove the certainty and simplicity of the method. Not only does this treatment obviate the necessity of prolonged rest and of serious neglect of work, but its duration until complete cicatrization of the ulcer seems in most cases to be shorter than that required for other methods of treatment in which the patient is kept in bed.

The employment of the rubber bandage has been found very useful by the author in the treatment of other affections of the lower extremities. Cases are referred to which show its utility in simple chronic eczema. It was found that, in cases of long-standing ulceration of the leg with eczema and infiltration and hypertrophy of the surrounding skin, the bandage acted very favourably on the general condition, and that, as the ulcer healed, the scaly and thickened skin became smooth, clean, and soft. The application of caoutchouc in the treatment of the different forms of eczema was long ago advocated by Hebra, but it was used by this physician simply as a water-proof material, with the object of raising the temperature of the affected surface, and of macerating the epidermis by retained perspiration. Martin's bandage not only fulfils these indications, but also exerts elastic compression of the skin, an action of much importance and utility for effecting absorption of infiltration and controlling any varicose condition of the superficial veins. Dr. Bruns is of opinion that this treatment is likely to be attended with very good results in cases of obstinate and relapsing chronic eczema of the lower limb, due to disturbance of circulation and nutrition. The advantage of applying compression in cases of varicose dilatation of veins, associated with infiltration of the cellular tissue, is universally recognized, and hence the common use of elastic bandages and stockings. The use of Martin's bandage has this advantage, that the degree of compression may be readily and easily controlled, and that the rubber is a durable material. There is frequently difficulty in procuring a well-fitting stocking; and with both stockings and the ordinary elastic bandages the material is apt to lose its elasticity, and so to become useless. Dr. Bruns states that he has attained very striking results from the use of the rubber bandage in the palliative-treatment of varicosity. The patient no longer complains of pain on standing or walking, and the sensation of heaviness and weariness is absent even during active labour. One case is quoted in which a good result was obtained, although on the first application of the bandage the varix was on the point of bursting. Cases have been reported by Martin and others in which a radical cure of varicose veins had been attained by the prolonged employment of the rubber bandage, but Bruns is of opinion that such a, result is hardly to be expected in instances of varicosity of extreme degree.

The employment of the rubber bandage is also indicated, Dr. Bruns thinks, in cases of elephantiasis of the lower extremity. In slight forms of this affection good results have been attained through elevation of the affected limb, and firm and forcible application of flannel bandages. The thickness of the limb has thus been reduced even to the normal size, but usually relapse occurs after the patient has ceased to maintain continuously the horizontal position. A double advantage might fairly be expected from the employment of the rubber bandage. In consequence of the compression of the limb being more regular and forcible, the duration of the treatment might be shortened, and the period of necessary continuous rest in the horizontal position reduced ; and, besides, the habitual wearing of the bandage might prevent the occurrence of relapses. In two cases, treated by Dr. Bruns, of chronic ulceration of the leg, associated with thickening and degeneration of the skin, of the nature of elephantiasis, this latter condition was completely removed after the application of the rubber bandage, although the patients were not confined to bed.·

The rubber bandage, on account of the perfect elasticity of its material, is the most fitting of all known agents for compression in cases of joint-disease. With regard to the indications of its employment, Dr. Bruns states that he has attained excellent results from its employment in cases of articular distortion. He has applied the bandage in cases both of recent and of chronic distortion of the wrist, knee, and ankle. In recent cases the swelling caused through intracapsular effusion is kept within bounds, and in late stages absorption is accelerated by the compression of the bandage. By continuous wearing of the bandage, which serves as an effectual support to the affected joint, the utility of the limb is restored in a short time.

In two cases of hæmarthrosis recently under the care of Dr. Bruns, and treated by the application of the rubber bandage, the extravasated blood was absorbed in a much shorter period than one might expect to suffice with the use of an ordinary bandage. In a case of fracture of the patella with hæmarthrosis, also treated by the rubber bandage, the abundant effusion of blood was absorbed within eight days. As an agent for bringing together and fixing the fragments of a broken patella, this bandage acts more effectually than strips of plaster.

Dr. Bruns has not hitherto had any experience of the use of the bandage in the treatment of acute hydrarthrosis, but he refers to cases reported by Byrne (*Lancet,* 1879, p. 645), in which striking results were attained from its employment in acute synovitis. The rubber bandage is particularly useful in cases of hydrarthrosis. The main difficulty in .the treatment of this very troublesome affection consists, not in procuring absorption of the effusion, but in the extraordinary tendency to relapse, which usually occurs sooner or later after use of the affected limb. The bandage has been applied by Dr. Bruns in three cases of chronic hydrarthrosis of the knee with very promising results, and by its long-continued application the tendency to relapse seems to have been permanently obviated. In one case the effusion was absorbed in two days on forcible compression, and in the other two cases in four and six days on gradual and slight compression. The bandage in each case was then worn night and day for two months. No relapse occurred in two of these cases after an interval of four months, and in the third case after one year. In the use of the elastic bandage in cases of this kind, Dr. Bruns thinks it well to apply a weak and continuous rather than forcible compression. The application of forcible compression demands some care when the elastic bandage is used instead of a flannel bandage. The former, even when not applied very firmly, exerts through its great elasticity an equable and permanent compression, and acts with much greater effect than a firmly applied inelastic roller. Instead of reducing the intra-articular effusion through forcible compression of the joint, Dr. Martin removes the fluid by aspiration, and then applies the rubber bandage, which is worn night and day for at least six weeks. A similar treatment has been carried out with much success in cases of prepatellar hygroma.

The rubber bandage, as it can readily be cleaned and disinfected, is a better agent than the bandage made of elastic webbing for producing artificial anæmia of a limb before operation, and also for retaining in position antiseptic dressings. When applied over a gauze dressing it insures absolute occlusion, and at the same time exerts equable compression, a condition favourable, in many cases, to healing of a wound by first intention.—*London Med. Record*, October 15, 1880.

Medicine.

Hemorrhagic Diathesis, in relation to Leukæmia and Allied Conditions.

Professor Mosler, in a contribution to the *Zeitschrift für Klinische Medic.* (Band i. Heft 2, p. 265 *et seq.*), discusses the relation of the hemorrhagic diathesis to the considerations which should guide the surgeon in undertaking operations in cases of leukæmia and allied conditions. At the beginning of his paper, he relates the history of the disease in a patient, aged 40. After this patient had suffered from various diseases, the last of which was an obstinate anomalous intermittent fever, a splenic leukæmia developed itself. It was diagnosed in 1877. The relation of the white to the red blood-corpuscles was as 1 to 5. After a long treatment, the patient (who was a medical man) desired that splenotomy should be performed; but Dr. Mosler, as well as Dr. Péan, of Paris, dissuaded him from the operation. The patient suffered, at the same time, from old hæmorrhoidal patches, and an inflammation had developed itself around the anus, without any distinct cause. When the abscess was opened, free bleeding occurred, which, notwithstanding all the means applied, lasted for several days. There was severe collapse. After an application of the thermo-cautery, the bleeding ceased on the fourth day, but recommenced subsequently to the evacuation of hard fecal masses. The patient could not be chloroformed, on account of his extreme weakness, and for the same reason, the thermo-cautery could not be applied; digital compression was employed, and pressure was made on the wound, from one to nine o'clock in the evening, a tampon of cotton, saturated with chloride of iron, being pressed on the wound. At the end of eight days more the bleeding recommenced, and was arrested after digital compression for an hour and a half. The patient recovered slowly; but four months afterwards death occurred, in consequence of retroperitoneal hemorrhage, the source of which could not be ascertained at the *post-mortem* examination.

The patient attributed his illness to the obstinate intermittent fever, as well as to excessive anxiety and mental exertion. The pains from the sternum were most important in the symptomatology of the medullary leukæmia. The severe bleeding, after slight operative proceedings, afforded evidence that account must always be taken of the hemorrhagic diathesis, in relation to leukæmia. In such circumstances, Mosler indicates solid ground for rejecting splenotomy. He relates short notices of twelve other cases, in which bleeding complicated the disorder; most frequently bleeding from the nose, but also from the stomach and bronchi. In 150 cases collected by Gowers, there were hemorrhages in 80 cases.

Mosler observes, that the operation of splenotomy can only be tolerated when there is a perfectly normal condition of the other organs; when the splenic tumour is not extensively adherent, and is of hard, firm consistence; and when hemorrhagic diathesis is absent. This diathesis shows itself, not only in the later stages, but sometimes, also, at the commencement of leukæmia, and is especially liable to complicate hypertrophy of the spleen. Mosler considers that the hemorrhagic diathesis, which always shows itself in pseudo-leukæmia, where there is no distinguishable increase of the white blood-corpuscles, depends on the poverty of the blood in functionally active red blood-corpuscles, and on the weakness and friability of the arterial walls, through deficient nutrition.—*Lond. Med. Record*, Nov. 15, 1880.

—

Cold Baths in Cerebral Rheumatism.

Dr. WOILLEZ has read an able paper upon this subject at the Academy of Medicine (*Union Méd*, October 14). After adverting to the former fatality of the disease, he states that since 1870 it has become more and more evident that it may almost always be successfully treated by the application of cold, the cold bath at 20° C. (68° F.) being the form of using it which he prefers, repeating it every three hours, until the cessation of the delirium and the reappearance of the swelling of the joints. Generally the cessation of the cerebral accidents only lasts for a short time after the first immersion, but gradually increases in duration after the subsequent ones, a refreshing sleep succeeding the period of agitation. When the baths cause shivering they should be discontinued. In no instance in which they have been employed have they given rise to mischievous effects; and even when, owing to their defective application, they have not prevented death, they have prolonged life. They may be prescribed under the following conditions: 1. When to the delirium there are added diminution or disappearance of the swelling of the joints and a temperature of 40° C. (104° F.) and above. Under this combination, the baths may be said always to succeed in procuring recovery at all periods of the disease, whether there be only delirium, coma, or imminence of death. 2. We should have recourse to them if with the delirium there is no diminution in the articular symptoms, but the hyperthermia exists. 3. The bath should be replaced by revulsives when merely delirium prevails, the articular disease pursuing its course, and no hyperthermia being present. Dr. Woillez observes that it is an error to regard the hyperthermia as the sole indication for the employment of the cold bath, the articular fluxion requiring also to be taken into consideration, since, in a certain number of cases, revulsive treatment having caused this fluxion to reappear, a cure has resulted. Although so strong an advocate for the cold bath in cerebral rheumatism, he does not regard it as opportune in all general diseases with high temperature, and especially in typhoid fever, in which he considers it as ineffectual and injurious.—*Med. Times and Gaz.*, Oct. 23, 1880.

—

Recovery from Symptoms of Organic Brain Disease.

Dr. HUGHLINGS JACKSON at a late meeting of the Medical Society of London (*Lancet*, Oct. 23, 1880) read a paper on a case of recovery from symptoms of organic brain disease. The case was one of supposed hysteria, double optic neuritis with nearly complete blindness, severe headache, no vomiting, loss of smell; no deafness; reeling gait; absence of patellar-tendon reflex; doubtful lightning pains. Recovery under mercurial inunction, except of anosmia and absence of patellar-tendon reflex.

The patient was a well-nourished woman, twenty-two years of age, admitted into the London Hospital on Dec. 22d, 1879. Menstruation was regular; there was no evidence of syphilis. In August, 1878, she was run over by a cart, her legs being injured above the ankles. In May, 1879, she went into service, and was quite well except for a "weakness in her legs." This "weakness" increased, and two days before admission she could not stand at all, and took to her bed. During the week before admission there was a weakness of the right arm, which would "go and come;" afterwards "pins and needles" in this limb, and then weakness of the left arm set in. Her sight began to fail two or three weeks before admission.

Symptoms of local gross organic disease: (a) double intense optic neuritis (with mere perception of light); (b) intense headache, from the misery of which she was silent and very quiet. On her recovery it was ascertained that smell was entirely wanting. She averred that she used to smell well before her illness. Dr. Jackson was doubtful whether anosmia was in her case a localizing symptom or not. It may have been owing to pressure, direct or indirect, on the olfactory bulb; or, what is quite hypothetical, to an olfactory neuritis.

Localizing symptoms: (a) absence of patellar-tendon reflex—an exceedingly important symptom, especially as her gait was abnormal, without paraplegia: The reflex was still absent when she left the hospital on March 25th. It may have been so long before she had the other symptoms, but of this nothing could be learnt. (b) Pains in limbs. At one spot a little above the left knee she had occasionally a dart of sharp pain, followed by a dull aching; it would come and go. She had no severe pain except in the head. It could not be averred that the pains were those characteristic of posterior sclerosis. (c) Reeling gait. This was noted carefully. When admitted she could scarcely walk at all, and not without help. Her gait then was not like that of locomotor ataxy. As she improved a little it could be better analyzed. It was evidently a reel—a drunken-like walk. Apparently she had good power in her legs, and, using popular language, though inexact, there was "disorder" of coördination without "paralysis." (d) Other symptoms. There was some slight weakness of the left arm, with a slightly feeble grasp. These symptoms were very slightly marked. Some tenderness of the lower part of the spine was found. No very local tender spinal spot was revealed, either by the application of a hot or cold sponge, or by manipulation. There was no spinal curvature, no atrophy of any muscles, no defective sensation, and no vesical trouble of any kind.

Progress: rapid recovery. Iodide of potassium was at first prescribed in doses of five grains three times a day; but on January 4th mercurial inunction was ordered in addition. The dose of the iodide was smaller than that usually given in such cases. Under this mixed treatment she rapidly improved. From what was practically blindness she became able to read on January 26th No. 1 of Snellen at six inches with her left eye, but with the right only No. 3. On the day of her leaving the hospital, March 23d, she could read No. 1 very easily with her left, and with slight difficulty with her right eye. Practically her sight was quite good. She felt well, and except that the patellar-reflex was still absent, and that she could smell nothing, she was considered to be free from symptoms.

Dr. Hughlings Jackson then considered the case from several points of view. He referred to cases of recovery from symptoms induced by tumour of the brain; cases in which after little illness there was post-mortem evidence of tumour. He discussed also the question of syphilis, pointing out that a syphilitic tumour sometimes gave rise to symptoms similar to those produced by glioma or other "foreign body." He did not think that the mere fact of his patient's recovery under anti-syphilitic treatment necessarily overruled the conclusion that the intra-cranial disease was syphilitic. He spoke of the importance of the routine use of the ophthalmoscope, both as sometimes negativing the diagnosis of hysteria, and also as leading to early treatment.

Dr. ALTHAUS said the great difficulties in diagnosis of brain disease could be traced to two classes of cases—viz., those in which coarse lesions, as hemorrhage, softening, abscess, atrophy, and tumours were found after death, yet no symptoms had existed during life; and others in which the gravest symptoms, pointing to severe organic changes, were observed, and the patients recovered under treatment. He alluded to hemi-anæsthesia occurring from disease of the posterior part of the internal capsule, and the same affection as occurring in Charcot's hystero-epileptic women, in whom the disturbance was purely functional. He also related a case resembling in many points that described by Dr. Jackson, and in which he had made the diagnosis of tumour in the right cerebral hemisphere. In this case the administration of mercury and iodide of potassium led to recovery, although the patient had never shown any symptom of syphilis.

Dr. BROADBENT remarked upon the interest and value of the communication, the case affording Dr. Jackson an opportunity for the refinements in diagnosis which he had placed so clearly before the society. He had, no doubt, seen many instances of recovery from far more serious symptoms of organic disease of the brain, as had Dr. Broadbent and others; and in this case the symptoms formed a distinct category, indicating the seat of the disease, and no one would doubt his diagnosis of a coarse lesion in or affecting the cerebellum. Dr. Broadbent thought the course of symptoms and rapid recovery were best explained by supposing the lesion to be syphilitic, and he cited a case of a young woman, recently under his care, suffering with headache, vomiting, convulsions, double optic neuritis, and paralysis of the left third nerve. She had certainly not acquired syphilis, but there was a scar on her forehead of a suppurating node (which had not healed until she took iodide of potassium), and no doubt she was the subject of hereditary syphilis. She rapidly recovered under large doses of the iodide; but about twelve months after was readmitted with paralysis of the right sixth and seventh nerves. He had also under treatment a case of hemiplegia in a young man, obviously due to inherited syphilis. The loss of patellar-tendon reflex was presumptive evidence of syphilis; for, as Dr. Gowers had recently stated, probably 75 per cent. of cases of locomotor ataxy were due to syphilis; and this case might be one of incipient ataxy. With regard to optic neuritis, he confirmed from many cases the fact so often insisted upon by Dr. Jackson, that this may exist without noticeable affection of sight; and in the present case he was inclined to attribute the blindness to pressure on the optic tracts or nuclei by the disease in the cerebellum. He held the view that optic "neuritis" was really ischæmia, due to strangulation of the nerve and its vessels just behind the eyeball, by effusion into its sheath; and he believed the neuritis, with numerous hemorrhages (not, of course, the ordinary albuminuric retinitis) seen in some cases of renal disease, had the same causation.

Dr. Dowse asked whether Dr. Jackson had met with the absence of patellar-tendon reflex when no actual posterior sclerosis existed; and said that in his opinion the phenomenon might be due to inhibition.

Dr. Jackson replied in the negative.

Lead-Paralysis.

Kast (Centralblatt für Nervenheilkunde, April, 1880) has made some experiments with a view of testing the accuracy of Mason's statement (American Journal of Med. Sciences, 1877). The latter said that the electrical reactions in frogs dipped in weak solutions of lead-salts proved the presence of degenerative atrophy in their nerves and muscles. The author's results were in direct opposition to this; in no case could he find any trace of the reaction of degeneration. Kast adds a few remarks on a case of saturnism, in which the muscles of the left thenar, though functionally almost normal, did not react to faradism directly or indirectly applied. The anodal closure contraction was obtained much more readily than the cathodal, and presented the typical sluggishness and persistence noticed in cases of degenerative atrophy.—London Med. Record, Oct. 15, 1880.

Neurotic Atrophy.

Professor Virchow had the good fortune this summer to be able to demonstrate to the Berlin Medical Society two cases of the rare affection to which he gives the above title. Without entering into much detail, we think it may not be unprofitable just to ask attention to the principal points in each case, and to the view Virchow takes of the disease. The first case is remarkable as having been under Romberg's care more than twenty years ago, when Virchow saw it and made notes of it. It was chiefly on it that Romberg based his theory of the tropho-neuroses. The patient, a man named Schwahn, is now aged forty-two, and the onset of his disease dates from his ninth year, when he is believed to have had a severe tonsillitis accompanied with swelling and abscess in the left cervical and submaxillary region. Whether post hoc or propter hoc, the whole left side of the face has suffered more or less atrophy, especially along the course of distribution of the branches of the fifth nerve. The left side of the face is smaller than the right, the affection having begun during the time of active growth of the bones. The difference between the two halves of the under jaw is particularly marked, the chin having been pushed over to the left some way beyond the middle line by the superior growth of the right half of the jaw. The tongue is also much atrophied on the left side, but, curiously enough, only in its middle portion, and not at the root or tip. A very striking feature in the case is the condition of the bloodvessels. While the surrounding tissues from the skin inwards are wasted and shrunken, the veins and arteries of the part appear absolutely unchanged, the larger even projecting above the surface of the skin. By stimulating the part they dilate as in a normal individual; in fact, they appear to be altogether excluded from the surrounding atrophy ; and Professor Virchow expresses his opinion that any idea of the atrophy being dependent on vaso-motor influences must be entirely given up. Again, the sensibility of the part shows scarcely any deviation from the normal, nor can there be said to be any paralysis of its muscles ; what remains of them contracts, but their nutrition has been terribly reduced. The most striking feature of the affection, in Virchow's eyes, is the curious and inexplicable way in which the disease leaves parts of a nerve-trunk intact, and skips as it were from one section to another. It is common to all this class of cases. He says—"This fact has a special additional interest for me, owing to the possibility of the occurrence of analogous processes also in the interior of the body, so that perhaps many changes in internal organs, which we are inclined to interpret quite differently, should be referred to similar alterations of the nerves to those met with here."

Before dismissing Schwahn's case we should say that Professor Virchow has not been able to convince himself, after comparing the patient's present state with that described in his notes taken twenty-one years ago, that any material alteration has occurred in the atrophic parts ; in fact, he regards the disease as having long ago become stationary. The point is an important one, as many authors regard the affection as inevitably progressive.

The second case exhibited by Professor Virchow was that of a woman, aged forty-one, also with atrophy of the left half of the face, but without atrophy of the bones, as she was twenty-five years old when the illness which appears to have excited the atrophy occurred. She is the subject, however, not only of an atrophy involving the branches of the fifth nerve, but also of one which, commencing in some of the dorsal cutaneous nerves of the scapular region, affects the musculo-spiral nerve from its origin in the axilla, passing down the arm and forearm, and attaining its greatest development in the region of the radial nerve in the forearm and hand. The appearances are practically the same as in Schwahn's case : thinning of the skin, absolute atrophy of the subcutaneous adipose tissue, intense atrophy of the muscles without paralysis, great prominence of the bloodvessels, and no marked alteration of sensibility. The patient sometimes suffers from stabbing pains in the eye and arm, as well as from numbness in the atrophic region. She attributes the disease to an attack of what was probably erysipelas following her confinement, but it also appears that a fall on the back of the head in the street, which occurred about the same time, may have had some connection with it. Professor Virchow has seen a third case in a girl of eighteen, where the atrophy was supposed to have followed dental inflammation when she was twelve years old. In many of the recorded cases, however, no cause for the atrophy could be assigned.

As to the exact nature of the disease, of course nothing definite is known, but Virchow distinctly lays it down that the affection of the nerves is here peripheral, and not central. He believes, however, that a primary process being once set up in the nerve-trunks, owing to inflammation of the surrounding tissues, may then extend upwards to the spinal and basal cerebral ganglia. If so, the disease has a certain analogy to herpes zoster. The way in which the nerve districts are unequally attacked finds a parallel also in the various forms of lepra and in morphœa, though we are equally unable to explain it in these diseases as in Virchow's "circumscribed neurotic atrophy." "What we want," says Virchow, "to clear matters up is an adequate anatomical examination of the nerves and central organs in one of these cases, so that we may know for certain what takes place. There are few phenomena in the field of nerve pathology which excite such a desire to explain them as the affection before us, and in which nature seems to perform such a test experiment for the isolation of the different kinds of fibres in the peripheral nerves."—*Med. Times and Gaz.*, Oct. 9, 1880.

An Epidemic of Hystero-Epilepsy.

A recent outbreak of nervous disturbance in Italy, which has been described in the *Annales d'Hygiène* by M. Léon Colin, indicates that the conditions which gave rise to some of the most remarkable epidemic phenomena of the Middle Ages are not yet extinct in the country in which they were then chiefly prevalent. On Dec. 11, 1878, the governor of the district of Tolmezzo informed the Prefect of Undine that for three months some forty females, living in the commune of Verzegnis, had been attacked by religious mania. In consequence, Drs. Franzolini and Chiap were delegated to examine the outbreak. From their report it appears that the first case was in the person of a woman named Marguerite Vidusson, who had been the subject of simple hysteria for about eight years. In January, 1878, she began to suffer from convulsive attacks, accompanied by cries and lamentations. She was regarded as the subject of demoniacal possession, and on the first Sunday in May was publicly exorcised. Her affection, however, increased in severity; the attacks were more frequent and more intense, and were especially provoked by the sound of church bells, and by the sight of priests. Seven months later, three other hysterical girls became subject to "convulsive and clamorous" attacks. Here, again, an attempt was made to get rid of the supposed demon. A solemn mass was said in the presence of the sufferers, but was followed only by a fresh outbreak. At the time of the visit of the delegates eighteen were suffering, aged from sixteen to twenty-six years, except three, whose ages were respectively forty-five, fifty-five, and sixty-three years. Similar symptoms had also appeared in a young soldier on leave in the village.

During the attacks the patients talked of the demon which possessed them, stated the date on which they were seized by it, and the names of the persons who were possessed before them. Some boasted of being prophetesses and clairvoyants, and of having the gift of tongues. In proof of the latter they pronounced incomprehensible sentences, which they affirmed to be Latin or French. In all the sound of church bells caused attacks, and religious ceremonies appeared not only to aggravate the disease in the sufferers, but also to cause its extension to those not previously attacked. The reporters referred the outbreak to pre-existing hysteria, aggravated by the fanatical zeal of certain preachers, and to the frequency and exceptional impressiveness of the religious services which were being held as a means of cure. Their effect was to recall to the memory of the hysterical women the legends of demoniacal possession and of sorcery, and the exorcism of the priests deepened their conviction as to the nature of the affliction. Dr. Franzolini draws special attention to certain old establishments long of repute for the efficacy of the exorcisms practised at them. He cites especially the sanctuary of Clanzetto, an odious vestige, as he terms it, of the barbarism of the Middle Ages.

M. Colin points out that the soil was particularly favourable for the development of an epidemic of this nature. The population of Verzegnis is backward in education, and most superstitious, and functional nervous diseases are common among them. Dr. Franzolini has, however, ascertained that they possess a practical immunity from alcoholism and from pellagra, and also from diseases due to general insanitary conditions. He appears to be inclined to ascribe some share in the production of the disease to an obscure pathological influence derived from the French race, since he notes that the inhabitants pronounce the letter "r" as it is pronounced in France, and not as in Italy—the suggested inference from this circumstance M. Léon Colin is naturally unable to discern. It appears, further, that the inhabitants of the village are a good deal cut off from intercourse with the adjacent country in consequence of comparative inaccessibility, and the frequent interruption of communications by storms and floods. Moreover, craniometric observations on twelve of the inhabitants seem to show that the brachycephalic form of skull predominates, and that the development of the cranium is slightly below the average.

M. Colin points out, with much truth, that the relative sequestration of the inhabitants of a town must tend to favour the spread of such a nervous malady, if it does not assist in its production. The reciprocal impressions of the inhabitants are little varied, and hence, in spite of differences in age and social position, the members of the community come to bear a close mutual resemblance in psychological constitution. Consanguineous marriages will be common in such a population, and will contribute to the deterioration of the masses, and to the development of any common morbid predisposition. If such a predisposition results, in one individual, in actual disease, many others are probably not far from the same morbid state, ready to undergo fuller development by imitative contagion.

The epidemic at Verzegnis has proved extremely obstinate. Since the commissioners visited the place, new cases have occurred, which have rendered energetic measures necessary—even a military occupation of the district (!)—while seventeen of the "possessed" have been compulsorily removed to the hospital at Undine. Such an epidemic constitutes a rare event in modern Europe, but it reminds us closely of some historical epidemics with which all are familiar. Even in our own day, in some backward races, as of Norway and New Caledonia, similar outbreaks have been observed.—*Lancet*, Oct. 16, 1880.

Puncture in Pleural Effusions.

GOLTDAMMER, at a recent meeting of the Berlin Medical Society (*Berl. Klin. Wochenschrift*, Nos. 19 and 20), laid before the members certain results of his rich experience at the Bethany Hospital with regard to this question. He has operated in all on 123 cases, and performed 200 punctures on them. Of these 123 cases, 19 were cases of purulent exudation, 49 cases of primary pleurisy with sero-fibrinous exudation, and 55 were cases of secondary exudation and transudation (in phthisis, pneumothorax, typhus, tuberculosis, carcinoma, and hydrothorax, and in affections of the heart and kidneys). In purulent exudations, Goltdammer thus far considers incision to be indicated without exception; he makes the opening generally at the angle of the scapula, and, at the same time, performs resection of a piece of rib. For the first time, on the 18th February, shortly before his communication, he had employed the puncture with antiseptic washing out, recommended by Baltz in a case of purulent exudation, and was very well satisfied with it. The exudation did not collect again, and at the end of seven weeks, the patient recovered with the lung perfectly expanded. Goltdammer divides sero-fibrinous exudation of primary idiopathic pleurisy in otherwise healthy infants, into two groups: the first includes the abundant effusions, which displace the whole contents of the thorax, the heart, and liver; in the second group, he reckons the smaller and average effusions. In the first group, in which he counts 22 of his 49 cases of sero-fibrinous exudation, puncture had the most excellent results. In several cases (8 times) one puncture succeeded in giving direct impulse to resorption; diuresis increased, and in from nine to fourteen days the residual fluid disappeared. In seven cases, the puncture needed to be repeated. It may be considered a rule that the level of the fluid rises a few days after the puncture in the intercostal spaces; this Goltdammer explains partly by the return of the displaced organs to their normal position. Puncture must not be delayed until dyspnœa becomes dangerous, but must anticipate such a condition. The degree of the phenomena of displacement determines the period for puncture. Fever does not contra-indicate it; it usually disappears after a few days. The author evacuates the fluid to the extent of from $1\frac{1}{2}$ to $3\frac{1}{2}$ litres with a trocar, protected against the admission of air, and generally in the median line. In the small and median effusions, he makes the puncture with Dieulafoy's aspirator with capillary canulæ. Delay of absorption, that is to say, when, about eight days after the cessation of fever, no resorption could be ascertained—indicated puncture in 27 cases. In these cases usually from 500 to 600 cubic centimetres were evacuated, sometimes a litre. All the cases of sero-fibrinous effusion recovered, both those with abundant and those with scanty effusion. No suppurative change in the exudation occurred in any case. The cases of pleurisy treated with puncture in no case gave rise to any considerable retraction. In cases of secondary exudation, as well as of transudation, he finds an indication for puncture principally in dyspnœa, and has always seen some, and often a very considerable, palliative result; and occasionally in heart disease, a considerable improvement in the primary affection. In pneumothorax, also, the removal of the fluid exudation relieves the patient. On five occasions, he found the effusion serous and not purulent. He aspirates with Dieulafoy's apparatus, puncturing in cases of slight exudation at the seventh or eighth intercostal space below the angle of the scapula, in more considerable effusions at the fifth or sixth space in the axillary line. Absolute cleanness of the instrument, of the place of puncture, etc., is to be looked after with the greatest care. Finally, he refers to the disagreeable incidents and occasional dangers of the method. Laceration of the lung by aspiration he considers to be impossible, with a little care; so soon as dragging pains occur, or the well-known paroxysms of coughing, induced by the re-admission of air to the collapsed part of the lung, the aspiration is stopped. Suppurative change of the exudation is also unknown, according to Goltdammer's experience, when the operation is performed carefully. He has seen such a thing once only, in a case in which the flow of fluid through the trocar was stopped, and in which he drew out his needle to clear it, and thus introduced germs of infection (drops of oil, etc.). In cases in which this suppurative change is believed to have occurred through puncture, either there has previously existed a slightly turbid exudation, or germs have been introduced, through unclean instruments. In a correctly performed puncture, sero-fibrinous exudation is never changed to a suppurative one.—*London Med. Record*, Oct. 15, 1880.

—

Traumatic Hœmothorax.

The following are the general conclusions given in a recent work by Dr. CH. NÉLATON, of Paris (*Des Epanchements de Sang dans les Plevres consecutifs aux Traumatismes*, Paris, 1880): 1. Effusions of blood into the pleura result either from a lesion of the vessels of the thoracic wall, or from wounding of the intrathoracic vessels. In the latter case, the pleural hemorrhage is usually derived from the vascular divisions accompanying bronchi of the second and third order. 2. Thoracic aspiration favours the flow of blood. The bleeding is speedily arrested by the accumulation of blood in the pleura. 3. The blood effused into the chest coagulates immediately and throughout almost its whole mass, and so becomes divided into two portions: coagulum and serosity. 4. If the effusion be not very abundant, the serosity is reabsorbed by the third or fourth day; and when the phenomena of inflammatory reaction supervene, they remain localized in the region around the clot. This irritative process serves to establish encysting of the clot. 5. If very much blood have been effused, the serosity exuded during coagulation has not time to be all absorbed before the appearance of phenomena of reaction. The serosity then becomes altered, and its presence gives rise to bad symptoms. 6. The symptoms and prognosis of traumatic hæmothorax vary in these two classes of cases. In the former, the prognosis is favourable; in the latter, it is grave. The rules of treatment are thus formulated. 1. In cases of stabbing, immediately after the injury to close the wound. This occlusion to be made either with gutta-percha tissue or with wadding and collodion. 2. If the symptoms of dyspnœa and the fever diminish gradually, to leave the patient at perfect rest and to avoid any interference. 3. If inflammatory symptoms be suspected between the eighth and twelfth days, to treat these by blistering and local bleeding. 4. But if the oppression of breathing and the fever, instead of diminishing rapidly, remain stationary or increase in intensity, it is necessary to act at once, and to evacuate the effused fluid. The surgeon should at first make a capillary puncture; if the effusion consist simply of dark coloured serosity, this method will be found the best; it will suffice to empty the pleura, and is not so grave a procedure as that requiring a counter-opening. If, however, the effused fluid have already undergone a change, and have become purulent and fetid, it will be necessary to evacuate the effusion, as in a case of empyema, in order that by frequent injections such phenomena of putridity as are presented may be effectually dealt with.—*London Med. Record,* Oct. 15, 1880.

—

Remarkable Heart-murmur Heard at a Distance from Chest-wall.

Numerous cases of heart-disease are on record in which a murmur could be heard at some distance from the chest. The following instance, reported by Dr. WILLIAM OSLER, Physician to the General Hospital, Montreal (*Med. Times and Gaz.,* Oct. 9, 1880), is remarkable from the absence of any evidence of serious cardiac disease, and from the exceedingly variable nature of the murmur:—

J. W., aged twelve, a well-nourished young girl, was sent to Dr. Osler in May last by Dr. Buller, who had noticed a remarkable whistling sound while examining her eyes. The mother states that she has been a healthy child, though never very robust. Had inflammation of the lungs at eighteen months, measles at the age of three, and scarlet fever three years ago. When stripped, and sitting quietly on a chair, the following facts are noted: Posture slightly stooping; shoulders rounded, chest long, ribs oblique, sternum short, and xiphoid cartilage tilted forward. Expansion of chest equal on both sides. Apex-beat is seen in fifth interspace in normal situation. No protrusion over heart, or irregularity in the attachment of the ribs to sternum over cardiac region. Heart's impulse is forcible, but not heaving. Area of dulness not increased.

Auscultation.—As she sits upright in the chair the heart-sounds at apex and base loud and clear; no murmur. When she stands, a loud systolic murmur is heard at apex, high-pitched, somewhat musical, of maximum intensity in fifth interspace; it varies a good deal, being loud for three or four beats, and then faint for one or two succeeding ones, due to influence of respiration. On removal of ear from the chest-wall the murmur can be distinctly heard at a distance of several inches. It disappeared quite suddenly, and could not be detected on most careful examination. She was then asked to run about the room and up and down stairs. On sitting down after this the heart's action was very forcible, but the sounds were perfectly clear. The child then suggested that she heard it most frequently when in the stooping posture; and on causing her to lean forward and relax the chest the murmur was at once heard, and with greatly increased intensity. It was distinctly audible at a distance of three feet two inches by measurement, and could be heard at any point on the chest and on top of the head. Pulse 96.

On May 28 she was shown at the Medico-Chirurgical Society of Montreal, and most of the members heard the murmur. A day or two before the meeting Dr. Osler called at her mother's house and satisfied himself of its presence, though it was very variable.

On July 13 he saw her again at her home, and failed, after prolonged examination, to hear the murmur. She stated that she had not heard it herself for some time. There was nothing special to note about her condition, which seemed unchanged; she enjoyed good health. The stooping posture had no influence in developing the murmur as at the first examination.

July 21. Came this morning for examination. While she remained sitting, heart-sounds clear, impulse tolerably strong. When she stood up, the murmur at once became evident, presenting the same characters as before described, but not so loud, nor could it be heard at such a distance from the chest-wall. It was not much influenced by posture, though somewhat intensified when the shoulders were brought well forward. It persisted for a short time after she sat down, and then disappeared. Running up and down stairs did not cause its return, but a minute or two after it again became audible. For two or three beats it was loud, and then diminished in intensity, but there was no constancy in these variations. The rhythm is distinctly systolic; the first sound of the heart is not effaced by it, though not so sharp as in its absence. During an examination extending over twenty minutes the murmur was present four or five times, and for a brief interval only—less than a minute each time.

August 31. Saw her again, and failed to hear a murmur in any posture, after a prolonged examination. Heart-sounds clear and sharp. Has been very well. Says she has not heard the murmur for some time; does not know that there is any special time when she hears it most distinctly. Is not very short of breath after running up stairs. Heart's impulse certainly appears stronger than normal, though not heaving. Pulse 100, of good volume.

Remarks.—The points of interest in this case are, as stated above, the absence of signs of grave heart-disease, and the extreme variability of the murmur. In aortic-valve disease, particularly stenosis, it is not very uncommon to have such a loud murmur that it may be heard at a distance of several inches from the chest-wall. Dr. Osler has had two such cases under his care lately; in both the murmur was audible at about three inches from the sternum; in one of them, sent by Dr. James T. Munro, the murmur was stated to have been heard several feet off. The subject is dealt with very fully by Professor Ebstein,[1] who has collected records of numerous cases. In his exhaustive review of the literature of the subject he has only found three or four instances of such murmurs unaccompanied with serious disease of the heart or large vessels. Two of the cases are reported by Stokes:[2] one a weak, nervous woman, the other a chlorotic girl; in both it disappeared. The third case occurred in the person of Professor Baum, a colleague of Dr. Ebstein's, who, from 1854 to 1857, had a murmur synchronous

[1] Deutsches Archiv f. Klin. Medicin, Bd. xxii., 1878.
[2] Diseases of the Heart, page 154.

with the heart's impulse, which was so loud that it could be heard at a distance from the chest. It was most marked at night time. The symptom disappeared completely, and does not seem to have interfered in any way with Dr. Baum's health, as at the date of Dr. Ebstein's writing he had reached the age of seventy-eight. Dr. Baum had met with a somewhat similar case in a clergyman, in whom also it finally disappeared. The case here reported would appear to belong to this group, as there is no indication of serious disease of either the heart or vessels. The apex-beat is in the normal situation, and though the impulse is increased in force, the evidences of an hypertrophy dependent upon organic disease are very slight. If the murmur originated in a stenosed aortic orifice—the lesion in most of the cases—there would be symptoms of this condition, increased area of cardiac dulness, etc., and, moreover, it would be, in all likelihood, persistent; not, as this one, extremely variable. The remarkable way in which the murmur appears and disappears is the most singular and puzzling feature. Dr. Osler thought after the first examination that it was only developed in the relaxed condition of the chest, with the shoulders well forward and the head bent, in which position there might be slight pressure exercised by the sternum or costal cartilages on the aorta or the pulmonary artery. Subsequent examinations, however, proved this to be erroneous. Evidently the murmur is diminishing in intensity, and is not heard so constantly. Dr. Buller states that on the first occasion on which he saw her it was audible half-way across the room, at a distance of six or eight feet. She was at the time very nervous and much excited. Dr. Osler is not prepared to suggest an explanation of the cause of the murmur in this instance. It is worthy of note that in three of the five cases of this sort here mentioned the patients were women—two of them weak and anæmic; and the third (the girl under my care) delicately built and nervous, though not anæmic.

—

The Pathogeny of Pericarditis.

Professor ZENKER, of Erlangen, at the fifty-second annual meeting of Physicians and Naturalists at Baden-Baden, called the attention of practical physicians to a mode of origin of pericarditis, which, although no doubt it had not hitherto escaped attention, was, in his opinion, not yet recognized sufficiently often, in relation to what he believed to be its relatively great frequency. This is the causation of pericarditis, by processes of ulceration in the posterior mediastinum, whether these processes only reach the pericardium, or lead to actual perforation of it. These ulcerations are usually related to perforations of the œsophagus or bronchi, being caused either by such perforations, or the perforations in the œsophagus and bronchi, or in both, being secondary. In both cases, the communication thus set up with the external air readily gives rise to suppuration and to a further spread of the ulceration, in which the pericardium is easily involved. The pericarditis thus excited may be either fibrinous or suppurative, and also, where there is simultaneous perforation of the pericardium and of the œsophagus or bronchi combined with pneumo-pericarditis. *Post-mortem* observations have shown to Dr. Zenker the relative frequency of these processes, as well as the frequent recovery from the pericarditis thus arising. The insidious commencement and the almost entire absence of symptoms in the course of mediastinal ulcerations, as well as their obscure seat, explain the little observation which this subject has yet obtained either at the bedside or in the *post-mortem* room. Among the causes of mediastinal ulceration, perforation of diverticula of the œsophagus appears to play a prominent part. The possibility of making a more sure diagnosis of these processes, so as perhaps to act more effectively on them by therapeutic means, does not appear to be excluded, looking to the pro-gress in physical diagnosis which characterizes modern medicine. In any case, however, it will be possible to clear up by observation of these facts in pathologi-cal anatomy, many cases of pericarditis of which the pathogeny has hitherto remained concealed. Professor Wyss, of Zürich, laid stress on the practical im-portance of this communication, and remarked in a general way on the relations of the posterior mediastinum to the affections of the pericardium. He related a case of diphtheria with secondary suppurative inflammation of the mediastinum and an extension of the inflammation to the pericardium. In a second case a workman fell ill with dysphagia, which was followed after some time by pericar-ditis. He died with symptoms of tuberculous peritonitis. At the necropsy, there were found tuberculous peritonitis and pericarditis. The bronchial glands had undergone tubercular degeneration, and were adherent to the pericardium, which was perforated. He remarks on this, that not only fibrinous, suppurative, and septic pericarditis, but also the tubercular form of it, may take its origin from the mediastinum, especially from the bronchial glands.—*London Med. Record,* Oct. 15, 1880.

Abdominal Faradization in Ascites.

POPOFF (*Vratsch,* 1880, No. 22) describes a case of ascites, with enlargement of the spleen, treated by faradization of the abdominal muscles and of the spleen. He gives a table showing the effects of the treatment on the quantity of urine excreted. This rose on the first day from 1200 to 3500 cubic centimetres, and was always much greater on the days when the patient was faradized. The cir-cumference of the abdomen steadily diminished from 95 to 80 centimetres, whilst the size of the spleen fell from 10 × 8 to 7 × 5 centimetres.—*London Med. Rec-ord,* Oct. 15, 1880.

Surgery.

Nerve-stretching.

At the last meeting of the Society of German Surgeons in Berlin (*Med.-Chir. Centralblatt,* No. 31), Dr. CREDÉ, of Dresden, showed a patient on whom he had performed stretching and division of the third branch of the trigeminal nerve by a modification of Lücke's method. He made an incision down to the poste-rior surface of the upper jaw. The lower jaw had to be dislocated; he then penetrated beneath the periosteum as far as the foramen ovale, seized the nerve with a blunt-hook, and isolated the middle meningeal artery. He then stretched the nerve, and cut it through at the base of the skull. There was no febrile re-action; and the neuralgia was removed.

A long discussion followed on the usefulness of nerve-stretching. Opinions were divided. Esmarch had carried out nerve-stretching seven times with good results; once he had stretched the brachial plexus in tabes with success. Trende-lenberg was not so fortunate; he had employed nerve-stretching in six cases, with only one example of success. He was undecided whether nerve-stretching was indicated in tetanus or in tabes. Sonnenburg did not observe any success in teta-nus. Vogt laid emphasis on the point that the nerves must be very strongly stretched, and that only the large nerves could be treated. Langenbeck reported that in the cases which he had published of nerve-stretching in tabes, relapse had occurred; and so also in the case of intercostal neuralgia which Nussbaum, on his part, had reported.

In the *Voyenno Meditsinsky*, quoted in *New York Medical Record*, August, 1880, it is stated that Dr. A. GEN collected 73 cases of nerve-stretching used as a therapeutic measure. In traumatic neuralgia it was employed 6 times—cured 4, improved 1 (recovered entirely after neurotomy), no improvement, 1 ; in neuralgia from other causes, in 14 cases—cured 10, improved 3, 1 died from the hemorrhage; in clonic spasms and contractions, 6 times—cured 4, no improvement 2 (one cured by neurotomy) ; in peripheral epilepsy, once—cure ; in tetanus, 16 times—cured 7, symptoms improved, but disease terminated fatally in 6, symptoms did not improve and patients died, 3 ; in anæsthetic leprosy, 30 times, in all cases with marked benefit.

As the therapeutic action of nerve-stretching is not well understood, he performed some experiments in the laboratory of Prof. Tarchanoff with a view to determine it. Some of his conclusions are as follows: Not only mild stretching, but also the use of force equal to half what is necessary to rupture the nerve, may produce an increase of its irritability and conduction. Mild stretching has no effect upon the reflex irritability, but if the force used be great, it is diminished; this effect is also observed on the opposite side, indicating the central seat of the change in its effects. Hence the operation is not limited to the peripheral parts only of the nerve, as Vogt was inclined to think. Under the microscope, he found the traces of hyperæmia and capillary hemorrhages ; the axis-cylinders and myeline might be severed, but Schwann's sheath was intact. He found also peculiar constrictions in the medullary fibres. He considers that the diminution of the reflex activity is the main feature, and in the cases operated on was the condition called for.

Dr. POOLEY (*New York Medical Record*, 1880, p. 173), collects 37 cases, and adds two of his own. In the operations, as recorded in his table, the following nerves were stretched: the sciatica, sixteen times; the crural and the median, each five times ; brachial plexus and ulnar, each four times ; the tibial, three times ; the musculo-spiral, twice ; the supra-orbital, spinal accessory, facial, inferior dental, and peroneal, each once ; making a total of forty-four nerves stretched in the thirty-five cases.

In all the cases of neuralgia (six of sciatica and seven of other forms) except one, the operation has been beneficial, and in most of them the cure has been complete. In the exceptional case, it seems very probable that if the nerve which was subsequently excised with success had been stretched in the first instance, instead of the sciatic, the result would have been favourable. The special form of neuralgia known as sciatica has yielded excellent results from nerve-stretching, which may now be regarded as a thoroughly recognized procedure in obstinate cases. Professional opinion seems to be steadily advancing in favour of the operation in other forms of neuralgia. Especially in the traumatic variety is it likely to prove useful, as here there are more generally found adhesions of the nerve to surrounding tissues which stretching may break up. In such cases it has been found not only to cure the pain, but also the wasting shiny skin, and other trophic disturbances associated therewith.

The success of nerve-stretching is little less marked in local convulsive affections than in pure neuralgia. It is in this class of cases that the most extensive operations have been resorted to—stretching of several nerves, and on both sides of the body—but no ill consequences have resulted to diminish the value of the result.

In the twelve cases of traumatic tetanus for which the operation was done, seven of the patients died, four recovered, and in one the result is not stated.

There can be no doubt that, as the matter at present stands, a physician would be culpable who trusted to nerve-stretching alone in this disease, and it may be doubted whether the cases where it has been done as an adjuvant to other treatment show any better average results than from the treatment by chloral-hydrate and (?) Calabar bean.—*London Med. Record*, Oct. 15, 1880.

On the Detection of the Presence and Location of Steel and Iron Foreign Bodies in the Eye by the Indication of a Magnetic Needle.

Dr. THOMAS R. POOLEY, of New York, in an interesting paper on this subject (*Archives of Ophthalmology*, Sept. 1880) based upon a series of experiments, deduces the following conclusions.

1st. The presence of a steel or iron foreign body in the eye, when of considerable size and situated near the surface, may be determined by testing for it with a suspended magnet.

2d. The presence and position of such a foreign body may most surely be made out by rendering it a magnet by induction, and then testing for it by a minute suspended magnet.

3d. The probable depth of the inclosed foreign body may be inferred by the intensity of the action of the needle near the surface.

4th. Any change from the primary position of the foreign body may be ascertained by carefully noting the changes indicated by the deflection of the needle.

Scarlet Fever as a Cause of Ear-Disease.

The above subject is treated by Dr. BURCKHARDT-MERIAN, Professor at Basle, in an able lecture[1] in Volkmann's *Sammlung Klin. Vorträge*, No. 182. It is one which deserves the attention of our profession, owing to the frequency with which scarlet fever attacks the auditory apparatus, and the disastrous results which too often follow neglect of proper treatment in the early days of the affection of the ear. Of 1950 aural cases of his own, Dr. Merian found that 85, or 4.35 per cent., were due to scarlet fever. Yearsley found 4.77 per cent. of his cases dependent on the same cause. In 18 of Merian's 85 cases—that is, in 21.17 per cent.—the hearing was totally lost in one or both ears, and three of these patients were deaf-mutes. The statistics of deaf-and-dumb institutions speak strongly as to the causation of deaf-mutism by scarlet fever; Dr. Merian tabulates 4309 cases of acquired deaf-mutism, of which 445, or 10.32 per cent., followed that disease. These facts will suffice to impress the importance of this subject on our readers.

There has been a good deal of discussion as to the way in which the middle ear first becomes involved during scarlet fever. Dr. Merian believes that the inflammation of the fauces extends upwards through the Eustachian tube or tubes, and that the cases where perforation of the tympanum afterwards occurs are those in which this inflammatory process is of a *diphtheritic* nature, diphtheritic patches being present at the same time, though often overlooked, on the soft palate and in the pharynx. There are no doubt a number of mild affections of the middle ear, which have nothing to do with diphtheria, but depend on the extension of a chronic congestion of the pharynx to the mucous membrane of the tympanic cavity; but these often rapidly subside without permanent injury to the ear. With the diphtheritic form it is far otherwise. Dr. Merian thus describes its symptoms. In the majority of the cases they first appear in the stage of desquamation; there is often a rigor and always a fever, which remits in the morning, and may rise to

---

[1] Ueber den Scharlach in seinen Beziehungen zum Gehörorgan.

39.5° Cent. (102° Fahr.), seldom higher, at night. Severe earache is complained of, which may be replaced in a few hours, especially if spontaneous rupture of the tympanum takes place, by pains of a true neuralgic character involving the second and third branches of the fifth nerve. More or less complete deafness is the rule, and may come on very rapidly. The anterior and posterior auricular lymphatic glands, as well as the submaxillary and cervical glands, almost always enlarge, and their enlargement may precede all other symptoms of the middle ear. Sometimes the mastoid process is painful on pressure, and especially on percussion, without any consecutive inflammation happening. All these symptoms, with perhaps the single exception of the glandular swelling, may also occur in an acute inflammation of the middle ear not due to scarlet fever; but there is *one* symptom peculiar to the otitis media of scarlet fever, or at any rate only met with in connection with it and with diphtheria, namely, the rapidity with which the tympanic membrane becomes destroyed in whole or in part. In ordinary inflammation this generally takes years; in the otitis of scarlet fever and diphtheria, only a few weeks. How common the destruction of the membrane after scarlet fever is, the following statement will show. Dr. Merian found in his 85 cases that 13 had had one ear and 72 both ears attacked. The total number of ears involved in these 85 cases was, therefore, $72 \times 2 + 13 = 157$, and of these 54, or 34.34 per cent., had completely lost the membrana tympani. When we reflect further on the other consequences of the otitis media—the chronic profuse suppuration after perforation of the membrane, the loss of the auditory ossicles, the formation of polypi, and in the worst cases erosion of the carotid artery and of the transverse sinus at an early period, or cerebral abscess at a late period—the importance of early and appropriate treatment is sufficiently evident.

This treatment is not only to be curative, but prophylactic. Dr. Merian holds that the best preventive of aural mischief in scarlet fever is the arrest of the primary diphtheritic process in the pharynx. He therefore cauterizes all patches that can be discovered, at first twice, and afterwards once a day, with a 10 per cent. alcoholic solution of salicylic acid. A piece of cotton-wool of the required size is wound round the end of a small knitting-needle on which a double screw is cut, and the wool, soaked in the liquid, is gently pressed on the part. Some pain is caused, but it does not last long. Nausea is best combated by ice, and the taste of the spirit can be concealed by adding 1 or 2 per cent. of oil of wintergreen to it. For the back of the soft palate and for the pharynx curved instruments are, of course, required.

The second preventive measure is the use of the nasal douche once a day where the patient is intelligent enough to bear it. Following Tröltsch (*Archiv für Ohrenheilk.*, Bd. ix. S. 191), Dr. Merian provides a printed form of directions for its proper manipulation. The apparatus consists of an Esmarch's irrigator, with a tube two feet long, furnished with a glass nose-piece. A litre of warm water, in which seven grammes and half of common salt have been dissolved, is the liquid employed at first. Without the salt the water irritates the nares. Later on, one or two tablespoonfuls of salicylated spirit are added to each litre. It is very important that the douche be slowly administered, the patient breathing quietly with open mouth, and not speaking or swallowing. The irrigator must not be raised more than one foot above the level of the head, else water may easily enter the Eustachian tube and penetrate the ear, giving rise not only to pain, but possibly to tedious inflammation. Our space will not allow us to reproduce Dr. Merian's instructions more fully. Besides the douche he recommends gargling every two or three hours with a dessertspoonful of salicylated spirit in a small glass of water, and the application of an ice bag to the front of the neck from one mastoid process to the other. Pieces of ice are also allowed to dissolve in the mouth, but the patient is told to spit out the water formed from it. Very small children are excited to sneeze, and so temporarily clear their nares, by a snuff of pure salicylic acid, which for infants may be diluted with equal parts of starch-powder. Before leaving the subject of prophylaxis, Dr. Merian mentions that it has seemed to him that consecutive ear-affections have been most often met with in cases of scarlet fever treated by cold baths or the cold "pack," both of which tend to cause congestion of the head.

In treating the acute stage of the otitis itself he uses ice externally, protecting the very sensitive lobe of the ear from the cold by flannel or a piece of wadding. The pain is relieved by iodine paint, or by iodoform ointment (iodoform, ol. fœniculi, āā 1.0 gramme, vaseline 8.0) covered with gutta-percha tissue, and over it the ice-bag. Very severe pain yields to equal parts tinct. opii and water, ten to twenty drops being poured into the meatus. The intermittent pains occurring towards evening or by night, and which are very depressing to the patient, require quinine (0 20 to 0.50 gramme) internally.

As soon as the acute stage is over, air should be blown into the tympanic cavity with a Politzer's bag, to restore the equilibrium of the internal air with the external atmosphere, and allow the membrane, which has yielded to external pressure, to recover its position. If, however, in spite of these measures, the fever continues, the mastoid process is tender, and dull pain is felt over the whole head, paracentesis of the tympanum is indicated. The opening made should not be too small, and there is generally rapid relief after the operation. The escape of secretion from the middle ear should be aided by Politzer's bag. Syringing should be avoided the first day, and wadding, frequently changed, alone used to soak up the discharge. The patient is ordered to lie on the side of the affected ear ; and if, as often happens, great improvement follows the puncture, iodine and ice alone suffice for the cure. If, however, the discharge is copious and with difficulty checked, the ear is syringed with a 5 per cent. solution of sodic sulphate, which Dr. Merian has long preferred to all others for this purpose (see *Correspondenz-Blatt für schweizer Aerzte*, 1874, S. 566). The wadding he uses is boracic. The very destructive diphtheritic forms of otitis media require the membranes, which often fill the whole osseous meatus and obscure the tympanum, to be scraped away energetically with a curette or removed by a "Wilde's snare," and the parts to be daubed with salicylated spirit, or dusted with pure salicylic acid ; the ear must also be syringed several times daily with diluted salicylated spirit (one to two dessertspoonfuls to 100.0 grammes water). These proceedings are rather painful, but generally wonderfully efficacious. Profuse suppuration in these latter cases without fever is best treated by thorough syringing twice a day either with diluted salicylated spirit, carbolic acid (acid. carbol., sp. vini, āā, one dessertspoonful to 100.0 grammes water), or boracic acid (one to two dessertspoonfuls to water Oss.) By the adoption of these measures at the outset, Dr. Merian is convinced that the number of cases of chronic ear-disease after scarlet fever will be much reduced, as well as the danger to hearing and to life which is its too frequent consequence.—*Med. Times and Gaz.*, Oct. 30, 1880.

—

Nephro-Lithotomy.

Mr. HENRY MORRIS, at a late meeting of the Clinical Society of London (*British Med. Journal*, Oct. 30, 1880) read a paper on this subject, with notes of a case in which the operation was successful. By the term "nephro-lithotomy" was meant the removal through a lumbar incision of a renal calculus from a kidney in which the pelvis was not dilated, and which, but for the presence of the stone, was presumably healthy. It was to be distinguished from the numerous cases in which the kidney was cut for the evacuation of fluid 'accumulated within it, whether as the result of a renal calculus, of tuberculous disease, or some other cause, and to which, from very ancient times, the name "nephrotomy" had been applied; as well as from those cases, also numerous, in which a stone had been removed after it had been detected through a sinus in the loin. The opinion of writers upon the subject had been universally adverse to the attempt to remove a stone from the kidney, unless it could be reached through a distended pelvis—the chief reason urged being danger of fatal hemorrhage if the existing substance of the organ were cut or torn. The case described in the paper conclusively proved the feasibility of the operation; and, in answer to the question —Was nephro-lithotomy feasible, and, if feasible, was it safe? the author stated "that it was entirely due to his friend and colleague, Dr. Coupland, who advised the patient to undergo the operation, that an affirmative answer could now, for the first time in the history of surgery, be given with certainty to the question." The position of the question before this case occurred was reviewed; Marchetti's operation on the English Consul Hobson was referred to, and six cases in which the operation was planned, but in which it proved abortive, were mentioned. These six cases were considered encouraging, because all the patients recovered from the operation of exposing the kidney, and, curiously enough, obtained, at least for a time, relief from their symptoms.

CASE.—Maria M., aged 19, a servant-girl, of short stout stature, and with a remarkably rough scaly skin, had for eight years been subject at times to pain in her right side, accompanied occasionally with a feeling of sickness, and even actual vomiting. In September, 1878, these symptoms became more pronounced; her urine became dark-coloured, and the pains so severe that she had to give up her situation and go under medical treatment. In April, 1879, she was admitted, under Dr. Thompson, into the Middlesex Hospital, and, after treatment and rest, so far improved that she went again into service. A life of activity, however, brought back the old symptoms, and she was readmitted (this time under Dr. Greenhow) into the hospital. In less than a month she was again able to go out, but only to return a third time, with urine as dark as porter, and with the pains in the right loin and groin as severe as ever. When she was admitted, under Dr. Coupland, on December 29th, 1879, her urine was acid, and contained no other abnormal constituents than blood; there was some tenderness, but no swelling in the right loin. Again the urine cleared up, but the nephralgia was not relieved; consequently, on February 11th, chloroform was administered, and the right kidney exposed through an oblique lumbar incision. The right index-finger was then passed over the posterior surface of the kidney, and at once detected something faintly projecting over the renal substance near the hilus. The renal substance was incised at this spot with a probe-ended bistoury, and a mulberry calculus, of triangular shape, and weighing thirty-one grains, was extracted by means of a scooping movement of the finger-tip. There was no hemorrhage at any stage of the operation. The upper end of the ureter was not dilated in the least, and, as the stone could not be felt there, it was consequently not interfered with. No attempt was made to examine the front surface of the kidney. The wound was brought together with three sutures, and a drainage-tube was introduced between two of them. The patient made a good recovery; urine ceased to flow through the wound on May 4th, and at the present time there was nothing whatever the matter with the patient, excepting that a sinus of one and three-quarter inches still remained in the loin, and discharged about a drachm of pus daily.

This case showed that a calculus could be extracted from an *undilated kidney* by surgical operation, without more risk than was amply warranted by the sufferings and general disability which the operation was designed to remove. But before the success of one case was allowed to influence treatment in others, four questions required consideration. 1. Could the diagnosis as to the disease, and the organ affected, be made with certainty? 2. What were the prospects of being able to complete the operation when a stone was found? 3. What were the dangers of the operation? 4. What was the best result which could be hoped for from the operation if successful? Mr. Morris, in answering each of these questions, gave arguments in favour of nephro-lithotomy; and finally expressed his agreement with Mr. Charles Bernard, the author of an account of Marchetti's operation, described in the *Philosophical Transactions* of 1696, that many of the writers upon the subject of wounds of the kidney "ought not to have so magisterially exploded the operation;" and hoped the operation would once again receive the consideration of the profession.

Mr. Lucas said he had been looking for such a case, but had not found one. The experience gained, however, when the whole kidney was removed, was likewise available in such instances. Cutting down upon the kidney was, comparatively speaking, a trifling operation, though the risk of leaving a permanent sinus was considerable.

Mr. Golding-Bird had operated on one case, but had failed to find a stone. The boy suffered from intense pain in the bladder and about the kidney. The organ was cut down upon, and nothing found, but the pain was relieved. The pain returned, and the bladder opened, but nothing found. The end of the case was unfortunately unknown.

Mr. Barker said that a case had been reported, where a canula had been thrust down through a small opening and struck the stone; this canula had been allowed to remain in, and the wound afterwards dilated by tents until a lithotrite could be introduced, and the stone crushed and removed. He had recently had a case where a large branched calculus filled the cavity of the kidney. He was able to remove a part, but not the whole. He then endeavoured to remove the whole kidney. The patient died of shock.

Mr. Bryant said he would support Mr. Morris's view as to the operation in his case, though it was a dangerous one. Granting the presence of a stone, and a persistence of symptoms refusing all amelioration, the surgeon was justified in operating. Still, there were many cases where the stone would settle down in the kidney, and the patient survive many years, dying finally of something else. As regarded diagnosis, it was quite true that the stone might be struck by a needle thrust down upon it, but it was a question how far this plan should be tried. He suspected that the evil would exceed the good done.

—

Spasmodic Stricture.

Prof. Zeissl publishes in the *Allg. Wien. Med. Zeit.* (Nos. 23 and 24) the portion of his forthcoming report on his division of the Vienna General Hospital, which relates to spasmodic stricture of the urethra. After adverting to the difference of opinion which has prevailed upon the reality of its existence from the time of Hunter, who first described it, and finding that this is still denied by some observers, he thinks it incumbent upon him to state what has so frequently come under his own notice.

Every one, he observes, knows how sensitive the bladder and urethra are to external influences, whether these are of a thermic or a mechanical kind, and the action of psychical influences on their functions is no less remarkable. Many men, even with a well-filled bladder, are not able to empty it while talking or laughing; and the case of a young man is cited, who during a railway journey was unable to pass water, although the train stopped at several stations for five or ten minutes, because he was always in fear that it would go off without him. When this fear had ceased to operate at the end of the journey, he at once emptied his highly distended bladder. As to the etiology of spasmodic stricture, even a slight chemical change in the urine may induce it. A catarrhal condition of the urethra, excessive coitus, hard riding, taking imperfectly fermented drinks, and especially organic stricture of the urethra, may also induce the spasm and give rise to retention of urine. This is not infrequently met with during gonorrhœa. Patients suffering from this often drink large quantities of liquids containing free carbonic acid, and become the subjects either of catarrh of the neck of the bladder with very frequent passage of urine, or of retention of urine. When called to such cases, we find them with the most anxious expression of countenance, the brow covered with cold sweat, and the bladder distended so as to reach the umbilicus, no urine being discharged in spite of the strongest efforts. A catheter of the largest size corresponding to the diameter of the urethra can, with a little patience on the part of the surgeon, be passed in with ease. It has frequently happened to Prof. Zeissl to find that the passage of a large bougie or sound for the treatment of chronic gonorrhœa has been impossible in individuals on the first occasion of this treatment being adopted; but after the instrument has remained at the obstructing part (usually the membranous portion) for some minutes, and often for a quarter of an hour, it slips in of itself. After the patient has become aware of the painlessness of the procedure, and ceases to have any fear, the instrument, on the very next occasion, can usually be passed with ease. These facts show that the action of the muscular structure of the urethra may prevent the entrance of a bougie or the discharge of urine. These urethral spasms are of frequent occurrence, and are found in persons who are suffering from organic stricture. They are not confined to any definite part of the urethra, but may affect any part of it. These spasmodic strictures are often a serious hindrance to the treatment of organic stricture, the spasm being induced by the introduction of an instrument. Not only is the introduction of an instrument opposed by the spasmodic action, which, however, may be overcome with patience, but its withdrawal is delayed by the same cause, often for a very long time, which is a great inconvenience in private practice.

After relating some cases in exemplification, Prof. Zeissl observes that a series of similar facts have convinced him that the muscular structure of the urethra may exhibit spasmodic action, and that the consequences of this diseased contraction may, (1) in rare cases, induce retention of the urine, the spasm then attacking the muscular structure surrounding the membranous portion—the musculus transversus perinei profundus; (2) it very frequently prevents the introduction of an instrument for some minutes; (3) it may become so severe in any part of the urethra that for a time it may render the withdrawal of an instrument impossible; (4) it may give rise to prostatic discharges and frequent pollutions. In reference to this last point, he observes that sometimes patients present themselves complaining of very frequent pollutions. They perceive a kind of fulness of the penis, as if it were filled with fluid from before backwards, and this is accompanied by a sensation of contraction in the glans. When these sensations cease, a small quantity of grayish-white fluid, containing filaments, flows from the urethra. There is no obstruction to the flow of urine, but a few seconds after this has ceased, some additional drops are discharged. This last symptom would seem to indicate hypertrophy of the prostate, but as most of these patients are about twenty years old only, it cannot arise from that; and, in fact, the passage of a sound and examination of the rectum prove that no such hypertrophy exists. The endoscope exhibits no abnormality of the urethral mucous membrane, nor is there hyperæmia or tumefaction of the vera montanum. The symptoms are, however, easily explained if we attend to what takes place when a sound is passed. It will be found that a well-oiled instrument can only be carried forward irregularly and by starts, being sometimes arrested at certain points, and if held with a light hand it may be turned round on its axis. There is, in fact, throughout the whole course of the urethra, but especially at the prostatic portion and the anterior part of the canal, a spasmodic condition. We know, from the researches of Brücke and Svetlin, that the greater part of the prostate consists of muscular substance surrounding the tubular glands. This muscular substance contracts spasmodically, and forces the secretions of the gland into the urethra, filling the prostatic and membranous portions first; and as soon as the prostatic secretion arrives in the urethra, the muscular structure of this is spasmodically affected, especially at the anterior portion, so as to impede its exit and induce the sensation as if the urethra were filled with fluid. After some minutes the spasm ceases, and the retained prostatic secretion flows from the urethra. On examination of the fluid thus expelled, no spermatozoa are found. The discharge of some drops of urine a few minutes after the flow has ceased is explained as follows: The greater part of this fluid is discharged on the contraction of the bladder, but as it flows through the urethra it induces muscular contraction, and when this becomes stronger than that of the detrusor the discharge of urine is arrested for some minutes until the spasmodic action has subsided. With respect to the occurrence of the pollutions, we know that under sexual excitement the secretion of the prostate is quickly discharged; and when its muscular substance contracts spasmodically in sleep and discharges its secretion, the patient becomes the subject of lascivious dreams, and seminal emissions ensue. This form of spasmodic stricture is especially observed in spinal disease or as a forerunner of this; but it may also occur in individuals whose central nervous system is in a completely healthy condition.

With regard to the treatment of this disagreeable affection, which also in its last-named form may prove injurious to the entire system, we should first forbid all drinks which exert an irritating effect upon the bladder, especially champagne, cider, new wine, and beer. The most important point is the daily introduction of a moderately large instrument into the urethra, and leaving it there for only a few minutes. It is also very serviceable, when the spasmodic action of the urethra affects a person who is the subject of an organic stricture, to order for him, an hour before the introduction of the instrument, either a morphia or belladonna suppository or a small dose of morphia. At the end of an hour an amount of narcotism is often induced, under which a urethra that before was impassable admits with ease a large instrument. The belladonna suppository is preferable to the morphia, because while, like it, it counteracts the spasmodic action, it does not induce constipation. The patient should also keep as quiet as possible in a room of equable temperature, make warm applications to the perineum, and use a warm sitz-bath twice a day.

" The exact recognition of spasmodic stricture is, in my opinion, of the greatest importance, because every one who is aware of its existence, when he meets with an obstruction while examining a urethra, will not endeavour to overcome this with force, but will allow the instrument to remain quietly for some seconds at the obstructing point, which he will soon be able to glide over with ease if the obstruction is induced by spasm. These spasmodic strictures explain the frequency with which false passages are made, by imprudent exploration, in urethras which exhibit no organic strictures."—*Med. Times and Gazette*, Oct. 23, 1880.

Osseous Ankylosis of the Knee operated on by Barton's Method.

Mr. M. H. KILGARRIFF relates the following case in the *Dublin Journal of the Medical Sciences* for March, 1880. M. H., aged 30, the subject of faulty bony ankylosis of the knee, was admitted into Jervis Street Hospital on the 4th September, 1877. On examination, the leg was found to be bent at a right angle, the knee immovable, the anterior and lateral aspects being rough and irregular, and covered with a thin slate-coloured cicatrix. On the 16th September, assisted by his colleagues, Mr. Kilgarriff operated. Ether having been administered, he cut on the lower portion of the thigh a triangular flap, with the base on the outside, exposing the femur. He then passed carefully under the bone a curved metallic spatula, and with a saw removed a wedge-shaped piece of bone which had its base in front, and measured vertically three-quarters of an inch. He then straightened the limb without difficulty, and placed it in a splint, the outside piece of which reached the axilla while the inner part fell short of the groin ; the lower portion was a box, and joined the thigh part at a very obtuse angle. The dressing consisted of lint steeped in carbolized oil, and a solution of permanganate of potash was used to wash the site of operation. The wound suppurated for a few weeks, then closed in, and the divided surfaces of the bone were early united by a firm osseous band. In somewhat less than three months the patient was able to lean on the leg, and, aided by crutches, could without difficulty walk about the ward. The operation differed from Barton's in two particulars, which Mr. Kilgarriff regards as an advantage, viz., cutting through the bone, which left no spicula to pierce the fascia behind, and having the base of flap at the outside averted the possibility of bagging of matter, and made the wound more accessible for dressing. In Barton's method the bone posteriorly was uncut, and the flap was on the inside. In the above case there was no shortening, and the patient could walk well and discharge her duties as a servant.— *London Med. Record*, Oct. 15, 1880.

Case of Resection of the Patella.

In a recent contribution from Dr. E. ALBERT, of Innsbruck, to the literature of practical surgery (*Beiträge zur Operativen Chirurgie*, 1880), a report is given which, though referring to an operation performed nearly three years ago, may now be regarded as one of particular interest in its relation to the views that have since been published by Volkmann, as to the pathogeny of articular white swelling. Volkmann has reported (*Sammlung Klinischer Vorträge*) cases of coxitis, due to osteomyelitis of the head and neck of the femur, in which, after having chipped away the outer wall of the great trochanter, he removed an inflammatory deposit from the interior of the bone. Osteomyelitic deposits were also removed in like manner from the articular extremities of other bones, and the neighbouring joint, in each case, was laid open and drained. In his comments on these cases, Volkmann endeavours to show that the destructive articular disease known as white swelling has its primary origin, not in any pathological change in the synovial membrane, but in deposit, usually tubercular, in the medullary portion of an adjacent bone. It is suggested that the destruction or removal of such deposit should be attempted when practicable, notwithstanding the unfavourable experience of surgeons as to caries of bone, and the frequent occurrence of death soon after recovery from resection of a diseased joint.

The case recorded by Albert is one of well-marked fungoid disease of the knee, which evidently had its origin in caries of the patella. According to Volkmann, the internal condyle of the femur is most frequently the seat of tubercular deposit, which may give rise to an infection of the knee-joint and articular white swelling. As the upper surface only of the tibia is included within the synovial sac, a tubercular deposit here usually finds an extra-articular outlet, and so the joint is saved. In some cases the tubercular deposit exists, as in Albert's case, in the patella. Every surgeon of much experience must, it is stated, have observed an instance of a sinus over the anterior surface of the patella leading down to bare and carious bone. The joint, in such case, is usually swollen, and sooner or later destructive disease of the whole joint is developed. A case of this kind would seem to be one well adapted for the treatment suggested by Volkmann, since the tubercular deposit is very accessible, and, if allowed to remain, is likely to extend speedily in the direction of the joint.

The subject of Dr. Albert's case was a woman, aged thirty, who in childhood had been affected with keratitis and swelling of the cervical glands. In the autumn of 1876, destructive articular disease had commenced in the right ankle, and in the spring of the following year an abscess had formed over the patella of the same limb. The patient, when first seen by Dr. Albert in September, was suffering from extensive carious disease of the ankle, and presented a small fistu-lous orifice in front of the knee, through which a probe could be passed down to bare bone in the patella. After amputation through the leg in November, there was a considerable increase in the amount of discharge from this opening, and the knee enlarged and became very painful. As the affection of the joint was pro-gressive, and the symptoms were those of fungoid thickening of the synovial cap-sule ; and as the patella was evidently the starting-point of the mischief, it was decided in January, 1878, to remove the diseased portion, or, if necessary, the whole of this bone. A vertical incision having been made in front of the joint and through the fistulous orifice, the patella was exposed, and its inner half, the structure of which was bloodless, soft, and eroded, was removed by means of a chisel ; the outer half, as the structure seemed to be healthy, was left *in situ.* The cartilage of the patella remained, but was reduced in thickness and marked by streaks of yellow deposit. The joint contained about three ounces and a half of turbid fluid ; and the whole of the synovial sac was found to have been con-verted into a thick fungous mass. The articular cartilages of the long bones were smooth and white, and all the ligaments were intact. An incision was made into the joint on each side, and a drainage-tube passed through the articular cavity, which was finally cleansed by the injection of a five per cent. solution of carbolic acid. Profuse suppuration commenced in the joint very soon after the date of the operation, and the patient died two months later in a state of extreme anæmia, after breaking down of the left lung and rapid development of general tuberculosis. —*London Med. Record,* Nov. 15, 1880.

Excision of the Cuboid Bone.

The excision of the cuboid bone in confirmed and inveterate club-foot, advo-cated by Mr. DAVY, has been recently practised successfully by Poinset in a case which he related to the Society of Surgery on the 28th July. This was a case of left talipes varo-equinus in a young girl, on whom an operation was per-formed, at the age of eight months. The foot was placed in a suitable apparatus; this, however, having been broken some time afterwards, was not replaced, and the deformity was reproduced. Subsequently, at the age of twelve years, a subcutaneous section of the tendons, which kept the foot in its abnormal condi-tion, was performed ; but this operation not having succeeded in removing the deformity, M. Poinset decided on performing the extraction of the cuboid bone ; the foot was then placed on a gutter. As the result of this operation, which was performed under antiseptic precautions, complete cure was obtained ; some months later, walking was easy, and the foot in a good position.—*British Med. Journal,* Oct. 30, 1880.

Midwifery and Gynæcology.

On the Treatment of Puerperal Fevers.

Dr. J. MATTHEWS DUNCAN recently delivered a lengthy address upon this topic before the Midland Medical Society at Birmingham, for the reproduction of which, in view of the importance of the subject, and the well-known ability of the author, no apology is necessary.

Dr. Duncan said: Although only a few years ago it was far otherwise, the remark may now pass unchallenged, that there is no such disease as "puerperal fever," whose treatment is yet my subject for this evening. That name has been for a century in constant use, and indicates, though with deplorable lack of precision, a group of diseases for whose designation it may meantime be, for convenience sake, retained. Whatever designation we may adopt, we experience no difficulty in recognizing the diseases meant, and there is no hesitation in ascribing to them the highest place in importance to lying-in women who suffer and die, as well as to medical men who observe and treat. Their baneful influences, including their mortality, exceed those of any other group of diseases of childbed. It is truly said that childbearing proves fatal to every hundredth mother, and it may be added that, of this fatality, the far greater part is due to these diseases. How enthusiastic does the study of them become when we contemplate the reduplicated danger of mothers who have just borne a first child; how grave and awful when we regard the rapidly-increasing perils of mothers who count their children by numbers that rise higher and higher into the physiologically excessive.

It is misleading to estimate the importance of puerperal fever by death alone. The habit of doing so is easily accounted for. Mortality is a result, plainly and infallibly ascertained and numbered. The modern science of statistics, and the connected statistical arguments deal almost exclusively with death. In most writings it is implied that escape from early death is recovery—an error which it is only necessary to mention in order to insure its recognition. Death is a simple result, final, unconditioned pathologically—an end, to which various pathological routes may guide. So-called recovery is not its antithesis in practice, whatever it may be in theory. In many cases so-called recovery is anything rather than restoration to health; it is merely an escape, more or less narrow, from early death. The escape is generally into paths which lead to health ultimately; often it is into paths which lead to death more or less directly, more or less slowly, and after a lapse of months or even years. Recovery as antithetic to death is a very indefinite matter. Puerperal fever ends in death or in survival of the immediate attack. Such survival may be in good health or in wrecked health, or it may be in grave and progressive disease.

A good deal of undesirable mystery and much of positive error has been propagated on this subject by the long-continued and still persistent practice—a mere practice, now, without any rational basis—of regarding puerperal fever as occurring chiefly in epidemics. In its prevalence it has a seasonal variation, which Buchan and Mitchell have traced, and which closely resembles that of erysipelas; but it has no periods of epidemic raging; or, rather, none have been demonstrated. Individual epidemics of cholera, smallpox, scarlet fever, measles, and other diseases, have been well described; cycles of epidemics of these diseases have been pretty well traced, but no such demonstration or tracing has been made in the case of puerperal fever. Histories of many so-called epidemics have been written, but their descriptions fail to prove the reality of their epidemic character. Were this disease prevalent in epidemics so frequent as authors ask us to believe, we should be able to give from statistical data a complete account of them in their individual and in their grouped or cyclical characters, but statistics afford no evidence of the occurrence of any epidemic. The group of diseases called puerperal fever is ever with us, its frequency varying slightly, never rising very high, never sinking very low, always governed by an average. This average of deaths in every community is an average of awful calamity, which we struggle to diminish by treatment, glad to escape from the task of encountering the additional evil that would be raised by epidemic prevalence.

In a meeting of practitioners such as this I make these preliminary remarks as a mere exordium, well knowing that nothing is required to heighten your sense of the interest and importance of the subject. Medical studies do not blunt the sensibility or harden the heart. Who is there so callous as not to be moved by the enthusiasm of a physician when he stands at the bedside of a young wife suffering, and, perhaps, dying, in giving life and joy to others? All of us are frequently in this responsible position, and I dare to say that none of us feels quite satisfied in it. There is not the vacant, hopeless, observation of acute hydrocephalus, nor the melancholy soothing of cancer, but the restless care of a fever, the watching narrowly with a view to judicious interference, watching, well done in proportion to the depth of knowledge and the quickness of intelligence and the warmth of sympathy; interference, judicious in proportion to the wisdom and experience and skill of the watcher. The wisest feels most deeply the want of more knowledge. The most experienced feels most acutely how little power he has to govern a case, how often he is a mere looker-on.

Our topic this evening is the treatment of puerperal fever—how to interfere judiciously, how to govern a case, how to conduct mere management. My remarks are thrown into the form of an address, suited, I hope, in some degree, for this occasion. I do not propose to elucidate any special point, to drive home a scientific argument, to suggest a novel treatment. Such are the objects of the communications which will be laid before you during the session. Mine is to give an address according to the invitation with which you have honoured me, not to read a paper. An address has its own useful place in our meetings; but it is never to be forgotten that the work of our societies is not the hearing of addresses, but the attentive listening to, and careful scrutiny of, papers, generally short, and occupying narrow limits, embodying the results of original observation and reflection. An address may be, as this is, an attempt to review the past, and to sketch the present, condition of a great matter.

In puerperal fever, as in most diseases, practice is more based upon theory than upon our often too much vaunted experience. We condemn old practices chiefly because we have new theories. There can be no doubt that this is a just proceeding, if our new theories are not mere fancies but based on increase of knowledge; and accordingly I shall show the connection of our new treatments with our new theories. However flimsy these theories may be, they are our guides, and they delight and encourage the inquiring spirit of the human mind. Cullen and Heberden based their therapeutics on Hippocratic observation. The Hunters and Laennec on morbid anatomy. The moderns specially on histology and chemistry. Bacteria and sepsin rule us to-day, while mere inflammation has lost its supremacy. We do not see in our change of treatment evidence of any change in the disease, but the reflection of our increase of knowledge.

A great old obsolete plan of treatment is not to be regarded as erroneous or bad, and so contrasted with ours. Such plans were not the fruits of caprice, nor the *ipse dixits* of great and famous physicians, but represented the knowledge and wisdom of their times. I have lived long enough to see the gradual decadence of the antiphlogistic treatment of Gordon, with its venesection and leeching and blistering. Heat of skin, rapidity of pulse, and abdominal pain were the notes of inflammatory disease which was to be attacked and cured if possible. Since these days much confusion of doctrine has prevailed, and there have been many variations of treatment.   The view that the disease was a special fever occurring in many forms, such as are described by Ferguson, led to correspondingly various treatments, which were not materially affected by the great phlebitic discovery which in this country we associate with the name of Robert Lee.   Indeed, since the days of antiphlogistics, no great therapeutical plan has been common, for no great medical doctrine has prevailed.   The profession has relied much on special drugs in the hope of curing rather than treating the disease whatever it might be ; and latterly many have devoted themselves to treating symptoms.   Some years ago we heard much of medicines to make the pulse slower; now, in accord with our temperature diligence, we have great stress laid on reducing it.

Living among great physicians, and, as a young practitioner, willingly submitting myself to them, I have seen several changes of treatment.   In my earliest days, as a hospital resident and for some time subsequently, while bleeding was a decaying treatment, the great remedy was calomel and opium, and I well remember the improvement in the prognosis which was based on the fortunate but rare occurrence of ptyalism.   Gradually the calomel disappeared, because it almost always produced painful and debilitating diarrhœa, and it was replaced by blue-pill.   Then the mercurial disappeared entirely ; and, under the influence of the teaching of Graves, opium alone became the great resort ; and this medicine still keeps its place as a valuable adjuvant in treatment.   While its great utility is incontestable, I feel bound to record that I have often seen it act injuriously from its being used in far too large doses.   The last treatment which had a passing pre-eminence was the copious administration of food and alcohol.   I have been in practice during the whole existence of this modern and still-surviving plan—not a mere spectator or willing subject of older advisers, but taking an active part in the management of grave cases.   Experience has taught me that there is no more delicate work in practice than the arrangement of the food and drink ;   and no part of treatment have I seen so overdone, with the result of producing intense present discomfort, as well as an injurious influence on the progress of the cases.   This mismanagement has always been the excessive administration of alcoholic stimulants, apparently under the belief that if a little is good more is better, and that excess is scarcely attainable and not to be feared.   The practice was derived from London, and I hope London will have the honour of putting an end to it.   Stories of quantities administered, that are scarcely credible, are probably still in all your memories ; and I can testify from my own knowledge that they are not exaggerated.   Great practitioners boastfully narrated how much they had succeeded in pouring into their patients, and this when they were not in a short critical period of weakness ; and the brandy practice and boasting extended even to the treatment of babes !

Although I have seen no treatment by ipecacuanha, yet there have been in my time several "cures" introduced, which have fortunately passed quickly into oblivion.   The search for "cures" is, as yet at least, a wild-goose chase.   We have a long course to pursue in acquiring intelligence regarding the disease to be cured before we can hope even for a well-established plan of treatment.

It is not uncommon, nowadays, to confine the name of puerperal fever to septicæmia and pyæmia occurring after delivery.   It appears to me, however, to be better, even on mere theoretical grounds, to include all the ordinary diseases of the lying-in chamber, which are accompanied by fever, and which may be fatal. In practice we cannot meantime maintain the limitation to septicæmia and pyæmia, because in many cases we cannot be sure of our diagnosis, and because a case may begin as one case and be complicated with another as it advances.

In addition to septicæmia and pyæmia, which are the result of the growth in the blood of certain micrococci having the power of rapidly multiplying, we have sapræmia, or mere poisoning by the chemical products of putrefaction, and we have simple or traumatic inflammatory fever.

Simple inflammatory or traumatic fever is often very alarming on account of the severity of the symptoms, also on account of the extent of the inflammation. There seems to be in addition to the influence of traumatism, in some cases, a temporary inflammatory diathesis, the region of the womb being not the only one attacked, but, in addition, the kidneys or the organs in the chest, or the encephalon, all at once. Sometimes the inflammation attacks the remote parts, while the womb and its neighbourhood are unaffected by it. But most frequently the disease is a parametritis, or a perimetritis which may become so extensive as to form a general peritonitis.

In these cases, when pain is great, the pulse quick and hard, the skin hot and dry, there is generally much benefit derived from the old antiphlogistic regimen and treatment; but now the regimen and treatment are not used with what we may call the rigour and severity of our predecessors. Patients are generally allowed soup daily, in addition to the appropriate quantity of slops, that is, bread and milk and tea. Venesection is rarely practised. I have never used the lancet, nor do I remember hearing of its use for the last twenty years. Leeching is frequently resorted to, the site being above the groins on one or on both sides, that side of course being preferred in which there happens to be most pain. Not fewer than a dozen leeches are applied, and the bleeding may be encouraged to a loss, always only vaguely estimated, and varying according to the hardness of the pulse and the constitutional condition of the patient. The leeching may be repeated if necessary. It is generally followed by well-marked relief of pain and some improvement of the general condition.

While bleeding is most relied upon in the earliest days of the fever, blistering has occasionally a place in the later days. Poulticing is always used. The very painful turpentine stupe is a common application; but in some cases the blister is of great value. It gives much less pain than the turpentine stupe, often, indeed, very little pain, and its effects are not so transitory; besides it causes a copious transudation of serum and subsequently of pus. The blister should be large, even to covering the greater part of the abdomen between the umbilicus and pubes. It should be an old-fashioned rising blister, the emplastrum lyttæ; not such blistering as is nowadays much, and perhaps usefully, employed in other cases, where a blistering fluid raises very rapidly the epithelium, producing little irritation, the skin being only slightly and temporarily reddened. Great irritation and effusion of serum copiously are what is desired here.

Opium is almost always used, and there are great variations in the quantity given, and in the preparation that may be preferred. A good dose of one or two grains at bedtime, to procure sleep, is an almost constant prescription. Advantage is often also found in using the drug during the day if it does not stop the secretions, dry the mouth, and destroy the inclination to take and the power to digest food. In cases where there is much pain, and especially a state of nervous agitation of body and restlessness of mind, the repeated daily use of the drug is most valuable. Many rely upon the copious administration of opium, without any regard to the peculiarities of the case, considering the continued moderate narcotism it produces as the most favourable condition for the patient's recovery. I do not adopt this view of the utility of opium and its preparations, and, therefore, do not press its use as an object in itself, but use it freely when it does not disagree, as a stimulant narcotic to allay restlessness, to soothe pain, to procure sleep.

In severe cases, with much local peritonitic tenderness, a mercurial is advantageously combined with the opium. Many have a special confidence in the calomel, but I hold that it is generally best given as the simple blue pill, about six grains in the course of the day. Or the blue ointment may be applied on the abdomen or elsewhere. Should evidence of hydrargyrismus appear, the further action of the drug is checked by partial or complete discontinuance of it. Many eminent practitioners, especially in Scotland, make no use of mercurials in any form of puerperal fever.

Ever since I began practice there has been less, and still less, of what is, or used to be, called heroic practice in inflammatory cases; and now it is not uncommon to see them indiscriminately treated by opium and stimulants, with poulticing locally. My own judgment of this important practical matter is that a large number do well on this plan if it is conducted not heroically but gently; that, indeed, in many delicate women, with attacks of slight severity, it is the best plan of treatment. But the antiphlogistic regimen and treatment, as I have sketched it, is proper for the majority of cases, demanding of course such modifications as may adapt it to the peculiarities of each individual example.

The next class of cases, that of sapræmia, or of simple putrid intoxication—poisoning not by an organism multiplying in the blood, but by the passing into it of the chemical products of putrid decomposition—is one upon which much light has been recently thrown, and with the most beneficent results in practice. Like the other forms of the so-called puerperal fever, this I shall treat as a separate entity, and it frequently is so. But it may be combined with the traumatic fever of inflammation, and it is especially liable to be combined with septicæmia and pyæmia. Indeed it has long been, and still is, the habit to speak of septicæmia and pyæmia as diseases of putrefaction, but this is a mistake. Putridity of the discharges is not an essential part of these diseases at all, though it often accompanies them. The organisms which cause septicæmia and pyæmia probably take no part in putrefaction. They live in the discharges, and are conveyed or pass into the blood, where they multiply indefinitely. The organisms which cause putrefaction, whether the bacterium termo, or others in addition, may pass into the blood with the putrid fluids to produce sapræmia, but they do not survive, far less grow therein.

We have, then, in sapræmia, when uncomplicated, a very simple problem. Putrid ichor is absorbed or flows through the uterine sinuses, or otherwise, into the circulation. Its poisonous constituents are eliminated rapidly from the blood; for if the supply is stopped the sapræmic phenomena quickly disappear. When once in the blood it does not increase in it, ferment-like, independently of any further supply. Sapræmia is kept up by a continuous supply of the poison. It disappears when the supply from without is stopped. To stop the supply is the problem of cure.

Fetor of the discharges has to be searched for in all cases of puerperal fever. It may be easily discovered by its strength; or it may be concealed, especially if the patient is kept very clean, and if vaginal deodorizing washes are used. The finger, if there is suspicion, or even the whole hand, carefully carbolized, may be passed into the uterus, to find the fetor and its cause, and peradventure to remove them. There may be putridity of discharges alone, but generally there is some decomposing substance, and more than mere bloodclot, a patch of membrane, and probably of chorion, a small bit of placenta, or some hypertrophied decidual mass. Sometimes the putrid fluid is retained *in utero*, and it may be discharged in great gushes, flowing at successive intervals.

Sepsin, or chemical products of decomposition dissolved in water are absorbed by the extensive mucous surfaces of the vagina and uterus, with their lymphatics, and by the placental and other wounds in the genital tract. Or they pass freely into the uterine sinuses and thus into the general circulation. The result is quick pulse and respiration, high temperature, delirium, and often purging. If the poisoning is slight, symptoms are slight. If the poisoning is by a large dose the symptoms are urgent, and death may result, and this without any added septicæmia to produce the fatal event.

During the currency of the disease or poisoning there is the possibility of a cure, almost sudden, by removing the fetor or stopping the supply of the poison. Nothing is more striking or more gratifying in the whole practice of medicine than this sudden recovery; and, as it is often produced by art, it deserves the name of a cure. A patient in the most alarming condition, apparently within a few hours of death, is appropriately treated, and within a few hours alarm has entirely subsided. It is not in lying-in women alone that such cases are seen; but sapræmia is more frequently observed in them than in others, and the joy of recovery is greater because the foreseen danger is greater, for evident reasons.

An aggravated case of this kind was recently under my care in St. Bartholomew's Hospital, and I shall give you a sketch of it from the notes of Mr. Nall. The largeness of the retained placental mass made the cause of the disease evident and easily discovered; and in this respect it is not like the run of similar cases which are classed under the designation puerperal fever. The recovery in it was so great, so quick, and so nearly complete, as to be scarcely credible. The woman appeared to be at the point of death. It was apparently not worth while to disturb her by treatment. In a few hours after the treatment she was comfortable, and every alarming symptom had disappeared. Yet for some days there was slight recurrence of fetor and persistence of diminished symptoms, but not to such a degree as to cause any suffering or alarm for the ultimate safety of the patient. Were the case not a typical one I should not take up your time with it.

A. E. was delivered naturally of her second child on June 8th. Flooding occurred after the birth of the child, and slight blood loss continued for seven days. Then the lochia became fetid. On the eighth day she had rigors, which were repeated daily. She was brought into the hospital on the tenth day, and was delirious during the night. On the eleventh day of her lying-in, when I first saw her, she had no complaint of pain, was pale, sick, frequently vomiting, troubled with diarrhœa; the uterus tender; breath sweet; respiration hurried, 44; pulse 146; temperature 104.2°; copious flow of stinking lochia. A piece of placenta was removed from the vagina. Under the influence of chloroform the hand was introduced into the uterus, which was soft and easily admitted it, and adherent placental masses were removed, some small shreds being left after many had been separated by volsella. The whole genital tract was then washed out by copious injections of carbolic lotion (1 in 30). Ergot of rye was administered, and the uterus was washed out every four hours during the day. The report of the next day bears that she had a good night without delirium, that the bowels had been twice moved, the motions being thin, yellow, and offensive. The discharge was slight and slightly fetid; the breasts were tender and swollen; the pulse had fallen to 100, the respirations to 36, and the highest temperature was 101.4°. The whole aspect of the case had changed from despair to hopefulness. Ergot was continued for some days, and the carbolic washings as long as any trace of fetor was found. Recovery was uninterrupted; indeed, it may be said there was no process of recovery, there was only convalescence. Such a progress is not seen in any other form of puerperal fever. The theory of sapræmia accounts for the rapid cure, while the theory of the other forms of puerperal fever explains their gradual advance from bad to worse, or to recovery.

Sapræmia is treated earnestly, even heroically if necessary, with a view to its own cure, and with a view to the prevention of the complications, inflammatory, septicæmic, or pyæmic, which it is very likely to. bring in its train. Heroic treatment may be required to reach the remotest part of the genital tract in search for decomposing matter, or to ascertain that there is nothing but putrid lochia in the case. Mere vaginal washing may suffice, or intra-uterine washing, or the volsella may be passed into the uterus to grope for the decomposing structure, or with the same view a finger or fingers may be passed, or even the whole hand; and it may be necessary to dilate the cervix preliminarily. Most of this may be done without an anæsthetic, but where the hand is to be introduced into the vagina, the previous induction of anæsthesia is desirable.

The lotion which I always use is the carbolic, of the strength of 1 in 40, or occasionally 1 in 30. It is used tepid or warm. In conducting the operation it is necessary to be very gentle, to avoid the introduction of air into the passages, and to see that the fluid runs out freely. If the os uteri externum and internum are not widely open, a pipe with double current should be used. The whole proceeding should cause little or no pain, and, for an ordinary washing, a pint or a pint and a half may be passed. But if the discharges are copious and fetid, more may be required, and the rule is to continue the injection so long as it comes away foul or perceptibly fetid. Of course, a bowl is to be so used as to receive all the lotion as it is discharged, in order to save the bed-linen from being wetted. When the uterus is washed out the medical attendant conducts the operation, but vaginal washings may be left to the nurse. The washings are to be repeated from twice to four times a day if the fetor persists in the discharges. After the fetor is suppressed twice a day is sufficient. If the discharges become natural, and if the symptoms of sapræmia disappear, the washings are stopped. In any case they are required only for a few days.

These antiseptic washings constitute the great or essential treatment of sapræmia—a treatment, as already said, so direct in its action, and so successful, that is may be called a cure. Though these washings have been described by ancient authors, and though they were recommended by Harvey and by Baudelocque, it is well known to you that no such practice was in use among us till the antiseptic theory of treatment was promulgated. Yet they are not covered by the antiseptic theory, for you know it was based on the presence of bacteria which passed into the blood, and the antiseptic treatment was planned to destroy them or prevent them reaching the wounded surface. Here we use antiseptics not with these views, but to remove and arrest putrefaction, with a view to stopping the supply of a chemical, not a living, poison, the product of putrefaction, which enters the blood and endangers the constitution.

Besides the washings out, a case may demand many attentions, and cares too varied and too uncertain of occurrence for me to enter on them here. But to one I must allude as probably directly useful. It is the administration of ergot. A drachm of the liquid extract, in divided doses, should be given daily for a few days. The object of its use is to induce permanent contraction of the uterus or uterine retraction. This diminishes the uterine cavity, in which the discharge accumulates; it thus also lessens the surface absorbing the putrid poison, and the contraction of the walls of the organ may to some extent prevent the passage of the fetid fluid along the vessels into the circulation. Of course, should it be desirable, the drug may be given hypodermically, ergotin being used instead of the liquid extract.

Perhaps I have made the pathology of sapræmia too simple; for, in addition to what I have said, it is necessary to add that fetid lochia do not always poison the constitution. They generally do so, but not invariably. They may flow in intense putridity, and yet be apparently not absorbed, as is generally the case. Why the putrid ichor is in some cases not absorbed I shall not here attempt to explain.

I know no reason why septicæmia and pyæmia should be called *real* puerperal fever, yet this is a common mode of speaking. The simple inflammatory fever, and the sapræmic fever, are not less really fever, nor less really puerperal. Probably the notion arises from the fact that grave cases of fever after delivery are for the most part septicæmic, or pyæmic, and that the great majority of the deaths in childbed is produced by these diseases. There has always, indeed, been a tendency to regard puerperal fever as desperate, or almost certainly fatal. I can remember well the saying of an eminent physician, with whose retrospective diagnosis many agreed, that if a case recovered it was not one of real puerperal fever. Probably he did not mean his words to be held as strictly true, but to express his sense of the hopelessness of such cases. This disheartening opinion should not be entertained, for it is not based on ascertained truth, and it induces despondency and feebleness in treatment which are prejudicial to the thorough management of a case. The pyæmic cases with their embolism, inflammation, and abscess, are more dangerous than the septicæmic, but even in pyæmia there are numerous recoveries. Every one has heard of rare and marvellous convalescence in pyæmia, even after several joints have suppurated; but these are very far from being the only instances. Many less severe cases survive the disease.

I may consider simultaneously the treatment of these two diseases. They are often combined, and their treatment is identical, if we except such surgical interference as is sometimes required in cases of pyæmia, a department into which I do not propose to enter. I have said that pyæmia and septicæmia may be combined, and while this is probably a frequent occurrence, it should also be remembered that all the forms of puerperal fever may be simultaneously present in one case. The separate consideration of simple inflammatory fever and of sapræmia is demanded by their utterly different pathology, and by their distinct indications of treatment. For the inflammatory fever we have some modification of the venerable established antiphlogistic method. For the sapræmia we have the arrestment of the putrid poisoning. For the septicæmia and pyæmia we have no treatment in any sense antidotal or curative in the humblest meaning of that word.

Cases of pyæmia and septicæmia are to be managed rather than treated. The word treatment implies too high an estimate of the physician's powers; or if not too high, at least a too definite view of them. We cannot arrest or even moderate the storm, but we may guide the bark through it. When the organisms producing these diseases are in the blood we cannot kill them, nor do we know any means of certainly controlling their growth. But we may wisely consider the constitutional and local circumstances of the patient, and judiciously interfere to modify them with a view to the patient's survival.

One unsound tree in a forest may be covered with lichen and fungus, and the tree may slowly die, or be killed. But it may survive, and becoming healthy, throw off the morbid growth which endangered it. The organisms of pyæmia and septicæmia find a favourable nidus for development in the weak, the unhealthy, the hopeless, the ashamed, the sad—in those who have been exhausted by a long labour or injured in the course of a severe one. But the attacked do not certainly die. The organisms may grow and grow, and cause death, but they are not necessarily fatal; their growth may be arrested, and they may all disappear. Debilitating and depressing conditions favour their development. Health and strength favour their disappearance. These principles are the foundation of our management; and experience, daily increasing, confirms the conviction that the foundation is not laid on sand.

Good nursing, careful feeding, prudent stimulation—these are the great points. In all of them there is now progressive improvement. While it is impossible to appreciate with any exactness what we owe to these, no one will deny the comparatively great advantages we now gain by them. It would be out of place to enter upon the subject of nursing here. It is no peculiarity of cases of septicæmia and pyæmia to require good nursing, and the subject is specially referred to in connection with these diseases because, in default of any direct treatment, we specially consider what remains for us to attend to.

On feeding and the use of stimulants I might content myself by making the same remarks as on nursing; but I wish to insist on the great necessity for more attention being paid to the niceties of these important departments. The food and drink should not be left altogether to the nurse. In quality, quantity, and time they should be regulated ; and this cannot be done by previously fixed rules, but by directions modified according to the observations daily or hourly made in each individual case. Milk and beef-tea are the staple of the patient's diet, and they may be varied almost indefinitely, to suit minor emergencies as they arise. In regard to food, the general rule is to give as much as the patient can take without evident disorder arising from it. It is seldom that too much is taken, for a common difficulty lies in overcoming the aversion to food.

The use of stimulants requires a little more discussion. At present the favourites are brandy and champagne, and I adhere to the general voice in preferring them—on one condition, that they be really good. At the same time I make no objection to other wines and spirits. Brandy and champagne are common and simple, and, for me at least, it would be only an affectation of refinement to appraise the merits of different wines and different vintages. But I am sure that, in regard to all stimulants, our aim should be to use as little as possible. Often, at least for a time, none at all is required. Occasionally, but rarely, in a crisis of weakness, brandy is to be administered largely. Always the principle holds good that too much will do more harm than too little. I am sure that it is a common error to give too much. Excess of food may be passed along the primæ viæ without entailing any considerable injury ; not so excess of alcohol. Food is rarely desired by the patient, while she often wishes alcohol; because, as it is given, it assuages thirst for a time and produces at once an agreeable excitement.

A sketch of the treatment of septicæmia and pyæmia would be bald and imperfect if it were confined to the paramount matters—nursing, food, and stimulants. Great attention has to be paid to the general condition and to the state of health as indicated by prominent symptoms. Iron and quinine are now frequently administered, and with great advantage ; and what a change of view does this imply if we look back to the days of Gordon, or even of Fergusson? I can well remember the astonishment and unsettlement of mind produced by the recommendation of Hamilton Bell to use the old tincture of the muriate of iron in erysipelas, and I frequently witnessed the earliest employment of the same remedy in the cognate diseases now under discussion, chiefly by the advice of the elder Begbie. It was always the custom to combine bitters with the iron, but now the regal bitter, quinine, is used, not only as a stomachic vehicle, but with the direct purpose of reducing the temperature whose regular observation helps so greatly to guide us now—a chart unknown in the days of Bell and Begbie. Besides quinine and salicin, the influence of cold is now familiarly resorted to to reduce temperature when it rises above 102° or 103°, and this is done with the result of giving comfort and securing probably real gain. Many physicians, Schrœder, Osterloh, and Spiegelberg, in Germany, and especially Playfair in this country, have used the

cold bath to reduce temperature when it is very high ; but I have no experience
with it.   Temperature does not long remain high in this disease, varying greatly
and often rapidly; and for keeping it moderate, quinine or salicin, in large doses,
with regulation of the heat of the room, of the bedclothes, and of tepid sponging,
are generally sufficient.

Ice is often taken internally against thirst, and it is a delicious mouthful ; but
the craving thirst is not relieved.   The dose is repeated and repeated in vain.
For the relief of thirst, the old remedies, such as toast-water, have more real
value.   But the urgency of thirst is minimized by the proper management of the
case.   At least, I can have no doubt that in the days of what I call the excessive
use of wine or brandy, or of opium, we heard a deal more of the suffering from
thirst than we do now.

Ice is much used to arrest vomiting, which is so common a symptom of the
peritonitis of puerperal patients, and it is sometimes effectual.   For this distressing symptom remedies are numerous, and their largeness of number is evidence
of their uncertain action.   The best is of course that most used—the hydrocyanic
acid and bismuth mixture, without or with morphia.

With or without sickness and vomiting there may be flatulence, and it is sometimes so great as to embarrass the heart and lungs.   In extreme cases relief has
been afforded by letting off the air by a small trocar and canula, but of this proceeding I have little experience.   The remedies which I have found of most use
are charcoal, in teaspoonful doses, given in water once or twice daily ; or turpentine, in ten-drop doses, given in water or some simple vehicle, three or four times
daily.

The hot linseed-meal poultice is almost always a grateful and useful application to the hypogastric region, relieving pain and promoting the lochial flow.
Besides, when the skin is hot and dry, it is a valuable diaphoretic.

Opium in some form is invariably administered, and almost always with advantage.   Occasionally, indeed, it produces great mental disturbance and uneasiness,
or vomiting, or dryness of tongue ; and, in such cases, if a change of the preparation does not bring better results, the medicine may have to be given up, or
used only to produce sleep.   Indeed, apart from any injurious effects, it is often
a good plan, when pain is not urgent, to give it only to secure a good night.
But generally it is given repeatedly during the day, either to relieve pain or with
a view to its soothing and supporting rather than narcotizing action.

Opium and other remedies are also often used against diarrhœa, and in this
way much good may be done.   But it is necessary to pay much attention to this
purging, generally of thin highly-coloured dejecta, for undoubtedly it often should
be encouraged rather than checked ; and, perhaps fortunately, it is often not easy
to check it.   The physician should see all the motions, so as to justly estimate
their quantity and character, and he should not regard it as his duty to try to
check free and even copious evacuations, or to get the stools in a formed state.
He will be guided in his judgment on this point by the strength of the patient
and the amount of food consumed.

During the whole course of the disease the regular flow of the lochia is anxiously
looked for ; and, should they be suppressed, an attempt is made to bring them
back by hot fomentations to the vulva and hypogastrium ; for it is naturally
regarded as desirable that there should be lochial discharge, and that it should
not be retained.   But, besides its mere flow, the character of the discharge,
especially as to fetor, is scrutinized.   If there is fetor there is probably sapræmia
complicating the septicæmia or pyæmia, and this fetor is treated by antiseptic
lotions, as already described.   But fetor of discharges forms no part of septicæmia
or pyæmia.   The bacteria or micrococci of these diseases flourish when there is

no fetor. At present, however, such is the enthusiasm for antiseptics, that it is considered desirable to have the womb well washed out once or twice daily by carbolic lotion, even when there is no fetor; and meantime I consider it good practice to do this twice daily while there is urgency, if the discharges are not quite healthy in all respects. The intra-uterine washing cannot work upon the infected blood circulating everywhere in the body, and carrying with it the baneful organisms, but it can keep the wounds clean; and, if the womb or vagina is a nursing-ground for further supplies of these organisms, then by the antiseptic washing the nursery is destroyed. The further supply of the contagium vivum is stopped, for the micrococci are killed by the carbolic wash.

Such, gentlemen, is an outline of the treatment of a group of terrible diseases. How imperfect it is, no one can feel more strongly than I do. It is not a fixed treatment, but the treatment of to-day. Were I the wisest therapeutist, and had I the best rhetoric, my description would still be imperfect; for no one can describe, with a near approach to perfection, what is imperfectly known and very dimly understood. But the variations of health and constitution, of complications, and of other conditions, are so numerous that a perfect theory or system of treatment would not carry with it directions for every individual case. Boundless scope, after all, would be left for intelligent interference of the practitioner warmed into zeal by a kindly sympathizing heart.

Meeting with these puerperal diseases, the practitioner dare not fold his hands in apathy and inaction on account of the incompleteness of his knowledge. No one would listen to him were he to proclaim that all our experience and all our laboriously acquired information had yielded no fruit for the benefit of suffering women. He is face to face with great and terrible danger, yet his position is not one of imminent peril to himself as in the case of a soldier, who, like him, has to meet unexpected combinations and unforeseen difficulties, and who, whether he has little or much knowledge, must act and that at once, for in boldness there is safety, in delay there is only disaster; and experience has amply demonstrated that no case is to be utterly despaired of till the moribund state supervenes, however severe and complicated it may be.

We have said that puerperal fever affects especially the weak, the unhealthy, the hopeless, the ashamed, those who have been exhausted by a long labour or injured in the course of a severe one; and there is no need to expatiate on the great field here opened up for the beneficent activity of the physician. To strengthen, to heal, to encourage, to console, to manage labour, to reduce injuries to a minimum, are all objects to be kept in mind; not indeed with a view only to the treatment of puerperal fever, but in order to its prevention. It is a trite saying that prevention is better than cure, and I think there can be no doubt that more suffering is avoided and more lives saved on this principle than by treatment; and I feel impelled to say a few words on this subject.

The prevention of simple inflammatory and of sapræmic fever demands no special consideration here; it is the prevention of septicæmia and pyæmia, or of contagious puerperal fever, that is generally in view when prophylaxis is spoken of, and few subjects are at present more discussed. The late trials of midwives for spreading puerperal fever, and the reiterated attacks on maternity hospitals, are familiar to all; and I believe all will admit that we want much more light and more wisdom in our dealings with these matters. They are not identical, for the propagation of puerperal fever in a hospital involves considerations which have no place in its propagation in a private or out-of-door dispensary practice. Hospitals are the seat of endemics of fearful character. The house becomes tainted, and every lying-in woman in it is in great danger from the infection. Fortunately, the infection does not become so intense as to affect all, but such a degree of intensity is quite conceivable. In an ordinary dairy no vessel of milk escapes the action of the bacterium lactis; every dish becomes curdled. In home practice the infection reaches patients only sporadically; the disease, however. occasionally dogging the footsteps of an individual practitioner. There are no epidemics, no prevalence of the infection over countries. A lying-in woman can easily find a safe home. The analogy of the curdling of milk does not apply here, for it is difficult to find a place where there is no bacterium lactis where milk does not curdle.

Against the dangers of both hospital and home practice we find some degree of protection in antiseptic midwifery, a great practical subject which I have discussed in an address lately given to the Medical Society of London. Antiseptics have, as yet at least, but little to do with the treatment of the infectious forms of puerperal fever; they avail greatly in the prophylaxis. This has been well exemplified in the case of hospitals. In private practice the protective power is not so easily demonstrated; yet I believe the plan is there also invaluable, rendering the patient comparatively safe and practically excluding all danger of infection by the careful accoucheur.

Ventilation and cleanliness were, up to the present time, the great resorts of medicine against endemics of puerperal fever, and they had little and only temporary effect. They are, however, even now justly valued very highly; but, with antiseptics, we come into closer quarters with the enemy we have to subdue, and have a weapon of greater potency, and consequently we have more success. In spite of all our prophylaxis, however, puerperal fever prevails. The enemy succeeds in the attack and the physician has to make every effort to rescue his patient by treatment.

Although we have at present no prospect of being able to stamp out the infectious forms of pueperal fever or of reducing them to comparative insignificance, there is yet, even as to the attainment of these great ends, some ground for hope arising from the success of scientific investigations. Vaccination seems destined only to a brief further protraction of its splendid and useful isolation and of the mystery of its operation. The results of Pasteur's researches on the cholera of the domestic fowl and of Toussaint's and Greenfield's on anthrax show how a contagium vivum may have its potency diminished, or nearly annihilated, by methods having a strong analogy with those employed to reduce the potency of the variolous contagion. If one contagion can be so modified, we are led to ask, Why may not also that of puerperal fever be likewise? There are other researches by Greenfield and Buchner which justify the philanthropic hope that with lapse of time the deadly characters of the organisms of septicæmia and pyæmia may be changed into others more innocent. Such anticipations are little more than mere indulgence of the scientific imagination; but they are far from being useless or foolish, though to the merely practical man they may appear so.

The idea suggested by the researches of Pasteur, of Toussaint, of Greenfield, and Buchner may prove to be mere *ignes fatui*, but may, on the contrary, prove to be true guides. It is by following out such ideas, verifying or disproving them by new investigations, that progress is made in science. Progress in science is a fountain of purest pleasure to its promoters and of widespread beneficence to mankind.

The Society whose new session I have the honour to inaugurate is devoted to the advancement of science, and I dare in conclusion to suggest to every busy medical man here that he should make some department of it, perhaps a very small department, his peculiar study. By so doing he will keep a special perennial joy in his life of toil; he will be, if not a discoverer of new truth, at least a diffuser of it; he will be a useful and honoured member of this Society, he will contribute to the elevation of medicine into a more and more useful profession, and of his medical brethren into a higher and higher position.

The healthy and diseased human body is not the greatest matter in the universe of things. Our profession acknowledges that there are others to whom, in respect of the value and grandeur of its aim, it willingly bows. But medicine offers more than sufficient scope for the greatest efforts of the greatest minds. It is for us to contribute to its prosperity and progress. *Floreat res medica.*—*Lancet*, Oct. 30, and Nov. 6, 1880.

———

On the Treatment with Alkalies of a little known Cause of Sterility.

CHARRIER, of Paris, calls attention (*Bull. Gén. de Thérap.*, Nos. 11 and 12, 1880) to an acid condition of the utero-vaginal mucus as a cause of sterility. He states that many women who are quite healthy, whose genital organs are perfectly normal, and who are married to healthy husbands remain sterile. The cause of this is frequently an acid condition of the uterine and vaginal mucus, which may be proved directly by the use of litmus paper. This condition is an absolute prevention of conception, because the spermatorrhœa die immediately. Accordingly, if the woman's mucous secretions give an acid reaction, she continues sterile. By treatment with alkalies, alkaline drinks and baths (Vichy water), and alkaline injections (1000 parts of water, sulph. of soda 90 parts, white of egg 1 part), the disease may be removed and conception follow. This, according to the author, explains the frequently incomprehensible results and numerous strange successes that follow the use of alkaline springs in sterile women. Two successful cases are given in illustration of the author's views. Professor Pajot also expresses himself as in agreement with the author's views.—*Edinburgh Med. Journal*, Nov. 1880.

———

Congenital Abnormality of Uterus simulating Retention of Menses.

Dr. BRAXTON HICKS related at a late meeting of the Obstetrical Society of London (*Lancet*, Nov. 27, 1880), the history of a patient, aged twenty-four, who had never menstruated. About twelve weeks ago she had severe pain in the right hypochondrium, lasting about six weeks. About the same time she noticed an increasing swelling in the lower abdomen, and recently tension had become severe. On admission a tumour was felt reaching above the umbilicus, tense and semi-fluctuating, causing distress and œdema of the legs. She had not distinctly suffered from monthly increase of distress. The vagina was nearly of normal length, ending in a kind of transverse depression, beyond which was felt the tumour, exactly resembling the uterus distended with menses. The author had had such a case, apparently exactly similar, the very extremity of the vagina and os uteri being closed. The patient was therefore placed under chloroform and a trocar plunged in, where a depression like a dilated os beyond the closure could be felt. Nothing but a little bloody serum flowed. The sound was then passed up into the centre of what seemed to be the uterus, but still no sign of menstrual fluid. Further interference was then abandoned, the tapping having been done antiseptically. In the night she became feverish, and died about thirty hours after the tapping. Post-mortem examination showed that there were neither uterus nor ovaries, but a large cyst attached to the upper end of the vagina; walls very irregular within, smooth without. It was half filled with a cheesy white matter, and the rest with dark grumous material. The wall above was thinned and perforated in two or three places, where the contents, in a fetid condition, had escaped into the peritoneal cavity. The trocar had passed through two layers of peritoneum. Probably the operation had only hastened the rupture.

A report by Dr. GALABIN on the Microscopic Structure of the Cyst was appended. The outer wall of fibrous tissue was only about one-twelfth of an inch thick. The soft material within was made up of round cells, longer than leucocytes, having a fibrillar reticulum amongst them. It was to be regarded as a soft sarcomatous growth.

Dr. ROUTH said that the practical point which came out was, that in another case the aspirator should be used to see the nature of the fluid, if any, before a trocar was employed.

Medical Jurisprudence and Toxicology.

Antidotes.

The following collection of antidotes is taken from the *Allgemeine Wiener Medizinische Zeitung :—*

Morphia. Sulphate of copper, 1 gramme; distilled water, 40 grammes, for an emetic; half to be taken at once and the remainder in five minutes, if necessary. To be followed by strong coffee, and then every five minutes by tablespoonful doses of a mixture made by dissolving 4 grammes of tannic acid in 50 grammes of simple syrup.

Opium. As for morphia.

Veratria. As for morphia.

Savine. As for morphia.

Fungus-poisoning. As for morphia.

Stramonium. As for opium. May be followed by a hypodermic injection of morphia.

Nicotine. For the sickness resulting from tobacco-smoking, vinegar, 50 grammes; simple syrup, 50 grammes; water, 200 grammes; half to be taken at once, and then a tablespoonful every five minutes. For accidental poisoning by nicotine, same as for morphia. Also tannic acid, 4 grammes; syrup, 50 grammes; distilled water 200 grammes; a tablespoonful every five minutes.

Phosphorus. Sulphate of copper, 1 gramme : distilled water, 40 grammes; half to be taken at once, the rest in five minutes, if necessary. Then oil of turpentine, 30 grammes; white and yolk of two eggs; simple syrup, 50 grammes; peppermint water, 250 grammes, for an emulsion, to be well shaken; one tablespoonful every half hour until a fourth part has been taken, and then a tablespoonful every hour.

Burns by Phosphorus. Nitrate of silver, 2 grammes; distilled water, 20 grammes; to be used as a lotion.

Petroleum. Oily and mucilaginous drinks to be taken frequently.

Lunar Caustic. Common salt, 20 grammes; water. 300 grammes; half to be taken at once, then a tablespoonful every half hour with oily mucilaginous drinks.

Strychnia. Tannic acid, 3 grammes; syrup of marsh-mallow, 60 grammes; distilled water, 140 grammes; a tablespoonful every five minutes. Then chloral-hydrate, 4 grammes; distilled water, 100 grammes; a tablespoonful every half hour.

Sausage Poisoning, and Poisoning by Decomposing Meat. Sulphate of copper, 1 gramme; distilled water, 40 grammes, for an emetic; half to be taken at once, and the remainder in five minutes, if necessary. With this may be given ether, 2 grammes; tincture of opium, 10 drops; distilled water, 150 grammes; a tablespoonful every half hour.

Ergot. As for sausage poisoning.—*London Med. Record*, Oct. 15, 1880.

MEDICAL NEWS.

Milk as a Carrier of Disease.

The tireless inquisition which sanitarians are ceaselessly prosecuting into nature's methods of propagating disease has seldom been rewarded with a more valuable discovery in a more unpromising field, than that in regard to the portability of certain infectious maladies by means of milk ; a fluid which from prehistoric times has formed so large a part of the food of juvenile humanity, and has as a rule, except on the score of aqueous dilution, been implicitly trusted by mankind.

The peculiar readiness with which milk absorbs disagreeable odours and flavours has long been a matter of common observation, but it is only within the past ten or twelve years, that its power of taking up the germs or disease poisons of several contagious affections and transplanting them from their original site to the congenial soil of some uninfected human organism, where they could flourish with renewed vigour, was detected. Doubtless much of this capacity for evil which is possessed by milk is due to the very circumstance of its obtaining access to infants and young children who have not been protected by previous attacks of scarlatina or enteric fever, but its chemical constitution being that of a dilute watery solution of highly complex nitrogenous matter, renders it almost as favourable a medium for the growth of bacteria as Pasteur's fluid itself, so that believers in the germ theory of disease contend its natural composition is peculiarly favourable on this account to the extension of its sphere of deleterious influence. Be this as it may, however, there is no question that more than a dozen localized epidemics of typhoid fever, scarlet fever and diphtheria (some of them affecting hundreds of individuals), the origin of which would otherwise have been shrouded in mystery, are now satisfactorily traced to dairy farms occasionally many miles from the scene of their deadly operations. In most instances the milkmen have strenuously denied that any typhoid fever poison could have found entrance to milk from the wells in which it was proved to have existed upon their premises, except during the process of washing out their milk cans, but knowing as we do how profitable and how difficult of detection is moderate aqueous adulteration, it requires all an optimist's faith in poor humanity to give credence to their statements.

We are led to call public attention to this subject at the present time by the fact that several recent English medical journals come to us bearing accounts of new epidemics, attributable to the infection of milk tainted with the poisons of typhoid fever, scarlatina, or diphtheria. Thus, for example, at Southport, one case of typhoid after another was announced to the municipal authorities until in about two weeks a total of twenty-eight was reached.   Such a rapidly invading epidemic demanded of course energetic measures for its repression and a careful inspection of the various dwellings in which the victims had been attacked was undertaken.   The health officers found, however, to their surprise, that with two trifling exceptions these premises were all in good sanitary condition ; but further investigation disclosed the fact that in every instance milk had been served to the families in which the typhoid fever had occurred from a particular dairy some miles distant, and upon the grounds of this dairyman was discovered a well horribly polluted with soakage from a filthy cess pit near it.   In the words of the chairman, " chemical analysis showed that it was nothing but liquid sewage and calculated to spread disease wherever its influence extended," and the proof that this foul infecting material had been accomplishing the work for which it was so well " calculated," is met with in the circumstance that on stopping the milk supply from this dairy the epidemic ceased to spread, although not before two of the cases previously attacked had resulted fatally.

The infectious material, when scarlatina and diphtheria are conveyed by milk, probably falls into the fluid whilst standing in open vessels, or is rubbed off, attached to the epithelial cells of the epidermis during the process of milking in such a way as to gain access to the milk.   In an example of this kind, recently the subject of judicial action in England, a medical officer of health stated before the magistrates that seven cases of diphtheria had occurred in his own practice, and that during inquiries made for the purpose of tracing the origin of the disease, he had heard of other instances, all of which as well as his own had been supplied with milk from the same establishment.   Acting upon this hint he proceeded to examine the dairy from which the milk was obtained and found that a child was dying from malignant diphtheria on the premises, so that this case was, it seemed highly probable, the starting-point of the whole outbreak of the malady.

Still another fresh illustration of the dangers we are now considering is reported from the town of Dundee in Scotland, where an extended epidemic of scarlet fever is stated to have arisen among families supplied from two particular dairies.   On careful investigation scarlatina was found to have been actually prevailing in the families of the dairymen in charge of these establishments before and at the time the other cases made their appearance.

Of course the only way to obtain a reasonable security for our families against this form of poisoning would be to follow the example of our English cousins and establish by law a system of thorough inspection of dairy farms, dairies, and cow-stables having special reference not only to the health of the animals and of their care-takers, but also to the state of the wells from which the water for washing out the milk cans, pails, etc., is derived. How common it is to see even on well-kept farms the water supply for these and similar purposes obtained from the barn pump which for convenience in cold weather stands under the cow shed or inside the farmyard, where it is at all times liable to furnish a liquid dangerously contaminated with excrementitious matters from both man and beast. As a substitute for such legal supervision the most feasible plan would probably be for citizens to unite together into limited associations, which could employ experts to investigate and keep watch over the sanitary surroundings of dairy farms patronized by their members. Although such undertakings might be at first rather expensive, yet when the mere cost of a dozen cases of typhoid fever is considered, there is no doubt that the outlay would be a truly economical one, even if looked upon from a pecuniary point of view only, without estimating the far more important saving of human life and suffering. In cases where such co-operative societies could not be organized, or whilst travelling, it would be advisable to use only milk which has been thoroughly boiled for a considerable length of time.

Symmetrical Neuralgia in Diabetes.—Dr. Worms, of Paris, has called attention to the occurrence of symmetrical neuralgias in an advanced period of diabetes. He has recorded two examples—one affecting the sciatic nerve, and one the inferior dental—and believes that the symmetry of the affection is a characteristic of this form, as also is its peculiar severity. It does not yield to the ordinary treatment of neuralgia—quinine, morphia, bromide—and the pain varies in intensity with the amount of glycosuria.—*Lancet*, Oct. 30, 1880.

Simultaneous Fracture of both Patellæ.—M. de Beauvais related at the Paris Société de Médecine (*Union Méd.*) an example of this rare occurrence. A man, thirty years of age, and apparently in good health, was engaged in the game of leap-frog, and, having struck the ground with his feet, when on the point of springing forwards he felt as if he had received a blow on the legs, and heard a crackling sound. He fell on the ground, believing that some one had struck him. On his being carried to the hospital, a transverse fracture of each patella, with a separation of not more than two centimetres, was found to exist. This was effected by the violent contraction of the extensors. The patient had had rheumatism with cardiac complications formerly.—*Med. Times and Gaz.*, Oct. 9, 1880.

A New Method of Preserving Raw Meat.—A new and apparently most valuable method of preserving raw meat, discovered by Prof. Artimini, of Florence, bids fair to supply a long-felt want, and to have an appreciable effect upon our markets. According to a report by Professors Barff and Mills, of Glasgow, and Dr. Stevenson, of Guy's Hospital, meat six months old was found to be perfectly sound and good, the muscular fibres unchanged, and the nutritive properties unimpaired. The material employed is stated to be less expensive than salt, and not only wholesome, but pleasant to the taste.—*Med. Times and Gaz.*, Oct. 9, 1880.

A Triple Ovary.—Dr. Keppeler, on the occasion of his sixth ovariotomy (all successful), found a third ovary, with its corresponding tube, completely developed. According to Rokitansky and Klebs, no such circumstance has hitherto been observed.—*Med. Times and Gaz.*, Oct. 9, 1880, from *Allg. Wien. Med. Zeit.*, Sept. 7.

—

Chian Turpentine and Cancer.—The Medical Committee of the Middlesex Hospital recently passed unanimously the following resolution: "That, as the results of a prolonged and careful trial of Chian turpentine in the treatment of cancer prove the drug to be quite useless as a cure for that disease, directions be given to the dispenser not to obtain any more of the drug for the cancer patients." —*Med. Times and Gazette*, Nov. 27, 1880.

Mr. Henry Morris, Surgeon of the Cancer Out-Patient Department of the Hospital, in a contribution to the *Lancet* (Nov. 27 and Dec. 4, 1880), on his experience with the use of the drug says he is "not able to report that there is a single symptom over which the drug seems to exercise even frequently, not to say constantly, an influence. It cannot be relied upon to assuage pain, to diminish or alter the character of the discharges, to check hemorrhage, or promote the destruction of the growth by ulceration or sloughing," and that the conclusion is forced upon him "that as a cure for cancer Chian turpentine is utterly valueless."

—

Medical College of Virginia.—This institution has just sustained a serious loss in the resignation of its talented Professor of Surgery, Dr. Hunter McGuire, of Richmond.

—

New Sanitaria.—A new winter resort for invalids has been recently established at Lakewood, a village on the line of the New Jersey Southern Railroad, about nine miles from the ocean and fifty from either Philadelphia or New York. The village is situated on the edge of extensive pine woods through which have been constructed numerous excellent roads. The soil is dry and sandy. The house is new and handsomely furnished and the cuisine is unexceptionable; each bedroom has an open wood fire. For the benefit of invalids in winter the verandas have been inclosed in glass.

A sanitarium has also recently been opened at Monterey, about 125 miles from San Francisco. The "Hotel del Monte" is a large building, with all the modern appliances of a first-class hotel, and accommodates 400 persons. It is situated in a grove of 106 acres of oak, pine, spruce, and cypress trees, and is within a quarter of a mile of the Bay of Monterey, with a fine sloping, sandy beach, admirably adapted for bathing. The climate is represented as charming, corresponding to our "Indian summer," with an equable temperature varying in the winter months from an average of 49° to 55°, and with a summer temperature averaging about 6° higher. It offers, in addition to beautiful and varied scenery, boating, fishing, and hunting to the sportsman.

—

Mr. Lister.—The Royal Medal of the Royal Society has been conferred on Professor Lister, in recognition of his important physiological services, and the advance in surgery due to his studies and application of antiseptic principles.

Mr. Lister is spoken of as the next President of the Clinical Society of London.

A Veteran Professor.

M. Chevreul has completed his fiftieth annual course of lectures on the Application of Chemistry to Organized Bodies, at the Museum of Natural History. M. Chevreul is in his ninety-fifth year and is still an indefatigable worker in the laboratory. His father attained the advanced age of one hundred and ten. The American Association for the Advancement of Science, during its recent session in Boston, sent a congratulatory telegram to the eminent savant, expressing the hope that he may be enabled to continue his labors until the end of the century.

—

Langenbeck's Seventieth Birthday.

In Berlin, on the 9th of November, a highly interesting celebration was held on the occasion of Professor.Von Langenbeck, the distinguished German surgeon, on that day reaching his seventieth year ; and, both from the military and the civil authorities, and from friends both near and far, he received an ovation which falls to the lot of few. The day began by a *reveillé*, played before his door by the band of the Third Regiment of the Imperial Guard. Soon afterwards arrived private letters of most affectionate greeting from the Emperor of Germany and the Empress. The Crown Prince sent a telegram of congratulation from Wiesbaden, in his own name and that of his wife. The Emperor of Austria sent the Grand Cross of the Order of Francis Joseph ; the King of Saxony, that of the Order of Albert. The Medical Faculty of the University of Berlin appeared as a body, and addressed Langenbeck through their Dean. A deputation also waited on him from the Frederick-William Military Medical School, whose Director-Surgeon-General (Schubert), in presenting a laurel wreath, addressed to Langenbeck the following words : "Ever since your arrival as Professor, in Berlin, our institution has rejoiced in your instruction, and we have all sat at your feet. In peace time, as in war, you have been our guiding star ; and there is scarce a single doctor, either in our army or our marine, who is not personally indebted to you for surgical knowledge and power." A number of his former pupils, now professors in the universities of Germany, presented an elaborate address. Amongst those present were Professor Esmarch of Kiel, Billroth of Vienna, Schönborn of Königsberg, Lücke of Strasburg, Trendelenburg of Rostock, Hueter of Griefswald, and others. Count Moltke paid personally his respects, as well as a host of other distinguished persons. A few cordial and appreciative words, engrossed on vellum and signed by the President of the Royal College of Surgeons of England and a number of prominent British surgeons, reminded Professor Von Langenbeck of the high appreciation in which he was held in England.

—

Health of Charleston.—This city is now reported to be very healthy. The dengue had pretty much expended its force before the cold weather set in ; since the appearance of ice (November 25) the disease seems to have completely disappeared. A few cases of influenza have been observed—one of them attended with sweatings, but it is doubtful if these were cases of dengue. As far as can be learned, the dengue originated in the northwestern portion of Charleston, about the end of June, and gradually extended. It may have exhibited itself earlier in Key West. It made its appearance at a later date in Summerville, Columbia, and other small towns on the line of the South Carolina Railroad—reaching Wilmington, N. C., where it appeared to a very slight extent and in a very mild form. Augusta, Savannah, Port Royal, and Beaufort were invaded in August and September. None of the Charleston cases, which were uncomplicated, proved fatal.

Diphtheria, which prevailed in Charleston for several years past, has almost entirely disappeared.

—

International Medical Congress, London, 1881.—We have received circulars informing us that the following subjects have been proposed for discussion :—

In Section V. (*Surgery*): 1. Recent advances in Abdominal Surgery ; 2. On the surgical treatment of certain diseased conditions of the Kidney ; 3. On the recent advances in the method of extracting Stone from the Bladder ; 4. On the treatment of Operation of Wounds ; 5. On the treatment of Aneurism by the elastic bandage ; 6. On the comparative advantages of early and late resection in Diseases of Joints.

In Section VII. (*Diseases of Children*); Medical : 1. The real position of the so-called Rubeola, Rötheln or German Measles, and its relation to Scarlatina and Measles ; 2. Syphilis as a cause of Rickets ; 3. On the different kinds of Spinal Paralysis and Myelitis in children ; 4. The conditions governing the occurrence of Albuminuria and of Paralysis as attendant on Diphtheria, or as Sequelæ ; 5. The relationship of Chorea to Rheumatism, with especial reference to the nature of the heart-murmur which so frequently attends Chorea ; 6. The forms of Acute Tuberculosis other than ordinary Tubercular Meningitis. Surgical : 1. The surgical treatment of Croup and Diphtheria ; 2. The surgical aspect of Tapping for Empyema ; 3. Pathology and treatment of Genu Valgum ; 4. The treatment of Diseases of the Joints, especially with a view to the prevention of deformity ; 5. Treatment of Spinal Curvature, with special reference to Sayre's method ; 6. The nature of the so-called Surgical Scarlet Fever.

In Section X. (*Otology*): 1. On the value of operations in which the Tympanic Membrane is incised ; 2. On morbid growths within the ear and their treatment ; 3. On loss of hearing where the external and middle ears are healthy.

In Section XIII. (*State Medicine*), first day : 1 Measures by which to prevent the Diffusion of different Communicable Diseases from country to country, or within the limits of any single country—*e. g.*, (1) yellow fever, cholera, plague ; (2) enteric fever, scarlet fever, measles, whooping-cough, diphtheria ; (3) syphilis ; (4) glanders, hydrophobia, anthrax. Second day—2. Influence of various articles of Food (not including water) in spreading Parasitic, Zymotic, Tubercular, and other Diseases. Third day—3. Conditions to be imposed on the legally qualified practitioners of one country who may seek authority to practise in another country. 4. Precautions to be taken in medical nomenclature and classification to guard against false statistical conclusions.

These lists are only provisional, and subject to modification. The final lists will be published at an early day. Abstracts of papers to be read before the Sections will be published in May, 1881, in English, French, and German for the convenience of the members.

The Lord Mayor of London has expressed the satisfaction he shall have in doing everything in his power officially to promote the success of the International Medical Congress to be held in London next August, and his intention to tender to it an official welcome on the part of the citizens of London. It is understood to be the intention of the Lord Mayor to open the Mansion House for a State reception of the members of the Congress.

—

To Readers and Correspondents.—*The editor will be happy to receive early intelligence of local events of general medical interest, or which it is desirable to bring to the notice of the profession. Local papers containing reports or news items should be marked.*

CONTENTS OF NUMBER 458.

FEBRUARY, 1881.

CLINICS.

MONTHLY ABSTRACT.

MEDICAL NEWS.

THE

MEDICAL NEWS AND ABSTRACT.

VOL. XXXIX. No. 2.   FEBRUARY, 1881.   WHOLE No. 458.

CLINICS.

Clinical Lectures.

ON THE TREATMENT OF CLUB-FOOT. PARTICULARLY THE CONGENITAL FORM.

DELIVERED DECEMBER 18, 1880, AT THE PENNSYLVANIA HOSPITAL.

By THOMAS G. MORTON, M.D.,

SURGEON TO PENNSYLVANIA HOSPITAL, FELLOW OF THE ACADEMY OF SURGERY, ETC.

[Reported by Frank Woodbury, M.D.]

GENTLEMEN: Several cases of club-foot, which happen to be in the hospital now, afford me a good opportunity of bringing before you the subject of the treatment of this deformity; and I will therefore devote a part of my hour to the discussion of this topic, and in my remarks I will give you my reasons for expressing views which are somewhat different from those generally held.

In my experience, this deformity is met with quite as often in the female as in the male, or nearly so. Club-foot may be found at birth, or it may result in after-life from injury or paralysis of a muscle or group of muscles; thus, the affection may be congenital, or it may be acquired. Thus, of 46 cases of club-foot which came under my care this year, 21 were congenital, and 25 were acquired. It will simplify the subject under consideration if I briefly point out to you at once the varieties of club-foot and their relative frequency. There are four principal deformities known as talipes or club-foot; and as many secondary forms: thus we have Talipes Equinus, Calcaneus, Varus, and Valgus. These typical forms may be combined or associated so as to form T. Equino-Varus, Equino-Valgus, Calcaneo-Varus or -Valgus. I will illustrate these abnormal conditions upon the foot of our patient upon the table. When the heel is drawn up so that the subject walks upon the phalanges and ends of the metatarsal bones, we have the condition of *Equinus;* when the toes are elevated and the heel supports the weight of the body we have *Calcaneus.* *Varus* refers to a lateral deviation of the foot inward, the outer edge being that part upon which the patient walks; while *Valgus* denotes a contrary condition, the soles being turned outward. When the heel is drawn up and the patient also walks on the outer side of the foot, there is represented *talipes equino-varus;* or, if on the inner border, *talipes equino-valgus;* in a similar manner *Calcaneus* may be associated with both forms of lateral deflection making *talipes calcaneo-varus* and *calcaneo-valgus.*

Morbid Anatomy.—All these deformities, considered under the generic term *talipes,* depend upon the contraction of muscles or tendons, or paralysis of antagonizing muscles. · Sooner or later the bones of the foot, which are not greatly altered at birth, become much distorted and changed in their mutual relations; the astragalus often being most affected, and it may even be congenitally malformed.

Etiology.—Theories the most contradictory have been advanced in regard to the etiology of congenital club-foot. Accept which view you choose, the fact still remains that the condition is due to *an arrest of development* from some efficient cause, which invariably continues to exert its influence through life, upon the subsequent growth of the limb.

Treatment.—In the treatment of club-foot we should have in mind not only the deformity but the causes which have produced it, and for these reasons we employ manipulation, including massage, galvanism, and stretching, these alone, or combined with the section of tendons, and the application of carefully constructed mechanical appliances.

In considering the treatment of individual cases, it is well to remember that we should not use the knife if it is possible to obtain a ready cure of the deformity without it, and never in congenital club-foot until the child is able at least to walk, *i. e.,* about the end of the first year or so. Nevertheless, it must be acknowledged that we may now and then materially shorten the treatment, occasionally even in children, by the judicious division of a tendon or of the plantar fascia. Each case must be a study in itself; and the surgeon will find his best guide in the conditions attending the individual case. There are certain rules, however, in regard to congenital infantile club-foot which have been laid down by surgical authorities; these I think are so erroneous that it is to this subject that I shall especially direct your attention.

History.—Let me say a word or two in regard to the history of tenotomy. The earliest recorded case of club-foot where operation was performed, was about 1784. Delpech after this performed subcutaneous division of the tendo Achillis, but to Stromeyer of Hanover is generally awarded the credit of successfully introducing, in 1830, subcutaneous tenotomy as it is now generally performed. Since that period a number of surgeons have, from their combined influence and favourable experience, placed tenotomy among the regular operations of modern surgery.

Operation.—In performing tenotomy, we use a small, sharp, and a blunt pointed knife; the former to puncture the skin, the latter to divide the tendon; if the surgeon be a dexterous operator he can continue the operation and divide the tendon with the same instrument; but it is usual to relinquish the pointed blade, substituting the probe-end knife to complete the operation; the knife being passed under the tendon, it is divided from below upwards. Many prefer the probe-end tenotome, especially for the tendo Achillis, on account of the proximity of the posterior tibial artery and the veins. In many cases, when the division of the tendon is effected, the sound of the sudden yielding can readily be heard, and when the foot is then put into a normal position, a gap occurs, making a depression which can be seen and felt between the divided ends of the tendon: before making the section, I need hardly say that the tendon should be placed on the greatest tension. In the course of a few days the interval of separation between the divided ends becomes filled by exudative material, which subsequently becomes organized and finally becomes converted into tendon; in fact the method of union is the same as in soft tissues or bone. At the expiration of about six weeks the union has become so intimate that if the tendon be tested it would more likely yield elsewhere than at the point of union by the adventitious tissue. This early and firm repair in the divided tendon has an important bearing upon the question of the after-treatment, as to the immediate rectification of the deformed foot; thus, shall a club-foot be allowed to remain in its original position, as some advise, for some days after the operation, before an attempt is made by gradual stretching to correct the deformity? I would lay down the rule, that, in all cases without exception immediately after tenotomy, the foot should be restored as nearly as possible to its normal position. The plastic material encompassing the cut tendon bridges the space between the two ends, in the course of a few weeks any excess of new material is absorbed and carried away just as in the provisional callus of bone, and thus the tendon is left permanently lengthened as desired. This is, therefore, an important point, not to permit the deformity to continue after tenotomy, but to reduce it by manipulation and stretching, while the patient is still under the influence of the anæsthetic. The operation of tenotomy is an easy one, requiring but ordinary care and little skill, although I have known of more than one fatal result following from erysipelas, and sloughing, and hemorrhage in this apparently trifling subcutaneous operation. The after-treatment, however, requires attention and careful management to prevent a recurrence of the deformity; should the latter occur, it would have been far better if no operation had been performed, for subsequent surgical treatment is much less satisfactory than if the case had been left quite alone.

Age for Operating.—There is another very important point: How early should you divide tendons in the treatment of club-foot? The very first case you may have to treat in your practice may be one of congenital club-foot. You turn to the authorities to learn the time for operating, and you find that Holmes in his "System of Surgery" says, that, "If at the expiration of the fourth week distinct contraction of the tendons remains in spite of assiduous efforts to overcome the deformity by manipulations, frictions, and steady but gentle employment of splint and bandage, or if benefit proportionate to the attention bestowed be not realized, or if the case unequivocally belongs to the second or third degrees of varus, the aid of tenotomy will be required to effect restoration."

Gross[1] says: "When the distortion is considerable I invariably employ the knife as a preliminary measure, and this may always be done with the most perfect safety even within the first four or five weeks."

Ashhurst,[2] in speaking of tenotomy, says: "In cases of ordinary severity tenotomy should be resorted to, the best age for the operation probably being between the second and third months of life." With the views just expressed, though with sincere respect for these authors, I cannot agree, and I shall presently give you my reasons, and at the same time show you in support of my views the practical results of another kind of treatment.

In discussing the varieties of congenital club-foot we will find that seve-

---

[1] System of Surgery, 5th ed., Phil. 1872, vol. ii. p. 1047.
[2] Principles and Practice of Surgery, p. 634, 1878.

ral can be readily disposed of, after which I shall devote my remarks particularly to the deformities which require the greatest care and attention on the part of the surgeon to insure complete success.

Talipes equinus is caused by the shortening of the common tendon of the gastrocnemius and soleus muscles, the tendo Achillis. It is seldom that this deformity if marked can be cured by any other means than the division of the tendon, yet I advise you never to operate until the child can stand or walk, then you get the best result possible, for in the joint motion the tendon and muscle are constantly stretched, which is not the case if the tendon is cut during infancy when the heel surely will become elevated. The tendo Achillis is divided just above its insertion, the heel is at once brought down by force if required, and the foot is held down by the band across the instep which is attached to the usual apparatus. In many cases of acquired club-foot there is not only a weak condition of the ankle, but it is well to bear in mind that more or less atrophy of the bones and muscles exists; in congenital club-foot this atrophy also exists, so that a brace affords the necessary lateral support not only to the ankle but for the entire limb. It is all-important to have the heel in good position, and this is done by pressing the foot well down in the shoe while lacing it up, then carrying over the strap before alluded to across the instep. The instrument consists essentially in a padded and well-fitting shoe, fastened in a steel frame, which has two bars running on the inner and outer side of the leg up to the thigh (in some cases only to the knee) united by a transverse bar below the shoe, having hinges opposite the knee and ankle-joints, and bands above and below the knee. (See Fig. 1.)

Fig. 1.

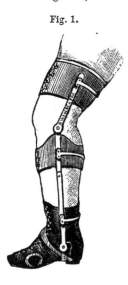

Talipes Calcaneus, a rare form of congenital club-foot, generally acquired as a result of infantile palsy, requires division of the tendons of the tibialis anticus, the common extensors, long extensor of the great toe, and the third peroneal (peroneus tertius) muscles. The apparatus required is the same as that for equinus just described.

Talipes Valgus (or splay-foot) is common as an acquired affection and occasionally requires division of the peroneus longus and brevis, and sometimes, the tibialis anticus and tendo Achillis; such cases also need the same form of apparatus as described for equinus and calcaneus to keep the foot in good position, and forcible stretching is often required before the apparatus is applied.

Talipes Varus, the most frequent and important of the club-foot deformities, is generally associated with a greater or less degree of elevation of the heel, forming that variety known as talipes equino-varus. I lay more stress upon this form because probably more than ninety per cent. of all congenital cases belong to some form of varus, and because its treatment is often most wretchedly mismanaged; of the twenty-one cases of congenital club-foot which I have already referred to, all were examples either of varus or equino-varus.

Varus and equino-varus, if examined soon after birth, will show more mobility of the tarsal articulation and foot pliability than you might be led to expect. The muscles at fault in varus are usually only the anterior and posterior tibials, and in equino-varus in addition to those named the tendo Achillis. But in most cases of varus you will find all the structures including the bones very susceptible to manipulation, so that the tarsal arch with all the other parts associated in the deformity may be pressed and stretched into a normal position. *All* cases of congenital varus and many cases of equino-varus can be cured by persistent stretching without any operation; therefore in these cases it is necessary that the treatment should commence at birth, and the nurse or attendant of the infant should be instructed how to daily manipulate the foot. I now show you an infant with double equino-varus, and, asking the mother to perform this simple operation before you as she is accustomed to do it, you observe that pressing in the prominent tarsus with the thumb, the rest of the mother's hand securely grasps the foot at the inner side, and by a steady outward movement and partial rotation the foot is at once brought into a normal shape; but it often happens, as in this case, that the equinus can only partially be overcome; this can readily be rectified by cutting the tendo Achillis when the child is ready to walk. It is sometimes well in stubborn cases of varus to keep up for some hours daily a continuous outward stretching, and this can be accomplished by the use of the shoe (see Fig. 2) which by the aid of the ratchet side motion, the foot being well secured, can be thoroughly everted; still this shoe should not be relied upon solely, for the foot of an infant confined in any apparatus necessarily brings about a want of circulation, atrophy, and often excoriations which retard, if not stop temporarily, all treatment.

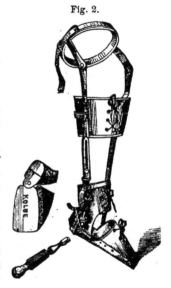

Fig. 2.

Unless we have the weight of the body upon the foot as in walking, the equinus is likely to return. Even with a shoe, if the child does not walk, it is practically impossible to keep its heel properly down; it will be drawn up, and defeat your object. But if you defer tenotomy of the tendo Achillis until the child is able to walk or until it is one or more years old, if the elevation is not too great, you will on the contrary have the best results. When you have corrected the varus and the child is ready to walk, an apparatus is required to overcome the tendency to a recurrence of the deformity; years ago I commenced using a modification of the ordinary Scarpa's shoe, which simply allows a hinge motion at the ankle but in no wise everts the foot. To give this outward ankle-motion, the apparatus is arranged as follows: Taking an ordinary leather shoe, which should lace up in front, with the lateral steel supports running up above the middle of the thigh, with transverse braces and bands, a hinge is placed opposite the external malleolus, and opposite this point on the inner steel rod a portion has been taken out and replaced by a toggle joint, or double antero-posterior hinge (Fig. 3), which enables it to yield when the child bears its weight on the inner side of the foot; the hinge on the outer side allows the foot to turn outward (Fig. 4). This I look upon as a valuable addition to the apparatus for children and one well worthy of your attention.

Fig. 3.

Fig. 4.

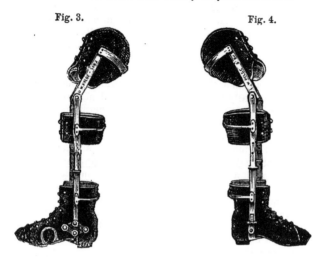

CASE I.—This boy, aged five years, which I now present to you with such admirable feet, so perfect that you would never suspect him to have been a subject of the worst form of equino-varus, was placed under my care shortly after birth with the request from the family physician that I would perform tenotomy; explaining the process of stretching and the value of such persistent efforts to his parents, and with their hearty co-operation; at the end of a year I had the pleasure of seeing the left foot entirely cured both as to the equinus as well as to the varus; in the right foot at the age of three years there was an equinus remaining, so I divided the tendo Achillis, the varus having been entirely cured. When this child was ready to walk, I told the father, Mr. W. P. Thomas, of this city, who has had considerable mechanical experience, that if he could arrange, as he first suggested, such a joint at the inner ankle as would give to the parts an outward motion as the child placed the foot on the ground, I thought it would be of even more service than the daily stretching which the child had been subjected to; he at once constructed the toggle joint which I have just shown to you; this I have been using ever since with excellent results. It has been suggested that the treatment by stretching is very slow, and that much time might be saved by tenotomy. To this I answer that unless even more care is devoted to an infant's foot after tenotomy, than in the simple stretching process, the results will be far from satisfactory, and that a club-foot neglected after operation is far less amenable to treatment than a club-foot that has never been treated at all. It is not well to keep constantly upon a child recovering from club-foot an apparatus after a good position has been obtained. I am in the practice of allowing the child to wear for an hour or two daily a pair of slippers, in order that the ankle-joint shall have all kinds of motions during the child's play; this I look upon as important: and, in regard to the use of mechanical apparatus at night, I am quite convinced that, as it is unwise to use any such apparatus for the infant, so it is unnecessary for the child;

the limb develops better, and a good stretching before the child is put in bed is far better than any apparatus which confines the limb during sleeping hours and retards the circulation and growth.

In considering the unyielding, rigid equino-varus which we often see in after years as the result of want of care after operations, and in those cases in adults where no operation has ever been performed, we find that the section of tendons and fascia, although accomplishing with apparatus considerable, is not by any means sufficient to insure a cure of many deformities, and for years past I have been in the habit of poulticing such stiff, rigid feet for a fortnight or so before operating, in order to thoroughly soften them, and it is wonderful how much is gained by this simple procedure. Then, under an anæsthetic after the division of all the tendons involved in the deformity, I apply either the "foot stretcher" (Fig. 5) which I devised some years ago, or the one gotten up at my suggestion by Kolbé, and with either of these force the unyielding bones at once into as correct a position as possible; and this operation may be repeated as often as may be necessary. The apparatus is simple: it consists of a block of wood on which there is fastened an inverted and well-padded horse-shoe, into which the heel of the foot is secured by straps passed through the slots, over the instep; a pad draws strongly upon the projecting tarsus by means of a powerful screw, another band and screw is connected with the forward part of the foot, and makes traction in the opposite direction; an immense

Fig. 5.

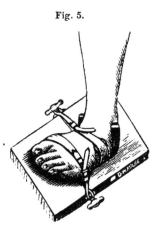

force is thus brought to bear upon the deformity; flexion and rotation of the foot is readily obtained by moving the wooden block. The apparatus is applicable to either foot. The other stretcher is a more powerful apparatus, and can be used upon either foot; a glance at it shows you its applicability (Figs. 6, 7). I have never known any injury result from this method of treatment, and I say to you that without some such apparatus, you will not be able to cope with many of the old deformities to which I have referred.

It is in most cases necessary to divide the plantar fascia; this you can readily do by a division of the tense tissue readily felt running lengthwise on the inner and under side of the foot. In illustration, I now show you several other cases bearing on my statements in regard to the plan of treatment of congenital club-foot by stretching or combined with division of the tendo Achillis.

CASE II.—This little girl, eight weeks old, was born with bad equino-varus of both feet; by continued daily stretching by the hands of the mother she has very much improved, the varus is readily rectified and the equinus is improved; when the child is ready to walk the tendo Achillis may require section; the parent is directed to continue the manipulations, and to present the child every month or so for inspection.

CASE III.—This infant three months old has, on account of a double congenital equino-varus, been subjected to stretching since birth; the positions of the feet are nearly normal, and I think that manipulation alone will be sufficient. You will notice the excellent position of the tarsus, and my ability to get rid of the equinus with a moderate force.

Fig. 6.   Fig. 7.

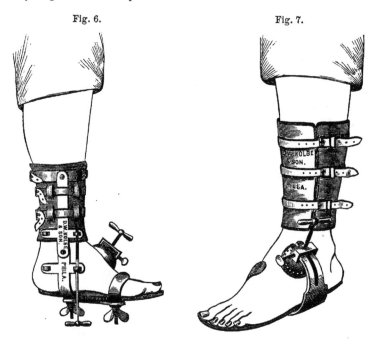

CASE IV.—This boy, now seven years of age, was born with double equi-no-varus, and is a brother of the child last presented to you. He now has perfect feet, and all this has been accomplished without tenotomy, by the lad's mother, and from her success with the boy she is thoroughly satisfied that her efforts with her infant will be successful. He now has no need for any brace, which indeed he has not worn for more than a year.

I need not now adduce any other cases in support of my practice, but may say to you that I have brought a large number of similar instances before the Philadelphia Academy of Surgery during the present year to show the importance of the treatment by stretching.

CASES V. and VI.—Of the two cases I have for operation this morn-ing, the first is this lad Eugene D., aged six years, who was born with equino-varus; when nineteen months old the varus was cured by manipu-lation, but he subsequently required division of the tendo Achillis for an equinus. He has an excellent foot, with a tendency to varus, which a shoe will not rectify because the plantar fascia is the cause of the inversion. This must be divided, which I now do, the patient being etherized. He shall now wear this shoe (Fig. 8). At its outer edge, an elastic band is attached which is connected to the apparatus below the knee. This draws the foot upward with each step, and tends to evert it at the same time. I have spoken to you of neglected club-foot, and here you have an example. This girl, of seventeen years of age, has congenital equino-varus; she was admitted into the hospital, Dec. 13th, with an exceed-ingly rigid foot. She has walked so long on the outer side of the foot that the tissues from the constant pressure are very dense. The heel is also drawn up. Now such a case would yield but slight results from a tenotomy operation alone.   The foot has been enveloped in a flaxseed poultice day and night for the past week, and the good effect of this course is here shown.   The skin and subcutaneous tissues are now very pliable.   In order to relieve the equinus, I place the foot on the stretch and divide the tendo Achillis and the separation between the ends of tendon is at least an inch, and I divide the plantar fasciæ, overcome the varus, and, with force, rupture the unyielding tarsal tissues, and at once rectify the malposition.

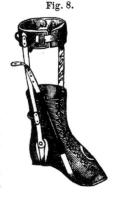

Fig. 8.

I frequently, especially in adult cases, where much force has to be used, apply for the first week or so a right angle posterior felt (Fig. 9), pasteboard or tin splint; if the latter, there should be a good opening for the heel; the splint should be carefully padded so as to avoid excoriations; after a time the regular walking shoe is substituted.

From the remarks I have made to you this morning, it will be evident that my object has been to discourage tenotomy in infantile life; that talipes equinus, calcaneus, and valgus can be readily and successfully overcome and seldom give rise to difficulties in their treatment; that all cases of congenital varus can be cured without operation if attended to early, and that the equinus, which is so often associated with varus, not infrequently requires division of the tendo Achillis, but that this operation should *never* be done until the child is ready to or has commenced to walk, for at this time you have to aid you in the cure, the constant flexion and extension of the foot, which must necessarily occur with every step.   Then the use of the toggle joint, as I have described to you, will overcome the disposition to a recurring varus, which has to be guarded against for a long time.   Then again, I have urged the importance of not confining children's feet too long during the day in any apparatus, for club-foot is essentially due to an arrest of development, and our efforts should be to encourage the growth of the limb, by the means already referred to, and that excellent results are observed in a freer ankle motion if the child be allowed to play for an hour or so each day without any apparatus.

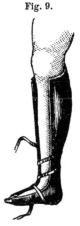

Fig. 9.

I have thus briefly given you my experience in the treatment of club-foot, and I am quite sure that if you will give the subject your careful consideration, you will abandon the use of tenotomy, at least in the very early treatment of this deformity, and trust rather to the various methods which I have endeavoured to impress upon you.

LECTURE INTRODUCTORY TO THE STUDY OF THE ARTHRITIC DIATHESIS.

Delivered at the London Hospital.

By JONATHAN HUTCHINSON, F.R.C.S.,
Senior Surgeon to the London Hospital.

IT is my purpose, Gentlemen, to bring under your notice the peculiar and very important group of diseases to which our forefathers applied the term arthritic. You are well aware that although this term, used according to strict etymology, means any inflammatory affection of a joint, yet that, conventionally, it has been restricted to certain morbid conditions in which a remarkable tendency is shown for many joints to suffer, and to suffer repeatedly. An arthritic person is one who over and over again suffers from inflammation, more or less transitory, of his joints, and who is so liable to it that he knows what are the influences which are likely to produce an attack. It is thus quite clear that a tendency to arthritis in this sense is a constitutional one. Other diseases of joints may be local, but true specialized arthritis, although often excited by local causes, always has in the background a constitutional peculiarity as its source. To this constitutional peculiarity we give the name of diathesis; and when we say of any one that he is the subject of the arthritic diathesis, we mean that he is in that bodily condition—of that organization—which renders him liable at some time, and under suitable provocations, to become the subject of active arthritic manifestations. It by no means follows that an arthritic man is always, or even often, suffering from arthritic maladies, any more than that the witty man is always brilliant; it is sufficient in each case that the basis qualification, the potentiality, be there. In each it is quite possible that the possessor of such qualification may go through life, and transmit to his successors his possession, without having ever himself exhibited it in an unmistakable form. Now, although liability to joint inflammation is the feature which gives its name to the arthritic diathesis, I must warn you against the notion that it is the only phase by which that diathesis manifests itself. It would be strange, indeed, if such were the case, and if it were possible that a constitutional state could exist which should give proclivity to inflammation of the joints, and should exempt wholly the other tissues. Although the joints suffer chiefly, and present the most prominent symptoms by which we recognize the diathesis, yet they take simply the first rank, and by no means an exclusive one. There is no structure in the body that may not be attacked. We have, possibly, arthritic dyspepsia, arthritic renal disease, arthritic pneumonia and bronchitis, arthritic affections of the skin; it is certain that we have many arthritic affections of the fascia, muscles, nerves, and eye. Hence, in part, arises the great importance of the subject to which I invite your attention.

Here we may suitably pause to assert that arthritic inflammations, whether strictly arthritic in the sense of attacking joints or otherwise, have a peculiarity of type. This peculiarity is such that by it alone their true nature may often be guessed in cases where other points of evidence are defective. They are, as a rule, remarkable for suddenness of onset, rapidity of development, and certainty of decline. If, however, there is a strong tendency to spontaneous decline, there is also one equally strong to future recurrence. There is about them all a here-this-week,-gone-the-next,-certain-to-come-again-some-time quality, which is most characteristic. As a rule, they are all, when at height, attended by very severe pain, and relatively to the intensity of the inflammation there is but little tendency to disorganize. Above all, in strong contrast with other inflammations, they show no tendency to cause suppuration. Lymph effusions there may be, and adhesions may result, slow alterations in the forms of bones and in the texture of ligament and cartilage may take place, but these are unusually trivial in proportion to the apparent intensity of the inflammation. It is a matter of astonishment to every one who watches these cases how surprisingly good reparation is when the attack passes off. In many cases it is not perfect, but in almost all it surpasses the expectations formed even by well-skilled spectators. I leave aside for the present certain forms of what are called arthritis, in which the malady appears to persist, and to produce, by slow, uninterrupted processes, great ultimate disorganization. These are very exceptional as to number, and far less so as to character, than they have been supposed, and they by no means invalidate the general statement that arthritic maladies are, as a rule, paroxysmal in character and remarkable for the excellence of the recovery which follows. If you hear of a man having had repeated and violent attacks of pneumonia, from each of which he has recovered perfectly; if of another that he is laid up every spring with severe iritis, yet every summer appears to see nearly as well as before; if of a third that he is frequently the subject of joint inflammations, whilst yet he never becomes disabled, you may in each case make a safe guess that the malady in question was of the arthritic type. The knowledge of this tendency to spontaneous recovery is of the utmost use to us in prognosis.

I have been hitherto speaking of the arthritic diathesis as if its existence were acknowledged by all nosologists, and it is time that I should admit that this is in the present day by no means the case. The term is a decidedly old-fashioned one, and if I venture to ask you to employ it, the duty devolves upon me of defending it and of showing that it is one based upon clinical fact. In the present day we are taught to speak of gout and rheumatism as essentially different maladies, yet both come into the old category of arthritis. Respecting rheumatic gout and the various forms recognized under the name of chronic rheumatism, although there is much difference of opinion and many contradictory statements extant, yet I believe I am right in stating that the balance of authority is in favour of the belief that they stand distinct, both from gout on the one hand, and acute rheumatism on the other.

Let me here attempt a brief glance at the kind of facts with which in the following lectures we shall have to deal, and at the terms by which they may most appropriately be designated. Let me also beg of each one of you to be most careful in defining his terms, for there will be no hope of our getting to the bottom of a complex question like the present one unless we are studious, on the one hand, to get clear and vivid conceptions of facts, and on the other, to use words in reference to them which we all employ in the same sense.

The time-honoured name of "gout" is one which is well understood, and of which the equivalent has been used from the days of the Romans, with singularly little difference of opinion as to the cases to which it is applicable. If the case be well characterized every one can recognize gout, for its symptoms are most definite, and almost every one, lay as well as medical, knows what they are. All that we have said as to the peculiarities of arthritic maladies finds a most definite realization in the case of gout. It is paroxysmal with a vengeance, and in it suddenness of onset and of decline, persistency of liability, and comparative freedom from local disorganization, find emphatic illustration. To these general characters we may add that gout usually attacks the smaller joints first, giving, indeed, primal preference to that of the great toe, that its acme is marked by . great swelling of the parts external to the joint, by a glossy skin, which pits on pressure, and which desquamates when the attack is past, by the most intense pain, and by great disturbance of health, more especially of the nervous system. Modern pathological research has given increased prominence to another symptom long well known. I allude to the secretion of chalk, or of a substance which looks like chalk. This salt, the white lithate of soda, is formed so constantly in gout that its presence or absence may, I think, be taken as the line of demarcation between true gout and rheumatic gout. Unfortunately, it is only in the latter stages of the malady that the presence of this salt can be proved during the lifetime of the individual. In advanced cases of gout we may find concretions about the affected joints or in various other parts, more especially in the cartilages of the ears. The researches of Dr. Garrod would tend to show that the examination of the blood during the paroxysm, and the detection of lithic acid in excess in that fluid, is always a pathognomonic and reliable symptom. It is unfortunately, however, one difficult of application, and in a majority of cases not available. The valuable researches referred to, supported as they are by a multitude of pathological data previously and since recorded, have, however, enabled us to place this symptom in the foremost rank in reference to the diagnosis. I believe I am giving you a definition which all will accept when I say that we count as gouty all manifestations which occur in connection with a state of health in which lithic acid is present in excess in the blood, and in which there is a tendency to the deposit of its salts in the tissues. You will note that we by no means require absolute proof of the presence of lithate of soda at any given time, or in any given case. If you have succeeded in making yourself and others believe that certain symptoms are essentially connected with a state of health which usually has for its result the excessive production and depositing of this salt, then you have succeeded in convincing yourself that those symptoms are in essential nature gouty. Perhaps not in one case in twenty in which we diagnose gout do we prove lithate of soda, but we ground our opinion upon the close resemblance of the symptoms to those in other cases in which lithates were demonstrably present. And mark again, I by no means join with those who regard the presence of lithate of soda as the true beginning of gout, or even as an essential phenomenon. It is only one of many concomitant results of a special state of the system—special as regards inherited organization, as regards digestion, assimilation, and excretion— but it is one so definite and so frequently present that it may be very suitably selected as the characteristic on which to base a conventional name. I have already implied, and shall assert more explicitly soon, that I regard the attempt to separate rheumatic gout from true gout by an abrupt line as a violence to sound pathological doctrine. It is very desirable, further, that you should not narrow your conceptions of the meaning of this important word. It is incorrect to say of any man " he has got the gout," in the same sense that we should say " he has got syphilis," " he has caught the measles." There does not exist any such abstraction as " the gout," or perhaps I ought to say there is no such entity. A man may *become gouty*—that is, his assimilation may have been slowly changed, and all his tissues modified in character, so that they may be liable to inflammations of the gouty type—but he cannot receive into his system *de novo* the malady " gout," for the simple reason that no such entity exists. I repeat that a clear conception on this point is essential, for unless you have it you will never make due allowance for the modifications which the gouty diathesis is so prone to undergo. It is precisely because it has been built up as the slow result of numerous complicated and prolonged influences that no two cases are precisely alike, that although the well-marked examples of it are very peculiar and utterly beyond all dispute, there are others, the recognition of which will task to the utmost the skill and insight of the physician. Nothing is easier in the cases I refer to than for equally well-informed and candid observers to become involved in an interminable war of words. Recollect, then, that our definition of gout is a conventional one, and that it applies to the better-marked states of system which are susceptible of the most multifarious complications and of endless modifications in degree. Thus it is quite fair, quite consistent with probable truth, to say of any given case, This is not gout, but it is closely allied to it—a phrase which, in the instance of a syphilitic malady, would be simply nonsense.

Having thus attempted to define the class of maladies which we may properly call gouty, we will now turn to the subject of chronic rheumatism or rheumatic gout. This malady, like true gout, has long been recognized, and many have been the debates as to what name it ought to receive. It presents even greater varieties as to form and severity than gout itself, and hence many discrepancies in authors respecting it. We will again endeavour to take pathological results as the basis of our definition. The results of rheumatic gout to the joints affected are very peculiar. There is no deposit of lithates, but there is a change in all the textures of which the joint is composed. The synovial membrane thickens, and its fringes become developed, from which pedunculated or loose cartilages at length result. The ligaments soften and stretch, and the cartilage becomes fibrous and splits up or wears away. But whilst these changes are going on in the soft parts, yet more characteristic and permanent ones are happening in the ends of the bones themselves. These, in mild cases, have rows of little nodosities developed on the line of junction between periosteum and cartilage, whilst in more severe ones these nodosities become confluent, and constitute projecting lips, often of very considerable size. In the worst cases all the ends of the bones alter remarkably in form, and become expanded to twice their original size. In some cases there is great expansion, with but little evidence of wearing away; in others the bone eburnates instead of expanding, and retains its form, but becomes polished and fluted by friction. In aggravated cases great crippling and great deformity is the result, and hence one of the names by which this disease is known on the Continent—*arthritis déformans.* But here let me raise protest that it is not every case of rheumatic gout which is deforming—not the majority, rather a small minority, and those chiefly in patients who are elderly. Rheumatic gout is a very common malady, far more common than true gout, and if, before we pronounce on its existence, we wait for the manifestation of visible deformity, we shall miss the diagnosis of all the milder cases. I have often taken occasion in this theatre to warn you against the too common mistake of selecting for study and for record only the most exaggerated and intense forms of a malady. Endless are the misconceptions which have resulted from this error, and few subjects have suffered more from it than the one under consideration. If every subject of the gouty diathesis would be kind enough to carry about specks of chalk in his ears, the recognition of gout would be easy enough; and in like manner we could easily tell rheumatic gout if all its subjects had their limbs crippled and deformed. But it is not so, and in each instance we are, in a majority of cases, thrown upon our ingenuity for the discovery of other and less obvious guides to the knowledge of our patient's real state.

Of the peculiarities presented by joints which have suffered from rheumatic gout, two stand out before all others in their value as means of diagnosis—I allude to the dry grating caused by the removal of cartilage, and the development of lips. We may venture to assign the chief place to the second of these, for it is the one which is earliest to be found. Grating is never present excepting at an advanced stage, and although very characteristic then, its value becomes, of course, much limited by that fact. Nodosities and lips, on the contrary, are amongst the very earliest of the products of this malady, and are often, indeed, present before the patient is aware that he has had any inflammation in the joint concerned. Nor have we, so far as I know, any reason to think that they occur to any characteristic extent in association with any other causes.[1] On the contrary, I believe that their diagnostic value is as great in rheumatic gout as is that of chalk concretions in true gout. Our differential definition of rheumatic gout may then, I think, be based on these peculiarities, and we may say that any form of joint disease which tends to the production of lip-like outgrowths at the margins of the cartilages has a claim to be placed in this category. I have already hinted that there are many varieties, some of them probably of considerable clinical importance, which are grouped under this head, and that in a certain large group, occurring in patients under middle age, whilst removal of cartilage is common, outgrowths of bone are rare, and if present usually small.

For the last few years I have been in the habit of using these outgrowths for the purpose of diagnosis in a somewhat novel way. I had often been struck by the remarkable prominence of these rheumatic lips on the condyles of the femur in museum specimens, and it occurred to me that they ought to be perceptible during life. I examined the knees of a few patients who had the disease in an advanced stage, and found that I could detect them very easily. Afterwards, with some practice, I found that I could appreciate their presence even in comparatively early stages, and also that they are frequently present when the patient has no external deformity whatever. By degrees, and after the examination and comparison of a great number of patients, I have come to rely with much confidence on this symptom. If you wish to employ it successfully, you must first practise carefully on healthy joints. In many, if not in most, there is a ridge at the part referred to, more or less resembling the pathological lip. The distinction between health and disease can only be acquired by practice. In examining a knee, I prefer to place myself in front of my patient, and to employ both hands at once. I place the finger-tips of one hand flatly over the edges of the one condyle, and those of the other on the opposite, and then direct him to bend and extend the joint slowly several times in succession. In this way you may find the edges and appreciate their elevation without risk of error. I much prefer to use the fingers flatly at first, and not to employ their tips, as I think there is less risk of error in estimating elevation; but afterwards I use the tips in order to determine whether the lip overhangs. In well-marked cases it curls outwards.

These condyloid crests, as I have already observed, are not to be expected in all cases. As a general rule they are present only in those who have passed middle life. You must not expect to find them in the young. In the latter, absorption of cartilage without osseous outgrowth is the rule. In the aged, however, these crests are invaluable as symptoms. I have very often recognized them in cases in which the patients were not aware that the knees had ever suffered. I have often been able by their aid to say which knee had suffered most frequently, and have found the patient's statement confirm my inference. The symptom is of especial use in those cases in which we are consulted, not on account of joint affections, but for iritis, or lumbago, or a skin disease which we suspect to be of arthritic origin.

I have hitherto said little or nothing as to clinical peculiarities of rheumatic gout, beyond a hint that they are by no means the same in all cases. I intend in a subsequent lecture to consider them in detail, but for my present purpose I

---

[1] I have just seen a case somewhat exceptional to this statement. A young woman under the care of my colleague, Mr. McCarthy, had her limb amputated on account of a myeloid tumour in the tibia. She had never been rheumatic, but there were present small lips on the edges of the condyles. No doubt the joint-changes had been induced by the proximity of the tumour.

must here give a short sketch in order to contrast them with those of gout. In many cases rheumatic gout begins insidiously, the patient being simply liable to attacks of aching in one or more joints. It affects large and small joints almost indiscriminately. It is remarkably prone to produce synovial effusion. Almost all cases of so-called hydrops articuli belong to it. Unlike gout, and unlike acute rheumatism, it but rarely causes redness of the skin, and the shiny surface and œdematous pitting are scarcely ever present. Its paroxysms are often prolonged or of indefinite duration, but in some cases, contrary to the general belief, I must assert that they are as short and definite as those of gout itself. In other cases —and these are those more nearly allied to rheumatism than to gout—the first attack sets in severely and affects many joints. In these, instead of getting well at the end of a month or five weeks, as acute rheumatism is in duty bound to do, the disease lapses into a chronic form, and the patient may perhaps become an invalid for the remainder of his life. Still, even in these persistent cases there are generally observed remissions and paroxysmal recurrences. The pain which attends rheumatic arthritis never rises to that extreme severity which character- izes gout, but it is often bad enough.

Rheumatic gout presents great difficulties as to diagnosis in two different direc- tions: there are cases which the physician can scarcely tell from acute rheumatism ; there are others, and very different ones, which it is almost impossible to distin- guish from true gout. My own belief is that in each of these instances the difficulties are insuperable, for the simple reason that the maladies in question do really merge into each other. and that the features characteristic of each exist in union.

On the third great subdivision of the arthritic family I shall not now speak. It is that of rheumatic fever or acute rheumatism.

Here then, gentlemen, to recapitulate, we have glanced at the three large sub- divisions of the arthritic family ; we have seen that gout is peculiar in having deposits of lithate of soda, rheumatic gout in having in the young ulceration of cartilage, and in the old absorption of cartilage with outgrowths of bone, and acute rheumatism in having synovitis without permanent articular changes, and in being very prone to damage the heart. Our next question is, Are these three maladies really related or not. and if so, to what do they owe their individual peculiarities ? Let me insist that it is a question of relationship merely, not of identity. No one denies that there are most important differences between the three—differences which it is wise and convenient to recognize by distinctive names. Still, however, the question of relationship remains a most important one. I may here conveniently admit to you, as, indeed, I have perhaps already done, that all three depend upon the same diathesis or constitutional state, and that their differences are due to the varying conditions as regards age, sex, tem- perament, habits of diet, exposure to climate, etc., to which the possessors of this diathesis are exposed. You will easily, I think, see that it is of great prae- tical importance to answer this question correctly. If relationship be admitted, there is little doubt that our opinions as to the treatment of each will receive some modification. It is not, however, as regards the principles of treatment that most is to be anticipated, for the differences between the three when in actual existence are quite sufficient, however they may have been acquired, to make it probable that great differences in treatment will be necessary. As regards pre- vention, as regards the general management of health in those in whom the diathesis is as yet latent, or in those who are known to be descended from arthritic subjects, much more may be expected. Very probably we may find that the same general measures which prevent the one will also ward off attacks of the other. There are also other important and common maladies respecting which our notions will be much cleared if we can decide whether there does or does not really exist an arthritic diathesis which is the common parent of gout, rheumatism, and their allies. I allude to such maladies as brow-ague, lumbago, sciatica, recurrent iritis, gonorrhœal rheumatism, and certain skin diseases. In trying to ascertain whether any one of these is really dependent upon an arthritic diathesis, we are at once met with the difficulty—What constitutes proof of that diathesis? If one patient with recurrent iritis tells me that his mother was crippled with "rheumatic gout," but never had "gout," and another that his grandfather was a martyr to "chalk-stone gout," how am I to interpret the facts? Am I to say that the two histories, referring to totally distinct maladies, help me not at all to an explanation of iritis, or am I entitled to assume that in both the facts imply the existence in the family of the arthritic tendency? Such questions meet us every day in practice, and the advice which we give our patients is based upon the opinions respecting them which we chance to hold. I need say no more to enforce upon you the importance of the investigation which I propose to commence.

We must next ask, How shall such a question be set at rest? On what data can we determine the relationship or non-relationship of any given maladies? On this point I must confess I have not been able to find much information in the works which I have consulted. Although the question has been much debated and with great ability, yet I cannot help thinking that it has never been stated with sufficient precision. The proofs of relationship between any two given diseases must be of the same character as those by which we should prove alliance of any species in animals, and first among them stands, Are they the offspring of a common parentage? First cousins or even brothers may be of very different aspect; but prove their descent, and you prove their relationship. In respect to gout and rheumatic gout, it appears to me that physicians have been far too much concerned with the examination of differences, and have almost forgotton to ask, Are they not producible by the same causes and influenced by the same circumstances? I fully admit that the investigation of the cause of these maladies is surrounded with difficulties, but nevertheless much has been, and much more may yet be, effected, not only by the critical investigation of individual patients, but by ascertaining whether any given races, or any given climates or occupations, are particularly prone to produce them. If, for example, it be found that gout and rheumatic gout prevail in excess always in company, —that the same race, the same climate, the same sex, and similar ranks in society, are liable to both,—the inference as to identity of cause would become strong. Then, again, we have data of great value derivable from the history of hereditary transmission. If I succeed in making it probable that gout and rheumatic gout prevail in the same families, and that of the children of a gouty father some suffer from rheumatism and others from true gout, I feel sure that your inference from the fact will be that it is probable that the diathesis is the same, and that it derives its peculiarities in each instance from some other special conditions in each sufferer—sex, temperament, etc.

Thirdly, we have the test of hybridism. Is it possible to mix up gout and rheumatic gout together, or rheumatic gout and true rheumatism, so that the characteristic features of the two shall be blended? Of course it is very possible for two quite distinct maladies to prevail by mere chance in the same person at the same time; but if we find that this admixture is common—that it is, in fact, the rule rather than the exception—then, I think, most will agree that such easy blending is strongly in favour of prior relationship.

MONTHLY ABSTRACT.

Anatomy and Physiology.

A Spinal Root of the Optic Nerve.

STILLING, of Strasburg, showed preparations to the International Ophthalmological Congress at Milan, in September last, which he believes demonstrate the existence of a spinal root of the optic nerve, which brings the retina into direct connection with the medulla. This root passes from the external corpus genieulatum, in a winding course, deep between the bundles of the crus cerebri, and can be traced into the pons; and it appears to course down in the direction of the medulla, although its further progress cannot be demonstrated. The existence of this branch is interesting on account of the light it throws on certain physiological relations between the medulla and the retinæ, and may constitute the hitherto undiscovered link between certain diseases of the spinal cord and of the optic nerve.—*Lancet*, Nov. 27, 1880.

The Effect of Exertion on Temperature.

Dr BONNAL, of Nice, has been experimenting on the effect of muscular exercise on·the temperature of the body. The observations were made on four individuals, the temperature being taken in the axilla, popliteal space, groin, foot, hand, mouth, and rectum. The investigation has been prosecuted during four years, and the conclusions reached are the following: All muscular exercise, even if of short duration, raises the temperature of the rectum, rarely, however, to a point exceeding 101° F.; but the rise occurs invariably, at whatever hour the exercise is taken, whether before or after rest, and independently of age, sex, and meteorological conditions. The effect bears no relation in degree to the duration of the exercise, or to the apparent fatigue. The influence of the same exertion, under identical conditions, varies in different individuals, and in the same individual at different times. The physical altitude, the state of the atmosphere, and the amount of clothes, exercise, as might be anticipated, a marked influence on the degree, and especially on the rapidity, of the rectal rise in temperature. On the other hand, however, the absence or abundance of perspiration has no appreciable influence on the variations in temperature during movement. Rest, after a given exercise, always determines a fall in the rectal temperature, more considerable and more rapid the shorter the exercise. All exertion which causes a great acceleration of the pulse and respiration lowers the peripheral temperature (mouth, axilla, groin), but the fall is immediately recovered from on rest, the rectal and peripheral temperatures becoming equalized, or resuming their normal difference —about two-thirds of a degree Fahrenheit. The greatest elevation by exercise which was met with amounted to 103.2° F., in the case of a celebrated runner, aged thirty-one years, who had just run eleven miles in an hour and a half without stopping, and without any other effect than an elevation of the pulse to 145. If the rectal temperature is below 98.6°, a moderate exertion, such as a gentle walk of a mile on level ground, raises the temperature up to the normal, even though the necessary rise amounts to 1½° F. But if the temperature is already above 98.6°, the same exercise will not raise the temperature more than .4° or .8° F. In a rapid ascent the greatest elevation of temperature almost always occurs during the first half hour; if the ascent is continued, the temperature may remain stationary, may be raised .2°, or may fall .2° or .3°. Some other observations which corroborate the fact that gymnastic exercises cause a rise of temperature are not of special interest. The account of the investigations has been communicated to the French Académie des Sciences.—*Lancet*, Dec. 4, 1880.

Materia Medica and Therapeutics.

Anæsthesia by Application of Chloroform to the Skin.

Dr. BROWN-SÉQUARD, who has recently brought before the Society of Biology an extremely interesting series of observations (see MEDICAL NEWS AND ABSTRACT, Jan. 1880, page 17), indicating the somniferous and anæsthetic influence of chloroform, when applied to the skin of guinea-pigs, showed, at the sitting of November 20th, that the effects are not produced through the blood, but through the nervous system; since, after division of the spinal cord, the effects were found to be absent when the chloroform was applied behind the seat of the medullary lesion, but to be present when it was applied in front of the lesion.—*British Med. Journal*, Dec. 18, 1880.

Eucalyptus Oil as an Antiseptic.

Dr. BASSINI contributes to the *Annali Universali di Medicina e Chirurgia*, September 1880, an exhaustive article on eucalyptus oil as an antiseptic. He was induced to experiment on this substance by some suggestions made in the *Centralblatt für Chirurgie*, 24th January 1880, in which it was proposed to supersede the use of carbolic acid by the above disinfectant. Eucalyptus oil is an ethereal preparation, citron colored, possessed of a penetrating odor, and mixing easily with alcohol or paraffin. The most practical method of using it, however, was found to consist in mixing the oil with a small quantity of carbonate of magnesia, after which it could be made to readily dissolve in water in the proportion of about 1 per cent. The author's experiments extended over six cases of intentional wounds in animals, and six surgical operations in the human subject, comprising removal of a breast, opening of a chronic abscess in the neck, hydrocele (two), removal of a fibro-lipoma, and a large incised wound of the leg. The observations were not continued further, the result obtained having been considered very unsatisfactory. The author thus sums up his conclusions. 1. Eucalyptic dressing (10 parts of eucalyptus oil as above prepared to 100 parts of wax or paraffin spread on gauze) causes intense annoyance to the greater number of patients by its disagreeable and penetrating odor. 2. Infiltration takes place much more readily with this dressing in the lips of the wound and surrounding tissues, and consequently there is a greater tendency to suppuration. 3. In certain cases, on removing the dressings, an odour of putrefaction was perceived, which showed that the antiseptic qualities of the substance could not be great. 4. The frequency with which eczema appeared on the parts covered by the dressing leads the author to suppose that this substance must have some specific action on the skin.—*London Medical Record*, Dec. 15th, 1880.

Tripolith—a Substitute for Plaster of Paris.

Prof. VON LANGENBECK introduced a new material for fixative dressings at a recent meeting (November 7th) of the Berlin Medical Society. Tripolith, so called on account of its hardness and power of resistance, was discovered by Mr.

B. von Schenke, of Heidelberg, in the course of last summer; and was exhibited, and obtained a premium, at the Exhibitions in Brussels and Mannheim. It was originally intended for stucco and decorative purposes, for which, on account of its greater lightness after drying, and its power of withstanding damp, it is said to be better adapted than plaster of Paris. Its mode of fabrication is not known, but its chief constituents are calcium and silicium, with a minute portion of iron oxide. Tripolith forms a gray powder, which to the touch is finer and softer than plaster of Paris, although of the same weight in the rough condition. An unfortunate accident in Berlin first led to its introduction into surgical practice. The local agent of Messrs. von Schenke broke his arm, and Professor Krönlein, who treated him, applied a plaster-of-Paris dressing. In due course, the dressing had to be changed, and the patient then remarked that he knew of something which would prove better than the plaster of Paris, and accordingly a tripolith dressing was applied. It answered so well, that since this time it has constantly been used at the Royal Clinical Hospital and also in private practice. Tripolith bandages are prepared and applied exactly in the same manner as their plaster prototypes. After the limb has been wrapped in a flannel bandage, gauze bandages filled with the powder are soaked in water and applied in the usual manner. A little thin solution of tripolith is then rubbed in. The charged bandages must not remain too long in water, nor must the mixture be made too thin, nor stirred too much. The advantages of tripolith over plaster of Paris are the following: 1. Tripolith appears to absorb moisture from the atmosphere less freely than plaster, and its power of setting is not lost even after long exposure to the atmosphere. The first lot received from Heidelberg was forwarded in a common sack, in which plaster of Paris would infallibly have been ruined. 2. Tripolith bandages are lighter, and therefore pleasanter to the patient. Thus an equal volume of liquid plaster of Paris, fresh, weighed 604 grammes; of liquid tripolith, 568 grammes. When dried the plaster weighed 470 grammes, the tripolith 413 grammes. Thus tripolith is about 14 per cent. lighter than plaster of Paris. 3. Tripolith dressings harden more quickly than plaster. While a bandage made with the best plaster requires ten to fifteen minutes before it is quite set—and in wet weather often remains soft for hours—tripolith sets completely in three to five minutes. On the other hand, it gives off vapour for many hours, and even after twenty-four feels moist to the touch. 4. Once hard and dry, tripolith absorbs no more water. A piece of dried tripolith dressing undergoes no change when laid in water. It would be possible, therefore, to allow a patient to bathe in his tripolith dressing, provided means be taken to prevent the water getting up inside it, by means of an India-rubber covering; while as regards plaster it is necessary to paint it with dammar varnish in order to make it waterproof. 5. Tripolith is a trifle cheaper than plaster of Paris.—*Med. Times and Gazette*, Nov. 27, 1880.

—

Vesical Irritation from Blisters.

At the Paris Société de Médecine Pratique (*L' Union Med.*, Nov. 23, 1880), M. JULLIARD observed that it had been recommended, in order to prevent the action of cantharidine on the bladder, to mix some bicarbonate of soda with the emplastrum lyttæ, but that this was difficult to do in Paris, where the blisters are spread on plaster; but the same end is obtained by adding some liquor potassæ of the British Pharmacopœia. He also recommends, on the application of a blister, that some alkalized mineral water should be drunk. M. Aubrun believed that the irritation is produced by allowing the blister to remain on too long. He thinks that the addition of camphor is useless. He is in the habit, when he applies a blister, to have the skin first well rubbed. The blister will then take at the end of five or six hours as well as it would otherwise have done in twelve hours; and when he has acted in this way he has never met with vesical irritation.—*Med. Times and Gaz.*, Dec. 11, 1880.

Pilocarpine in Skin Diseases.

Prof. PICK, of Prague, communicates to the *Vierteljahrschrift für Dermatologie und Syphilis*, I. 1880, an interesting paper on this subject. Various salts of pilocarpine were employed, especially the muriate, about ⅓ grain being administered by the mouth or subcutaneously. When protracted sweating was desired, the remedy was taken twice a day, the patient being confined to bed. In other cases confinement in bed was not insisted on; and when warm weather exercise out of doors was permitted; the best time for giving it seemed to be one or two hours after the morning and evening meal. When the remedy had been continued three or four weeks, the effect became less marked, and the dose had either to be increased or the medicine intermitted for some days, when the same dose was again quite efficacious. An important difference in the order of appearance of the physiological effects was seen in some instances. Of 30 individuals, in 21 the internal administration caused first increased flow of saliva and afterwards sweating, while subcutaneous injection induced sweating first, then salivation. In the remaining 9 both methods caused salivation first. Continued use of pilocarpine exerted an important influence on the oiliness of the hair and on its growth. The skin became softer, more pliant and satiny; comedos and papules of lichen pilaris could be more easily pressed out or got rid of, the scurfiness of the scalp became less or disappeared, the hair was less brittle, the new growth of lanugo hairs changed more rapidly into dense, properly pigmented ones. Under employment of the drug for months the general condition of the patient was not impaired; indeed, the appetite improved, and he was better nourished. In prurigo (of Hebra) pilocarpine alone had little effect, but this was otherwise when its use was combined with that of woollen clothing, so as to induce free sweating, which was at first manifest only in the sound parts, after a time also in the portions of the body affected with prurigo. Clinical experience agreed with that of the patients themselves when they declared that when, after a few days' use, a material amelioration of their condition declared itself, the itching also continually grew less, in the end entirely to disappear. The other symptoms also underwent improvement, such as the glandular enlargements, the dry and thickened condition of the skin. The average period required to attain this result was sixty-five days. The effect was more rapid when the employment of pilocarpine was combined with that of other remedies found useful in prurigo, as tar, Vleminx solution, glycerine of starch, etc. As to the curative influence of pilocarpine, the disease recurred at longer intervals after its use than after the employment of other measures, and the outbreaks were less severe when they did occur. While not absolutely curative, therefore, it is possible to attain by its use a more favourable result than when purely local treatment is made use of. Whether, if long continued, the disease would be finally worn out remains unsettled. Pilocarpine exerted no influence on psoriasis, though observations were made in 25 cases. In eczema it produced a deleterious influence when employed during the moist stage or too soon after its cessation. It caused a return of the weeping, and even a spread of the eczema to new parts. In chronic cases, however, where there was little more than scaling, itching, and infiltration remaining, the use of pilocarpine caused these to disappear more rapidly than they would have otherwise done. Subcutaneous injections of pilocarpine cured two cases of pruritus senilis, causing disappearance or lessening of the itching for some hours, thus rendering sleep possible and imparting both physical and mental strength. A case of chronic urticaria which had resisted other remedies yielded to pilocarpine. From what has been said as to its effect on the condition of the skin and growth of the hair, as might be expected, it seemed to hasten recovery from the baldness of alopecia areata, while in ten cases of alopecia pityrodes (seborrhœa) the results were even more favourable.—*Edinburgh Med. Journal*, Nov. 1880.

Medicine.

Case of Combined Measles and Scarlatina.

Dr. DE GIOVANNI records (*Gazetta Medica Italiana*, October 9th) an interesting case of measles and scarlatina occurring synchronously. The patient was a girl aged 10 years, and the symptoms of measles were, on the whole, the predominant ones during the course of the attack. On the third day after measles had been diagnosed, a bright red rash diffused itself over the abdomen and legs, presenting all the appearances of scarlatina. A curious feature in the case was that the upper part of the body was throughout covered with a distinct morbillous rash, while in the lower the rash was that of scarlatina; at the confines of the two eruptions, they were more or less merged in each other. On the eighth day there was paralysis of the bladder, and the urine was for several days albuminous. The patient became convalescent about the twelfth day. The author remarks that the presence of the one exanthem did not in any way appear to affect the course which the other would have pursued had it occurred alone.—*London Medical Record*, Dec. 15th, 1880.

Ear and Eye Disease on Relapsing Fevers.

In a recent epidemic of relapsing fever at Königsberg Dr. LUCHHAU has investigated the frequency of ear and eye complications. Since no less than three hundred cases were treated in the town hospital, the field for observation was unusually favourable. Only one hundred and eighty cases were specially examined as to the existence of ear complications, and these were found in fifteen only, and in all the middle ear was the part affected. In most cases there was suppuration, and the pus was evacuated through the tympanic membrane. In most cases of disease of the middle ear in acute maladies the inflammation appears to arise by extension from the throat; but it was found that, in relapsing fever, pharyngeal catarrh is absent, as a rule, in the cases in which the middle ear suffers, and there was no evidence of disease of the Eustachian tubes. The prognosis is not unfavourable if prompt treatment is adopted.

Only six cases presented eye symptoms out of the hundred and eighty examined ($3\frac{1}{2}$ per cent.) In three there was iritis, which was unilateral in every case. All these cases did well. In one case, however, some weeks later the patient complained of failure of sight, and opacities were discovered in the vitreous. In two other cases optic neuritis occurred. In one the affection was discovered in the first relapse. The second relapse was severe, and some time afterwards there was atrophy of the optic nerves, and vision was reduced to $\frac{1}{15}$. In the other case the neuritis also occurred during the second febrile attack; a few days after it had ceased the swelling of the optic papilla was discovered, dirty-red in colour, with arteries narrowed, and veins distended and somewhat tortuous. Vision was reduced to $\frac{1}{3}$ in one eye and $\frac{1}{4}$ in the other. Another patient came into the hospital during the first relapse with iritis and hypopion. The ocular trouble healed completely, but after the relapse the patient insisted on leaving the hospital, and passed though the second relapse at home, under-very unfavourable conditions. When it was over he returned to the hospital with double iridocyclitis. Numerous thick flakes were seen in the vitreous, the fundus was very indistinct, but the papillæ were seen to be red and swollen, and there were numerous retinal hemorrhages. The account of these cases is published in the October number of Virchow's *Archiv.—Lancet*, Dec. 11, 1880.

Nerve Stretching in Locomotor Ataxy.

Hitherto, little success has attended the employment of the various therapeutic measures designed to arrest the progress or relieve the symptoms of locomotor ataxy. Of all its symptoms, the most urgent in their demand for relief are the darting pains which characterize its early stages, and frequently accompany its entire evolution.

Encouraged by the success which has followed the operation of nerve-stretching for neuralgias of various origins, Langenbeck, more than a year ago, stretched both sciatic nerves, and afterwards both crurals, with the result not only of obtaining complete disappearance of the pains, but also cessation of the motor incoordination. A second case was reported by Esmarch, who stretched the nerves in the axilla for pains in the forearm ; and, in this case, too, the motor incoördination disappeared completely. A third case has been published by Erlenmeyer, in which stretching both sciatic nerves failed to influence beneficially either motion or sensation.

A fourth case was shown recently to his class by M. CHARCOT, at the Salpêtrière, an account of which is published in *Le Progrès Médical* (No. 50). The patient was under the care of M. DEBOVE. He was in an advanced stage of the disease, having been bedridden for eighteen months. The pains were very severe, preventing sleep, situated in the upper as well as the lower extremities ; and had required constant injections of morphia, in large doses. The motor incoördination was limited to the lower extremities ; the patient could not stand at all. The patellar reflex was absent on both sides ; there was extreme myosis, without visual defect, in both eyes. Cutaneous sensibility was deadened ; there were no anæsthetic patches. There was loss of the sense of the position of his lower limbs. The left sciatic nerve was selected for operation, on account of the pains being more severe on the left side. It was exposed in the middle third of the posterior aspect of the thigh, and violently and suddenly elongated. The wound was dressed antiseptically. The operation was performed without chloroform, as experiment has shown that pinching a nerve violently causes momentary arrest of the circulation and respiration ; and it was feared that this arrest might be dangerous to a patient under chloroform. However, the patient did not suffer much pain, owing to the extent to which he was saturated with morphia. The results were very remarkable. The darting pains had ceased completely, and the motor incoördination had nearly disappeared ; but the tendon reflexes and the myosis remained unaltered. The patient could touch M. Charcot's hand with either foot when held a couple of feet above his bed ; and, when assisted, could stand upright, and even walk a few paces.

M. Charcot remarked that we do not know how this operation effects this result ; but this matters little. The point of importance is, that nerve-stretching appears likely to be an operation of much service to the unfortunate sufferers from ataxy.—*British Med. Journal*, Dec. 25, 1880.

Spinal Paralysis in the Newly-Born.

In the *Archiv für Gynäkologie*, Bd. xvi. s. 87, LITZMANN makes a contribution to our knowledge of this subject. He appends his observations to an account of a case observed by him in Kiel. The presentation was breech. The pelvis was not particularly small, the diagonal conjugate measuring $4\frac{3}{16}$ inches, leading to an assumed conjugate of $3\frac{1}{2}$, the type being justo-minor. The extraction of the body required to be hurried on account of absence of pain and arrest of the circulation in the cord while the body of the child was passing through the pelvis. The child, on being delivered, was deeply asphyxiated. The delivery required no great amount of force to be exerted upon the spine. The asphyxiated child was quickly brought round, and cried loudly. It cried a great deal in the course of the forenoon, and was very restless. Inspirations were irregular and crampy. In the afternoon both legs were completely paralyzed, sensation and reflex sensibility were arrested; the belly muscles were also more loose than usual, and the belly distended. Other symptoms of paralysis were detected. The child shortly improved somewhat, however; but in spite of care and prolonged application of electricity, direct and indirect, there remained considerable permanent paralysis. After a review of the literature of the subject, in which special attention is directed to the work of Little, the author maintains that during severe deliveries which are accompanied with deep asphyxiation of the child, extravasations frequently take place into the meninges of the brain and into the brain tissue, as also into the membranes of the cord, during the delivery, which present themselves in the early years of life as paralyses more or less severe in character. He insists upon greater attention to cases of the kind, and considers that those extravasations may take place quite independently of any force used at delivery.— *Edinburgh Med. Journal*, November, 1880.

———

Some Points in the Clinical History of Effusion into the Pleural Cavity.

At a late meeting of the Medical Society of London (*Lancet*, Dec. 11, 1880), Dr. BROADBENT read an interesting paper on this subject, of which the following is an abstract. He first enumerated and explained the relative importance of the physical signs of pleural effusion, and pointed out that the curved line of dulness was due to the manner in which the lung shrinks around its root, and as the fluid rises the vocal resonance and vibration become exaggerated over that part of the chest-wall where the lung is still in contact. When the cavity is full of fluid the respiratory murmur may be conducted for a short distance across the back from the unaffected lung. Sometimes, however, the lung was prevented from collapsing by adhesions, by consolidation, or congestion: and he believed the persistence of bronchial breathing in such cases was due to imperfect collapse of lung, although the fluid was in large amount.

The chief point he wished to urge was that while the ordinary signs of effusion into the pleural cavity—dulness, extinction of vocal fremitus, diminution of vocal resonance, and limitation of bronchial breathing to the region of the root of the lung—show that the lung retreats and shrinks before the fluid, loud tubular breath sounds at the base of the lung posteriorly and over the lateral and anterior aspect of the chest show that the lung has not entirely retreated, but that it retains a certain volume, and is more or less deeply immersed in the fluid. The patency of the bronchi and the partial condensation of the lung favour the transmission of sonorous vibrations. It is in these circumstances that ægophony is heard most distinctly and widely—from the thin layer of fluid intercepting some vibrations and transmitting others—conditions which ordinarily exist only in the earlier stages of effusion. In some of these cases there may occur some degree of vocal vibration at a period when the amount of fluid is sufficient to give dulness on percussion over the entire lung. Paracentesis would be of comparatively little value in such conditions, for the quantity of fluid is small, and the consolidation of the lung would persist after its removal; and most cases of this sort get well without resort to paracentesis. In one such case only thirty ounces of fluid could be withdrawn. The conditions are met with in the pleural effusion of renal disease, often accompanied by congestion, and partial consolidation of the lung preventing its collapse; also, in effusions which rapidly become purulent, as in empyema in children. Apart from these cases, the signs indicative of a large congested lung deeply immersed in the fluid are prognostic of rapid absorption, and Dr. Broadbent had seen this now in a sufficient number of instances to enable him to predict with considerable confidence the recovery of the patient without paracentesis and in a comparatively short time. One of the first steps towards recovery is a rather sudden disappearance of the tubular breathing and the substitution of the more ordinary signs of simple effusion; and it is probable that the congested lung has relieved itself by diffusion of serum into the pleural cavity, and that the amount of fluid there is actually increased.

In conclusion, Dr. Broadbent stated the rules which guide him in recommending paracentesis. It should be resorted to at once when there is serious continued or paroxysmal dyspnœa; but in the absence of urgent symptoms a week or ten days may be given after one side of the chest is full, on the chance that absorption may set in, and a longer period still, when the lung has not greatly shrunk. Old age, phthisis, or a phthisical tendency, are reasons for early tapping, as also is the existence of disease of the kidneys. The spot for puncture is the eighth space, in a line with the angle of the scapula, and he had come to prefer the common trocar and canula, with antiseptic precautions, to the aspirator. The whole of the fluid should never be removed, or attempted to be. Where the effusion has lasted some time, frequent partial emptyings are to be preferred.

Dr. C. T. WILLIAMS referred to a case of pleural effusion with presence of marked bronchial breathing and vocal vibration, and alluded to the valuable aid in diagnosis rendered by the use of a hypodermic syringe.

Dr. DE HAVILAND HALL mentioned a case of sarcomatous growth filling the pleural sac and collapse of lung, yet with presence of vocal fremitus. In one case he had withdrawn 107 ounces of fluid, and he asked the author as to the amount he would recommend to be withdrawn.

Dr. HABERSHON spoke of the various forms of pleural effusion—e. g., in renal and in cardiac disease, secondary to pneumonia or due to primary pleuritis. He recalled a case of Dr. Addison's where a small area of bronchial breathing existed, surrounded by complete dulness and absent breath-sounds. The autopsy revealed a portion of lung adherent to the chest-wall at that spot. He pointed out that many cases recover if left alone. If there were high temperature, hectic fever, and tendency to tubercular disease, and if dyspnœa were present, he would advise paracentesis, especially if empyema were suspected.

Dr. HARE said the physical signs were often misleading, especially in children; the presence of vocal fremitus and respiratory murmur on the affected side was only to be accounted for by conduction from the healthy side, through the compressed lung and fluid.

Dr. WHARRY asked how far vocal fremitus and tubular breathing were indications of the existence of uncollapsed lung in the fluid. He had seen at least one such case where these signs were absent. What were the author's reasons for assuming that exudation took place from the lung into the pleura in certain cases?

Dr. GILBART SMITH agreed with Dr. Hare as to the difficulty of diagnosis in children. He instanced a case where the lung was wholly collapsed, notwithstanding presence of fremitus and tubular breathings, and asked whether a purulent effusion did not conduct vibrations better than a serous one. He also asked whether the disappearance of these signs would not be better explained by an increase in the effusion and pressure on the lung than by an exudation from the lung itself.

Dr. BROADBENT, in reply, said he had not seen cases of vocal vibration and bronchial breathing with collapsed lung, nor could he explain such. The persistence of vesicular breathing implied the existence of a non-collapsed lung. He did not consider that increase of pressure explained the disappearance of bronchial breathing, for almost invariably improvement quickly followed—ushered in by returning apical resonance. He had not practised injections into the chest in serous effusions, but had frequently and with benefit employed solutions of iodine in cases of empyema. He now preferred to use the simple trocar inserted near the angle of the scapula; this allowed of the withdrawal of the right amount of fluid, while the entrance of air did no harm. If the aspirator were used it was his practice to stop as soon as the patient became distressed or attacked with cough. Eighty-four ounces was the largest amount he had ever drawn off.

———

Sudden Death in Pleuritic Affections.

Dr. LEICHTENSTERN (*Deutsches Archiv für Klin. Medicin.*, Band iv. 4 Heft) discusses a number of cases recorded in medical literature of pleuritic patients, in whom severe syncope and sudden death have occurred, with the view of explaining the causes; and he arrives at the following conclusions. Sudden death or severe attacks of syncope in cases of pleuritic effusion have sometimes their origin in embola of the pulmonary arteries. In other cases, no pulmonary embola exist, but voluminous and far-extending thrombi in the right auricle and ventricle, and in the superior vena cava. The generally prevailing view that left-sided effusion has a greater effect in disturbing the circulation than effusion on the right side, is incorrect. On the contrary, extensive exudation on the right side causes greater disturbance of the circulation by pressure on the large vessels, and on the right auricle and ventricle than does considerable effusion on the left side. And the opinion that cases of sudden death and severe syncope are more frequent in left than in right exudations, is contradicted by statistics. Of fifty-two cases, in thirty-one the exudation was on the right side, and in twenty-one on the left. Cases of sudden death, apoplectic attacks in pleuritic effusion, sometimes arise from embolism of an artery of the brain, or its consequences. In a great number of sudden deaths with pleuritic exudation, we are not yet in a position to explain the cause. The fatty degeneration of the muscles of the heart, the anæmia of the brain, and the œdema of the lung do not suffice for an explanation. To anæmia of the brain as a cause, those cases only can be assigned in which the raising of the sick person from the horizontal position has been followed by severe syncope ending in death. Various causes which sometimes quite interrupt or impede the flow of blood to the left heart, such as a severe paroxysm of coughing, vomiting, lifting heavy burdens, may give rise to a suddenly fatal anæmia of the left heart, and secondarily of the brain. The anæmia of the lungs or brain found in many cases is only of secondary importance. It frequently happens after thoracentesis with aspiration that an anæmia is induced in the partially distended lung; and this may lead to death by asphyxia. In sudden death, during or immediately or a short time after thoracentesis by aspiration, the cause is anæmia either of the heart or of the brain.

In cases in which severe syncope and sudden death are observed during the irrigation of the pleural cavity, the cause is either direct mechanical concussion of the easily exhausted heart by the stream of water thrown in, or shock. The washing out of large empyemic cavities with strong solutions of carbolic acid may cause severe collapse, and perhaps death, due to the rapid absorption of large quantities of the acid.—*London Medical Record*, Dec. 15, 1880.

Retarded Signs in Pneumonia.

Dr. Tyson (of Folkestone), at a recent meeting of the Clinical Society of London (*Lancet*, Dec. 18, 1880), read notes of cases of acute pneumonia, in which the usual physical signs of the disease appeared late in the case.—Case 1. A man, aged sixty-four, caught cold whilst driving on April 4, 1880, and next day was compelled to give up work. He was seen for the first time on the 8th, when he complained of pain in the chest, and expectorated some tenacious mucus. There were no abnormal physical signs. Temperature 103; pulse 88; respiration 30; urine albuminous. On the 11th slight dulness appeared at the base of the left lung; fever was high. On the 12th (eight days after the chill) there was well-marked dulness, bronchial breathing, and bronchophony. He was very feeble, and died on the 15th.—Case 2. A female, aged twenty-five, in Guy's Hospital under the care of Dr. Pye-Smith, taken ill three days before admission, when the temperature was 104°. Signs of pneumonic consolidation appeared on the sixth day, and death took place on the seventh. There was gray hepatization of the right upper lobe. — Case 3. A male aged fifty, in whom no dulness was discovered till the sixth day. Death occurred on the tenth day. In two other cases Mr. Tyson had marked the absence of physical signs until the fifth day. He referred to the statement made by Dr. Bowles, that in asthmatical subjects attacked with pneumonia dulness often did not develop till four or five days after the seizure. After quoting passages from Ziemssen's Cyclopædia and Trousseau's lectures to show that such a late development of physical signs was not generally acknowledged, he concluded by stating that this retardation of signs occurred more frequently than was generally supposed, and might be attributed to the central parts of the lung being primarily affected. In such cases the onset of the attack, the pyrexia, and the altered pulse-respiration ratio should be relied on as diagnostic points.

Dr. F. Taylor confirmed the author's statement as to the relative frequency with which the physical signs appeared late in the disease, and quoted a case which came to the out-patient department with a history pointing to pneumonia. The physical signs were not apparent, although it was about the fourth day; but the patient coughed up some rusty sputa and was admitted. Soon afterwards physical signs became developed. In another case the delayed signs appeared before the rusty expectoration.

Dr. Andrew Clark said the paper was an important contribution to the literature of the subject, for anomalous and capricious cases of pneumonia were imperfectly recorded; but he did not think it added much to the knowledge of experienced men. He was constantly meeting with cases in which the constitutional evidence of pneumonia long preceded the appearance of local signs. He would mention three such cases. One was a case of a gentleman he saw in consulation with Dr. Stephen. After a slight rigor the temperature rose to 101°, and for seven days there was no evidence of the disease, except the general distress, rapid breathing, and altered pulse-respiration ratio. The physical signs of pneumonia appeared on the eighth day. Another case was that of a gentleman, aged eighty, at Southsea, seen with Mr. Potts and Sir W. Gull. After a chill there was a period of ten days marked by irregular pyrexia, malaise, and hurried breathing. On the eleventh and twelfth day slight friction was heard below the angle of the right scapula, followed by dulness and tubular breathing. The patient recovered. A third case was one he saw with Dr. Buzzard, when the patient had been ill for six days with pyrexia without the local signs. He did not think it necessary to have all the physical signs present to diagnose pneumonia ; and that in cases of central pneumonia the disease was too far removed from the surface to yield these signs. With a history of chill, with distress and prostration, with fever, and a disturbed relation between pulse and respiration, one may be absolutely certain that the case is one of pneumonia.

Dr. HABERSHON concurred that in some cases the general symptoms, with hurried breathing and rusty expectoration, without physical signs, must be taken as sufficient for diagnosis. No doubt such anomalies were explained by the disease being deep-seated, so that the physical signs are obscured, just as a severe pleurisy may involve the surface of the diaphragm without any friction being audible. When the physical signs do become manifest, the pneumonia has probably extended to the periphery.

Dr. ANDREW CLARK added that pneumonia might be diagnosed from the general conditions; because in a large number of cases there is neither cough, nor expectoration, nor pain in the side.

Dr. DE H. HALL, some five or six years ago, had recorded two cases of apical pneumonia marked by severe head symptoms. One was a man, aged nineteen, who was comatose for six hours ; the other a child, who had repeated convulsions ; and it was only on the fifth or sixth day that distinct tubular breathing appeared. One reason for the severity of these cases, as compared with those which ran a more typical course, might be found in the greater amount of lung involved in central than in peripheral pneumonia.

Dr. BURNEY YEO said that such cases suggested the question whether the lung condition was not secondary to a constitutional disorder.

Dr. GOODHART observed that the question was a complicated one, so many conditions occurring under which the physical signs varied. In old people the late appearance of these signs was attributable to the presence of emphysema. At the same time he agreed with Dr. Yeo that blood-poisoning might be the primary condition to which the pneumonia was secondary. Some years ago he examined the body of an old man, who died three or four days after taking a chill. There was only a slight amount of pneumonia, and the only interpretation he could put on the case was that the chill, arresting the function of the skin, had caused blood-poisoning, and that sufficient time had not elapsed for true pneumonia to be fully developed.

Mr. TYSON replied, that all his cases ultimately developed the signs of ordinary pneumonia. The last case he had seen was in a child, five years of age, with high temperature for six days, without pneumonic symptoms. He had written the paper because all the authorities he had consulted did not mention the proportion of cases in which this delay in the development of physical rigors occurs ; although many state that they have seen such cases.

The Production of Phthisis by Inhalation.

In 1877 Dr. TAPPEINER[1] published an important series of observations on the production of tubercular disease in the dog by the inhalation of the sputa of persons suffering from phthisis. He has lately extended his investigation by an

---

[1] See Monthly Abstract, 1878, p. 252, and 1879, p. 15.

attempt to ascertain whether the inhalation of material from scrofulous glands is capable of producing the same effect, and the results have been published in Virchow's *Archiv*. If scrofulous diseases are indeed identical with tubercular processes, as it is fashionable now to assert, the effect of inhalation of gland-pus ought to be the same as that of phthisical pus. The material for the experiments was pus from a scrofulous boy, five years of age, with suppurating glands. Half a gramme of pus was obtained daily, mixed with 100 grammes of water, and the dogs were made to inhale the atomized mixture for a quarter of an hour during about ten days. For purposes of comparison, two dogs were similarly treated with phthisical sputa. These two, and one of the dogs treated with the gland-pus, were killed and examined twenty-three days later. The organs of the latter were found to be perfectly normal, although the animal had presented a cough and loss of weight. In the two dogs treated with phthisical sputa, tubercular nodules were found in both lungs and spleen; their nature, from the microscopical characters, was beyond doubt. The two other dogs treated with gland-pus were killed and examined thirty-three days after the commencement of the inhalation, and the organs were also found free from tubercle. The same negative result was obtained in the case of two dogs killed on the twenty-ninth day after the inhalation of gland-pus.

Further investigations were made as to the period of incubation from the commencement of the inhalation of phthisical sputa until the tubercles are distinct in the lungs. One dog was killed on the thirteenth day after the commencement of the inhalation; it had coughed for eight days, and had lost three-quarters of a pound in weight; no tubercle was found in the organs. In another dog, killed on the nineteenth day, also, no tubercle was found. It thus appears that the period of incubation is more than nineteen days. Another dog, treated at the same time and in the same way with phthisical sputa, was killed three months after the commencement of the inhalation, and abundant tubercles were found in the lungs and pleuræ.

By the suggestion of Professor Waldenburg, two other dogs were treated with sputa from simple chronic bronchitis, fifteen grammes daily for ten days; and they were killed on the twenty-eighth day after the commencement of the inhalation. The post-mortem examination showed both lungs to be perfectly normal, without a trace of tubercle. The experiments were made at Berlin, and the pathological results ascertained by Grawitz, Israel, and Friedlander, under the supervision of Virchow, so that the facts appear to be beyond question.

The conclusions drawn by Tappeiner from these experiments are: (1) The inhalation of phthisical sputa by dogs, even in small quantities, produces with certainty tuberculosis of the lungs, with or without general tuberculosis, especially of the spleen. (2) The stage of incubation is, in dogs, longer than nineteen days, but shorter than twenty-three days. (3) The inhalation of scrofulous caseous pus from glands produces no infection—a fact which indicates an essential difference between scrofulosis and tuberculosis. (4) The inhalation of the sputa from chronic bronchitis is equally ineffective.

The facts ascertained in these experiments are certainly of a very important nature. The period of incubation, however, can hardly be fixed from so small a number of experiments, since it may not improbably be subject to considerable variation. But these observations constitute experimental confirmation of the infection of phthisis, to which many clinical facts point, and they indicate the probable mode by which the infection is produced. The difference in the effect of scrofulous pus and phthisical sputa, if not entirely conclusive as to the difference between tubercular and scrofulous affections, indicates that we must still pause before we abandon the older view. That view rests, we must remember, on clinical facts, which were so well described long ago by Sir William Jenner; and these facts must be explained away if we are to accept, as Dr. Hilton Fagge would have the members of the Pathological Society accept, the results of inoculation experiments as conclusive evidence of the identity of the two conditions.—*Lancet*, Nov. 27, 1880.

—

Case of Gonorrhœal Endocarditis.

Dr. CIANCIOSI records a case of this rare complication in *Bulletino delle Scienze Mediche*, September, 1880. The patient, whose family history was good, contracted a gonorrhœa, which was checked almost immediately by strong astringent injection. The disappearance of the discharge was, however, quickly followed by an undefined feeling of malaise, which became aggravated, and finally accompanied by intense cephalalgia and pyrexia. Auscultation showed at this period a systolic murmur most distinctly heard at the apex. Respiration, 28 ; temperature, 39° centigrade (102.2° Fahr.). The diagnosis of endocarditis was arrived at, of which no other explanation seemed possible than that it was dependent on the suppression of the gonorrhœal discharge. This shortly afterwards became re-established, and the patient eventually recovered. The author, in explaining the etiology of the attack, exhausts various hypotheses, but eventually adopts that suggested by Klebs in certain cases of rheumatism, viz., an actual emigration of micro-organisms. In this case such organisms found their way into the blood, whence they may have been deposited on the valves of the heart, or in its stroma, with the result of exciting interstitial inflammation, accompanied by the usual train of symptoms.—*London Medical Record*, Dec. 15th, 1880.

—

Two Cases of Intestinal Occlusion Treated and Cured by Electricity.

BOUDET de Paris (*Progrès Médical*, August, 1880) gives two cases of intestinal obstruction successfully treated by electricity. In the first, the patient, aged 15, had just recovered from an attack of peritonitis, when she was suddenly seized with all the symptoms of obstruction, due probably to the entanglement of a loop among the freshly formed adhesions. The usual means having failed to give relief, the faradic current persistently applied externally was tried, but without any result. The patient was in a very critical condition, bringing up everything that was given her by the stomach. During the next forty hours the continuous current was applied about every three hours for half to one hour at a time ; the negative pole was in the rectum, and with the positive the abdominal walls were dabbed so as to produce interruptions. During these applications the intestines were noticed to be the seat of lively muscular contractions, and eventually desire of going to stool was experienced. At last an evacuation was obtained, and from this moment convalescence was established. In the second case, the author had to do with fecal accumulation due to habitual constipation from deficiency of muscular power. Electricity, in the shape of internal galvanization as above, and abdominal faradization, was resorted to as a last resource. The result was most gratifying. From the first, intestinal contractions were obtained, and on repetition large quantities of excreta were expelled   The author remarks that he has collected fourteen other cases where electricity has proved useful in obstruction. He shows that the superiority of the galvanic current, where paralysis of the intestine exists, is due to the fact that it stimulates much more powerfully the unstriated muscular fibres. The interruptions must be slow, because the contractions of these fibres are not sudden but gradual. Care must be taken not to electrolyze the rectum by using a moderate current. The author used from 8 to 14 Leclanché's.—*London Med. Record*, Oct. 15, 1880.

Double Cystic Kidney with Renal Calculi.

Dr. L. A. AMAN and AXEL KEY relate the following case (*Hygeia*, 1879: and *Nordiskt Medicin. Arkiv*, Band xii.). The patient, a man aged 37, had first voided a renal calculus in 1871, and another in the autumn of 1872. Since that time his health had been good; but sometimes he had a feeling of weight in the loins and discharged a little gravel. On July 1, 1879, he took cold, and soon noticed that the daily quantity of urine diminished until the 8th, when there was suppression. He was admitted on July 9th, into the hospital at Linkoping: his bladder was then empty. In the course of the next night, he voided about seven ounces of urine with his stools. He complained only of soreness in the region of the right kidney. The urine could not be examined until the 15th, when it was found to contain much albumen. On that day, symptoms of uræmia set in, and he died on the 16th. At the necropsy the mucous membranes were found to be œdematous, and the brain hyperæmic. The kidneys were sent to Dr. Axel Key for examination. They were both greatly enlarged, the left, however, more than the right; and both presented almost complete cystic change. The renal parenchyma remaining in the interspaces between the cysts had a yellow-gray turbid appearance. The pelvis of the right kidney was much dilated, and contained a large nodulated calculus, the lower part of which was rounded, and covered in the orifice of the ureter, which was dilated. The left ureter, at a distance of about two inches from the kidney, was completely blocked up by a calculus of moderate size; below this, the canal was completely strictured by indurated connective tissue, scarcely allowing the passage of a fine sound. Above the stone, the ureter was dilated, and the pelvis and calyces especially were greatly expanded. Dr. Key thinks it remarkable to find such extensive changes in the kidneys of a person who had enjoyed relatively good health up to a fortnight before his death. He regards the cystic change as having been principally congenital, and as having no connection with the formation of the renal calculi and the consequent obstruction to the flow of urine. The renal parenchyma which was found between the cysts had been sufficient for the function of the kidneys. When the renal concretions began to be formed, hydronephrosis was gradually developed, and in connection with it a chronic nephritis with interstitial and parenchymatous changes, which went on for a time without producing any marked disturbance, until at last an acute exacerbation set in and rapidly caused death.—*Brit. Med. Journ.* Oct. 30, 1880.

Sciatica caused by Aneurism of the Abdominal Aorta.

In this case, reported by GAREL (*L'Union Médicale*, p. 951), the pains of sciatic neuralgia absorbed the attention both of patient and medical men so entirely, as to leave absolutely unnoted symptoms of aneurism until the day when the patient succumbed rapidly after its rupture. This fact teaches that, in the presence of obstinate sciatic neuralgia, the course of the abdominal aorta should always be minutely explored. Lebert, in a work published in 1865, asserts that pain in the kidneys is often one of the first signs of aneurisms of the abdominal aorta. [See particulars of a similar case shown by Dreyfus to the *Société Anatomique de Paris*, in 1876; other cases cited by Samuel Archer, in the *Dublin Medical Journal*, 1878; and Lediard, in the *British Medical Journal*, 1878.] M. Garel's case also presented an important symptom, a diastolic souffle at the base of the heart, which was not due to insufficiency of the aorta, since the other rational symptoms of this affection were absent. It remains an ascertained fact that aneurism of the abdominal aorta may give rise to the production of souffles in the region of the heart—diastolic or systolic souffles in no way connected with a lesion of the aortic orifice. Moutard-Martin's cases (*Société Anatomique*, 1845), those of Lepine and Falzer (*Société Anatomique*, 1877), and of Archer (*loc. cit.*) show that these souffles are due to the propagation of sounds produced at the level of the tumour.—*Lond. Med. Record*, Oct. 15, 1880.

Surgery.

Carbolic Acid in Facial Erysipelas.

Dr. ROTHE observes (*Betz. Memorabilien*, 1880, No. 9), that, however efficacious the subcutaneous injection of carbolic acid proves in arresting the course of erysipelas, it is not suitable when the face is the part attacked, for not only does it give rise to considerable pain, but induces a swollen and painful condition of the periphery. For some years past he has been in the habit of using the following application: Acid. carbolic., sp. vini., āā one part; ol. terebinth. two parts; tinct. iod. one part; glycerin. five parts: pencilling the inflamed skin and its vicinity with it every two hours. No pain or sense of burning is produced, and the skin is usually next day pale and wrinkled. The further progress of the disease is more effectually arrested than by any other remedy, any new patches being rapidly effaced, so that in three or four days the facial erysipelas is usually at an end. The pencilled places should be covered by a very thin layer of wadding. When febrile action is present the ordinary internal measures must also be resorted to.—*Med. Times and Gazette*, Dec. 4, 1880.

Peritomy.

At a late meeting of the Ophthalmological Society of the United Kingdom (*Lancet*, Dec. 18, 1880), Mr. CRITCHETT read a paper on Peritomy, and gave the following reasons for introducing the subject to the notice of the meeting: First, that during a long career many cases of vascular opacity with granular lids had come before him in which the disease had remained for many years unrelieved, although the patients had been under treatment for considerable periods at various institutions; and secondly, because the operation of peritomy had fallen into unmerited neglect, and was seldom practised. He then proceeded to give a brief sketch of the leading symptoms of the disease, and alluded to the type of patient in whom it most frequently occurs, he having found that it is most prevalent in young adults who had been ill-nourished and neglected; and that it is frequently propagated by direct transmission, so that constitutional defects and local causes contribute in varying degrees to its development. It often exists in a more or less aggravated degree for many years; and the treatment is, as a rule, directed to removing the granular condition of the lids. This may be partially effected by the application of caustic and astringent lotions, but such treatment is rather palliative than curative, and not unfrequently during its progress the case will relapse and the symptoms become even more intensified.

Mr. Critchett recommended—although it might seem contrary to the pathology of the disease—that curative treatment should in the first place be directed to the vascular web, which in these cases covers the upper third or upper half of the cornea, since he believed that the exciting cause of the relapses lay rather in this morbid condition, and that the granular state of the lids was kept in activity by the existence of the above-mentioned vascular membrane. He, therefore, in every case initiates his treatment by performing the operation of peritomy, since he finds that when sufficient time has been allowed (usually from four to six months) for the resulting cicatrix to become dense, white, and atrophied, thus cutting off the vascular supply to the partial pannus, the web gradually disappears, the cornea becomes transparent, and the granulations either take their departure or become much more amenable to ordinary treatment. He was anxious to dwell upon this last point, because for a certain period after the performance of the operation no benefit, but rather the contrary, would usually be observed, and it is only on the completion of the last atrophic stage of the cicatrix that the curative influence is established. He earnestly commended the operation to the attention of his colleagues. Three cases were shown illustrating the effects of treatment at different stages. Mr. Critchett said that he extended the peritomy beyond the pannus—i. e., right round the eye.

Mr. HIGGENS has performed peritomy in many cases without result, and had therefore abandoned it. Possibly he had not observed the case long enough afterwards, and after Mr. Critchett's advocacy he would again perform the operation.

Mr. STREATFEILD asked whether any treatment was adopted for the granular lids ?

Mr. CRITCHETT said all the cases had granular lids, but he began by the peritomy, and in a large number of cases the granular condition subsides when the vascularity of the pannus is cured. In other cases the granular lids require additional treatment.

Mr. JAMES ADAMS had long been in the habit of performing peritomy, and was satisfied with the benefit resulting from it. He thought the cases should be selected. He had found that the pannus was not always dependent on granular lids, but the cornea was vascular from the first.

—

Case of Hemiglossitis.

An example of this affection (which, like all similar cases on record, occupies the left side) has been recently treated in the Lariboisière. An œdematous swelling occupied the anterior two-thirds of the left side of the tongue, and a deep-seated lump was sensible to palpation. All the neighbouring parts of the mouth and the teeth were in good condition, there being only present a little redness in the pharynx and a painful swelling of the submaxillary glands. The functional disturbances consisted in difficulty of speech, nasal intonation, fetid breath, and abundant salivation. It is remarkable that there was no pain in the part, the face or the neck. The exact localization of the disease became more and more obvious in its progress, and while the side affected was divested of its epithelium and appeared of an intense red, the right side retained its natural aspect, its whitish colour contrasting strongly with the other half of the tongue. Under the use of emollient gargles and the chlorate of potash internally, the disease was cured in eight or ten days.—Med. Times and Gaz., Dec. 11, 1880, from Gaz. des Hôpitaux, Nov. 27, 1880.

—

Anæsthesia of the Larynx by a New Method.

Dr. ROSSBACH (Wiener Med. Presse, No. 40, 1880), being dissatisfied with the ordinary method of producing local laryngeal anæsthesia by the administration of bromide of sodium, on account of the greater difficulty in operating when the patient is listless and drowsy under the influence of that drug, has of late followed another method, which he finds perfectly practicable and more convenient.

His object is to influence the sensory portion of the laryngeal nerves, so as to interrupt conduction through them for a time, and thus induce complete anæsthesia of the larynx. The sensory portion of the superior laryngeal nerve is most easily reached at the point at which it passes through the thyro-hyoid membrane into the interior of the larynx, immediately below the extremity of the greater horn of the hyoid bone; here it is so superficial that a subcutaneous injection of about $\frac{1}{14}$ grain of morphia on each side, at the spot indicated, will produce full local anæsthesia. A simpler method of obtaining the same result is to direct the ether spray from a Richardson's apparatus on the above described points, which can be done on both sides simutaneously, with a double pointed nozzle; in one to two minutes complete anæsthesia is established.—*Glasgow Med. Journal*, Dec. 1880.

Thyrotomy in a Child aged Eighteen Months.

The subject of intra-laryngeal new growths is one of sufficient interest, on account of the intrinsic difficulties of diagnosis as well as treatment, to make all contributions concerning it both welcome and instructive. Dr. NAVRATIL, of Pesth, contributes an interesting paper to the *Berliner Klinische Wochenschrift*, No. 42. After some preliminary remarks concerning some former communications on the same subject, he relates the following case : A male child, who appeared from the history to have been hoarse from its birth, when eight months old got whooping-cough ; after the cough had subsided, the hoarseness became more marked. A peculiarity in the voice, and a noisy, laboured respiration, had been noticed, and in the course of the last two months, especially at night, the child had suffered from occasional attacks of dyspnœa. Treatment, which had been of an " anti-catarrhal" kind, had proved quite unavailing. In consequence of this failure, but especially because an extensive ulceration had broken out on the scars of the previously healed vaccination places, a possible syphilitic origin for the dyspnœa was taken into consideration, and anti-syphilitic remedies were accordingly ordered. They proved, however, quite unavailing. Meanwhile, the dyspnœic attacks increased in severity to such an extent that the parents sanctioned a more radical method of treatment. At this time the child was exceedingly emaciated; it presented no signs of syphilis, but it was cyanosed and its breathing was hard and laboured. Tracheotomy was now performed ; and although the operation barely lasted two minutes and a half, respiration ceased. After the subcutaneous injection of ether, and other means had been tried, the child gradually revived. Contrary to Dr. Navratil's usual custom, and led thereto chiefly by the child's exhaustion, further operative means (the extirpation of the growth) were not undertaken at this time. Not until four weeks later was the general condition sufficiently improved to warrant any further attempts. A vertical incision was then made over the middle of the thyroid cartilage, which was thus laid open. But between the lower extremity of this incision and the tracheotomy wound, a narrow bridge of tissue was left untouched. The object of this was to secure a more exact adaptation of the edges of the wound and of the vocal cords, and for the better holding in place of the canula when sewing up after completion of the operation. Instead of finding the papilloma, the operator found a cavity lined with mucous membrane, in the form of a shut sac ; he therefore passed a bent probe upwards from the canula into the larynx, and in this manner established that the mucous sac (above mentioned) was not the larynx. The sac was then slit up, and the papilloma discovered. It was as large as a medium-sized strawberry, and almost filed the laryngeal cavity. The growth was removed with the hæmostatic forceps, and the place from which it had sprung was then touched with the galvano-caustic ; for, owing to the small size of the larynx, even when widely expanded with sharp hooks, it was found impossible to cut off the mucous membrane itself, which seems to be the best prophylactic against recurrence. The edges of the thyroid cartilage were then brought together (a proceeding which was greatly facilitated by the little bridge of tissue already mentioned), and the wound was covered with carbolic gauze. It may be remarked that there was very little hemorrhage, and that there was not the slightest need to plug the trachea. The after-proceedings were not altogether untroubled, for the edges of the wound separated and became very unhealthy, and there was fever for several consecutive days. On the sixth day (after the operation) fluids came out of the tracheal wound: this was considered as probably due to injury to the posterior wall of the larynx and the adjoining wall of the œsophagus by the cautery. But after two weeks this ceased. The child now began to grow and develop in a remarkable way. Its voice—on stopping the canula—was clear; it could whistle and breathe through the mouth, though only for a short time. The growth, however, began to recur after a period of ten weeks. A metal probe was coated with nitrate of silver, and this was applied twice weekly. The new growth rapidly disappeared under this treatment (but whether permanently or not is not stated). The recurrent growth was much firmer than the original one; and Dr. Navratil considered this a good omen. A similar appearance has been observed in other cases. As a rule, the softer the growth—presumably from greater abundance of the cellular element—the more probable its recurrence after extirpation, and the greater the necessity for excising the basement membrane on which it rests, with a view to prevent this recurrence. This form of growth is very unusual in children. Thus this author had only seen three other cases, aged three and a half, five, and seven years respectively. The case may be regarded almost as unique in so young an infant as the present instance.—*Med. Times and Gazette*, Dec. 25, 1880.

<hr>

Œsophagism.

Dr. ELOY concludes (in the *Gaz. Hebdomadaire*, December 10) an elaborate paper on œsophagism in these terms: "As a result of the consideration of all the cases which we have cited, we come to the conclusion that the most efficacious means for combating this affection, when existing independently of all functional disturbance—that is, œsophagism from a nervous cause, whether local or general —are the employment of catheterism (with or without dilatation) as a mechanical agent, the hypodermic injection of morphia as an analgesic, and the bromide of potassium (either by the mouth or as an enema) as a moderator of the reflex power. Moreover, this last agent will facilitate catheterism, by imparting a greater toleration of the mucous membrane to the contact of instruments."— *Med. Times and Gaz.*, Dec. 18, 1880.

<hr>

Extirpation of a large Retro-peritoneal Fibroma, and of the left Kidney and Supra-renal body which were adherent to it.

Dr. F. B. BUSCHMANN reports this case. The operator was Professor Billroth. The patient was aged thirty-five. The belly was distended; no distinct masses could be felt; palpation gave a feeling of firmness and elasticity, but no distinct fluctuation; the percussion dulness passed without interruption into that of the liver and spleen. The tumour seemed fixed, and no connection could be made out between it and the uterus, which was apparently normal. The size and weight of the tumour caused much suffering, and there had latterly been rapid wasting. There was some bronchial catarrh, but with this exception the other organs were normal. The incision made was twenty centimetres long.

The tumour, which felt as if it contained fluid, was punctured, but nothing came. As the size of the tumour therefore could not be lessened, the incision was prolonged ten centimetres. The tumour was then separated from the surrounding peritoneum by numerous ligatures. The left kidney and supra-renal body, which were quite healthy, were lying in the true pelvis, and were firmly adherent to the tumour, attempts to separate them producing great hemorrhage. The vessels in the hilum of the kidney and the ureter were therefore tied, and it and the supra-renal body removed with the tumour, which weighed eighteen kilogrammes (about 39¾ lbs.). The growth was not pediculated; it had sprung from between the folds of the broad ligament, and grown upwards behind the mesentery. The uterus and both ovaries were normal, and not connected with the tumour. The wound was closed with twenty-nine sutures, and four drainage-tubes put in. Every antiseptic precaution was observed. Symptoms of peritonitis appeared next day, and the patient died in collapse on the fifth day. There was no autopsy. The tumour was found to be a fibro-myoma.—*Obstetrical Journal of Great Britain*, Nov. 15, 1880.

—

Accident to a Lithotrite.

At a recent meeting of the Medical Society of London, Mr. COULSON read notes of a case of lithotrity (Bigelow's operation), in which an accident of an unrecorded kind occurred to the lithotrite. The patient was sixty-eight years of age and had suffered from symptoms of calculus for about seven years. The operation was performed on the 11th inst. The meatus urethræ having been previously incised, a large stone about two inches in diameter was caught and crushed with Bigelow's lithotrite. The stone offered much resistance to the instrument, and the fragments separated with a loud crack. Three or four fragments had been successively crushed when it was found that the screw and two pins by which the lithotrite is fastened to the shaft had given way, so that the two portions of the instrument became separated. No means for connecting the handle with the shaft could be extemporized. By percussion, however, upon the handle the blades were freed as much as possible from the débris, and the instrument removed from the bladder, some injury being inflicted on the neck of the bladder and urethra in its withdrawal. The operation was completed by the fenestrated lithotrite, and fragments weighing 500 grains removed by the tube and aspirator. The operation occupied two hours and ten minutes, a delay of twenty minutes being caused by the accident. No bad symptoms followed, and this was attributed to the complete removal of the fragments having been effected. Mr. Coulston remarked on the enormous power of the blades of the instrument, and the inadequate resistance to the force applied by the screw, due to the imperfect manner in which the handle is connected with the shaft.—*Lancet*, Nov. 27, 1880.

—

Removal of Villous Growth from the Bladder.

Mr. DAVIES-COLLEY, at a recent meeting of the Clinical Society of London read notes of a case of villous growth of the bladder, successfully removed by perineal incision. Henry W., aged thirty-two, a shipwright, had suffered from hæmaturia for eight years. At first blood was passed only occasionally, and in small quantities. Latterly the flow had increased, and he had become so weak that for sixteen months he had been unable to work. He was admitted into Guy's Hospital last March. His family history was good. He was strongly built and fairly nourished, but very anæmic. There was a continual desire to micturate, and a feeling as if something always remained behind in the bladder. Blood was passed, sometimes at the beginning, sometimes at the end of micturition. No stone could be detected, and all efforts to find villous masses in the urine failed. No tumour could be felt per rectum. On April 16, he was placed under ether. Mr. Davies-Colley then opened the bladder by the usual incision for lateral lithotomy. At first nothing could be felt. Then a slight projection was made out on the left side of the fundus, and a cord-like process running from it. In a short time the free end of this process, with a soft pinkish tuft of villi attached to it, was seen at the deeper part of the wound. This was seized with the forceps, drawn out, and the pedicle cut with a pair of scissors close to the wall of the bladder. No other growth could be felt. There was but little hemorrhage during the operation, and some which occurred in the evening was readily arrested by the injection of iced water into the bladder. He made a rapid recovery. In two weeks the urine ceased to flow from the perineum, and soon afterwards the wound healed. When last seen, two months after the operation, there had been no return of the hemorrhage. The irritability of the bladder had ceased, and he was in the enjoyment of perfect health. The tumour grew from the posterior wall of the bladder, at a point about three inches from its neck, and one inch to the left of the middle line. It consisted of a fibrous stalk one-sixth of an inch thick and two inches long, terminated by branching filaments from half an inch to three-quarters of an inch long. These filaments contained capillary loops, invested by many layers of epithelium of a cylindrical shape.

Professor HUMPHRY has recorded in the *Medico-Chirurgical Transactions* a case in which he successfully removed a fibrous polypoid growth from the male bladder. He mentions a similar success in Professor Billroth's practice. The chief difficulty in the male subject is to ascertain the presence of a tumour as the source of hemorrhage. In the present case the diagnosis depended solely upon the long continuance of the bleeding and the absence of other causes. Perhaps the fact of blood passing sometimes at the beginning, and other times at the end of micturition, may assist in the detection of growth. No doubt the villi were in this case sometimes washed into the prostatic part of the urethra, where they were squeezed, so as to give rise to a flow of blood before the urine ; while at other times hemorrhage into the bladder was set up by the pressure of its muscular walls upon that part of the growth which lay in its interior.

Mr. CLEMENT LUCAS said that in these cases operative interference was justifiable and reasonable. He had thrice performed cystotomy in chronic disease of the bladder with great relief. The diagnosis of villous disease was not assured until a small portion of the growth could be obtained and detected by the microscope. These cases often went on for years without much effect upon health. He had a case under his care for two years ; astringent injections afforded some relief. Mr. Durham attempted the removal of a growth from the bladder a few years ago.

Dr. HABERSHON said that the patient on whom Dr. Davies-Colley had operated was very weak and prostrate on admission into the hospital, and it was evident that the hemorrhage came from the bladder, and not from the kidneys. There was often great difficulty in the diagnosis of these cases. He remembered a case in which the symptoms were attributed by one to calculus in the bladder, by another to calculus in the kidney, and by another to cancer. The patient suffered from hæmaturia, and at times intense pain in the penis. After three or four years' suffering a portion of a villous growth was passed per urethram, and all the symptoms ceased. Some pain returned after many years' interval. In other cases hemorrhage continues ; and in the presence of such cases it was a great advantage to know that operative interference might be undertaken with relief.

Dr. A. P. STEWART said that about twenty years ago he sent in to the Middlesex Hospital from the out-patient room a woman who had suffered for many months from intermittent hemorrhage from the bladder, at times very profuse, then ceasing for weeks, and then returning. Mr. De Morgan made a digital examination of the bladder, but found nothing. The urine continued to contain blood at intervals, and ultimately the patient died. The bladder, with a pedunculated villous growth, is now in the hospital museum. The reason why it had not been detected by Mr. De Morgan was, that it was attached to the front wall of the bladder immediately under the pubes.

Mr. TEEVAN congratulated Mr. Davies-Colley on the ease ; the first and only case of successful removal of a villous growth by the knife. Civiale had removed one by the lithotrite. Villous growths were usually attached to the posterior wall of the bladder, whereas polypi were fixed to its neck. The diagnosis of such cases was difficult ; and he mentioned one which he had lately seen with Dr. A. Clark, when in catheterism clear urine flowed at first, followed by pure blood and some shreds of villous growth. The patient was old and paralytic, so that attempt at removal of the growth was out of the question. Incision into the bladder for cystitis was done largely in America, and he himself had practised it four times, making the median incision. Perhaps an external urethrotomy would suffice ; villous disease was not always fatal. He had seen a case where the mass was spontaneously extruded with recovery.

Mr. BARKER asked whether in the cases operated on by Professor Humphry and Professor Billroth the growths were as pedunculated as in Mr. Davies-Colley's case. In some cases the villous disease is distinctly sessile, and involves a large surface of the fundus of the bladder. Supposing a growth of that variety were cut down upon, it would be difficult to know how to deal with it.

Mr. DAVIES-COLLEY, in reply, said that the tumours removed by Professors Humphry and Billroth were not of the villous kind. Prof. Humphry's was a case of polypoid fibrous growth from the mucous membrane. In his own case had the growth been sessile, no doubt great difficulty would have been experienced, but still, by tearing and scraping much might be removed, and the hemorrhage checked at least for a time. It was generally possible to entangle a small portion of a villous growth in the eye of the catheter, and thus extract it for diagnostic purposes ; and lately he had employed the washing bottle used in litholapaxy very effectually for the same purpose.—*Lancet*, Dec. 18, 1880.

—

Washing out the Bladder.

Dr. FISCHER, in a paper on this subject in the *Berliner Klin. Wochenschrift* for November 29, objects to the ordinary double catheter, because, as the stream of fluid always enters the bladder on one side only, the other side of the bladder may not be sufficiently cleansed. To obviate this defect he has modified the instrument as follows : The fluid passes into the bladder at the extremity of the instrument, which is somewhat bulbous and perforated with holes, and it escapes through a slit near the curve of the catheter. The instrument is disinfected in a three per cent. solution of carbolic acid before being introduced. In injecting the fluid he uses the irrigator, and thus the fluid is introduced in a continuous equable stream, and not in jerks as when it is pumped in. He washes out the bladder in cases of chronic catarrh, in order to remove the mucus, etc. He also advocates the injection of cold water into the bladder in cases of atony of that organ. At the commencement of the injection the water must be tepid, but it is latterly introduced quite cold. The cold stimulates the bladder to contraction, and after these injections have been employed for a few times the organ begins to regain its power. In destructive inflammation of the bladder he washes it thoroughly out before introducing any medicaments. Indeed, he thinks that continual irrigation with diluted remedies might in some cases be desirable.— *Med. Times and Gaz.*, Dec. 18, 1880.

Varices in Pregnancy.

M. Budin, of Paris, has written an interesting monograph upon the varices of pregnancy. The most common varices are, of course, those of the leg. M. Budin points out that the signs and symptoms of varicosities of the superficial and of the deep veins are quite distinct. Those of the superficial veins are familiar to every one. In the case of deep varices there is nothing to be seen wrong with the affected leg, except that it is increased in size. The patient complains of severe pain in the calf, in the popliteal space, and in the sole of the foot ; and there is increased perspiration of the affected limb. If such symptoms as these are rapidly relieved by rest, it is probable that a varicose condition of the deep veins is their cause. These varices are not constant in their mode of appearance. Sometimes they only become troublesome after several pregnancies, and then not till the last months of gestation ; but in some women they are noticed in the first three or four weeks ; one patient commonly first became aware of her pregnancies by the development of the varices. M. Budin also describes the varices of the internal and external genital organs, of the anus and rectum, of the urethra and bladder, and of the trunk and upper extremities. Hæmorrhoids often cause a good deal of trouble during pregnancy, but not danger ; they commonly disappear after delivery. If fissure coexist, it will be best treated by forcible stretching. Varices of some kind occur in from twenty to thirty per cent. of all pregnancies.—*Med. Times and Gaz.*, Dec. 18, 1880.

Peripheral Neuroganglioma.

Dr. Axel Key, of Stockholm, describes, in the *Hygeia* for 1879 (*Nordiskt Medecin. Arkiv*, Band xii.), the microscopic structure of a nerve-tumour removed from a journeyman tailor, aged 31, who was discharged cured after a stay of fourteen days in hospital. The tumour had commenced as a small knob in the soft parts in the neighbourhood of the left ala nasi, and had grown in the course of a year to the size of a plum. The extirpated tumour was encapsuled ; it was not adherent either to the skin or to the subjacent bone ; it was grayish-red in colour, homogeneous, and rather soft. After hardening in Müller's fluid, it appeared to be of tolerably firm consistence ; it was sharply defined, with smooth round projections, and was of somewhat irregular flattened shape. To one of the projections were attached some shreds, like connective tissue. Macroscopically, it was like a sarcoma, and had been diagnosed as such in the hospital. The microscope, however, revealed an entirely different structure ; namely, very large cells, which completely resembled ganglion-cells, and were inclosed in perfectly developed capsules, the interior of which had the same appearance as the capsules of ganglion-cells. The cells were apolar ; and not only one, but two or three, or even more, were contained in the same capsule. In the shreds connected with the tumour was found a nerve broken up into fine fibres of unequal size, probably a portion of the infra-orbital. On examining these branches of nerve, it was clearly seen that the large ganglionic elements of the tumour were developed from the nerve-fibres. Thus there was in this case a true ganglioma, which throws light on the hitherto unsolved question, whether a tumour of this kind can be developed on a peripheral nerve. Only one case of ganglioma is described in medical literature, viz., by Loretz in Virchow's *Archiv;* but the tumour, which was of the size of an egg, had proceeded from a pre-existing ganglion, and was thus a simple hyperplastic new growth. The case reported by Professor Key renders it certain that a ganglioma may be developed from a peripheral nerve, altogether independently of preceding ganglionic formations; and hence, in order to avoid all misunderstanding, Dr. Key calls this new growth, "neuroganglioma verum periphericum."—*British Med. Journ.*, Dec. 11, 1880.

—

The Plaster-of-Paris Jacket for the Treatment of Fracture of the Spine.

Sayre's jacket meets, as is well known, with a varying amount of approval in the hands of different surgeons. Those, however, who use it most frequently will, we believe, allow that its indiscriminate use will not lead to invariably satisfactory results; and not only so, but that some promising cases appear to go progressively from bad to worse notwithstanding the application of the jacket, while others in which its employment has seemed at first likely to be of doubtful utility have, contrary to expectation, been much benefited by it. We can call to mind two cases—one of a boy with an early condition of spinal caries in the dorsal region (just the case, it might be said, for the treatment), who, in six weeks after his jacket was put on, had a large psoas abscess; and another sickly child, with disease in the same part of the spine, and marked fulness in one iliac region, who, nearly a year after the plaster of Paris was applied, had a tolerably strong back, but in whom no abscess had shown itself. The use of this apparatus has long been suggested—and, we believe, practised—for fractured ribs, and from its employment for this purpose it is difficult to imagine any evil result following; but our German brothers have recently been using it for another object, in which, as might have been expected, a very varying amount of success has been attained.

In No. 7 of the *Centralblatt für Chirurgie* for this year is a paper by Professor König, of Göttingen, on the application of the "Thorax Gypsverband" for fractures of the spine, which recounts three cases, in all of which, although considerable displacement was present, very slight, if any, nervous symptoms had arisen. In each of these three instances the patients were suspended sufficiently to correct the deformity, and a long jacket reaching down to the trochanters was put on; and every one of them made a complete and rapid recovery. On the other hand, in No. 46 of the same journal we find a paper by Dr. W. Wagner, of Königshütte, which tells of two similar cases in which, after the application of the jacket, such intense pain in one instance, and paralysis in the other, set in, in the lower extremities, that it was necessary to remove the apparatus. In one it was re-applied later, with comfort to the patient. Both patients recovered. Professor König, after pointing out that all the cases treated by him in this way were recent and simple, adds that it is obvious that if extensive injury of the spinal cord is present, especially if the injury be of some standing, and bedsores have perhaps already developed themselves, it cannot be expected that the case will be benefited by the treatment; but, as he says, the diagnosis of the degree of injury is not, as a rule, a very difficult one. For uncomplicated cases the plan seems likely to prove of great service, and is undoubtedly an improvement on any of the older methods of treatment now in vogue; but the moment of suspension can scarcely fail to be one of anxiety to the surgeon, as it is easy to understand how the correction of a deformity may cause pressure on a cord which has previously escaped injury. This danger is very likely more hypothetical than real, and is probably exaggerated in our minds by the cautions that have been impressed upon us, as students, against attempting to rectify deformities so produced—the practice of " letting sleeping dogs lie " having commended itself to our fathers as, on the whole, the safest.—*Med. Times and Gaz.*, Dec. 18, 1880.

Fracture of the Sacrum.

By its position and structure the sacrum is peculiarly free from liability to fracture except from bullet wounds, and, although it is sometimes found fissured, or even comminuted in severe crushes of the pelvis, simple uncomplicated fracture of this bone is a very rare accident. Erichsen has seen one such case, the injury being a blow from the buffer of a railway carriage, and proving rapidly fatal. Agnew says that simple transverse fracture of the sacrum is usually accompanied by fatal injuries to the pelvic viscera.

A remarkable case has recently been put on record in Paris. A woman, thirty-six years of age, was brought into the St. Lazare Hospital with the history of having fallen about eight feet on to her buttocks. She fainted, and when she was conscious was quite unable to sit. A slight transverse depression corresponding to the middle of the sacrum was readily felt from the back, the part was very tender, and pressure gave fine crepitus; extensive ecchymosis quickly occurred over the whole sacrum. From either the rectum or vagina the line of fracture was readily felt, and the projection forwards of the lower half of the sacrum verified, this part of the bone was easily moved with crepitus. Reduction was easily effected by the finger pressed back from the front, and displacement did not recur. A bandage was applied firmly round the pelvis and the patient kept in bed. Defecation gave intense pain, and the woman was unable to lie on her back for a fortnight, but sat up in bed on the twenty-eighth day, and got up in the ward on the forty-second day. There were no signs of pressure upon or other injury of the lower sacral or coccygeal nerves.

In cases where there has been a tendency for the displacement to recur, various mechanisms in the rectum have been employed to keep the bone in position, such as a plug of wood, a stuffed silver canula which could be opened to allow the passage of feces. The ease with which in the above case the reduction was effected shows that the displacement was due to the direction of the fracturing force, and not to the action of the muscles attached to the lower fragment. The main difficulty in the treatment of these cases where the fracture is the sole injury is the intense pain in defecation, and the local disturbance it induces. Some have, by means of opium, kept the bowels confined and then cleared the rectum by an enema every week or ten days. It is still better to diet the patient very carefully with a view to the production of the smallest possible quantity of feces, which may then be easily and almost painlessly removed by means of an enema every three or four days.—*Lancet*, November 20, 1880.

Tight Rings.

Treatises on operative surgery are absolutely silent on the constriction, by rings, of fingers swollen from one cause or another, and on the method of removing them. The accident is, nevertheless, of common occurrence, causes great pain, sometimes gives rise to great uneasiness, and may even threaten the safety of the finger itself. As a rule, in these cases of constriction, the ring is cut unnecessarily, for want of a simple method of removing it, notwithstanding the popular plan which comes to us by tradition, and is thus described by Oribasius, vol. iv. p. 251, Daremberg's edition. He writes: "Sometimes the finger is constricted by a ring ; and it is necessary to remove the ring without delay, by giving it a rotatory motion ; bathing at the same time the finger with warm water, and greasing it with some kind of fatty matter. If the ring do not yield to these efforts, the following operation is recommended. A thick and twisted thread is sharpened at one end in the same way as cobblers sharpen their threads, and passed between the finger and the ring, whilst the rest of the thread is rolled round the finger. When this thread is unrolled, the ring moves towards the tip of the finger, whence it can be removed. If the ring resist this treatment, it is then necessary to cut it." Aetius, who lived at the end of the fifth and the beginning of the sixth centuries, repeats the recommendations of Oribasius. A writer in the *Concours Médical* suggests some improvements on the plan, so as to reduce the volume of the finger by ischæmiatizing it, in the same way as ischæmia is produced with Esmarch's bandage. In the first place, the finger is coated with fatty matter; then a thin thread, about a yard and a quarter long, is taken; one end is placed under the ring, and passed above it with a pair of pincers to the length of about three inches. The end of the thread being thus fixed by the ring, the rest of the thread is taken to the top of the finger, round which it is rolled in close overlapping lines, not leaving any space between them. This done, the second end of the thread is also passed under, and brought up above the ring. Then, this end being taken between the fingers, the rest of the thread is unrolled resting on the ring, which is thus gradually brought up to the point, where it is easily removed. If a first trial do not always succeed. it is rare for the ring not to yield to efforts twice or thrice repeated. Should this be the case, the ring, of course, must be cut on a canulated sound with a file or divider.—*British Med. Journal*, Dec. 18, 1880.

Midwifery and Gynæcology.

On Listerism in Gynecology and Midwifery.

FRANKENHAUSER (*Centralblatt f. Gynaek.*, No. 22, 1879) thinks that the principal agent in producing infection is impure air. He, therefore, performs all his operations under the spray, and limits the number of students at his ovariotomies to four or five, who take off all unnecessary articles of clothing before coming into the operating room. On the other hand, he looks on the prophylactic intra-uterine injections *post partum* as carrying with them more danger than they avoid. If the hand has to be introduced into the genitals, it is always done under the spray, which is even used when making an ordinary examination, for he thinks it is much easier to prevent the entrance of impure air than to wash away septic material once it is formed.

When reporting Frankenhäuser's paper, Oeri says that for some years back, in Bischof's clinique, the spray is always used when the hand has to be introduced into the uterus, the perineum to be sewn up, as well as during many gynecological operations. Even during the time, however, when the antiseptic injections alone were made use of, it was usual to find patients recovering after protracted labours, manual removal of the placenta, or decomposition of the ovum, without any feverish symptoms.

In the report of the obstetrical clinique of Prof. WEBER RITTER VON EBENHOF, in Prague, for the year ending Ap. 30, 1879 (*Centralblatt*, No. 26, 1879), a description is given of the precautions that are taken for avoiding septic infection during labour and the lying-in state. No student is allowed to make any examination who has any sort of sore on the hands, or whose nails are long or dirty. Even after the most thorough washing of the hands the students are obliged, before making an examination, to rinse them first in a two per cent. solution of carbolic acid, and afterwards in a solution of permanganate of potash and weak hydrochloric acid. The finger is then covered with a five per cent. solution of carbolic acid in glycerine. As soon as a new patient is admitted her vagina is washed out with a two per cent. solution of carbolic acid, and the parts about the vulvæ thoroughly washed with soap and carbolic acid solution. If the labour be long delayed after the escape of the waters, the vagina is washed every two hours with carbolic acid solution. In order to prevent the entrance of air into the vagina a wad of cotton steeped in dilute liq. chlori. (1 to 3) is laid before the vulvæ. After the expulsion of the placenta the vagina is washed out by the head midwife with carbolic acid solution, and if the labour has been a protracted one, the fœtus decomposed, or any operation been undertaken, the assistant himself must wash out the uterus with a three per cent. carbolic acid solution. All fissures of the genitals are closed with carbolized catgut, and ruptured perinea with carbolized silk. If the vagina has been much bruised a wad of cotton-wool saturated with camphor is passed into it immediately after the removal of the placenta. In all natural labours the child is born under the hand-spray, and all operations are performed under the steam-spray. The placentæ, till removed from the ward, are placed in a solution of carbolic water. All dead children are at once removed, and closets for soiled linen are disinfected with chloride of lime. To prevent infection after labour the vagina is washed out every two or three hours with lukewarm two per cent. carbolic acid solution, which has previously been boiled. If fever is present a carbolic acid decoction of chamomile flowers of the same strength is used. All the old tin injection tubes have been replaced with glass ones. In all cases where the passage is injured or there are puerperal ulcers, a wad of cotton is laid before the vulva, impregnated with carbolic acid or camphor. The nurses are made to wash their hands in carbolic solution after having in any way come in contact with the genital tract of a lying-in woman. It is of great importance to treat the first indications of fever promptly by injections of three per cent. solution into the uterus, and the administration of purgatives. Nine mothers died out of 925 mothers thus treated, being a mortality of less than one per cent.

Of late years it has been proposed, with a view of lessening the chance of puerperal infection, to wash out the vagina, cervix, and uterus of every lying-in woman with a three per cent. solution of carbolic acid immediately after the child is born. HOFMEIER (*Centralblatt f. Gynaek.*, No. 5, 1880) found that of 260 cases treated thus prophylactically by him in the University Lying-in Hospital in Berlin, 16 per cent. were attacked with fever, 8 of them very severely, while of 249 patients not so treated only 8 per cent. got ill, only 1 case being serious. Hence he concludes that such treatment of ordinary cases does more harm than good.

It is very different, however, when we have symptoms of putrefaction or decomposition taking place during labour, accompanied by the formation of gas in the uterus and elevation of temperature in the patient. Stande found that 57 per cent. of such cases were attacked with fever, and that 50 per cent. died. It is evident, therefore, that we should endeavour to remove and render harmless every particle of decomposing matter, for which purpose it will be necessary to use a tolerably strong solution (at least five per cent.) of carbolic acid. Of 27 such cases, with temperatures reaching above 106° F. and pulses up to 144, that were thus treated *post partum*, 6 only died, or 22 per cent., and 18, or 60 per cent., made an uninterrupted recovery. The wonderful contrast between the threatened danger and the undisturbed convalescence can only be properly appreciated by a perusal of the whole history of such cases which Hofmeier hopes shortly to publish.—*Dublin Journal of Medical Science*, Nov. 1880.

Absence of the Vagina; Uterus distended by retained Menstrual Fluid; Operation; Recovery.

At a late meeting of the Obstetrical Society of London (*Lancet*, Nov. 27, 1880), Dr. C. H. CARTER stated the case of a patient, aged sixteen, who had never menstruated. Pain had begun two years previously, and recurred almost daily. The urethral orifice was found large, the vagina absent. By rectal examination the finger felt the sound in the bladder with only a thin layer of tissue intervening. About one and a half to two inches up the rectum a rounded elastic mass was felt, reaching up half way to the umbilicus, about the size of the uterus at the third or fourth month of pregnancy. On July 25th the operation was performed for making an artificial vagina. After slight longitudinal and lateral incisions, the passage was chiefly torn by finger and director. Nothing like os or cervix uteri could be detected. The uterus was first punctured with the aspirator, and the opening then enlarged with a bistoury. About ten ounces of treacly matter escaped; several ounces of treacly fluid were afterwards expelled, and the same evening the dressings were soaked with fresh blood. The next day syringing out the uterus with carbolic lotion (1 in 80) was commenced. For about ten days there was some elevation of temperature, and a rapid pulse, 112 to 130, but the disturbance then passed off. When the patient went out on Oct. 11th, the new vagina had narrowed a good deal, and only admitted the finger for about three-quarters of an inch. Thick sounds were passed occasionally to keep open the passage into the uterus, and menstruation took place regularly after the operation. In October of the following year an examination was made, and it was found that the ordinary sound could not be passed into the uterus, but a small-pointed sound could be passed into it three inches and a half. The author expressed to the mother his opinion that marriage was inadmissible, since delivery could not take place *per vias naturales*.

Dr. GALABIN's experience was, that the difficulty of keeping an artificial vagina in a condition fit for married life and parturition was considerable. He had had a similar case, in which also no trace of os or cervix could be detected. An artificial vagina was successfully made, and the patient afterwards menstruated naturally; but the attempt to keep the passage of full size was defeated by the fact that the pressure of the dilator repeatedly caused an opening into the bladder, though without producing any continued incontinence of urine.

Dr. ROUTH said that in his own case the patient had not died from the operation, but from the rupture of another cyst. He believed that in most of these cases the vagina had originally existed, but became subsequently adherent. He thought so in his own case, from the ease with which he tore it open. He thought that the passage could be kept dilated by using sponge-tents, and subsequently Sim's dilators. The dilators should not be too large, and should not be worn more than a few hours at a time; they then would not cause inflammation. He mentioned a case in which Mr. Baker Brown had made a good artificial vagina, and the girl subsequently went upon the town and consorted with Life Guardsmen.

Dr. BRAITHWAITE said there were two classes of cases of atresia, one being incomplete, a fistulous track existing. From the presence of mucous membrane in this contraction was less likely. When the atresia was complete he thought that mucous membrane might be transplanted from the vulva or from an animal, to prevent the tendency to contraction. In a difficult case, the urethra might be dilated and the finger kept in the bladder, and the thumb in the rectum, during the operation.

Dr. GODSON said that he had that morning seen a young woman for whom he had reluctantly made an artificial vagina two months since. There was no retention of menses, but she had married in ignorance of her deformity. Though a fortnight ago there was a capacious canal, it would now barely admit a penholder. He believed that such failure was inevitable, and would not again operate unless there were retained menstrual discharge.

Dr. AVELING thought that Dr. Carter was quite right in dissuading his patient from marriage. He did not agree with Dr. Routh that the majority of cases of absence of vagina were due to inflammatory adhesion. In the three cases he had seen it was evidently congenital, as the uterus was also absent, though the ovaries were present.

Dr. CARTER, in reply, said that Dr. Emmet stated that the tendency to close depended upon the passage being made by cutting rather than by tearing. He did not think that the tendency to contract depended altogether upon the absence of mucous membrane, but rather upon the contractility of the tissues, since in his case a mucous membrane like that of the labia minora was noted in the new passage. He agreed with Dr. Galabin that it was better to defer washing out the uterine cavity a short time. He did not recommend marriage in his case, because the end of the new vagina was closely attached to the margins of the opening into the uterus. No natural dilatation of this opening could occur in labour, and Cæsarean section would probably be necessary.

The Mechanical Dilatation of the Uterus.

FRITSCH thinks (*Die mechanische Uterus Dilatation, Centralblatt f. Gynaek.,* No. 25, 1879) that where our only object is to dilate the uterus we should entirely abandon such means as the sponge-tent, laminaria, or tupelo, in favour of rapid instrumental dilatation, by which we can so entirely avoid all risk of septic infection. He uses for this purpose graduated steel sounds, seemingly very similar to those proposed by Peaslee in 1870. The thickest is about the size of a thick finger; the smallest is somewhat larger than a thick sound (0.5 mm.). He first introduces one of the smaller sounds to the inner os, and then grasps the uterus externally, and presses the fundus down over the sound. This often requires an amount of force which would be quite unallowable if applied only from within, without the control of the hand externally. The danger of septic infection can certainly be avoided by using frequent injections, and it is much safer than the metrotome. He has made use of the method in multiparæ to remove retained portions of an abortion, mucous polypi, and to enable him to use the curette. As to its efficiency in cases of dilatation of the inner os he has no experience.

It is only when we wish to produce artificial infiltration of the uterus that the slow process is indicated. If we wish to strengthen a flabby uterus, to give tone to the circulation, or increase the power of contraction, then we should make use of the laminaria. If we only want to open the way into the uterus, then we should use rapid instrumental dilatation.

This paper has elicited one from Professor C. SCHROEDER, of Berlin ("Sind die Quellmittel in der gynaekologischen Praxis nothwendig?"—*Centralblatt f. Gynaekologie,* No. 26, 1879), in which he says that he does not think that in private practice he has made use of the slow method of dilating the uterus for more than one and a half years, and even in hospital it is now only rarely that he does so, and when he finds it necessary he uses the tupelo tent. Many years ago he procured a set of graduated sounds, such as Fritsch advises, but uses them only very rarely. Nor can he say that he has been led to abandon tents from finding their use too dangerous, for he thinks such accidents as have occurred might be certainly avoided in the future by following Schultz's antiseptic method, which has, however, the disadvantage of most wearily lengthening the whole process. He has, however, been led to abandon them, partly because, in many cases where he formerly used dilatation for the purpose of diagnosis or treatment, he can now attain his object by means of the sharp scoop, which can be passed through the undilated os, and part or all of the mucous membrane of the uterus so removed. When, however, he requires to pass the finger into the uterus, he now first incises both sides of the cervix as far as the roof of the vagina on both sides, and then forces the finger into the cavity, either by pushing down the fundus from above, or drawing the cervix over the finger by means of a Museaux' vulsellum. In some cases it is quite surprising how readily this may be done; in difficult cases we will generally rupture some of the fibres of the inner os. These slight ruptures, if not infected, heal readily, and when we have finished our diagnosis or treatment we can close the cut sides of the cervix with sutures.

Though a very large number of cases come annually before him, he has in this way been led almost entirely to give up the use of tents for dilating purposes.

In the number of the same paper for April 24th of this year, Dr. FRANCK gives an account of the results obtained by using Prof. Schultz's dilator—the essential conditions for its use being that the cervical canal should measure at least 6 mm., and that there is no inflammatory process going on in either the uterus or its appendages. The instrument, after being thoroughly cleansed and disinfected, is passed into the uterus and the branches separated. The amount to which this is possible varies greatly with the condition of the uterine tissue and the varying amount of pain experienced by the patient. The instrument is then withdrawn to see what size the passage is, and before it is again introduced the uterus should be carefully washed out with warm water to prevent infection. With such precautions it is absolutely without danger, and it has the great advantage that it produces the same amount of dilatation in a few minutes that laminaria tents do in about eight hours. In cases where the woman has not borne a child, or where the cervix has not the diameter of 6 mm., it is necessary to begin with a single laminaria tent. He says the patient after the dilatation must remain lying for at least an hour, but need not necessarily be confined to bed. If the spasmodic pains still continue she should have an opium suppository and warm stupes to the abdomen. He thinks that this dilatation repeated at intervals has a powerful effect in curing subinvolution and flaccidity of the uterus. It also causes the expulsion of portions of retained placenta or membranes, and retroflexions may also be cured thereby, provided there are no adhesions present. Stenosis of the inner, but not of the outer, os will yield to this treatment.

In *The Lancet* for Nov. 1, 1879, Mr. LAWSON TAIT gives twelve cases in which he dilated the cervix by continuous elastic pressure. He says: "I have had such unsatisfactory results from all kinds of tents in dilating the cervix uteri that I have long desired to get something which would accomplish this more safely, more speedily, and with less pain. Having been struck by the ease with which an inverted uterus can be returned by continuous elastic pressure, I applied this method for the purpose of dilating the cervix, and my results have been so completely satisfactory that I hasten to narrate my experience of the first twelve cases in which I have used it." The advantages of the plan are that it is absolutely free from smell and septic risks, and almost free from pain. It produces more complete dilatation of the whole canal than that obtained with tents. The dilators are made of vulcanite, and are sold in sets of four sizes to screw into a common stem. "The only precaution necessary in their employment is to use extremely gentle pressure." In this paper Mr. Tait does not, however, enter into any details as to how the continuous elastic pressure is to be applied.

Just as we were going to press we received one of the series of *Volkmann's Clinical Lectures*, by Dr. LEOPOLD LANDAU, on " The Various Methods of Dilating the Uterus" (*Ueber Erweiterungsmittel der Gebärmutter*), which treats the whole subject in a most exhaustive manner.—*Dublin Journal of Medical Sciences*, Nov. 1880.

On the Treatment of Ruptures of the Uterus.

Dr. FROMMEL, Assistant Physician to the Gynecological Clinique in Berlin, publishes two interesting cases of this accident in No. 18 *Centralblatt für Gynä. kologie*, 1880. Case I. refers to a patient 40 years old, who had given birth twelve times previously, and who suffered from slight contraction of the pelvis— diagonal conjugate being 4 inches. The labour had been a prolonged one, and had suddenly become arrested, when the assistance of Dr. Hoffmeier was obtained. He removed without great difficulty, by version, a dead full-grown child, and discovered an almost complete transverse rupture of the uterus between the lower segment and the cervix, only a bridge of tissue about 2½ inches broad to the left and anteriorly remaining to connect the two. The peritoneal investment of the uterus was quite entire ; but as the child had passed out through the rent in the uterine tissue, it was almost completely separated from the uterus, so that now a large cavity shut off from the peritoneal cavity existed. Dr. Hoffmeier caused the patient to be immediately brought to the hospital, in which a thorough irrigation of the cavity with a warm two per cent. solution of carbolic acid was performed under chloroform, and a thick drainage tube introduced through the vagina into the cavity. This was secured in position. An ice bladder was put upon the abdomen. The condition of the patient was after this satisfactory. No vomiting ; pulse strong, regular, 84. The highest temperature which she reached was 100° on the evening of the sixth day. This was also the only time that an antiseptic injection was made through the drainage-tube. For the first few days the patient got only a little fluid nourishment. From the eighth day gradually more nourishing food was administered. During the first days a tolerably copious bloody fluid was discharged from the drainage-tube, which after a few days became less bloody, and, finally, purely pus. On the twenty-sixth day, no further discharge appearing, the drainage-tube was taken out. On the twenty-eighth day the patient was allowed to rise, and on the thirtieth day she was discharged. On internal examination an opening several centimetres deep was found to exist anteriorly to which the finger could penetrate up to the peritoneum. On the right there was a considerable amount of exudation ; the uterus somewhat dislocated towards the left and retroflected. General condition good. The second case was that of a patient 30 years old, who had suffered from rickets in early life, and had three times been delivered naturally. In her fourth confinement, in consequence of the labour proving tedious, the midwife administered four powders of ergot. A medical man who was called prescribed morphia, and, having obtained the aid of another medical friend, diagnosed rupture of the uterus, for which laparotomy was decided upon. The execution of this operation was prevented by the opposition of a drunken husband, whereupon the patient was taken to the hospital. On examination under chloroform the parts of the child were to be felt directly under the abdominal wall. Internal examination discovered the child situated with its head presenting, quite movable, at the pelvic brim, the whole child and placenta having passed into the abdominal cavity. The body of the uterus was almost entirely torn from the lower segment and cervix, except for a small connecting part on the posterior wall, and lay powerfully contracted, pushed upwards and backwards. Professor Schroeder delivered at once, by version and extraction, a fresh, full-grown female child, whereupon the abdominal cavity was washed out with two per cent. carbolic acid, and a thick drainage-tube introduced as high as possible into the peritoneal cavity, which was secured likewise by suture to the posterior commissure. On the abdomen a bandage was so applied that the uterus was pressed firmly backwards and downwards, and also the cavity compressed. Thereby a great accumulation of blood in the abdominal cavity was prevented. In addition an ice-bladder was put on the abdomen. The condition of patient thereafter was wonderfully good. The pulse was somewhat frequent and irregular, but powerful ; the temperature not elevated. This case also ran a favourable course. During the earlier days a copious bloody fluid was discharged through the tube, which became purulent after ten or twelve days. The temperature only once rose to 101°. As often as it exceeded 100°, which it did on several evenings, a two per cent. carbolic solution was injected into the cavity through the drainage-tube, which readily flowed out past the tube. For the first few days attempts were made, by the administration of opium, to prevent peristaltic action of the bowels, so as to allow the formation of adhesions around the torn part. The pulse, which from the first was frequent, ultimately settled down to about 100, but was strong and regular. On the seventeenth day after delivery the drainage-tube was removed, when the opening was found only large enough to hold the tube, and secreted a small quantity of laudable pus. On the nineteenth day the patient got up, felt well, and complained of nothing. Two days afterwards she was discharged. To the account of these interesting cases the author adds a few words in recommendation of the practice.—*Edinburgh Med. Journal,* Nov. 1880.

———

Hyperpyrexia after Listerian Ovariotomy.

At a late meeting of the Royal Medical and Chirurgical Society, Dr. BANTOCK read a paper on this subject which elicited one of the most animated debates upon Listerism which has yet occurred in London. Dr. Bantock stated that Mr. Lawson Tait had already questioned, before the Society, the advantages attributed to the Listerian precautions in the operation of ovariotomy. The absence of pyrexia has been claimed as one of the best results following such precautions. In this paper the fact that pyrexia is absent in cases treated antiseptically is disputed on clinical evidence. In the author's own experience, the Listerian method in a series of thirty-six cases shows in its favour a difference of but 0.4°, compared with the same number of cases undertaken without complete antiseptic precautions ; the very lowest temperature occurred after a non-Listerian ovariotomy. Volkmann admits a condition of poisoning from absorption of carbolic acid, and terms this accident "aseptic fever." Thiersch has encountered instances of great irritation from this agent, and now employs salicylic acid in its stead. Keith finds very little difference in the temperature of series of cases undertaken under the old and the new method. In three Listerian cases the temperatures were the highest he had ever seen. Before adopting antiseptics he never found the ice-cap necessary for the reduction of pyrexia, excepting in one acute case of septicæmia. On the other hand, Mr. MacCormac asserts that the rise of temperature in Listerian cases is slight or absent, and when present is due to other causes ; Mr. Spencer Wells has found that, contrary to Mr. Tait's experience, pyrexia is subdued by antiseptics. Mr. Thornton has observed no fever at all, as a rule, after antiseptic ovariotomy. When, however, an operator is disposed to support Listerism, he may readily attribute to other influences ill results, of which it alone can be the cause. It is easy to explain how pyrexia follows "antiseptic operations." Carbolic acid is an irritant ; its great advocate introduced the "protective" to counteract its irritating qualities. It is also a poison. It has caused death when inhaled, and has produced very serious symptoms when absorbed; this is illustrated in cases related by Lister, Lightfoot, Hanhorst, and the author, who describes at length two cases of poisoning from prolonged action of carbolic spray in complicated ovariotomies. In both, the kidneys were affected by this medium. Agostini relates a case of poisoning from carbolic acid solution injected frequently into an abscess cavity. Thomas Smith and others have noted the bad effects of this acid in operations upon children. The author observed albuminuria and temporary suppression of excretion of sulphates in the urine of a young girl after antiseptic ovariotomy. Sonnenburg, Lightfoot, and others have also found that sulphates disappeared from the urine in similar cases, whereas in the author's patient that excretion did not become dark. Hence carbolic poisoning is not always indicated and exposed by discoloration of the urine, as is generally believed. Keith admits that evil effects may result from prolonged action of spray. The hyperpyrexia which follows is due not solely to reaction, but also to carbolic intoxication. The whole merit of Listerism lies, not in the supposed good effects of carbolic acid, but in the cleanliness which it promotes. By greatly reducing the strength of the solutions used in operations, the author has gained excellent results with absence of pyrexia.

Mr. ERICHSEN remarked upon the local anæsthetic effect produced by the carbolic spray. It produced a numbness of the hands, and he thought this showed that the carbolic action had some action on the peripheral nerves.

Mr. KNOWSLEY THORNTON said, that no one had claimed that Listerism was never followed by pyrexia, unless it were Mr. Tait himself, who, in his paper published in the recent volume of the Transactions, says (page 133) : "As the temperature and pulse-curve are uniformly admitted to represent the course of any case involving febrile action, if the antiseptic system makes its claims justly, ovariotomies performed under its precautions ought to indicate a more even and less febrile course of recovery than the non-antiseptic cases, and this should occur independently of all other details of the operation." Obviously more fever must follow a difficult operation than a simple one. In the debate on that paper Mr. Holmes remarked that the whole question was one of "impressions," and he (Mr. Thornton) resolved now to state facts ; and to contrast the temperatures of non-antiseptic and antiseptic ovariotomy. Of the former he had had twenty-five successful cases with an average stay in hospital after operation of 26.3 days, and of the latter 150 successful cases with an average stay of 20.5 days. In twenty-five non-antiseptic cases the ice-water cap was used seventeen times, or in 68 per cent. ; in 150 antiseptic it was used thirty-one times, or 20 per cent. It was used to reduce temperature in twelve non-antiseptic cases, or 48 per cent., and in fourteen antiseptic cases, or 9 per cent. On this point he saw from a letter from Dr. Bantock in the *Medical Times* that he agreed with him. In the remaining cases the cap was put on to prevent high temperature—viz., 20 per cent. of the non-antiseptic cases, and in 11 per cent. of the antiseptic cases ; but of late he had limited its use to the reduction of temperature only. In the non-antiseptic series the temperature never rose above 100.4°—i. e., there was no fever in but two cases, or 8 per cent., in the antiseptic—forty-five cases, or 30 per cent.; and if the cases in which there was a slight additional rise of 1° or 2° for a few hours be included, the figures would be 32 per cent. of the non-antiseptic series, as against 75 per cent. of the antiseptic recovering without fever. Dr. Bantock should not have styled his cases as Listerian ovariotomies at all, and the number (thirty-six) was too small to draw such large inferences as he had done. Although he himself had practised antiseptic ovariotomy in 200 cases, he felt he had yet much to learn in the application of the method, and he generally found that when a case went wrong some detail had been omitted. In his last 100 cases, with a mortality of 7 per cent., three patients died from septicæmia, a result which he was sure would not have occurred had he thoroughly acted up to the theory of Listerism, and in Dr. Bantock's cases the drainage-tubes were often changed by the nurses during the night, a practice certainly *not* that of Listerism. Recently Dr. Bantock had (in *The Lancet*) published statements of practice which he styled Listerism, but which only proved that he was not in a position to carry out that practice, so contrary were they to Lister's express teaching.

The occurrence of nephritis could not be attributed to carbolic acid poisoning, for long before antiseptics were introduced into ovariotomy deaths occurred from suppression of urine, etc., and quite lately he had such a case, in which death took place within twenty-four hours after the removal of a tumour weighing 88 pounds, there being chronic Bright's disease. Septicæmia, too, was often fatal from failure of the kidneys to act, and comparison of the post-mortem records of such cases before the days of antiseptics showed no difference in the lesions observed in them and in those cases attributed to poisoning by carbolic acid. A German surgeon had recently said that in his country they had become so convinced that septicæmia had been banished by Listerism that deaths formerly attributed to this cause were put down to the toxic effects of carbolic acid. It was one thing to use the method and another to act up to Lister's practice and theory, and it would be far better if those who did not accept the theory would cease to practise the method, since their failures were no proof of the falsity of the theory. When studying under Professor Lister, at Edinburgh, he had repeatedly seen the urine darkened by carbolic acid without any other effects. He failed to see on what principle Dr. Bantock used a 1 per cent. solution of the acid, which Dr. Bantock said was no longer germicide. If so, why trouble to introduce this 1 per cent. of an "irritant" and a "poison?" Was it done to increase the cleanliness of the water? Dr. Bantock's results at the Samaritan Hospital were the same as those obtained by Mr. Spencer Wells without antiseptics at all, and using chiefly the extra-peritoneal method.

Mr. TAIT says that the advantages claimed for Listerism are really due to the adoption of intra-peritoneal method. But was this so? He had compared the statistics of the Samaritan Hospital for periods of six years with this result. Mr. Spencer Wells, from 1872 to 1877 inclusive, had 191 cases (extra-peritoneal) with a mortality of 20 per cent. ; Dr. Bantock, from 1875 to 1880, inclusive, had 136 cases (intra-peritoneal and modified antiseptics) with a mortality of 17.64 per cent. Mr. Thorton in the same period had 181 cases (intra-peritoneal and antiseptics), with a mortality of 11.6 per cent. These differences were due to the more thorough use of the antiseptic method. In the present year, Dr. Bantock, using his *very modified* antiseptic method had had forty cases with a mortality of 12 per cent. ; Mr. Thornton with pure Listerism, had fifty-four cases with a mortality of 7.4 per cent., including two deaths from septicæmia, which he attributed to failure in carrying out the method. Still, Mr. Wells in the last two years of his hospital practice had only a mortality of 10 per cent. in intra-peritoneal cases, a result largely due to the use of the ice-cap and drainage. In his own last 100 cases, Mr. Thornton had a mortality of 7 per cent., twenty-seven of these being private cases, with one death—a case of unusual difficulty. All this went to prove that with every case the mortality without Listerism could not get below 10 per cent. ; and if by the adoption of the method the mortality could be lowered by three or four per cent., that end was alone worth the extra trouble and difficulty entailed by the method.

Mr. Lawson Tait was surprised that Mr. Thornton should have quoted the passage from his paper in the sense he did, and regretted that there did not seem to be a clear understanding as to the meaning of Listerism; since it had just been stated that it was no part of the Listerian theory to avert septic fever. Hitherto he had thought that the whole aim of the theory was to eliminate this surgical fever after operations. If this were not its aim, what was it? In fatal cases of ovariotomy the temperature rises steadily to the end. He could not then concur in any of Mr. Thorton's remarks. As to the duration of stay in hospital, there was a great difference between cases in which the clamp was used and those in which it was not.

Mr. Thornton said he had excluded all clamp cases from this reckoning.

Mr. Tait, proceeding, said that he had a series of 137 abdominal sections, in which 48 were done with *extreme* Listerian precautions, and the remainder successively by the elimination, one after another, of these precautions; so that after reducing the strength of the carbolic spray to 1 in 150, he had finally conducted the whole of the process under a spray of water alone! And so far as the temperature went, it had diminished in proportion as the amount of carbolic acid was lowered. In the 48 pure Listerian cases there were 5 deaths; in the 91 "modified" cases, 6 deaths; and he did not know if any better result could be obtained than that. With Listerian precautions the wounds never heal by first intention, but always with formation of pus; and Dr. Savage who practises Listerism, remarked that in his cases the wounds did not heal so well as Mr. Tait's without it. Mr. Tait had had one case in a young woman, from whom he had removed both ovaries—no adhesions—in which the temperature rose to 112°, and remained at that height for forty-eight hours. She recovered perfectly, and there was nothing in the case but carbolic acid poisoning to account for the remarkable rise in temperature. The ice-cap could not be cited as a criterion; he himself had never used it. He once used Dr. Richardson's "collar," invented many years ago; but the case proved fatal, and he never used it again. Success depended more on personal care and experience than on anything else. Mr Thornton had had the great advantage of being associated for many years with Mr. Spencer Wells, and this must be taken into account in comparing his statistics with those of others. He (Mr. Tait) lost nineteen out of his first fifty cases, and he did not think he would have had such a mortality had he had the opportunity of seeing, and assisting at, the operations of so distinguished a master.

Mr. DORAN having examined after death forty-one cases of ovariotomy, found that the kidneys were normal in only seven, and in one of that number death, was due to tetanus, in another to pleurisy. Of the renal disease six were cases of dilatation of ureter and pelvis on one side. The rest exhibited various degrees of subacute and chronic Bright's disease. In many cases there were lesions of other viscera, mostly diagnosed before operation; but the renal disease was nearly always latent; and this fact should be borne in mind before pronouncing on the statistical results of operations by different methods; and until it became possible to ascertain the existence of such disease there must always be room for fallacy in the comparison of such statistics. Albuminuria alone would not contra-indicate operation, for it might be due to pressure, which the operation would relieve. Diminution in the quantity of urea might be due to diminished quantity of food: and sometimes in renal disease there was an excess of urea. Dr. Bantock had remarked upon the diminution of the sulphates as evidence of carbolic acid poisoning. Dr. Parkes has shown that thirty-one grains of sulphuric acid are eliminated by the kidneys in twenty-four hours. After a severe operation the call on the kidneys must be very great, and if they be diseased great risk was added to the patient's chances of recovery.

Mr. SAVORY said that the only point on which there seemed to be agreement, was that as experience increased the mortality diminished. He asked if this did not point to the question being one of the man rather than the method; and did not such a reflection vitiate all conclusions derived from statistics of the first twenty cases compared with the second twenty, and so on?

Mr. SPENCER WELLS would meet Mr. Savory's argument by the experience of the same surgeon in a successive series of years. No doubt the mortality diminished with increasing experience, but after a time the mortality reaches a level below which it will not fall, until the introduction of a new method leads to further improvement in the results. It had so happened with him. At first the mortality gradually fell from 34 per cent. to 28, to 24, and so on, until it reached a level beyond which it did not fall, and the question came whether it was possible to reduce the mortality still lower. This caused him to adopt the antiseptic treatment, and at the beginning of 1878 he commenced to follow Listerian methods. To be sure, the cases in which he applied it were all in private patients, but he had when in hospital practice found no difference in the results of the two classes of patients; nor was it due to the intra-peritoneal method, for before he used antiseptics he had been less successful with this than with the extra-peritoneal. Since adopting Listerism he had had 131 cases, with 13 deaths—a mortality of 10 per cent.; which was precisely the same mortality he had in the last two years of his hospital practice—viz., 7 deaths in 71 cases. These figures alone might be quoted to show there was no advantage gained by Listerism. But there were very real advantages. He was surprised to hear Dr. Bantock, Mr. Tait, and Mr. Thornton find such rises in temperature after Listerian ovariotomies, for he never saw them; it was rare to see the temperature over 100°. The method did not involve trouble—it greatly saved it. Formerly a case had to be closely and personally supervised; but all this trouble and anxiety were saved in treating a case antiseptically. Again, in forty-nine cases out of fifty so treated the wounds heal by first intention; and it was quite a matter of surprise to him to find, as he did lately in a case, any pus in the wound. In that case its appearance was explained by development of boils in other parts of the body. In reply to Mr. Tait, Mr. Wells added that when the pedicle was short he used the ligature in preference to the clamp.

Mr. HOLMES said that after all they had heard that evening from the advocates and opponents of Listerism he was ready to withdraw his former observation that the grounds urged in favour of the method were based only on "impressions"; and he would like to put it to the Society, whether, after these definite details, there were such characteristic differences between cases treated with and without the method, as would be the case were its theory true. Recalling the claims urged for the theory when it was first promulgated, he would ask whether it was at that time thought that 130 cases treated under the theory would show the same result as those treated otherwise? Whether, if one was not told, one would perceive any real essential difference between the cases which were treated on the basis of the germ theory and those without this basis? He was not a partisan of any one method. He had sat at the feet of Lister, and had tried to master the details of his method, which in the early days were far simpler than at present, for they had been so modified that he confessed he did not understand them, and he was sure Mr. Thornton did not understand them, since he attributes his fatal cases to a lack of mastery of these details. Did Mr. Lister himself even understand them? Was the theory itself understandable? When a case is lost, the failure is put down to failure to understand the theory; when a case is saved, then the theory is triumphant. If this were all it came to, and after the method had been so long in use there was still a quarrel as to its advantage in 1 per cent. of the cases, it might fairly be said that the theory was "not proven."

Dr. BANTOCK, in reply, said that the local anæsthesia produced by carbolic acid was well known to him. He quoted from a paper written by Mr. Thornton to show that that gentleman attributed two deaths from pleurisy to the chilling produced by the spray, and one from suppression of urine to the carbolic acid: and in another paper spoke of extreme congestion of the kidneys as due to carbolic acid. In his own practice he had treated thirty-six cases with true Listerian precautions, with eight deaths, one patient dying on the operating table. With a solution of carbolic acid, 1 in 50, he had treated forty-one cases with a mortality of three; one of these cases was *in extremis* when operated on; another died from acute nephritis, and a third from tetanus, on the eighth day, and apparently independently of the operation. In two of these cases he had used the ice-cap, and he found that in proportion as the strength of the solution was reduced to 1 in 60, 1 in 80, to 1 in 100, the results improved, the ice-cap never being required since he had used the weaker solution. He had had many cases in which there was disease of the kidneys—a most unfavourable condition, owing to the little or no power of elimination. He quoted recent statistics of an Italian surgeon, showing that in his practice ovariotomy with Listerism in 100 cases gave a mortality of 37 per cent., and in a second series of 100 cases without Listerism a mortality of 36 per cent. Mr. Bryant had recently published facts showing that pyrexia in surgical cases was considerably less than supposed, without undue antiseptic precautions being taken. Mr. Spencer Wells had stated in his book that he never used the ligature when the clamp could be used, and it was not therefore surprising that the ligature should compare unfavourably with the clamp. The merit of using a solution of carbolic acid of 1 per cent. strength lay in its not causing hyperpyrexia; he had not once to use the ice-cap in cases treated with this solution, and out of twenty-nine cases had lost eight, two deaths being from shock. The great point was strict attention to cleanliness, and in this respect the modern practice differed from that formerly in vogue. Mr. Heath was the first to put this principle into practice, and combined with free drainage, found that Listerism did not add to the measures, although it added to the risk of subsequent pyrexia. The dread of injuring the peritoneum had disappeared before Listerism was taught, for it was shown that fever decreased in proportion as effectual drainage was practised, and the causes of irritation of the peritoneum avoided. Patients still died even under the strictest Listerism. He would not follow Galezowski, who said that since he had used antiseptics (!)—viz., solution of carbolic acid of 1 in 1000—his operations on the eye were markedly successful; and, whilst according full measure of praise to Mr. Lister's teaching, he could not admit the truth of those exaggerated pretensions claimed for his method by his disciples with a zeal which outran discretion.—*Lancet*, Dec. 18, 1880.

Medical Jurisprudence and Toxicology.

The Law of Slander as Applicable to Physicians.

The importance of a clear understanding of this subject to the practising physician is so great that we feel justified in reproducing, from the *American Law Register* (August, 1880), the following paper on the subject from the pen of Mr. W. H. WHITAKER, of Cincinnati:—

There is, perhaps, no class of professional men more subject to abuse, and, it is believed, more powerless to obtain redress, than physicians. About clergymen the law has thrown its protecting arm, and public opinion has been wont to overlook, if not to pardon, their short-comings. The clergyman is a sort of privileged person, whose character is tried before and whose conduct is regulated by ecclesiastical tribunals to which the courts of law have relegated it. Lawyers can take care of themselves.

For alleged professional misconduct, incapacity, or ignorance, for rumored unskilful treatment of diseases, physicians who choose may have recourse to legal proceedings. But to cowhide the editor or sue the newspaper for the circulation of a libel, may be said in either case to be social suicide. The physician must grin and bear it. But if he braves public opinion and asserts his rights, if he endeavours to obtain satisfaction at law, the chances are, to say the least, uncertain. It is doubtful, as the law now stands, what charges of misconduct in a physician in a *single* instance are actionable. One court (*Camp v. Martin*, 23 Conn. 86) has held that words spoken of a physician, charging him *merely* with ignorance or misconduct in the treatment of a particular case, were not actionable *per se*. The words were, "If Dr. C. had continued to treat her, she would have been in her grave before this time. His treatment of her was rascally."

Another court (*Secor v. Harris*, 18 Barb. 425) has adopted a contrary view in a similar case, where the words were: "Dr. S. killed my children. He gave them teaspoon doses of calomel: it killed them; they died right off, the same day." This last is no doubt a more aggravated case, but it is difficult to understand the grounds upon which the principle was distinguished in the two cases. The court said in the last instance that in the rendition of its judgment it was borne out by the authorities, while in the first case the court was equally confident, after having examined the authorities, that none could be found analogous to the case at bar, to justify an action for damages *per se*. Both, however, united on one case (*Sumner v. Utley*, 7 Conn. 257), as being in point, and it is amusing to observe what different constructions the two opposing tribunals gave to a case which must certainly have decided one way or the other. The Connecticut court said it thought that the case referred to, so far from varying the rule as they had given it, intended to sanction it, and quoted at length from C. J. HOSMER, as follows: "I readily admit that falsehood may be spoken of a physician's practice in a particular case, ascribing to him only such want of information and good management as is compatible with general knowledge and skill in his profession, and that when such a case arises, unless some special damage exists, his character will be considered as unhurt and no damages will be presumed. But, on the other hand, it is indisputable that a calumnious report in a particular case may imply gross ignorance and unskilfulness, and do him irreparable damage. A physician may mistake the symptoms of a patient, or may misjudge as to the nature of his disease and even as to the power of the medicine, and yet his error may be of that pardonable kind that will do him no essential prejudice, because it is rather a proof of human imperfection than of culpable ignorance or unskilfulness. On the contrary, a single act of his may evidence gross ignorance and such a deficiency of skill as will not fail to injure his reputation and deprive him of general confidence."

Now the New York court, on the other hand, said that the doctrine laid down in the cases of *Poe v. Mondford*, Cro. Eliz. 620, and *Foot v. Brown*, 8 Johns. 64, both of which were adopted as authorities by the Connecticut court, had been repudiated. In the former, defendant charged plaintiff with having killed a patient with physic, and it was held that the words were not actionable *per se*, and that the law only gave an action for words affecting a man's credit in his profession, as charging him with ignorance or want of skill in general. In the latter the words were spoken of an attorney: "F. knows nothing about the suit, he will lead you on until he has undone you;" and it was held, on the authority of the former, that, no special damage being shown, the action would not lie. Rejecting these two cases as unauthoritative, the New York court also quoted from the case of *Sumner* v. *Utley, supra,* as follows: "As a general principle it can never be admitted that the practice of a physician in a particular case may be calumniated with impunity unless special damage is shown. By confining the slander to particulars, a man may thus be ruined in detail. A calumniator might follow the track of the plaintiff and begin by falsely ascribing to the physician the killing of three persons by mismanagement, and then the mistaking of an artery for a vein, and thus might proceed to misrepresent every single case of his practice until his reputation should be blasted beyond remedy. Instead of murdering character by one stroke, the victim would be successively cut in pieces, and the only difference would be in the manner of effecting the same result."

It is good to beat your adversary with his own weapons, and while the case of *Sumner* v. *Utley,* decided in effect that slanderous words spoken of a physician were actionable *per se,* the court in *Camp* v. *Martin, supra,* notwithstanding, drew a favourable conclusion for holding that in its case slanderous words were *not* actionable *per se.* It is true that the case of *Sumner* v. *Utley* was somewhat stronger than either of the other two, and may have furnished grounds for the distinction that was drawn between gross ignorance in a single instance, and gross ignorance generally in the treatment of diseases, but there seems to us to be little, if any, difference between a case where the words were that a doctor killed his patient, and one where they alleged that if he had continued to treat the patient she would have been dead by this time, so far as the presumption of incapacity is concerned. In *Sumner* v. *Utley* the words imputed gross ignorance generally and particularly. The defendant said of the physician: "He has killed three and ought to be hung—damn him. They all died through his mismanagement. I have understood that he left an after-birth, and the man that would do that ought to be hung;" and on another occasion, addressing himself to Mrs. H., who had employed plaintiff as her physician, said: "He was the means of her sickness by cutting an artery in her head—damn him; you ought not to pay him a cent; if Mr. H. had taken him up for it, it would have cost him $400. It ought to be put in the newspapers." The rule may be said to be as Chief Justice Hosmer put it, though it does not appear to be very clear: "This then is the correct principle, that the misrepresentation of a physician's practice in a particular case, if it does not warrant the presumption of damage is not actionable, unless special damages are averred and proved; but if from the nature of the calumny damages are inferable, the words are actionable."

The question still remains, when do the misrepresentations of a physician's practice in a particular case warrant the presumption of damage? It is allowed that slanderous words alleging gross ignorance generally, or such ignorance or thorough incapacity as unfits him for the proper exercise of his profession, are actionable *per se.* To say of a physician that "He is a quack" (*Pickford* v. *Gutch,* Dorchester Assizes, 1787); or "He is an empiric and a mountebank" (Vin. Abr. Act. for Words, S. a. 12); or "He is a quack; if he shows you a diploma it is a forgery". (*Moises* v. *Thornton,* 8 Term Rep. 303); or "He is no doctor; he bought his diploma for $50" (*Bergold* v. *Puchta,* 2 Thomp. & C. (N. Y.) 532); or "He is a drunken fool and an ass, and never was a scholar". (*Cawdry* v. *Tetley,* Godb. 441); or "He has killed six children in one year" (*Carroll* v. *White,* 33 Barb. 615); or "It is a world of blood that he has to answer for in this town through his ignorance. He was the death of J. P. He killed his patient with physic" (*Tutty* v. *Alewin*, 11 Mod. 221); or "I wonder you had him to attend you. Do you know him? He is not an apothecary; he has not passed any examination. He is a bad character; none of the medical men here will meet him. Several have died that he has attended to, and there have been inquests held upon them" (*Southee* v. *Denny*, 1 Ex. 196). In all these cases it has been held that damages are inferable without proof; but to say of a physician, "He is so steady drunk that he cannot get business any more" (1 Ohio, 83, n.); or "He is a two-penny bleeder" (*Foster* v. *Small*, 3 Whart. 138); or to charge an allopathic physician with having met homœopathists in consultation, and that in the opinion of the profession it was improper to do so and against etiquette, and, further, that in the opinion of the profession it was disgraceful to meet a homœopathic in consultation (*Clay* v. *Roberts*, 8 L. T. N. S. 397); or to charge him with adultery not necessarily touching him in his profession without showing that it was connected with his profession (*Ayre* v. *Craven*, 2 Ad. & E. 2), have been held not actionable *per se*.

While the authorities are generally agreed as to charges of gross ignorance or incapacity in the exercise of the duties of the physician, it is not easy to determine what words are actionable in themselves in special instances. In analogous, and even in precisely similar, cases, the courts are divided. Where the words were: "He killed my child; it was the saline injection that did it" (*Edsall* v. *Russell*, 4 M. & G. 1090); or "He has killed my child by giving it too much calomel" (*Johnson* v. *Robertson*, 8 Porter, 486), they have been held actionable *per se*. And, on the contrary, the words, "He has killed his patient with physic" (*Poe* v. *Mondford*, *supra*), or "In my opinion, the bitters A fixed for B were the cause of his death" (*Jones* v. *Diver*, 22 Ind. 184), or "He gave my child too much mercury, or he made the medicines wrong through jealousy, because I would not allow him to use his own judgment" (*Edsall* v. *Russell*, *supra*), have been held not actionable in themselves.

In the examination of these cases, it will be found that where the physician is charged with killing his patient, the words have been held actionable on account of the imputation of crime which they import, and the only case in which such language has been held not actionable, is that of *Poe* v. *Mondford*, of an early origin. This case was rejected by the court in *Secor* v. *Harris*, on the ground that it was decided at a time when the doctrine of *mitior sensus* prevailed. And as for the case of *Jones* v. *Diver*, the court held that the words were not actionable, because they did not import a charge of murder; that if the defendant had said that "the bitters Dr. D. gave John Smith caused his death; there was enough poison in them to kill ten men," he would have been held guilty of the charge, and the words would have then been actionable.

How such words necessarily import the crime of murder or manslaughter, in the absence of any expression of intention, is not quite clear. This was not the ground of the decision in a case of a non-professional, charged with having destroyed the life of a patient by mistaken, but well-meant, efforts to save his life (*March* v. *Davison*, 9 Paige (N. Y.), 580). But even if the words do not import the charge of crime or of gross incapacity generally, there seems to be reason for holding that they should be actionable. It is true, as was said in a former case, that a physician might make a mistake in his treatment of a disease, because it was rather a proof of human imperfection than of culpable ignorance, but the consequences are often as fatal to him as though the charge was a general one. His mistake might be of "that pardonable kind" which would do him no injury in his profession, but the public might not pardon it. And what if he is not guilty of the charge? What if he has done his duty towards his patient, and has adopted every means in his power, and such as were recognized in the profession as suitable for the case, to restore him to health? The consequences, so far as the public are concerned, are the same, with the additional mental suffering which every man must undergo whose conduct and whose actions are grossly misrepresented before the community at large. True, the law does not deny him his remedy, if he chooses to take it. Perhaps it would be more fatal to resort to legal proceedings in any case. If he does, he is compelled to show special damages, for none will be inferred. This alone would cause many to hesitate before bringing an action. The difficulty attendant upon proving damages, the length of time intervening between the publication and the consequences of a slander, would deter many from the prosecution of the slander.

As the cases now stand, you may bring almost any charge of misconduct against a physician in a particular case, without subjecting yourself to an action for damages *per se*, provided it does not come within the category of a statutory crime, or impute to him general incapacity.

—

On the Elimination of Lead by Iodide of Potassium.

At the instance of Prof. Vulpian, M. POUCHET has examined quantitatively the urine of patients suffering from saturnism, in order to estimate the effect of the administration of the iodide of potassium on the elimination of lead (*Archives de Physiologie Normale et Pathologique*, 1880). The methods were electrolytic. The quantities of urine examined always measured from five to ten pints, quantities sufficiently large to permit the detection of even the smallest traces of lead. During the period of aggravated symptoms, the urine contained an average of one milligramme of metallic lead to the litre of urine examined. Under the influence of iodide of potassium in doses of from four to six grammes daily, the elimination of lead increased quickly, but again decreased at the end of from six to ten days, when it became less marked than before the treatment was instituted. During the first days of treatment there occurred a rapid desaturation of the system, which was more or less decided according to the intensity of the morbid phenomena. Thus, in the case of a patient who was gravely affected, the quantity of lead passed by the urine, immediately after the administration of the iodide, rose to five milligrammes per litre. After the continuous administration of the salt for more than two weeks, the elimination of lead ceased almost altogether, so that in fifteen litres of urine only a trace of lead was discernible. But when, after withdrawing the remedy, the patient was allowed to rest some days, prior to the readministration of the iodide, small quantities of lead were again eliminated with the urine. Hence arises the therapeutic indication of employing the iodides for a long time, instituting, however, intervals of repose, during which the remedy is not to be administered. M. Pouchet also analyzed the urine of a patient treated exclusively with the bromide of potassium without detecting any increase of the lead eliminated. From this, he deduces the inefficiency of bromide in the treatment of lead-poisoning.—*London Med. Record*, Nov. 15, 1880.

MEDICAL NEWS.

Food Adulterations.

Some recent and valuable researches in regard to the intentional and accidental impurities in our various articles of diet, become especially interesting when we remember that a healthy adult male takes into his stomach during every year, on the average, about four hundred pounds of meat, five hundred pounds of bread, three hundred pounds of potatoes and other vegetables, ninety pounds of butter and fats, and one hundred and fifty gallons of tea, coffee, and water; because obviously in this large quantity of nutriment, impurities or adulterations to the extent of a single grain to the pound might eventuate in the introduction of an absolutely large amount of poisonous material into the human organism.

Foremost among these investigations are to be ranked those of Dr. Charles Smart, U. S. A., undertaken under the direction of the National Board of Health, and reported in the Supplement No. 11 of its valuable *Bulletin*. From a purely sanitary point of view, Dr. Smart's experiments are quite reassuring, since they demonstrate that with such exceptions as the use of alum in bread and baking powders, of sulphate of lime in the sophistication of creamor tartar, of water in the dilution of milk, and of the injurious colouring matters entering into certain kinds of confectionery, prevalent adulterations affect the pocket of the consumer rather than his health, and cannot therefore be characterized as deleterious, but only as fraudulent. Dr. Smart's conclusions are based upon the examination of 713 samples, of which 304 were obtained from sources (such as the proprietors of first class stores, who knew their goods were to be tested, from the Commissary-General of the Army, etc.) where their purity was probable, and 409 were specimens the origin of which might be considered suspicious. Of the former of these two groups about 8 per cent. were impure, whilst of the latter nearly 45 per cent. were so far sophisticated, that under a law similar to that enforced in Great Britain, for the punishment of fraudulent adulteration, the dealers from whom they were derived might have been prosecuted with a fair prospect of success. As pointed out, these percentages give us no exact idea of the prevalence of food adulteration, since of certain articles, such as lard and corn meal, which were found to be genuine, but few specimens were tested, whilst had the examinations of classes of articles such as the ground spices, which are seldom unadulterated, been more numerous, the proportion of impure articles of food in our markets would be represented as much greater.

In illustration of the details of these useful researches, it may be mentioned that 109 specimens of imported teas were examined, 90 of these
being presumably pure and 19 from suspicious sources. In no case was
any leaf met with which was not derived from the tea plant, and of the
90 samples in the first group all were approved, although 5 of the 19 from
suspected origins were found to be so deteriorated that an analyst would
be warranted in reporting them as fraudulently dealt with. The mixture
of glucose with brown sugar appears to be not infrequent, as out of 38
samples purchased for examination, nine were adulterated with glucose,
which, although not injurious, has an economic value inferior to that of
cane sugar. As our author suggests, glucose properly prepared from
starch, and sold under its own name, at the low rate for which it could
be furnished, would be a great blessing to the poor, who now use large
quantities of it, in the sophisticated cane sugar, for which they pay an
unreasonable price. Creamor tartar, which is important in this connection, on account of its extended use in culinary processes, was found to
be largely adulterated, only 6 out of 18 specimens examined being of
satisfactory purity. Eleven of these samples contained sulphate of lime
in quantities varying from 17 to 90 per cent., and two mixtures consisted
of sulphate of lime and phosphate of lime, alum, and starch, without a
trace of the tartaric acid salt. The results in regard to spices of various
kinds were lamentably unfavourable; for example only 1 out of 26 samples
of ground cinnamon was found to be pure, the adulterations in the remainder
being powdered corn, wheat, beans, allspice, almond-shells, and turmeric;
two out of 18 specimens of ground cayenne pepper, were met with of
satisfactory purity, the only gratifying point respecting the 16 fraudulent
mixtures, being that they contained no red lead, reported by Dr. Hassall
some years ago, as occurring in nearly half the English red pepper.
Mustard, which is even more important as a medicinal agent, was almost
equally unreliable, only 6 out of 17 samples being honest in their character,
the fraudulent admixtures being chiefly wheat flour, or starch, and turmeric,
although corn starch, rice, cayenne pepper, and sulphate of lime were also
used. Almost the sole really poisonous adulteration detected was that observed in the yellow coloured confectionery, which was found to be tinted
in 3 out of 5 instances with pigment containing lead. In one of the remaining samples the yellow material was composed of antimony, and in the other
of turmeric. These results confirm the more extended series of observations made by H. B. Hill of Harvard College, who reports that 19 out of
21 yellow, and 11 out of 12 orange candies, contained lead. Dr. Smart
found that 13 specimens of red confectionery owed their tint to cochineal,
and were therefore unobjectionable on the score of their colouring material.

Dr. Smart concludes, from his investigations, that food adulteration is
now practised in this country to as great or even a greater extent than it

was in England when an effort was first made, some twenty-five years ago, to suppress this fraudulent and dangerous practice by stringent legal measures. The corn meal and lard we obtain, as well as our wheat flour, are pure, although bakers introduce alum into our bread. Sugars are less commonly sanded than formerly, but adulteration with glucose is becoming increasingly frequent. Thanks to our American fashion of grinding coffee at home, this important beverage may generally be secured pure, but our spices are very generally sophisticated, and some kinds of confectionery, especially those of a yellow or orange colour, are so apt to be poisonous that they should be studiously avoided.

The dangers to health arising from unsound and infected meat, such as of trichiniasis from diseased pork, and of phthisis from tuberculous beef and milk, etc., call for prompt and earnest consideration, which, however, must be reserved for some future occasion.

—

Listerism in Paris.—One of the most thorough disciples of Listerism in Paris— where the antiseptic method, slow to take root, is now the subject of an ardent and convinced propaganda—is M. Richelot, Professor *agrégé* of the Faculty of Paris. M. Richelot took the place of M. Richet at the Hôtel-Dieu, during a three months' holiday of the latter. The remarkable successes which he achieved were the subject of much observation, and produced a great impression on those who were able to contrast his results with the surrounding state of things. M. Richelot has published a *Note sur les resultats du pansement de Lister*, which is very interesting and satisfactory.—*British Med. Journal*, Nov. 27, 1880.

—

Deaths from Chloroform.—A writer in a recent number of the *Lancet* (November 6, 1880) states that during the past twelve months no less than twenty-five deaths from chloroform have been reported, and in comment says, "It is not for me to say that a grave responsibility rests on the surgeon who employs chloroform when a safer anæsthetic is available, but I think it cannot be long before the voice of the profession (if not of the public, as in America) demands some explanation for the use of an agent whose victims are numbered by hundreds."

—

Sheep's Tallow for Carbolic Acid Ointments.—HERR NUELCK, a Berlin apothecary, recommends, in the *Berliner Klinische Wochenschrift*, No. 30, the substitution of sheep's tallow for the ordinarily used oils as a menstruum for diluting and applying carbolic acid. Sheep's tallow has a much higher melting point than lard or oils; and thus remains as a soft, bland, and consistent salve, when the heat of the skin would melt the usual ointments, and convert them into flowing and irritating fluids. He gives formulæ for preparations and dressings made with carbolic sheep's tallow.—*British Med. Journal*, Dec. 18, 1880.

—

The Gross Surgical Prize.—The Philadelphia Academy of Surgery offers through its President, Dr. S. D. Gross, a Prize of Five Hundred Dollars for the best Essay on the Surgical Pathology, and Treatment of Tumours or Morbid Growths of the Testis, Scrotum, and Spermatic Cord, to be open exclusively to American Surgeons.

1. The Essay must be founded solely upon original investigations, be illustrated by suitable drawings, microscopical, and other, and be written in scholarly English.

2. The Essay must comprise an amount of matter equal to 250 pages octavo.

3. It shall be the property of the Academy, which shall, at its option, permit the author to publish it at his own risk or expense.

4. Each Essay must be accompanied by a motto, and by a sealed letter containing the author's name.

5. The award will be made at the meeting of the Academy in January, 1884, by a committee of five of its Fellows, consisting of D. Hayes Agnew, M.D., Wm. Hunt, M.D., R. J. Levis, M.D., John H. Packard, M.D., and J. Ewing Mears, M.D., Secretary, 1429 Walnut St., Phila.

Essays should be forwarded to the Secretary of the committee on or before October·15, 1883.

———

University of Pennsylvania.—Dr. William Pepper, Professor of Clinical Medicine, was, on the 12th ult:, elected Provost of the University. The duties of the Provost were at the same time modified, and the supervisory and disciplinary functions of the Vice Provost and Deans of the various faculties were enlarged. We understand that the Trustees are desirous of having the University's needs actively brought to the attention of the public; and it is believed that Dr. Pepper's well-known energy and executive ability will largely conduce to this end.

Mr. Henry C. Gibson, of this city, with great liberality has offered the University Hospital to erect at his own expense a new wing for incurables, with accommodation for one hundred beds. The plans are now in preparation, and a permanent endowment fund for the support of the ward is being raised.

———

Bequest to Yale Medical College.—The late Dr. David P. Smith, Professor of Medicine in the Medical School of Yale, bequeathed his medical library, instruments, and two-fifths of his estate to Yale Medical College. The pecuniary bequest is for the endowment of the chair of Theory and Practice of Medicine.

———

Midwifery in Cincinnati.—It is stated that seventy per cent. of the labour cases in Cincinnati are delivered by midwives, who are for the most part ignorant and uneducated.

———

The Library of the College of Physicians of Philadelphia.—The annual report states that this library now contains 23,288 volumes, an increase of 1259 in the past year. We regret to learn that ill health has compelled Dr. Robert Bridges to resign the office of Librarian, which he has held for many years.

———

Library of the New York Academy of Medicine.—At the annual meeting of the Academy, in January, it was reported that the library contains over 17,000 volumes, and is in receipt of 122 current American and European medical journals. Mr. John Jacob Astor has recently given $500 for the improvement of the journal and circulating department of the library.

———

New York State Medical Society.—This Society will hold its annual meeting at Albany on the first day of February.

International Medical Congress, London, 1881.—The following subjects, in addition to those announced in our last number, have been proposed for discussion.

Section VIII. (*Mental Diseases*).—Anatomy: 1. Modes of Preparation of Nervous Tissues; 2. Morbid Appearances due to Modes of Preparation; 3. Minute Structure of Special Parts of Brain. Physiology: 1. Relation of Cerebral Localization to Mental Symptoms, as Hallucinations; 2. Hypnotism. Pathology: 1. Of Idiocy, Morphological and Histological Changes; 2. Relations of Insanity to Gout, Renal Disease, Exophthalmic Goître, and to Coarse Brain Disease. Clinical: 1. "Folie à Double Forme"; 2. Influence of Intercurrent Diseases on Insanity; 3. Insanity due to Toxic Agents. Therapeutical: 1. Use of Baths, of Narcotics, of Chloral Hydrate, of Opium, and of Alcohol; 2. New and Unusual Remedies. Asylum Administration: 1. Cottage and Village Treatment; 2. New Legal Codes—Austrian, Italian, English Projects. Civil Relations of the Insane: 1. Marriage, Wills; 2. Insanity and Aphasia. Criminal Relations of the Insane: Special Asylums for Insane Criminals.

Section XIV. (*Military Surgery and Medicine*).—1. By what arrangement can the practical difficulties in the way of employing antiseptic surgery (Listerism) in the treatment of wounds inflicted in the field in time of war be most readily overcome? [The discussion to include (*a*) the system on which the treatment can be most efficiently carried out; and (*b*) the fittest material means to be employed in it, under the circumstances in which armies are placed while on actual service.] 2 To what extent, and in what special directions, has conservative surgery advanced in field practice, as shown by statistical results of the treatment adopted for gunshot wounds during the wars of the last ten years? and what indications have been afforded, if any, by the experience gained during this period for making further advances in the conservative treatment of such injuries? 3. What are the most reliable, and at the same time practicable, means of immobilizing the parts involved in gunshot fractures of the Spine, Pelvis, and Femur in field practice? 4. On improvements in field hospital and transport equipment, for use with armies moving in uncivilized or partially civilized countries, suggested by the experience gained during the recent military operations by British troops in South Africa. 5. On the prevalence and prevention of Typhoid Fever among young soldiers in India.

—

International Exhibition of Hygiene.—It is proposed to hold during the International Medical Congress at London, an exhibition at South Kensington of sanitary and medical apparatus, under the auspices of the Executive Committee of the Parkes Museum of Hygiene. It is intended that the scope of the exhibition shall be broad, and all branches of sanitation will be included. In addition to sanitary apparatus there will be classes devoted to the exhibition of: 1, hospital construction and arrangement; 2, surgical instruments and apparatus; 3, appliances of the ward and sick-room; 4, drugs, disinfectants, and medical dietetic articles; 5, electrical and optical apparatus; 6, microscopes and other apparatus used in the investigation and relief of disease; 7, appliances used for the treatment of sick and wounded in time of war.

—

Allgemeine Wiener Medizinische Zeitung.—At the close of December, Dr. B. Kraus celebrated the "twenty-five years jubilee" of this able journal, of which he has been the editor since its foundation. With the offer of our congratulations on the occasion we couple the hope that many years of prosperity and usefulness may await the journal and its learned editor.

Professor Milne-Edwards.—The *Revue Scientifique* publishes the following notice : "Professor MILNE-EDWARDS, having recently completed his 'Leçons sur la Physiologie et l'Anatomie Comparée de l'Homme et des Animaux,' a committee has been formed to present a public testimonial of gratitude to the acknowledged master who, after more than half a century of personal research, has summed up in this work the past and present of the zoological sciences. The intention of the committee is to strike a medal bearing the effigy of M. Milne-Edwards, and, convinced that in every country there will be found men happy to associate themselves with this manifestation, it appeals with this object to foreign as well as to French *savants.* The committee is composed of M. Dumas, perpetual secretary of the Academy of Sciences; the members of the Zoological Section of the Academy ; all the professors of zoology, anatomy, and physiology of the great establishments of public instruction in Paris ; and M. Masson, the publisher of M. Milne-Edwards' works. Subscriptions and lists of subscribers may be forwarded to M. Maindron, at the Secretary's Office of the Institute, Paris." —*Med. Times and Gazette*, Dec. 4, 1880.

Literary Notes.

Messrs. J. B. Lippincott & Co. have just published Dr. H. C. Wood's Smithsonian Contribution on the Study of Fever.

Mr. H. K. Lewis has recently issued "Elements of Practical Medicine" by Dr. Alfred H. Carter, Physician to the Queen's Hospital, Birmingham, and a "German-English Dictionary of the Medical Sciences" by Dr. Fancourt Barnes.

Mr. David Bogue, of London, announces a translation of Fournier's lectures on "Syphilis and Marriage."

Among new journals we notice *Archives d'Ophthalmologie,* edited by Prof. Panas and Drs. Landolt and Panas, which promises to become the leading Paris journal on its specialty.

The *International Journal of Medicine and Surgery* is a weekly published in New York, and devoted to translations of abstracts of articles appearing in Continental journals.

L'Encephale is a forthcoming serial on mental and nervous diseases, to be edited by Prof. Ball and Dr. Luys.

The Annals of the "Anatomical and Surgical Society," of Brooklyn, has met with such deserved success that its editors feel themselves justified in increasing its size and widening its scope. It will be hereafter known as the *Annals of Anatomy and Surgery.* The journal has been conspicuous for the excellence of its original matter, the ability of its editorial management, and the attractiveness of its typographical appearance, and in its enlarged form we have no doubt its field of usefulness will be increased.

The English *Publishers' Catalogue* contains an analytical table of the books published during the past year, from which it appears that during 1880 medical and surgical literature has been enriched by the addition of 202 volumes (54 being new editions), as compared with 189 (53 new editions) in 1879. It is interesting to observe that of the fourteen sections into which the subjects of the books are divided, in point of number of works issued, only three, viz., those of "Law, Jurisprudence, etc.," "Poetry and the Drama," and "Belles Lettres, Essays, etc.," fall below that of "Medicine and Surgery."

To Readers and Correspondents.—*The editor will be happy to receive early intelligence of local events of general medical interest, or which it is desirable to bring to the notice of the profession. Local papers containing reports or news items should be marked.*

CONTENTS OF NUMBER 459.

MARCH, 1881.

CLINICS.

CLINICAL LECTURES.

HOSPITAL NOTES.

MONTHLY ABSTRACT.

ANATOMY AND PHYSIOLOGY.

MATERIA MEDICA AND THERAPEUTICS.

MEDICINE.

Vol. XXXIX.—9

MEDICAL NEWS.

CLINICS.

Clinical Lectures.

ACUTE TRICHINIASIS, MARKED BY CONTINUOUS FEVER AND SEVERE MUSCULAR SYMPTOMS.

A CLINICAL LECTURE DELIVERED AT THE PENNSYLVANIA HOSPITAL,

By J. M. Da COSTA, M.D.,

PROFESSOR OF PRACTICE OF MEDICINE IN JEFFERSON MEDICAL COLLEGE, AND PHYSICIAN TO THE PENNSYLVANIA HOSPITAL.

[Reported by Frank Woodbury, M.D.]

GENTLEMEN: The case now before you is a striking one from more than one point of view. It presents a typical illustration of a disease which I have rarely had the opportunity of presenting before the class. It is interesting in its causation and the question of possible prevention. It is instructive in the accuracy of which the diagnosis admits.

In narrating the history of the case I shall tell you particularly of the condition of the patient when he entered the hospital, for it was a little different then from his present state. His name is Richard E.; he is a German, 20 years of age, a machinist by occupation. He stated positively that he had always been in very good health up to the beginning of his present illness. For a week or two before admission into the hospital, which was on the 7th of December, he suffered from cold in going to and returning from his work. But as he had no underclothing and only wore his overcoat on Sundays, it might be naturally supposed that want of proper clothing was the cause of the chilliness. However this may be, he says that about four days before admission, and following the chilliness of which he complained, he had headache and muscular soreness; he was also very restless, the skin was covered with perspiration, his extremities were cold. This discomfort increased rapidly, became attended by fever, loss of appetite, and constipation; on the day before he came here he had a spell of vomiting. There had been no convulsions, no active delirium, and no signs of brain disorder beyond a dull headache, with confusion of ideas. Now it was in this state that he sought admission into the hospital. When I saw him I was much struck with the appearance of his face. It was flushed, and had a bloated look; the fulness was not confined to the eyelids, but was general, diffused, and had changed the expression of the entire face. His eyes were clear, the pupils rather dilated. He was, when I met him, wandering in an aimless sort of way at the hospital gate. His face gave me the impression that he was a case of typhoid or rather of typhus fever, though it was not so deeply flushed as we find it in this complaint. His joints were not affected; they were not markedly swollen and certainly were not discoloured, nor were they the seat of special heat or pain. He persisted, however, in calling our attention to the general muscular aching, the stiffness, and the tenderness, at least so far as he spoke of anything, for he was very dull in his mind. Though he was stupid, he was at the same time extremely restless; the muscular soreness was so great that he could not rest, and he did not seem to be able to make himself comfortable in any position. His tongue was red and slightly coated; the breath very fetid; the abdomen swollen; the feet were also a little swollen, but there was no pitting upon pressure. The general surface seemed more or less bloated and pale, there was no eruption of any kind. The urine was of the specific gravity of 1026, acid in its reaction, and contained an excess of urea and of urates, but neither albumen nor sugar. He had a temperature of 104° in the axilla; his bowels had been constipated for several days. He was purged with castor oil, he had quinia given to him, and subsequently muriatic acid, and various means were tried to relieve the muscular soreness. The redness of face soon passed off, and it became pallid and looked swollen; but it did not remain so, the puffiness disappeared in a few days. A slight œdema of the lower extremities, shown especially by the pitting on pressure at both ankles, also passed off in a few days.

The tongue, as you see, has remained red; his appetite is better, indeed it is very good; the fetor of the breath has measurably disappeared; he still complains greatly of the muscular pains. All this time he has had a fever temperature; in the first six or seven days after admission it did not pass below 101°, and ranged between this point and 104°.

Abdominal soreness he has not got. There is some tenderness in the muscular wall, especially is this noticed in the chest, and there is soreness too in the muscles of the extremities, though by no means so much as it was some time since. The respirations have never exceeded twenty-six in the minute, have been more generally twenty-two, and regular. The heart sounds are distinct, evidently no valvular lesion exists, but towards the left base can be found a faint anæmic murmur. The respiratory murmur is everywhere well heard. Now, what is the matter with the patient? Is it muscular rheumatism? Dengue, or breakbone fever? Is it typhoid fever? We concluded that it was not a case of muscular rheumatism, not breakbone fever, and not typhoid. The muscular rheumatism view had a good deal in its favour; his exposure to cold and his insufficient clothing, the great muscular soreness, the chills. But I could not account in this view for the continued fever, the stupor, the expressionless bloated face. The view of typhoid or typhus fever had much to commend it; the continuous character of the fever, with only slight remissions in the morning, his nervous symptoms, his flushed, pallid face, all looked like a low fever. The absence of enteric symptoms was against typhoid but not against typhus; but the absence of eruption was strongly against typhus. Dengue, not being a disease of this time of the year, and not belonging to this latitude, I need not discuss; the symptoms, moreover, appeared too grave for it.

If not any of these affections, what was it? It occurred to me that it was a case of trichiniasis, a disease produced by the introduction into the system of the trichina spiralis in immense numbers, from partaking of ham, sausage, and other forms of infected pork.   The view of trichiniasis gained upon me, I may say upon all of us, for these reasons.   Trichiniasis gives rise to a fever that is very similar to that of typhoid fever; we have, in this case, you remember, a low form of continued fever.   What also arrested my attention was this: the face looked stupid, swollen, flushed, and then pallid; without there being any albumen in the urine, and the swelling passed off in a few days.   This also belongs to the history of acute trichiniasis; this swelling particularly is characteristic, and in most cases is even more decided than in this one before you.   But, above all was the great muscular soreness which I was unable to account for as a symptom of continued fever.   Nor could it be accounted for as a muscular rheumatism; because the sustained temperature was not that of rheumatism as it occurs in the muscular system, nor in rheumatism do we find the entire muscular system involved, but rather the pain and tenderness limited, especially to certain groups of muscles.   Therefore, having all this in mind, I diagnosticated trichiniasis.   I put the diagnosis to the test, and after some delay, occasioned by attempts to procure instruments for examining muscles—which were found not to work—we etherized the patient, and cut out a small piece of his deltoid muscle.   Placing it under the microscope, it was found swarming with living and most active trichinæ.

We have then here a case of trichiniasis; and I have told you by what steps we arrived at the diagnosis, which was finally confirmed by the actual inspection of the muscles.   You see that it was chiefly reached by exclusion; although there were, as I shall presently explain to you, one or two features in the case, in themselves of direct significance.

But has this patient had all the features of acute trichiniasis?   No; a number were wanting, others indistinct.   In acute trichiniasis from the introduction into the stomach of infected pork, we have generally much more marked symptoms of gastro-intestinal irritation than were here presented; the parasites in the stomach and bowels occasion them.   He had great fetor of breath, and vomiting on the day before admission; but only on that occasion, and there was no diarrhœa, the intestinal symptoms were absent, loss of appetite in the early stage certainly existed, but he recovered his appetite better and much more quickly than most of the cases do. Again in pointing out to you anomalies of the early stages, let me tell you that he denied being fond of pork, ham, or sausage, said that he rarely ate it, and that there was not a single one of his friends in the boarding house where he lived that had similar symptoms or had complained of any signs of gastro-intestinal irritation.   Generally the history of several persons being stricken at the same time and being seized with cramps, with vomiting, with purging, is a strong element in the diagnosis of this perilous affection.

Looking now at the chief symptoms of the case, we are first struck with the character of the *fever*.   It was essentially a continuous fever; the highest temperature reached was 104°, and though in the first ten days there were at times quite marked differences between morning and evening, the temperature subsequently became more and more uniform.

Here is the record kept from the day of admission, so slight are the variations between morning and evening that we may take it as illustrating the course of an ordinary continued fever of long duration.   With this elevation of temperature he had the accelerated pulse corresponding to the rise of bodily heat. There was indeed little about the continuous fever that would have arrested our attention as being different from any other fever of the type, except the remarkable absence of cerebral symptoms. Apart from the headache which existed, the fever was marked by the want of hebetude and of hallucinations of every kind, the mind at first dull, became brighter and quite clear, although the fever persisted.

Secondly, what arrested our attention in connection with the febrile state was the unusual *appearance of the face*—the features swollen, the face later pallid, but at first the cheeks and forehead flushed—looking like the face of typhus fever, but not associated with any marked dulness of expression of the eye, nor with that hebetude which is so thoroughly characteristic of the physiognomy of typhus.

Now while we are examining this swelling of the face, which, let me add, was a passing symptom, and which subsided leaving for a time moderately swollen eyelids, I will call your attention to the fact that for three or four days, for even a shorter period therefore than the swelling of the face existed, he had some œdema around the ankles, but without a particle of albuminuria. The slight dropsical symptoms were therefore not among the earliest symptoms, nor were they late symptoms, since they were noticed not long after the patient was admitted to the hospital, and I think existed markedly about the middle of the second week of the disease, and swelling of the face occurred prior to this. The œdema did not pass away in consequence of any profuse sweating, for almost throughout absence of sweating has been a remarkable and unusual feature of the case, unusual because profuse sweats are quite common in trichiniasis.

But after all the most striking symptoms of the case were the *muscular symptoms*. The phenomena were those of a most extended muscular rheumatism. The pains affected the muscles all over the body, and were present whether motion was made or not, although they were very much aggravated by motion; the muscles were also nearly everywhere sore to the touch, and some felt swollen. None were contracted, but some were so much affected that certain muscular movements could not be effected; for instance, our patient could not stoop. The muscles responded to the faradic current; the sensibility of the skin over them seemed normal. The muscular symptoms are directly due to the migration of the trichinæ into the muscles, and to the irritation and havoc in the fibrillæ, and to the inflammatory changes in the sarcolemma, by which the capsule that stops their mischievous career is finally formed. Many of the trichinæ we found were very large and very vigorous; indeed, muscular trichinæ are generally large and vigorous; and it is said that they may live or reproduce themselves for years in the muscles of their unwilling possessor.

The muscular symptoms are said not to happen before the tenth day of the disease; but unless we are utterly misinformed here as to the duration of the case, they began to be noticed in the first four or five days of the illness. Let me add, that of the many local means that were tried for the relief of the local distress but one seemed to be of any benefit, and that was a liniment containing about one ounce of chloral to four of camphorated oil. Let me also again impress upon you that attending the muscular symptoms was an amount of prostration and low fever, which was entirely unlike what occurs in ordinary rheumatism; and that, on the other hand, the muscular pains were greatly in excess of any which would happen in a continued fever.

January 15th, 1881. Gentlemen, after the lapse of three weeks, I show

you this patient again; and now it is clear that he is approaching convalescence. Indeed, when you look at the good colour of his lips, his improved general nutrition, the fact that he can perform a number of
movements well, which previously stiffness and pain prevented him from
executing, all demonstrate the correctness of this conclusion. Accepting
it, let us discuss what has become of the trichinæ. Under the treatment of
moderate doses of quinia and of tincture of iron, under good food, and
after the diagnosis of trichiniasis was made, under carbolic acid, under
anodyne liniments, and occasional hypodermics of morphia, the symptoms
have much ameliorated; some of them have passed entirely away. To
what shall we attribute the striking change? I should like to say to the
carbolic acid, but I cannot think it would be a truthful inference. I think
that he would have recovered without it, because improvement had commenced before he began to use it. I believe his recovery was due to a
good constitution, good nursing, and good food, enabling him to withstand
the shock of the mishap until time had brought about certain curative
processes, which I shall presently explain to you.

You will ask me what is the ordinary course of the disease, and is
recovery from trichiniasis the rule? Also, under what plan of treatment
does recovery most often take place? Gentlemen, the course of the disease is very uncertain, being influenced by the accident of the intrusion of
the disease into internal organs impossible to foresee, but the duration of
the disease is generally very protracted, the muscles being affected in
their movements for a long time by the multitudes of trichinæ which
become deposited in their structure. Until the parasites become encysted
or encapsuled in the muscular fibre, more or less irritative fever persists,
the patient begins to recover only when the trichinæ become incarcerated.
Subsequently these living worms, after a certain lapse of time, thus far
undetermined, perish, and their cysts undergo calcareous degeneration, or
it may be that calcareous deposits take place in the capsule, and the parasite becomes choked up with the earthy salts. While this is going on the
fever gradually declines, and the muscular soreness and stiffness are gradually relieved, but the impairment of muscular power is much more permanent. In the present case, you have observed a continuous fever lasting over four weeks, and you see that it is only in the last week that the
temperature has reached the normal. There is a steady decline from the
time of admission; but it did not really descend to the norm until four
days ago. It is a continuous fever, varying slightly from week to week,
and gradually lessening; but for all this it does not reach the healthy
standard until the fifth week, going hand in hand with this process of
encapsuling; which, however, is far from complete, for in a specimen of
muscle just examined we still find some very lively trichinæ. But does
recovery always take place? By no means; of course it does not where
the nervous system is invaded or prominently implicated, or the respiratory muscles attacked, and their functions crippled, or where long-con-
tinned diarrhœa exists. But even in cases such as this, chiefly marked by the
muscular symptoms, and presenting these in a striking degree, the patient
often dies from the universal presence of trichinæ in the muscular system,
and the irritation they cause. Moreover, although this was not here the
case, frequently recovery is impeded or altogether prevented by very
decided coexisting affection of the gastro-intestinal tract, producing long-
continued vomiting and purging. While this renders the diagnosis much
easier, it is a bad thing in point of prognosis, because, in these cases of

gastro-enteric irritation, there is not only an element of additional exhaustion thus acting, but they leave behind them dysentery, diarrhœa, and chronic bowel complaints, or affections of the stomach.

Is recovery complete in those muscular cases where, as here, a cure is apparently obtained? Will this man recover entirely? I think yes. The chances are that every trichina will become encapsuled; I see no reason why this should not occur. At the same time, I will not say that a man in whom exist many millions of trichinæ imbedded in his muscles, as I believe is the case in our patient, would ever be as strong as he was without them. But we may tell him that he will recover completely to all intents and purposes, be fully able to earn his livelihood.

The treatment, as you are aware, was conducted mainly—excepting the carbolic acid—upon the general principle of supporting strength and relieving pain; the great object being to keep up the patient's strength until the parasites became encysted and harmless. But you may inquire, Is there nothing specific to cure trichiniasis by killing the trichinæ? I tried carbolic acid in this patient; but, as I told you, I cannot claim that it was very effectual, because recovery had already begun before it was administered; still it was well borne, and I think the patient improved more rapidly under its administration than before. I shall, in other cases, try it again. It does not disturb the stomach, and on account of its destructive action upon low forms of life, it may, if we can get enough into the system, poison the parasite. Let me add that under the field of the microscope the trichinæ we found live less than a minute on addition of a concentrated solution of carbolic acid.

Benzine, given internally, has been highly recommended for the purpose of their destruction; but the German physicians, who have the greatest opportunities for studying trichiniasis, have abandoned the use of benzine; and so with picric acid, urged for a time as a valuable remedy, it has now entirely fallen into disuse; and calomel, oil of turpentine, and electricity have proved very disappointing. The treatment now followed by several distinguished authorities, consists in giving large doses of glycerine, based upon the observation that when the living trichina is placed in glycerine, it quickly shrivels and dies. We have ourselves tested the matter here, and Dr. Jiminez, the resident physician, found, no matter how active the trichinæ under the microscope, that they perish at once when brought in contact with a drop of glycerine. I would advise you to try glycerine early in a case; at all events it will kill most likely the trichinæ in the stomach and intestine, without being injurious to the patient. Whether it will kill those in the blood and in the muscles is a different question, and I doubt much whether any amount of glycerine given by the mouth will accomplish this. But laying aside the administration of glycerine and of carbolic acid, the main treatment is, I regret to say, nothing better than to support the patient's strength until the encapsuling is accomplished.

Let me say, in conclusion, a few words about the way in which we got at the trichinæ. We had, as I told you, to cut down upon the muscle after etherizing our patient. This, you will admit, is not a pleasant method of diagnosis, but we were obliged to do it; for we found that the ordinary Duchenne trocar, and the harpoon made for the purpose would not work. They fill with blood; they do not extract the muscle. Nor was another appliance, sent by an instrument-maker, more successful. It was very large; a kind of a cross between a bullet extractor and an obstetrical forceps. Dr. R. N. Hart, one of the resident surgeons of this hospital, then came to our assistance, and has invented an ingenious instrument for the object of extracting muscle for microscopical examination, which promises to be very valuable. I here show you the instrument, which we have now used several times with great ease, and which I shall describe to you in Dr. Hart's own words.

The instrument consists of a small trocar and canula, with a supplementary trocar bearing a peculiar-shaped point (see fig.), the object of which is to secure and remove a small portion of animal tissue for examination. After the plain trocar and canula are inserted into the interior of the muscle or tumour, the trocar is withdrawn, leaving the canula in place. The stylet or cutting portion of the instrument, consists of a steel stem, of the same diameter as the first trocar, at the end of which is a contracted portion, and terminates in a cutting screw edge. By a few rotations of this instrument a fragment of tissue can be secured and removed through the canula. If the first attempt is unsuccessful it can be re-introduced, and any number of successive specimens removed without the necessity of a second puncture, as would be required in using Duchenne's instrument.

Feb. 15. I add a short note concerning the further progress of the case. The man walks about the hospital yard, and looks like a well man. His colour is excellent; he is plump. The pupil has lost all dilatation, and he sees clearly. His eye, examined with the ophthalmoscope, showed nothing abnormal. He is capable of performing almost any motion, except that he still stoops with difficulty. The muscles of the calf are harder than normal and their electro-muscular contractility is impaired; elsewhere the muscles all act well to the faradic current. He has lately complained a little of headache and of some stiffness and pain at the back of the neck; but for these lingering symptoms he would have been discharged from the hospital. All trichinæ are not, however, encapsuled in his muscles, a few in a piece taken out from the forearm with Hart's trocar were still found alive. But the great majority were encapsuled, and the capsule was full of cretaceous salts.

ON TUBERCULAR PERITONITIS IN CHILDREN.

A Clinical Lecture delivered at St. Bartholomew's Hospital.

By SAMUEL GEE, M.D., F.R.C.P. LOND.,
Physician to the Hospital.

GENTLEMEN: There are three kinds of tubercular abdominal disease occurring in children: chronic peritonitis, decay of the mesenteric glands, and ulceration of the intestines. These diseases are sometimes associated in different ways, sometimes they happen each alone by itself. They constitute a condition which the common people call "consumption of the bowels," although this term also includes the chronic enteritis which is not tubercular.

My topic to-day is tubercular peritonitis, or, what in the case of children is almost the same thing, chronic peritonitis.

I. *Pathognomonic Signs.*—They are discovered by physical examination of the abdomen, and are of two kinds: indurations and suppurations.

1. *Indurations* are detected by palpation. They have the form of bands and patches, or of lumps and knots. They certainly are present in most cases at some period or other of the disease. They begin to appear within a few weeks

of the onset of the illness. They are more or less obscured by coexisting tympanites; and for this, or some other reason, they are not felt equally well at all times in the same patient. When the abdomen is very tender or resisting, I usually administer chloroform to the child before proceeding to the examination; and I strongly advise you to do the same thing in a doubtful case. The *bands* which I spoke of are commonly transverse, stretching right across the belly, or confined to one side of it. They are felt above the navel, on a level with the navel, or below it—for instance, parallel to Poupart's ligament. They are sometimes remarkably hard. They are mostly about the breadth of the finger, or rather more. The *patches* of induration, like the bands, may be met with anywhere; in a boy now in the hospital, they are felt in the hypogastrium. The *lumps* and *knots* are sometimes very numerous, sometimes there are only one or two. Their size is very different, they often feel like nuts or pips. They differ very much in situation; there is no rule in these matters. The distinction (not always possible) between peritoneal and glandular lumps is to be found in the fact that the former are as a rule more superficial, less deeply seated than the latter.

2. *Suppuration.* Discharge of pus from the navel, due to a local peritoneal abscess, is likewise characteristic. Sometimes there is nothing more than an appearance of pointing, which afterwards subsides, and never goes on to discharge. The navel looks red and swollen, not merely protruded, but its tissues swollen. This sign I believe to be no less characteristic. The pus is sometimes mixed with feces. This is a condition which indicates ulceration of the intestine, and is a very much more dangerous affair than the discharge of pus alone.

Physical examination will also discover signs of either or both of two other abdominal lesions in most cases of tubercular peritonitis. *Tympanites* to a less or greater degree is a symptom almost always present at some period or other of the disease. *Ascites* is less common. In one case of this kind a diagnosis was made possible by the coexistence of phlegmonous scrofulides on the leg, otherwise there was nothing but ascites.

II. *Onset of the Disease.*—Tubercular peritonitis is usually idiopathic, that is to say, it constitutes the disease in and by itself. This is the only case which I consider on the present occasion. I pass by the chronic peritonitis which is secondary to manifest tubercular disease of the lungs, intestines, or other parts.

1. The onset of protopathic tubercular peritonitis is mostly *gradual.* The belly becomes tender, painful, and large; at the same time the health of the child fails; there are emaciation, loss of appetite, and in many cases slight fever. At the beginning examination of the abdomen discovers nothing but more or less tympanites, sometimes associated with a little ascites. The tympanites usually remains moderate, but in some children it becomes excessive, so much so as to cause permanent dyspnœa. The ascites of the onset is small in quantity, and mostly goes away in a few weeks. Afterwards the indurations which I spoke of begin to appear.

2. The onset is sometimes *sudden*, and attended by very great tympanites. The tympanites is sometimes the only abdominal symptom. Sometimes it is associated with vomiting. And sometimes there are also all the signs of acute gastro-enteritis. In my lecture on tympanites last session I narrated a case of this kind—a child suddenly attacked by infantile cholera; violent vomiting and purging, with collapse, algidity, and tympanites. This was the beginning of chronic tubercular peritonitis.

III. *Course of the Disease.*—Suppose the chronic peritonitis established, you will most likely be able to detect one or other of the pathognomonic signs which I spoke of at the beginning. I will now speak of the symptoms which are attendant upon the confirmed disease.   Emaciation from the first; appetite bad; vomiting now and then.   Action of the bowels uncertain.   Diarrhœa, occasional or even more continual, is no proof by itself of the coexistence of intestinal ulceration.   Constipation is common, and it goes on in a few uncommon cases to absolute obstruction of the bowels.   This obstruction is either temporary, giving way at length to the remedies employed, or it is permanent, and causes the death of the patient.   The latter course is well illustrated by a case published by Dr. Wolston in the 10th vol. of the Clinical Society's Transactions.   Obstruction of the bowels, although it may have been relieved, is apt to recur.   Pain in the belly is sometimes severe, and is sometimes felt on heavy pressure only. The movements of the bowels are sometimes visible, whether there be much tympanites or not.   Fever is present at first, but is seldom high; it often ceases altogether after a week or two; sometimes a low degree of fever is constant throughout the whole course of the disease.   So that, at the time you see your patient, it may happen that there are no fever or other symptoms of disease, except the emaciation and the abdominal signs already spoken of.

IV. *Termination of the Disease.*—1. *Recovery* from tubercular peritonitis is common.   In the course of months, or a year or two, the tympanites disappears, and the indurations cease to be palpable.   The patient is left pale and weak, and may continue so for the rest of life.   On the other hand, he may regain his original state of health.   The most positive proof of recovery from tubercular peritonitis is afforded by Mr. Spencer Wells's case,[1] in which the ascites of that disease resembled an ovarian cyst.   Abdominal section was performed; the peritoneum was seen to swarm with tubercles; the intestines, for the most part, were adherent together.   Acute peritonitis followed the operation, but the patient recovered, and six years afterwards she was stout, hearty, and well.

2. *Death* from tubercular peritonitis occurs in several ways.   A slow exhaustion is common, especially when other forms of tubercular disease come to complicate the case.   Increasing and great ascites may be the cause of death.   You remember a girl who died in Mary ward after paracentesis for ascites ?   In her, tubercular peritonitis was associated with highly-marked cirrhosis of the liver, and this is a combination of lesions which I have seen before.   Obstruction of the bowels is an uncommon cause of death.

When suppuration has occurred there is an additional danger.   Mere pointing sometimes goes away without any manifest discharge of pus from the navel or any other part.   When actual discharge of pus from the navel has occurred recovery is still possible.   But when there are signs of a fistulous opening into the bowel the case is hopeless, as I said before.

V. *Therapeutics.*—The first thing to mind, in the treatment of tubercular peritonitis, is to keep the abdomen at rest.   This can be done only by keeping the patient in bed.   I have known a boy, who was slowly recovering whilst he was in bed, undergo a fatal relapse of his disease by being taken up and dressed against orders.

Another part of the treatment consists in putting a flannel bandage round the belly, so as to reach from the hips to the ribs.   Much pain in the abdomen is alleviated by hot and moist fomentations, as hot as the patient can bear ; linseed meal poultices, flannel fomentations, or, what is usually best, a flannel bag full of bran or camomile flowers, which can be heated in hot water or an oven as often as needful.   You may sprinkle the fomentation with laudanum; or you may smear the abdomen with a liniment composed of equal parts of extract of belladonna and glycerine.

---

[1] Quoted by Dr. Fagge, Guy's Hospital Reports, third series, vol. xx. p. 203.

I need not say much about the necessity of allowing none but the most easily-digestible kinds of food; in short to feed the patient very much as you would feed a baby. Cod-liver oil, if it can be taken, is sure to do good.

For the ascites you may try copaiba resin cautiously, beginning with three or four grains, made into an emulsion, with an equal quantity of compound traga-canth or almond powder, and some water. If this mixture disagree with the stomach you must discontinue it.

When suppuration has set in, the proper treatment is assiduous poulticing.

Hospital Notes.

Hysterical Spinal Affection of Two Years' Duration; Cured by Corrigan's Iron.

Mr. J. D. T. RECKITT, House-Surgeon at the Newark Hospital, records (*Lan-cet*, Jan. 15, 1881) the notes of the following interesting case:—

Alice D——, aged twenty-five, dressmaker, and single, was first seen on May 20, 1878, when she stated that until two years before, when she had a fall, sprain-ing her back a little, she had always enjoyed good health. She was first attended at her home. She kept her bed, but had a healthy appearance, though the ex-pression of her countenance was melancholic. She had.been treated in the hos-pital, and had also been under treatment at home for what she stated was spinal disease, the treatment including blisters to the spine, various liniments, and, lastly, crutches; but all to no purpose. The nature of the case was suspected to be hysterical, and in answer to inquiries the patient said she had severe pains almost everywhere, not excepting even the ends of the finger-nails, and added to this, a sympathizing mother dilated very largely upon the extreme suffering the patient underwent. She had not been able to walk for several months, but her appetite had continued pretty good. She slept badly, and had much headache. It was therefore determined to apply the actual cautery, and the patient was assured that she would be able to walk in two months' time.

On May 25th, assisted by Mr. J. Sheppard, Mr. Reckitt made six impressions —three on either side—in the spinal fossæ, from the commencement of the dorsal region downwards. The patient complained of considerable pain, and she nearly fainted. It was decided to reapply the iron in a week's time if there was no improvement.

On June 2d she appeared so depressed and reluctant to have a re-application, that it was deferred a week; and accordingly, a week later, six more impressions were made on either side, but below the former. She was ordered to get up.

On the 16th she felt a little better, but still had a little pain and slight head-ache. She was ordered to try to walk with help.

On the 23d she said she was improving slowly. She was told that probably another application would be necessary.

On July 7th she was downstairs, and had walked several times with help.

On August 20th she presented herself at the hospital, having walked up a dis-tance of half a mile with her sister's aid. Much better, and walked fairly.

On the 30th so much improved that she was discharged.

Remarks.—The apparent total inability of the girl to walk when first seen, and the rapid effect of the heroic measure adopted, would appear to prove that hys-teria—or rather, perhaps, malingering in a hysterical subject—was the main fea-ture in the case; and also that the treatment, though somewhat cruel, was the only means to make such an obstinate individual use her ambulatory powers, and to assure her of her ability to do so.

MONTHLY ABSTRACT.

Anatomy and Physiology.

The Circulation in Marrow of Bone and Cerebral Meninges.

KOLLMAN, in a series of investigations into the circulation in the medulla of human bone, has corroborated the statements of Hayer and Rindfleisch that this circulation is not continuous through vessels, but that the minute veins open into the interstices of the tissue. In spite of this interruption, the circulation goes on with perfect regularity. Aqueous solutions of Berlin blue find their way from the veins to the arteries as readily as from the arteries to the veins, and, what is still more remarkable, they find their way from the sub-arachnoid space of the spinal cord, to the spongy structure of the skull, into the sinuses of the dura mater, and into the veins of the skull and of the face. It is conjectured that the communication between the sub-arachnoid spaces and the veins is by means of the Pacchionian granulations. The sub-arachnoid and subdural spaces of the brain are not in direct communication, but the injection readily passes from the subdural space into the periphery of the Pacchionian granulations and so into the venous sinuses. There are also fissures in the inner surface of the dura mater which are openings into the lymphatic canals.—*Lancet*, Jan. 29, 1881.

Some Points in the Anatomy of the Ear.

In a paper which has just appeared in the *Archiv für Anatomie*, by Professor RETZIUS, he states that as the great work of the anatomy of the ear on which he is engaged will take a long time to complete, on account of the trouble and expense of the engravings which are to accompany it, he desires to publish provisionally some of the new facts which he has discovered. In the first place, he some years ago found in the auditory labyrinth of teleostean fishes two small plates on the floor of the utriculus, near the canalis communicans, on which two branches of the cochlear nerve terminate. He considered this structure to be the first indication of the "pars basilaris cochleæ." Hasse acknowledged its existence in fishes, and thought it to be the rudiment or "pars initialis cochleæ." Further researches satisfied Retzius that it was present in the plagiostome fishes, and still more recent researches have enabled him to trace it through the amphibia, through many reptilia, in which it is less developed than in the amphibia, and through the birds, where it is smaller and more rudimentary than in the reptilia, appearing only as a small spot with a few nerve fibres distributed to it, situated on the floor of the ampulla frontalis. No trace of it can be found in the rabbit, cat, or dog, amongst mammals. He has, therefore, changed his opinion, and no longer regards it as the rudiment of the cochlea, but has named it the "macula acoustica neglecta," and the branch of nerve supplying it the "ramulus neglectus." How, then, he asks, does it stand with the true pars basilaris cochleæ—the most important part of the organ of hearing? Since this nerve termination does not represent it, it may be settled that there is no pars basilaris; they only possess the lagena cochleæ. The first traces of the true pars basilaris occur in amphibia.

A second point to which Retzius has directed his attention is the mode of division of the acoustic nerve. He quotes the descriptions given by Henle, Hyrtl, Luschka, Krause, Quain, and Turner. In the works of all these authors the auditory nerve is stated to divide into two chief branches—a ramus vestibularis and a ramus cochlearis. Some authors admit that the vestibularis nerve divides into four branches, which supply the sacculus hemisphericus and the cochlea. Others consider that the cochlear nerve only supplies the cochlea, and that the vestibular nerve gives off five branches. Neither of these statements is correct. The anterior of the two main divisions of the auditory nerve—that is to say, the vestibular nerve—which, by the twisting of the parts really lies posteriorly to the other, divides into three branches, which supply respectively the recessus utriculi, the ampulla sagittalis, and the ampulla horizontalis. The posterior main branch—i. e., the cochlear nerve—divides into three branches, which supply the ampulla frontalis, the sacculus, and the cochlea.—*Lancet*, Jan. 1, 1881.

The Mucous Membrane of the Anus.

In the *Journ. de l'Anat. et Phys.*, G. HERMANN has recently published some observations on the structure of the anal mucous membrane. He includes in this term a circular rim from 5 to 12 mm. in depth, reaching from the narrow white ano-cutaneous line pointed out by Hilton, to the ano-rectal line above—a portion corresponding to the internal sphincter and analogous to the red free border of the lips between the skin and true mucous membrane. After pointing out that with the exception of a serous coat on the outside, the structures of this region are the same as those met with in the upper part of the intestine—two layers of muscular tissue, mucous membrane, Auerbach's and Meissner's plexuses, —he enters into fuller detail as to the structure and development of the mucous membrane. The epithelium is squamous and stratified, but columnar in the depressions between the columnæ recti of Morgagni. At the sides he finds pouches and duct-like tubes lined with simple or stratified epithelium, which dip down to the depth of one centimetre into the subjacent muscle and there sometimes branch at their extremities. He considers these to be analogous to the glands found in this situation in animals. It is also suggested that these depressions, duct-like tubes, and the closed follicles found between them play an important part in the production of anal abscess and fistula.—*Lancet*, Jan. 29, 1881.

Rigor Mortis.

M. RICHET, in a lecture delivered as one of a course auxiliary to that of the Faculty of Medicine of Paris, has just given a very full and complete résumé of the present state of our knowledge of rigor mortis, which has engaged the attention of observers from the time of LOUIS, who in 1752 wrote an essay upon it, in which he pointed out that it was one of the principal signs of death. NYSTEN, in the early part of the present century, demonstrated that cadaveric rigidity is due to the condition of the muscles, since if the ligaments of the joints, the fasciæ, and the aponeuroses, are all divided, rigor mortis persists, whilst it is removed or prevented by division of the muscles or by the separation of them from their attachments. BROWN-SÉQUARD and KÜHNE next examined the phenomena in question minutely, the former showing that it could be removed by the injection of blood into the vessels, and the latter demonstrating that it was essentially a chemical action. It may be stated generally that rigor mortis is never absent; the few cases in which reliable authorities have believed that it has not occurred having probably been instances where it has occurred extraordinarily early or late. It occurs in all animals, both vertebrated and invertebrated. In fishes it takes place almost instantly after death, whilst in frogs, if due precautions be taken, it does not occur until after the lapse of eight or ten days. It has no relation, therefore, to the temperature of the blood of the animal. The first muscles to undergo rigor mortis appear to be those raising the lower jaw, as the masseter, temporal, and pterygoid, which are very irritable muscles. M. NIDERKORN finds that in 113 subjects rigor mortis was complete at the fourth hour in 31, at the sixth hour in 20, at the fifth in 14, at the third in 14, at the seventh in 11, at the eighth in 7, at the tenth in 7, at the ninth in 4, at the thirteenth in 2, at the second in 2, and at the eleventh in 1. It commences about two hours after death, and in the human subject is usually complete about the fourth hour. It may supervene whilst the animal is still warm, as is seen in those which have been hunted to death. On the other hand, its appearance is retarded by cold, whilst its duration is almost indefinitely retarded by it. A muscle which has become rigid after death becomes still more rigid if exposed to a temperature of 120° F. This increase, according to KÜHNE, is due to the coagulation of the serine and caseine contained in the muscular juice. Mere congelation of a muscle does not cause it to lose its irritability, but it very rapidly becomes rigid when thawed.

The remarkable positions sometimes assumed by men killed on the field of battle have been described by many observers, and demonstrate that rigidity may supervene at the moment of death. BROWN-SÉQUARD has, indeed, recorded a case of adynamic typhoid fever, in which the jaws and limbs became fixed, whilst the heart still continued to beat; and quite lately the same thing has been recorded by M. BOCHEFONTAINE in dogs poisoned with salicylate of soda, and M. RICHET has observed it in animals poisoned with medium doses of strychnia. In these cases all the muscles were rigid and unexcitable, with the exception of the heart; and artificial respiration could only be maintained with difficulty owing to the rigidity of the chest. Division of the nerves supplying a muscle appears to have little or no effect in accelerating the occurrence of rigor mortis, and according to HERMANN, neither exposure to oxygen nor to the vacuum of an air-pump exerts any influence.

In becoming rigid, muscles slightly diminish in volume; they shorten less, at least with moderately heavy weights, than muscles in contraction; they entirely lose their irritability, and their elasticity is greatly impaired. Heat is eliminated whilst rigor is being established.

In regard to the cause of rigor mortis, which is an extremely interesting point, M. RICHET is of opinion that, as KÜHNE originally maintained, it is a chemical process; but this process is a phenomenon not of life but of death. The myosine of the muscle coagulates. The acids, which are constantly being formed and as continuously removed during life, accumulate after death in the muscle, and gradually effect the solution of the myosine, and then the azotized matters undergo decomposition and develop ammonia, which, in its turn, dissolves the myosine, and thus occasions the disappearance of the rigor. Speaking generally, rigor mortis is a chemical phenomenon, characterized by the coagulation of the myosine, and may be considered as the commencement of the death of the elements of the muscle.—*Lancet*, Jan. 22, 1881.

Materia Medica and Therapeutics.

Maize and Maizenic Acid.

The following are the conclusions drawn by Dr. VAUTHIER, in a brochure entitled, *Etude sur le Maïs (Zea Maïs) et l'Acide Maïzenique (Archives Méd. Belges*, August, 1880): 1. The action of Zea maize is always favourable in all affections of the bladder, whether recent or chronic. 2. Maizenic acid is the active principle of the stigmata of maize, and it alone contains the therapeutic properties. 3. The diuretic action is not constant; it is met with in cases of acute traumatic cystitis, and in cases of retention, but here the improvement in micturition is due to the recovery of the affected organs, and not directly to the action of the maizenic acid. 4. The best results are observed in uric and phosphatic gravel, in acute cystitis, whether simple or due to gravel, and in mucous or muco-purulent catarrh. 5. In the cases observed by the writer, the ordinary remedies for these affections had already been employed without benefit, while the maize never failed to effect a cure. In connection with the maize, simple and medicated vesical injections were employed. 6. Maizenic acid, moreover, has the power of dissolving calculi by its chemical action; and not only vesical calculi, but also all the other calcareous concretions that are met with in the human system. Hence its use seems indicated in cases of gout and rheumatism, as well as in affections of the urinary organs. The preparations used by the author were the infusion (10 parts of corn-silk to 100 of boiling water, with syrup *ad libitum;* dose, a tablespoonful every two hours), the extract in doses of one and one-half to three grains, and maizenic acid in doses of one-eighth of a grain in pill or mixture.—*London Med. Record,* Jan. 15, 1881.

Anæsthesia by the Application of Chloroform to the Skin.

We lately described the interesting experiments of Dr. BROWN-SÉQUARD on the effect of the application of chloroform to the skin on the functions of the central nervous system. It has been objected that the effects might possibly be due to the inhalation of some of the chloroform vapour. He has therefore repeated his experiments, and with the precaution of making the animal breathe air from another floor of the laboratory than that in which the experiments were made, its head being placed within a tube. The results obtained were the same as those already described, the only difference being that the period of excitement which usually precedes that of complete resolution, was a little longer than in the experiments already published. During this period, which is frequent, although not constant, the respiratory and cardiac movements are more rapid and more energetic. The animal cries and is disturbed—it appears hyperæsthetic, and its rectal temperature is raised a fifth or a quarter of a degree Centigrade.

Dr. Brown-Séquard, in a fresh series of experiments, has ascertained that the influence of chloroform on the mucous membranes is, as a rule, much more rapid and energetic than when applied to the skin. In these observations also the animals (dogs, cats, rabbits, and guinea-pigs) were made to breathe, by means of a tube fixed in the trachea, air coming from a distant part of the laboratory. Inhibition of the heart and respiration was invariably produced in a very brief, though variable time. Moreover, the loss of sensibility, of reflex action, and general resolution, with arrest of the exchange between the tissues and the blood, were frequently observed almost immediately after the application of the chloroform to the mucous membranes of the nose and larynx, or when it was poured into the mouth of guinea-pig or rabbit. But, strange to say, the application of chloroform to the posterior part of the mucous membrane of the mouth of the dog. or to the surface of the pharynx, always produced the opposite effect to the inhibition observed in the other animals. Respiration is greatly augmented, one dog, for instance, breathing 160 times a minute. Thus the effect in the same animal is altogether different when the chloroform is applied to the laryngeal mucous membrane, than when it is applied to the adjacent mucous membrane in the pharynx and mouth.

The influence of chloroform poured into one nostril upon the diaphragm and phrenic nerves is exactly the same as that produced when it is applied to the side of the thorax or to the shoulder.   There is a loss of the equilibrium between the action of the two halves of the diaphragmatic apparatus ; the phrenic nerve and the half of the diaphragm on the side corresponding to the nostril irritated become more energetic both in the degree and in the duration of their action, after the thorax has been opened, while those on the other side present the opposite condition.

Chloral hydrate, even in the most concentrated solution, when applied to the skin, does not usually produce any of the anæsthetic or other effects which follow its injection into a vein or beneath the skin.   This is, however, not true when a large area of the skin is irritated by anhydrous chloral.   The effects of this are perfectly analogous to those of the application of chloroform.   The only differences are that the chloral acts more slowly, but causes death more readily ; that it causes pulmonary, renal, and intestinal hemorrhages more frequently than chloroform, and that it produces abundant secretions from various abdominal glands, and so causes diarrhœa, an effect which is never produced by chloroform. Chloral seems to cause glycosuria, which chloroform never does, and is apparently absorbed by the vessels of the skin to a much greater extent than chloroform.   Inhalations of anhydrous chloral or its application to the skin, do not produce anæsthesia except at the moment of death.   In the guinea-pig especially, which is rendered anæsthetic so readily by the inhalation of a very small quantity of the vapour of chloroform, the inhalation of chloral has very little anæsthetic effect.—*Lancet*, Jan. 29, 1881.

—

Gelsemium as a New Antipruritic Remedy.

Dr. L. Duncan Buckley recommends (*New York Medical Journal*, Jan. 1881), gelsemium as an adjuvant for the relief of itching in certain cases, especially eczema in adults.   He gives it in increasing doses, repeated every half hour or every hour, until the pruritus is relieved.   He begins with ten drop doses of the tincture and has often found some measure of relief after the first or second dose.

—

On the Action and Uses of Certain Remedies employed in Bronchitis and Phthisis.

Dr. T. Lauder Brunton makes the following interesting communication to the *Lancet* (Jan. 1, 1881), on this subject :—

In both bronchitis and phthisis the first symptoms that attract notice are cough and expectoration, and the first remedies that claim our attention are the so-called sedatives and expectorants.   Cough consists in deep inspiration, closure of the glottis, and violent expiratory effort, by which the glottis is forcibly opened by the compressed air, which carries with it, in its exit, mucus or other matters which may have lodged in the lungs or respiratory passages.   The nervous centre for this act lies in the medulla oblongata.   It is bilateral, and situated on each side of the central raphé.   It is excited into action reflexly by irritation of the respiratory branches of the vagus distributed to the glosso-epiglottidean folds, to the whole interior of the larynx, to the trachea, especially at its bifurcation, and to the bronchi, and the substance of the lung itself, as well as the pleura when it is inflamed.   Irritation of the internal auditory meatus at the point to which the auricular branch of the vagus is distributed also causes coughing, and so also may irritation of the liver and of the spleen.   As coughing is a reflex act, excited by irritation applied to a sensory nerve, and reacting through a nerve centre upon the respiratory muscles, it is obvious that it may be lessened, either by removing the source of irritation or by diminishing the excitability of the nervous mechanism through which it acts. Both methods are employed in medicine. One of the commonest is that of lessening irritation by the use of glutinous and saccharine substances. These have in themselves little or no action upon the nervous mechanism. They do not pass down to the bronchi, or lung substance, so that they can have no direct effect upon the mucous membrane there, nor have they, so far as we know, any effect upon it after they have been absorbed into the blood; and yet one of the commonest observations is that glutinous and saccharine substances have a very great power to allay cough when applied to the back of the throat, even in cases where we know that inflammation and consequent irritation exist in the respiratory passages below the glottis, at a point which the mucilaginous substances cannot reach. The probable explanation of this action of such substances as marshmallow lozenges, jujubes, consisting of gum and sugar and Spanish liquorice, is that the irritation which occasions the cough exists at the root of the tongue and around the fauces, as well as in the trachea, bronchi, or lungs, the combined irritation rendering the cough worse than either the one or the other alone would do; and, therefore, if we soothe the tongue and fauces we relieve the cough, even though the irritation in the bronchial tubes or lung may remain as before. The power of such substances as those mentioned to relieve cough depends, no doubt, to a great extent either on their covering the inflamed and irritable surface directly with a mucilaginous coat, and thus protecting it from the action of the air or from irritation by other substances passing over it, or by exciting an increased flow of saliva or mucus, which has a similar effect. At the same time we cannot deny the possibility of their having other actions, though with these we are at present unacquainted. The use of the mucilaginous substances containing opium or other sedatives, which we know under the name of "linctus," is a more complicated one. In them we have the soothing action of the mucilaginous compound, combined with the local sedative action of morphia, chloroform, or hydrocyanic acid upon the inflamed or irritable mucous surfaces at the root of the tongue and back of the throat, and this renders even their local action more powerful than that of a mucilaginous substance alone. Such drugs as opium, hydrocyanic acid, and chloroform have a certain amount of local action upon the peripheral ends of sensory nerves, and lessen their sensibility to impressions. When they are applied to the ends of the nerves only for a very short time, as they are when we swallow these drugs in a liquid form, their local action is comparatively slight. It is much greater when they are taken in a mucilaginous vehicle, which, adhering to the irritated mucous membrane over which it passes, keeps the sedatives in contact with it for a longer time, and thus allows them to exert a more powerful action. But the sedatives which we give to relieve cough are not unfrequently administered in the form of solution, and then, though their local action must be comparatively slight, they still lessen a troublesome cough. Their action here is a different one from that which we have just discussed, but it is possessed by the sedative whether given in the form of linctus or of solution. In either way it is swallowed by the patient, absorbed from the stomach and intestines into the circulation, and carried by the blood to the medulla oblongata, and also to the inflamed mucous membranes, in which the blood circulates freely, just as well as in other parts of the body, although here its action is likely to be very much less than if it were applied for a length of time directly, as in the shape of the linctus; but, as we have mentioned, the linctus can only be applied to the back of the tongue and throat, and the source of irritation of the afferent nerves may be in the bronchi or in the lung itself. Here, no doubt, a linctus cannot penetrate, but we may to a certain extent act locally upon the nerves by the use of spray and inhalation. Some of these, such as the vapour of conium and the vapour of hydrocyanic acid, are intended to ·lessen the irritability of the sensory nerves in the respiratory passages, and thus lessen cough. Others, such as the spray of ipecacuanha, and inhalation of essential oils and terebinthinous substances, have probably a different action, and do not lessen the irritability of the sensory nerves in the respiratory passages, but alter the nutrition of the mucous membrane in such a way as to diminish the irritation which the abnormal condition of the membrane exerts upon the nerves. When the irritation is situated in the larynx, as in cases of laryngeal phthisis, one of the best means of relieving it is by applying the sedatives locally, whether by means of a brush, or, what is perhaps still better, by blowing it, in the form of a ·powder, directly upon the irritated surface. A useful application in laryngeal ·phthisis consists of a mixture of· morphia and starch, in the proportion of about ·one-sixth of a grain of morphia to two grains of starch. This mixture is introduced into a glass tube, of a proper shape, and is blown down the throat at the instant that the patient takes a deep inspiration. The powder is thus distributed over the interior of the larynx, and exerts its local sedative influence upon the irritated surface, as well as a general sedative effect upon the central nervous system after its absorption.

· This brings us to the second mode in which sedatives relieve cough. After their absorption into the blood, in whatever manner they may have been applied, they are carried to the medulla, and there lessen the excitability of the nerve centre through which the reflex act of coughing is produced. In large doses their sedative effect may be so great as to endanger life, and the caution is given in every text-book, and by every teacher, that respiratory sedatives such as opium should be carefully administered to persons suffering from bronchitis with profuse expectoration, lest the irritability of the medulla should be so far diminished that it will no longer respond even to a powerful stimulus from the lungs, and the secretion may consequently go on accumulating until when the patient awakes the respiratory passages are so clogged with mucus that no effort which he can make is sufficient to clear them, and he dies of suffocation. ·By administering them ·in smaller quantities, however, the effect of respiratory sedatives may be graduated so as to diminish cough without any risk of· causing death, and their effect would be exceedingly· beneficial if ·they acted only upon· the respiratory centre. Unluckily, however, this is not the case, and the most powerful of all— viz., opium—not only influences the respiration, but the digestion. It·diminishes the cough, but sometimes, also, it diminishes the appetite. and may interfere with the proper action of the bowels. · When this is the case, we áre obliged carefully to steer between two dangers: (1) the injurious effects of the cough itself, and (2) the injurious effect of disturbed digestion. If we leave ·the cough alone, it exhausts the patient, for the muscular exertion involved in a violent fit of coughing is very·considerable indeed, and the muscular effort exerted by·a patient with a bad cough during the twenty-four hours is really more than equivalent to that of many a man in a day's work. . Nor is this all. Any one who watches the face of a patient during a violent fit of· coughing will see the skin become flushed, and then dusky; the veins in the forehead and in the jugulars swell up, and becomé so tense that they seem as if about to burst; so that there is both venous engorgement and interference with the respiration. But what we see in the face takes place elsewhere. ·· The same tension which we see in the jugulars is also ·present in the right side of the heart, in the vena cava, and in the portal system; for the portal vein has no valves, and the increased tension is transmitted backwards to the veins of the stomach, spleen, and intestines. By and by this· all begins to tell upon the heart and upon the digestive system, as well as, to some extent;

upon the kidneys. The stomach becomes congested, and we have loss of appetite, nausea, and vomiting. The patient, too, is kept awake, and we have nervous exhaustion, or loss of sleep, added to the weariness caused by the muscular exertion, and to the depression occasioned by digestive disturbance. These are what we have to fear: on the one hand, continuous coughing; on the other, we must avoid the digestive disturbance produced by our sedatives; and the duty of the physician is, so far as possible, to relieve the cough without disturbing the digestion. Numerous combinations have been devised, and are found to be, empirically, of very great service. If we take one of them and attempt to analyze it, we shall find that its components are such as to diminish the excitability of the respiratory centre, and at the same time to lessen the injurious effect of the sedatives upon the stomach. Such a one is the following mixture: Solution of hydrochloride of morphia and dilute hydrocyanic acid, of each eighteen minims; spirit of chloroform and dilute nitric acid, of each one fluidrachm; glycerine, three fluidrachms; infusion of cascarilla or infusion of quassia, two fluidounces; a sixth part to be taken three or four times a day.

In this mixture, which in its essence was much used by the late Dr. Warburton Begbie, of Edinburgh, to relieve the cough in phthisis, we find the sedatives morphia, hydrocyanic acid, and chloroform, to lessen the excitability of the respiratory centre; we find glycerine, which will tend to retain the sedatives for a longer time in contact with the back of the throat, and will also act to some extent as a nutrient. We have combined with these nitric acid and infusion of cascarilla or of quassia, which have so-called tonic (?) action upon the stomach. In what this effect precisely consists we cannot at present say, but we may imagine that it will in some way partially counteract the effects of the congestion which the cough produces, and at the same time we know that they have the power of exciting appetite, and they will thus in a great measure counterbalance the injurious effects of the morphia upon digestion. Nor is this all. The nitric acid, as I shall shortly have to mention, has a very definite effect indeed upon the secretion in the lungs themselves; and this brings us to the consideration of another part of our subject—viz., the effect of drugs upon the secretion and nutrition of the lungs, by which they tend to restore the healthy condition of the bronchial and pulmonary tissues, and thus diminish coughing.

First of all, then, we must consider those drugs which lessen congestion. If a person, hastily eating or drinking, get a crumb of bread or a drop of fluid down the larynx, or into the wrong throat, as it is termed, he suddenly begins to cough violently, and the cough continues until the source of irritation has been removed. If the irritation has been violent he may give a few coughs after the crumb has been coughed up, although the primary source of irritation—namely, the crumb —has disappeared; but the congestion which it occasions still remains for a short time, and acts as an irritant. If a person suffering from disease of the mitral valve makes any sudden exertion, he is very likely to bring on a cough, which, however, quickly subsides after a short rest. The cough here is not due to inflammation of the mucous membrane, but simply to congestion, and when the congestion disappears the irritation goes with it. In cases where we have inflammation of the respiratory vessels actually present, as in persons suffering from bronchitis, the congested condition of the membrane is a source of considerable irritation, and we frequently notice that such persons, on going out into the cold air, may cease to cough, but again begin to cough violently when they return from the cold air into the warm room. The reason of this is that the cold air has acted upon the congested vessels of the respiratory passages in a somewhat similar way to what it does upon the vessels of the face; it causes them to contract, and the congestion being thus diminished the cough is lessened. When the patient goes into the warm room the face, which may have been pale while he was exposed to cold, flushes up with the heat, the vessels of the respiratory passages also became engorged, and the increased congestion causes irritation, bringing on the cough. In other cases, again, we notice that, just as the face becomes pale when exposed to cold, it shortly afterwards becomes flushed, although the application to cold continues. A person suffering from bronchitis, on going into a cold room, will begin to cough violently, the cold here increasing instead of diminishing congestion.

The pulmonary capillaries have great contractile power. Ten years ago I made some experiments, which I have not yet published, on the subject. I found that on the application of cold to the lung of a frog, when placed under the microscope, the capillaries would contract to two-thirds of their former diameter. We have, however, very few observations on the action of drugs upon the pulmonary circulation, the difficulties in the operative procedure being very considerable. I have observed that muscarin appears to have a power of contracting the pulmonary vessels, and that this effect is abolished by atropia. I am unaware, at present, of any other observations on the action of drugs upon the pulmonary circulation. Circumstances have prevented me from studying the recent researches on this subject in the way I should have wished, while drawing up this paper. From its power of contracting the vessels in other parts of the body, we should expect that digitalis would have a similar action upon the lungs; and we find, in looking over Beasley's "Book of Prescriptions," that digitalis has been used in pulmonary affections—as for example, in the following draught, employed by Sir A. Crichton in acute phthisis: lemon-juice, half an ounce; carbonate of potash, to saturation; decoction of sarsaparilla, ten drachms; tincture of digitalis, ten to thirty minims; acacia mucilage, ten drachms; to be taken every sixth hour. In such a prescription as this we have the tincture of digitalis, which will, in all probability, by contracting the vessels, diminish the pulmonary congestion and lessen cough. It is combined with carbonate of potash, and the effect of potash upon the lungs is very marked indeed. For my knowledge of its action I am indebted to Dr. Andrew Clark. Its action is perhaps best noticed in a patient suffering from consolidation and softening of a limited portion of one lung. When such a patient is in ordinary health, one may observe, on a stethoscopic examination, crepitant râles, limited to one spot. When he catches cold, one may hear, in addition to those, dry râles extending for some distance around the irritated spot, and the cough at the same time becomes more frequent and troublesome, while there is very little, if any, expectoration. If potash be now given alone, or, still better, in combination with a vegetable acid, the dry râles subside, and are replaced by moist ones, which in the course of a day or two, as the potash is continued, alter in character, giving one the impression of their being caused by less viscid fluid. At the same time the expectoration becomes more copious, and the cough less frequent and less troublesome. Now is the time to alter the treatment, and for the potash to substitute nitric acid. If this be given too soon the cough, which had begun to get easier, will again become drier and harder, but it it be administered at the proper moment the cough becomes still less troublesome, the expectoration diminishes, and the moist râles disappear from the neighbourhood of the consolidated part of the lung, although they may still remain, as before, in that part itself. Potash, then, has a very marked effect in rendering the pulmonary secretion more fluid and abundant, while nitric acid has an opposite effect. As in many cases we wish to diminish the secretion rather than increase it, it is nitric acid rather than alkalies which we employ for long periods in the treatment of phthisis, as we have already seen in the modified formula of Dr. Begbie's phthisis mixture.

One of the most powerful expectorants is simply a little warm food in the stomach, and in cases of chronic bronchitis, in which the patients complain of violent coughing immediately after rising, one of the best expectorants is a glass of warm milk, either with or without a little rum, and a biscuit or a piece of bread about a quarter of an hour before they get up. A little warm beef-tea will have a similar effect. After taking this for a short time they generally tell you that the sputum comes away much more easily than before, and they are not so much exhausted by it. But perhaps the remedy, *par excellence*, not only in cases of phthisis, but in chronic bronchitis, is cod-liver oil. Persons suffering from long-standing chronic bronchitis will often come to the hospital to beg for cod-liver oil, saying that it eases their cough far more than any cough mixture. Other oils or fats have not this power to the same extent as cod-liver oil. We cannot say positively what the reason of this may be, but I think there is no doubt about the fact. My own belief is that cod-liver oil is more easily assimilated than other oils, and not only so, but more easily transformed into tissues themselves. Whether it owes this property to its admixture with biliary substances, or to its chemical composition, we cannot say. In his book on "Fat and Blood, and how to make them," Dr. Weir Mitchell quotes a remark made by an old nurse, that "some fats are fast, and some fats are fleeting, but cod-liver oil fat is soon wasted." By this she meant that there were differences in the kinds of fat accumulated under the subcutaneous tissues of men, just as there are differences in subcutaneous fats which accumulate in horses. The horse fed on grass soon gets thin by hard work, while fat laid on when the horse is feeding on hay and corn is much more permanent. Persons fattened on cod-liver oil soon lose the fatness again, and this, I think, points to the power of ready transformation which the oil possesses. Supposing that it does possess this power, we can readily see how very advantageous it will be. In chronic bronchitis, and in catarrh and pneumonia, we have a rapid cell-growth, but want of development. The cells lining the respiratory cavities are produced in great numbers, but they do not grow as they ought to do. They remain, more or less, lymphoid cells, instead of developing into proper epithelium. They so rapidly form, and are thrown off so quickly, that they have not time to get proper nutriment, and if they are to grow properly we must supply them, not with an ordinary kind of nutriment, but with one which is much more rapidly absorbed, and is capable of much more rapid transformation in the cell itself than the usual one. This power is, I believe, possessed by cod-liver oil, and to its quality of nourishing the rapidly-formed cells in the lungs in cases of bronchitis and catarrhal pneumonia I believe its great curative power is owing.

The next subject we will consider is the action of some drugs in the vomiting associated with cough. The action of vomiting, like that of coughing, is reflex; the nervous centre for it is also in the medulla oblongata, closely associated with the respiratory centre, and it is excited by various afferent nerves, the chief of them being the branches of the vagus distributed to the stomach. When congestion of the stomach is present, these become irritated, and we get loss of appetite, nausea, and vomiting. Like coughing, vomiting may be prevented by the removal of the irritant. For example, where the irritant is indigestible food, the vomiting ceases after the ejection of the offending substances. When the irritation depends on inflammation of the walls of the stomach, it may be soothed by sedatives having a local action upon the nerves, such as ice and hydrocyanic acid, or by drugs having the power of lessening the irritability of the nerve centre of the medulla, such as opium. In the chronic vomiting of phthisis, all these drugs may be employed, but there is one other which has been useful in this affection, and which probably has no effect either upon the nerve centre or the nerve ends

This is alum. Its mode of action probably is that by its astringent power it contracts the vessels of the stomach, and thus lessens the congestion and consequent irritation produced by the continued coughing in the manner already described.

Eruption Produced by Chloral.

Dr. Gee, Physician to St. Bartholomew's Hospital, has recently had under his care in the wards a girl, seventeen years of age, with chorea, for which chloral hydrate in frequently-repeated doses was prescribed. During the third week of its administration, a papular eruption of a dusky hue, surrounded by much cutaneous redness, was produced on the forehead, face, chest, and extremities, in arrangement partly crescentic and partly confluent. The eruption consisted essentially of a combination of lichen and erythema papulatum, and was attended with some increase of temperature.—*Lancet*, Jan. 1, 1881.

Medicine.

The Treatment of Diphtheria.

This is a subject of almost exhaustless interest, and therefore any well-observed facts in connection with it deserve notice. Some recent numbers of our contemporary, the *Berliner Klinische Wochenschrift*, contain papers which treat of it; and as the remedies proposed are simple and readily obtainable, and more especially as they appear to have been very efficacious, we shall briefly analyze the papers for the benefit of our readers.

Dr. G. GUTTMANN, of Cannstatt, proposes the use of pilocarpin. He reports in No. 40 of the *Berliner Klinische Wochenschrift* that he has used it during the past fifteen months, and, as the result of his present experience, is inclined to regard it almost as a specific. He feels unable to decide whether the local or the general manifestations of diphtheria are the primary. He inclines, however, to the belief that the local symptoms precede and give rise to the subsequent general condition, for, as a rule, and with few exceptions, the general disease is in proportion to the severity of the local lesion, pharyngeal or otherwise, and, moreover, recovery sets in as soon as the local signs of the disease begin to abate. And professional attention has long and largely been devoted to the means by which false membranes and other local conditions may be got rid of; hence the use of paintings, caustics, gargles, and inhalations. Unfortunately their application is not always easy, and often increases the local irritation. The knowledge of the physiological action of pilocarpin has led Dr. Guttmann to try it in diphtheria. As is well known, it increases bronchial secretion, and it was thought that in this manner the diphtheritic membrane would be loosened and got rid of. The result seems to have been extremely satisfactory. In April, 1879, Dr. Guttmann was called to attend a family of nine persons ill with diphtheria, of whom three were in a serious condition. Pilocarpin was ordered in medium doses, so that about one grain was taken during the day (gramme 0.05). Within a few hours a copious salivation was going on, and "the diphtheritic membranes swam away in the flowing saliva." Quinine was ordered internally, as well as a gargle of lime-water and pepsine. All these nine cases recovered within two to four days.

During the following fifteen months he treated sixty-six cases of diphtheria on the same plan. Of these fifteen were very severe cases (under other methods of treatment he considers that at least two-thirds of the patients would have died), eighteen were slight, and the remaining thirty-three of medium severity. *They all recovered;* the most severe cases only lasting eleven days, while the majority were cured within two or three days. The earlier cases of this series had other treatment at the same time—quinine, etc.—but the later cases were treated solely with the pilocarpin. In speaking of the cases as diphtheria, Dr. Guttmann took especial care to exclude other forms of disease; in most of the cases there was a clear history of infection, and as diphtheria was constantly occurring, he would be quite familiar with it; thus we may take it for granted that there is no error as far as diagnosis is concerned. Many professional colleagues in his own neighbourhood tried the remedy and found it efficient. The drug was administered internally; within a short time it produced an active flow of saliva, by means of which the false membrane was loosened, the inflammatory infiltration also lessened, and the intense redness gave place to a more normal colour. His formula for children is as follows: ℞. Pilocarpini muriatici 0.02–0.04, pepsini 0.6–0.8, acid. hydrochlorici gtt. ij, aquæ destill. 80.0; a teaspoonful every hour. For adults the dose is about double. If the physiological action of the drug does not manifest itself within a short time, increase the dose.

Dr. Bosse, of Domnau, relates in No. 43 of the same journal how the accidental administration of a spoonful of turpentine to a child in the last stage of diphtheria apparently saved its life, all other remedies having previously failed. This led him to make further trials with the drug; and he reports that he found it very serviceable. His first case was a boy, ten years of age. Carbolic acid had been placed in a saucer in the room for the purpose of disinfecting the air; but the odour was intensely objectionable to the boy's parents, and so turpentine was substituted. In the hurry and excitement attendant on the illness, a tablespoonful of the turpentine was given to the boy instead of his proper medicine. Both were contained in very similar phials. The turpentine does not appear to have caused any very great discomfort, and as the mistake was quickly perceived a quantity of milk was given in order to palliate it. After a while the boy became quieter and fell asleep, his breathing having previously been extremely laboured. On the following morning he appeared very much better, and he finally recovered; there had been no ill effects from the dose, either on the intestinal canal or on the urinary system. The circumstance produced a vivid impression on Dr. Bosse, who at first rather feared that the effect might be *post* rather than *propter hoc.* However, being placed in a district where diphtheria was endemic, he decided to put the treatment to the test, and in the course of a short time he tried it in twenty-three cases, all children from two to twelve years of age. The younger children took two drachms, the elder ones three drachms, of rectified turpentine. It was given pure, and forced down if necessary. The children were allowed as much milk afterwards as they cared to drink. In only one case was there vomiting; in all the others the oil was well borne. Dr. Bosse's usual treatment (chlorate of potash in lime-water with syrup of Peruvian balsam, and locally painting with Peruvian balsam) was continued after the turpentine. Within twenty-four hours, on examination, the false membranes were found broken and loose and raised. In four cases a second dose of turpentine was given. The whole of the twenty-three cases were well within forty-eight hours of the appearance of the diphtheritic patches. Of sixty-three other patients so treated, four died; but as they were all at a distance, Dr. Bosse was not only unable to control the treatment, but also to report very accurately on the cases. He says, "If sceptics might wish to argue that the above twenty-three cases were all of a mild variety, there was proof at least that the remedy considerably shortened the duration of the disease."

In the same number of the journal, Dr. Annuschat, of Liegnitz, after reporting on the uselessness, in his hands, of the ordinary remedies (chlorate of potash, salicylic acid, benzoate of soda, inhalations of lime-water, and of lactic acid) in several cases of severe and very typical diphtheria, among children for the most part, refers to a case in which the first local appearance was in the vagina; it was accompanied by severe constitutional symptoms. The following is the case: The pharynx was normal; proceeding from the right side of the vagina, and involving the thigh, there was a diphtheritic ulcer eight centimetres broad; the surrounding parts were œdematous, while the edges of the sore were raised and rigid, the sore itself being correspondingly depressed; it had a white, glossy appearance. Solid nitrate of silver was applied, but the sore continued to extend very widely. Under these circumstances it was felt necessary to try other measures: cyanide of mercury was decided upon—two grains of the mercury in three ounces and a half of peppermint water, of which one teaspoonful was given every hour throughout the day and night; water dressing was applied locally to the vagina. Within twenty-four hours a remarkable change took place, and on the third day the sore was granulating healthily. The mercury, which had been taken regularly, was then discontinued. Two other successful cases of vaginal diphtheria are likewise reported. Shortly after the occurrence of these cases, an outbreak of pharyngeal diphtheria took place, affecting some 120 children under fifteen years of age. They were all treated with cyanide of mercury internally, and a spray of benzoate of soda solution locally. Stimulants also were freely prescribed. Of the 120 patients, 106 recovered, and 14 died.

The preceding records are certainly not a little remarkable; but diphtheria, in a typical as well as severe form, is known to occur in certain districts of Prussia, and thus the practitioners of those districts must be well acquainted with its clinical features, and are not likely to be misleading in their statements. We have transcribed them as we have found them, and must leave it to those whom it concerns to verify them or otherwise. This much we are all aware of—that diphtheria is a very serious disease, and that our most approved remedies (so called) not infrequently fail to produce any effect upon it. In such cases it would, no doubt, be hard to try new remedies, and failing, to condemn them as useless; but if, tried as an *ultimum refugium*, they should prove of service, it would greatly enhance their claims to further and more extended trials in less desperate cases.—*Med. Times and Gazette*, Jan. 22, 1881.

—

The Temperature in Tubercular Meningitis.

Dr. JULES TURIN, in an interesting article on Tubercular Meningitis, in the *Jahrbuch für Kinderheilkunde*, vol. xvi., sums up the question of temperature as follows: 1. Tubercular meningitis is always accompanied by a rise in temperature in one or other of its stages, but very seldom during its entire duration. (The stages are given according to Dr. Wyatt, who, as is well known, first described the disease.) 2. In a few cases only does the disease begin with a sudden rise of the bodily heat, as in some forms of acute disease. 3. The thermometric results are extraordinarily variable, so that it is quite impossible to establish any typical temperature curve. 4. In uncomplicated cases of tubercular meningitis the temperature rarely exceeds 102.2° F.; it generally varies between 100° F. and 102° F., but it may also sink some degrees below the normal. 5. The most common type is the remittent, with the usual day fluctuations. The variations within twenty-four hours are normal, or more than normal; sometimes they are very irregular, with more or less sudden rise or fall at any stage and at different periods in the twenty-four hours. 6. If the tubercular meningitis is the terminal affection of some previously existing febrile disease—as, for instance, a coxitis, or any bone- or other joint-lesion,—the average temperature will be higher than in other cases; but, in other respects, the course of the disease will be unaffected. 7. In the cases with acute general miliary tuberculosis the febrile exacerbations are more considerable and the variations more marked.—*Medical Times and Gazette*, Jan. 15, 1881.

Epilepsy and its Differential Diagnosis from Hystero-Epilepsy.

In view of those not infrequent cases of hysteria closely simulating epilepsy, and of epilepsy occurring in hysterical patients, we think our readers will peruse with some interest a short account of an address delivered on the above subject by Professor von STOFFELLA, of Vienna, to the Medical Society of Vienna. Professor von Stoffella employs the term epilepsy as a collective expression for the sum of certain symptoms. Following Nothnagel he believes that essentially it consists in a peculiar condition, "a change *sui generis*," in the central nervous system, which change is characterized by increased irritability, more especially of the pons and the medulla oblongata, the reflex vaso-motor and muscular centres situated in these portions of the brain reacting to the slightest stimulus. This epileptic condition or "epileptic alteration" (Nothnagel) is to be distinguished from the prolonged comatose condition of rapidly consecutive epileptic attacks—the *status epilepticus*, or *état epileptique, état de mal* of French writers. Loss of consciousness more or less complete is an absolutely constant symptom of epilepsy; while, on the other hand, the tonic and clonic convulsions may fail, as in the *petit mal* of French writers, which is undoubtedly epilepsy.

Trousseau speaks of certain cases, which he would designate by the term "partial epilepsy," where the epileptic convulsions are confined to the spot in which the aura originates, and there is no loss of consciousness; and to this class he would refer many cases of angina pectoris. Professor von Stoffella practically refuses to admit these cases into the category of epilepsy, and recognizes no fundamental analogy between angina pectoris and epilepsy. Proceeding with his definition, Professor von Stoffella remarks that epilepsy is in its nature a chronic disease; and it therefore does not include those cases where epileptiform convulsions are caused by an irritation—*e. g.*, the eruption of teeth in children, —and subside at once on the removal of that irritation. So also it does not include those cases of epileptiform convulsions resulting from cerebral anæmia or hyperæmia caused by coarse cerebral disease, such as profuse cerebral hemorrhage, large tumours, acute hydrocephalus, emboli, etc. Such epileptiform attacks are distinguished from epilepsy by the frequent absence of a stage of tonic spasm, by the longer duration of the convulsions, and sopor, and by the frequent absence of laryngeal spasm.

In epilepsy no coarse change is found in the pons or medulla oblongata; and possibly, as Schröder van der Kolk says, the dilated capillaries, the granular albuminous exudation, and corpora amylacea are the results rather than the anatomical causes of the disease. This we must note, however, does not imply that coarse brain disease may not lead to the "epileptic alteration" above mentioned, for affections of the cortex, and more especially tumours of the convexity of the cortex frequently cause a unilateral epilepsy.

In the differential diagnosis of pronounced epilepsy and hystero-epilepsy, the loss of consciousness in epilepsy is not absolutely distinctive, for there are undoubted cases of hystero-epilepsy where the consciousness is clouded or even entirely lost. The following are important points of distinction: 1. The aura of hysteria is generally the *globus hystericus*, a feeling as of a ball pressing on the umbilical and epigastric regions, and rising gradually to the throat, where it causes a feeling of constriction. We may notice that this is no imaginary feeling, but is really a spasmodic constriction of the œsophagus passing gradually upwards to the pharynx. The aura of epilepsy is described in various ways, like a breath of wind or like formication. However short the hysteric aura may be, it is of longer duration than the aura of epilepsy, which is of lightning rapidity. 2. The hysteric attack is more noisy; the movements more extensive, not confined principally to one half of the body, as is frequently the case in epilepsy; and the attack frequently ends in a fit of weeping or laughing. An epileptic, on the other hand, after the cry with which the attack usually begins, is absolutely silent, and rarely moves from the spot where he drops down. 3. Charcot has observed that in a tonic hysteric attack, even if slight, the temperature rises just as in an epileptic attack, about 2° Fahr. But in a case of repeated epileptic attacks (e. g., fifteen to twenty in twenty-four hours) the temperature will rise to 41° Cent. or higher (105.8° Fahr.); while, however often the epileptiform hysteric attacks occur, the temperature does not rise above 38° Cent. or thereabout (100.4° Fahr.). For example, in a case of hystero-epilepsy recorded by Charcot, where the attacks lasted over two months, numbering one day as many as 150 to 200, with complete loss of consciousness, the rectal temperature throughout was 37.8° Cent. (100° Fahr.), with short exceptions of 38.5° Cent. (101.3° Fahr.). In only one fatal case of hystero-epilepsy recorded by Wunderlich did the temperature rise immediately before death to 43° Cent. (109.4° Fahr.). 4. Romberg mentions that the pupils in hysteria are sensitive to light, while in epilepsy they are absolutely insensitive; and Hasse notes that the hysteric attack lasts longer than the epileptic. 5. In addition to these, Professor von Stoffella remarks on a peculiarity in the pupils of epileptic patients (one or both sides) which he has lately observed, and which we do not remember having seen elsewhere noticed. They are either abnormally wide or abnormally narrow, and exceedingly slow in reacting to light. In the cases in which he has observed this peculiarity—numbering four—it has disappeared under the use of bromide of potassium. He explains the condition by the persistence of the temporary disturbance of circulation in the corpora quadrigemina which causes the insensitiveness of the iris to light during an attack; and remarks that, should the symptom turn out to be constant, it will give a valuable means of diagnosing the nature of the disease in an interval before seeing an attack.—*Med. Times and Gaz.*, Jan. 15, 1881.

Eye Symptoms in Locomotor Ataxy.

At a late meeting of the Ophthalmological Society of the United Kingdom Dr. J. Hughlings Jackson read an interesting paper on this subject. He first alluded to the great number of very different symptoms in this disease, better called tabes dorsalis, since the gait might be normal. He referred to the fact that some of the symptoms were occasionally found in other diseases. At present we have to study the symptoms as they occur in association or in sequence. In this paper three well-marked non-ocular tabetic symptoms were taken and considered in connection with certain ocular symptoms. Twenty-five cases in different stages furnished the material for the communication.

a. Non-ocular symptoms. (1) *The "Lightning" pains.*—There is a succession of sudden, small, severe short pains in batches. As Pierret and Buzzard have pointed out, these pains may occur about the head, although they occur mostly in the legs, trunk, and arms. Charcot and others have observed eruptions in the parts seized by pains. Buzzard has published the case of a patient (whom he permitted the author to see) who, with every batch of pains, has a small crop of herpes; this patient has double optic atrophy and Westphal's symptom (absence of so-called patellar tendon-reflex), 'as well as the pains; he walks well. An interesting feature in this case is that the patient had for several years crops of herpes before batches of pain, and then always both together. It is most important to note that pains are denied by some patients, who, nevertheless, have them. Many patients see no relation betwixt their pains and their amaurosis or ataxy, especially if the pains come years before. This one patient strenuously denied having any pains, but it came out, as it were accidentally, that he had had sciatica ; really he had had true lightning pains. He had optic atrophy and Westphal's symptom. Many of those who deny pains will admit that they have long been subject to rheumatism or neuralgia, or to "flying gout," and will describe these things so that it is certain they are lightning pains. It is often difficult to get a patient to fix his mind upon his pains. A patient, aged fifty-four, had recently continuous severe pain in the toes and sides of his feet. This he admitted to be one of the symptoms of his disease, but ignored lightning pains, which he had, on and off, for twenty years; those pains were, he would have it, "only gout." It was difficult to get him to attend to questions about them. He had had incontinence of urine nine years; difficulty in walking, according to his account, six months according to his wife, slightly for about eighteen months earlier; his gait was only slightly ataxic. There was Westphal's symptom. The ocular symptom was that his pupils, which were small, did not contract to light.

It is to be insisted on that a patient may have for very many years the pains before any of the striking symptoms of tabes dorsalis. "I have recently seen a patient, about sixty years of age, who had pains which I concluded to be 'lightning' for about twenty years. His gait was normal; by most careful testing I could find nothing the matter with it. The patient had besides, of late years, attacks of what he called sickness, but really faintness, with intense depression for hours. That these were slight gastric crises I could not be sure; they possibly depend on derangement caused by very large quantities of opium he had taken for relief of pain. The narcotic taking was evidence of the severity of the pain; he began this practice many years ago. Hearing his account of pain, I looked for Westphal's symptom, and found it. He had an ocular symptom, too. The pupils did not contract at all to light, and, I thought, very sluggishly, during accommodation. I do not in the least doubt that this is a case of posterior sclerosis; Charcot and Bouchard report a case in which pain had been the only symptom; the necropsy showed commencing sclerosis of the posterior columns."

(2) *Westphal's symptom* ("absence of knee phenomenon," "loss of patellar tendon reflex").—"Everybody knows that smart tapping just below the knee in healthy people makes the leg jump up. As Westphal and Erb point out, this does not occur in the great majority of cases of tabes. There is no doubt of the correctness of this statement. The jumping up upon the tapping is usually called patellar tendon-reflex, but as this name involves a theory much disputed and not accepted by the discoverer of the symptom, I will call the loss of this so-called reflex 'absence of the knee phenomenon,' or Westphal's symptom. It is by no means easy to be sure of the absence of the knee phenomenon. We should bare not the knees only, but the legs, let the trousers down, and take off tight drawers; then we should make the patient sit on the edge of a table with his legs hanging loose, and hit carefully both with the hand and a hammer. I am quite certain that the knee phenomenon is said to be absent when it is not. It is admitted that in cases which are evidently not cases of tabes, Westphal's symptom is present. Thus in atrophy of the quadriceps the knee phenomenon cannot, for obvious reasons, occur. Buzzard has published a case of diphtherial paralysis, in which there was Westphal's symptom. On the patient's recovery from the

paralysis the knee phenomenon returned. I have seen it absent in a case of diphtherial paralysis, but have not heard of the progress of the patient."

(3) *The ataxic gait.*—Under this head the author gave briefly the explanation of the gate of tabes dorsalis, which he gave in the *Lancet*, Jan. 30th, 1875, and the *Medical Times and Gazette*, July, 1873. He believes the so-called disorder of co-ordination to be a double condition—paresis of some movements and over-action of others. He illustrated by the duplex effects of paralysis of ocular muscles. A similar explanation has since been given by Pierret.

b. Three eye symptoms.—"One great question of interest is as to the frequency with which eye symptoms are the earliest symptoms. Since the Argyll Robert-son's symptom does not inconvenience patients, it is hard to say whether it is ever first or not. I was never consulted for that symptom, although, as I shall mention shortly, I was once consulted for a condition somewhat like it. Excluding from consideration for the moment Argyll Robertson's symptom and Westphal's symptom, since we cannot learn anything of them from the patients' accounts, I found in nineteen cases that the earliest symptoms were as follows: in ten cases pains, in six double vision, in one abnormal gait, in one optic atrophy, in one mental symptoms; probably the last was a case of general paresis. The pains are often neglected in taking note of the earliest symptoms; manifestly this puts all wrong; makes the case seem to begin months or years later than it really does."

(1) *Paralysis of parts supplied by oculo-motor nerve trunks.*—Several cases were alluded to under this head. "A man aged sixty-three, who twelve months before had had paralysis of parts supplied by the left third nerve. I could find no symptom of tabes with one very important exception: this was Westphal's symptom. Not very long ago I should have had to say that he had no symptom of tabes. I could only have guessed tabes. Thanks to Westphal, I now feel sure that this patient is tabetic. It is important to say expressly that this pa-tient's pupils acted well to light and during accommodation; he had no pains of any sort anywhere. He complained only of a heaviness in his head."

(2) *Alterations of pupils.*—The common condition described is what is called the Argyll Robertson pupil; the pupil does not act to light, and does not act during accommodation. This has been observed in tabes by Hempel, Vincent, Erb, Hutchinson, and others. It is a double condition, negative and positive, and in this way resembles the so-called disorder of co-ordination of locomotor movements. Erb calls the condition of inactivity of the pupil, "reflex pupillary immobility," and advances an hypothesis as to its fundamental community of character with Westphal's symptom. That hypothesis, however, had been pre-viously made by Buzzard; he points out that both in Westphal's symptom and in the Argyll Robertson symptom there is loss of a reflex movement when the more voluntary movement is retained. Buzzard's hypothesis seems to harmonize with the explanation suggested as to the peculiarity of the gait. It must be remem-bered that we have not merely an affair of light and pupil. It is well known that brisk cutaneous irritations cause the pupil to enlarge; pinching a comatose man will often enlarge his pupils. Erb tells us that the pupils inactive to light in cases of tabes are not affected by such procedures; he says, too, that they are not affected during lightning pains. Frequently the tabetic pupil when inactive to light is myotic also. We have in all cases to consider the size as well as the immobility of the pupil; we must remember in this regard that the senile myotic pupil contracts to light. "Although much impressed by Buzzard's generaliza-tion already mentioned, I adopt no theory on the duplex condition of the pupil. I show a diagram copied from a paper by Erb (Seguin's *Archives of Medicine*, Oct. 1880) which gives that physician's view of the central conditions correspond-

ing to the double pupillary condition. ' The following case is, in my experience, a very rare one : A woman, aged twenty-six, was sent to me simply because her right pupil was larger than the left. It had been so three years. The right pupil was dilated, and absolutely motionless to light, and also during accommodation. Yet her ciliary accommodation on this side was perfect. This was severely tested by Mr. Couper. She could read No. 1 Jaeger from fourteen inches up to five, or by effort to four. The field was perfect. The fundus was normal, except that the veins were large, and convoluted at the disk, probably physiological; the media were clear. Her sight with this eye was perfect. The pupil of the left eye was most active, and of normal size; the left disk was slightly paler than the right; the veins as on the right; macula normal; doubtful slight limitation of nasal part of field. She could read Jaeger No. 2 with the left eye, but the centre syllable of a long word seemed blurred. This case puzzled me. She seemed to be in perfect health except for the ocular abnormalities mentioned. It occurred to me to test her knees. Neither I nor Mr. Couper found the smallest trace of the knee phenomenon. Several times did I re-examine into this, and pertinaciously inquire for other symptoms of tabes ; there were no other symptoms of any kind. Except for the two things mentioned she is in seemingly perfect health.'' It is not said of Argyll Robertson's symptom that it is peculiar to tabes. It may be found in general paresis of alienists, at least reflex pupillary immobility, less frequently is there myosis, and the size of the pupils is more often unequal. Erb has found the pupillary condition in patients who had no other nervous symptoms, as well as in nervous affections which could neither be classed as tabes nor as general paresis. Again, it is not said that the action to light may not be present in very well marked cases of tabes. A man sixty-five had, as he was told by Pagenstecher, paralysis of the right external rectus in 1874 ; there was a return of double vision from some cause in 1876. He was subject to pains in his legs, his gait was ataxic; there was Westphal's symptom. He was obliged to carry a catheter to draw off his water. This patient's pupils do act to light. This was observed by Mr. Laidlaw Purves also, to whom the patient was sent for deafness. The following statement refers to cases from the pupil point of view. There were thirteen cases in which there was no optic atrophy. In ten of them the pupils did not act to light (in one case the pupil on but one side was inactive and was so in all ways). In nine of the ten cases of inactive pupils there was Westphal's symptom. Now as to paralysis of the oculo-motor nerves in the same thirteen cases. In one case with normal pupils and Westphal's symptom there had been paralysis of the third nerve. In one case of inactive pupils with Westphal's symptom there had been temporary double vision. In another case with inactive pupils and Westphal's symptom there was paralysis of one sixth nerve.

(3) *Optic atrophy.*—Tabes dorsalis is a disease which, like general paralysis, rarely occurs in women. '' When clinical assistant at Moorfields, about twenty years ago, I was struck with the fact that many of the men who had ' white atrophy' of the optic disks had also pains in their legs—the pains were lightning pains. Later on, making a distinction as to the kind of atrophy, I concluded that the pains were a symptomatic link betwixt ' uncomplicated amaurosis' and locomotor ataxy. This relation had been previously noticed. In the *Medical Times and Gazette* of Sept. 1st, 1866, I wrote : ' We have (1) amaurosis without pains in the legs ; (2) amaurosis with pains in the legs only ; (3) amaurosis with pains in the legs and difficulty in co-ordinating the legs ; (4) pains in the legs and difficulty in co-ordinating the legs, without amaurosis ; (5) amaurosis without pains in the legs and with difficulty of co-ordination.' I could now put five patients in a room showing the above sets of symptoms.' The term ' amauro-

sis' meant then atrophy which did not follow neuritis. I mention what I observed not with any view to priority, having none, but because what I then said, some fourteen years ago, was denied, and the authority of Duchenne, that the amaurosis in locomotor ataxy presented quite the ordinary features of atrophy of the optic nerve as it occurs from other causes, was quoted against me.'' The atrophy is now more particularly described as gray degeneration, and is supposed by Charcot and others to be parenchymatous. The peculiar limitation of the field of vision in cases of the atrophy in tabes is significant when we consider that the developed disease is in great part one of the locomotor system. The limitation would seem to correspond roughly to certain ocular deviations from cerebellar disease, in the way that hemiopia does to lateral deviation of the eyes from cerebral disease. In all cases of optic atrophy we should inquire for the pains, test the knees whether the gait be abnormal or not. The pains are often bridging symptoms, betwixt so-called uncomplicated amaurosis and tabes. Charcot says that so far back as 1868 he pointed out that the great majority of women admitted into La Saltpétrière for amaurosis have sooner or later manifestations of tabes. He mentions one case in which the amaurosis preceded the pains ten years. Gowers has seen a case of tabes in which optic atrophy preceded other ataxic symptoms twenty years. In the twenty-five cases mentioned there were twelve of optic atrophy. In two there were also ocular paralysis, and in one a history of it; in nine there was Westphal's symptom. In one of the three without this symptom there had been no pains; gait was slightly ataxic. In the second there had been double vision ten years ago; there is now paresis of the left third nerve; this patient had pains; his gait was normal. The third case was one of atrophy of one disk, with limitation of the field outwards and downwards; this patient saw green as gray, and red as reddish-brown; he had pains; his gait was good.

. Dr. GOWERS stated that he had examined a number of cases of ataxy with myosis and loss of reflex action to light, and he could confirm Erb's statement that in this condition the pupils did not dilate on stimulation of the skin. He thought, however, that we must hesitate in regarding this phenomenon as strictly analogous to the loss of other reflex actions in the disease, which were due ·to a lesion of the sensory structures or reflex-centres. It might be the result merely of the motor paralysis of the sympathetic fibres for the dilator pupillæ. This view was confirmed by one case which he had seen, in which, although there-was loss of reflex action to light, there was not myosis, and the pupils did dilate on cutaneous stimulation.—*Lancet,* Dec. 18, 1880.

—

The Influence of Menstruation in the Progress of Pulmonary Consumption.

Dr. DAREMBERG, of Mentone, has been writing in the *Archives Générales de Médecine* upon this subject. There is no question that disturbances of the menstrual function very commonly accompany phthisis; and the view of their relationship to one another which is commonly accepted in this country, is that the latter is the cause, and the former the effect. Dr. Daremberg has seen reason for thinking that the state of the menstrual function has a distinct influence upon the lung-disease. His experience leads him to make the following statements upon this subject : Menstruation is sometimes a cause of phthisis; in the sense that women become phthisical who would not have done so had they been free from the monthly loss of blood. When phthisical changes have begun, the menstrual function may lead to attacks of congestion, either around old foci of disease, or in healthy parts of the lung, which may go on to hemorrhage or to inflammation. When the catamenial flow is suppressed, the ovarian molimen being still present, these congestions are liable to become more intense and more dangerous. If the discharge should persist after ovulation has disappeared, it becomes simply a cause of anæmia, but does not provoke reflex congestions. When the two functions, uterine and ovarian, are suppressed—that is, when the menopause has completely taken place—menstrual congestions are no more to be dreaded. After delivery, similar pulmonary congestions of reflex origin are to be feared. The abrupt suppression of the menses cannot *per se* bring about tuberculosis; but it may cause its development in women predisposed to it. From these pathological generalizations he draws the following principles of treatment. In phthisical women the lungs should be carefully watched during the menstrual period, and at the least sign of mischief the nervous and vascular excitement should be calmed by the moderate use of digitalis, bromide of potassium, and quinine; absolute rest should be advised, and the pulmonary organs should be acted on by energetic revulsives (blisters, croton oil, etc.), and this during several successive periods. If the menstrual flow should cease while the ovarian molimen continues its course, the same treatment should be carried out, with the addition of external means to bring back the discharge (blisters, friction, hot baths, leeches to the lower extremities); and if these do not succeed, then the careful employment of purgatives and internal emmenagogues (general stimulants, such as alcohol and acetate of ammonia; local excitants, as rue, savin, aloes, uva ursi, apiol, ergot of rye, borax; and tonics, viz., strychnia and quinine). These measures, he holds, will do good, even if they should not re-establish menstruation. When the discharge persists after ovulation has ceased, we should with caution endeavour to diminish it, bearing in mind, that its sudden suppression may be dangerous; and the same remark applies to leucorrhœa. When both functions (uterine and ovarian) have disappeared, we should keep from seeking to re-excite the flow, for it will then be useless and cause anæmia. When, after a long absence, the menses reappear, without any great improvement being evident in the local and general condition, it is necessary to be very cautious about giving a favourable prognosis; for this apparent return of menstruation often indicates grave disturbance of the circulation, and is the precursor of serious mischief.—*Med. Times and Gazette*, Jan. 8, 1881.

—

The Muscles in Phthisis.

Two years ago FRÄNKEL, observing how many patients with phthisis presented hoarseness without any corresponding laryngoscopic changes, investigated the condition of the laryngeal muscles in order to ascertain whether any changes in them explained the symptom. In a considerable number of cases, both those in which there were ulcerations in the mucous membrane and those in which the naked-eye appearances were normal, he found constantly an atrophy of the striated muscles. The contractile substance was broken up, the striation indistinct, and a granular opacity had replaced the normal translucence, while in the fibres in which the process was more advanced there was an actual molecular destruction, and ultimate disappearance of the proper tissue. The connective tissue between the primitive bundles also presented a marked cell-formation, and the muscle nuclei were so increased in number as to constitute cellular sheaths to the fibres. This increase seemed to have produced additional damage to the muscular fibres, since these in places were apparently destroyed by the pressure of the groups of cells.

These observations have been confirmed by a series of investigations on forty phthisical subjects by Dr. POSADSKY of St. Petersburg, which show that the changes found by Fränkel in the muscles of the larynx exist also in other muscles examined—viz., those of the upper and lower limbs, flexors and extensors, the intercostal muscles, and the diaphragm. The muscular fibres were pale, and exceedingly friable, so that they broke across with undue readiness, and could with difficulty be separated into longitudinal fibrils. This was found in two-thirds of the cases; in the remaining third the muscles were perfectly healthy. The microscope showed a granular degeneration of the fibres in all cases in which the naked-eye changes were observed. In many cases the transverse striation had entirely disappeared. Many of the fibres were strikingly narrowed, and some empty sarcolemma sheaths were seen. Fibres which were not degenerated also showed the tendency to break up into transverse segments which had been noted in the naked-eye examination. Why these changes should be so conspicuous in some cases of phthisis and absent in others it is difficult to say, since the cases with and those without the change presented nearly the same conditions and nearly the same visceral changes. The changes in the interstitial connective tissue described by Fränkel were not found by Posadsky.—*Lancet*, Jan. 22, 1881.

—

Passive Congestion of the Spleen.

At the suggestion of Virchow, the histological changes in the spleen which result from passive congestion have been studied very carefully by Dr. R. NIKO-LAIDES. In the indurated organ, the naked eye can detect a thick white layer around the vessels, which renders the tint of the section a paler red than might be expected. Under the microscope the walls of the bloodvessels, and especially those of the arteries, are seen to be enormously thickened by an increase of the adventitia and the adjacent zone of tissue, which passes gradually into the neighbouring reticulum of the splenic pulp. The trabeculæ are thickened, and the contiguous cells of the pulp undergo atrophy, just as do the outer cells of the acini of the liver in cirrhosis. These changes are more or less marked in all congested spleens, and confer upon the organ its increased density. Their degree appears to depend upon the slowness with which the mechanical congestion is developed. Besides these changes, alterations occur also in the intima of the vessels. They are most marked in the arteries, and are only found in the veins in very chronic cases. In the veins the change consists in merely fatty degeneration; but the inner coat of the arteries presents an overgrowth of all the connective tissue layers—a true end-arteritis, similar to that which Virchow has described in the veins of some other organs, as the lungs and liver, in passive congestion. It is difficult to say whether the muscular coat of the vessels is thickened or not; but Nikolaides believes that there is a considerable increase in the circular muscular fibres. Not only is this conclusion suggested by histological examination, but it is remarked that the mechanical congestion of the spleen never entails the degree of hyperæmia met with in other organs, as the liver and the kidney, in spite of the fact that the circulatory arrangement of the spleen is highly favourable to the occurrence of such hyperæmia. This fact is regarded as supporting the view that in congestion the muscular walls of the arteries contract, overgrow, and lessen the hyperæmia. The evidence on this point seems scarcely conclusive. Some share in this effect might be ascribed to an overaction of the muscular fibres proper to the splenic pulp, since it is difficult to understand, without such overaction, how the blood could be lessened in an organ, like the spleen, destitute of capillaries, by contraction of the arteries, if there exists an obstruction to the exit of blood. The splenic follicles, Nikolaides believes to take no part in the overgrowth of tissue which results from passive congestion.—*Lancet*, Jan. 29, 1881.

*

The Treatment of Abscess of the Liver.

In a recent communication (*Bulletin de l'Académie de Médecine*, No. 43, 1880), M. J. ROCHARD describes the treatment of hepatic abscess by free and direct incision, combined with the practice of Lister's antiseptic method. Three cases are reported, in which this treatment was carried out with complete success by Dr. STROMEYER LITTLE, of Shanghai.

Abscess of the liver, M. Rochard states, when not treated surgically, causes death in about 80 per cent. of the cases. The old methods of surgical treatment have not reduced this rate of mortality to any great extent; certainly, in cases of large abscess, to not less than 68 per cent. Consequently, surgeons have not been eager in interfering, and some, with Dr. Maclean, in consideration of the prolonged suppuration resulting from the opening of a large hepatic abscess, and of the putrefaction of pus and the gangrene consequent on the penetration of air into the large cavity, have declined to intervene. Most surgeons who have to deal with cases of this kind, think it right to open the abscess, but, before doing so, wait until œdema and redness of the abdominal wall have indicated the point to which the pus is making its way, and often whilst waiting lose their patient, or find that the abscess has burst internally. Finally, in cases where such practice is successful, the cure is attained at the price to the patient of many months of suffering and danger. A method which would permit the surgeon to act in good time, to operate with certainty, and to effect a cure within one month, must be regarded as constituting considerable progress. That such progress has been made seems, according to M. Rochard, to be proved by the results of the treatment carried out in the three recorded cases. Dr. Little had previously treated twenty cases of hepatic abscess either by frequently repeated puncture and aspiration, or by incision without any antiseptic precautions. All the patients died with the exception of one, in whom a small abscess with a chronic course projected into the epigastric region, and was opened there without any bad results. In his three recent cases, Dr. Little had recourse to the method described and discussed in M. Rochard's communication. This method consists in determining, with as much precision as possible, the seat of the purulent collection; in verifying the diagnosis by puncture and aspiration; then using the needle as a conductor, making a free incision into the abscess, clearing out all the contents, and, finally, preventing consecutive mischief by antiseptic injections, drainage, and Listerian dressings. The diagnosis of abscess of the liver, M. Rochard points out, is not easy. Local pain is not manifested until the pus has reached the surface of the organ, and perihepatitis has been excited. This symptom is often absent, even in cases of very large hepatic abscess. Reflex pain in the right shoulder, also, is very frequently absent. The only symptoms on which reliance can be placed, are increase in the size of the organ, digestive and respiratory disturbances, and fever. In most of the cases, the hepatitis succeeds dysentery or dysenteric diarrhœa. When, in a subject who has suffered from either of these affections, fever occurs, the digestion becomes disturbed, and the liver enlarges, it may be concluded that hepatitis has been developed. If the fever present a remittent character, with evening exacerbations, preceded by rigors and followed by sweating, the formation of an abscess should be expected, and steps at once taken to test this diagnosis by puncture and aspiration. The abscess is situated in the right lobe in seven out of ten cases, and in most cases projects at the convex surface of the organ. The dulness then extends towards the nipple, and is bounded by a curve with its convexity upwards. The patient is troubled by cough, dyspnœa, and pain during inspiration, and occasionally auscultation and percussion reveal the signs of diaphragmatic pleurisy. In a case of this kind, the most favourable seat of an exploratory puncture would be the eighth or ninth intercostal space, in a line with the anterior border of the axilla. When the purulent collection projects at the concave surface of the liver, the false ribs are expanded, and the extent of the swelling may be made out by palpation. The spontaneous pains, when they occur, radiate towards the iliac fossæ and the sacral region. Vomiting is a frequent symptom. An exploratory puncture in such case is best made below the margin of the eighth rib, and at the point where there is tenderness on pressure.

The preliminary puncture is made by Dr. Little with a needle about three millimetres in diameter, the instrument having been dipped in carbolic oil, and the integument of the right hypochondrium washed with a 5 per cent. solution of carbolic acid. It is often found necessary to introduce the needle several times before pus can be obtained. These repeated punctures of the liver, as has been proved by the observations of Jaccoud and Lavigerie, are absolutely free from danger.

When the presence of pus has been made out, a free incision through the whole thickness of the abdominal wall is made by the side of the needle, and parallel to the ribs. The evacuation of the fluid contents of the abscess is facilitated by the introduction of forceps between the lips of the wound, and by expansion of the blades, and also by the transmission of manual pressure through the abdominal wall to the inferior surface of the liver. The cavity of the abscess is then washed out with a weak solution of carbolic acid, until no traces of pus, of flakes, and of portions of slough, can any longer be seen in the returning current of the injected fluid. A piece of drainage-tubing of very wide calibre is then passed to the bottom of the cavity, the outer portion of this being cut off on a level with the wound. Application is then made of the ordinary antiseptic dressing of gauze with protective and jaconette, which dressing is maintained by means of an elastic bandage. This dressing is changed daily, and at the same time the protruded portion of the drainage-tube is cut away. The results of this treatment in the three cases treated by Dr. Stromeyer Little were most satisfactory. The operation in each instance was immediately followed by improvement in the general condition of the patient. There was also immediate disappearance of fever, and complete absence, during the subsequent treatment, of any febrile reaction. In two cases, complete cure was attained within one month, and in the third case, in which a second operation was necessitated through relapse, the patient was able to travel on the seventy-sixth day.—*London Med. Record*, Jan. 15, 1881.

Jaundice in New-born Infants: Icterus Neonatorum.

There are many points of interest in the jaundice to which young infants are peculiarly liable. As age advances, they of course become liable to jaundice from exactly the same causes which produce it in adults. It occurs too, sometimes, as an epidemic, and would then seem to be dependent on some cause which might be either infection or one more or less widely spread and more or less uniformly acting within a given area. The etiology of the disease in new-born infants is difficult to study, owing to the nature of the circumstances; and thus at present we have hardly passed the stage of hypothesis on this point, although the disease is very common.

The latest summary of our present knowledge is from the pen of Dr. ALOIS EPSTEIN; it is published in Volkmann's *Sammlung Klinischer Vorträge*. It would seem desirable to exclude from this consideration all cases of more or less congenital jaundice, due to any malformations. Thus, obliteration of the larger ducts would offer an impediment to the flow of the bile; and this would lead to jaundice. Occasionally there is found an absence of the gall-bladder also, though this, except the ductus communis was also absent or closed, could never cause jaundice. Then, again, there may be congenital disease of the parenchyma (interstitial hepatitis), or occasionally cirrhosis, due to syphilis. Finally may be mentioned the pyæmic hepatitis, spreading along the umbilical vein, which, though rare, is nevertheless sometimes met with. With such cases we are not at present occupied, for there are anatomical grounds quite sufficient to account for the morbid condition.

Icterus neonatorum is *characterized* by an abnormal deposit of yellow pigment in the skin and mucous membranes. Many authors consider this jaundice as physiological and normal. They regard it as one of the transformation phases of the bright-red colour of the integument of new-born babies, which set in shortly after birth, and which they consider due to the altered temperature of the surrounding medium in which a child lives after intra-uterine life is over. It seems difficult, says our author, to accept such a theory, because so many children are born healthy and strong who yet never show a trace of this yellowness. Neither does the intensity of the colour stand in any constant relationship with the intensity of the previous redness; and further, children who are pale when born become jaundiced, while those of a deep red colour not infrequently change to a normal tint without evincing any yellowness at all. We must also remember that an erythema (redness) of several days' duration is itself very often a sign of impaired respiration and circulation. For these reasons we are bound to regard the icterus as a pathological condition.

The *frequency* with which jaundice is found will never be very accurately made out, owing to the difficulties of collecting the cases from private practice. But it would seem that the disease is much less common in the country and in private generally than among infants born in public lying-in institutions. This deduction is entirely found on the statement of mothers, who have already had children which were not jaundiced; but it must be counterbalanced by others, which go to prove without doubt that many exceptions to this rule occur. Dr. Charles West states, in his work on Children's Diseases (sixth edition), that jaundice seldom occurred in the Dublin Rotunda, while few children escaped it in the Paris Foundling Hospital. He believes that this was due to the excellent sanitary arrangements of the former, while those children which get into the Foundling Hospital in Paris have to contend largely with the ill effects of bad air as well as of cold. Seux, in Marseilles, found it present in 15 per cent. of the children; Scanzoni, in Würzburg, in 58 per cent.; Porak, in the Cochin Hospital in Paris, in 80 per cent.; and Kehrer, in Vienna, in 68.4 per cent.

The jaundice generally *comes on* during the first week of life, and in a majority of cases on the second or third day after birth; from this time, as age advances, the cases become rarer. It usually *lasts* from six to eight days, so that among children two weeks old it is rare to meet with any having a yellow skin. In premature children, in whom the physiological processes (the falling-off of the navel-string, the exfoliation of the epidermis, etc.) are somewhat retarded, so also the pathological take place less rapidly, and hence the jaundice may be protracted for two or three days longer. The *intensity* of the colour varies, among other things, with the complexion of the child, from a pale straw-yellow to a bright lemon or yelk-yellow. In cases the prognosis of which is bad, due to plugging of peripheral ducts, the yellow assumes a bluish or greenish tint—cyanosis icterica, in fact. The *distribution* of the pigment is not always uniform; thus the conjunctiva, though often yellow in colour, may be free, or not tinted to the same extent as other tissues. The same also applies to the subcutaneous connective tissues. On the whole, it may be said that the yellowness depends chiefly on the amount of blood in a part, and on circulatory conditions of individual parts, and that the various shades which can be detected in new-born children would seem to be best explained by the transparency of the epidermis. At the approach of death, not infrequently the jaundice suddenly disappears from the integuments; and a conjunctiva which has shown palpable signs of icteric pigmentation during life, may be found quite free from it after death.

As regards *symptoms*, it will be best to emphasize those which do not occur in the jaundice of adult life. Pain in the region of the liver, and palpable enlargement of the organ, are not as a rule present, although the edge of the gland may just be felt if the abdominal walls are fairly flaccid. Slowing of the pulse is not present, nor is there any appreciable change in respiration. The function of the intestinal tract is normal; there is generally no constipation. On the other hand, any catarrh which may happen to be present cannot be attributed to the jaundice. The feces are always bile-stained, never, as in adults, clay-coloured, neither is there any obvious excess of fat present in them. The urine, even in intense forms of the disease, is often free from colour, and generally only light yellow; very rarely is it darkly stained as in adults, and when it is there are for the most part blood-corpuscles or blood-products to be found at the same time. Fairly often there is albumen in the urine, the presence of which, however, during the first few days of life does not seem to be very uncommon. It may also be mentioned that dark-coloured urine in children the subject of this complaint, on being tested, does not always contain bile-pigment; and even when it stains the linen yellow, it is not always to be put down to the presence of bile, as is too frequently done.

Epstein's method of obtaining the pigment is as follows: He collects the urine (with a catheter if necessary), and precipitates any albumen, if present; it is then shaken up with lime-water; the filtrate is washed in alcohol, and sulphuric acid added. The sediment thus produced consists of amorphous masses of uric acid together with the characteristic crystalline, or grains of, pigment. The pigment is easily distinguishable from the uric acid by its yellowish or yellowish-red colour. On adding caustic soda and acetic acid, the uric acid forms urate of soda, while the pigment remains unchanged. On microscopic examination, the pigment is found in the form of fine, tuft-like needles, or in tables, or sometimes as an amorphous deposit. It may likewise be found in the kidney-tubules and epithelium, and in the bloodvessels and interstitial connective tissue. Besides these places, this same pigment may be found more or less richly in the blood and in the other organs, chiefly in the neighbourhood of the vessels. Epstein has repeatedly found it in the brain, in circumscribed patches. It occurs also in the liver, but it is not found there more abundantly than in the places just mentioned. There is still some uncertainty as to the exact *nature and source* of this pigment in icteric children. Meckel and Neumann regard it as bilirubin, while Virchow and Buhl consider it as hæmatoidin; but, seeing that some chemists regard these two substances as almost identical, further research will be necessary before the point can be definitely settled.

The *etiology* of the condition is one of difficulty, and it must be by the way of exclusion rather than by direct means that we approach it. Most authors, if not all, and until quite lately, have not unnaturally associated it with changes in the liver, and regard it as hepatogenic—*i. e.*, as resulting from absorption of formed bile into the blood-circulation. Frerichs sought to explain it as a result of the altered blood-pressure in the liver which commenced at the moment of birth, when the navel-string was tied. But, though very clever, this is merely hypothetical, for we are in complete darkness as to whether any alteration in the blood-pressure really does take place; if it were so, the condition at once becomes physiological, and it should be found, to a greater or lesser degree, in all children. Virchow, as long ago as 1846, pointed out the probable hæmatogenic origin, but a little later he withdrew from this opinion, and came to regard the jaundice as catarrhal and due to mechanical causes. Virchow's name secured for the catarrhal doctrine a wide acceptance. Epstein has bestowed special attention to the elucidation of this point, and has been unable to accept Virchow's teaching, for in most cases the ductus choledochus is found to contain bile along its whole length, the feces are bile-stained, and the liver, as regards size, colour, and consistence, is always normal. Other authors have sought for the source of this pigment in the integuments. Billard thought it due to congestion, and to the consequent transudation of blood-colouring matter. West also adopted this view. But, considering that the intensity of the jaundice, no less than its occurrence, seems to be quite independent of hemorrhages, such as occur after the use of forceps, or cephalhæmatoma, one is led to doubt this theory of mere congestion and transudation. On the other hand, there is much to confirm a hæmatogenic source from other causes than transudation—viz., an autochthonous formation of abnormal pigment resulting from the decomposition of fœtal red blood-corpuscles in the bloodvessels, and quite independent of the liver. The view is upheld by the well-known occurrence of jaundice in many of the acute infectious diseases and in hæmoglobinuria. Kühne has shown that the injection into the blood of a variety of substances (water, gallic acid, ether, ammonia) gives rise to the presence of bile-pigment in the urine. Gubler, in the year 1857, described a form of jaundice under the term "ictère hémapheique" in adults, resulting from a rapid destruction of red corpuscles. He distinguishes it from mechanical jaundice (ictère bilipheique) by its lighter colour, the absence of retardation of the pulse, and of itching in the skin. In the next place, are there any facts which confirm the occurrence of a destruction of blood-cells? Microscopic examination, as well as an enumeration of the blood-cells, largely confirm this view. According to Neumann and Kölliker, the blood of full-term infants contains a number of pigment granules, which after a while disappear; and further, there are observations which show that infants' blood is specifically heavier and richer in hæmatoidin than maternal blood. Spectral analysis also confirms this latter observation; while Hayem has shown that during the first fourteen days of life, and from day to day, the corpuscles present obvious and remarkable differences both in number and form. This being the case, we next inquire what should lead to such destruction of the red blood-cells. In answering the question, we naturally think of the altered conditions under which the child begins to live after intra-uterine life has ended, and of the important physiological changes by which this is brought about. Thus it seems probable that a large quantity of red corpuscles are called suddenly into use for respiratory purposes when the breathing medium is no longer the half-oxidized blood of the uterine sinuses, but the air directly inhaled into the lungs. Moreover, the blood corpuscles must be formed in a new way—not as in the fœtal state, from maternal fluids, but from the products of digestion. Thus it may be that the fœtal corpuscles may differ in certain respects from those of independent life. All things considered, then, this seems to be by far the most probable explanation of the occurrence of bile-pigment in the skin of young infants; it is favoured rather than otherwise by the fact that this so-called jaundice is most common in prematurely born infants and in those which are born weakly. Unfavourable hygienic circumstances will naturally react, and with proportionate power, on weakly children; and thus will be accounted for the large percentage of cases met with in public institutions, which are chiefly for the use of the poor and needy, as compared with those placed in more favourable circumstances.—*Med. Times and Gaz.*, Dec. 4 and 18, 1880.

A Case of Acute Fibrinuria.

Dr. BAUMÜLLER (Virchow's *Archiv*, Band lxxxii. Heft 2) describes the case of a woman who, after several attacks of hæmaturia, extending over a period 'of three years, passed white slimy masses, and thereafter improved and recovered. On examining these masses, they were found 'to consist of casts of the calyces, pelvis, and ureter. Under the microscope the urinary deposit showed numerous pus-corpuscles, and many tiny crystals of triple phosphates, but no ephithelium. The coagula consisted of very fine granules in a homogeneous basis substance, with here and there disintegrating red blood-corpuscles. The granules disappeared on treatment with ether. The urine was clear yellow, turbid, neutral; specific gravity of 1014–15; it gave a precipitate on boiling and adding acid, which dissolved in excess. Further examination showed it to contain serum, albumen, and paraglobulin. The coagula were insoluble in water, alcohol, ether, chloroform, alkalies, and concentrated mineral and organic acids, both at ordinary temperatures and on boiling. In caustic potash, concentrated solution of sodium chloride (less in dilute hydrochloric acid), and concentrated acetic acid, there was some swelling to be observed; also after longer action of dilute hydrochloric acid, lime-water, solution of sodium chloride, acetic acid, and alcohol. In alcohol, after two or three days, the swollen masses broke up into ragged shreds. Attempts to digest the masses with gastric juice, obtained from a fistula in a dog, or with artificial gastric juice, failed. He considers the phenomena to have been due to an acute fibrinuria, such as Vogel has described (Virchow's *Handbuch der Specieller Path. und Therapie*, Band vi. 2 Abtheilung, sec. 542), and which is derived from a purulent catarrh of the pelvis of the kidney.—*London Med. Record*, Jan. 15, 1881.

Surgery.

The Catgut Ligature.

There is no part of the surgical practice instituted by Mr. Lister that has excited more interest and attention than his reintroduction of an animal ligature. In spite of many experiments, and much clinical experience, the opinion of the profession is far from unanimous in favour of carbolized catgut. Imperfections in its preparation, and its use in unsuitable cases, may explain a part, if not all, of the failures and accidents that have attended its employment, but its most ardent advocates, we believe, will grant that some improvement in its preparation is still demanded. A recent contribution to our knowledge of the action of catgut ligatures is found in a memoir entitled "Contribution à l'Étude de la Ligature dans le Traitement des Anévrismes," by Dr. G. F. Arnaud. Dr. ARNAUD ligatured the carotid or femoral artery of dogs fourteen times, using carbolized catgut, and examined the parts from four to sixteen days afterwards. In nine cases the ligature had entirely disappeared, or was only scarcely appreciable; in two it was partially absorbed, with destruction of the knot; and in three it was little altered. In one of the latter only four days had elapsed from the application of the ligature, which may be held to account for the fact; in the other two, examined on the ninth and sixteenth days respectively, there was an absence of inflammatory reaction and clot, and the ligature was encysted, while for its ab-sorption a rather abundant outpouring of lymph, or development of "granula-tions," is held to be necessary.   In twelve of these cases the outer coat of the artery was found quite unaltered, not having been severed by the ligature; in two it was partially ulcerated, in neither case completely.   In twelve cases, the inner and middle coats of the vessel were completely divided, as happens in the use of a silk or hempen thread; in one they were entire, and in one other it was doubtful whether they were partly divided or not.   The clot, where not absorbed, was very small, and the obliteration of the artery was complete and firm.   Senf-tleben has stated that internal clot rarely forms with catgut ligatures, but the evidence of these experiments, as well as of others, points to an opposite con-clusion.   Arnaud concludes that the effect of catgut on the artery is like that of hemp, except—a most important exception—that the outer coat is not ulcerated, the knot of the ligature softening before that occurs.   It was noticed, in cases where a strand of catgut was left in the tract of the wound, that there was much more active cell-growth round the ligature than around these strands, with corre-sponding difference in the rate of absorption.   The "absorption" of catgut is thus again fully corroborated, and still more the fact that the use of catgut liga-tures is not necessarily followed by the complete severance of the artery, with the attendant risk of secondary hemorrhage, as always follows the use of hemp or silk.—*Lancet,* Jan. 22, 1881.

—

Gouty Cataract.

Dr. GALEZOWSKI (*Recueil d'Ophthalmologie*, Sept. 1880) records four cases of cataract recurring in gouty subjects.   These cataracts belong to the secondary stage of gout; that, namely, in which all the tissues have become thoroughly saturated with the poison.   While occupied in looking for glucose in diabetic cataracts, Dr. Galezowski accidentally found that in many cases uric acid salts were present in the crystalline lenses of gouty subjects.   Gouty cataracts appear most usually from the ages of 50 to 70, and are generally hard, though he has also seen them in younger subjects of a more or less soft consistence.   Gout often acts as the predisposing cause, after operation, of various inflammatory affections of the iris, sclerotic, and less frequently of the choroid.   In the gouty diathesis, cataracts often become adherent, and are complicated with synechiæ and narrow-ing of the pupil.   The best chance of success in these cases is to place the patient for some weeks before operation on a strictly anti-arthritic regimen, and to give large doses of salicylate of soda.   In some of these cases, some days after opera-tion, a collection of blood forms in the lower part of the anterior chamber; in others, it remains suspended in the aqueous humour, rendering it turbid.   This blood transudes from the iris or ciliary circle, and is a very constant manifestation of the gouty diathesis.   In some cases it would appear that the gouty manifesta-tions in the eye were due to the irritation of the wound, and hence were, in their origin, traumatic.   In such cases, local remedies are powerless, but the symptoms at once yield to large doses of salicylate of soda internally.—*London Med. Record,* Jan. 15, 1881.

—

Syphilis in Cataract.

Dr. GALEZOWSKI (*Recueil d'Ophthalmologie*, Sept. 1880) considers that syphilis may cause cataract in the adult primarily, or predispose to it hereditarily. He gives details of a case of kerato-irido-choroiditis in a child of four years of age affected with syphilis from its birth.   In this case, a cataract became developed, and the eye was enucleated.   The author has seen, in all, nine cases of congenital cataract in children born of syphilitic parents. As regards the effects of syphilis in the adult, he has frequently seen cases of monocular cataract affecting an eye in which there was syphilitic choroiditis, while in the other eye the lens was perfectly transparent. He gives details of a case of syphilitic choroiditis attacking one eye, followed by the development of soft cataract six months afterwards in the other.—*London Med. Record*, Jan. 15, 1881.

Examination of Vision in Railway Employés.

The conclusions of the Committee, WARLOMONT and MOELLER, appointed by the Minister of Public Works in Belgium to report upon the vision of railway employés, with special reference to the detection of Daltonism, have recently been made public (*Annales d' Oculistique*, September–October, 1880). The committee recommends that in future all persons employed on the State Railways should, as regards their visual and chromatic acuity, be placed after examination in one of the following classes, viz., "very satisfactory," "satisfactory," and "unsatisfactory," the latter class being inadmissible into the public service. The requirements of the first class are laid down as follows: 1. Eyes and eyelids healthy, and free from all habitual irritation or congestion; 2. Normal acuity ($= 1$); refraction perfect within the dioptric; 3. A normal field of vision; 4. The power of distinguishing colours to the extent of $\frac{4}{4}$ at least; 5. Complete freedom from cataract or other disease. For the second class the conditions are the same, except that in one of the eyes visual acuity must be normal, in the other it may be $\frac{1}{2}$, and the perception of colour must in one be at least $\frac{3}{4}$, in the other at least $\frac{2}{4}$. In the report is included the instructions for the examining medical officer, which are as follows. Holmgren's colour-test is the one recommended, the candidate being required to match all the shades of several given colours selected at random. Refraction is to be tested by Loiseau's optometer, which is constructed on the principle of finding the reading distance of the patient when using a lens of known focal length. Visual acuity is to be determined by the use of a series of three test types prepared *ad hoc ;* the limits of the field of vision by the movements of the hand, held at the distance of 1 metre.—*London Med. Record*, Jan. 15, 1881.

Treatment of Aural Polypi.

Although Professor POLITZER (*Wiener Medizin. Wochenschrift*, July 31, 1880) finds the action of alcohol, as recommended by Löwenberg, excellent in some cases of chronic otorrhœa, he considers that, in regard to the frequency of its good effect, it is inferior to boracic acid, as recommended by Bezold, whilst, in the rapidity of action, it ranks second to the caustic method of Schwartze. In the treatment of polypoid growths, however, the author strongly recommends its use in the form of rectified spirit. This is applied either pure or (if this produces much pain) diluted with an equal quantity of water, and is poured thrice daily, warm, into the meatus, being allowed to remain there from ten to fifteen minutes. The indications for its use are, he considers, as follows: 1. In the treatment of remains of polypi in the meatus, on the membrana tympani, or in the tympanic cavity, which are not removable by operation; 2. In cases of multiple granulations in the meatus, or on the membrana tympani; 3. In diffuse hypertrophy of the tympanic membrane; 4. In cases in which mechanical impediments in the meatus prevent the removal of polypi by instrumental means; 5. It may be employed experimentally in order to avoid an operation if possible in very nervous persons and in young children. The author relates a case in which, after partial removal of a polypus growing from the meatus, a portion of the size of a pea still remained ; but, as the patient had to leave the town on business, alcohol drops were prescribed. When he presented himself again after several months, the remains of the polypus had entirely disappeared. Other cases illustrative of the good effects of alcohol are also described. The author, it may be noted, expressly states that this treatment often requires to be continued for weeks or even months, and mentions that one of its chief advantages is that it can be employed with good effect by any surgeon, no especial skill in manipulation being required, as in the case of the application of strong caustics.—*London Med. Record*, Jan. 15, 1881.

Epithelioma of the Tongue.

A paper read by Prof. VERNEUIL at the Société de Chirurgie (*Bulletin*, November 10, *et seq.*), "On the Inutility and Danger of Pharmaceutical and Topical Treatment of Surgical Epithelioma," gave rise to a prolonged discussion. He observed that he addressed his observations not so much to the members of the Society as to practitioners at large, for while he did not believe that any of his colleagues had any faith in the medical treatment of epithelioma, unfortunately the great mass of practitioners are of a different opinion. He has scarcely ever seen a case that had not previously been treated by iodide of potassium, or even by mercury, while some caustic substance or chlorate of potash has always been used. "At the commencement of my practice, I also, on the faith of others, did what I now condemn." How comes it that a practice which is inefficacious and injurious has become so diffused and tenacious? 1. There is a very general belief that the iodide is a good means against neoplasms. It is, however, a great error to suppose that it is useful in true neoplasms; for, however useful it may be in tertiary syphilis, in scrofulous pseudo-plasms, or in chronic inflammations, it is of no avail in epithelioma or cancer. 2. The tongue is sometimes the seat of syphilitic manifestations, curable by mercury or the iodide, and as lingual syphilis is but ill known, and lingual epithelioma at its commencement still less known, the specific treatment is employed with the vague hope that the medicine will find out what it is suitable for. A cure may in this way be accidentally effected, but can be no rule why mercury should be given in all cases. The diagnosis is the great thing; and since the writings of H. Fournier the diagnosis of a tertiary glossitis is easy. There are, indeed, occasionally hybrid cases in which epithelioma occurs in a syphilitic subject, but this is of little consequence, as the prognosis and treatment of such a case is that of epithelioma. As in the immense majority of cases the diagnosis is easy, the practice of giving mercury or the iodide in epitheliomatous affections of the tongue should be abandoned. 3. Internal remedies are given to seem to be doing something, and not to alarm the patient by announcing the necessity of an operation, which also there may be inability to perform—it being also thought that there will always be time to seek the aid of a surgeon. This fear of alarming the patient about an operation decuples his danger, for this epithelioma, like all those which invade the mucous membranes, is a very dangerous one, although it may sometimes be cured when taken in time. Prof. Verneuil has met with four such cases, but then in these the epithelioma did not exceed the nail in size and was not deeply placed. But when more than a third of the tongue is invaded, when the floor of the mouth is seized, when the glands have degenerated, and the disease has lasted for more than a year, the case has become deplorably serious. The operation might have succeeded at the time when medicines were being given, but no chance of success remains at the late period when the surgeon is consulted. 4. The idea prevails that cauterization is useful for ulcerations, and these ulcers of the tongue are tormented by caustics, forgetting that this method is useful only when destructive and not merely modificative. 5. When there is but little illusion as to the curative effect of medicines and cauterizations, it is still believed that these means are, at all events, innocent. This is a great error; not only is precious time lost, but the iodide of mercury and the chlorate may aggravate the conditions of the disease.

In the discussion which followed the paper, Dr. ANGER, in confirmation of Prof. Verneuil's views, stated that in a large number of 260 cases of cancer of the tongue which he had collected, he had found that the disease had been aggravated by the administration of the iodide, and especially by mercury. He did not think that the diagnosis was quite so easy as stated by Prof. Verneuil, and in doubtful cases a morsel of the tumour should be examined by the microscope. As a local treatment he had sometimes found interstitial injections of salicylic acid calm the pain, and especially the sympathetic pain of the ear. They even seem to arrest the progress of the disease. Dr. DESPRÈS also believed that Prof. Verneuil makes too light of the diagnosis, for among other affections of the tongue, psoriasis may be confounded with it. In doubtful cases he is in the habit of cauterizing gently with the nitrate of silver, and if after some days the ulceration undergoes a favourable modification, he feels certain that he has not to do with an epithelioma. When, after an operation, the case persists for ten years or more, we have had to do with a simple psoriasis, for epithelioma of the tongue always relapses within the space of two years. Prof. TRÉLAT observed that this communication of Prof. Verneuil's led to such useful and practical conclusions that he desired to adduce his own personal experience in support of it. In 1876, while drawing the attention of surgeons to the transformation of lingual psoriasis into epithelioma, he had insisted especially on the great advantage of operating early and on the efficacy of such operations. But patients and practitioners seem to do all they can to prevent these early and inoffensive operations, and only apply when the operation required has become extensive, and success nearly impossible. For the last five years Prof. Trélat has refused to perform these dangerous and useless operations. Of many patients who have consulted him when the epithelioma has been operable and success highly probable, he has never been able, by persuasion or alarms, to induce one to submit to it at that stage. The diagnosis should be made as early as possible, and in doubtful cases it is far better to perform an unnecessary operation than to leave the patient to the probability of an early death. All are agreed, in fact, as to the desirability of early operations, as must be the case when the results following these, as regards the prolongation of life, are contrasted with those which are observed in patients left to themselves. Prof. LE FORT, while agreeing that a cancroid which is limited should at once be operated upon, believes that when the disease has greatly extended, relapse takes place so rapidly that it is better to abstain from operating in these cases. Prof. Verneuil, however, differed from this view, believing that palliative operations which relieve the patient's sufferings, and may prolong his life for awhile, are justifiable. They must, however, be on a large scale, when they may give very great relief, and render life supportable for some months. M. GUYON expressed himself with more reserve as to these palliative operations—so rapid is the relapse in such cases. M. LABBÉ maintained that it was the right and duty of the surgeon to intervene even in these desperate cases, but he must intervene boldly, and proceed far beyond the disease itself, however far this may have reached. He ties the two linguals, and removes the part by means of large scissors, which enable him to effect this much more exactly than by any other means.

Prof. VERNEUIL afterwards drew the attention of his colleagues to the importance of extensive operations for epithelioma as a security against relapse, referring especially to the numerous cases of total extirpation of the tongue published by Billroth and Schepffer. By means of extensive operations great success has sometimes been obtained in apparently very desperate cases. It might be thought that in far less formidable cases even more success would be obtained; but this is far from being so. The operations are too parsimonious, and a prompt relapse occurs, the relapse always occurring at one of three points—the stump of the tongue, the soft parts of the floor of the mouth, or in the cervical glands; and the rapid and inexorable relapse takes place because the operation has been incomplete. The glands in the vicinity of the epithelioma require to be removed; and since Röcher, of Bern, has removed even those that seemed unaffected, his operations have been much more successful than before.—*Med. Times and Gaz.*, Jan. 8, 1881.

—

Cases of Tracheotomy for Diphtheria in Children, Tumours of the Larynx, and Stenosis of the Larynx and Trachea.

Dr. KOERTE reports in the *Archiv für Klinische Chirurgie*, Band xxv. Heft 4, that no fewer than 149 tracheotomies for diphtheria (membranous croup) were performed in the Bethanien Hospital during the epidemic of diphtheria in Berlin in the year 1878. Of these, 34 recovered, and 115 died. In the latter months of the year the epidemic increased, not only in extent but in malignancy, so that against 56 tracheotomies with 30.3 per cent. recoveries in the first half of the year, there were 93 tracheotomies with only 18.2 per cent. recoveries in the second half of the year. The epidemic was at its height in October, November, and December; and of 62 children tracheotomized during that time, only 12 per cent. recovered. The patients were generally admitted at an advanced stage of the disease. In many, the diphtheritic affection had extended from the throat to the nasal passages; in such cases the prognosis was most unfavourable. Many cases were associated with measles, or with scarlet fever, and were then especially liable to terminate fatally. The greatest mortality occurred in children under 3 years of age. In the first year of life no operation was performed; but in the second year there were 29 cases with 3 recoveries, and in the third year, 27 cases also with 3 recoveries. The percentage of recoveries increased with the age and capacity of resistance of the children. Dr. Koerte regards croup and diphtheria as different degrees of the same affection; and considers that they cannot be distinguished clinically, although they present certain pathological differences, the nature of which, however, he does not state. With regard to the after-treatment, inhalations of weak solutions of lactic acid, when membranes were present in the trachea, of common salt or alum, when there was much muco-purulent secretion, were administered every two or three hours. Internally, chlorate of potash, wine, and camphor, were given. No remedies were applied locally to the throat, except when the mucous membrane was deeply affected. With the exception of cleansing the canula, and clearing the trachea of membranes by mopping it out with a feather, Dr. Koerte does not regard the after-treatment as having had any appreciable influence upon the course of the disease. The relief that is obtained by inhalations is to be attributed to the steam rather than to the medicaments. He thinks that the results, fatal or otherwise, depend entirely upon the severity of the epidemic, and not upon the treatment; as, during the year 1877, when the epidemic was much less severe, with 40 per cent. of recoveries, and during the first half of 1878, with 30 per cent. of recoveries, the treatment was the same as that pursued when the epidemic was at its height, during the second half of the year 1878, with only 18 per cent. of recoveries. Most of the deaths occurred within three days of the operation, the cause of death being in some cases collapse, but in the majority dyspnœa from the extension of

the membranes into the smaller bronchial tubes, for the clearing of which inhalations appeared quite inoperative; indeed, in these cases, little seemed to be
gained from the performance of tracheotomy. [It does not appear, however,
that the suction method, strongly recommended by Mr. Parker, for removing
membranes from the bronchi, was resorted to.] The deaths that occurred more
than three days after the operation, were generally due to broncho-pneumonia
and infection of the wound. When the wound became infected, disinfectants,
and occasionally cauterizations with chloride of zinc, were resorted to. In one
case, albumen appeared in the urine, and suppuration of the shoulder-joint occurred. The patient recovered after the shoulder-joint had been opened antiseptically. In another case, diphtheria occurred for the second time. Tracheotomy was performed on each occasion, and the patient recovered. Three cases
of papilloma of the glottis are reported. Case 1. A child, aged 8 years, had for
a year suffered from hoarseness, and sometimes dyspnœa. The larynx was
almost filled by papillary masses growing from the vocal cords. Three months
later, the larynx was opened by dividing the cricoid cartilage, crico-thyroid
membrane, and the lower portion of the thyroid cartilage in the middle line;
the growths were then removed with the scissors and a sharp spoon, and their
bases cauterized. Cicatrization of the wound was followed by a slight narrowing of the larynx. Four months after the operation, bougeal dilators were used
and Dupuis' tube introduced. The tracheal canula was removed, and the wound
allowed to heal. The patient was discharged with the voice hoarse. Both vocal
cords were involved in the cicatrization; they were shortened and their movements much impaired. Case 2. A woman, aged 30, had, for six months, had
difficulty in breathing. Tracheotomy was performed. The right vocal cord was
found normal, but the left was almost covered by a tumour with a broad base,
which nearly occluded the lumen of the glottis. An operation was not allowed,
and the patient was discharged, wearing a canula. Case 3. A woman, aged 47,
had often suffered from hoarseness, and for six weeks had had great difficulty in
breathing. Beneath the vocal cords, papillary masses were perceived narrowing
the lumen of the larynx. Tracheotomy was performed, and shortly afterwards
the larynx was opened, the masses removed with the scissors and knife, and the
actual cautery applied to the base of the growths. The wound in the larynx and
in the thyroid cartilage cicatrized; but the patient could not dispense with the
canula. Dr. Koerte remarks that these three cases belong to that class of tumours
which, from having a broad base and penetrating deeply in the mucous membrane, can only be removed by opening the larynx and seizing them from the
front. It is very easy to open the larynx when the trachea has been incised;
an incision of part of the thyroid cartilage being sometimes sufficient to make the
glottis entirely accessible. Two patients were treated for syphilitic stenosis of
the larynx, and one for stenosis of the trachea following diphtheria. In one of
these patients, in whom the vocal cords were completely destroyed and speech
was lost, an artificial vocal apparatus in the form of a tube provided with a vibrat-
ing tongue, was introduced into the larynx by the mouth. By means of this the
patient was able to speak, but it failed to be of any permanent use, in consequence of the metal tongue becoming clogged by particles of food, which could
not be prevented on account of the loss of the epiglottis, from entering the tube.
In the case in which tracheotomy was performed for diphtheria, stenosis of the
trachea occurred, in consequence of ingrowing granulations immediately above
the tracheotomy wound, so that on the cessation of the diphtheria the canula
could not be dispensed with. The granulations were removed by scraping; and
dilatation of the constriction with various curved bougies completely relieved the
patient. The tracheotomy wound was then allowed to heal. The stenosis re-

curred in a month's time; tracheotomy was again performed, and the constriction successfully dilated as before. The wound again healed, but within a week or two asphyxia suddenly came on, the tracheotomy and dilatation were repeated a third time, and when the report was published, the patient was still under treatment.—*London Medical Record*, Jan. 15, 1881.

On Rapid Lithotrity.

In a paper entitled "On Lithotripsy and Poisoning by Chlorate of Potash," read before the Vienna Medical Society (published in full in the *Wiener Med. Wochenschrift*, 1880, Nos. 44 and 45), Prof. BILLROTH stated that he felt some embarrassment in bringing the subject before those who had had so much more experience in the operation than himself, inasmuch as it was not until the end of his fourteenth year of clinical practice that he had performed the operation at all. The results of his operations from 1867 until last year, when he adopted the new method, were as follows: Deducting two cases in which after the first sitting lithotomy was resorted to, there were 41 patients, for whom 120 sittings were required—these sittings, which at the commencement of his practice of the operation lasted from three to five minutes each, being soon afterwards extended to from ten to fifteen minutes. Of these 41 cases, 9 terminated fatally, or 7 per cent., reckoning each sitting as an operation. In 7 instances death followed on the first sitting, and in 2 on the second—resulting from periurethritis, pericystitis, diphtheria of the bladder, and pyæmia. The mean number of sittings for each stone was three and a half.

After adverting to the prolongation of the sitting which took place after the employment of anæsthetics became general, until at last Bigelow[1] astonished the world with his one-sitting operations, some of which lasted for three hours, Prof. Billroth states that he is able only to refer to six such cases in his own practice. These are of different import as regards judging of the feasibility of the method, in consequence of the very different size and hardness of the stones in the six cases. 1. In a man fifty-nine years of age, the operation lasted forty-three minutes, the stone consisting of uric acid and the urates, and measuring three centimetres in diameter. 2. A phosphatic stone in a patient aged forty-five measured two centimetres, the operation lasting twenty-three minutes. In the third and fourth cases, the stones, both of uric acid, were three and a half and four centimetres in diameter, the operations lasting fifty-five and one hundred and twenty minutes. The fifth case was that of a phosphatic calculus of two centimetres and a half, the operation lasting thirty minutes; and in the sixth case the operation lasted fifteen minutes, the calculus measuring one centimetre and a half. The diameters of the calculi are derived from measurements with the lithotrite, and it is not easy to judge of the size of the stone by means of the fragments that are discharged, it being generally much under-estimated. A tolerably near idea of its size may be attained by allowing all that is washed out of the bladder to pass through a calico filter—the fragments thus collected, pressed together, and compared with the diameter already obtained, furnishing an approximative representation of what the calculus must have been. But Prof. Billroth has often been struck with the small size of the stone as estimated by the fragments, giving rise at first to the belief that all these could not have come away. All the cases recovered, and in all the febrile reaction was insignificant. In the case which lasted two hours, shivering ensued, but this was only of a purely nervous character, such as frequently occurs in operations upon the bladder. Some of

---

[1] Am. Journ. Med. Sci., Jan. 1878.

the patients were dismissed cured in ten or twelve days. With respect to the possibility of fragments being left behind, all the cases four or five days after the operation have been carefully examined, and again this has been done three times with two days' interval, always with negative results. There can be no doubt that this operation is a great progress.

Prof. Billroth is convinced that, setting aside bad cases of cystitis and cysto-pyelitis, the unfavourable chances in all operations for stone do not arise from the danger of purulent inflammation or of hemorrhage from injury done to the mucous membrane, but from the large amount of ammonia, free or combined with carbonic acid, in the urine, and of the diphtheriticoseptic character of the inflammation of the bladder that is set up in such cases. So dangerous is this ammoniacal fermentation that is set up, that Prof. Billroth believes lithotrity in general, and especially lithotrity at a single sitting, is contra-indicated unless some means of counteracting its influence can be employed. The danger of the generation of ammonia in the structures, and especially in the bladder, has been long since shown in Prof. Billroth's own experiments, as also in those of the late Gustav Simon and Menzel. The question is, therefore, How is the formation of ammonia in the urine to be prevented? Prof. Billroth has found the alkaline condition of the urine in paralyzed persons capable of removal by repeated in-jections of muriatic acid; but as most patients object to the frequent introduction of the catheter for this purpose, he tried the daily administration of a drachm of phosphoric acid: and the urine can in this way be rendered acid; but after a few days such acidity of the stomach was produced that it had to be given up. The same may be said of muriatic and nitric acids. Under these means the urine was changed in appearance from intense yellow to the clearness of water, as if the acid had exerted an influence on the colouring matter. Patients who were suffering from cystitis and pyelitis found acids aggravate their suffering. In general, when the carbonate of ammonia disappears from the urine, the pa-tient obtains great alleviation of suffering, the vomiting, fever, and penetrating smell of the urine disappearing, and the introduction of the catheter being much better borne. The chlorate of potash in a five per cent. solution, five grammes being taken in the course of the day, was next tried, and acted more promptly on the urine than did the acid. Prof. Billroth had hitherto believed that the statements which were published concerning its occasional poisonous effects had been exaggerated; for, when these related to diphtheritic children, he called to mind how many of such he had seen die from paralysis of the heart, without having taken any of the chlorate. He has, however, now met with a case in which he is convinced that death resulted from the use of this remedy. To a man aged sixty-four, who was admitted with urinary derangements of fifteen years' standing, the urine containing ammonia, much pus, and blood, the chlorate was ordered for three days in doses of five grammes (77½ grs.) per diem, the bladder being also washed out with diluted muriatic acid. The urine was acid on the second day, and on the third was clear, so that lithotrity, which lasted fifteen minutes, was then performed. After the operation the catheter had to be introduced several times, and the chlorate was continued. On the evening of the second day, when lying apparently asleep, he was found dead. At the autopsy the heart and large vessels were found filled with fluid blood of a very peculiar brown colour. This colour was quite remarkable; and Prof. Ludwig expressed the opinion that it was highly probable that the man died poisoned by the chlorate, although no trace of it was discoverable in the blood. After the death it was ascertained that fifteen instead of five grammes had been given daily, so that the patient had thus taken altogether from forty to forty-five grammes (620 to 700 grs.).

At the discussion which followed the reading of the paper (*Allg. Wien. Med.*

Zeit., Nos. 44 and 45), Prof. DITTEL, after referring to two cases in which Bigelow's operation was performed by Sir H. Thompson at Vienna, and eight others which he had operated upon himself, spoke highly in favour of the new procedure. The aspiration which was employed did not cause the hemorrhage of the bladder that was feared by some, while it enabled us to be assured whether there were still fragments in the bladder or not. This operation also in many cases may prevent the occurrence of a cystitis. A patient may have a stone in the bladder for years without excessive suffering; but no sooner is he lithotrized than several sharp-pointed fragments are suddenly produced, and cystitis is at once set up. But by this operation, in which the stone is completely crushed and removed at a sitting, he is preserved from this occurrence; while impactment of fragments in the urethra, which sometimes gives great trouble to the surgeon, and may even give rise to fatal results, is also avoided. So also for operations on the paralytic bladder, this is the only possible method. The number of cases has been as yet too small to allow of a final judgment being passed as to the amount of reaction produced, but, generally speaking, it has been not greater than under other modes of operating. Taken altogether, this new method can only be regarded as a very considerable progress.

With respect to the alkalescent condition of the urine, Dr. ULTZMANN observed that this may be caused either by fixed alkalies or by the carbonate of ammonia. In the former case, as often met with in diseases of the nervous system, it is secreted from the kidney in this alkaline condition; and here the internal administration of acids is of utility, especially carbonic acid, which transforms the amorphous and crystalline lime and magnesia salts of the urinary sediments into easily soluble bicarbonates. It is entirely otherwise when the alkalescence of the urine is brought about by the fermentation of the urea, an abnormal condition of the mucous membrane of the bladder, or the presence of micro-organisms. Here the change takes place in the bladder itself, the urine being secreted acid or normal in the kidney, and becoming alkalescent only in the bladder. When the urine has been for some time alkalized by carbonate of ammonia, we may be certain that the bladder itself or the parenchyma of the prostate has undergone change. It is in cases in which an incomplete discharge of the urine takes place that this ammoniacal condition of the urine occurs, and it is much more effectually treated by local applications than by the internal administration of acids. Prof. Dittel observed that in many cases of obstinate alkalescent urine in old vesical catarrh the bladder exhibits hundreds of diverticula, which resemble cavities of abscesses, with narrow orifices, and in such cases it is quite impossible to wash the bladder clean out so as to remove all the alkalescent urine. Prof. Drasche stated that as the result of numerous experiments he had found that two grammes of salicylic acid with glycerine and alcohol, or three grammes of salicylate of soda, may be given with advantage in vesical catarrh, these substances preventing the decomposition of the urine. They cannot, however, be given in these doses for a long time, and small doses are of no use; but they furnish a medicinal substances that proves efficacious for a time in affections of the bladder attended with rapid fermentation of the urine.

In reference to the influence of chlorate of potash taken internally, Dr. MARAZEK stated that when he was clinical assistant in the department for syphilis he had administered the chlorate in cases of cystitis and cysto-pyelitis arising from gonorrhœa. Altogether there were forty hospital and thirty out-patients who took daily five grammes, dissolved in 100 grammes of water with two drachms of cherry-laurel water added to it. Most of these persons took it for twelve to fourteen days, and several for a longer time, so that in most cases as many as sixty grammes were taken. Acid reaction commenced in the urine from the second day, and the triple phosphate disappeared from the sediment, which became diminished in quantity and less viscid. The quantity of the urine remained the same, but the urgency for passing it was diminished. When it contained blood at the time the chlorate was given, the quantity of this was increased. No ill consequences resulted from the use of the chlorate, in spite of the fact that most of the patients were in a bad condition of health, and some of them the subjects of tubercle and syphilis. The chlorate must therefore be regarded as a valuable aid in treating this form of cystitis and cysto-pyelitis. Of the forty cases treated in hospital, twenty-eight completely recovered, and several others were much improved.

Dr. ENGLISCH observed that he had often administered the chlorate in affections of the bladder, and had found it useful in acute cystitis, but in chronic and obstinate cases it proved of no advantage. He gives from five to seven grammes daily during a month, and has never met with any ill consequence resulting from its use.

Prof. LUDWIG, referring to Prof. Billroth's fatal case of poisoning with chlorate of potash, stated that the blood, the contents of the stomach, and the urine were examined. The urine was turbid, with an acid reaction and very abundant sediment; it was albuminous, and contained a few blood corpuscles and granular cylinders. The blood had undergone great change, leaving the hæmatin free; but neither in it, in the contents of the stomach, nor in the urine, was any of the chlorate perceptible. This, therefore, had been completely reduced in the economy, and had passed into the condition of chloride of potassium—a remarkable circumstance, quite in contradiction to the views hitherto held by chemists. Binz was the first to show that organic substances (as yeast, blood, fibrin), when passing into a state of putrefaction, may decompose chlorate of potash; and it is now no longer doubtful that the chlorate, under certain circumstances, that we are at present ignorant of, may become wholly or in great part reduced within the body. As regards the mischievous influence of this, it would seem to be twofold. On the one hand, it operates like arsenic or phosphorus, the blood corpuscles being destroyed during the conversion of the chlorate into chloride of potassium. Secondly, it is decomposed into its base and acid by the weak acid urine in the kidneys, and the violent effects of the chloric acid have full play. The examples of strong acids being separated from their combinations by weaker acids are on the increase, so that it is not surprising that the weak acid urine is able to decompose the chlorate of potash.

Prof. HOFFMANN observed that as the effects of chlorate of potash on the blood can be demonstrated in a test-glass, it is only to be expected that the same changes would take place in the circulating blood.—*Med. Times and Gaz.*, Jan. 15, 1881.

On the Radical Cure of Varicocele.

At a meeting of the Royal Medical and Chirurgical Society (*Lancet*, Jan. 15, 1881), Mr. HENRY LEE read a paper on this subject, of which the following is an abstract.

The operation advocated in this paper is that of removing a portion of the anterior skin of the scrotum, and subsequently dividing the veins which are to be obliterated. All the steps of the operation are conducted through the wound made by the removal of the skin. The veins are compressed temporarily, so as to prevent hemorrhage, and then divided. The cut orifices of the veins are sealed with the black hot cautery, which if of proper temperature, is allowed to adhere to them for five or six seconds. The ligatures and needles used in compression are then removed, and the edges of the skin brought into apposition from below upward by carbolized sutures. Union by first intention takes place more or less perfectly, and the patient is allowed to follow his usual avocations in three or four days.

Mr. PEARCE GOULD described an operation that he had performed for the radical cure of varicocele during the last two and a half years. It consisted in passing a loop of platinum wire round the spermatic veins subcutaneously, and then connecting it with a galvanic écraseur, and making it burn its way through the veins. In all he had performed it eleven times, two of the cases being incomplete, the other nine having resulted in cure without accident. The advantages he claimed for it were its safety, simplicity, painlessness, and efficiency, and the fact that the operation is limited to the diseased parts. He considered Mr. Lee's operation as more complicated, and held that the wound of the scrotum was liable to œdema, and even suppuration; and being closed by the continuous suture, there was no outlet for any effused serum. The removal of part of the scrotum has been shown to be ineffectual for the cure of varicocele, and he doubted if it were needful if the occlusion of the veins were satisfactorily secured. He thought it hardly safe to allow patients to get up and move about so soon as three or four days after such operations on veins, but preferred to wait until the clots were firmly adherent, and the divided ends of the vessels securely closed.

Mr. LEE, in reply, said, that, although he had now employed the actual cautery in a very large number of cases, he had never had a case of septic poisoning following its use. He attributed this to the complete closure of the veins—the small as well as the large—effected by it. It also effectually sealed the arteries; and if the operation is fairly done there is no oozing whatever. The wounds heal without any sloughing. His object in interfering with the scrotum was to prevent any return of the varicocele.

—

Case of Tying the Left Common Carotid Artery after Tonsillotomy.

In this case (*Hygeia*, Band xlii. April, 1880; Schmidt's *Jahrb.*, Band clxxxvii. No. 8, 1880) extirpation of the left tonsil had been performed by LIDÉN in the usual manner for excessive hypertrophy. The hemorrhage was not very great after the operation, but it did not cease after gargling with cold water, and became more and more abundant in spite of preventive means. After cauterization with lunar caustic, and application of perchloride of iron, it stopped for an hour, then recommenced, the clots becoming larger and more frequent. There was no arterial bleeding. Bladders of ice laid on the neck, and ice in the mouth, diminished the hemorrhage for a time; but afterwards it came on afresh and more violently. The patient's strength was failing, the pulse 130, weak and irregular. Three hours after the tonsillotomy, the common carotid artery was tied with carbolized silk, and immediately afterwards the bleeding from the mouth stopped. There was no pain felt on tying the carotid, nor pain in the head afterwards. Recovery was very slow, the patient not leaving her bed for three weeks. She had always been weak and chlorotic; and had always experienced strong pulsation of the left side of the neck, and very rapid action of the heart. There were no signs of hemophilia either in the patient or in her family. Dr. Lidén thinks that an abnormal ramification of the vessels was the cause of the bleeding. [A very simple method of arresting hemorrhage after excision of the tonsils, and one that does not seem so often resorted to as it deserves, is by pressure with a pad of lint on the end of a short stick.—*Rep.*]—*London Med. Record*, Jan. 15, 1881.

—

Dislocation of the Spine.

In the July number of the *Revue Mensuelle*, MM. A. POUSSON and F. LA-LESQUE give a detailed report of three cases of dislocation of the spine, observed in the Saint André Hospital at Bordeaux; and to this report they attach an interesting review, with regard both to clinical and to physiological data, of the effects produced on the spinal cord through displacement of the bodies of the vertebræ. The first case, the subject of which was a male aged forty, was one of fracture of the laminæ of the eleventh dorsal vertebra with consecutive dislocation of this in front of the twelfth; contusion of the cord; ascending myelitis; and death on the eleventh day. In the second and third cases, the cervical portion was the seat of injury. One was an instance of partial dislocation of the fifth cervical vertebra, causing death on the third day, in a male aged twenty-four: and in the third case, which terminated fatally within thirty-six hours, there was luxation forwards of the fourth cervical vertebra and rupture of its inferior cartilaginous disk. The patient in the last case was a man aged thirty-eight.

These cases present no special point of interest with regard to the character of the injury. The chief value of the contribution is due to the very rigorous analysis of the pathological facts made by the authors, with the view of testing the results that have been attained by experimental physiologists as to the functions of the spinal cord. With the exception of acute pain at a fixed point of the spine, which was noted in all three cases, and of mobility of the eleventh dorsal spinous process in the first case, the local signs were very obscure. In the third case, there was not any appreciable distortion of the spine at the supposed seat of injury, and the movements of the neck were preserved. The lesion in each of the cases of injury to the cervical region was beyond the reach of a finger introduced into the pharynx. In severe injury to the spine and cord, the activity of the brain may be suspended for a time, as one of the results of the general disturbance known as shock. In two of the above cases there was temporary loss of consciousness, and in the third case an inability to articulate. In each of the three cases, there was motor paralysis in the region supplied with nerves by the segment of the cord below the seat of injury. In the first case, as the seat of injury was near the origin of the first pair of lumbar nerves, the parts supplied by the lumbar and sacral plexus were paralyzed, and voluntary motion of the lower extremities was abolished. In the other two cases, the brachial plexus had been cut off from the upper part of the cord, and therefore the upper extremities as well as the inferior were paralyzed. In the second case, the motor paralysis of the upper extremities was not complete, and the loss of movement affected only certain groups of muscles, in consequence, probably, of integrity of certain channels of conduction in the midst of the disorganized parts. There was, in the third case, complete and immediate paralysis of motion. This seems to be exceptional; for, according to Gurlt, in cases of dislocation below the third cervical vertebra, complete and immediate motor paralysis has rarely been observed.

In cases of injury to the spinal cord, the area of lost sensibility usually corresponds very closely to that of motor paralysis. This might be expected, from the fact that the anterior and posterior roots emerge from the cord at the same level. In the first case, there was anæsthesia of the lower extremities and of the abdominal wall as high as the umbilicus. In the second and third cases, the area on the trunk of anæsthesia was limited by a line drawn through both nipples. There was loss of sensibility in the upper limbs in the third case, but not in the second case. Here there was persistence of sensibility, which, together with freedom from motor paralysis in certain groups of muscles, indicated that there was but incomplete disorganization of the cord at the seat of injury. When all kinds of sensibility—to pain, touch, and temperature—are abolished, as was made out in the first and third cases, it may be concluded that the whole thickness of the spinal cord has been involved in the injury. Marked hyperæsthesia, with intense pain just beyond the paralyzed region, was noted in the second and third cases. In the first case, there was exaggerated reflex motion in the lower extremities. The phenomena observed in the other two cases were not in accordance with the theory that, whenever a portion of the spine is cut off from the encephalon, the excito-motor power of this portion, provided it remain sound and intact, becomes intensified. In the second case, not the least movement of the lower extremities could be excited by active stimulation of the integument. In the third case, the extensor muscles of the lower limbs contracted when the soles were touched, but over all the other paralyzed parts the excito-motor action of the medullary exit remained indifferent to every kind of excitation. In these two cases, however, death occurred early and before the effects of shock had passed off. Besides, in each case the lower portion of the spine below the chief seat of injury was not quite sound, and hence the conditions of experimental physiology were not fulfilled. Contraction and immobility of the pupils were noticed in the second and third cases, in which the lesion of the cord existed at the lower part of the cervical region. Neither palpebral stenosis nor injection of the conjunctiva was observed in any of the cases.

The penis was found to be turgescent in all three cases, and in one case, the third, there was marked erection. Voluntary micturition was abolished in every case, and it was found necessary to relieve the bladder by catheterism. The urine remained normal as to quantity; and in one case only, the first, did the physical and chemical characters become altered. In the other two cases, however, death occurred very soon after the date of injury. Changes in the quality of urine, which take place in cases of injury to the spine, though they come on suddenly and progress with much rapidity, do not usually occur until after an interval of some days. In the above case the excretion became turbid and alkaline, and had an ammoniacal odour, for the first time, on the fourth day; on the fifth day it was purulent.

Tympanites was observed in all the cases, and was excessive in the second, so as to interfere with respiration. This condition is due, not only to paralysis of the muscular fibres of the intestine, but also to failure of contractility of the abdominal muscles, which then offer no effective resistance to gaseous distension of the intestinal canal. Intestinal paralysis is usually manifested also by absence of stools. Fecal incontinence, in cases of injury or disease of the spine, is to be regarded as a very unfavourable symptom. In the second case, involuntary discharge of fecal matter commenced a few hours before death.

In all the cases the breathing was diaphragmatic, and both the thorax and the abdominal wall moved but passively and under the influence of the play of the diaphragm. The seat of the injury to the spinal cord accorded perfectly, in the second and third cases, with the symptoms that were observed. The lesion existing at the level of the fourth and fifth cervical vertebræ paralyzed all the muscles of respiration save the diaphragm, supplied by the phrenic nerve emerging above the fourth cervical vertebra. In the first case, another reason must be found to explain the modification in the normal type of respiration; it is to be attributed, on the one hand, to paralysis of the abdominal muscles, and, on the other hand, to violent pain experienced by the patient in the right hypochondrium. In pleurodynia and pleurisy the patient, in order to obtain relief, instinctively keeps at rest the painful side of the chest.

In cases of serious injury of the spinal cord there is paralysis of the vaso-motor nerves, determining a diminution of the arterial pressure, and giving rise to certain modifications in the character of the pulse. These changes were observed in each of the cases reported by MM. Pousson and Lalesque, and in the second case particularly remarkable changes in the pulse were made out on the second day, and when the effects of shock had passed off. It was noted that the radial pulse was strong, and that with each blood-wave there was a forcible impulse, but that at the same time the vessel was compressible. This impulse was still more marked in the larger arteries, as the femoral and the abdominal aorta. The sensation of a strong pulse is due to sudden variation of the arterial pressure in the vessel which is under the surgeon's finger. There is a feeble pressure in consequence of the vaso-motor paralysis, which, at the periphery, allows a ready flow of the blood from the arterial into the venous system; and this condition of feeble pressure passes suddenly into a condition of forcible pressure at the moment of the ventricular systole. The sphygmographic tracing presents, with pulse-modifications of this kind, a very high and vertically ascending line, and a concave and prolonged descending line. With regard to the number of cardiac beats, no deduction could be drawn from these cases. According to M. Marey, the movements of the heart in a given time are the more frequent, the less obstruction there is to overcome in the accomplishing of the ventricular systole. In these cases, therefore, as there was certainly diminution of the arterial pressure, and consequently a more ready flow of the blood-stream, an increase in the number of cardiac pulsations would have been expected. But in the first case only was there an acceleration of the pulse (112 to the minute): in the other two cases the pulse was 88 and 60. These facts, however, it is pointed out, do not really invalidate the law of Marey, since, in the second and third cases, the spinal lesion had involved the cervical enlargement and the region from which are derived the accelerator nerves of the heart. The authors failed to make out any precise results as to the temperature in these cases of spinal injury, in consequence of the disturbing influence of shock and consecutive inflammation. In conclusion, it is reported that, beyond some sloughing over the sacral region, in the first case, no indications of any trophic disturbance were observed.—*London Med. Record*, Jan. 15, 1881.

Midwifery and Gynæcology.

Cystic Degeneration of the Chorion with a Living Fœtus.

It has been maintained with much plausibility that cystic degeneration of the chorion results from the death of the embryo. A case, therefore, which completely negatives this view is both of interest and importance. Such a case has been put on record by Dr. C. BREUS (*Wiener Medizinische Wochenschrift*, No. 36, 1880). It occurred in the private practice of Professor Braun. It was the patient's first pregnancy after ten years' marriage. Gestation went on without any unfavourable symptom until the fifth month, when metrorrhagia came on, so severe as to oblige the patient to keep her bed. A week afterwards labour-pains began. The uterus then reached to the umbilicus. The fœtal heart could not be made out, but fœtal movements were perceptible. The child and placenta were expelled naturally and easily. The child corresponded in development to five months' pregnancy; it weighed 440 grammes (1 lb. 1½ oz.), and lived for three hours. It presented no abnormality, and death appeared to take place simply from its having been prematurely born. The placenta and membranes weighed 320 grammes (10 oz.).· The placenta showed in parts clusters of thin-walled vesicles of different sizes, the largest being as big as a hen's egg; at other parts it presented the general appearance of healthful placental tissue, but nevertheless, on close examination, vesicles of the size of a pin's head or a hemp-seed could be seen in it. Microscopical examination showed, even in the least altered placental tufts, a pronounced increase of embryonic connective tissue with abundant intercellular substance. That this disease of the placenta did not lead to the death of the child, the author explains by supposing that it did not begin till later than usual, and that sufficient of the placenta was left in a tolerably healthy state to allow of the nutrition of the fœtus. He believes that had not the child been expelled prematurely, the progress of the disease must have led to its intra-uterine death.—*Med. Times and Gazette*, Dec. 25, 1880.

—

Induction of Abortion as a Therapeutic Measure.

The discussion of a paper by Dr. PRIESTLEY, on the Induction of Abortion as a Therapeutic Measure, at the last meeting of the Obstetrical Society of London, leads us to offer some remarks thereon. Dr. Priestley's paper was, of course, an ably written one. But it did not attempt to extend the boundaries of knowledge: it aimed rather at a temperate judicial summing-up of the conditions which may justify the artificial termination of pregnancy at an early stage. As to the soundness of the conclusions set forth, little doubt could have been felt. But no new facts were brought forward, either in the paper or in the debate. The *raison d'être* of the paper was, not that the author had any fresh information to communicate, but, to use his own words, because "the indications for the induction of abortion . . . had never been laid down with sufficient precision in this country." And the debate also was a somewhat barren one, the only speaker who recognized the wide bearings at issue being Dr. Barnes.

Dr. Priestley set forth seven sets of conditions in which he considered artificial abortion justifiable. In two of them the objection to it is what is called a "moral" one. These are (1) "pelvic deformity so great as to preclude the birth of a living child," and (2) "narrowing of the genital canal by tumours, cicatrices, or cancer, so as to prevent the passage of a viable child." The existence of these conditions is seldom found out until the end of the first pregnancy, when a dangerous operation is needed to effect delivery. Then, if the patient become pregnant again, the question presents itself, "Is it not right to empty her uterus before its burden has got too big to pass through the narrow strait which is its sole communication with the outer world?" The so-called "moral" objection is, that the woman knew what would be the natural result of a second pregnancy, and ought not to have incurred the possibility of it; she having done so, the medical man ought not to destroy a child to save her from the penalty to which she has voluntarily submitted herself. We agree entirely with Dr. Barnes in thinking this doctrine a barbarous one. "Who art thou that judgest another?" is the text we would commend to the consideration of those who hold that the turpitude of a poor deformed wife's offence in becoming pregnant after she is aware of her deformity, is only to be expiated by her running a risk of death considerably greater than if she had been condemned to capital punishment in the Old Bailey dock. In these cases the woman is not a free agent; and, as Dr. Barnes said, if pregnancy under such circumstances be really a crime calling for punishment at the hands of the medical man, there is a measure, at once penalty and preventive (which need not be mentioned), and which would fall with more justice upon the other side. The life of a healthy young wife and mother ought to outweigh in the balance that of any number of immature fœtuses.

In the second set of conditions the indications for artificial abortion stand upon different grounds. These include diseases which are believed to be so aggravated by the coexistence of pregnancy as to endanger life. Dr. Priestley specified (3) obstinate vomiting of pregnancy; (4) eclampsia; (5) irreducible retroversion or retroflexion, endangering life; (6) hemorrhage; and a seventh class included the remainder.

The point which seemed to us too much overlooked, both in the paper and in the discussion (except by Dr. Barnes), was this: that it is not yet a question of this or that symptom, or collection of symptoms, calling for the termination of pregnancy. It is first and chiefly a question concerning the *natural history of disease.* We want to know what is the natural history of the vomiting of pregnancy, of eclampsia, etc., if the pregnancy be let alone; and then, what is the effect of abortion upon them. Till there is some certainty upon these points, nothing definite can be said upon the indications which denote, in each case, the necessity of abortion. Take, for instance, the vomiting of pregnancy. We know that it is usual for this to be troublesome during the first three or fourth months of pregnancy, and that then it generally gets better. But this typical course is widely departed from in particular instances, and we know hardly anything of the conditions which lead to such variations. But until we do, it is useless to dogmatize upon the effect of remedies. One speaker mentioned cases in which, after various modes of treatment had been tried without success, and abortion was thought necessary, the use of a favourite remedy of his own was followed by cessation of the sickness. We have little doubt that each man in the room could have also narrated cases in which his own pet drug had done good after others had failed. The explanation is, that probably in most such cases the vomiting would have ceased whether the medicine had been given or not; and the remedy which the patient happened to be taking, when the sickness naturally stopped, was given the credit of the cure. The induction of abortion has this advantage over all other remedies, that by it cure is certain. Sickness solely dependent upon pregnancy must cease when the pregnancy ceases. Dr. Priestley's cautious indications for abortion in these cases practically amounted to this: that if the patient be dying from incessant vomiting, abortion should be induced. We rather agree, however, with Dr. Barnes, that if it is to be done at all, it should be done earlier than this. But the point we want to insist on is this: that the indications for inducing abortion in cases of intractable vomiting of pregnancy cannot be formulated with any precision until the natural history of such vomiting is better known.

The induction of abortion in eclampsia does not stand upon such sure ground as in the case just mentioned; for it is not at all certain that in uræmic convulsions occurring in the early months of pregnancy, the evacuation of the uterus will benefit the patient. In retroversion of the gravid uterus there is the same uncertainty as to the need of abortion. There is no doubt not only that a retroverted pregnant uterus may right itself (and generally does, if the bladder be kept empty), but that even if it do not, pregnancy may go on as usual, and delivery be effected by the natural efforts. Dr. Priestley did not specify what are the cases in which retroversion of the gravid uterus may endanger life if abortion be not induced. We know that when these cases end fatally, it is usually through the bladder and kidney changes which are caused by the retention of urine—cystitis, pyelitis, rupture of bladder, sloughing of its mucous membrane, etc.—diseases which can be prevented by careful attention to the bladder, and which, when once set up, would probably not be much modified by the presence or absence of pregnancy. Dr. Priestley stated that he did not regard the mere fact that the displacement was irreducible as sufficient reason for inducing abortion. We may add, with reference to the cases that have been recorded in which the uterine contents were discharged by ulceration of its wall, that very competent critics have thrown doubt on the accuracy of the diagnosis in these rare instances. The other indication which Dr. Priestley specified—viz., (6) hemorrhage—requires no comment.

The author's last group (7) was a very general one: "in certain other diseases where the complication of pregnancy is undoubtedly endangering life." Heart-disease, chorea, and insanity, were the conditions chiefly dwelt upon in the discussion. It is in these cases that our present contention applies with the greatest force. In the conditions named there are not yet materials for formulating the indications for artificial abortion. This question cannot possibly be settled until the more fundamental one has been elucidated: What is the effect of pregnancy upon the course of these diseases? It was Dr. Priestley's opinion that gestation has probably little influence on the progress of the malady; and therefore his practical advice was to "treat the morbid condition, and let the pregnancy take care of itself." Dr. Barnes took the opposite side, and went so far as to say that the disease depended upon the pregnancy. Whether in this statement he be correct or not, there can be no doubt that the point of view from which he treated the question is the only one which at present can help us to sound rules of practice. Little has been done, or rather little definite is known, as to the effect of pregnancy upon chorea or insanity. Cases have been recorded in which chorea or insanity coexisting with pregnancy ceased when the pregnancy was put a stop to; but others have been seen in which the artificial interference with gestation only made the patient worse. In heart-disease, thanks to the laborious and able work of Dr. Angus Macdonald, we are on surer ground; but even here much remains to be done.

We will conclude these remarks by repeating again the principle which we wish remembered in this connection; viz., that the question of the artificial induction of abortion for the relief or cure of morbid conditions of other parts is essentially one of the natural history of disease. We want to know more of the effect of pregnancy upon disease: and until we do, no scientific indications for the induction of abortion under such circumstances can exist.—*Med. Times and Gazette*, Jan. 8, 1881.

—

Treatment of Mammary Abscess.

Dr. HIRAM CORSON, of Conshohocken, Pa., strongly urges (*Am. Jour. Obstetrics*, Jan. 1881) the local use of ice in the treatment of mammary abscess. He puts the ice into a bladder with just enough water to form a water cushion that will adapt itself to the inflamed part.

—

Narrowness of the Uterine Orifices in relation to Dysmenorrhœa and Sterility.

In an interesting article on stenosis of the external os uteri (*Annales de Gynecologie*, Dec. 1880), Professor PAJOT relates three cases in which an extremely small os uteri was present, with the usual dysmenorrhœa and sterility in young married women. In all three cases the os uteri was gradually dilated by means of an ordinary uterine dilator. Pregnancy ensued in all three cases, although in the first case the os uteri was invisible to the naked eye, and almost invisible in the second case. Professor Pajot is opposed to incision of the external os uteri as a means of removing the stenosis, and prefers gradual dilatation. He draws the following conclusions. In the same way that any obstacle to the facile flow of menstrual blood may cause dysmenorrhœa, stenosis of the external orifice may cause it. When stenosis appears to be the cause, enlargement of the orifice is indispensable. The opening of the uterine orifices by cutting instruments exposes the patient to serious dangers—septicæmia, pelvic peritonitis, and metritis, and even to death. Sponge and laminaria tents also frequently lead to serious complications, such as perimetritis and septicæmia. Dilatation, carried out by means of graduated dilators, for several minutes at each sitting, is, in the absence of proof to the contrary, absolutely free from danger. In cases of sterility depending on stenosis, it is only necessary to dilate the external os uteri; and where this has to be done, transverse dilatation appears to be more favourable to subsequent impregnation than circular dilatation.—*London Med. Record*, Jan. 15, 1881.

On the Operative Treatment of Cancer of the Cervix Complicating Pregnancy.

The above is the subject of a contribution in the *Zeitschrift für Geburtshülfe und Gynäkologie*, bd. v. s. 158, by Dr. RICHARD FROMMEL of Berlin. His observations are suggested by two cases of the complication, the histories of which are given at some length. The cases were severe, the affection having dated back to a period before conception in both. In the first, as natural delivery was plainly impossible, Cæsarean section was performed with antiseptic precautions. A deeply asphyxiated child was delivered, which, however, came round and lived for three months. The placenta and membranes, being adherent, had to be removed, and a drainage-tube was then introduced through the vagina and cervix. The uterine wound was closed by seven deep and several superficial silk sutures. The patient died in two days. On post-mortem examination it was found that the silk stitches had all come loose. The carcinoma was very extensive, affecting the cervix to the os internum, the parametria on the right side, the bladder and upper part of the vagina, and completely filling the entrance of the true pelvis. In addition there was hemorrhagic peritonitis, interstitial Bright, and commencing endocarditis. The second case came under treatment five days after the waters had come away. The child was then dead, and the presentation a cross one. That being so, an attempt was made to remove manually the degenerated tissue so as to open a channel for the extraction of the child. This was effected without injury to adjoining organs or any bleeding worthy of the name. A foot was pulled down, and the dead, slightly macerated, full-grown child delivered. After this there was only very slight bleeding; the placenta was removed by expression, and the uterus contracted fairly. The operation was well borne by the patient, and she continued tolerably well for a few days. She suffered greatly from pain, for which large doses of narcotics were administered, and lived for a fortnight, during which time rapid advance of the carcinoma was observed. No post-mortem could be obtained. The author then proceeds to discuss the question when and by what sort of operation carcinoma, when complicating pregnancy, ought to be dealt with. This he holds depends chiefly upon the degree of advance of disease. Provided the case be seen at a time when the whole diseased tissue can be removed, the author recommends this to be done irrespective of the stage of pregnancy or of the risk of abortion resulting. He maintains, however, that the latter is not likely. But if the extent of the disease is such as to render its complete removal impossible, Dr. Frommel recommends Cæsarean section with antiseptic precautions, in the interests of the child chiefly, provided the fœtus is alive and viable. But if the child be dead, he would follow the plan of treatment adopted in his second case. In discussing the question of diagnosis of early cancer, the author considers Spiegelberg's view in regard to the fixation of the mucous membrane to the subjacent tissues as doubtful, since Ruge and Veit have shown that carcinoma of the cervix has only seldom those ingrowths of epithelial tissue assumed by Spiegelberg to be present in all cases. He comes to the conclusion that accuracy of diagnosis can only be obtained by removing a small portion of diseased tissue and subjecting it to microscopic examination. The operative interference for complete removal he recommends is the wedge-shaped excision of both lips of the os after Simon's method.—*Edinburgh Med. Journal*, Dec. 1880.

Cancer of the Uterus in the Seventeenth Year of Life.

That cancer of the uterus is exceedingly rare in early life every one knows. A few cases under the age of twenty have been recorded, but none in detail. Those that occur in old authors have, indeed, been rejected by later and more critical writers as instances of 'mistaken diagnosis; and a case of so rare a kind, mentioned without confirmatory details, must always be open to this suspicion. A case, therefore, that occurred in the clinique of Professor Späth, and is reported by Schauta in the *Wiener Medizinsche Wochenschrift* (Nos. 37 and 38, 1880), is of much interest. The patient was a weak and delicate girl, but no inherited tendency to carcinoma could be made out. She began to menstruate shortly after the completion of her fifteenth year, and the function was regularly performed without pain, but the flow was always abundant. In October, 1878 (the patient having completed her sixteenth year in December, 1877), a sanious watery discharge began to appear, accompanied with pain in the lower abdomen, so severe as to oblige her to keep her bed. In November an attack of profuse hemorrhage led her to seek medical advice. On examination, a rounded tumour, of the size of a walnut, uneven on the surface, was felt in the vagina. It seemed as if it grew from within the uterus; its pedicle passed through the os uteri. From its consistence, and from its being covered with adherent fibrin, it was at first suspected to be a placental polypus which had followed an early abortion. The uterus could not be made out to be enlarged, and the patient denied all possibility of a miscarriage. An attempt was made to remove the tumour with a Simon's sharp spoon; but the stalk was found too strong to admit this, and it was therefore cut away with curved scissors. It was found to grow from the right half of the vaginal portion of cervix; and on section and on microscopic examination was found to have the characters of malignant disease. The removal of the new growth was completed with a Sims's knife. The patient recovered, and remained well till January, 1879. Then some small nodules, at first of the size of millet-seeds, but subsequently getting larger, were discovered in the neighbourhood of the cicatrix. They were removed with the knife; but after this others appeared, which were destroyed with Paquelin's cautery. At the end of March a tumour as large as an egg was felt in the right parametrium. It was rounded, and not connected with the uterus. It grew so fast that at the end of April it reached to the umbilicus and filled both iliac regions. On May 12 bits of tissue microscopically shown to be malignant in character were discharged in the urine, proving that the bladder was now involved. On May 15 the patient died. The autopsy was made by Dr. Chiari. A mass as big as a man's head was found in the pelvis—the lower part of the ileum, the cæcum, lower part of ascending colon, and sigmoid being adherent to the mass. The uterus was small, and pushed to the left. The posterior wall of bladder and right vaginal fornix had been destroyed by the growth. Secondary growths were present in the lumbar lymphatic glands and in the lungs. The growth was very vascular, soft, grayish-red in colour, and exuding a milky juice on section. It was examined microscopically by Prof. Heschl. His report concerning the growth was, that it was a malignant adenoma; that no definite distinction could be drawn between a growth of this kind and a true cancer, and it must be looked upon as a transition form to the latter disease.—*Med. Times and Gazette*, Jan. 1, 1881.

MEDICAL NEWS.

Short-Sight in Relation to Education.

In an address recently delivered to the Birmingham Teachers' Association, Dr. Priestly Smith has given the results of the examination of the eyes of school children and college students, with reference to the existence and increase of myopia. 1636 pupils of the board schools and 357 students of the colleges in which young men and women are trained as teachers were examined. The ages of the former ranged from seven to thirteen, and of the latter from eighteen to twenty-three. Five per cent. of the school children were found to be short-sighted, and twenty per cent. of the college students. Though the number of the older subjects is not large enough to make the statistics at all conclusive as to the effect of education upon myopia, Dr. Smith's observations, so far as they go, confirm the results of previous more extended examinations. Ware, in a paper read before the Royal Society (London), seventy years ago, established the fact of the much greater prevalence of myopia among the educated classes than the uneducated. No precise observations based upon the careful examination of large numbers of eyes, however, were made until Cohn, of Breslau, in 1867, published the results of his now well-known researches.

The interest excited by these remarkable observations stimulated others to similar work, and many thousand examinations have been made, particularly of the eyes of school children, in this country as well as in Europe. The testimony of all the statistics thus collected, though varying in degree, is in the same direction, and shows a great excess of myopia among those who use their eyes in near work, and an alarming increase of the defect during school life. Dr. Siggel, among 1600 German soldiers, found that only 2 per cent. of those from the country were short-sighted, 4 per cent. of those who had been labourers in large towns, 9 per cent. of artisans, 44 per cent. of tradesmen, clerks, etc., and 58 to 65 per cent. of those who had been university students. Cohn examined the eyes of more than 10,000 school children, and found a constant progression in the percentage of myopia, as the classes advanced from year to year. The following are his figures.

Elementary schools	6.7 per cent.
Intermediate schools	10.3 "
High school	19.7 "
Colleges	26.2 "

In the high schools, 50 per cent. of the first class were found to be myopic, and 55.8 per cent. of the first class in the colleges. Erismann among 4358 school children in St. Petersburg found 10.2 per cent. of those under eight years of age, and 40 per cent. of those over twenty years of age myopic. No wonder, in the face of such startling revelations, that Dr. Loring, of New York, seriously discusses the question whether " the human eye is changing its form and becoming near-sighted under the influence of modern education," and that a recent French author exclaims in alarm that the whole civilized world is growing myopic.

Almost all the published statistics of school children have been obtained by the simultaneous examination of numbers of pupils in different stages of education, and nothing has yet been done on an extensive scale towards recording the history of individual cases. Indeed, this seems scarcely practicable unless by some systematized plan in connection with the public schools. Jaeger, years ago, recognized the importance of such records, and announced his intention of following the course of refraction in the same persons through their whole lives ; for which purpose, Donders wished him " long life and faithful patients."

Dr. Hasket Derby is doing some good work in this direction at Amherst. He examined the Freshman class in 1875, with the intention of following at least four successive classes through their college course. This will test the truth of the general opinion, that there is comparatively little increase of myopia after twenty years of age, but can shed no light on the mode of its origin or the rate of its increase in the earlier stages. According to Javal, myopia rarely commences after eight or ten years of age, and, if this opinion is correct, its connection with the process of education might be somewhat complicated with the question of coincidence.

The literature of myopia has grown to be very voluminous, but, even in its more recent chapters, contains sufficient diversity of theories to show that many of the most important points connected with it are still far from settled. That its anatomical condition is a prolongation of the antero-posterior axis of the eyeball is almost the only point of universal consent; whether increased pressure or diminished resistance is the essential factor in producing this condition, and what may be the exact pathology of either, may, perhaps, be considered as open questions. Sclerotico-choroiditis posterior is generally abandoned as a prime cause, and the idealized plates with a convenient local bulging at the outer side of the optic nerve are no longer satisfying. Some authorities place their faith in hereditary weakness of the sclerotic, others assign to this cause a secondary role, and some are bold enough to discard it altogether, or even to set up race peculiarities in its place. Some charge the ciliary muscle with all the mischief and find hope only in atropia, while others accuse convergence and set the ciliary muscle to work with concave glasses. Perhaps, however, but few ophthalmic surgeons will refuse their consent to the following articles of belief voted by the Ophthalmological Section of the International Medical Congress held at Geneva in 1877.

I. "The ordinary causes of myopia are heredity and eye work, the influence of which may be separate or combined.

II. "Hypermetropia may be transformed into true myopia, under the influence of near work, passing through emmetropia.

III. "The progress of civilization, and particularly of school education, tends to increase the extension of myopia.

IV. "The predisposition to myopia is often but not always hereditary. The influence of race upon this predisposition is still an open question.

V. "In use of the eyes for near work, three principal factors concur, with predisposed individuals, to produce the anatomical lesions of progressive myopia. These are, in the order of their importance, accommodation, convergence of the visual axes, and oculo-cephalic congestion.

VI. "The conditions of age, attitude, light, and duration, under which eye work is performed, as well as the character of the objects used, and the state of the visual apparatus itself, have a powerful influence in the development of myopia.

VII. "The prophylaxis of myopia requires a combination of individual, school, and domestic hygienic measures, in great part attainable by the cooperation of physicians, educational bodies, and the authorities. Among these measures should be included the use of convex glasses by hypermetropes."

———

Desiccated Ox-Blood and Hæmoglobine.—Dr. LE BON, in the *Journal de Thérapeutique* (November 25) protests against the claim which Dr. Andrew Smith and others in America have made of having invented this preparation, the full description of which he had published five years since in the *Comptes-Rendus* (1875), and notices of which were given in all the French medical journals. It has now, he states, been well tried at the Paris hospitals, and especially at the Children's Hospital, and has been found most efficacious in all cases in which reconstituents are required. It is indicated wherever iron, raw meat, or the phosphates are useful. Hæmoglobine, Dr. Le Bon says, is difficult to prepare, and in some modes of desiccation of blood all hæmoglobine is lost. He has had it prepared by a skilful chemist, and it is now in the trade. It is almost completely soluble in water, giving to this a magnificent red colour. It may be given in this way or with chocolate, or in the form of powder. The American plan of adding alcohol is chemically bad, as this precipitates the albumen. Dr. Le Bon observes that all the elixirs or wines sold containing any of the essential principles of blood or meat are an entire delusion, as they cannot contain an atom of the albuminoid principles which give to meat its nutritive properties.—*Med. Times and Gazette*, Dec. 4, 1880.

———

Guy's Hospital.—The *Lancet* (Dec. 25, 1880), in its summary of the events of medical interest during the past year, gives the following temperate but brief sketch of the recent troubles at Guy's Hospital which have during the past few months attracted a large share of professional attention in Great Britain.

"In the present year we have to mention with regret a disturbance of the harmony of one of our large endowed Metropolitan Hospitals, which threatens even yet to mar its historical usefulness and fame, and has already produced the resignation of its two senior medical officers, Dr. Habershon and Mr. Cooper

Forster. This discord began in an attempt on the part of the Treasurer and Governors to make fundamental changes in the nursing system of the hospital without previous consultation with the medical officers, who are as vitally interested in the efficiency and subordination of nurses and nursing as in the quality of the quinine or of the chloroform which they prescribe. As if to accentuate the scandal of a nursing system acting independently of the medical staff, two cases came to light which greatly shocked public feeling. One, that of a patient with chronic phthisis, who was subjected to a cold bath for an hour by one of the nurses, partly apparently with a penal view, and with a slight notion that it would do no harm therapeutically. Very shortly after symptoms of acute mischief in the head appeared, and soon proved fatal. The nurse was found guilty of manslaughter. In a later case a man was brought to the hospital after a fall, with a slight scalp wound. He was seen and the wound dressed *by a nurse slightly*. The next day he was brought back to the hospital and found to have fracture of the skull, of which he soon died. The controversy which took place between the Treasurer and the Governors, upholding the new nursing system on the one hand, and the medical men on the other, has occupied most of the year. On the part of the Treasurer and Governors it has been disrespectful and highly unmindful of what was due to the medical faculty of a hospital which has been made famous at home and abroad by its medical faculty. On the part of the medical staff there has been a want of decision, strength, and, we had almost said, self-respect; but it would be more proper to say respect for the profession they represent. Although, however, the senior medical officers have resigned, the public scandal remains of a great hospital so badly administered financially that it is deeply in debt, that nearly a hundred beds have had to be closed, and that by a system of self-election on the part of the Governors medical men have gradually been ousted from the Board of Management, and that the admission of two is now conceded as a sop to public and professional indignation. Clearly, we have not got to the end of the crisis at Guy's, which discredits the year 1880. But good will yet come out of it."

Rupture of the Vermiform Appendix.—The subject of this case was a robust soldier, forty-five years of age, who had been in good health until a week before, was brought into the hospital with the symptoms of peritonitis, and died two days afterwards. On examination, a large quantity of purulent fluid was found in the cavity of the abdomen, and the vermiform process, nearly five times its natural size, exhibited a large aperture, while its communication with the intestine was obstructed by a long bean-shaped concretion of a greenish colour. On cutting through this, there was found as its nucleus at the centre a piece of husk of rye, around which had formed deposits of phosphate and carbonate of lime, the calculus having attained a centimetre in diameter before it caused rupture of the process. The case differs from most of those on record in having caused rupture by distension, instead of by ulcerative process.—*Med. Times and Gaz.*, Jan. 8, 1881, from *Petersburg Med. Woch.*, 1880, No. 40.

Instantaneous Rigor Mortis.—Dr. J. EWING MEARS writes to us that "In a copy of the *London Times* of November 7, 1805, which has recently come into my possession, I find the following paragraph, forming a part of a description of the memorable naval engagement between the English and allied French and Spanish fleets off Cape Trafalgar:—

"'A man was so completely cut in two by a double-headed shot, that the whole of his body, with the exception of his legs up to his knees, was blown some yards into the water; but, strange to tell, his legs were left standing on the deck with all the firmness and animation of life.'

" As I do not know of any report of this remarkable case in surgical works, it has occurred to me that it would be well to record it at this time."

The retention in death of the last attitude of life as the result of instantaneous rigor, accompanying sudden and violent death, has attracted but little attention. A very interesting paper on the subject, illustrated by some remarkable cases observed in the War of the Rebellion, was published by Dr. John H. Brinton in the number of the *American Journal of the Medical Sciences* for January, 1870, p. 87.

Listerism in Japan.—Miss Isabella Bird, in her recent charming work, "Unbeaten Tracks in Japan," describes a visit to a native hospital at Kubota, under the charge of Dr. Kayobashi, who "is fresh from the medical college at Tôkiyô, and has introduced the antiseptic treatment with great success." Miss Bird says: "the odour of carbolic acid pervaded the whole hospital, and there were sprays enough to satisfy Mr. Lister! At the request of Dr. Kayobashi I saw the dressing of some very severe wounds carefully performed with carbolized gauze, under spray of carbolic acid, the fingers of the surgeon and the instruments used being all carefully bathed in the disinfectant."

Société Medico-Psychologique of Paris.—Dr. John P. Gray, of the Utica Asylum, has been elected an Associate Member of this Society.

An Ingenious Suggestion.—A French philanthropist proposes to diminish the mortality amongst the wounded in war by tattooing on the soldier's body the principal points where compression may be made in cases of hemorrhage. Life may be lost in a few minutes by a wound of a large artery, and it is thought that the soldier might often escape if he knew where to command an artery whilst waiting for help.

Ovariotomy during Pregnancy.—KARL SCHRŒDER (*Zeitschrift für Geburtshülfe und Gynäkologie*), on the strength of seven successful ovariotomies during pregnancy performed by himself, and fourteen performed by Olshausen, with only two deaths, considers that ovariotomy, during pregnancy, is an operation not to be feared especially, and only to be avoided when especial contraindications are present. It improves the prognosis, he considers, for the mother, and probably does not injure it for the child. The operation is best performed during the earlier months of pregnancy; later, the broad ligaments are so full of dilated veins, that the treatment of the pedicle becomes more difficult and more dangerous.—*British Med. Journal*, Dec. 25, 1880.

Peritoneal Transfusion of Blood.—The transfusion of blood into the peritoneal cavity recommended by Ponfick, and supported by the experiments of Bizzozero and Golgi, has been recently practised in Italy with marked success. The case is reported in the *Annali di Ostetricia* of June last. The patient, who was moribund from hemorrhage after parturition, was transfused with 200 *grammes* of defibrinated blood taken from a man by venesection, and injected into the peritoneal cavity. There was no reaction; and the patient made an excellent recovery. The method is one which seems to deserve trial in this country.—*British Med. Journal*, Dec. 25, 1880.

Medical and Surgical History of the War.—A bill is now before Congress for the printing of fifty thousand copies of the four volumes which have been already

issued of the "Medical and Surgical History of the War of the Rebellion."
'Should the bill become a law, these books will be distributed gratuitously by
Members of Congress, and consequently early application should be made by
constituents desiring them.

———

The Introduction of Vaccination into America.—Dr. HENRY A. MARTIN, of
Boston, gives in the *North Carolina Medical Journal*, for January of this year,
a very interesting sketch, with fac-simile letters, of the efforts made by President
Jefferson to extend the introduction of vaccination into this country at the beginning of the century.

———

International Medical Congress, London, 1881.—The following subjects, in
addition to those previously announced, have been proposed for discussion:—
Section IV. (*Medicine*).—1. Localization of Disease in Brain and Spinal
Cord, so far as pathognomonic and diagnostic; 2. Trophic Changes of Nerve-
origin; 3. Vascular Changes, Functional and Organic, in Disease; 4. Primary
Diseases of the Lymph-system; 5. Gout, Rheumatoid Arthritis, and Rheumatism; 6. Forms of Renal Disease (Bright's Disease); 7. Methods of Physical
Diagnosis; 8. Therapeutic Methods: Revulsions, Blood-letting, Diet-cure,
Uses of Heat and Cold, Drug-cure, etc.
Section I. (*Anatomy*) will receive communications relating to any of the fol-
lowing subjects: 1. Human Anatomy, descriptive, microscopic, and topographical; 2. Embryology and Teratology; 3. Anatomical Anthropology and Anthro-
pometry; 4. Comparative Anatomy in so far as it illustrates structural changes
in Man; 5. Improved Methods of Instruction in Anatomy, and of preparing and
preserving Anatomical Specimens.
Section XI. (*Diseases of the Skin*).—1. The Relation between Constitutional
Diseases and Diseases of the Skin; 2. The Nature and Treatment of Lupus
Erythematosus; 3. The Influence of Climate, Difference of Race, and Mode
of Living upon the Development and Character of Diseases of the Skin.

———

Louisiana State Medical Association.—The fourth annual meeting of this
society will be held at New Orleans, on March 30, under the presidency of Dr.
C. M. Smith, of St. Mary.

———

Statistics of Medical Journalism.—On the authority of M. DUREAU, one of
the librarians of the Académie de Médecine, the present number of medical
periodical publications for France and its colonies is 147, 95 of these being published in Paris, and 52 in the departments. The Germanic Confederation publishes 133 journals, Great Britain 69, Austria 54, Italy 51, Belgium 28, Spain
26, Russia 26, Holland 16, Switzerland 10, Sweden and Norway 9, Denmark 5,
Portugal 4, the Danish Principalities 4, Turkey 2, Greece 1—the total for Europe
being 583. In America there are 183 journals, in Asia 15, in Oceanica 4—the
total for the various continents being 785. The number of medical journals created
since 1679 exceeds 2500.—*Med. Times and Gazette*, Jan. 22, 1881, from
Lyon Médical.

———

To Readers and Correspondents.—*The editor will be happy to receive early
intelligence of local events of general medical interest, or which it is desirable
to bring to the notice of the profession. Local papers containing reports or
news items should be marked.*

.CONTENTS OF NUMBER 460.

APRIL, 1881.

CLINICS.

MONTHLY ABSTRACT.

MEDICAL NEWS.

THE

MEDICAL NEWS AND ABSTRACT.

VOL. XXXIX. No. 4. APRIL, 1881. WHOLE No. 460.

CLINICS.

Clinical Lectures.

ON FRACTURE OF THE PATELLA. RELATIVE VALUE OF BONY AND FIBROUS UNION IN TRANSVERSE FRACTURES.

A CLINICAL LECTURE DELIVERED AT BELLEVUE HOSPITAL, DEC. 1880.

By FRANK H. HAMILTON, M.D.,
SURGEON TO BELLEVUE HOSPITAL, NEW YORK, ETC.

GENTLEMEN: Last year I presented to the medical gentlemen and students assembled here fourteen cases of fracture of the patella, which had united by fibrous tissue. Some of these were quite old cases, and some quite recent cases; some with a short fibrous union, and in some the bond of union was quite long;, but the patients were all able to walk very well, and in some the flexion and extension, and all the functions of the limbs were completely restored. At the same time I presented an analysis of 127 cases, 64 of which had been more or less under my personal observation and care. In the analysis of these cases it was found that in a large majority the union was known to be fibrous, indeed, that not in more than five or six cases was there a suspicion that bony union had taken place, and in not one was its existence proven. Subsequently these 127 cases were published in detail, with the results of the analysis, embodying certain other conclusions and inferences; and my remarks to-day are intended chiefly to supplement the observations then made, but especially in reference to the relative value of a fibrous and bony union.

First, I will repeat what was said by me on the occasion alluded to, namely, that the evidence presented by the study of cases which had come under my observation was well-nigh conclusive that a fibrous union is as useful as a bony union, and probably less liable to a renewed separation. The same was substantially shown by the cases brought before the gentlemen for their inspection. I shall pursue this subject to-day more in a theoretical point of view than by an actual study of cases.

Suppose it were possible to make a transverse fracture of this bone to unite by bone—remember that nearly all of these fractures are transverse—with the fragments in actual contact. What evidence has been presented, and what reason can be assigned why it should be any stronger than if the

union were fibrous ? The ligamentum patellæ, although much more slender
than the patella in its transverse and antero-posterior diameters, does not
break once where the patella breaks ten times; yet it is subject to the same
strains as the patella.   In the last (6th) edition of my work on "Fractures
and Dislocations," I have recorded a case seen by me in which the patella
having been broken the second time by muscular action, the separation
took place, not through the newly-formed fibrous ligament, but through
another portion of the bone itself, proving conclusively that the new ligament, of half an inch in length, at the end of five or six months, was
better able to resist the cross strain and muscular action than the original
bone.

In the preceding remarks, gentlemen, I have supposed the fragments to
have united by bone, while they were in actual or nearly actual contact,
although no evidence has yet been presented to me that this has ever happened in the case of a transverse fracture.   I see no reason, however, why
it might not occasionally happen when the fragments have been broken,
but not actually separated from each other through their entire thickness;
nor, indeed, that it might not happen whenever the fragments having
been completely separated are again, and at an early day, brought into
contact, and maintained in absolute contact for a sufficient length of time.
I am not disputing the possibility of close bony union, under certain possible conditions.   I am only comparing the value of that close bony union
with an equally close fibrous union, and the conclusion is that the fibrous
union is likely to be the strongest, and, therefore, the best.   A fibrous
ligament here, as everywhere else in the body, is stronger than a bone of
equal size, and will especially resist more successfully a cross strain.

Let us now make another supposition, namely, that the fragments have
united by bone, *but with a separation of half an inch or of an inch.*
Here is a specimen of that kind of union.   The fragments after a transverse fracture have united by a slender bridge of bone of about one inch
in length.   The argument will be the same whether its length is more, or
somewhat less.   It is a bridge of solid bone, but of less than half the
thickness of the original bone.   The bridge is defective in the centre,
presenting here a pretty large oval space, which was closed in before it
was cleaned by a fibrous tissue.   A glance will convince you that this
bridge of bone could not have resisted any considerable cross strain, and
that any effort to bend the knee to a right angle must almost inevitably
have snapped it like a pipe stem.   The bone was sent to me, and its history has not yet been obtained, but the presumption seems to be inevitable
that it was taken from an anchylosed limb.   In my attempt to clean it, I
broke, as you will see, one side of the bridge, and it is certain that no
portion of it could have withstood a bending of ten degrees, while the
quadriceps retained its normal power of contraction.   It requires very
little mechanical or physiological learning to understand that a fibrous
band of the same dimensions would have been much stronger, and, therefore, more useful than this.

If the bond of union is to be bone, then, we argue the union must be
accomplished with the fragments in absolute, or nearly absolute contact;
and I have no satisfactory proof that this has ever been done, nor does it
seem to me that it is possible that it ever will be done, except in those
rare cases in which the fracture has occurred without complete separation
of the fragments; as, for example, where the anterior margins of the line
of fracture are separated, and the posterior remain in contact, so that the

joint is not actually opened. This is a possibility, as this experiment upon the cadaver will illustrate. With a broad chisel and hammer, my assistant has cut or broken the patella transversely, but the thin cartilage covering its posterior surface has not been torn, and the joint is not exposed. So that while in front the fragments can be separated one-quarter of an inch, they remain in contact posteriorly. If this were the condition of the fragments from the beginning a bony union would be very possible, or quite probable. If they are separated an inch or even one-quarter of an inch completely, posteriorly as well as anteriorly, the union of bone would be accomplished under great difficulties, and probably not until after the lapse of several months, during which the joint must be kept in a state of complete immobility. It is my opinion that in all of the cases in which an examination of the specimens after death has shown that the fragments have united by bone with a separation of half an inch or more between the fragments—and the specimens of this kind of union known to exist are very few—the knees of the patients from whom they were taken, were anchylosed. Certainly it could not have been formed when the knee was in motion, and probably in all these cases there has been first a ligamentous bond, which has been gradually changed into bone.

Notice what difficulties exist in the way of union by bone. The fragments are not usually in absolute contact immediately after the accident, and experience has shown that they can seldom be brought and *maintained* in absolute contact subsequently. There is no bone in the body which under such circumstances is ever expected to unite by bone. If it does it is a rare and exceptional event, and does not occur until after many months or years of confinement of the limb. Why should it happen with the patella and not with other bones? There is no reason why it should; but there are several reasons why it should not, which do not apply in the cases of most other bones. The disadvantages under which it labours in this regard are peculiar, and nearly or quite equal to those which exist in the case of an intracapsular fracture of the neck of the femur. The synovial fluid is greatly increased in quantity, and pressing forwards occupies the space between the broken surfaces, and by distending the capsule actually increases the separation. There is very little soft tissue either in front of or behind the patella. Posteriorly the thin plate of cartilage is torn entirely across, except in those rare instances which I have supposed possible, but the existence of which has not been actually proven, where the fragments may be supposed to have separated in front, but not posteriorly. You must not forget that this fracture is almost invariably caused by great muscular action, and if under this immense strain the bone has given way, the thin and delicate cartilaginous plate posteriorly would offer only a feeble resistance to the action of the muscles and the separation would be completed. In this fracture made upon the cadaver with a chisel the synovial membrane was not torn and the joint was not opened, but the circumstances are different from those in which a fracture usually occurs in life; in this fracture produced by a chisel there was no muscular action, and the fracture could be limited to any point. You see then how difficult, if not impossible, it is to supply the bony material. There is absolutely nothing left behind the line of fracture from which repair of any kind can proceed.

In front again the periosteum is torn entirely asunder, and so also are the few scattering fibres of the tendon of the quadriceps. Even the posterior wall of the bursa patellæ is probably torn in most cases, and nothing is left in front of the line of fracture but a thin tegumentary layer, the posterior surface of which, corresponding to the fracture is, in case the bursa has been torn, a synovial surface, which I need not tell you is unfitted for the process of repair.   In the case of ordinary fracture of the long bones there is always an abundance of soft tissue to aid in the repair, and there is also in almost every case a considerable portion of periosteum which is untorn, and which bridges over a part of the chasm and contributes very largely to the future callus ; the fragments are also in most cases in actual contact ; and yet even under these most favourable circumstances bony union sometimes fails. ·

If the fragments are not therefore in actual contact there is usually, I will repeat, no source of supply for reparative material but this thin tegumentary layer in front and the lacerated fibres of the tendon of the quadriceps on the inner and outer margins of the patella, of which two, it is probable that the latter furnishes the chief supply.   An examination of the lesions in the aponeurosis, which hug closely the lateral margins of the fragments, would lead us to conclude that this must be the chief source of the supply ; and the fact that the new fibrous bond is usually more abundant or stronger on the margin of the fracture sustains this opinion.

In order that you may comprehend the difficulties fully in this case, where the fragments are not in actual contact, I must again call your attention to the fact that the synovia, always increased in quantity, presses up between the fragments, bathing the broken surfaces, and washing away the reparative material almost as fast as it is deposited.   You will see that nothing but absolute and firm contact, such as will prevent the admission of the synovia between the fragments, can encourage a hope that the repair will be effected by material supplied by the broken surfaces themselves.

Let us not lose sight of the statement made in the opening of this lecture—namely, that a fibrous union is probably as useful as any bony union which can be obtained.   No one has ever claimed that it is not easy to get a strong fibrous union where the original separation is not very unusual; and my purpose is to congratulate you on this fact, inasmuch as it is so difficult, and in most cases impossible, to maintain absolute contact and thus secure bony union.

Now we will consider some of the extreme, or, as they think, more certain expedients to which some surgeons resort to obtain a close bony union.   Regarding a bony union as essential to the most perfect success or as required in order that the limb may hereafter be the most useful— an opinion which I do not entertain—they have sought to insure immediate bony union by the use of mechanical appliances which operate directly upon the fragments, and not indirectly through the integuments; with steel points or wire they propose to place the fragments completely under their command.   Of which measures I affirm my belief that they have not in general, if ever, accomplished their purpose; that they are more or less dangerous to the limbs and lives of the patients, and that inasmuch as the other methods which insure a fibrous union, which will be as useful as a bony union, in all recent cases, are perfectly safe, surgeons cannot be well justified in adopting either one of them.

Let us first consider what is known as " Malgaigne's method," or the method of holding the fragments by metallic hooks.   The instrument which I show you is the instrument invented and used by Malgaigne. His experience with these hooks, as related in his "Treatise on Fractures," is contained in four cases. (Although Druitt says, I do not know on what authority, that he had in 1858 treated eleven cases by this method satisfactorily.)

In two of these cases the hooks loosened and slipped, tearing the flesh and had to be removed after a short time. In one case, that of a boy eleven years old, the patella was *thought* to be united by bone; in one the union was thought to be partly bony and partly ligamentous; in one the character of the union is not mentioned, and in the fourth case, in which the hooks were not employed until after three months, the fragments were at first supposed to be united by bone, but it was soon found that no union at all had taken place. No evidence is presented that either of these patients had any more useful limbs than is usually obtained by other modes of treatment. Nor is there any substantial evidence that any of these had united by bone; no more indeed than is often presented after other methods of treatment, but in which the lapse of time or the autopsy has almost constantly proven that it was not united by bone.

I will now read to you what Malgaigne himself says of the value of bony union.

"On the whole, ossific union, taking place in the majority of cases with some separation of the fragments, the bone remains elongated and deformed; and I am not sure that this deformity does not interfere as much with the functions of the knee as union by fibrous tissue would. Boyer relates a case of this kind; the patella was elongated by about six lines; the patient was obliged to use a cane for a year, and thirteen years afterwards the flexion of his knee was still limited. I have myself published a case of bony consolidation obtained by M. Blandin; the increase in length of the patella was estimated during life at eight lines; at the end of the fourth month the leg could hardly be flexed five or six degrees. I sought in vain to find this man subsequently."

In both of these cases the bony union resulted in all but complete anchylosis. Certainly these examples do not argue much for bony union as compared with fibrous union.

Here is another paragraph which I will read you from Malgaigne; speaking still of bony union, he says " I have sometimes seen it myself, but what is very essential, never in simple transverse fractures. There was always at least one small splinter broken off from one of the fragments."

Speaking of the difficulty of adjusting and maintaining the hooks in position a long time, he says he has not been able to remedy it, and he alludes with his usual frankness to the cases of M. Roberts who failed completely with his (Malgaigne's) hooks to approximate the fragments; and finally he refers to one of his own cases in which, for some reason not stated, he removed the hooks and substituted pressure, "but the little wounds became inflamed, and erysipelas ensued."

Hear what Volkmann has recently said on this subject: " That Malgaigne's hooks, have caused ulceration of the joints and death of the patient in a number of cases, is only too true; I myself know of two which occurred in the practice of friends, and which were never published, and another sad experience met with in my own clinic a number of years since, of which I shall speak directly." Gross says they are apt to cause an erysipelatous inflammation. Erichsen speaks of their causing pain and irritation. Bryant says they are objectionable for the same reason. I have myself heard of a case in one of our city hospitals in which serious results followed the use of these hooks.

Agnew, in his excellent "Treatise on Surgery," has spoken very emphatically in regard to Malgaigne's hooks. I quote from the first volume, p. 980, of his recent publication.

"Once I have seen death follow the use of this infernal machine from an erysipelatous inflammation extending into the joint and giving rise to abscesses both within and without the articulation. No advantage whatever results from the close contact of the fragments accomplished by the instrument; it is rather a disadvantage, as the tendency to refracture is increased by the very closeness of the tension, the intermediate bond not being as strong as the ordinary fibrous tissue which fills the gap when the pieces of the bone are a short distance apart. Three times I have seen the union broken a few weeks after the patients treated by this method had been discharged from the hospital."

The only decided advocate of Malgaigne's hooks known to me in this country is Dr. R. J. Levis, of Philadelphia, who has modified the hooks, substituting two points for the four in the original instrument. The principle remains the same. In the *Medical and Surgical Reporter* for 1878, he has reported four cases, one of which was treated by Malgaigne's hooks, and the result was a separation of the fragments to the extent of half an inch. It is not stated that it united by bone, but he calls the result "good." The other three cases were treated by his own modified hooks. In one there is said to be "some separation"; one was refractured soon after he left the hospital, and in the third an abscess resulted which he thinks might have been due to the original injury. In one of the four cases the union is said to be ligamentous and in none is it declared to be bony.

Perhaps Dr. Levis has published other cases, but I cannot see in these four any thing to remove the prejudice which most surgeons, in common with myself, entertain towards this instrument. It is not sufficient for any surgeon to say that he has adopted this method in four cases without any disastrous results; nor indeed that he has had no mishaps in 20 or 25 cases. Other surgeons have met with them much oftener than this, and a method which exposes to suppuration of the joint, and death as a consequence solely of the apparatus employed, cannot be commended even if these results do not happen oftener than once in fifty cases; and especially when there is no satisfactory evidence that the average results are any better than by other and perfectly safe methods.

There are many other methods which have from time to time been suggested and practised, for the purpose of effecting a bony union of the fragments; a result which, you will remember, I have in the opening of my remarks to-day declared to be undesirable, and therefore certainly not to be sought for at the risk of life. Most of the plans I shall now refer to are in a greater or less degree attended with this risk.

Severinus, an Italian, proposed to make an incision into the joint, exposing the fragments, and then to freshen the broken surfaces and bring them together. This was nearly 300 years ago, when surgeons did not pretend to have any specific for preventing inflammation after wounds of large joints, such as Mr. Lister thinks we possess to-day. It certainly was a very bold or rather I would say a very foolish and reckless suggestion, and it is gratifying to know that he never practised it himself. It has, however, been actually done lately by Van der Meulin, Cameron, and Rose, with antiseptic precautions.

Dieffenbach is said to have cut the rectus femoris and ligamentum patellæ, the operation resulting in some improvement; but so good a surgeon and anatomist as he, ought to have known that the cutting of the rectus femoris alone would not affect materially, if at all, the upper fragment. It would be necessary to cut the whole of the quadriceps; and to cut the ligamentum patellæ would be to substitute an ununited ligament for an ununited patella. The joint would in all probability be entered and the most disastrous consequences might ensue. Malgaigne doubts the faithfulness of the report of this case, and I doubt it also. Gould has more recently cut the quadriceps alone; at least we are told so, but I do not know the result.

Surgeons have occasionally, in the case of old, ununited fractures, introduced a tenotome subcutaneously and roughened the broken surfaces. This I have seen two or three times myself, but there has been no result whatever, so far as the union was concerned; nor is it probable, considering the peculiar conditions under which the fracture exists, that any benefit can be obtained from this expedient.

MM. Ollier and Goujon have recently injected fresh marrow cells between the fragments, and Dr. Wyeth, of this city, has repeated the experiment in old, ununited fractures; but neither of these gentlemen have obtained any results; nor do I very well see how they can reasonably expect any result, since the osteogenic materials must be placed, not actually between the fragments, for that would be in the joint itself, but only in the very thin tegumentary covering over the point of fracture.

Prof. Kocher, of Berne, Schede, and Volkmann, have recently advocated and practised opening the joint, with antiseptic precautions, for the purpose of letting out the blood, and for the purpose of securing bony union; but Kocher thinks this cannot be accomplished satisfactorily when the blood has become coagulated. He advises, therefore, that it be done immediately, or as soon as the fracture comes' under the surgeon's observation.

The objections to this method are, first, that it is dangerous despite antiseptic precautions; second, that blood in any considerable quantity is seldom effused into the joint; third, that we can never be sure of being able to remove any but a small portion of the blood; fourth, that even if successful, we have in only a slight degree removed the obstacles in the way of bony union; and finally, that bony union is not desirable. As to the danger of suppuration from the presence of blood in the joint, I have not in a very large experience seen such a result from such a cause. Yet I can conceive of a case in which the extravasation may be so great as to render the evacuation of the blood advisable to prevent suppuration. But such cases must be exceedingly rare, and considering all the objections which exist, you will probably do better if you never adopt the suggestions of these gentlemen. There is more danger in this indiscriminate opening of joints than in omitting to open the few cases in which it might possibly prove serviceable.

I think it was Schede who first proposed and practised, for the purpose of effecting bony union, introducing a large needle, armed with a silver wire, through the joint; introducing it below the lower fragment, and bringing it out above the upper, and then drawing the fragments together. The operation being done antiseptically. He says he has done it three times and obtained bony union—a statement, the correctness of which Kocher ventures to doubt.

Kocher has modified this operation by first making incisions through the skin, above and below the fragments, and then introducing the needle and silver wire. He says he has done this twice, but he confesses that he did not prevent separation of the fragments, and he does not pretend that the union was bony.

Volkmann, as I have already told you, confesses to having had a sad experience with Malgaigne's hooks, still however seeking for some mode of obtaining bony union he has employed what he calls the "tendon suture." A common ligature was passed through the tendon of the quadriceps and of the patella, and by these means he tied the fragments together. In one case he thinks he had bony union, in one a "satisfactory result," in one it was "all that could be desired," and in one the patient died! Although in this case the ligature was in place only one quarter of an hour, but the ligature had, as the autopsy showed, penetrated the joint.

Such are some of the expedients for the purpose of procuring bony union to which surgeons have from time to time, and especially of late, resorted. I confess, gentlemen, it does not increase my respect for the judgment of surgeons who adopt any or most of these methods. Their performance does not exhibit simply a rudeness of conception as to what it is desirable to accomplish, but some of them an absolute lack of appreciation of danger in surgical operations. They seem to me to be the devices of mechanics and not of surgeons.

Dr. Hamilton's Method of Treatment.—In nearly all cases the adjusting retentive apparatus may be applied at once. If exceptions occur it will be in those cases in which the patella has suffered from a direct and severe injury, and the swelling and tenderness are unusual. The single inclined plane recommended by me in the earlier editions of my work on "Fractures and Dislocations" I now very seldom use. It is in all respects sound in principle, but it is unnecessarily cumbrous for ordinary cases. A light splint and a cotton roller are the only essential parts of a proper apparatus.

Here is a patient to whom this dressing has been applied. The best materials for a splint now known to me, in the case of a fracture of the patella, is gum shellac cloth, made of about six thicknesses of cotton cloth saturated with gum shellac. It is made by the hatters, and can always be obtained from the instrument makers in this city at a moderate cost. The same material can be used for splints in the case of most long bones. It is not patented. . The splint must be long enough to extend from above the middle of the thigh to near the ankle, and wide enough to envelop half the circumference of the limb. This being moulded to the back of the limb, must be covered by a complete sack of cotton or woollen cloth, after which it is to be laid against the back of the limb ; and first a roller is applied just below the knee by several circular turns, including both splint and leg ; second, the roller is carried obliquely above the patella, and then around the limb and splint in a circular manner. In short, by oblique and circular turns the fragments are to be gradually drawn together—the integument being meanwhile, as far as possible, kept from doubling itself between the fragments—and the oblique turns gradually approaching each other in front of the patella until the whole is covered in. Third, a separate roller is applied to the lower part of the limb and splint, and a third to the upper part. Fourth, all the turns of the rollers are carefully stitched to each margin of the cover of the splint. Fifth, the limb is laid in bed with the foot resting upon a pillow so as to raise the foot about six inches. If you deem it necessary, the foot may be secured in this position by some permanent apparatus, or by being placed in a swing ; only that the importance of keeping the foot permanently elevated during the first two or three weeks must be recognized.

The limb must be examined daily, and as soon as the bandages about the knee have slackened from the subsidence of the swelling or from any other cause, with a large needle and strong linen thread, they must be tightened by overstitching; and especially must the oblique turns which pass above and below the fragments be thus tightened. This may have to be repeated every day for several days, but it will seldom be found necessary to remove and reapply the bandages within the first two or three weeks. At the close of the second or third week the dressings should be removed and the limb examined, when it will generally be found that the upper fragment is nearly or quite immovable, unless considerable force is applied; it is therefore no longer liable to be drawn up by the ordinary action of the rectus or quadriceps, and we can give to the joint a little motion without in any degree increasing the separation of the fragments; but to avoid all danger we may press down the upper fragment while we move the joint gently.

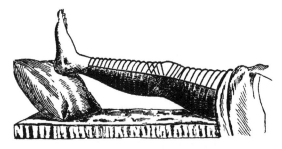

The same dressings are then to be reapplied and with the same care. From this time forward there can be no objection to the patient's being about on crutches, since the anchylosed or semi-anchylosed condition of the upper fragment will prevent its being influenced by the ordinary action of the rectus; but regularly at night, or at least every second day, the splint should be removed and slight passive motion employed.

Ordinarily we may discharge the patient at the end of six or eight weeks from our immediate care, but with instructions to continue to wear the splint or some equally firm substitute eight weeks longer. It may be removed, however, whenever he is in bed. The necessity of wearing the splints so long is found in the great frequency of refractures during the first month or two after the dismissal of the patient; that is to say, after the splint has been removed, and within four months from the date of the receipt of the injury. Laced or elastic knee-caps do not give the required support; they give way under any considerable strain upon the joint, as experience has shown in several instances. And the same accident would be just as liable to occur if the fragments had united by bone, or even more so. Remember that we cannot apply the same rules here that we do in fractures of long bones. When these latter bones have united, and the limbs are put into use, the point of fracture is not subjected to the enormous cross-strain to which united fractures of the patella are subjected —I speak particularly of fractures of the shafts of long bones—and we can generally permit these patients to go about safely without splints at the end of eight weeks. It is very different, as you must see, with the patella.

Please, gentlemen, remember all the details of the treatment which I have recommended to you. They all contribute to the best results, and no one of these details can be safely omitted. If you wish to avail your-selves of the results of my experience, you must follow minutely my direc-tions. Do not use compresses, or adhesive strips, or elastic bands, or metallic, or other hard adjusters, or plaster-of-Paris, or any other form of immovable dressings. Do not let the patient get up on crutches in less than two or three weeks. I have good reasons for advising you thus, some of which I have given, and others of which I have not time now to give. Avoid every method, whether new or old, which endangers in any degree the limb or the life of the patient, since there is before you a simple and perfectly safe method, which assures to your patients as good and probably better results than the dangerous methods.

There is one thing more which I had almost forgotten to say: when, at the end of four or five months from the time of the original injury, the splint is wholly laid aside, do not apply a knee-cap or any bandage to the limb, but let the patient use the muscles of his leg freely, so that they can recover their normal strength and size. It is surprising how much the ability of flexing the limb and to sustain the body is improved under free and unrestrained use of the muscles.

The anchylosis of the upper fragment soon disappears under use; and the anchylosis of the knee-joint itself disappears gradually, in the same manner. Under no circumstances is it proper to seek to overcome it by force.

ABSTRACT OF A CLINICAL LECTURE ON THE TREATMENT OF SOME FORMS OF EPILEPSY.

Delivered at the Hospital for Epilepsy and Paralysis.

By J. S. RAMSKILL, M.D. LOND.,
Junior Physician to the Hospital, Consulting Physician to the London Hospital.

GENTLEMEN: The boy I show you (L——) says he is eight years of age, and that he has been ill eight months. He looks his age, and is fairly intellectual. He had been at school for five years before the accession of the fits. The shape of his head is good, and there is no particular vaulting of the roof of the mouth. I always examine the mouth both with a view of ascertaining the height of the roof and the state of the teeth, both as regards caries and overcrowding. About the age of puberty the latter condition is not a very rare cause of epilepsy. And it is always well to exclude every source of irritation arising from that most reflex nerve of the body, the trigeminus.

We have no neurotic family history, and no account of any previous illness to note. Examination of the heart and lungs reveals nothing, neither does the ophthalmoscope. The abdomen seems full, some gurgling sounds are heard on palpation, and it is more doughy than natural; but on account of a certain amount of superficial fat, the state of the colon and viscera can hardly be made out. Now, about a month before the commencement of the fits, the boy complained of a bad cramp in the left wrist and upper half of the hand. In remained only a few seconds, but recurred at different intervals: sometimes twice or three times a day, and next day only once. About the end of a month he was knocked down by a blow on the left side of the head. He did not lose consciousness, nor was he sick, neither had he subsequent headache.

Next morning he had a fit, and several during the next fourteen days; then he was free for a month. They then returned, but only by night; but during the following month they came both by night and day. We learn from the parents that the character of the fits is as follows: He first has the cramp in the left hand and wrist, screams, and also, sometimes, bites his tongue; is universally convulsed, but most so on the left side. The fits last only a few seconds. He occasionally has one in the day, but usually eight or ten every night. It is observed that if he falls asleep during the day he has a fit. There are no sequelæ of note to the attacks.

Such is the aspect of the patient and the history of the case. The first point to decide is this: Is the patient epileptic? and, if so, is the disease idiopathic and primary, or is it secondary or sympathetic? It would be waste of time to argue the first question. The case is clearly epileptic; but it is quite a question as to whether it be idiopathic or not. Modern science would at once say it is centric, and the particular part of the brain most involved was the right ascending frontal convolution, an explosion from which spreads upwards, downwards, and backwards, involving an area which might be mapped out by the presence of convulsion or spasm in the muscles engaged. The aura does not consist of an irritation going to the brain, although a ligature above its seat may stop the fit. You all know aura may exist with some coarse centric disease, and a ligature may still stop the accession of the fits. This, I say, is the received opinion; but I am not sure of its universal truth, especially with regard to unfelt aura, which we must suppose to exist. An unfelt aura seems a contradiction in terms; but it is not so, for, as far as I can make out, in the case of a patient who one day has a fit with an aura, and next day another of exactly the same extent and character without any, there must have been a similar, or the same, cause in both.

I think, perhaps, the explanation lies here, that the spread of the discharge was too quick, that the patient had not time to perceive the aura before the attack became general, or before consciousness was lost. But we find on examination the boy has often the aura without a fit. Then I look on his aura as a fit—a minor and localized one. A greater question to my mind is this, Are not most epilepsies eccentric rather than idiopathic and centric at first? Does the existence of an aura really settle everything? Neither physiology nor pathology helps us, but I think practice can. If you prevent both aura and fit, by slight treatment, which cannot reasonably be presumed to have any influence on the cerebro-spinal centres, it is a fair supposition that the cause is not centric, but originates within the sphere of action of your treatment. But I do agree to this opinion, that eccentric soon passes into centric idiopathic epilepsy, or perhaps, that you may, after one has generated the other, have both forms of disease in the same subject. Be this so or not I am inclined, and I dare say you are, to say with the celebrated Trousseau, " Good heavens, gentlemen, a little less science—a little more art." The question then is what line of treatment shall we pursue. This is the programme we adopted.

(a) To see if we could find any source of irritation in the abdomen, "for of all the regions of the body there are none which reflect more strongly on the brain than the intestines and visceral organs."

(b) To give what remedies we know are able to allay the reflex, excitability and force of the cerebro-spinal centres.

With the first object in view, vermifuge aperients, santonine and castor-oil, is the usual combination for children, to be given sufficiently long to make sure of the result.

In our case the result was *nil*. Had a worm been expelled the fits might have vanished; but this is not the rule, unless your treatment has commenced very early in the case after the first attacks. The lumbricus may be dislodged, but the central excito-motor region has taken on morbid action, and the epilepsy remains. Still, in these cases, I always think there is most hope, and most room for treat- ment; for if the irritation of a lumbricus could by a certain route in the nervous system produce a morbid result on the centre, some remedy acting through the same route may lessen, deaden, and finally stop that morbid process in the same centre.

Let us continue our examination of the abdomen. I want to know the con- dition of the colon. We have found the abdomen full—that is, tumid, bigger than it should be, but, without chloroform, we cannot make out anything beyond gurgling.

By the light, then, of experience we make the assertion, that there is probable defect of the colon, as to secretion, spasm, contraction, and alternate dilatation of its calibre. In a post-mortem of an epileptic by Vanderkolk he says: "We found in the abdominal cavity the colon and sigmoid flexure very much dilated and lengthened, the latter ascending to the transverse colon. Above and beneath the sigmoid flexure were many constrictions, which higher up alternated with dilatations; the cæcum, too, was very dilated." This is a severe case; but one cannot help observing in the records of post-mortems the frequent occurrence of a strictured and dilated colon.

What cases of mental depression, of melancholia, have we not all seen asso- ciated with loaded, and probably sacculated, colon! In one series we seem to get an irritant; in the other an inhibitory action on the nerve centres. I recol- lect an old practitioner saying (before the advent of bromide) that a daily morn- ing dose of beaume de vie was of more service in epilepsy than all the medicines in the Pharmacopœia.

To recur to our patient, we kept him in the hospital ten days without treat- ment, beyond the prelude of aperients, to see his exact condition as to the kind, number, and duration of the fits.

On Oct. 13th he had 5 fits; 14th, 7 fits; 15th, 15 fits; 16th, 13 fits, and one in the afternoon, when he had fallen asleep; 17th, 9 fits; 18th, 6 fits; 19th, 7 fits; 20th, 15 fits; 21st, 9 fits; 22d, 15 fits. The fits turned out as described. On Oct. 23d we ordered thirteen grains of bromide of potassium, three grains of iodide of potassium, and eight grains of carbonate of ammonia, three times daily, with this result: Oct. 24th, 9 fits; 25th, 7 fits; 26th, 11 fits; 27th, 9 fits; 28th, 13 fits; 29th, 9 fits; 30th, 9 fits; 31st, 10 fits. The same rate continued until Nov. 4th, when we added more ammonia in the shape of ammoniated spirit. The rate began to diminish, as for the consecutive days we got 7, 6, 6, 7, 2, 8, 6, 5, 6, 5—plus one in the day—then 5, 6, 9, 5, and about the same rate until Nov. 27th. On that day a mixture of equal parts of chloral, camphor, and vase- line was ordered, a portion equal to a small teaspoonful was to be rubbed into the scalp every night. The mixture of bromide, iodide, and ammonia, to be con- tinued, and a pill containing equal parts of aloes, valerianate of zinc, and extract of conium, given every night.

The result of this treatment was, that we had no recurrence of fits of any kind for more than five weeks. Then we had one fit each night for three nights, and I confess that I was glad to see them return. Vanderkolk quotes some cases showing the danger to life which may arise from the prolonged freedom from fits. And, as a general rule, it may be said that in chronic epilepsy the longer you manage by treatment to prolong the interval between the attacks the more severe the following fit will be. Death occurs from asphyxia or from congestion of lungs and coma. It is astonishing that apoplexy is not frequent, but to me it is simply unknown as a result of the most violent and prolonged attacks.

I have had experience only of three fatal results ; all occurred after a so-called cure had been made ; all in the night, and the patients were found dead in the morning. What I wish you to remember is that after a prolonged interval of freedom you must apply some counter-irritant, such as a seton, issue, or leeches, to prevent or to break a too violent explosion.

To return to our case, To what is the improvement due? What is the rationale of the action of the means employed? Perhaps we should do best to see these points illustrated in another case.—*Lancet*, Feb. 26, 1881.

Hospital Notes.

BELLEVUE HOSPITAL, NEW YORK.

(Service of Dr. AUSTIN FLINT, Sr.)

Acute Articular Rheumatism.   Treatment with Salicin and Alkalies.

(Specially reported for the MEDICAL NEWS AND ABSTRACT.)

Robert C., æt. 26, Irish, porter ; admitted Feb. 22, 1881. The patient confesses to the occasional excessive use of alcoholics. He has been employed in the kitchen of a hotel, where he was subjected to frequent alternations of heat and cold. On Feb. 18, he was attacked with acute pain in his left ankle, accompanied by heat, redness, and considerable swelling. The right ankle was next attacked and both knees, both shoulders and the fingers of both hands were subsequently, successively, involved in the inflammatory process. On his admission, Feb. 22d, all the above-named joints presented the signs of acute inflammation. A soft, blowing systolic cardiac murmur was heard at the apex, and was not transmitted to the left. There was no cardiac enlargement. Temperature 103°, pulse 98, respiration 28. Inasmuch as the blowing endocardial murmur was regarded as the evidence of endocardial inflammation it was decided to employ salicin rather than salicylate of soda. Two-hourly doses of salicin, grs. xx. with acetate of potassium, grs. xxx. were prescribed. No other remedies were administered. At the beginning of the treatment the urine was acid and high coloured, with a specific gravity of 1032. It contained no albumen and no sugar.

Feb. 23d. Pain in the joints has been considerably relieved. The urine still remains acid. Temperature, A. M., 103°; P. M., 102¼°.

24th. The pains, redness, and swelling of the joints have markedly diminished. The urine is alkaline. Temperature, A. M., 102°; P. M., 102°.

25th. The joint symptoms have almost disappeared. The urine is alkaline. The cardiac murmur still persists. No pleuritic or pericardial complications have appeared.

March 1st. The acute inflammatory symptoms have disappeared. The temperature has remained at about 100° since the last note. The alkali is now discontinued, but the salicin is still administered, as before, and has occasioned no gastric disturbance.

3d. All febrile symptoms have ceased. Temperature 98½°. Only slight stiffness of the limbs remains. The cardiac murmur is indistinctly audible.

Hystero-Epilepsy ; Phases like those described by Charcot ; Obstructive Dysmenorrhœa ; Treatment by Dilatation of the Cervix Uteri.

A fairly intelligent Roman Catholic aged twenty-one was admitted into Dr. SANSOM's ward in the London Hospital, on Aug. 20th, 1880. She lived from the age of thirteen to seventeen in Canada. Her mother's father died of consumption, but there was no neurotic family history. As a child she had good health, but whilst in Canada, and even after, she had suffered much from headaches, and from frequent attacks of vomiting. She first menstruated at the age of eleven; had always been very irregular; her menses were scanty, lasting never more than three days, and always accompanied by severe pain, both constant and paroxysmal, referred vaguely to the back and to the front of the abdomen, and coming on at the commencement of the flow, and lasting till it ceased.

She was first taken with fits in April, 1880, in which she lay for about five minutes in a rigid condition, and with her eyes shut. She at the same time had great impairment of memory. These fits came on about once a day on an average till the middle of July, when they became much more frequent, and of a more violent character.

She had five fits on the first day of admission, lasting from a quarter of an hour to an hour, and several similar fits on many days following. A fit could at any time be excited by pressure on the ovaries, and during its manifestation pressure on the ovaries would either arrest it or alter its character. Pressure on other parts of the body did not produce a fit. They were most frequent about the time of a menstrual period, and she also seemed to be more liable to them after being visited by the priest. Between the fits she seemed cheerful and intelligent, but suffered a good deal at times from headache, which, she said, felt as "though nails were being hammered into her head."

The fit consisted of a series of stages: 1. They began by her head being thrown up, and inclined slightly to the right, while her eyes were turned up and to the right, and her mouth widely open. Her limbs were placed in a position approaching that of crucifixion, her legs extended and lying together, while her arms were held out straight nearly at right angles to the trunk, her fingers being over-extended, bent back towards the dorsum of the hand. 2. After lying quite still in this position for a short time she began to make lateral and to-and-fro movements with the tongue, and to froth at the mouth (she never bit her tongue). Her head began to move slightly from side to side, then more violently, till at last her whole body was implicated in a violent side-to-side movement. 3. These movements were soon exchanged for violent and extreme extension and flexion of the trunk; at one moment she bent forwards so that her head almost touched her feet; the next, threw her head violently back on to the bed. 4. She then again assumed the crucifixion position, and on some occasions arched her back in a rigid opisthotonos. 5. Finally, she drew several long breaths, her limbs relaxed, and she turned on to her left side, placed her hand over her heart, and began to cry; she then sat up, smiled, and said she felt tired and weak. During the fit the corneæ were insensitive, and pricking her with a pin caused her no pain in any part of the body.

Treatment was directed to the relief of the dysmenorrhœa, which Dr. Herman considered to be due to a narrow cervix. On Sept. 27th bougies Nos. 4 and 5 were passed; their passage excited a fit. On Oct. 5th bougies Nos. 6, 7, and 8 were passed; a fit again occurred. On Oct. 18th bougies Nos. 8, 9, and 10 were passed; a fit occurred afterwards. She at the same time took one grain of valerianate of zinc three times a day. Her fits soon began to diminish in frequency, till by the middle of October she did not have more than two a week. Her menstruation also became easier, and the pain was much lessened. Pressure on the ovaries produced much less effect. She menstruated on Nov. 30th and Dec. 1st without pain for the first time in her life. She had no fits after that, and when she left the hospital on Dec. 7th she had not had a fit for more than a month.—*Lancet*, March 5, 1881.

MONTHLY ABSTRACT.

Anatomy and Physiology.

The Vessels of the Retina.

Professor His, in the third part of his *Archiv* for 1880, gives an interesting description of his observations upon the distribution of the vessels in the retina of man and some animals. He makes this communication *à propos* of a paper by Dr. Hesse, who has demonstrated the existence in the retina of the rat of an internal arterial and an external venous layer of capillaries. Professor His depicts the arteria centralis in man as running in the nervous fibrous layer, and giving off from either side lateral capillary branches, which he names the arteriæ afferentes. These leave the main trunk almost at right angles. After a short course they divide and subdivide dichotomously, and form a tolerably distinct network of arterial capillaries, the individual vessels passing in and out through the spaces of the inner granular layer, where they form the deeper-lying or more external venous plexus. These, again, transmit the blood they contain into the venæ efferentes. The arteria centralis retinæ possesses a muscular tunic whilst it is still imbedded in the optic nerve; but this coat becomes thinner as the artery approximates the lamina cribrosa, and loses itself after the artery has traversed that lamina. In the retina itself the arterial branches are surrounded by a tunica adventitia, which gradually becomes thinner. There are no horizontally running capillaries in the molecular layer. All the vessels here have a radiating direction. Another point which he believes he has made out, though he is not quite certain, is that the portion of the optic nerve which is situated distally to the lamina cribrosa is provided with a very close network of large capillaries.—*Lancet*, Feb. 26, 1881.

The Atrophic Lines on the Abdomen in Pregnancy.

The appearance of silvery, riband-like streaks on the abdomen, the result of atrophy of the skin, as a result of stretching of the integument, after pregnancy, or distension of the abdomen otherwise brought about, is not merely familiar to medical men, but to patients; and the minute anatomy and conditions of origin of this change have been pretty well worked out, thanks chiefly to the labours of Credé, Schultze, and Hecker. Drs. Krause and Felsenreich have investigated them from a new point of view, viz., as an index of the tension of different parts of the abdominal wall, and a measure of the degree to which they regain their former state when that tension is removed. The best anatomical researches into this form of atrophy of skin which had been made previously are those of Küstner. He has shown that the change is often not merely in the epidermis, but that there is a solution of continuity in the deeper layers of the skin also. At the lines of atrophy, the cells of the horny layer of the epidermis are arranged more in rows which are regularly transverse to the course of the atrophic striæ than in the healthy integument; and the minute depressions and elevations of the natural skin are here smoothed out. Länger has also investigated the subject, and has shown that the bundles of fibrous tissue, which in the reticular layer of the normal corium cross one another so as to make the interspaces between them rhombic in shape, run transversely and nearly parallel to one another, across these atrophied parts. The papillæ also are here set in transverse rows; but if the band be a broad one—that is, if the stretching have been considerable—they may be so distant from one another as to make it difficult to perceive what is their arrangement. The bloodvessels also run transversely, instead of forming the usual network.

This was the state of the subject when Krause and Felsenreich applied themselves to its further investigation from the point of view we have indicated. They took as the field of their researches women pregnant for the first time, because in them the changes due to stretching of the skin would of course be seen at their maximum. Their method was this. They used a wooden stamp to imprint upon the abdomen a circular mark about an inch in diameter. The marks were made with aniline blue, which, after a trial of many other pigments, they found to be that which would best and longest resist friction and moisture. Being made with a stamp, the marks were of course all exact in shape and equal in size. A circle was marked, having the umbilicus as its centre; and from this as a starting-point rows of circles were imprinted, running up to the ensiform cartilage down to the symphysis pubis, transversely from side to side across the abdomen, and obliquely on each side to the right and left anterior superior iliac spine. These marks were made before labour; and on the ninth and tenth day after delivery (this day being taken because it was the last of the patients' stay in hospital) they were again examined. The diminution in size of these circles showed, of course, the amount of contraction of the skin at each place, and the alteration in their shape the direction in which contraction had occurred. The first thing found was that the post-partum contraction was not regular; the vertical row of circles, instead of being, as when made, a perfectly straight line, now was undulating and zig-zag. The amount of shortening of the line connecting the umbilicus with the symphysis pubis was from half an inch to two inches; of that joining the navel to the ensiform cartilage did not amount to more than half an inch. The lines going from the umbilicus to the iliac spines were at most only shortened an inch, and there was often more than half an inch of difference between the two sides, even when before labour their length had been identical. The diminution in the circumference of the belly at the umbilicus varied from about five to seven inches. By comparison of the circles forming the lines mentioned it was found that along each line the amount of post-partum contraction of the skin increased as the umbilicus was approached. It was greater along the lines radiating from the umbilicus than in the direction perpendicular to them. An exception to this, however, has to be made in reference to the linea alba, in which the contraction was less in the vertical than in the transverse direction. A comparison of the circles showed that, although the contraction of the linea alba above the umbili-cus was less than that below, yet that in other parts of the abdominal wall there was more contraction above than below the navel—a fact which the authors sup-pose due to the great stretching of the parts below the umbilicus having deprived them of their elasticity. It results from these observations, that above the um-bilicus the contraction of the abdominal walls after delivery is greater in a direc-tion transverse to the linea alba than parallel with it, the direction of maximum retraction being a line running downwards and towards the linea alba. At the level of the navel the contraction takes place towards that point; and below this line the direction of its maximum is indicated by a line running upwards and to-wards the linea alba. The reason why the contraction is less in the direction of the linea alba than transverse to it is a simple one. It is this: that such contrac-tion is effected by the fibrous bundles coming to cross one another at more acute angles. In the linea alba the fibrous bundles are already nearly parallel, and therefore there is little room for this change to take place. According to Länger, the fibrous bundles of the skin of the abdomen form rhomboidal meshes, the long diameter of which is parallel with the ribs. It will be seen that the statement of Länger explains the changes observed by Krause and Felsenreich.

Immediately around the navel contraction takes place equally on all sides and towards that point. The course of the atrophic lines is this. Near the linea alba they run parallel to it. Close round the umbilicus (over the area in which contraction takes place uniformly towards it) they form a confused network around that point, striæ crossing one another in all directions and at all angles. Further outwards they run concentrically around the navel. Comparing the course of the striæ with the lines described as those of maximum retraction, it will be seen at once that the former are at right angles to the latter. The atrophic striæ therefore indicate the directions in which, during pregnancy, the greatest tension has been put upon the abdominal walls.

So far as the particular facts themselves go, which Krause and Felsenreich have thus ascertained, they are not of much practical moment. The chief interest and importance is that which they suggest, viz., the relation between the lines of greatest tension, the direction of the atrophic striæ, and the texture of the tissues concerned. It remains to be seen, by equally careful examination of other parts, whether similar conditions in other parts of the body are the result of the same concurrence of causes.

The work of Drs. Krause and Felsenreich is an example of that patient labour bestowed upon apparent trifles, for which we so often have to thank our German brethren. Unimportant as they may seem to the self-styled "practical" man, investigations like these yet fill crevices in the edifice of scientific truth, and are of more value than nine-tenths of the literature which is concerned only with the production of so-called "cures."—*Med. Times and Gazette*, Jan. 29, 1881.

Materia Medica and Therapeutics.

The Antagonism of Atropia.

Dr. ROBERTS BARTHOLOW, in his third Cartwright Lecture, summarizes the conclusions of his studies upon the antagonisms of atropia as follows:—

Antagonism of Atropia and Physostigma.—1. That physostigma or eserine, and atropia are antagonistic in their effects on the pupil. 2. That they act differently, but probably not antagonistically, on the heart, unless we accept the views of Köhler and Bezold and Bloebaum—the former maintaining that physostigma paralyzes the accelerator nerves of the heart, and the latter that atropia stimulates these nerves. 3. That they are opposed in their action on respiration, physostigma paralyzing, and atropia stimulating, the respiratory function. 4. That they are not opposed in their action on the cerebrum, atropia producing delirium, and physostigma having no effect on the cerebral functions, while both cause more or less carbonic-acid narcosis. 5. That they act differently and not in an opposed manner on the spinal cord and nerves, both producing paralysis, but atropia does, and physostigma does not, impair the irritability of motor nerves. As regards the sensory nerves, physostigma augments their irritability, while atropia seems rather to lessen it, if any effect is produced. 6. That they act oppositely on secretion, physostigma stimulating and atropia arresting the secretions in general.

It follows from these conclusions that the lethal effects of physostigma, due to paralysis of respiration, are overcome by atropia by sustaining the respiratory function. The Committee of the British Medical Association assert that "the antagonism exists within very narrow limits," but 'this happens to be sufficient to avert death, when doses little more than lethal have .been administered; still, the use of physostigma against the lethal effects of atropia ·is of doubtful propriety. The paralyzing effect of physostigma on respiration may, doubtless, be successfully overcome by the suitable application of atropia.

Belladonna and Pilocarpine.—Belladonna and pilocarpus are antagonistic in their action: 1. On the secretions, especially of sweat and saliva, pilocarpus promoting, and belladonna arresting, them.   2. On the heart and arterial system, pilocarpus slowing and enfeebling the heart and depressing the vascular tonus—belladonna stimulating the cardiac movements and raising the arterial tension.   3. On the eye, pilocarpus contracting the pupil, inducing spasm of accommodation, and approximating the nearest and most remote points of vision—belladonna dilating the pupil, paralyzing accommodation, and making the vision presbyopic.

On the brain there is no real antagonism.   The excitement, the delirium with hallucinations and illusions, and the subsequent coma, caused by atropia, are not affected by any of the actions of pilocarpin.   The soporose state brought on by the latter, as I have pointed out, is a secondary effect, the result of exhaustion and cerebral anæmia.—*New York Med. Journal,* Jan. 1881.

Physiological Action of the Active Principle of Piscidia Erythrina—Jamaica Dogwood.

Dr. Isaac Ott, describes (*Archives of Medicine,* Feb. 1881) some experiments which he has lately performed to ascertain the physiological action of the Jamaica dogwood—a drug which has recently been introduced as a narcotic.

His conclusions are—

1. That piscidia (the active principle) is a narcotic.

2. That it does not paralyze or excite the motor nerves.

3. That it does not act on the extremities of the sensory nerves, but their central connection—the sensory ganglia of the spinal cord.

4. That it produces convulsions, partly by stimulation of the spinal cord and partly by heightened excitability of the voluntary striated muscles.

5. That it reduces the frequency of the pulse by an action on the heart itself, probably on its muscular structure.

6. That the arterial tension temporarily rises by stimulation of the monarchical vaso-motor centre; that it soon falls, due to a partial paralysis of this centre and the heart itself.

7. That it at first contracts and then dilates the pupil.

On the Catgut Ligature.

Upon the occasion of his taking the Presidential chair at the Clinical Society at London, Mr. Lister delivered the following address on the catgut ligature, which is full of interest for every practical surgeon. He said :—

The catgut ligature has in some respects exceeded my original hopes. I feared that its advantages would be limited to wounds in which putrefaction was avoided, and that if septic suppuration took place in a wound in which it was employed for securing the vessels the ligature would sooner or later come away like little sloughs. Such, however, has not proved to be the case. Whatever be the progress of the wound, we never see anything of the catgut, so that even surgeons who have not adopted strict antiseptic treatment have been led to employ the new material in ordinary wounds. Under other circumstances, however, the catgut has often led to disappointment. We hear of cases in which Cæsarean section has been performed, and all has gone on well until the knots of the catgut with which the uterine wound was secured have given way, and the patient's death has been the result. Again, in ligature of large arterial trunks in continuity several surgeons have met with bitter disappointment, the case ending in disaster from secondary hemorrhage or the treatment proving abortive through the channel of the vessel becoming opened up again at the site of the ligature. Hence many surgeons have been induced to return to silk, even though using strict antiseptic treatment, rendering the silk aseptic by steeping it in suitable lotion and cutting the ends short. This practice has, however, by no means proved uniformly successful. As an instance of unsatisfactory result, I may mention a case which was recorded by Mr. Clutton in the last volume of our *Transactions*. He tied the external iliac artery under strict antiseptic precautions, and the wound healed within a week ; but, as I learned from a letter which he was good enough to send me at the time, six weeks after the operation a little blister formed and fluid began to escape, forming a small scab, and in three months the loop which had been placed around the artery came away. Such a result was not at all surprising to me, seeing that what induced me to try the animal ligature was the discovery of a small abscess about the remains of a partially absorbed silk thread which I had applied in the same manner as Mr. Clutton, and, as it so happened, to the same artery. It can hardly be doubted that suppuration proceeding from the immediate seat of the ligature must be a source of danger. As an illustration of the mischief which a ligature of ordinary material may do, I may mention a case of goitre in a young woman on which I operated on January 28 last year. It was of moderate dimensions, but the effect on the respiration was considerable, and I determined to operate by Dr. Patrick Heron Watson's plan of preliminary deligation of the thyroid vessels circumferentially to the tumour (if this is effectually done the operation is bloodless) ; so that, as the laryngoscope, applied by Dr. Felix Semon, who had recommended the case to my care, showed that the trachea was pressed backwards considerably by the growth, I adopted a measure which I believed would, in all cases of removal of the thyroid, prove advantageous—namely, I divided the tumour in the first instance in the middle line, so as, in the case of adhesions to the trachea, to be able to remove the two halves of the growth at leisure, to dissect it off from the trachea. But in order that the carbolic ligature may be secure it is essential that the material should be very strong, so that the tissues round about the tumour, including the vessels, may be securely tightened up. I possessed no catgut which I felt was strong enough to bear the full strength of my hands, and therefore I was compelled to use the hempen ligature, after of course carefully rendering it antiseptic by means of the carbolic lotion. Six of these hempen ligatures were used—three on each side. During the first eight days everything went on in a typical fashion according to the antiseptic method. There was a small serous effusion rapidly diminishing, and we looked to the wound being healed in a few days more ; but on the ninth day there was seen to be a little something of a purulence mingled with the discharge ; the pus became thicker—always in small quantity ; a small quantity could be pressed out from each side. In a month one of the hempen ligatures made its escape. In six days more four other of the hempen ligatures came away altogether unaltered, as may be seen on the table, where I have exhibited the hempen ligatures which came away from this case. I submitted them to careful examination. They had a sour odour, and, applied to litmus paper, gave an acid reaction—that is to say, the natural alkaline reaction of the blood-serum had been changed to acidity by some peculiar species of fermentation, inasmuch as putrefaction would have, if possible, made the blood-serum still more alkaline. On examining them with the microscope, I found the interstices of the threads of the hemp loaded with a little organism, to which I believe I happened to be the first to direct attention as to its mode of growth, and to which I gave the name of granuligera, occurring in groups of twos, threes, fours, and so forth, as distinguished from the chains in which ordinary bacteria occur, and of which one form at least has been since shown by Mr. Cheyne to occur very frequently in cases treated antiseptically without any interference with the antiseptic process. I found that the interstices of the threads of the hemp were leaded with these little micrococci. It so happens I have had an opportunity within the last few days of obtaining a sample of these micrococci, thanks to Mr. Cheyne's kindness. He brought this bottle of a pure and perfectly transparent infusion of meat to a case which I had operated on a fortnight before by excision of the ankle. The skin was unbroken; we were able therefrom to operate antiseptically. The case pursued a perfectly typical course. The wounds, which were left gaping at the time of the operation, were filled with blood-clot, which remained unaltered in appearance, though undoubtedly becoming organized by that time—more or less. A little piece of the blood-clot from one of these wounds was introduced with careful antiseptic precautions into the flask of clear fluid, and you will see it is now turbid. But though, under ordinary circumstances, these micrococci may be present—as Mr. Cheyne has abundantly shown, and as the case I have referred to illustrates—without causing any evil, yet there may be circumstances in which they may prove mischievous, and the case which I have been relating appears to have been one of these. The micrococci developing in the interstices of the hempen ligature produced an acid fermentation of the serum in its most aggravated form. The acid serum became a cause of irritation, and thus the ligatures which otherwise being unirritating would have been capsuled, and in due time absorbed, became causes of suppuration. One of the six ligatures still remained unaccounted for. In due time we sent the patient home with a small sinus remaining, a little pus always discharging from it; but it was not until the middle of September last that the last ligature came away altogether unaltered. Now, gentlemen, there is no doubt whatsoever that if I had had a ligature of catgut which I could have trusted for the operation, the catgut ligature would have been disposed of within two or three weeks. Here, then, we have an illustration of the great disadvantage which may arise, even under antiseptic treatment, from the use of the ordinary forms of ligature.

Animal ligatures of another kind have been provided by Mr. Barlow in order to remove these difficulties, namely, strips of the mingled yellow elastic and unstriped muscular tissues which constitute the arterial wall, obtained by spirally cutting the aorta of one of the larger animals. But though fully admitting the efficiency of these ligatures in his hands, I cannot but feel that it is unsatisfactory, if it can be avoided, to have a special material for this particular purpose, and it will be better, if possible, to have the catgut in a thoroughly reliable condition. Catgut, of which I have samples here, is to be had all over the world in abundance. It is beautifully strong and smooth; it is prepared of various sizes, admirably adapted for all the purposes of the surgeon, and is extremely cheap. Wholesale it is sold at 12s. per gross, that is to say, 1d. per hank. But, as it comes from the maker, it is entirely unfit for the purposes of the surgeon. However beautiful it is in the dry state, it becomes soft and pulpy soon after it has been placed in blood-serum. In one of these glasses is a piece of unprepared catgut which was placed in warm blood-serum this morning—the blood of a cow—and within half an hour it was in the condition in which it is at the present time—swollen, soft, and pulpy. A knot tied upon it would hold as little or scarcely better than a piece of intestine from which the catgut is derived in the dead-house—an utterly unsatisfactory material, soft and slippery, the knot not holding in the least. It is essential, in order to fit catgut for the purposes of the surgeon, that it must be altered in its physical constitution, so as to be no longer liable to this softening effect by the serum of the blood. This is a remarkable circumstance, that the blood-serum softens catgut more than even water does. I confess I should have thought, *à priori*, that in the case of a colloidal substance like albumen, a solution of albumen would have been much less likely than water to permeate and soften an animal tissue like catgut; but it is otherwise, and therefore we cannot trust the trustworthiness of catgut by steeping it in warm water as I formerly used to do. In order to be sure that a given specimen of catgut will answer the purpose in so far as the knot is concerned, that it shall not slip, it is needful that we should steep the catgut in blood-serum, a somewhat troublesome process, as it involves sending to the slaughter-house for blood. The method which I published long ago answers the purpose very well for ligature of arteries in continuity, provided certain conditions in its preparation be complied with; such, at least, is my own experience. This indeed has not been very extensive, but it has been sufficient to deserve consideration. I have tied altogether nine considerable arteries in continuity with prepared catgut. Of these one was a case of ligature of the carotid in a young woman, aged twenty-two, with a pulsating tumour below the angle of the jaw, in the situation of the carotid aneurism, and with all the symptoms of that disease. The application of the ligature reduced to a certain degree the pulsation and the dimensions, but the further cure which we hoped for did not take place. She left the hospital with a pulsating tumour, and I heard only yesterday from the medical man under whose care she is in Scotland, that this tumour, for which I had tied the carotid artery in 1874 still exists as a pulsating tumour, if anything rather on the increase. But though, as regards the cure of the disease, the ligature was unsatisfactory, nothing could be more beautiful in its effect as respects the healing of the wound without suppuration.

A case of traumatic arterio-venous aneurism of the temporal artery may be mentioned in the category, partly because the greatly dilated condition which the naturally small artery had assumed brought it up towards the dimensions of a large trunk, and partly because the concurrent ligature of the largely dilated veins would, without antiseptic means, have been justly regarded as of considerable danger. The others were all cases of ligature of the femoral. Six were popliteal aneurisms, four of which presented nothing deserving of special remark. One was a diffuse aneurism, extending up to the junction of the lower and middle third of the thigh. One was an enormous diffuse aneurism reaching up nearly to Poupart's ligament. It was necessary for me to tie the femoral artery about the situation of the ordinary origin of the profunda, and even there my incision opened into the aneurismal clots. The last was a case of a large arterio-venous aneurism of the upper part of the femoral of idiopathic origin. This case was of such special interest that I hope on a future occasion to make it a subject of a paper before this Society. In all these cases except two the catgut ligature prepared by the old method was employed, and in all these nine cases the result was satisfactory, and recovery perfect, except as regards the poor young woman who has still the pulsating tumour. Why, it may naturally be asked, has my own experience been more satisfactory with the catgut ligature than that of many other surgeons? There are, I believe, two reasons for this. One is, that I have never ventured to tie an artery of considerable size in its continuity without having taking pains to ascertain that the catgut was of thoroughly reliable material; and the other reason is, that I have adopted strict antiseptic means of treatment not only during the earlier stages of the case, but to the last. So long as any sore exists unhealed, antiseptic treatment of the strictest kind ought, I believe, to be employed.

Even though the sore may seem to be superficial, there may still exist a sinus leading down to the site of the ligature, and if ordinary treatment as distinguished from antiseptic be employed down this sinus, the septic process may advance and invade the ligature, and lead at last to disaster from hemorrhage. I know that this has actually taken place.

But although the catgut prepared upon the old method answers very well if it be of proper quality, there is this great objection to it—that this method requires a long time in order to produce this quality. At least two months are needed to make the ligature at all trustworthy. It is better at the end of six months, and still better at the end of a year. I possess catgut prepared in this way twelve years old; I have brought here a sample of such catgut, which has been steeping in warm blood-serum since this morning, and it will be seen that it remains trans-lucent, and is comparatively firm, instead of being opaque and soft like the unprepared catgut in the same serum.

Now, this length of time that the present method requires is a very serious objection. It makes the surgeon who has not prepared the catgut for himself, and kept it for a long time, at the mercy of the person who supplies it; and the person who supplies it, not being aware of the enormous importance of the time for which the catgut has been prepared, if he happens to have run out of that which has been long prepared, will sell what has been prepared for a short time, and is in consequence altogether unreliable. A case illustrating this point occurred last year in my practice at King's College Hospital. A patient was admitted who had met with a severe wound on the ulnar side of the forearm, the anterior aspect. The ulnar artery had been divided. This had been secured by my house-surgeon. He had also tied with catgut the corresponding ends of the various tendons that had been divided. But when I saw the patient the next day I found that he could not feel with his little finger and the adjacent side of the ring finger, and therefore it was evident that his ulnar nerve had been divided, and my house-surgeon had not thought of attending to the ulnar nerve. I there-fore said, "We must open up the wound, search for the ends of the ulnar nerve, and tie them with catgut." I thereupon cut the stitches in the skin, and pro-ceeded to explore the deeper parts of the wound, and I found that every one of the ligatures, which were numerous, by which my house-surgeon had tied the various ends of the tendons together, were lying absolutely loose; the knots had slipped within the twenty-four hours; and yet this catgut had been supplied by our ordinary instrument-maker as reliable catgut. He had supplied what had not been sufficiently long prepared. This, then, is a sufficiently serious objection to the present method of preparation; and one great object which I have had in view in a series of experiments on this subject, with a view of improving the preparation of the catgut ligature, has been to devise a means, if possible, of preparation within a short time. These experiments—it may seem almost ludi-crous to say so—have occupied two years of my leisure time in the past, some time ago, and, after having been interrupted, have been continued in a merely desultory manner since; but at length I feel myself justified in bringing before you a new mode of preparation, by which the catgut can be prepared in a short time, and at the same time in a perfectly reliable condition.

But before I allude to these experiments, which I must endeavour to do in a short compass,—I should weary you if I were to bring a large proportion of my facts before you, though I may say, out of the hundreds of experiments I have performed on the subject, I have never performed one which has not added something to my knowledge on the subject,—before referring to these experi-ments, I wish to say a few words as to what catgut is. Catgut, as you are doubt-less all aware, is prepared from the small intestine of the sheep. The small intestine of the sheep is treated in what seems an exceedingly rude manner for so delicate a structure. It is scraped with some blunt instrument, such as the back of a knife, over a board, and by this means, as the people express it, the dirt is scraped out. That which these people call the dirt is the exquisite and complicated structure of the intestinal mucous membrane. The intestinal mucous membrane is scraped out by means of the back of the knife. But while the mucous membrane is scraped out from within, there is also scraped off from without, or from more external parts, the circular coat of the muscular fibres. The circular muscular fibres are disposed of, and the result comes to be that the intestine is converted into a comparatively slender material of two parts, the one consisting of the peritoneum and some longitudinal muscular fibres; when the mesentery is stripped off by the butcher, the peritoneal coat contracts into a narrow band, and this, with some longitudinal fibres, constitutes one of the two parts to which the intestine is reduced by this process of scraping. The other part is the essential part from which the catgut is prepared, and this is neither more nor less than the submucous cellular coat of the intestine. When I first visited a catgut manufactory I was astonished to find that after this scraping process the intestine could be blown up still as a continuous tube, as you will see here. This structure is a beautiful anatomical preparation, made, though in this rude fashion, by these preparers of the catgut. The submucous cellular tissue or submucous cellular coat of the intestine which is in the sheep has this extraordinary toughness, and is the material out of which catgut is prepared. For what the manufacturer terms the "ones"—the thicker form of ordinary catgut—all that is done is to twist the gut by means of a wheel, like a rope in a ropewalk, up to a considerable degree of tightness, and then allow it to dry. It is then exposed to the fumes of burning sulphur, and for some more special purposes it is somewhat bleached by the application of potash. But the essential thing is the twisting and drying. It can be prepared without the use of sulphur as well as without the use of potash. Some specimens which I have here are prepared by water only, without the use of any other ingredient. This exceedingly beautiful structure, as I think we must consider it, as fine as a horse-hair, is prepared without any ingredient whatever, nothing but an animal tissue twisted and dried. For the finer kinds the tube of the submucous coat is split up by means of razor-blades, more or less numerous according to the degree of splitting required, connected with a conical piece of wood which is pushed along the tube.

Such is the catgut. It is composed of the submucous cellular tissue. The first of the more recent experiments which I performed was one with a view of ascertaining, if possible, what part the water had in the material used for the preparation by our old method. If I steep unprepared catgut in a mixture of carbolic acid and oil, however long it be so steeped—it will be of course abundantly antiseptic—it is utterly unfit for the purpose of the surgeon, a knot upon it would still slip. But if, instead of using carbolic acid in the crystalline state, we use carbolic acid which has been liquefied by the addition of a little water, we get in course of time a properly prepared catgut. I wished to ascertain how much water was required. The carbolic acid would enable oil to dissolve a certain amount of water; would that amount of water be sufficient which carbolic acid enables oil to dissolve? Accordingly I prepared some jars, some containing the full amount of water we had used hitherto, some the smaller quantity, and some none at all. In due time I proceeded to examine the result by taking portions of gut and putting them into warm water and leaving them for a certain time in order to ascertain how the knots would hold. To my great surprise I found that which had been steeping in the carbolic acid and oil without any water was just as good as that which was in the carbolic acid and oil with the water. It was contrary to distinct previous experience. Reflecting on the matter made me see that the only possible explanation could be that the catgut was, so to speak, prepared before I put it into the liquid. Now, it so happened that the catgut I had used was several years old: it turned out that the mere age of the catgut prepares it—that in proportion to its age it is rendered less liable to be softened by water or by blood-serum, and a knot tied upon it will hold better. And thus I had for the first time, I believe, scientific evidence of the truth of what is popularly spoken of as the "seasoning" of various articles made of animal products. I asked a person who sold violin-strings if there was any result from keeping the strings a long time. He said, "No," the only result he knew was that they would probably get rotten. But it so happened just about that time there came an old fiddler to amuse the patients at the Royal Infirmary of Edinburgh at Christmas-time. They happened to have wet weather, and he said that his fiddle would not work properly because the fiddle-strings were not properly seasoned. So that he was aware that fiddle-strings, which of course are catgut, are liable to seasoning, and require it. This is a very important fact—at least, it was extremely important to me, because it served to explain the success that I had had in my earlier experience with the catgut, before I knew at all the proper modes of preparing it. I look back almost with horror at some of my early procedures with catgut. I have operated, for example, on an irreducible ventral hernia, opened the sac, divided the adhesions, returned the protruding intestines, stitched up the mouth of the sac with the catgut, and then applied stitches at considerable intervals in the skin. All went perfectly well, but the mode of preparation that I then used, if I had worked with catgut recently made, must have ended in utter disaster; the knots must have slipped in a few hours, and the intestines must have been protruded through the wound. I need hardly say that this mode of preparation, interesting though it is, would not be satisfactory; it would only have, in a more aggravated form, the inconvenience of the extremely long period required which our old method has; and, besides that, it by no means provides all the conditions that are required for a perfectly satisfactory state of the catgut for surgical purposes. These conditions I may mention. In the first place, I have spoken of a short period of preparation. This is very desirable. Then it is essential that the catgut should have the proper strength, so as to bear any reasonable strain that the human hands can put upon it in the thicker forms, as when used, for instance, in such cases as the ligature of the thyroid vessels, in the removal of a thyroid tumour, or in ovariotomy. But it is not sufficient that it should be strong to start with—it is easy to get catgut strong in the dry state—it is necessary that it should be strong after steeping in blood-serum for a while. Suppose, for example, in the case of tumour of the thyroid I had passed the various ligatures. I passed in that case six, and in a former case, where the tumour was larger, I thought it prudent to pass as many as eight so as to subdivide the mass that had to be tied; but it is not convenient to tie each of these ligatures as soon as it is passed. The process of passing takes a considerable time, and it would be a very sad thing if the residence of the catgut among the tissues soaked with serum for a few minutes, or even a quarter of an hour, should render the catgut so soft that it should give way when we put the strain of the hands upon it. That, then, is another point that is essential if it is to be useful for the purpose for which it is devised. Then, again, it is necessary that a knot tied upon it should hold it with absolute security—not merely in the first instance, but after soaking for an unlimited time in blood-serum. It is further necessary that it should not be too rigid; that it should not be over-prepared, for, as we shall see immediately, it may be over-prepared, so that it may remain almost like a piece of wire among the tissues, in which case it may come away in consequence of the irritation which it produces as a mechanical object, as a hard mechanical substance. It is necessary that it should be somewhat soft, so as to be mechanically unirritating; and yet while it must be soft it must not be too rapidly disposed of by absorption. If it is to do duty for the ligature of an artery in its continuity in the immediate vicinity of some large branch, it must remain for a considerable time of good firmness, unabsorbed, and when it is at length absorbed it is desirable that it should be absorbed in such a manner that while it is reduced in thickness it should still, as long as any of it remains, retain its firmness.

Now, these are a series of conditions which, I assure you, it is not easy to comply with. I have in various experiments complied with some of them easily enough, but failed in others. Sometimes I have complied with all but one, and failed in one. I have used various materials in experiments, as you will naturally suppose. One material that suggested itself was tannic acid, so as to convert the catgut into leather. I succeeded well enough in some respects with tannic acid in different ways modified, but in this respect I did not succeed. I have not obtained by means of tannic acid a kind of catgut that is not too speedily absorbed. I tried at last a piece of kid leather cut into a suitable shape, and I found that this, after being rendered antiseptic, and applied as a stitch, became too rapidly absorbed. Chromic acid was another substance which I very naturally used, knowing as I did how it was employed for hardening tissues. Chromic acid in itself does not work very well, but I found that the addition of some other substance to it aided its action very greatly. By the addition, for instance, of a little glycerine, thus producing a reducing action on the chromic acid, we get a different sort of material which acts much more energetically on the catgut. I was highly delighted with the results of the action of a mixture of chromic acid and glycerine. Just about this time it so happened that Mr. Alfred Pemberton, of Birmingham, applied to me for a piece of catgut for the purpose of ligaturing an external iliac artery in a remarkable case of three aneurisms in one limb—two in the femoral, and one in the popliteal. I thought I could not do better than send him my recently prepared chromic catgut. I did so. He wrote to me soon afterwards, saying that nothing could be more satisfactory than the result. He had operated antiseptically; the wound had united by first intention, and a month afterwards, so far as the case could go well, all had gone well. There was, indeed, gangrene of the lower part of the leg, which Mr. Pemberton predicted, in consequence of the existence of the obstructions of the ligatures of three aneurisms in the course of the arterial channel; but the case, by proper management, was doing well, and ultimately the patient recovered, though with an amputated limb. But four weeks later Mr. Pemberton wrote to me again, telling me that soon after his last report the patient had begun to show signs of suppuration about the seat of the wound. After awhile the abscess opened in the cicatrix, and the ligature which he had put on was discharged. It is now on one of the cards before you —an over-prepared ligature which had come away, rigid and wire-like, making its way out as a piece of glass might have done, by mechanical irritation. This opened my eyes for the first time to the possibility of having catgut ligatures over-prepared. It is by means of chromic acid, however, that I have arrived at the ultimate result which I have to bring before you. I may mention that the over-preparation by means of chromic acid is, I believe, to be found illustrated in a large German school at the present time. I have been told by an American physician who has lately been in London that at that school catgut ligatures invariably come away from all wounds. They count the ligatures as they put them on, and invariably see them all before the case is done with. The ligatures have been over-prepared.

Before speaking of the present method, I wish to say a few words with regard to the old method. To what is it that it owes its virtue? Here we have some catgut which has been in our old preparing liquid, viz., one part of carbolic acid which has been liquefied by means of water, to five parts of olive oil. Here we have some catgut which has been the same length of time, since April last, in a solution of carbolic acid and water. Water will only take up one-twentieth part of its weight of carbolic acid, but the effect produced upon the catgut is very much greater. In the one case, as you can see, the catgut is almost black, a sort of purple black, while the other is completely pale, very little. altered from its original colour. This circumstance shows two things. In the first place the effect of the watery solution of carbolic acid upon catgut explains the efficacy of the water in our old method. It is the watery solution of carbolic acid in the liquid of the old method that is the effective agent. But, while that is the case when this watery solution is mixed with oil, the fact that it is so mixed limits and checks its operation, whereas if we have it in the watery solution only, there seems to be no limit to the degree of continuous preparation of the gut, so that it becomes more and more dark in colour, and more and more difficult to absorb by the tissues. It is otherwise when the watery solution is blended with the oil. Though the process does go on for many months, there arrives a time when it comes to a standstill. You need not fear that the catgut prepared by the old plan is over-prepared at the end of two years. I have a specimen here which at the end of twelve years is as limp after steeping in blood-serum as it would have been at the end of a single year. Therefore we possess in the carbolic oil a means of checking any mode of preparation that we may adopt, keeping it from that time forward not materially further prepared; while at the same time this large proportion of carbolic acid to oil insures the catgut being perfectly aseptic.

The method which I have found, after various trials, to be that which may be recommended is the following: I take one part of chromic acid, 4000 parts of distilled water, and 200 parts of pure carbolic acid or absolute phenol. In other words, I use a one-to-twenty carbolic acid solution, only that the carbolic acid is dissolved not in water, but in an exceedingly dilute solution of chromic acid. This small quantity of chromic acid has a very great effect upon the gut. Into a solution of that composition I introduce catgut in weight about equal to the weight of the carbolic acid. If you have too large a proportion of catgut, it will not be sufficiently prepared; if you have too small a quantity it may run the risk of being over-prepared. This liquid seems really to answer the purpose, and to comply with all our conditions. At the end of forty-eight hours catgut steeped in such a solution is sufficiently prepared. It is then taken out of the solution and dried, and, after drying, placed in one-to-five carbolic oil; it is then fit for use. I have here a sample of the prepared catgut by the new method. Although it has been steeped in warm blood-serum since this morning at eleven o'clock, it is still firm and translucent, and a knot upon it holds with the most perfect security.

The strength of the catgut depends upon different circumstances. In the first place, sheep differ as to the strength of their intestines, and the catgut-maker, if he be a good one, will insist upon having sheep of the proper kind. In the next place, the intestine must not be allowed to putrefy—it must be taken fresh. For these things you must of course rely upon the maker of the catgut. In the next place, whatever method you adopt, the liquid will probably cause a certain amount of swelling of the catgut, and this will tend to produce a little uncoiling of the twisted gut. It is of very great importance that this should not occur, because, if you have uncoiling, you may have uncoiling of different degrees in different parts, and this may lead to weakness at some part which you cannot foresee, and the gut may give way when you subject it to a strain. The catgut, then, should be prepared on the stretch, both when it is put to soak and when it is put to dry.

I need not enter into the mode in which this can be done by the manufacturer. I may only say this, that the private surgeon who wishes to prepare it himself may do it in different ways. For instance, he may take two large test-tubes, one a little larger than the other, and he may wind the catgut on the smaller tube, fixing one end by sealing-wax, winding round, and then bringing it up again, and fixing the other end with sealing-wax at a higher level than the liquid will come to, putting sufficient liquid into the larger test-tube, and putting in the smaller test-tube with the catgut wound round it, with a little shot to keep it down in the liquid. After forty-eight hours he takes out the smaller test-tube, and leaves it till the catgut is completely dry. I merely mention this as an illustration, and also as furnishing a hint to some surgeons in private practice who may desire to prepare the catgut themselves. Or a couple of gallipots, one larger than the other, will do just as well.

So much for strength in the dry state. As to strength in the condition after steeping in blood-serum, I confess it is only this very day that I have obtained evidence that catgut prepared by this method is really all that we can desire in that respect. The catgut of the hank from which this specimen was taken in the dry state measured 2¼ hundredths of an inch in diameter, and broke at 13 lbs. A piece 2⅔ hundredths in diameter broke at a strain of 13 lbs. 6 oz. I found by experiment that 10 lbs. is the utmost strain that my arms are able to put upon a cord. 13 lbs. 6 oz., then, is amply sufficient, while at the same time the catgut is not at all too large for going into the eye of an aneurism-needle. Having obtained, the other day, some fresh blood of a cow from the slaughter-house, I took some of the serum to-day, and put two pieces of this same hank of catgut, prepared after this new method, in the serum, and I put this in my warm box in a stoppered bottle. The temperature of the box was 98° Fahr. After more than half an hour I tested the breaking strain (I must not stop to explain how that is done), and I found that the breaking strain of the same catgut, which in the dry state has broken at 13 lbs. 6 oz., was 11 lbs. 4 oz.—that is, though suppled by the serum, it had only lost in strength 2 lbs. out of 13 lbs. I think that is really all that can be desired.

As to the behaviour of the catgut among the tissues, I wish to say a few words on this point before I conclude. It has been said of late by various persons that the catgut is dissolved by the serum. I must confess that this is entirely contrary to my own experience. I have already said that in order to test the quality of catgut you must have it steeped in blood-serum. I have tested catgut prepared in various ways in this manner. The serum has sometimes been putrid, sometimes it had no smell at all, and sometimes it had a little odour. This serum has been kept about the temperature of the body, but I have never seen the slightest indication of any chemical solution of the catgut. Then, again, as to the behaviour of the catgut in the body, suppose we use it as a stitch, if the catgut were disposed of as a matter of chemical solution we should expect that when it is employed as a stitch and a piece of our protective is put over it, which is always kept moist with serum perpetually oozing from the wound, the outer parts of the stitch, the parts outside the skin, as well as the parts among the tissues, would show signs of diminution. It is never so. The diminution is always absolutely limited to the parts within the tissues. Then it is still more striking, perhaps, as was suggested to me by Mr. Cheyne, to consider the case of the catgut drain. There its very function is to drain out the serum, and it is perpetually washed with it. You might suppose that the stitch would get a little dry. Here there can be no mistake; the serum from the wound is perpetually flowing; yet, as in the other case, we find the diminution of the catgut is absolutely limited to the part within the tissues. This seems to me sufficient evidence that it is not a question of the mere chemical solution of the catgut, but a question of the disposal of the catgut in some way or other by the living textures. Then, again, if we examine catgut in the process of diminution we find that it may be effected in one of two ways. If the catgut has not been properly prepared, the substance of the catgut becomes converted in the course of a very few days into a soft, pulpaceous mass, which, when we examine it by a microscope, we see consists of remains of the old cellular tissue of the submucous coat, and the interstices among these fibres filled with cells of new formation. The catgut tissue is infiltrated with cells of new formation, and it is obvious it is this infiltration which is the cause of the softening. But, on the other hand, if we find that the catgut is properly prepared, instead of being infiltrated by the cells of new formation it is only superficially eroded. I have on one of these cards a pretty example of catgut that has been served in that way by the tissues. You will see that there remains a very slender residue of the catgut, all the rest having gone; but that slender residue has continued firm and translucent, still retaining its firmness, showing not even a superficial infiltration—in short, having exactly the characters that we desire for catgut required for the ligature of an artery in its continuity, that till the last, even though reduced in dimensions, it shall retain its firmness and its tenacity. We know that antiseptic treatment has shown that a piece of dead bone may be absorbed provided it be not putrid : the granulations that overlap it superficially may, so to speak, erode it. It is not necessary for us to consider how that may be done, but certainly in some way or other the granulations do what mere steeping in that serum, whether putrid or non-putrid, never would do. Never would the bone be dissolved by the serum. Just as a non-putrid sequestrum is served by the tissues, so is a well-prepared specimen of catgut ; it is superficially eroded. I have here a stitch that I removed to-day from a wound made for stretching the anterior crural nerve, which was stretched, as well as the sciatic, in an aggravated case of sciatica ; and you may see that as yet it shows no signs of erosion. We know by experience that if it were left three or four more days we should find it largely eroded, as these specimens show ; but until nearly a fortnight has elapsed erosion does not begin. It proceeds gradually, and the thicker the catgut the slower does it proceed. We may fairly consider that a fortnight or three weeks is long enough for the persistence of a ligature upon an artery in its continuity.

I have brought with me the carotid artery of the calf in which I first established the fact of the substitution of new living tissue for the dead old tissue of the catgut. If any gentleman will examine the specimen he will see the ligatures of new formation incorporated with the external cellular coat of the artery. I am sorry that I am not able so to express myself in the English language as to make my meaning understood. I have been strangely misrepresented as having conveyed the idea that the catgut, when it becomes organized, comes to life again. Gentlemen, such an absurd notion certainly never entered into my head, any more than when I have spoken of the organization of a blood-clot, I have meant by that expression to convey the idea that the blood-clot becomes organized by its own inherent virtue. I found the term organization ready to my hand ; it was no term of my own invention. It was used with reference to lymph. Now, pathologists, in speaking of lymph as becoming organized, did not, I suspect, mean by that expression to imply that it was the lymph substance that had the power of self-organization as distinguished from any influence that surrounding tissues might exert upon it. So, in the same way, when we speak of the vascularization of lymph, that was the term used when it was universally believed by pathologists that the bloodvessels were formed only by loops from pre-existing bloodvessels. Nowadays a different view may be taken, but the term "vascularization of lymph" was used without any idea that the lymph itself created the bloodvessels. And so, when I spoke of the organization of the blood-clot or of catgut, I certainly never meant to convey the idea that either the one or the other did the work itself. With regard to the catgut, I think if gentlemen would refer to my original paper in the *Lancet* they would see that I stated very explicitly that new tissue forms at the expense of the old, that the old tissue is absorbed by the new, and that as the old is absorbed, new is put down in its place.—*Med. Times and Gaz.*, Feb. 5, 1881.

Medicine.

Diphtheritic Albuminuria.

The albuminuria which occurs so constantly in diphtheria was long believed to be a direct effect of the altered blood-state, without any renal lesion. Lancereaux and Brault, however, have described certain organic changes in the kidney. They found the epithelial cells swollen, badly defined, infiltrated with granules of protein, and the lumen of the tubules obliterated in many points by colloid or granular masses. These lesions are analogous to those described by M. Cornil in acute poisoning by cantharadin.

The nature and mode of production of this diphtheritic nephritis is the subject of a recent communication by M. E. GAUCHER to the Société de Biologie. It may be *à priori* expected that the lesion would be due to the same mechanism as that which produces the similar changes which have been found in some other infectious diseases. In the nephritis which sometimes occurs in typhoid fever, for instance, there is a similar granular infiltration of the epithelial cells and a similar obstruction of the lumen of the tubules by diffused material or globular masses. These alterations have lately been ascribed by Bouchard to the infiltration of the kidney by bacteria. In a case of malignant diphtheria in which the urine contained a considerable amount of albumen, M. Gaucher, adopting all precautions to prevent the access of external germs, was able to demonstrate without difficulty the presence of bacteria in both the blood and the kidneys. The urine was collected in a glass, washed with alcohol and heated, and, examined immediately, was found to contain a large quantity of spherical or punctiform mobile bacteria (monads or micrococci). There were no rods or chains. In the blood the same organisms were found, less numerous, but perfectly distinct. The patient died seven days after the onset of the disease. The kidneys, examined in the fresh state, were found crammed with bacteria similar to those which had been found in the urine and the blood during life. The epithelial cells of the urinary tubules were filled with highly refracting granules, strikingly similar to the micrococci found in the urine. In sections which had been hardened in osmic acid the same granules were found. From these facts Gaucher concludes that diphtheritic nephritis is of parasitic origin, and that the albuminuria is the result of the passage of the bacteria of the blood through the kidneys. The albuminuria is thus to be regarded as an effort at the elimination of the poison.—*Lancet*, March 5, 1881.

Syphilis and Tabes Dorsalis.

WESTPHAL (*Archiv f. Psych.* xi. p. 230) concludes that an etiological relation between syphilis and tabes is unsupported either by clinical or pathologico-anatomical facts. In 75 cases, whose histories were comparatively well ascertained, he found chancres in 14, chancres and secondary symptoms in 11. Nineteen out of 20 cases occurring in women had no history of chancre, and the twentieth case was a doubtful one. In one case only were secondary symptoms present whilst the patient was under observation. Of 16 cases that came to autopsy one only showed evidences of syphilis, and in another the appearances were doubtful. Further, Westphal has never seen a case of gray degeneration of the posterior columns cured by anti-syphilitic remedies. Remak (see *Centralblatt ,f. d. med. Wissensch.* 1880, No. 43) obtained a history of syphilis in 25 per cent. of his cases of tabes, nevertheless he does not admit a direct causal connection between the two. Bernhardt admits that syphilis may produce tabes, but it is not nearly so potent a cause as is often supposed.

Westphal reports a case in which, besides other lesions of a syphilitic nature, there was disease of the posterior columns in the upper cervical region. The medulla of the nerves had disappeared, but the axis-cylinders were intact, and in some places seemed larger than normal. The vessels were dilated and their walls thickened. There was no increase of connective tissue or proliferation of nuclei, no corpora amylacea, no cells with fatty granules. The changes were evidently due to a peculiar parenchymatous affection. A gumma was found in the posterior part of the corpus callosum. Westphal compares this case with one recorded by Schultze, in which there was a tumour of the anterior part of the corpus callosum and degeneration of Burdach's columns down to the lower dorsal region. In Burdach's columns the nerves had lost their axis-cylinders, but for the most part retained their medulla. The neuroglia was normal.— *Brain*, Jan. 1881.

—

On the Early Stage of Locomotor Ataxy.

An early recognition of ataxic tabes is of the highest importance, as it is only at the earliest stage of the disease that we can hope to do much good by our remedial measures. The ocular symptoms are frequently the earliest; and among them the author draws attention to a sudden and transitory paralysis of accommodation of one eye. This may be the only trouble present, but is often accompanied with mydriasis paralytica. These symptoms may precede the actual invasion of the disease by some years. Then dissociated paralyses of the third, of the fourth, and sixth nerves may intervene, as well as spinal myosis, which is characterized by absence of reaction to light, but not to the accommodative impulse. Or, again, mere sluggishness or absence of reaction to light may be present. Charcot has well described the progressive optic atrophy; the papilla presents the appearance of a flat depression according to MÜLLER, and the vessels gradually become smaller. The field of vision diminishes concentrically in the two eyes unequally, the region of dimness has the shape of sectors having (not the fovea, but) the papilla as centres; and this diminution is much more readily appreciated on indirect vision. Achromatopsia may occur, first to green, then to red. In disseminated sclerosis the sense of colour is preserved. The author recommends Doucet's perimeter as the most convenient to test these defects in practice.

The lancinating pains present various peculiarities which need not be dwelt upon here; the various other defects or alterations of sensibility are also well known. Berger has shown that there may be deficient algesia to powerful stimuli, whilst weaker ones are responded to. Retardation of transmission of sensations is not very common. The sense of pressure is often deficient at an early period.

The well-known "tendon reflex" may coexist with ataxia (in 2 cases among 82: Berger). Certain facts lead the author to suspect a period of heightened reflex preceding its abolition.

[I have now under observation a somewhat doubtful case, in which there are shooting-pains in the left leg with very diminished tendon reflex, and markedly increased reflex in the right. The right hand is the seat of progressive muscular atrophy.]

Erlenmeyer has prominently brought forward the early gastric symptoms of tabes; they either take the form of nervous dyspepsia or actual catarrh. These symptoms have the characteristic suddenness of many tabetic symptoms.

The genito-urinary organs present numerous forms of disturbance. We may note here urethral and rectal neuralgias, causing spasmodic contraction of the bladder, and tenesmus.

The well-known crises gastriques may constitute for a long time the chief feature of the disease, and may require care in their diagnosis from other stomach ailments. The pneumogastric may be affected differently, and give rise to tremendous fits of coughing. The "crises néphritiques" need only be mentioned here.

Arthropathies and osseous fragility may appear early. The pulse is usually frequent. The sweat, increased at first, becomes deficient later on, and is not readily induced by pilocarpine in the diseased regions. The ataxic symptoms are usually pathognomonic of the second period. The author has noticed two cases of early peroneal paralysis.

The treatment of tabes at this initial stage consists, first, in a strict hygienic mode of life; second, in the administration of ergot and nitrate of silver, a mild course of hydrotherapy (the water to range between 20°–25° centigrade) and electricity. The latter is to be applied centrally by means of large electrodes (2×6 inches), using a current strength of 8–11 milliwebers; and may be also usefully applied symptomatically for relieving the ocular troubles, the gastric pains, etc. Against the latter and the shooting-pains Chapman's bags may also be used with success.

The author next discusses the anti-syphilitic plan of treatment, and condemns it—first, because it is useless; second, because he does not consider the syphilitic nature of the disease as demonstrated. Several instructive cases bring Dr. Müller's valuable paper to a close.—*Brain*, Jan. 1881, from *Mittheilungen des Vereines der Aertzte in Steiermark*, 1879.

———

A Case of Chronic Vomiting in which no Food was taken, except Koumiss, for Sixteen Months.

At a late meeting of the Clinical Society of London (*Med. Times and Gazette*, Feb. 26, 1881), Dr. H. SUTHERLAND related this case. The patient, a girl, aged twenty-four on admission, had been for five years under his care at St. George's, Hanover-Square, Dispensary. One year and seven months ago the vomiting commenced, the attack coming on at first only once a fortnight, but lately it had occurred always once, and sometimes five or six times a day. As far as could be ascertained, there was no organic disease of the stomach, no tenderness on pressure, or cachexia, nor any other constitutional symptom. Every known remedy was tried to allay the vomiting—bismuth, opium, hydrocyanic acid, creasote, carbolic acid, hyposulphites, etc.—without any satisfactory result. All attempts to cure the case by dieting had failed, and the patient could keep nothing on the stomach as food except koumiss, which she had taken for sixteen months. She is, however, able to retain a quinine-and-orange mixture, and also sherry in small quantities, for brandy makes her sick immediately. The uterus was not displaced. The object in bringing the case before the Society was to ask if members could suggest any remedies or mode of treatment in this distressing case.

Dr. JAGIELSKI had found that koumiss could often be retained and do good when nothing else would. The case just recorded was probably unique, inasmuch as koumiss was required for eighteen months, and that the patient had decidedly improved under its use. Often, koumiss could be borne when milk could not. This might be because the casein had been broken up by the carbonic acid in the process of production.

Dr. BROADBENT inquired whether the patient had been engaged in any kind of work or been entirely idle during the period referred to. The case was in all probability one of hysteria, as indicated by the nervous condition, the irregular menstruation, and the regular morning and evening vomiting. It belonged to the fasting-girl class.

Dr. B. O'CONNOR mentioned a case where he had used various forms of milk and Valentine's beef extract with success. He found that, in some cases, the upper portion of the milk after standing suited best.

Dr. WILBERFORCE SMITH said that in such cases the stomach could not digest nitrogenous substances, and that therefore he would recommend cream and fat boiled with water-biscuits as an alternative diet.

Dr. DOWSE asked how much koumiss was given in the twenty-four hours. The case was evidently a nervous one, and he would suggest that solid instead of liquid food be tried.

Dr. SUTHERLAND said the patient lived at home and did no work. The case was not, he thought, hysterical, but the patient was bad-tempered and inclined to suicide.

Post-mortem Emphysema from Gastric Ulcer.

Among the causes of subcutaneous emphysema ulcer of the stomach is one of the rarest. An instance has, however, lately been reported by POENSGEN in the *Deutsches Archiv für Klin. Med.* The patient was a man aged thirty-seven years, who had for three years presented the symptoms of gastric ulcer. He had been treated by washing out the stomach by a douche, and was relieved. A fresh attack of vomiting occurred, and he died suddenly on his way to the hospital. A short time after his death, the abdomen, chest, neck, head, face, arms, and the left leg were gradually invaded by enormous subcutaneous emphysema, which was also found after death in the connective tissue of the mediastinum and beneath the peritoneum. In the smaller curvature the wall of the stomach was perforated by an ulcer, and on the inner surface of the abdominal wall was another ulcer, which had apparently corresponded to the perforation in the stomach, and through it the gas from within that organ had seemingly escaped into the cellular tissue.—*Lancet*, Jan. 22, 1881.

Nature of the Green Vomit.

The chemical and microscopical nature of green vomit has been made the subject of recent investigations by Dr. F. BETZ (*Mémorabilien*, Oct. 6, 1880). It was supposed that the green vomit (*vomitus æruginosus*) was the result of a greenish discoloration of brown biliary pigment, caused by the acid action of the gastric juice. The supposition received corroboration from the bitter taste of the vomited matter, associated with its acid reaction. Dr. Betz concludes, however, that the green colour is not invariably due to the presence of bile. The colour often varies from a yellowish-green or grayish-green, to a grass-green or dark-green, in accordance with the greater or less amount of the green "substance" and other admixtures.　If green vomit be allowed to stand in a vessel, the greater part of the greenish substance will sink, whereas a small portion, containing slime and fatty matters, will float on top.　Shaking with water shows that the green substance is heavier than water and insoluble in it, a proof that bile is not the cause of the colour.　Agitation with chloroform or ether likewise demonstrates this, for neither fluid takes up the green substance.　It may, however, be isolated by shaking with ether in a test-tube.　This manipulation results in the appearance of three strata, an upper one consisting of ether, a middle one composed of the green substance, and a lower one containing the gastric mucus. Strong sulphuric acid produces a red colour, strong nitric acid leads to a yellowish discoloration of the green substance.　Acetic acid develops and fixes the green colour very completely.　Tincture of iodine produces a yellowish-brown, and not a blue tint.　Alcohol dissolves the green substance.　In some respects, it resembles the chlorophyll of plants.　The alcohol dissolves it, and even retains the green colour when boiled.　The green vomit may be kept for months and during the hot season, without spontaneous putrid fermentation taking place—a fact which militates against the possibility of its biliary or even animal nature. Dr. Betz also states that sometimes the green vomit has a neutral or alkaline reaction.　Microscopical examination shows the green substance to consist of an amorphous, finely granular greenish mass.　Discoid heaps, or rounded colonies, are commonly observed.　But the green substance may also form a lining over epithelial cells, salivary corpuscles, etc.　From these facts Dr. Betz infers the vegetable nature of this substance, and he adds that it is probably derived from punctiform algæ, which he calls *chlorococcus*.　He denies any relation of this low fungus to other microphytes, such as the torula cerevisiæ, sarcina ventriculi, or oïdium.　Finally, the author remarks that, apart from all other considerations, the frequent occurrence of copious green vomits would go to show that bile could not find its way into the stomach in such erroneous quantity.　The bitter taste of the green vomit receives its explanation in part from the frequent admixture of some bile, but is also in part due to the presence of a bitter principle in the chlorococcus.—*London Med. Record*, Feb. 15, 1881.

Treatment of Infantile Diarrhœa by Charcoal in the Milk.

For children belonging to families in easy circumstances, M. J. GUÉRIN mixes a certain quantity of Belloc's powder of charcoal with each milk meal—half a teaspoonful only at each meal.　For the children of the working classes, Belloc's powder, which is a little dear, is replaced by very finely powdered, farina-like, ground bakers' charcoal.　This powder mixes readily with milk, and children drink the mixture as though the milk were pure.　In a very short time, sometimes on the first day, the stools change in consistence and odour, and instead of being green, become blackish-yellow.　At the same time that this addition is made, M. J. Guérin dilutes the milk with one-third or one-half of sweetened water, and the children take it without repugnance or vomiting.　M. Guérin has frequently seen children, exhausted by seven or eight days' uncontrollable diarrhœa, regain in two or three days the expression of health.—*Lond. Med. Record*, Feb. 15, 1881, from *L'Union Méd.*

Causes of Contracted Kidney, and on the Diagnosis of Different Forms of Nephritis.

ZIEGLER (*Deut. Arch. für Klin. Med.*, Band xxv., sec. 586) says the chief factor in the causation of granular kidney is not the degeneration of the parenchyma, but the non-occurrence of its regeneration which can restore it to its integrity. Simple fatty degeneration, which occurs in various diseases, in anæmia, and may be caused experimentally, has not succeeded in affording any explanation of granular atrophy. He starts with the investigation of senile atrophy of the kidney, in which, obviously in consequence of generally diminished nutrition, there occur enfeeblement of the circulation, wasting of the glomeruli, first at the periphery, then disappearance of the tubules connected with them, and finally more or less extensive small-celled infiltration. The arterio-sclerotic form of granular atrophy stands next to this. Here, the most important changes are wasting of the glomeruli, collapse and atrophy of the tubules, and finally, hyperplasia of connective tissue. Fatty degeneration occurs secondarily, but the cells become smaller, like those of the looped tubes; most contain cylinders. The vessels are widened, and this seems to be the cause of the increase of urine. The embolic form is similar to the latter. By obstruction to the greater circulation, and increase of the heart's action, the same changes take place in the kidney, which apparently originate in wasting of the glomeruli, perhaps in consequence of exudation into the capsules. Great interference with the nutrition of the kidney of different sorts may lead to extensive degeneration of the parenchyma; but regeneration takes place if the glomeruli have not been involved, or if the destruction be not too great or continued. When the latter occurs, atrophy results; as occasionally happens, for instance, in acute jaundice. It may also follow parenchymatous degeneration, as seen in the small patches of atrophy on the surface of the large white kidney; but generally atrophy occurs only rarely. The glandular degeneration, in all those forms which he groups together as interstitial indurative nephritis, is of secondary importance. The atrophy of the tubules is the result of their abolished function, of the destruction of the glomeruli, which latter depends upon fibrous hyperplasia of the capsules, or on a concomitant disease of the arterial system. Besides the form of atrophy from compression, he gives three groups of atrophy of the kidney. The first, of which the type is the arterio-sclerotic form, is dependent on simple interference with the circulation, and must be distinguished from the inflammatory forms. In the second, he classes all the degenerative processes which are followed by destruction of the epithelium (embolism, temporary ligature, chemical irritants), excluding regeneration. In the third group (interstitial nephritis), there is a combination of epithelial degeneration with other processes—cellular infiltration, proliferation of the epithelium of the capsules and glomeruli, wasting of the vascular tufts. Both the latter groups—which differ only quantitatively, not qualitatively, as in both there are epithelial degeneration and hyperplasia of connective tissue—are, nevertheless, to be kept distinct, as there is no "identical pathological principle," as Weigert thinks.—*London Med. Record*, Feb. 15, 1881.

Post-scarlatinal Nephritis.

The greater part of the contribution of Dr. HAJEK (*Archiv für Kinder*, vol. 1. pl. 10) agrees with the majority of articles to be found in German periodicals, in consisting almost entirely of an enumeration of the names of every one who has had anything to say on the subject in question, coupled with a partial criticism of their views, and concluding by leaving the question still in doubt, or only augmented by some trifling additional information. As articles of reference to what has been said, such papers are invaluable. Whether all that has been said is worth being referred to, is perhaps doubtful. With the uncertainty that exists as to the cause of the complex symptoms included under uræmia, this title is rather to be regarded as provisional; and the further question of the exact connection of nephritis with the acute exanthemata, especially scarlet fever, is still uncertain.   Uræmia is a constant accompaniment of diffuse inflammation of the kidneys; and researches on uræmic eclampsia have disclosed affections of the brain and cord, such as œdema, and even hemorrhage into the meninges and nerve-substance, which, according to Traube, by producing a capillary anæmia leads to convulsion, a theory at variance with what is usually held.   Frerichs attributes the symptoms of so called uræmia to carbonate of ammonia, derived from urinary salts, whilst Voit regards the retention of all or some of the products of decomposition within the body as the cause, and compares the result to the extinguishing of a fire by accumulation of ashes.   Caffer (1878), by injections of carbonate of ammonia into the blood, found that the corpuscles by the retention of this salt are materially changed in their structure and power of absorption of oxygen, and their number considerably diminished.   Jaksch and Treitz suggest the decomposition of materials in the intestine as a supplementary source of ammonia.   Mantegazza has seen muscular convulsions from injection of urinary matter as well as from the immersion of portions of muscle in urinary sediment.   Perles and others speak of the quantity of kreatin and kreatinin in the blood in Bright's disease.   In short, the connection between retention of urine in nephritis, and the appearances of uræmia or ammonæmia is yet so imperfectly defined, that Thomas, in Gabault's *Handbook of Children's Diseases*, says that uræmia arises upon some disturbance of the urinary secretion, and is probably occasioned by it. To the question, what is the pathological connection between nephritis and scarlet fever?   the answer is, the long-continued, more or less complete, suppression of the perspiration.   The constant results of complete or partial covering of the skin with oil, varnish, etc., are albuminuria, and diminished quantity of urine, fall of temperature, dyspnœa, convulsions, coma, and death.   Corresponding *post mortem* to these symptoms are diffuse nephritis, pneumonia, myocarditis, and hepatitis.   Some observers consider that death is due to increased radiation of heat from the distended superficial capillaries ; others attribute it to uræmia, and the crystals of triple phosphates which are found in the bodies of animals so treated are products of urinary decomposition   Lang clearly explains the uræmia as being caused by disease of the looped renal tubules ; since excretion of water by the skin is stopped, and the lungs cannot compensate, the tubules are blocked up, and retention of urine brings about the uræmia.   Lassar supposes that the sudden determination to the internal organs of blood very much cooled at the surface of the lung, is itself a cause of inflammation.   An identical train of symptoms follows extension of superficial scalds.   The identity in symptoms and *post mortem* appearances between primary or scarlatinal nephritis, and those brought about by artificial suppression of cutaneous secretion, however-produced, justifies the conclusion that in scarlet fever the same causes, viz., the suppression of perspiration, induces the same effects, viz., nephritis and uræmia.   Barthez and Rilliet put forward the idea, in which they were supported by Baginsky, that the albuminuria depended upon the non-conversion into epithelium, for which it was destined, of certain albuminous matter in the blood, which was, therefore, excreted by the urine.   Bohn opposed this view, and showed how the function of the skin is impeded by the œdema of the cutis, and the dead and stiffened epidermis.   From this point of view the scarlatinal nephritis would seem not to be a local expression of the primary disease, and still less due to taking cold (that scape-goat of etiology, as Bartels says) during the desquamation stage, but to be a direct consequence of the fever from the conditions of the skin.—*London Med. Record*, Feb. 15, 1881.

Surgery.

Lister's Antiseptic Treatment in Surgical Wounds.

BOECKEL (*Gaz. Méd. de Strasbourg*, Dec. 1, 1880) gives a table of statistics of major amputations performed by himself, some with and some without antiseptic precautions. Fifteen amputations of the thigh were performed antiseptically with four deaths, and seven were treated otherwise with three deaths; eighteen amputations of the leg were treated antiseptically without a death, and nineteen treated in other ways with four deaths. In going into the causes of death, the author concludes that in neither case can the deaths be attributed to the method of dressing employed. Nevertheless, he thinks that the advantage is decidedly with the cases treated antiseptically, on account of the rapid healing, the absence of fever and of suppuration, and the rarity of the dressings in these cases. He mentions the occurrence of aseptic fever in a few cases, and, with Edelberg, he attributes this to absorption of blood from the wound.—*Lond. Med. Record*, Feb. 15, 1881.

Statistics of Congenital Colour-blindness in Denmark.

Dr. O. E. DE FONTENAY has explained (*Nordiskt Medicinskt Arkiv*, vol. xii., 1880) the progress which has been made in Denmark as to the relations existing between daltonism and the practical pursuits of life. The authorities have carefully examined all the persons engaged on the railroads in order to ascertain the proportion of daltonians (the colour-blind), and all candidates for employment on the lines are hereafter to prove that they are endowed with an adequate sense of the perception of colour. These requirements, however, have not yet been sanctioned by law in reference to the sailors of the navy or the merchant service, except so far that candidates of the school of naval officers are subjected to an examination such as that just referred to.

The author adopts the classification of cases proposed by Holmgren, namely, into (1) total blindness as to colours, and (2) partial blindness, subdivided into complete blindness to red, green, or violet, and incomplete blindness as to those colours. He gives a complete list of the results of his researches, founded on 217 cases, giving information as to the ages and social position of the persons affected, the colour of their eyes, and the degree and kind of daltonism in each In 9659 cases examined at all ages (beginning at eight), of all classes, and in the whole of Denmark, 217 were daltonians. As to social position, 1001 persons belonging to the superior classes presented 31 with defective vision, or about $3\frac{1}{2}$ per cent., while 3491 of the lower classes (workmen, small artisan, peasants, etc.) gave 134 daltonians, or rather less than 4 per cent. From some of Dr. de Fontenay's researches it would appear that females are less subject to daltonism than males, for out of 176 cases of daltonism only 11 were females, and of 632 females of the upper classes not one was daltonian, and 16 daltonian females were all of the lower classes. Out of 2714 children from eight to sixteen years of age, there were 41 daltonians, of whom 36 were males and 5 were females. Of 215 cases of daltonism, 56 were cases of red-blindness, 24 of green-blindness, and 135 were incomplete cases; whence it follows that in Denmark red-blindness is more than twice as common as that of green. In all the 217 cases of daltonism the author found that the two eyes were equally affected; but as to the relation between the colour of the eyes and the frequency of daltonism, the statistics showed that there was no special relation between the colour of the eyes and the affection in question.

As to the hereditary character of daltonism no very satisfactory or conclusive results have been obtained. In 34 cases where the family history was carefully examined, heredity was denied in 27. In two of the cases there was a daltonian father, and in both the daltonism of the father was of the same degree and kind as that of the offspring. One of the cases had normal parents, but a paternal uncle, two brothers, and his own son were daltonians. Other similar anomalies were observed, and one case offered four daltonian members in the family, namely, an uncle and a maternal cousin, the mother's grandfather, and a brother.

In another paper on the same subject, by Dr. E. J. Mellberg, the author states that he has examined, by the method devised by Holmgren with coloured wools, 227 pupils of the Helsingfors Lyceum, and discovered among them 10 cases of daltonism, of which 4 were cases of red-blindness, 1 of green-blindness, 2 of violet-blindness, and 3 of incomplete daltonism.—*Med. Times and Gazette*, March 5, 1881.

Bacteria in the Choroid.

The *Centralblatt für prakt. Augenheilk.* for October last contains a paper by the DUKE CHARLES of Bavaria on the discovery of bacteria in the choroid coat of two eyeballs. The eyeballs, which showed neither naked eye nor microscopical evidence of disease, were preserved in Müller's fluid. On examination the vessels of both the coarser and the finer vascular network of the choroid were found closely packed with bacteria. They were especially abundant in the larger capillaries just before their ultimate divisions and in the finest capillaries themselves, and least numerous in the small arteries and veins. There was no sign of decomposition of the eyes, nor were any organisms found in the Müller's fluid, in which they had been immersed, while other globes contained in the same vessel did not present any similar appearances. These, together with the fact that the bacteria were only in small numbers in the veins and closely packed in the capillaries, negative the supposition that they had originated *post-mortem.* The bacteria were cylindrical rodlets about half the length of the nucleus of a leucocyte, with a clearly defined outline, homogeneous, glistening, and structureless contents. Besides these, some bacilli from five to twenty times their length and some of the small rods undergoing division were found. They mostly resembled the forms of organisms seen in septic diseases and in decomposition, and they differed from the bacilli of splenic fever by their greater thickness and the slight rounding of their ends.—*Lancet*, Jan. 29, 1881.

Treatment of Cancer of the Tongue.

In the December number of the *Bull. et Mém. de la Soc. de Chir.*, is a report of a communication by M. VERNEUIL on the inutility and danger of any save operative treatment of epithelioma of the tongue. This disease, it is pointed out, has never been cured either by internal treatment or by topical applications. M. Verneuil states that he seldom meets with a case of lingual cancer which has not previously been treated by iodide of potassium. Such treatment, it is argued, cannot be justified. It is a gross error to think that iodide of potassium has any efficacy in instances of true neoplasm, for, as is well known, this agent effects no amelioration in cancers of the lip, cervix uteri, and other organs. The diagnosis of epithelioma of the tongue, in the majority of cases, should not be difficult; and, through the recent teaching of M. Fournier, this affection may be readily distinguished from tertiary glossitis. There are, it is true, hybrid cases in which the cancer occurs in a subject of old syphilis, and in which the objective characters of the epithelioma are modified by the constitutional affection. This condition does not indicate any alteration of treatment, for the hybrid affection in its course, termination, and prognosis, resembles pure epithelioma, and should be dealt with in a like manner. M. Verneuil asserts that medicinal treatment of cancer of the tongue is not only fruitless, but also hurtful. Surgical removal of the disease is postponed, and so much precious time is lost. Iodide of potassium often excites troublesome and obstinate glossitis, and mercury stimulates the growth both of the primary epithelioma, and of any affected cervical glands. Chlorate of potash is as useless in cases of cancer of the tongue, as it would be if given for the relief of cancer of the cervix uteri. Epithelioma of the tongue, M. Verneuil holds, if taken in time, may be cured by operation. Mention is made of four cases of complete cure. In three of these cases the growth was small and superficial; in the fourth case a relapsing growth, together with a degenerated gland, was removed. When more than a third of the tongue has become involved, when the floor of the mouth is also affected, and when the disease has been progressing for longer than a year, the case is deplorably grave, and cannot then be treated by operation with any chance of success. Removal of lingual cancer, it is asserted, is not a serious operation when it can be performed by the mouth, and when the disease is recent and not extensive. Of two hundred such operations performed under these conditions by M. Verneuil, one only was fatal; and, in this instance, the death was due to pneumonia, and not directly to surgical action. Operation at an early stage of the disease is strongly recommended; and it is stated that between the early and favourable stage, and the advanced and hopeless stage, there is a long interval, at any period of which the surgeon may operate without risk, and with some prospect of permanent success.—*London Med. Record*, Feb. 15, 1881.

—

Extirpation of the Pylorus.

Prof. BILLROTH makes the following contribution to the *Wiener Medicinische Wochenschrift* (Feb. 5):—

"We to-day register a triumph which surgical art has recently been enabled to celebrate. The important question which has so long engaged the attention of surgeons—whether the carcinoma which so frequently attacks the stomach, and for which all internal remedies are useless, may not be made amenable to operative surgery—would seem to be at once decided affirmatively. On January 29, Prof. Billroth performed a partial excision of the stomach on account of advanced carcinoma of the pylorus, which up to the present time has been attended with success. Already, seventy years ago, Karl Merrem had shown in a dissertation, by experiments upon dogs, that the pylorus might be excised, and recommended the procedure in incurable cancer. The conviction, however, that the vital processes in man and animals were the same, was as yet too little assured, and operative procedures too little advanced, for the operation to be ventured on. It is only during the last ten years that essential progress has been made in this province of surgery; and Billroth and his pupils have done much in that time to prepare the way for the operation. After Billroth had shown, in 1871, that portions of the œsophagus may be cut out in dogs, Czerny first performed this operation in man. Then followed Gussenbauer's and Winniwarter's excision of portions of the intestinal canal and stomach in dogs, and Martini and Gussenbauer's successful excision of a sigmoid flexure that had undergone cancerous degeneration. Gastrorraphy, successfully performed by Billroth in 1877, was another step in advance, and led him to make the remark that from this operation to the excision of a cancerous portion of the stomach required but one bold step. The first, however, who performed excision (in 1829) for cancerous pylorus in man was the Parisian surgeon Péan, so well known for his numerous laparotomies, but the patient died on the fourth day; and no suitable case came under Billroth's notice until the present one.

"The woman upon whom the operation was performed on January 29 was forty-three years of age, and previously in good health, having borne eight children. In October, 1880, she suffered from vomiting, and soon presented all the symptoms of carcinoma of the stomach and stenosis of the pylorus. During the six weeks prior to the operation the constant vomiting and the small amount of nourishment taken led to excessive pallor, emaciation, small and frequent pulse, and exhaustion; so that the patient, feeling her end approaching, consented to the operation proposed by Billroth. The preparation for the operation, which was performed in a temperature of 24° R. (86° Fahr.) under chloroform, consisted only in washing out the stomach with the ordinary tube. An incision about eight centimetres in length was performed over the tumour, which was readily movable under the thinned integuments. The tumour proved to be a nodulated carcinoma of the pylorus, which was in part infiltrated, and occupied more than the lower third of the stomach. The parts were carefully separated from the omentum and transverse colon, and, the vessels being tied before their division, very little blood was lost. The tumour having been completely brought on to the integuments of the abdomen, an incision was made through the stomach one centimetre beyond the infiltrated part—first only backwards, and then through the duodenum. An oblique incision through the stomach was next directed from above and inwards to below and outwards, always at a distance of one centimetre from the infiltrated parts. After uniting the oblique incision only sufficiently to allow of its being adjusted to the duodenum, the tumour was completely separated from the duodenum, one centimetre distant from the infiltration, by means of an incision parallel to that made in the stomach. The duodenum was adapted to the aperture left in the stomach, about fifty sutures of carbolized silk in all having been employed during the operation. After cleansing with a 2 per cent. carbolic acid solution, and the application of a guard-ligature, the parts were replaced in the cavity of the abdomen. The operation, including a tedious chloroformisation, occupied one hour and a half. The excised portion consisted of fourteen centimetres of the greater curvature of the stomach, and a quill could only be passed with difficulty through the pylorus. The form of the stomach was not essentially changed by the operation, the organ only being rendered smaller. After the operation there was neither vomiting nor pain. . . . From a communication of Prof. Billroth on February 13, it appears that the patient had continued to improve, so that the recovery then seemed assured. The result is indeed favourable beyond all expectation, and already suffices to show that such an operation is practicable, so that persons may now be successfully treated for a disease hitherto reputed incurable; and even when a relapse takes place, they will at least have received temporary alleviation."—*Med. Times and Gazette*, March 5, 1881.

—

Excision of the Initial Syphilitic Sclerosis, and on the Treatment of Syphilis.

In the *Wiener Med. Presse*, Nos. 27, 28, 29, 1880, Professor ZEISSL opposes the view that the initial sclerosis is only a local symptom whence the general infection takes place; he believes the initial lesion to be the first expression of the general infection of the patient's system. The author also relates five cases of excision of indurated sores, in all of which general syphilis followed, notwithstanding the removal of the initial lesion. In the treatment of syphilis the author speaks favourably of Zittmann's decoction, but states that he has not found benefit from pilocarpine.—*Lond. Med. Record*, Feb. 15, 1881.

Suprapubic Operation of Lithotomy.

Dr. PETERSEN (*Archiv für Klin. Chir.*, Band xxv. s. 752) considers that the dangers of the high operation for stone, which consists in injury of the perito-neum and infiltration of urine, may be prevented by modern methods of opera-tion. He has found, by observation on eleven bodies, that when Braune's method is followed by the gradual distension of the rectum, the full bladder is dragged further forward and upright, and the peritoneum thus rises considerably with its anterior fold, much more so than when this is not the case. Petersen, therefore, has recently always operated in such a manner that he not only fills the bladder to the utmost, but the rectum also, by the introduction of a rectal tube, and the gradual injection of water of the same heat as the body, so as to dilate it. In his last two operations, Petersen did not even see the peritoneum; while, in his earlier operations, he was obliged to push it upward. He considers that the danger of infiltration of urine may be overcome by careful suture of the bladder with fine catgut, under complete antiseptic precautions. The special indications for the high operation he sets out as follows: (1) The presence of a large hard stone; (2) encapsuled stone; (3) stone in diverticula, behind the prostate gland; (4) enlargement of the prostate gland; (5) hæmorrhoids; (6) fat subjects; (7) tumours of the bladder; (8) impermeable stricture (with the assistance of posterior catheterization).—*London Med. Record*, Feb. 15, 1881.

—

Simultaneous Ligation of Carotid and Subclavian for Aneurism of the Arch of the Aorta.

A case of successful ligature of the right subclavian and right common carotid arteries simultaneously, for aneurism of the arch of the aorta, under the care of Dr. J. MANSERGH PALMER, surgeon to the Armagh County Infirmary, deserves record. The patient, a woman aged fifty, was admitted to the hospital on Feb. 10th, 1880, having noticed a slight swelling close to the right sterno-clavicular articulation during the previous November. On the night of the 12th Dr. Palmer found her suffering from great difficulty of breathing, stridulous respira-tion, lividity of face and neck, coldness of extremities, and other symptoms which rendered an immediate operation absolutely necessary. She was removed to the operating room, the right common carotid artery was tied, and as the tumour did not appear to decrease and pulsation continued, the subclavian was also ligatured. On the 29th the carotid ligature came away, and on March 2d the subclavian. On April 27th she left the hospital, both wounds being quite healed. Early in June she caught cold and was readmitted to the Infirmary, but refused to take any medicine. On June 14th hemorrhage took place from the old cicatrix in the neck over the carotid vessel, being complicated with hæmoptysis, which also occurred on the following day, and on the 10th there was profuse hæmoptysis and death supervened 125 days after the operation. A post-mortem examination showed that the aneurism involved not only the arteria innominata, but also the arch of the aorta, while at the posterior and left side of the arteria innominata was an opening communicating with the left vena innominata, which latter com-municated with the trachea at one point and at another opened into the right lung.—*Lancet*, March 5, 1881.

—

Three Cases of Knee-joint Abscess in Children.

Mr. EDMUND OWEN, Senior Assistant-Surgeon to St. Mary's Hospital, at a late meeting of the Medical Society of London (*Lancet*, Feb. 12, 1881), ex-hibited three patients who happened to have been lately under treatment together, and are, indeed, the only instances in which he has recently had occasion to open the knee-joint for suppurative arthritis. Short as the series is, these cases offer, he thinks, "an interesting subject for discussion and criticism; and especially so as you have just had the opportunity of examining the present condition of the joint in each instance. The eldest child only was treated by me as an in-patient; the others were brought as out-patients to the Children's Hospital.

"Briefly, the line of treatment has consisted in free incisions into the joint and subsequent free drainage; in absolute and prolonged rest of the limb with compression of the articulation; in constitutional and dietetic support, and (need I say it?) in local cleanliness. But having remarked that I have employed cleanliness in the treatment of these diseased and opened joints, the conclusion that I adopted the high ritual of spray and the vestments of gauze would be both hasty and inconsequent. I wish it, however, to be thoroughly understood that I did my best to keep the articulations clean, both on the exterior and in the interior. I would like it to be understood also that by no means do I bear the spray and gauze ill-will; I even look upon them as a kind of safety-lamp which may well be carried by those who work in an atmosphere of surgical fire-damp, as well as by those who, trespassing in the seductive regions of speculative surgery, may on occasion require evidence of their having started on their excursion without neglect of approved precaution. To the great champion of cleanliness in our art I personally owe a boundless debt of gratitude, but to certain of his enthusiastic disciples who, to speak within bounds, seem to consider those who do not adopt their creed as wilfully obstinate or morally oblique, I will delicately put this question: Could any other method of treatment have obtained better results than those which we have now before us?

"Our medical journals are continually called upon to publish reports of cases, trifling and serious, which have recovered after 'antiseptic treatment,' that this short series out of the groove cannot now but be of interest. Possibly even they may help to show that *post* and *propter*, when employed in connection with a certain surgical practice, need not be confused even when half-obscured in a cloud of carbolized vapour.

"The first case is that of a girl of about four years of age. A little more than two years ago she was brought into the out-patient room in Great Ormond Street in a most pitiable condition. The left knee was red and enlarged from a collection of fluid in the interior. So painful had the joint been that appetite and sleep had left her. Moreover, she had had several attacks of convulsions—the rigors of childhood. Ten months previously, the mother said, the child had fallen off her chair, and directly afterwards the knee had begun to swell; but though the swelling had steadily increased, the child had been able to limp about until three weeks ago. The whole limb was red and swollen. She was at once put to bed, and the Registrar (Dr. Abercrombie) going round next morning noted that the leg and thigh were the seat of erysipelas, and that there were several blebs on the leg. The glands in the groin were enlarged and tender. Though there was a small sinus leading towards, or into the joint, from the inner side, from which a thin fluid was oozing, the patella was floated from off the femoral condyles. The temperature was just under 101° Fahr. On the third day after her admission—that was when I next saw her—chloroform was administered, and a free incision was made on each side of the knee, much thin pus escaping. The finger passed into the interior of the joint detected much thickened and pulpy synovial membrane, but no diseased bone. The joint having been thoroughly washed out with a weak solution of chloride of zinc, a drainage-tube was passed through it, and the limb was put up again on a slightly bent tin splint.

Nevertheless, the erysipelas continued to advance, and blebs now had made their appearance on the thigh, and the temperature went up two or three degrees. The child was taking quinine, iron, and wine ; in less than a week the temperature began to track the chart along the normal line. For convenience in the washings, which were daily performed by the house-surgeon, Mr. Kempe, the back splint was changed for extension by the stirrup, weight, and pulley. A month after her admission the joint was strapped, the drainage-tube still lying in the outer wound ; and at the end of another like period she was taken home in excellent condition, the wound, though steadily closing, still weeping a little. But at home she did not prosper, and in three weeks she was again in hospital for ten days. Since that time she has steadily improved, the limb being fixed upon a back tin splint. It is no exaggeration to say that in function and movement the damaged knee is now as good as the other. The child runs about on it all the week, and kneels upon it on Sundays. It is absolutely free of pain.

" The second case is that of a little boy. The mother says that the disease was started by a fall out of bed upon the knees, after which the right joint began to swell. At the beginning of last year he was sent to me by Dr. Goullet, of St. John's Wood, for an attack of subacute synovitis. The child was then under a year and a half old. We fixed the limb on a tin splint, and Dr. Goullet looked after the child until April, when, in spite of the treatment adopted, the inflammation had run on to suppuration. In this case only one incision was made into the joint, and that on the inner side. The solution used for washing was weak tincture of iodine. Three days after that operation it was noted that the child had lost its thirst, and that its nights were quiet. Previously it had been in the habit of starting in its sleep and awaking with a scream. Seven months later it was remarked at the side of the prescription-paper, under the date of Nov. 17 : ' Has been wearing the splint up to to-day. The wound has healed, but there is a good deal of eczema around its site. There is good flexion and power of movement in the joint, but there is still some fulness about the ligament of the patella from the old thickening of the synovial membrane. The health is excellent.' There is no tenderness at the knee, which can be bent, without disturbing the child, to less than a right angle. Though the skin over the old wound is not sound-looking it is serviceable enough, and the child cruises about the room without inconvenience.

" The last case is that of a baby of four months, who was brought as an outpatient from Hendon at the end of last June. Against his name in the case-book I then wrote : ' Subacute synovitis of the left knee-joint,' and fixed the limb on a bent splint with strapping and soft bandage. But by the tenth day it was evident that a purulent collection occupied the synovial pouch. Excessive pain in the part had driven away sleep, and the child had attacks of convulsions. The knee was red, hot, swollen, and very tender. By means of incisions, and injections of weak tincture of iodine and water, much thin sero-purulent fluid and flakes of thick and curded pus were washed out of the joint, and the limb was then packed round with vaseline lint and tenax, and fixed to a splint. Gradually the splint was straightened, and by the middle of September drainage was discontinued, and the wounds healed up. The child never had a bad symptom. In October last there was free movement in the joint, and the infant was flourishing ; and, as you have seen to-night, the child allows full examination of the capabilities of the joint to be made. He even flexes it of his own accord ; and, his mother says, tries to walk on it.

" I am well aware that there is nothing of an extraordinary nature in these reports and cases, unless it be the simplicity of the treatment adopted. A treatment somewhat similar to that described by Mr. Sampson Gamgee (*On the*

Treatment of Wounds, p. 101), with this exception—improvement, I will call it—that the pus is straightway washed out of the joint, instead of being allowed to ooze out.   So the joint gets a well-considered and fair start towards the goal of recovery.

"In conclusion, I will venture to express the opinion that the chief requisites for obtaining such happy results in the treatment of acute joint-abscess in childhood are the early employment of clean and free drainage and the prolonged continuance of absolute rest.   And these are conditions which are fortunately very generally obtainable."

—

A Case of Gangrene of the Arm from a Poisoned Wound—Amputation at the Shoulder, and Recovery.

Mr. HEATH reported this case at a recent meeting of the Clinical Society of London (Med. *Times and Gazette*, Feb. 26, 1881).

The patient was a nurse, aged thirty-four, who, in laying out the body of a lady who had died of puerperal septicæmia, pricked her thumb with a pin.   Notes of the puerperal case were given by the physician who had attended her, and it appeared that she was a primipara in good health, and was the first patient attended by the accoucheur after his holiday, and that strict antiseptic precautions were employed.   On the fourth day a rigor occurred, and the temperature was 105°, pulse 120.   Subsequently the temperature went up to 107°, but was reduced to 102° by an ice-cap and water-bed.   On the seventh day, however, the left pleura filled, and the patient sank.   A nurse in attendance pricked her finger on the day of the rigor, and had a sharp attack of lymphangitis, with recovery.   The second nurse carried out the attendance till the patient's death.   This nurse applied nitrate of silver to the puncture on the evening of the day she received it, and the next day the hand was swollen and painful.   She had no further advice until the fourth day, when she was admitted to University College Hospital with the whole arm swollen and tense.   Free incisions were made, but the next day the hand and forearm had gangrened.   At first, the gangrene seemed limited to the forearm, and the swelling of the upper arm decreased for a few hours, but a relapse taking place, Mr. Heath amputated at the shoulder-joint.   The patient made a rapid recovery, and was discharged in a month.   Mr. Heath remarked upon the virulence of the puerperal poison, and protested against the common practice of applying nitrate of silver to punctures received at post-mortems.   He believed that the application of belladonna was most useful in cases of local inflammation, coupled with free incisions when necessary.

Mr. HARRISON CRIPPS gave the history of the case referred to by Mr. Heath as occurring in St. Bartholomew's Hospital.   The patient was under the care of Mr. Holden, and was both healthy and temperate.   He had pricked his finger very slightly; next day it began to swell, and when seen the arm was black as far as the wrist, the forearm was red.   Free incisions were made in the hand, but only a little clotted blood and serous fluid came away.   The swelling and redness rapidly extended upwards.   It was consequently determined to amputate through the shoulder-joint, but some diseased tissue had to be cut through.   Next day the temperature had fallen and the pain gone.   Six days afterwards there was a severe rigor, and the neck swelled.   This was punctured, but nothing came away; his face subsequently became gangrenous, and the man died.   In Mr. Heath's case recovery was no doubt due to early operation.   It would be important to know when and where to operate in such case.

Mr. LISTER thought the cases only tended to confirm the old rule to operate at once in a case of spreading gangrene.   In these cases there was probably an organism at work, as in the case of the *Bacillus anthracis*. But in some the blood was specially affected, or, as in Mr. Heath's case, the tissues.

Mr. HEATH said, in reply, that the rule was not only to operate early in these cases, but also to operate high up.

The Treatment of Malignant Pustules.

M. VERNEUIL, in an important communication to the Académie de Médecine on this subject, reminded his hearers that the malignant pustule consists of three zones or regions: first, the slough or gangrenous zone with its characteristic vesicles; secondly, an indurated zone presenting on its surface other vesicles; and, lastly, the zone of œdema. Until recently surgeons have concentrated their attention on the central or gangrenous zone, have applied almost no treatment to the indurated zone, and always none to the zone of œdema beyond poulticing and leeching. According to M. Verneuil it is important to apply to each zone special and energetic treatment. These are—first, to destroy or excise the gangrenous part; secondly, to incise and cauterize deeply the zone of induration; thirdly, to disinfect, by antiseptic hypodermic injection, the zone of œdema; lastly, to employ general antiseptic treatment, such as the internal administration of iodine or some other efficient internal antiseptic. The experiments of Davaine have shown that iodine, even in small doses, has an efficient neutralizing action on the virus of anthrax, and it is possible, according to M. Verneuil, to introduce into the circulation a sufficient quantity of iodine to produce this effect. The hypodermic injections into the œdematous zone should also consist of iodine, ten drops of a one-half per cent. solution. The first case thus treated was one of malignant pustule on the arm, in which the actual cautery had failed, and amputation was contemplated; the treatment was perfectly successful. In another case the pustule was situated on the eyelid, inoculation having been effected by inadvertently scratching a pimple there. The eyelid was much swollen, and presented the characteristic vesicles and bullæ, and there was considerable œdema of the whole of that half of the head. The temperature was 103°; the patient was delirious, sleepy, and vomited continually. The pustule was destroyed by means of the thermo-cautery. In the zone of induration a series of punctiform cauterizations were made with the same instrument, to a depth of one-third of an inch, and then the solution of iodine was injected in the œdematous part at intervals of five centimetres. The temperature rapidly fell. The delirium, somnolence, and vomiting ceased as if by magic, and on the third day the patient was out of danger. In the discussion which followed M. Léon Labbé agreed with M. Verneuil as to the necessity of cauterization in the zone of induration, and employed it even in the œdematous region. He was inclined to attribute more importance to this measure, employed in an energetic and even, as it might seem, barbarous degree, than to the injections of iodine. M. Gosselin urged the importance, before applying the treatment to every pustule which had a malignant aspect, of ascertaining if it were really anthrax, by microscopical examination of the serum in the vesicles and of the blood. M. Verneuil, speaking from the standpoint of practical surgery, maintained that better indications could be drawn from the clinical aspect of the affection than from the presence or absence of bacteria. He had seen cases in which bacteria were found in the vesicles and in the blood, although the symptoms were benign, and others in which, in spite of the absence of bacteria, the augmenting gravity of the affection necessitated the use of the most energetic remedies.—*Lancet*, Feb. 19, 1881.

Midwifery and Gynæcology.

The Distance between the Fontanelles as an Index of the Size of the Fœtal Head.

Dr. J. MANDELSTAM has published in the *Archiv für Gynäkologie* the results of an investigation into the relation which the distance between the anterior and posterior fontanelles bears to the other dimensions of the fœtal head. This measurement—viz., the distance between the fontanelles—is one which may be estimated before the head has entered the pelvis; and if its relation to the degree of ossification and the size of the head be constant, it is obvious that it may be made to give us information of great value in deciding as to the best course to follow in the management of a particular labour. Fehling has shown that there is a relation between the size of the anterior fontanelle and the horizontal circumference of the head; but this knowledge is of little use in practice because the over-lapping of the bones during labour alters the size of the fontanelle. It has also been shown that there is a relation between the distance from the anterior to the posterior fontanelle and the length of the child; but the latter is not a very important factor in the mechanism of labour. Dr. Mandelstam has therefore set himself to ascertain whether the distance between the fontanelles bears the same constant relation to those diameters of the fœtal head upon which the ease or difficulty of delivery chiefly depends. As yet he has only commenced the subject. He very properly approached the problem in its simplest form. He measured children's heads three or four days after birth, when the overlapping of the bones and swelling of the soft parts had had time to disappear. He has examined ninety-eight heads, and the results lead him to the following conclusions: That there is a direct proportion between the development of the child and the size of its head, on the one hand, and the distance between the anterior and posterior fontanelles, on the other; if the distance between the fontanelles be great, a large head and a well-developed child may be expected. Should a larger number of observations confirm this statement, we shall have, in the distance between the fontanelles, a datum from which to judge of the amount of mechanical hindrance to delivery which the child will offer; and in the present uncertainty of all other criteria, this is not to be underrated. How far it is possible, at the bedside, to properly measure this distance, Dr. Mandelstam at present refrains from stating; but he believes that a practised accoucheur can in many cases, even when the head is high up, feel the sagittal suture in its whole extent, and therefore form a tolerably accurate judgment upon its length. We feel sure that all who are interested in obstetrics as a science will agree with Dr. Mandelstam as to the uncertainty attending the judgment we are at present able to form, in the early stages of labour, as to the size and compressibility of the head; and we hope that he will continue his researches, and give us definite criteria by which to go.—*Med. Times and Gazette*, Feb. 19, 1881.

Pregnancy and the Acute Infectious Diseases.

A recent clinical lecture of Dr. RUNGE has been devoted to a recapitulation of what is known as to the mutual relations of pregnancy and the acute infectious diseases. It may not be without interest and instruction to our readers if we glean from Dr. Runge's lecture its most important points.

The frequency of abortion, or premature labour, in the acute infectious diseases varies according to the disease (the prognosis for the child being worst in smallpox and in cholera), the character of the epidemic, and (especially in typhoid fever) the treatment. The process of abortion is much the same as when it takes place from other causes, except that in some diseases, notably typhus and smallpox, there is apt to be unusual hemorrhage. In the later stages of pregnancy, premature delivery is generally without complications.

In considering the causes of fœtal death in these cases it must in the first place be asserted that none of these diseases have any special lethal effect upon the fœtus. The death of the infant is due to the concurrence of a number of unfavourable conditions, some of which we know, others we do not know. First, the effect of temperature. In all conditions attended with fever the fœtus runs a risk which is proportional to the height and duration of the pyrexia ; and where these are extreme, it dies from what may with accuracy be called "heat-stroke." As the mother's temperature rises, the beats of the fœtal heart increase in frequency, and the child's movements become more active. A maternal temperature of 42° or 42.5° C. (about 108° Fahr.) appears to be absolutely fatal to the child. Risk begins at 40° C. (104° Fahr.). Dr. Runge has confirmed these clinical observations by experiments upon animals.

Next, the effect of asphyxia. It has been clinically ascertained that in diseases interfering with the respiration or circulation the fœtus often dies, and its death is preceded by retardation of the heart's action and discharge of meconium —signs which indicate death from asphyxia. Dr. Runge has performed some experiments on animals which afford exact demonstration of the fact that fœtal asphyxia is thus caused. He opened the abdomen of a pregnant rabbit, and took out one or more embryos, inclosed in their membranes and with their placentæ, and put them in a solution of chloride of sodium. Then, having closed the uterus and abdomen, he killed the animal by suffocation. He found that the embryos which had been taken from the mother and put in the chloride of sodium solution, lived ; while those still in connection with the mother while she was being suffocated, died. The inference he draws is, of course, that those taken out of the mother and put in the saline fluid were simply deprived of oxygen, and recovered when oxygen was given them ; while those retained in connection with the mother were not only deprived of oxygen, but were poisoned with carbonic acid. It has been found clinically that great anæmia leads to fœtal death. This is due to deficiency in the supply of oxygen.

The third condition which helps to bring about fœtal death is the direct transmission of infectious matter from the mother to the child. This is not so satisfactorily proved as could be wished. All the experimental investigations that have been made tend to show that no molecular contagion can pass the walls of the placental villi. In relapsing fever, for instance, the spirillum is never found in the fœtal blood, and mothers suffering from this disease often bear healthy children. On the other hand, patients with variola have borne children suffering from the same disease. It has also been asserted that when women advanced in pregnancy have been successfully vaccinated, the fœtus has proved insusceptible to the vaccine virus. This, however, needs further confirmation. Mothers suffering from ague have sometimes borne children with large spleens. With these exceptions, there is no evidence of the transference of any acute infectious disease from mother to child. Even in these such communication is rare.

As to the fourth mode in which these diseases affect utero-gestation—viz., by causing changes in the placenta—little is known. Changes in the endometrium occur in cholera and in typhus, and it is to be presumed that were a patient pregnant such changes would affect the placenta.

The conditions which lead to the premature expulsion of living children in these diseases seem to be the same. in kind as those which in some cases lead to fœtal death. It has been found, by experiment, that deprivation of oxygen, or cutting off the blood-supply, leads to uterine contraction ; and that prolonged pyrexia also increases the irritability of the uterus. The reason why in some cases the fœtus dies, but in others is expelled prematurely, though living, appears to be, that where the injurious conditions mentioned rapidly reach a great height, the fœtus is killed; but where their onset is slow, the infant is expelled before the state of things has become such as is incompatible with its vitality.

Hemorrhage into the decidua or placenta will occur to most as a probable cause of abortion in such diseases as are associated with a tendency to hemorrhage. But there is this difficulty about admitting it to be such: that we cannot yet separate the cases in which hemorrhage is a cause from those in which it is a consequence of abortion. Hemorrhagic inflammation of the endometrium, leading to destruction of that tissue, has been found by Slavjansky after death from cholera.

Dr. Runge concludes his lecture with a plea in favour of the experimental method of studying physiology and pathology, and laments that the majority of those engaged in the study of obstetrics and gynæcology busy themselves more with operative technicalities than with the microscope, with chemical analysis, or with the vivisector's knife. It is to be regretted that sentimental legislation obliges English workers in this and other fields to depend upon other countries for the invaluable information which is only to be obtained from experiments on living animals, and of which the experiments of Dr. Runge that we have just quoted are a sample. Dr. Runge's work cannot fail to be fruitful in practical results. He indicates some; but as they are only suggestions we refrain from quoting them.—*Med. Times and Gazette*, Feb. 26, 1881.

———

Spinal Paralysis in New-born Children.

LITZMANN has contributed to the *Archiv für Gynäkologie* a valuable paper on the above obscure subject. Attention was first drawn to the occurrence of deformities due to spastic rigidity of more or less extensive groups of muscles, and probably caused by lesions of the central nervous system during delivery, by Dr. W. J. Little. His cases, however, were mostly those of children from one to ten years of age, and therefore it was impossible for him to make any precise statement as to the cause or nature of the initial lesion. Since then little has been done at the subject. Litzmann records a case of his own, in which a full-term child presented by the feet in a slightly contracted pelvis. Some traction on the foot was needed to effect delivery. When this traction was begun, the reflex movements of the leg were active; but while it was being pulled upon, a slight cracking sound was twice heard, and the reflex irritability of the foot ceased. The child was born living; but both lower extremities were found to be paralyzed. On the tenth day movements of the toes were perceived. About two months after delivery, reflex irritability and sensation began to decidedly, though slightly, return; but talipes varus, which was present slightly after delivery, became more marked. No treatment was carried out (owing to the objections of the parents) till the child was eight months old. Nevertheless, movement and sensation gradually returned. At this age treatment by faradization was begun, and regularly carried out; but although the child continued to improve, yet the amelioration was not so rapid as to indicate a marked effect from the treatment. Dr. Litzmann believes that in this case the symptoms were due to a lesion of the lumbar enlargement of the cord produced during delivery. He refers to cases published by Seligmüller, Hennig, and Mauthner, which resembled his own in that there was paralysis following birth, and the children recovered. He also quotes others in which an autopsy was made. Parrot has published a case in which the spinal cord was found ruptured without discoverable injury of the spine. Gueniot and Ahlfeld record cases in which the spine was fractured. Ruge, out of 64 cases of delivery by the feet, found fracture of the spine in 8, mostly in the dorsal or cervical regions. Litzmann believes that in his own case the lesion was probably hemorrhage into the vertebral canal, due to disturbance of the circulation from pressure on the cord. He states that out of 161 autopsies on newly born children made in his clinique, the vertebral canal was opened 81 times, and in 33 of these hemorrhage into the canal was found, in 19 cases the extravasations being of considerable amount. In 23 the blood was wholly external to the dura mater, in 4 also in the arachnoid sac, and in 1 also in the sub-arachnoid space; it was 4 times only in the arachnoid cavity, and once only in the sub-arachnoid space; in none was there any injury to the canal itself. In the cases in which the blood was found in the arachnoid and sub-arachnoid cavities, there was also intra-cranial hemorrhage: 23 of these children were full term, 10 premature; 13 were born dead, and 20 (15 at term, 5 premature) were born alive—all of them head-presentations; 5 of these died within twenty-four hours (4 of them being premature), 12 between the second and tenth day, and the others at the fifteenth, sixteenth, and twenty-eighth day respectively. Extravasations in the substance of the cord were never found. Billard, however, has described changes (softening and disorganization) of parts of the brain and spinal cord in newly born children who were paralyzed.—*Med. Times and Gazette*, Feb. 26, 1881.

———

Vaginitis Exfoliativa and Dysmenorrhœa Membranacea.

Vaginitis exfoliativa, or exfoliation of the epithelial lining of the vagina, is not an affection frequently observed; yet several cases of it have been recorded, and in some of these it was associated with membranous dysmenorrhœa. In a paper in the current number of the *Archiv. für Gynakologie*, Dr. COHNSTEIN describes an interesting case of this disease which was associated with severe dysmenorrhœa, but apparently not of the membranous kind. The chief interest of the paper, however, lies not in this case, but in the part of it devoted to membranous dysmenorrhœa, and more especially in the attempt therein made to explain the etiology of this form of menstrual disorder. Like most disorders of which we possess little real knowledge, membranous dysmenorrhœa has been the occasion of much theorizing, rather more theorizing than observing—some of it baseless and purely fanciful, and some of it with a show of reason. The attempt made in the paper referred to is quite refreshing in these days, when attention is concentrated upon local changes and mechanism, for it looks for the cause of the disease, not in the uterus or ovaries themselves, but in the general conditions of the system. Indeed, the author maintains that membranous dysmenorrhœa is not the result of local changes but of general disease. In support of this view he brings forward, in the first place, reasons for not regarding membranous dysmenorrhœa as a local affection. They are: 1. In by far the greatest number of cases of metritis, chronic catarrh of the uterus, tumours, etc., there is no expulsion of membranes. 2. Women who present no discoverable change in the sexual organs suffer from membranous dysmenorrhœa. 3. Of sixty-two cases collected, the author finds general disorders three times more frequent than local disease. 4. Cases are known in which a decidua menstrualis has been extruded without suffering. Such cases indicate that a general cause brings about the condition, and dysmenorrhœa is often only incidental. 5. Local treatment of membranous dysmenorrhœa is usually not followed by any good result; sometimes it produces more evil than good. Having given the above reasons for regarding dysmenorrhœa membranacea as not the result of local change, the author proceeds to give his reasons for believing in a causal connection between hysteria and the disorder, and they are the following : 1. The frequent coincidence of a slight degree of hysteria with nervous dysmenorrhœa. 2. Dysmenorrhœa membranacea is not rarely associated with hereditary troubles. 3. In the course of hysteria the most various anomalies of secretion and excretion occur. 4. The occasional complete disappearance of the membrane, and its return after longer or shorter intervals ; such irregularity cannot be due to a disorder of the genital organs. 5. The vaginismus and the suffering lasting through or only coming on during the intermenstrual interval, without apparent disease of the sexual organs. 6. In sixty-two cases collected by the author, in twenty the expulsion of membranes was said to be due to a local cause, while in forty-two it was ascribed to general disorders—as hysteria, anæmia, chlorosis, chronic dysentery, etc. Heartily sympathizing as we do with the author in his attempt to elucidate the etiology of membranous dysmenorrhœa by having recourse to a wider base than the sexual organs, yet we cannot help feeling that with two exceptions the two sets of reasons given—those against regarding the disease as of local, as well as those for regarding it as of general origin—have no bearing upon the question. They prove nothing. The two exceptions are :—1. Women who present no discernible change in the sexual organs suffer from membranous dysmenorrhœa. Had we been able to state that women who present no change suffer, the author's first position would be proved, but it is well known that our means of investigation can discover only very coarse changes, while many even of these elude our search. 2. Were it true that two-thirds of the cases are due to general conditions, the author's second position would be a just inference—that is, that membranous dysmenorrhœa is due to general conditions. But, as a matter of fact, the general conditions presented by two-thirds of the cases were not those now described as the causes of the affection. In some of them, it is true, they may have been so described, but by no means in all. So long as our knowledge of the physiology of the female sexual organs remains in a state of uncertainty and doubt, we cannot expect that the pathology of the same structure will be better understood. The investigation both of the physiology and pathology of these organs is surrounded with peculiar difficulties, and this may be excuse enough for some theorizing upon them ; but we feel sure that we cannot arrive at a correct pathology until we arrive at a correct physiology, and any theory of the pathology or etiology of the uterus and ovaries which does not start from physiology will prove true, if at all, by accident only. Here we think Dr. Cohnstein has erred, and consequently missed his mark. We think with him that dysmenorrhœa membranacea has in many instances at bottom a general condition for a cause, though we do not believe it to be hysteria ; that condition produces dysmenorrhœa by organic changes in the uterus resulting from it, though these changes may elude our means of research.—*Lancet*, Feb. 12, 1881.

Chronic Complete Inversion of the Uterus.

Dr. ROGERS, at a recent meeting of the Obstetrical Society of London (*Lancet*, Feb. 5, 1881), related a case of Chronic Complete Inversion of the Uterus, successfully treated by sustained elastic pressure. S. B——, aged twenty-nine, had a child two years ago. Delivery was followed by great flooding, and menorrhagia has continued more or less ever since. On admission a tumour was felt in the vagina, as large as a turkey's egg ; a ring encircled its neck, but the sound could not be passed more than a line or two above this. On April 28, Dr. Aveling's double-curved repositor was applied, and adjusted by Dr. Aveling. After twenty-four hours the strings were tightened, the patient being very comfortable. About sixteen hours later she felt great relief ; something had given way, and the strings had become loose. On examination the repositor was found within the uterus high up, and was removed without difficulty. The uterus was completely restored.

Dr. AVELING stated that, since he invented his repositor last year, five cases had been successfully treated by it.

Medical Jurisprudence and Toxicology.

Diagnosis of Blood Stains by the Micrometric Method.

In a lengthy letter to *Gaillard's Medical Journal* (Jan. 1881), Dr. J. G. RICHARDSON presents the following summary of the final results of his studies upon the measurement of red blood corpuscles and its bearing upon the diagnosis of blood stains.

1st. That in unaltered blood stains as ordinarily produced by the sprinkling of drops of blood upon clothing, leather, wood, metal, etc., we can by tinting with aniline or iodine distinguish human blood corpuscles from those of the ox, pig, horse, sheep and goat, wherever the question is narrowed down by the circumstances of the case to these limits.

2d. By the method I have devised we can measure the size of the corpuscles and apply the two corroborative tests of tincture of guaiacum with ozonized ether and of spectrum analysis to a single particle of blood-clot weighing less than one fifteen-thousandth part of a grain, a quantity barely visible to the naked eye.

3d. Hence, when an ignorant criminal attempts to explain suspicious blood spots upon his clothing, weapons, etc., by attributing them to the ox, pig, sheep, or goat, or to any of the birds used for food, we can, under favourable circumstances, *absolutely disprove* his false statement and materially aid the cause of justice by breaking down his lying defence, even if twenty years have elapsed.

4th. But if the accused person ascribes the tell-tale blood to a dog, an elephant, a capybara, or any other animal in Dr. Woodward's list, it is useless to attempt to dispute his story, on microscopical evidence as to the size of the blood corpuscles.

5th. In cases of innocent persons wrongfully accused of murder, and really stained with the blood of an ox, pig, or sheep, testimony of experts founded upon measurement of the corpuscles would be valuable, but less conclusive, because under certain circumstances human blood corpuscles may *shrink* to the size of those of the ox, whilst under no known conditions do ox or pig corpuscles *expand* to the magnitude of those in human blood.

6th. In order to do away with ingenious objections of lawyers that the murdered person may have been affected with some disease which altered the size of his blood disks, or that the articles of clothing, etc., upon which the stains were deposited had produced chemically or otherwise some similar change in their magnitudes, it is very important to obtain promptly, stains from the fresh blood of the victim made in the presence of witnesses upon portions of the prisoner's clothing or weapons analogous to those upon which suspicious red spots are found when he is arrested. When this cannot be done spots of the murdered person's blood sprinkled on white paper, and fragments of his lungs and kidneys should be carefully preserved, the former by rapid drying and the latter by preservation in diluted alcohol. These little precautions, which may in any instance prove to be of infinite importance, should be earnestly impressed upon coroners, district attorneys, and policemen throughout the civilized world.

MEDICAL NEWS.

The Dangers of Diseased Meats.

At the present time popular attention is so generally aroused to the possiblity of infection from unsound meat, by the promulgation of a French edict against the importation from America of trichinous pork, and the rumored embargo upon our meat in England on account of an imaginary epidemic of "hog cholera," in the Western States, that the moment seems an opportune one for discussing what may prove a far more serious danger to ourselves from diseased animals used as food, viz., the transmission of consumption by the flesh and milk of cattle affected with tuberculosis.

Since it is estimated by competent authorities that only about one-fourth of the cases of phthisis in the human race can be traced to hereditary influence, it has long been supposed by medical philosophers that there must be some unknown predisposing cause to the formation of tubercle, which, acting in concert with the great exciting cause in our climate of atmospheric vicissitude, determines the advent of consumption in many of the instances which go to make up the remaining three-fourths of the mortality from this fatal disease.

The experiments of Villemin and Burdon Sanderson in 1865, seemed to show that (contrary to the previously received opinion) tubercle was easily inoculated, especially upon rabbits and guinea-pigs, but they were, as is well known, corrected by further observations which demonstrated the curious fact that the production of a suppurating wound by the introduction of an inert substance, such as a fragment of paper or India-rubber, beneath the skin of one of these animals, was often followed by general tuberculosis. Some more recent investigations of Prof. Chauveau, of the Lyons Veterinary School, are so devised as to eliminate this disturbing element of a surgical operation, and appear to indicate that tubercle can be readily conveyed by the ingestion of tubercular animal tissues. Chauveau purchased upon one occasion four healthy calves, made them each swallow about an ounce of tubercular matter from an old cow's lung, and repeated the dose to three of them at short intervals. Within a month these three presented a miserable aspect as compared with the fourth, which had escaped infection, and when killed, they showed on post-mortem examination a condition of general tuberculosis, the local lesions of the intestines and mesenteric glands, constituting *tabes mesenterica*, being particularly well marked. The lungs were studded with caseous nodules and the bronchial glands were involved, but the spleen and kidneys were not affected.

Prof. Orth, of Göttingen, so well known by his excellent work on Pathological Anatomy, has very lately published his opinion deduced from his own experiments, which corroborate those of Chauveau and others, that the transmissibility of tuberculosis from one creature to another in this way is now *proved* to occur, and that it is highly probable human beings have often been thus infected from the brute creation. In Prof. Orth's investigations, out of fifteen animals which were fed with tuberculous material from a diseased cow, nine were infected and four died. Autopsies of the diseased beasts revealed a general tuberculosis of nearly all the organs.

Nor is this dangerous infective property confined to the meat of diseased animals, for Prof. Bollinger, who is associated with Prof. von Pettenkofer in the celebrated Hygienic Laboratory of the University of Munich, asserts that the milk of such creatures has a pre-eminently contagious influence, and reproduces tubercular disease in others to which it is administered. According to his experiments even boiling the milk does not destroy its injurious properties in this respect.

With such a probability as these various investigations establish, that consumption, the most dreaded malady of northern latitudes, and the disease which leads the mortality lists of most large cities, is often propagated by the ingestion of meat and milk from tuberculous animals, it is surely time that energetic efforts should be made by our legislators for the prevention of traffic in food which is so dangerously diseased. Dr. Noah Cressy, V. S., of Hartford, Connecticut, several years since called attention to this important subject, and in a recent paper in the State Board of Health Report ably urges that steps should at once be taken to stamp out the affection from among our cattle, with the reasonable hope that by breeding only from stocks of acknowledged purity, combined with proper sanitary care of the animals (especially the utter abandonment of stall and swill feeding), we might afterwards be able to preserve our herds free from taint of this disease. Of course only the most earnest and persistent trial of this plan could be successful, and in many cases it would probably be advisable to completely destroy the stables which had become infected by sheltering animals suffering from the malady. A necessity for this extreme precaution is indicated by the results of observations made by Dr. Grad, of Alsace, who on visiting a farmer in his neighbourhood was informed that annually for five years one of his cows had died of consumption in a certain stall. In order to test the question of local infection, Dr. Grad, with the consent of the owner, selected a vigorous three-year-old heifer of perfectly healthy pedigree, and placed her in the supposed fatal stall. For a time the animal continued well, but after calving, a slight cough set in and this gradually increased, emaciation took place, until when inspected a year later the creature was a mere shadow of her former self, and presented all the symptoms of advanced tuberculosis. In this case it is naturally to be inferred that the malady was transmitted by the ingestion of tuberculous matter, which had been coughed up on the stall by animals which had previously occupied it. Nevertheless, it is highly probable that, in some instances at least, the infection is conveyed to a healthy creature from a sick one, especially in the latter stages of the complaint, by inhalation of the breath charged with tuberculous matter. Dr. Tappeiner's experiments, which are very instructive upon this important point, are as follows. He caused eleven puppies to inhale fine particles of tuberculous matter distributed through the air of the room in which they were confined, by the aid of a steam atomizer. Within forty days, when the animals were killed, ten of them showed well-marked miliary tubercle in both lungs, and, although such a series of experiments is alone by no means conclusive, its results are so corroborated by occasional events in the experience of most physicians of large practice in pulmonary diseases, that no system of prophylaxis against phthisis can at present afford to ignore their teachings.

—

Indiana State Board of Health.—A bill has passed the Indiana Legislature authorizing the Governor to appoint a State Board of Health.

—

Treatment of Extra-uterine Pregnancy.—At the meeting of the Medical Society of the County of New York held Feb. 28, 1881, Dr. WILLIAM T. LUSK read a paper upon this subject in which he advocated the use of the faradic current, according to the method proposed by Dr. Allen, of Philadelphia, for the destruction of the fœtus, which he prefers to leave for absorption, unless its presence excite too grave local and general symptoms, when laparotomy, conducted antiseptically, should be resorted to.

—

Index Catalogue of the Library of the Surgeon General's Office.—The final action of Congress, looking to the continued publication of this work, has resulted in the appropriation of $10,000 for the publishing of vol. ii., which will, it is estimated, about cover the cost of type-setting and stereotyping; for its issue we will have to possess our souls with patience until another appropriation can be had. In the mean time, much can be effected if the members of the profession will exercise their personal influence upon members of Congress in favour of liberal appropriations for the publication of this important work.

—

International Sanitary Conference.—The diplomatic sanitarians adjourned March 2d *sine die*. What they did is yet to be made public by the State Department; it is said that they did some good work, and held a number of dignified and protracted meetings. It will be interesting to see the result. If sanitation gets so mixed in an American Congress, what will it be in a Congress of diplomats? Diplomacy is not always healthy, and sanitary measures certainly must at times violate diplomacy to be effective.

—

National Board of Health.—Congress, after considerable discussion, during the last days of its session, appropriated $50,000 for the use of the National

Board of Health, but with the proviso that no other moneys heretofore appropriated and remaining unexpended should be made use of by the Board.

The Bad Odours of New York.—The committee of the N. Y. State Board of Health on effluvia and nuisances, has recently held meetings to inquire into the causes of the pestilential odours emanating from Hunter's Pt., Brooklyn.

At a meeting held Feb. 26, several bitter complaints were read from residents of Murray Hill and the adjoining fashionable quarters of New York. Dr. Chandler, President of the N. Y. Health Board, attributed the odours to the oil refineries, varnish, fertilizers, chemical, and ink factories, and to the sugar refineries. He believed such changes in the mode of manufacture could be introduced as would prevent the development of the bad odours.

At a subsequent meeting, held March 5, letters were read from a number of prominent physicians of the east side of the city complaining of the Hunter's Point nuisances. Residents of Brooklyn also testified to the offensive character of the odours. Dr. J. H. Raymond, Sanitary Superintendent of the Brooklyn Board of Health, said the Board would be glad to have the State Committee investigate nuisances, but that the Board would be capable as it was thoroughly desirous of effecting the necessary changes, if the laws defining its powers could be enforced.

Prosecution of Unregistered Practitioners in New York.—The New York County Medical Society has authorized its Censors to employ counsel for the purpose of prosecuting irregular and unregistered practitioners.

Graduates in Medicine in 1881.

Jefferson Medical College (Phila.)	205
University of Pennsylvania	110
Bellevue Hospital Medical College (N. Y.) . . .	117
University of the City of New York	191
University of Nashville and Vanderbilt University . .	168
Nashville Medical College	53
Indiana Medical College (Indianapolis)	85
College of Physicians and Surgeons (Baltimore) . .	154
University of Louisville	100
Louisville Medical College	54
Hospital College of Medicine (Louisville)	24
University of Maryland	73
Michigan College of Medicine (Detroit)	28
University of Buffalo	48
Medical College of Ohio (Cincinnati)	103
Cincinnati College of Medicine and Surgery . . .	30
Miami Medical College (Cincinnati)	34
Rush Medical College (Chicago)	172

Medical Society of the State of New York.—The seventy-fifth annual meeting of this society was held at Albany, February 1, 2, and 3, Dr. William H. Bailey, President, in the chair. A large number of excellent papers were read.

The following resolutions were adopted.

" *Resolved*, that the Medical Society of the State of New York advises the various county medical societies that form its constituency, to endeavour to secure the coöperation of the other incorporated county and district medical societies, throughout the State, in the enforcement of the 'Act to regulate the licensing of physicians and surgeons,' passed May 29, 1880.

"*Resolved*, that, in the opinion of this Society, it is desirable for the legislature to thoroughly amend and revise the laws of this State in regard to the office and duties of coroners, and that the Society would recommend, for their consideration, the recent statute act adopted by the State of Massachusetts.

" *Resolved*, that a special committee of five be appointed, by the President, to be designated a 'Committee on the Code of Ethics,' whose duty it shall be to consider the question of desirable changes in the code, and who shall present to the Society, at the annual meeting in 1882, such suggestions on this subject as they may decide upon."

The President appointed, as this special committee, Drs. Wm. C. Wey, of Elmira, C. R. Agnew, of New York, S. O. Vanderpoel, of Albany, Wm. S. Ely, of Rochester, and H. G. Piffard, of New York. A resolution offered by direction of the New York County Medical Society, to the effect that the State Society investigate the propriety of making a change in the law preventing the disclosure in court of any information obtained by physicians in their professional character from their patients, was referred to the Committee on Legislation with instructions to report in 1882.

The following officers were elected for the ensuing year: President, Abram Jacobi, M.D., of New York; Vice President, Dr. William Goran, of Stony Point; Secretary, Dr. Wm. Manlius Smith, of Manlius. Drs. T. F. Cock, of New York, and Jos. C. Hutchison, of Brooklyn, were appointed delegates to the International Medical Congress to be held in London, in August. The society adjourned to meet at Albany on the first Tuesday in February, 1882.

———

Primary Cancer of the Pancreas.—Dr. KENNIG reports, in the *Petersburg Med. Woch.* (February 5), a minute history of the case of this rare affection occurring in a woman aged fifty-three.

———

Gastric Remittent Fever.—In confirmation of the views respecting this disease advanced by Dr. F. Peyre Porcher in the January number of the *American Journal of the Medical Sciences*, we publish the following from Dr. D. I. CAM, of Asheville, N. C. :—

"The disease is essentially ' *gastric.*' The bowels, if at all, are only slightly involved. It is an *irritation, not* an inflammation. This is the true pathological state. My study of this disease, which has been deep and extensive, does not lead me to agreement with the view expressed, or at least suggested, by Dr. Charles West, that it is the child's typhoid fever. There is one sign of the disease which I consider as nearly *pathognomonic,* so nearly invariable is it. This is the child lying with the eyes obstinately closed, only opening them when aroused by being shaken or loudly spoken to.

"As regards the treatment, I yet pursue substantially the course which you mention; but I now use bismuth and oxalate of cerium every three or four hours, considering these as among the best means we have of allaying gastrointestinal irritation ; and I use injections of warm water and assafœtida p. r. n. to move the bowels—not insisting upon *purgation* as an important part of the treatment. The mortality must be infinitesimally small. If I have ever lost a case, I cannot remember it.

" The disease is as common *here* as it is on the seaboard or elsewhere."

———

University of Pennsylvania. Installation of the Provost.—On the 22d of February, at the Academy of Music, in the presence of a large and imposing assemblage Dr. William Pepper was duly installed, by the Governor of Pennsylvania, as Provost of the University. In his installation address Dr. Pepper considered the past progress and plans for the future of the University. In the evening a reception was given to the Provost by the Penn Club.

Vienna Medical Faculty.—Professor Czerny has been elected to fill the chair left vacant by Prof. Dumreicher, and Prof. Kaposi to succeed Prof. Hebra.

College of Physicians and Surgeons, Baltimore.—The faculty of this institution have decided to lengthen their curriculum to six months, and to obtain the doctorate a student must have read medicine under a preceptor for one year and have attended two six months' courses.

Value of the Dentaphone.—Mr. EDMUND TRIBEL, Superintendent of the Royal Asylum for the Deaf and Dumb in Berlin, has made a series of extensive and critical experiments with the dentaphone as an aid to hearing, with entirely negative results. He states (*Archives of Otology*, Dec. 1880) that where deaf-mutes are concerned, the dentaphone, in its present condition at least, cannot be put to any practical use, not even as a means of advancing articulation, and he believes that the instrument cannot give any noteworthy assistance to any one whose hearing is in the least defective. These results agree entirely with those obtained by competent observers in this country.

Health of New York.—The number of cases of contagious diseases reported to the New York Health Board, for Feb. 1881, are as follows:—

Smallpox	62
Scarlet fever	657
Diphtheria	402
Measles	169
Typhoid fever	23

Smallpox has somewhat increased during the last month. Eight cases were removed to the Riverside Hospital, Blackwell's Island, on March 10th, and seven cases were reported on March 11th. The officials of the Vaccinating Department of the New York Health Bureau are vaccinating large numbers in the tenement houses. The department vaccinated 48,000 persons in 1880. The virus employed is bovine, and comes from calves kept on a farm at Clifton, New Jersey.

The mortality of the present season is unusually large. On March 11th 122 deaths were reported, while the number for the corresponding week of previous years was below 100. Although the various contagious diseases, as well as pneumonia, prevail more extensively than is usual, the increased mortality can hardly be accounted for in that way. The computations of the Bureau of Vital Statistics rest upon the last census, while the present population of the city is believed to have been largely augmented by transient visitors, from West and South. The total mortality for the five weeks ending March 5th was 3520, and that for the five previous weeks 3540.

At a meeting of the New York Academy of Medicine, held March 17, 1881, Dr. A. L. Loomis called the attention of the Academy to the largely increased death-rate of the city. He said: "All of us have noted the increased malignity of diseases, both acute and chronic, recently, and we have been alarmed by the increase of the mortality rate in our city. Old diseases seem to have taken new forms of violence, and fevers of a new type have spread through the city, whose symptoms and development put them beyond our power of classification. Those who have had patients advanced in years who are suffering from illness of this new nature have been forced into the greatest anxiety, for what before was little feared now proves dangerous. What is the cause? Have the diseases themselves taken a new direction, or is there some new danger among us that deserves to be discovered and removed?

"It is our duty to answer these questions if we can, and to answer them promptly. From my personal inquiry into the subject I am led to lay down the following four propositions:—

"*First.* That the city must now be considered as in a malarial condition.

"*Second.* That our sewerage system is very defective.

"*Third.* That large quantities of animal and vegetable matter are undergoing decomposition in our streets.

"*Fourth.* That nearly all diseases are now more malignant and fatal than they have been in my experience in the last twenty years.

"I believe that the factors I have named are responsible for the low condition of the public health; nor does it seem strange to me at all that there is such a high percentage of mortality in this city. I predict that, if the causes referred to are not removed, an epidemic of great proportions will certainly result."

Dr. Loomis then offered the following resolutions, which were seconded by Dr. Austin Flint, and unanimously adopted:—

"*Whereas*, it is our opinion that the uncleanly condition of the streets of this city is an efficient factor in increasing the malignity of many diseases, and thus contributes to the present alarming death-rate:

"*Resolved*, that, acting under a deep sense of our responsibility as members of a profession whose chief duty it is to check the development of disease, we earnestly warn the public against the danger of allowing this state of things to continue."

———

Anti-vivisection Bill.—Mr. Bergh has again presented to the New York Legislature the same anti-vivisection bill which he endeavoured to have passed a year ago. The Committee on Public Health, to which it was referred, have reported adversely to it.

———

Convalescents' Home.—This home, situated at No. 433 E. 118th St., New York, was organized last year with the object of providing a temporary retreat for convalescents recently discharged from the hospitals but still unable to resume their usual occupation. 47 patients were treated in it during the past year.

———

Health of Charleston, S. C.—Dr. F. PEŸRE PORCHER, of Charleston, informs us, under date of March 18th, that a form of influenza prevails at present in that city and State. It is characterized by fever, catarrhal symptoms, cough, some pains in the head and limbs—sometimes by vomiting and redness of the tongue. He has noticed in two cases marked swelling and suffusion of the face. There is no eruption, and there is an absence generally of the severe pains and prostration which accompanied the Dengue of last summer. Sometimes the attacks are pretty severe, the fever being high, with some head symptoms, dizziness, etc. It has prevailed in Columbia and elsewhere, and we have heard of a number of cases on the Ashley River, ten miles from the city.

Scarlet fever exists to some extent in Charleston, and an occasional case of diphtheria, but the latter has almost completely disappeared. Though the children in the public schools are all being vaccinated, there is no smallpox.

Library of the College of Physicians of Philadelphia.—Dr. Frank Woodbury has been elected Librarian, vice Dr. Robert Bridges, resigned. The making
of the Card Catalogue has been placed in charge of an assistant to the Librarian,
and is now progressing satisfactorily.

—

Retrogression in Medical Education.—The Faculty of the Bellevue Hospital
Medical College introduced, for the session of 1880–'81, important changes in
the curriculum of instruction and in the requirements for graduation. The preliminary term was abolished, and the regular winter session was extended to six
months. Attendance upon three winter sessions was made obligatory. Students
were required during the two first years to attend all the lectures, didactic and
clinical, and at the end of the first and second years to pass examinations in
Chemistry, Anatomy, Physiology, Materia Medica, and Therapeutics. An examination in these branches having been passed, the third year was to be devoted
to the practical departments of Medicine, Surgery, and Obstetrics. These
changes were made by the Faculty with entire unanimity and with the expectation that a considerable pecuniary sacrifice would be demanded on the part of its
members, who were actuated solely by a desire to secure a higher grade of professional acquirements for the graduates of the college.

In a circular just issued, the Faculty states that "The experience of the session
of 1880–'81 has led them reluctantly to the conclusion, that to persist in the
requirement of attendance during three courses will be to incur a risk, as regards
the interests of the college, which they do not feel justified in assuming; and the
purpose of this announcement is to state that, after the present session of 1880–'81,
attendance during a third session will be optional and not obligatory. This college, like most American medical colleges, is self-sustaining; and the special
provisions for instruction, which have been and will continue to be maintained,
call for a large expenditure of money as well as of time and labour. With an
undiminished desire to continue the requirement of the three sessions, and with
not less willingness than heretofore to make whatever personal sacrifices may be
necessary, the Faculty feel obliged, by a proper regard for the prosperity and
usefulness of the college, to return to the requirements for graduation which were
in force prior to the session of 1880–'81. In making the changes introduced
during this session, it was foreseen that, a large proportion of the students in this
college coming from distant parts of the United States, the necessary expenses
of spending three winters in the city of New York would render difficult or impossible the attendance of many who would otherwise join the classes. Many
students, of course, would be led to attend other colleges which require only two
sessions for graduation. It was hoped, however, that the progressive movement
of the Bellevue Hospital Medical College would secure approval and co-operation on the part of the medical profession sufficient to render the change feasible.
In so far as a judgment can be formed from the present session, the profession is
not prepared to sustain the movement.

"In announcing a return to their original requirements for graduation, the
Faculty desire to state that all the new additions to the curriculum will be retained. It is not proposed to recede in the least from these. Students will have
the same opportunities for practical exercise in the different departments as those
enjoyed by the class of 1880–'81. For those who choose to attend during three
sessions, the provisions as respects examinations in the elementary branches at
the end of the second year, and an exclusive devotion to the practical departments during the third year, will be continued. To all students who are able to
do so, now, as hitherto, attendance during three years is strongly recommended;
and, from the number of those who have already matriculated with the expecta-

tion of attending three sessions, the Faculty entertained a belief that not an inconsiderable proportion of future classes will voluntarily follow their example."

Washington, D. C., Training School for Nurses.—This institution is now about completing its third session with a small but earnest class of nurses. It labours under many disadvantages in the want of funds and sufficient hospital accommodation for practical purposes, but has been recently encouraged by the interest which its active Board of Managers have succeeded in exciting among the residents of Washington, and which has resulted in an Art Loan Exhibition, the contributions to which are of a high order of merit—and which is conducted by a large number of those best able by their personal influence to insure success in the undertaking. The exhibition bids fair to prove a pecuniary gain, and a prize having been offered for the best essay on nursing, already 27 contestants have presented themselves.

A New Hospital for Washington.—A bill for the establishment of a general hospital that shall be independent of all private interests, or of sectarian influences, was accepted by the U. S. Senate Committee with a recommendation on their part to appropriate $125,000 for its benefit, but unfortunately was not put into proper shape until the last hours of Congress, and so died in travail. Its projectors, however, are sanguine of final success, and will be ready with their bill to push the matter at the opening of the next Congress.

Providence Hospital, Washington, D. C.—This hospital, which, up to the present time, has been for many years the only one possessed by the District, which could be made available for the general treatment of the better class of patients, is, it seems, controlled entirely by Sisters of Charity, the medical board occupying a very insignificant position in the exercise of its own authority in the treatment of disease, and none in the management of the hospital; holding their appointments at the will of the Sister-in-charge. As a natural consequence, a want of harmonious action on both sides resulted during the past winter in the enforced resignation of some, and voluntary resignation of others of the hospital staff, which fairly represented the best elements and interests of the local medical men, leaving but two men on the Board. A new staff was immediately organized which took their places—and, as a sop to Cerberus—one of the causes of complaint was removed, how effectually remains to be seen, by the appointment of a resident house physician; up to this time the rules of the Sisterhood would not permit one of the male sex to pass the night under their roof, unless he in some way required their care and attention. Sober young professional men with all their senses under control and prepared for emergencies, gave way to drunkards and debauchees.

International Medical Congress, London, 1881.—Arrangements for the approaching International Medical Congress are being energetically prosecuted by the Executive Committee. The Inaugural address will be delivered by Sir James Paget on the morning of August 3d. The following mornings will be devoted to the business of the various Sections; while the afternoons (with the exception of Saturday afternoon, which will be left free for garden parties, excursions, etc.) will be devoted to the general sessions of the Congress, at which four addresses will be given by four distinguished men of different nationalities, viz.: Prof. Huxley, on the "Connection of General Science and Medicine;" Prof. Volkmann, of Halle, on "Modern Surgery;" and Dr. John S. Billings, of Washington, on "Medical Literature;" the fourth address, to be given by a distinguished Frenchman, has not yet been definitely arranged.

The Executive Committee has announced the rules for the organization of the Congress, which " will be composed of medical men legally qualified to practise in their respective countries, who shall have inscribed their names on the Register of the Congress, and shall have taken out their tickets of admission. The subscription is fixed at one guinea, which amount is to be paid on inscription and before the commencement of attendance at the meetings. Each Member of the Congress will be entitled to a copy of the Transactions when published."

" Notices of papers, together with abstracts of the papers, to be read in any one of the sections must be sent to the Secretaries of that section before April 30, 1881. These abstracts will be regarded as strictly confidential communications, and will not be published until the meeting of the Congress. Any Member wishing to bring forward a subject not already on the programme must give notice of his intention to the Secretary-General at least twenty-one days before the opening of the Congress. The Officers of each Section will decide on the advisability of accepting any communication addressed to their Section, and also the time when it shall be made. No communication will be received which has been already published."

" No speaker is allowed more than ten minutes, with the exception of readers of papers and those who introduce debates, who may occupy fifteen."

The Reception Committee has decided upon giving an evening reception at South Kensington, and perhaps a second in the Albert Hall. The Lord Mayor of London purposes entertaining the members of the Congress at dinner at the Mansion House on August 4th.

—

Regulating the Sale of Proprietary Medicines.—We are informed that a bill has been drafted, which has received the official sanction of the New York Academy of Medicine and of the New York County Medical Society, and will be presented to the New York Legislature, requiring that the manufacture of proprietary medicines shall affix the fórmula of each nostrum to the bottle containing it, and designating a penalty to be inflicted for neglect of so doing.

—

A New Hospital for Brooklyn.—Mr. Geo. I. Seney has given $200,000 and land worth $70,000, at Seventh St. and Seventh Ave., Brooklyn, for the erection of a hospital constructed upon the cottage plan. A board of thirty-two trustees has been appointed who will superintend the erection of the new hospital.

—

Meetings of State Medical Societies will be held during the month of April as follows :—

Medical Society of Tennessee at Nashville, on Tuesday April 5th

Mississippi State Medical Association at Winona, on Wednesday April 6th.

Medical Association of State of Alabama at Montgomery, on Tuesday April 12th.

South Carolina Medical Association at Newberry, on Tuesday April 19.

California State Medical Society at San Francisco, on Wednesday April 20th.

Medical Association of Georgia at Thomasville, on Wednesday April 20th.

—

A Medical Knight.—Queen Victoria has announced her intention of conferring the honour of knighthood upon JAMES RISDON BENNETT, M.D., President of the Royal College of Physicians of London.

Literary Notes.

Henry C. Lea's Son & Co. have in preparation a "Treatise on Midwifery," by Dr. Theophilus Parvin, of Indianapolis. It will be a copiously illustrated octavo volume of about 500 pages, and will be the first systematic work on obstetrics which has emanated from an American author since the publication of the late Professor Hodge's great work in 1864. Also a "Practical Treatise on Impotence, Sterility, and allied Disorders of the Male Sexual Organs," by Dr. Samuel W. Gross. Sterility is generally ascribed to the female, and she is apt to undergo treatment therefor without consideration as to the possible existence of the defect in the male, but Dr. Gross gleans from prominent specialists in female disorders that about one-third of the cases of sterility are due to the male, and that an examination of the causes of this condition should include the male as well as the female before operations are performed upon the latter.

The same house promises early in April a volume of "Lectures on Diseases of the Nervous System, especially in Women," by Dr. S. Weir Mitchell. The subject includes the wide scope of nervous disorders of the hysterical and their treatment. The book will be illustrated with five lithographic plates, showing the intimate connection of temperature, season, and climate, with attacks of chorea. Also a "Practical Treatise on Electricity and its Applications to Medicine," by Prof. Bartholow. The scope of the work embraces electro-physics and electro-physiology as well as electro-diagnosis and electro-therapeutics.

J. B. Lippincott & Co. have just issued the second volume of Prof. Hayes Agnew's "Surgery." It is, like the first, a profusely illustrated volume of 1066 pages. The third volume, which will complete the work, is in process of rapid preparation.

William Wood & Co. have issued in their "Library Series" a volume on the "Materia Medica and Therapeutics of the Skin," by Dr. H. G. Piffard of New York; and announce a volume on the Continued Fevers, by Dr. J. C. Wilson of Philadelphia.

D. Appleton & Co. have just published the long promised new edition of Prof. Van Buren's "Lectures upon Diseases of the Rectum;" the book has been greatly enlarged and indeed largely rewritten; and announce as in preparation "The Applied Anatomy of the Nervous System," by Dr. Ambrose L. Ranney, Adjunct Prof. of Anatomy in Univ. of City of New York. The work is intended to present the latest knowledge in the anatomy and physiology of the nervous system, and to show its application in medicine and surgery.

Dr. W. F. Mittendorf, Surgeon to the New York Eye and Ear Infirmary, has issued through G. P. Putnam's Sons "A Manual on Diseases of the Eye and Ear." It forms an octavo volume of nearly 450 pages, and is illustrated with some very handsome chromo-lithographs.

A German translation of the last edition of Dr. Hamilton's "Treatise on Fractures and Dislocations" is announced by Vandenhoeclk and Ruprecht, of Göttingen.

—

Index Medicus.—Mr. F. Leypoldt, of New York, the energetic publisher of the *Index Medicus*, undaunted by the pecuniary loss entailed by its two years of publication, but with firm faith in the ultimate support of the student members of the profession, announces his intention of continuing the publication for another year, in the hope that by the expiration of that time it may be placed upon a self-supporting basis, for which it requires only two hundred additional subscribers. The *Index Medicus* is a monthly classified record of the current medical literature (including contents of medical journals and transactions) of the *world*, and is compiled under the supervision of Dr. John S. Billings, of the National Medical Library at Washington It forms, in connection with the magnificent Index Catalogue of the National Medical Library, a complete index of medical literature to date, and is of inestimable value to every intelligent student, teacher, writer, and practitioner in the profession. We trust that the members of the profession will recognize the importance of insuring the continuance of the *Index* by at once forwarding subscriptions ($6 per annum) to Mr. Leypoldt, since upon the encouragement which he *now* derives depends his ability to continue its publication after this year. The worth of the work has been so fully recognized by all who use it that its suspension could only be looked upon as a great calamity.

———

OBITUARY RECORD.—Died, at Washington, on the 23d of February, aged 50 years, GEORGE ALEXANDER OTIS, M.D., Surgeon U. S. A. Dr. Otis, who is widely known as an eminent writer on military surgery, and as the compiler of the surgical volumes of the Medical and Surgical History of the War, was born at Boston, Mass., Nov. 12, 1830; he graduated in the Arts at Princeton College and in Medicine at the University of Pennsylvania, in 1850. He then visited Europe and prosecuted his studies in London and Paris, and returning to this country he entered upon the practice of his profession at Springfield, Mass. He entered the army as surgeon of the 27th Massachusetts Volunteers in September 1861, and after the close of the war he entered the medical corps of the regular army.

Surgeon General Barnes announces his death in the following official circular:—

"It is with profound regret and a sense of loss, not only to his corps, but to the medical profession, that the death of George Alexander Otis, Surgeon and Brevet-Lieutenant-Colonel U. S. Army, is announced to the Medical Corps of the Army.   .   .   .   .

" Surgeon Otis, with his personal observations of the surgical collections abroad, brought indefatigable industry and untiring energy to the development of the surgical and anatomical collections of the Army Medical Muesum, which he has made the most valuable of their kind in the world. The compilation of the Surgical Volumes of the Medical and Surgical History of the War has placed Surgeon Otis confessedly among the most prominent contributors to surgical history.

" While on duty in this office Surgeon Otis wrote for publication no less than ten reports on subjects connected with military surgery, etc. ; among which are his most valuable and exhaustive reports on ' Excision of the Head of the Femur for Gunshot Injury,' and on ' Amputation at the Hip-joint in Military Surgery.' Of great culture, retentive memory, and with a remarkable facility of expression, he was, as a compiler and writer, conscientious in his analyses, giving his deductions from the facts before him with modesty, but decision. With such a record it is needless to speak of his zeal, his ambition, or his devotion to his profession and especially to the reputation of the corps of which he was so bright an ornament. While devoting himself to the preparation of the third and last surgical volume (now more than half completed) of the Medical and Surgical History of the War, he died in Washington February 23, 1881. His untimely death will be deeply deplored, not only by the Medical Corps of the Army, but by the whole medical profession at home and abroad.''

———

To Readers and Correspondents.—*The Editor will be happy to receive early intelligence of local events of general medical interest, or which it is desirable to bring to the notice of the profession. Local papers containing reports or news items should be marked.*

CONTENTS OF NUMBER 461.

MAY, 1881.

CLINICS.

MONTHLY ABSTRACT.

MEDICAL NEWS.

THE

MEDICAL NEWS AND ABSTRACT.

VOL. XXXIX. No. 5.   MAY, 1881.   WHOLE No. 461.

CLINICS.

Clinical Lectures.

ON AMYLOID KIDNEY.

A CLINICAL LECTURE DELIVERED AT THE GOOD SAMARITAN HOSPITAL, CINCINNATI.

BY JAMES T. WHITTAKER, A.M., M.D.,

PROFESSOR OF THEORY AND PRACTICE OF MEDICINE IN THE MEDICAL COLLEGE OF OHIO.

GENTLEMEN: You may almost read in the face of this little girl that she has chronic disease of the kidneys. The partial paraplegia which you see still exists, shows that she has also some lesion of the spinal cord, and as nearly all such lesions at this age depend upon caries of the vertebræ, that is, upon Pott's disease, you will recognize that she is the victim also of bone tuberculosis. For although we shall have a clear history of an accident in this case, you are aware of the fact that trauma alone is not sufficient to explain or account for the vertebral caries without the previous presence of tubercle in the blood. What the trauma does is simply to determine the deposition or the localization of the tuberculosis. But we will leave this subject to the surgeons, and take up the complication which has presented itself in the course of her disease; a new catastrophe, so to speak, grave enough in its import, to divert to it our whole attention.

One of the internes, Dr. French, who has had immediate charge of the case will first read us the main outlines of its history.

"Mary K., æt. 15 years, native of Philadelphia, resided before admission to the hospital, on Front Street amidst bad hygienic surroundings.

The family history is indefinite and unimportant. No hereditary predisposition to disease can be traced, and her health has always been excellent previous to the accident which led to her present illness.

On Nov. 20, 1879, she fell through a hatchway from the second floor to the cellar of an apple-butter manufactory where she was employed and alighted in a sitting posture. When admitted to the house she suffered from complete paraplegia with retention of urine. During the first six weeks, the catheter had to be used regularly in the morning, in the evening, and at midnight. Then the vesical paralysis suddenly disappeared. At the same time she began to recover from the paraplegia and continued to improve so rapidly that on Jan. 1, 1880, she was able to stand.

About ten days after her admission, there was discovered a prominent knuckle-like protrusion in the lower dorsal region of the spine and a plaster-of-Paris jacket was applied. . This treatment was continued until shortly before Christmas last, when the vertebræ seemed to have solidified, and she felt comfortable without artificial support. Strengthened as she was by the jackets, she was in a few weeks after the first application of them, able to walk. The motion of her limbs was carried on, however, wholly by the muscles of the gluteal region and thigh as the muscles of the leg and foot are still beyond her control. In order to maintain the equilibrium of her body, she has to partially flex her knees and she walks. by giving her body a swinging motion from side to side and by dragging her feet with the toes turned outward.

The improvement of sensation in the paralyzed limbs has kept pace with the improvement of voluntary motion. Since the middle of last summer the sensation above the knees has been good, but below the knees, from two inches downward, the feeling is so obtunded that the prick of a pin could not be noticed, and the nail of a toe was removed without inflicting pain. At present the tactile sense is a little more acute as far down as the ankles. She has at no time had involuntary contractions of any of the affected muscles.

At various times during her illness, she has suffered from dysentery and diarrhœa; indeed her bowels could never be said to have acted properly. About the 15th of December last, signs of suppuration were noticed about the nail of the great toe of her left foot. On the 20th, the toe was more than twice its natural size, and a small quantity of pus was evacuated by incision. The discharge then continued several weeks until the second phalanx was removed. The foot became swollen and œdematous. About ten days later she complained of pains in her sides, in the lumbar region—sometimes darting upward. Then there was noticed a fulness of the face, the bridge of the nose seemed flattened, and her lower eyelids were puffed. Upon interrogation it was found that she had to micturate very frequently, passing very small quantities with great pain. Her skin now had a pallid hue, she became very anæmic, lost her appetite, and was easily nauseated. Auscultation and percussion revealed no lesion of the heart or lungs.

Examination of urine resulted as follows: sp. gr. 1.012; reaction neutral; colour, deep red; odour, strong; blood and albumen present in small quantities. The microscope showed red and white blood-corpuscles, small round epithelium cells and one or two granular casts.

From this time until the 15th, the patient's condition grew worse, both feet and legs becoming œdematous. Then a profuse diarrhœa set in which lasted three days, whereupon the dropsy rapidly subsided. Examination showed no change in the urine except a slight increase in the specific gravity.

. During the last two weeks the only change worthy of mention has been the occurrence of obstinate and frequent vomiting.

Urinalysis to-day with the following result. Quantity in 24 hours, 20 ounces; specific gravity 1.010; colour dark red; odour strong; reaction neutral; albumen, less than 1 per cent.; blood, earthy phosphates, pus, colouring matter normal. Under the microscope are seen numerous white blood-corpuscles, round and pavement epithelium, pale hyaline casts, and . an occasional granular cast. In fresh specimens red blood-corpuscles can be seen. Examining the small quantities as they are passed. the colour is found to vary from a very pale to a deep red, but it is never clear. The amount of albumen varies also in different specimens from a mere trace to about one per cent."

I remarked to you, at the start, that you might read in the face of this little girl something of the nature of her disease. I had reference then to her almost unearthly pallor, and to the still evident puffiness of the face. If, now, you will simply recall the nature of the disease which preceded, and which probably produced the kidney affection, you will recognize also its form. The appearance of the patient, the history of the disease, above all, the condition of the urine, speak for amyloid degeneration of the kidneys.

Fatty degeneration we know very well as the commonest mode of the death of any cell. With calcareous degeneration we are as fully familiar in the coats of the larger arteries. Pathologists have made us familar with these tissue changes ever since morbid anatomy was especially studied. But amyloid degeneration is something new. Our definite knowledge of it dates from our own decade, and though we know of it already what it is, and when it appears, it must remain for another decade to inform us exactly why it occurs.

As might have been premised almost, our first knowledge of the amyloid process came from the study of the liver. The changes it produces in this organ are so gross, so palpable we might say, in life, as to have early attracted the attention of the pathological anatomists. So, some vague mention is made of it in the old writings of Stahl and Boerhaave, but their descriptions included all kinds of "Infarctions, Obstructions, and Engorgements" as they called them; conditions all supposed to be due to an accumulation of "altered, thickened, or corrupted blood within the bloodvessels."

Budd says of Laennec, who noticed everything, that he noticed also the "waxy" liver which he, however, considered to be a variety of fatty liver. The first mention of the condition with a distinct description was made by Antoine Portal, in 1813, who says that he "found the liver excessively voluminous, reduced to a substance like lard, both in colour and consistence, in the body of an old woman who had various exostoses and ulcerations about the genital organs." Nothing but unimportant and isolated observations, as by Budd, Andral, Graves, were then made in the history of amyloid degeneration, until 1842, when Rokitansky cleared up the field, so to speak, by showing that amyloid degeneration was a general process with local expression in different organs, and that it stood in close genetic relations to certain cachexiæ. Rokitansky was the first to describe amyloid degeneration of the kidney. Gairdner and Sanders next, 1854, demonstrated that the waxy condition of the liver and kidney also presented in the spleen, while Virchow and Meckel almost at the same time, 1853, had already discovered the iodine and sulphuric acid reaction by which we are enabled to distinguish amyloid matter in any organ, at any time. This reaction, it was, by the way, which gave it its name. For starch is also coloured, as everybody knows, by free iodine. The coloration of amyloid matter is not blue like starch, but violet, deepening to mahogany. So Virchow called it matter like starch or amyloid. Meckel, however, was not willing to surrender the term "lardaceous," or, more strictly, "bacon-like" (speckartig). But Meckel fell into an error too, for he believed it due to the development of cholesterine. Now we know of amyloid matter, that it is neither starch nor fat, but is a pure albuminous principle, and for this knowledge we are indebted to Friedreich and Kekulé, 1860.

After the nature of amyloid matter had been decided, the next point of interest was to determine whether it was a material circulating in the blood and deposited in the tissues where it was found, or whether it was a result of disintegration or retrograde metamorphosis of the tissue itself, in other words, whether it was a mere infiltration, or a true degeneration.

What seemed to lend special support to the infiltration theory was the place of its first deposit. Virchow and Recklinghausen more especially emphasized the point that amyloid matter is first found in the walls of the bloodvessels. Moreover, it was noticed that the most vascular organs, the spleen, the liver, and the kidneys, organs which stand in the most intimate relations with the blood, are the most frequently and extensively affected. But, it was maintained, on the other hand, amyloid matter has never been found in the blood. A substance present in such quantity as to duplicate the size of the liver, at times, and quadruplicate the spleen, ought certainly to be discovered in the blood. Nor could we explain with the assumption of this view the unequal dissemination or distribution of the amyloid matter in the organs mentioned. A distinct ring of it we sometimes see in the course of an arteriole while the rest of the vessel is free. It is especially in the kidney that we find parts of the Malpighian coil thickened and blocked while blood may still circulate through unaffected parts. Moreover, amyloid matter is not infrequently found in strictly circumscribed or isolated deposits, as a purely local change, and not as a local expression of a constitutional condition. Thus (I quote from a recent article by Birch-Hirschfeld) Billroth observed two cases in which individual lymph-glands had taken on amyloid change. Hirschfeld reported an amyloid degeneration in a single mesenteric gland after a case of typhoid fever; Kyber described cases of amyloid degeneration in inflammatory neoplasms; Oettinger, Saemisch, and Leber amyloid degeneration of the sclerotic, producing hypertrophic exuberations similar to those of trachoma; Burow a case of amyloid degeneration of a fibroid tumour of the larynx. Freidreich states that he got the amyloid reaction from the interior of old blood clots; Jürgens had the same results in thrombi of the endocardium; Virchow from the intervertebral, tracheal, and symphysial cartilages of old people; and, lastly, Zeigler describes—and these are cases of the greatest interest—amyloid tumours of the tongue and larynx that had developed in the immediate vicinity of old gummata which had run their course.

All these facts speak strongly in favour of a local change in the affected part; just such change as regards localization, as is seen in the rule in the transformations into fat and salts of lime, the so-called fatty and calcareous degenerations.

But, however the change is effected, the alterations it produces in time in the organ affected are sufficiently gross and coarse for ready recognition. We say in general terms that amyloid matter has four distinguishing characteristics, viz., a peculiar consistence (like dough or caoutchouc), a waxy lustre, a vitreous translucency, and a lack of colour. But neither the macroscopic nor microscopic appearances enable us to pronounce upon it without fear of error. The true test of amyloid matter is its reaction with iodine and sulphuric acid. The surface to be tested must be first washed free of blood, else a mistake is very easy, and then painted over with a brush dipped in an aqueous solution of free iodine. In a few minutes the amyloid matter is coloured violet or brownish-red, like the colour of mahogany. On the super-addition of sulphuric acid the mahogany colour changes to blue. The iodide and chloride of zinc show the same reactions, as do also the iodide and chloride of lime, and methylanilin is said to distinguish itself in this reaction by colouring the amyloid parts a beautiful red, while the unaffected parts assume a bluish or violet tint.

This much we must say of amyloid degeneration, in general, and all the more are we compelled to say it, because amyloid affection of the kidneys is always only a local expression of a condition more or less universally present in the body at the time.

And now we are prepared to study the affection or complication as illustrated in the case before us. Let us take up the points, therefore, in the order presented in the history of the case. And, first, as regards age, sex, and social state. The youthful age of our patient (15) by no means excludes amyloid disease, which occurs at all ages, and even congenitally as the result of hereditary syphilis. Frerichs found among his 68 cases three under the age of 10 years, and nineteen between the ages of 10 and 20; and from Wagner's 48 cases it is seen to occur in five cases under 10, and in five between 10 and 20. The male sex is two or three times more frequently affected; a singular fact, as Frerichs justly remarks, because the diseases which induce this degeneration by no means especially affect the male sex. Tuberculosis and syphilis have no regard either for social caste, hence this affection is no respecter of persons.

The next point in the history of our case bears upon the etiology of the disease. I do not think it necessary to more than state here that amyloid degeneration is always (there are exceptions enough to make it a rule and not a law) a secondary affection. It follows, in the rule, close upon the heels of some disease attended with persistent suppuration. Dickinson, by the way, proposed a very pretty theory to account for it, based upon this fact. Pus is alkaline, as we know, he said, and the long drain of pus dealkalizes the blood, and dealkalized fibrin is amyloid matter. The scientific treatment of the condition, therefore, is the administration of the alkalies. Unfortunately for this beautiful theory, there are typical cases of amyloid degeneration unattended by suppuration. Now, although there is no evidence of tuberculosis elsewhere, in this case, I take it for granted that the vertebral caries present is an indication of that disease.

Tuberculosis is the most prolific cause of amyloid degeneration. Wagner gives the percentage of cases at 56.25, Weber at 40.55, Hoff at 67.5; but aside from this question altogether, the bone caries present in the big toe is enough to account for it in this case. Bone caries is followed by amyloid degeneration, according to Wagner, in 23 per cent. of cases, according to Weber in 38 per cent., while Hoffman admits it as a cause in 7.5 per cent. of cases.

The next points in the history of this case bear upon the affection of the kidneys.

I have already tried to impress it upon you as a good routine system in the investigation of the symptomatology of disease of the kidneys to take up the study of them as offered first by the dropsy, second by the condition of the urine, and third by the nervous system.

There is no great amount of dropsy in this case, and that is the rule in amyloid kidneys. What there is, in the rule, shows itself in the lower extremities rather than in the face, as in our case, and is due not so much to the kidney affection as to the general hydræmia of a cachexia. Indeed, we might say this of all the symptoms offered by amyloid degeneration of any organ of the body. As Bartels puts it, "the issue of the forms of disease attended by amyloid degeneration of the kidneys depends much more upon the fundamental malady, and the simultaneous affection of other organs than it does upon the renal disease itself." Many cases of amyloid kidney show no dropsy from beginning to end. Grainger Stewart saw general dropsy only six times in one hundred cases. Œdema of the legs and ascites characterize the dropsy of amyloid kidneys; neither dependent upon obstruction in the kidneys so much as upon the general hydræmia, and portal obstruction from simultaneous affection of the liver. So, the obstinate diarrhœa and vomiting which occur in advanced cases of amyloid kidneys depend for the most part upon the block in the portal circulation, or upon amyloid degeneration of the walls of the alimentary canal. I have often seen this child start up suddenly from a sound sleep and forcibly eject from the stomach all its contents, and then quietly fall asleep again.

The quantity of urine is reduced more than one-half in our case, which is the exception and not the rule. For, in the rule, the quantity is increased above the normal, though never to the degree so characteristic of renal cirrhosis. I have often had patients with renal cirrhosis point triumphantly to a large vessel brimful of clear, limpid, urine, the accumulation of a single night, as an indication of the supposed healthy action of the kidneys. A quantity to be proud of is seldom passed from amyloid kidneys, though enough escapes to prevent the block and side outlet into the immense reservoir under the skin, as in chronic parenchymatous nephritis.

A small amount of albumen is present here, which is in accord with the rule, a few clear casts and white corpuscles, a like conformity, but also some red blood-corpuscles which is a decided exception. But we have to say of amyloid kidneys always, that this form of kidney disease is so often complicated by the others as to present the greatest variations in every respect of them all. Our endeavour is rather to ascertain which form predominates, than exclusively prevails.

Symptoms on the part of the nervous system, so frequent in the acute and chronic parenchymatous forms, as well as in renal cirrhosis, are distinguished by their absence in amyloid kidneys. Beyond a recent tendency to sopor, this child has shown no signs of uræmia at all. Bartels says that he knew but one case of amyloid kidneys to die of apoplexy. So this element of sudden danger is lacking in this form of Bright's disease.

The prognosis in all cases of amyloid disease is bad. It is most favourable, I need hardly say, when dependent upon syphilis, because for syphilis we have means of relief. Prevention is the greatest victory and this we may secure, at times, by free evacuation of pus, and destruction, or obliteration of pus-secreting surfaces. Amputations, resections, drainage, aspirations, these are the prophylaxes of amyloid disease. The treatment of syphilis continued long after the subsidence of manifest signs, the thorough neutralization of chronic malarial poisoning, resort to change of climate in phthisis pulmonalis, prevent the development of many a case of amyloid disease. So far as concerns drugs, from the standpoint of existing knowledge, there is but one worthy of trial in amyloid degeneration, and that is iodine. Whether its worth here depends upon its efficacy in syphilis and scrofula, the so frequent forerunners of the condition, is a question yet *sub judice*. We will push it with this child in the form of the syrup of the iodide of iron. From small doses of morphia in cherry laurel water frequently repeated, we have had the best results in combating the vomiting which was the most distressing and exhausting feature of this case. Moreover, we will ask the surgeons to cut out the carious bone at the toe, not in the hope of removal of the amyloid matter, which has already substituted structure in the kidneys and the spleen, the enlargement of which I readily detect, but of faintly helping (perhaps we ought to say, making a feint of helping), to prevent the continuance of the change. Every hope is in prophylaxis. Pitiful is the therapy of amyloid disease when at all advanced. The patient is already reduced by the disease which brought it on. Then it steals upon a prostrate victim like the jackals which prey upon the wounded on the field of battle.

REMARKS ON THE DIAGNOSIS AND TREATMENT OF PRURITUS VULVÆ.

A Clinical Lecture delivered at St. Mary's Hospital.

By ALFRED WILTSHIRE, M.D., F.R.C.P.,
Joint-Lecturer on Obstetric Medicine at the Hospital.

GENTLEMEN: The patient, an elderly woman, who is now before you, has brought this specimen of her urine at my request; our object in procuring it being the demonstration to you that it contains sugar. Its specific gravity is high—1040; and, on applying Fehling's test, with heat, you may observe that a copious precipitate of suboxide of copper is thrown down. We conclude, therefore, that it contains sugar—the influence of any other reducing agent, e. g., uric acid, being excluded.

Looking at the patient, probably a few of you would suspect that she is diabetic: she is neither notably thin, nor has she had, until recently, either thirst or a large appetite; moreover, the amount of urine voided when she first attended was not remarkable; now it averages seven or eight pints in the twenty-four hours. We were led to suspect the presence of sugar in the urine from her complaint of itching of the private parts, the symptom for which she sought relief; and at each visit we have found it to be loaded with sugar. The vulvar itching was at once greatly relieved by a borax lotion; and although there is no abatement of the glycosuria, yet the itching has scarcely troubled her again; in fact, she now makes no complaint of it.

I have availed myself of this case as illustrating an important form of pruritus vulvæ due to a general disease of great gravity, the first clue to which is sometimes obtainable through the symptom of vulvar itching long before the manifestations of diabetes commonly regarded as classical—e. g., wasting, thirst, voracious appetite, polyuria, etc.—have declared themselves. This symptom of pudendal itching—for males, though in a less degree, are subject to it—has repeatedly led me to the discovery of glycosuria. Observe that I use the word glycosuria rather than diabetes; for not all the patients whose urine contains sugar are diabetics, that is, they do not all have an excessive flow of urine, polyuria being manifested later, if at all. Clinically, it is important to recognize that glycosuria occurs in stout as well as in thin folk; otherwise, the malady may be long overlooked. The symptom of pudendal itching will direct your attention to the state of the urine, and may thus lead to the early detection of sugar. Before dismissing the patient, I will ask you to observe her teeth, and note the injection of the capillaries of her cheeks. Her teeth are being shed without decay, as the teeth of elderly diabetics sometimes are, apparently from shrinking of the sockets, the alveolar processes wasting. In some cases, the teeth become brittle and crumbly. The tendency to injection of the facial vessels seems to be part of a general proclivity to capillary erethism, for flushing of other regions of her skin is easily excited. Here is a photograph of another patient who was tormented with vulvular pruritus, a stout gouty diabetic; and, as the local condition in her case was typical, I will describe it.

The separated vulva looked pale, rough, granular, thickened, and sodden—in texture like the rind of a Seville orange, only dead white. Mark the absence of pigment: it is diminished or absent in many cases, just as in pruritus ani. This change I regard as neurosal. Very rarely there is increased pigmentation, a slaty hue overspreading the parts; or there may be suffused dusky redness, or a glazy redness, especially in the aged, mostly arising from acrid uterine discharges.

But the glycosuric or diabetic is only one of many forms of pruritus vulvæ; and, as the symptoms may arise from a variety of causes, we must review these together, in order that you may acquire a comprehensive knowledge of them. Broadly, they may be divided into two chief classes: the *local* and the *general;* but in some instances these overlap.

Local Causes.—These are as follows :—

a. Animal and vegetable parasites may infest the vulva, and excite itching. Among the former are pediculi, acari, and ascarides. Pediculi and ascarides are easily recognized, but the itch-insect may be overlooked. Ascarides are more common in girls than in women, but are by no means unfrequent in the latter. They crawl from the anus over the vulva, and thus annoy; sometimes provoking leucorrhœa also. (The same may be said of tænia, joints of tapeworm escaping *per anum* and exciting irritation in the adjacent parts; but this very rarely happens.) The vegetable parasites are of interest; for the itching appears in many cases immediately to depend upon the presence of certain low varieties, not only in the glycosuric cases, but also, it appears to me, in other instances, in which loss of pigment points to neurosal impairment. The *oidium albicans* (the thrush-fungus) has been met with, and also other low forms of vegetable life, as Friedreich, Hausmann, and others have observed. Sugary urine obviously supplies a most favourable pabulum for the development of lowly organized fungi. It is interesting in this connection to note that most of the successful remedies are parasiticides, as we shall see when discussing treatment. Parts whose innervation are impaired afford, as you are aware, a favourable nidus for the development of low forms of parasitic life, both animal and vegetable; and the flourishing of such organisms in the parts in question may be regarded as evidence of neurosal impairment, indicated, furthermore, by the occasional presence of leucoderma.

Among local causes, we have, further, several important affections, *e. g.*—

b. Diseases of the vulva (as vulvitis, abscess, carcinoma, oozing tumour, lupus, elephantiasis, etc.);

c. Diseases of the urinary system (urethra, bladder, and kidneys);

d. Vaginitis—gonorrhœal and other.

e. Diseases of the uterus (metritis, endometritis, senile catarrh, cancer, fibroids, polypi; acrid discharges arising from some of the foregoing, or occurring mainly in association with menstruation);

ƒ. Ovarian and other tumours, and pelvic effusions;

g. Skin-affections—eczema, ecthyma, herpes, urticaria, acne, etc.

As regards the latter, eczema may be associated with diabetes, producing terrible suffering; while urticaria suggests ovarian disease. Ecthymatous spots, with ashen-gray bases, may indicate grave cachexy (? syphilitic); while the herpetic vesicles are prone to crop out periodically in females of gouty parentage just before each menstrual period. The French attribute this to the herpetic diathesis. A pustular form of acne is sometimes accompanied by troublesome itching.

It is perhaps true, as a broad generalization, that syphilitic eruptions are not prone to itch; but I have met with marked exceptions to this in some syphilitic affections of the vulva, as in the patient of whom I show you a photograph illustrating elephantiasis of the clitoris and vulva, from whom I removed an hypertrophied clitoris weighing a pound and a quarter. Venereal warts may excite itching.

Malignant disease of the uterus and upper part of the vagina may provoke itching in two ways: first by acrid discharges; and, secondly, reflexly—the latter uncommonly. The same may be said of fibroids, polypi, sarcomata, etc. I have known pruritus to exist for a long time apparently as a consequence of pelvic effusions—e. g., hæmatocele, cellulitis, partly perhaps from venous obstruction, and partly from implication of nervous structures. Some discharges from the interior of the womb are virulently acrid, and excite excoriation of the parts over which they flow. These are revealed by the speculum.

Urethral and vesical affections—e. g., vascular growths, stone, incontinence, etc.—are sometimes complicated by vulvar itching. Careful local investigation, therefore, is obviously necessary in all such instances; and even when the predisposing cause is general, as in diabetes, the local condition may be significant and important, yielding, as has already been pointed out, valuable information.

General Causes.—Among the general causes of pruritus vulvæ, we find: (*a*) diabetes (glycosuria), (*b*) pregnancy, (*c*) gout (or lithiasis), (*d*) syphilis, (*e*) prurigo senilis, and perhaps (*f*) the dartrous diathesis of the French. (Diphtheria must be mentioned as an extremely rare cause.)

a. The patient whom you have seen is now a type of the diabetic causes. Such are not uncommon; but they usually escape detection until other symptoms obtrude themselves. I have shown you and met with many such; although usually among the middle-aged or elderly, yet also in patients under twenty, as in the case of a young woman who was under my care some years ago. She consulted me for severe pruritus vulvæ; and, on examination, I found extensive eczema. I at once examined her urine, and found sugar. She had then no other symptom indicative of diabetes, nor did she present any for many months; but she ultimately died of it; and I belive her brain is figured in Dr. Dickinson's able work on diabetes. We have had other cases here, as you know, notably one in which diabetes came on rapidly after severe mental trouble; the vulvar pruritus alone leading to its detection.

b. Pregnant women are liable to a severe form of pruritus vulvæ. It is usually accompanied by an irritating discharge—whitish, creamy, or yellow in colour, and occasionally very abundant. Sometimes aphthæ and erosions are seen upon the turgid labia or cervix, or there may be vaginitis granulosa. Most of the cases that I have seen have been accompanied by extreme venous turgescence. The distress experienced by some sufferers appears to be painfully augmented by the exalted nervous tension attending pregnancy. Parturient women seldom make complaint of pruritus; but I have seen a few instances in which it occurred, and it has been associated with hydroa or herpes gestationis.

c. The gouty form is not uncommon, but, fortunately, it is seldom intense or obstinate unless complicated with glycosuria. It may be seen in plethoric women, even when young, recurring before menstruation, when the urine is apt to be loaded with lithates. Sedentary habits, beer, and strong wines, aggravate it. Stout gouty women at the change of life are prone to suffer from vulvar irritation; some, doubtless, are examples of gouty glycosuria, in whom climacteric disturbance intensifies the mischief. Ordinarily indulgence in the pleasures of the table provokes itching, while abstinence alleviates. Obese elderly women are liable to vulvar irritation,· the secretions of the parts apparently possessing very irritating properties; but you will be amply repaid for your trouble by systematically examining their urine for sugar, for thus you may be enabled to detect latent diabetes.

d. As regards syphilis, it is seldom that the early or acuter manifestations of the disease excite itching. It is associated rather with later phenomena, as in the case of elephantiasis already mentioned; but chancres and venereal warts may provoke much irritation.

e. Sometimes intractable pruritus vulvæ appears to be part of a general affection, the so-called prurigo senilis, and is associated with general cutaneous hyperæsthesia. Klob says that there are little elevations of the skin, like goose-flesh, consisting of growths analogous to tubercular formations, and giving rise to violent itching. These cases are grave. Some are amenable to the bromides, which are advocated by Gueneau de Mussy, in the form of lotion or ointment, as well as internally. Arsenic and cod-liver oil are also indicated. Such cases are not to be confounded with senile pruritus arising, as commonly happens, from phtheiriasis.

f. A tendency to pudendal itching seems to prevail in those who have what the French call the dartrous diathesis. In them, fissuring of the affected parts is often observed, the skin presenting a glazy, cracked appearance. Renal disorder, notably oxaluria and inadequacy, may be associated with this condition.

All forms of pruritus vulvæ are subject to periodical exacerbation. Some patients suffer only at night, after becoming warm in bed, experiencing comparative freedom during the day. All who menstruate are conscious of aggravation at that time. Stimulants, as a rule, exert an injurious effect. Sedentary occupations aggravate pruritus: governesses and seamstresses, for instance, suffering much, as also do those who work treadle sewing-machines. Piles and hepatic disorders generally are conspicuous.

Treatment.—While in many cases vulvar itching readily yields to treatment, in others it proves obstinate and intractable, taxing our therapeutical resources to the utmost. Here, as in other affections, a clear diagnosis as regards causation is generally essential for successful treatment. It is obvious that a symptom owning so many and varied causes cannot be appropriately treated in a routine manner; search must made into the origin of each case, and treatment based upon the knowledge thus acquired.

Attention to cleanliness will often do much to allay irritation, and should always be enjoined. Demulcent washes are preferable to soap, unless carbolic or coal-tar soap be used, and usually even these are inadmissible. Almond-meal, strong bran-water, decoction of rice, marsh-mallow, slippery elm, or fine oatmeal, are suitable, especially the first, which, if pure, yields during use a marked odour of hydrocyanic acid, and appears to soothe materially.[1] The prohibition of friction may be required, some afflicted sufferers finding transient relief only during scratching, which may be indulged in to an extent involving serious consequences. Relief may be so frequently sought in this manner, as to exclude sufferers from society, and even from the family circle; while other regretable results, moral as well as physical, may ensue.

When pruritus is due to acari or pediculi, ointment of sulphur, white precipitate, or stavesacre speedily cures, by destroying the insects and their ova. If nits persist about the pubic hairs, a lotion containing bichloride of mercury and acetic acid will dissolve them. Ascarides are destroyed by a carbolic lotion (1 in 60);

---

[1] Experiment has proved that hydrocyanic acid is evolved.

but general, rather than local, treatment should be relied on for their eradication —iron, quinine, cod-liver oil, together with enemata of hamamelis, lime-water, iron, etc.

The vegetable parasites are very efficiently treated by unirritating parasiticides, e. g., borax, boracic acid, sulphurous acid, etc. Here I would again emphasize the fact that most of the favourite remedies for vulvar pruritus are parasiticides. It suggests that—whether from the sugary pabulum provided by diabetic urine, or from alteration in the nutrition of the parts from neurosal impairment, or from a combination of the two, when coincident—the immediate exciting cause of pruritus is, in numerous instances, the growth upon the implicated parts of low forms of vegatable growth.

Friedreich (Virchow's *Archiv*, Band 30, p. 476) alleges that the pruritus is due to the development of fungous organisms, and my own observations are certainly confirmatory of this view. It is a curious clinical fact, that patients are often freed for days from itching by a single application of a parasiticide ; I have observed this repeatedly in glycosuric cases, after the use of a strong borax lotion. It is best to use such remedies in a fluid form, for, when necessary, powerful combinations may thus be made in the unhappily intractable cases. In my experience, fatty preparations of drugs do not suit so well for local application as non-fatty; and yet great relief may be afforded by some ointments, as we shall see presently.

Many cases of pruritus vulvæ are promptly relieved by a borax lotion, and it is well to use this simple and efficacious remedy where not contra-indicated. A drachm to five ounces of warm water is a good standard strength, but a stronger solution is usually needed, seldom a weaker. Hydrocyanic acid may be added —say ʒj of the dilute acid to ʒx, or morphia (gr. ij), atropia (gr. ½), aconitia (gr. ½), or veratria (gr. ½). Infusion of tobacco (half an ounce to the pint) alone relieves some cases. and forms a good vehicle for borax or boracic acid. It is not well to use glycerine with the borax as a rule, as it is apt, owing to its affinity for water, to aggravate the irritation. Some find relief from chloral lotions, but the drug has not always suited. Strong decoction of poppy is a soothing vehicle for borax, etc. Ice alone will relieve some ; while others can get relief only from the use of very hot water. In excessively severe cases, the ether-spray might be tried.

Boracic acid is an excellent remedy ; but, being much less soluble in water than borax, is not so handy as a lotion. It may be combined with hydrocyanic acid, morphia, atropia, aconitia, veratria, etc. In the form of ointment, where fats do not disagree, it often soothes greatly. A non-rancid fat should alone be employed as the vehicle, e. g., freshly made spermaceti cerate, vaseline, fossiline, or purified benzoated lard, etc.

Lotions of iodine occasionally answer, e. g., two drachms of iodine in ten ounces of elder-flower water. Electricity may afford relief in neurosal cases. Probably faradism would be the preferable form.

In simple vulvitis, lead, borax, or carbolic lotions relieve. An ointment of calomel or bismuth is also good. Malignant affection of the parts call for appropriate treatment, such as ablation, where practicable ; but sedative applications (conium, opium, belladonna) alone are often all that we can employ.

Urethral caruncles should be removed ; and urethritis, gonorrhoeal or other, treated *in loco*. Cystitis, stone, and kindred vesical affections and renal diseases, must be treated according to their several indications. Success is unattainable if they be overlooked. Vaginitis, gonorrhoeal or otherwise, demands thorough treatment. The packing of the upper part of the vagina with a tampon soaked in glycerine, with carbolic acid, lead, tannin, chloride of zinc, or borax, seems the·most prompt method of cure; but injections of these agents may suffice, and may be preferable. When the itching is associated with chronic metritis, iodized tampons are useful; and so are copious irrigations of the parts with warm water.

When vulvar irritation arises from acrid discharges proceeding from the uterine cervix or cavity, the use of a tampon filling the top of the vagina is most efficient. Cotton-wool, iodized or carbolized, answers well. As glycerine is apt to excite a watery flux, it is not always admissible, but may now and then be required. Absorbent wool, dusted with iodoform, boracic acid, morphia, tannin, camphor, chloral, and such like, may be packed against the cervix uteri, so as to arrest and disinfect virulent discharges; the choice of drug being guided by the form of disease present. It is necessary to attach a string to each tampon to facilitate its withdrawal. Vaginal and pudendal pruritus, arising from acrid uterine discharge, .is mostly seen in elderly women, and may be accompanied merely by glazy redness around the ostium vaginæ. Search for uterine discharge may, therefore, be necessary. I have seen it in cancer of the fundus uteri, as well as in senile catarrh.

Local treatment by the tampon may be demanded in malignant disease of the uterus, and also in fibroids and polypi when accompanied by irritating discharge, e. g., in disintegrating calcified growths. Removal of the diseased structures is preferable where practicable; and the same may be said of cases dependent upon ovarian growths. Urticarious itching is the form of pudendal irritation mostly seen in association with ovarian tumours. A lotion of bicarbonate of soda, or one of borax with hydrocyanic acid, generally relieves. Magnesia internally is useful. When there is previous turgescence of the vessels of the part, as may be seen from stasis in some pelvic effusions, relief is afforded by the watery flux provoked by the presence of a well-soaked glycerine tampon; and a mercurial and saline purge is helpful when portal congestion is present. Eczema—often symptomatic of glycosuria, remember—may be very obstinate. Dusting freely with fine oxide of zinc answers well when ichorous weeping is abundant. If fissure be present, a poultice formed of the clot resulting from the addition of two drachms of liquor plumbi to ten ounces of new milk is most useful. Sometimes calomel ointment will alone relieve, as in certain instances of anal mischief; or bismuth may answer, dry or otherwise. Mercurial ointment suits certain cases excellently.

Angry ecthymatous spots appear to yield only to calomel, either dry, or in the form of ointment or of black wash. Opium is a valuable adjunct, both internally as well as externally.

Herpetic eruptions are benefited by a small mercurial dose followed by a saline purge, as the effervescent sulphate of soda, and the local use of borax lotion. If they be very severe, hydrocyanic acid and other local sedatives may be necessary; but it must be borne in mind that these herpetic manifestations generally run a definite course, the vesicles dying away completely. They are often accompanied by lithiasis, and may excite preputial herpes in the male.

It is unnecessary for me to dilate further on the importance of recognizing diabetes as a cause of pruritus vulvæ. When the parent disease is discovered, those restraints upon diet, drink, etc., which observation and experience have taught us to be necessary, should be strictly enjoined. Unhappily, we have no cure for confirmed diabetes, but much may be done by judicious treatment and management, alike for those who are threatened with glycosuria, as for advanced cases. Immense comfort may be secured by the habitual use of cleansing ablutions, and of borax or boracic acid.

Gouty diabetics may experience much benefit from a course of the Bath waters · and baths, or from those of Carlsbad, as I have seen there; but I doubt whether confirmed and advanced diabetics are so relieved. The insomnia of diabetic pru- .

ritus vulvæ sometimes shows a gratifying amenability to codeia, in the form of one-grain doses in pill. The bromides are also useful as hypnotics.

The distress that pregnant women sometimes experience, especially towards the latter months, may be terrible. When associated with aphthous ulceration, and the oidium albicans is present, nothing relieves more quickly than a lotion of sulphurous acid. Some prefer the hyposulphites, and in either case prolonged use is undesirable. As sulphurous acid is very volatile, it is best to mix a table-spoonful of the pharmacopœial solution with half a pint of warm water, barley water, or almond emulsion, freshly for each occasion. Another very useful lotion is formed by two drachms of bicarbonate of potash in half a pint of water. This should also be injected into the vagina; it checks the discharge, often alkaline, which seems to excite irritation. Borax is again a valuable agent, and so is lead.

In some cases, relief is only obtained after treating the cervix uteri; as when aphthous ulceration is seen around the os. Nitrate of silver, lightly used, suf-fices. Bromide of ammonium internally is highly serviceable. Attention should be paid to the state of the bowels, and to the hepatic and renal secretions, for in many cases elimination is defective. Turkish or hot-air baths exert a better effect over some of these cases than any ordinary treatment; and the same remark applies to certain other varieties of pruritus vulvæ, e. g., those seen in the obese, gouty, and (senile) pruriginous. Jaborandi may prove very helpful under simi-lar circumstances, by producing profuse diaphoresis. Diuretics—juniper, broom, potash, lithia, etc.—are often beneficial, as in gouty cases, especially when com-bined with colchicum. Restrictions as regards meat, beer, and wine, should be imposed on the subjects of lithiasis.

When vulvar pruritus appears to be part of a general prurigo senilis, besides the local applications already indicated, a lotion of bromide of potassium may afford ease, as has been shown by Dr. Gueneau de Mussy. The same drug given internally is helpful, the affection appearing to be part of a general nervous ere-thism. Arsenic exerts a controlling effect in some instances of senile prurigo, as well as in those due, as the French allege, to the dartrous diathesis.

Arsenic may be said to be indicated in the neurosal forms, and especially when there is marked loss of flesh. It has appeared to me to benefit most those who are the subjects of leucoderma.

It remains only to remark that, in the intractable cases, frequent changes of remedies may be inevitable for the relief of torment. Chloroform locally applied answers occasionally; it may be used in the form of vapour, liniment, ointment, or lotion. Bichloride of mercury, also a parasiticide, gives relief to some in the form of a lotion, but it requires caution in its use. Used in the proportion of gr. j to gr. v to ℥viij of mistura amygdalæ, it may afford great relief.

I have no experience of section of the pudic nerve in inveterate cases, nor am I aware that it has ever been practised; but Sir J. Simpson mentions that he once severed the skin from the subjacent structures, with considerable benefit.—*British Medical Journal*, March 5, 1881.

Hospital Notes.

BELLEVUE HOSPITAL, NEW YORK.
(Service of Dr. AUSTIN FLINT, Sr.)
Quebracho in Dyspnœa.
(Specially reported for the MEDICAL NEWS AND ABSTRACT.)

CASE 1. *Aneurism of the Ascending Arch of the Aorta; Cardiac Hyper-trophy. Great Dyspnœa. Treatment with Fluid Extract of Quebracho.*—Henry J., æt. 43, U. S., wood-carver; admitted December 8, 1880. The patient has not, habitually, indulged in alcoholics. In 1870, he had primary syphilis, for which he was treated. Secondary or tertiary symptoms never appeared. In 1872, he became affected, without apparent cause, with dyspnœa which was paroxysmal, but not severe. It has slowly increased in intensity up to the present time, and has become constant. He began to suffer from præcordial pain, paroxysmal in character, and increased by muscular effort, three years ago, since which time he has continued to experience it at irregular intervals. On admission, Dec. 8, 1880, he complained of great dyspnœa, of pain in the præcordium, and of debility. Physical examination revealed increased strength of cardiac impulse. The area of cardiac dulness was notably increased. The apex-beat was in the 8th intercostal space, and 1½ inches to the left of the *linea mammalis*. In the 2d intercostal space, near the right border of the sternum, pulsation, thrill and a double *bruit* were obtained. Dulness also existed. A mitral regurgitant murmur was present. Pulse 104; respiration 25. Temperature normal; urine normal.

Treatment.—Potass. iodid. grs. x, thrice daily, increased gradually until, on Dec. 29th, grs. xxx were administered thrice daily. The dyspnœa persisted during all this time, and was relieved, temporarily, by spts. ætheris comp. On January 12, symptoms of iodism having appeared, the iodide was discontinued.

Jan. 28. The præcordial pain and the dyspnœa being still unrelieved, resort was had to the fluid extract of quebracho bark, which was administered in doses of 30 minims every three hours.

29th. After the patient had taken two doses of the quebracho he was completely relieved of his *dyspnœa*, which has not returned. The pulse, which has averaged 100 since his admission, is now 86, and the respiration which has, hitherto, been hastened, is normal. Præcordial pain remains.

Feb. 3. The quebracho was discontinued.

5th. The dyspnœa having returned last night, the quebracho was readministered with the same result as that above recorded.

10th. The remedy has been given thrice daily, since the last note, and the dyspnœa has almost disappeared. Pulse and respiration are normal.

14th. The patient was discharged, improved.

CASE 2. *Asthma; Emphysema; Bronchitis. Treatment with Quebracho.*— Thos. S., æt. 63; Irish, pedlar; admitted February 8, 1881. The patient has suffered from attacks of asthma for a number of years, and has been harassed by chronic bronchitis in the intervals of the asthmatic paroxysms. For two years he has suffered from gradually increasing dyspnœa, which now hardly permits of any exercise. His asthmatic attacks recur every few days without apparent regularity. He has anorexia, and has become much emaciated. His dyspnœa is now continuous, but is much increased at the time of the asthmatic paroxysms. Physical examination shows great emaciation. The facies is anxious and cyanotic. The veins of the neck are turgid. The heart's impulse is felt in the epigastrium. The thorax is distinctly barrel-shaped. The percussion resonance is vesiculo-tympanitic. The expiratory murmur is prolonged and low-pitched. Sibilant, sonorous, and mucous râles are diffused over the chest.

Treatment.—The fluid extract of quebracho was prescribed in doses of 30 minims, at intervals of four hours, during the day-time.

Feb. 10. The constant *dyspnœa*, due to the emphysema, has been much relieved. The patient had an asthmatic paroxysm last night, but the shortness of breath attending it was less intense than usual, and its duration was shorter than is ordinarily the case.

20th. The patient has had two attacks of asthma, since the last note. Each was less severe and protracted than its predecessor. The constant dyspnœa which harassed the patient has almost disappeared under the continued administration of the quebracho thrice daily. Appetite and strength have so much improved that the patient was, to-day, discharged at his own request.

CASE 3. *Nephritis (Chronic). Dyspnœa. Treatment with Fluid Extract of Quebracho.*—Jno. M., æt. 51; English, printer; admitted January 24, 1881. The patient had always enjoyed remarkably good health up to the time of his present illness. Six weeks ago, after prolonged exposure to cold and wet, incident to a debauch, he was attacked with pain in the head, anorexia, and emesis. His ankles and legs became swollen. His urine was very scanty and high-coloured. These symptoms persisted a few days and then disappeared. Two weeks ago his feet, legs, and scrotum became swollen, he grew weak, lost his appetite, and took to the bed. The urine was dark and scanty. A week later, his abdomen also became swollen. On admission, Jan. 24, he complains of swelling of the abdomen and of the lower extremities, of dyspnœa, weakness, and loss of appetite. Ascites, with œdema of the scrotum, penis, and legs, are prominent signs. The thoracic and abdominal viscera are normal, as are the pulse, respiration, and temperature. The urine is scanty; its sp. gr. is 1014. It contains 50 per cent. of albumen (by volume), epithelial and fatty casts.

25th. Amount of urine passed, in twenty-four hours, is 16 ounces. The same clinical and microscopical characters present. *Treatment.*—Potass. acetat., ℨij; spirits æther. nitros., fl. ℨij, and infus. scopar., fl. ℨiij, every three hours.

29th. The patient now passes 30–40 ounces of urine daily, but it still contains fatty casts and much albumen. The *dyspnœa* which he had on admission is unrelieved. Fluid extract of quebracho was, to-day, ordered in doses of 40 minims, at intervals of three hours.

Feb. 2. The dyspnœa has much abated. Forty-four ounces of urine were passed to-day; albumen and casts are less abundant.

3d. No dyspnœa whatever is complained of. The quebracho is still administered, as before.

10th. The quebracho was discontinued several days ago. The dyspnœa has not returned.

17th. The patient now sits up. The sp. gr. of the urine is 1012; it contains some albumen and some fatty and granular casts.

March 2. The patient having regained his strength in large measure was discharged.

NOTE.—Quebracho has been tried by Dr. Flint in several cases of dyspnœa from phthisis and pneumonia without avail. In one case of extreme dyspnœa, from mitral regurgitation, it was very efficacious.

—

Atony of the Bladder; Recovery.

J. L——, aged fifty-seven, was admitted into Mr. PEARCE GOULD's wards at the Westminster Hospital, on August 10, 1880, suffering from retention of urine. He was a labourer with small but very firm muscles, no subcutaneous fat, bald and gray, and looked more than his age, and had marked arcus senilis. He had always enjoyed good health until twelve months before, when he found difficulty in passing his urine. This gradually increased until the night before admission, when after a hard day's work he was unable to pass a drop. He went to a medical man, who gave him some medicine and sent him into the hospital. The "difficulty" he noticed was a slow, feeble stream, and inability to empty his bladder, with frequency of call to micturate.

On admission the distended bladder formed a prominent tumour in the hypogastrium, reaching almost up to the umbilicus. The prostate felt from the rectum was hard and moderately enlarged. Mr. Gould passed without any difficulty an olive-headed catheter, No. 10 English scale, and drew off rather more than four pints of clear, acid, healthy-looking urine. The urine flowed slowly, falling vertically from the end of the catheter. The influence of respiration on the stream was evident. After the escape of about a pint the flow ceased, and the rest was forced out by the hand above the pubes, and when the pressure was relaxed air was heard to be sucked in through the catheter. The man was kept in bed on full diet, and his bladder was emptied by catheter night and morning. On August 15th a mixture containing five minims of tincture of nux vomica was ordered to be given three times a day. The catheter used was always carefully washed in carbolic lotion—5 per cent.—before being used, and lubricated with carbolic oil—10 per cent. This appeared to cause some irritation of the meatus, and vaseline was substituted for the oil, and the irritation quickly passed away. There was no sign of any vesical irritation; the urine remained clear, acid, free from mucus and albumen, and the bladder gradually regained its expulsive power. Thus, on August 15th, the patient could pass 4 oz. of urine by his own efforts, and on August 17th this had increased to 10 oz., and thus he improved until on his discharge from the hospital on September 15th there was only half an ounce of "residual urine" to be drawn off.

Remarks.—This case is an example of the extreme degree of atony of the bladder with complete retention of the urine, not unfrequently met with in connection with chronic prostatic enlargement. The daily use of the catheter has long been recognized as the proper mode of treatment for such a condition, but the occurrence of decomposition of the urine with subsequent chronic cystitis have too often prevented the attainment of a perfect result. The case illustrates one application of antiseptic surgery to urinary surgery, and its value in preventing the decomposition of the urine can hardly be overrated. The result of the daily emptying of the bladder in leading to a gradual and almost perfect recovery of the bladder's power throws considerable light on the way in which this atony of the bladder is originally produced. For it is clear that it is not by obstruction of the outflow of urine with retention and stretching of the muscular coat of the bladder, nor is it from any local action of decomposed urine; but rather, it seems, from a small primary "residue" of urine. A few drachms which the bladder cannot evacuate have a paralyzing influence upon the bladder muscle, which leads to the retention of a greater amount of urine; this, again, to further diminution of expulsive power, and so on until the stage of complete retention and atony is reached. The history of such cases before they come under treatment, as well as the results of catheterism, bear out this view. The symptoms often arising from a very small quantity of "residual urine" and the importance of its relief have been laid stress upon by Sir H. Thompson. The patient attends the hospital as an out-patient every month, and up to the present time (March 2d) his condition remains as on the date of his discharge; he continues to draw off the few drachms of "residual urine" every night. The quantity has not increased since he left the hospital.—*Lancet.* March 12, 1881.

MONTHLY ABSTRACT.

Anatomy and Physiology.

Calcification of the Spinal Dura Mater.

Professors HESCHL and LUDWIG of Vienna have described a pathological (or rather senile) condition of the dura mater of the spinal cord, which has hitherto been very rarely if ever noticed. The discovery was made during the *post-mortem* examination of an insane and paralyzed female, aged 65. The brain was small, especially the left hemisphere, and the convolutions were very narrow. In the spinal cord, especially the lumbar region, the ganglion-cells of the anterior cornua were much reduced in number and in size ; and indications of chronic poliomyelitis were present. No history of the subject—whose death was sudden —could be obtained. The spinal dura mater presented, along the whole length of the posterior aspect of its dorsal portion, a peculiar fine yellow dotting, arranged in rhomboidal figures, with their long axes lying in the direction of the longitudinal axis of the spine. The series began in the lower cervical region with an isolated group of yellow dots, four-sided, but with rounded angles, and about six-tenths of an inch in diameter. Immediately below this was a second group, rather larger, which was connected by a narrow bridge with a third. From this point, the groups became gradually closer, and the yellow dots more thickly arranged ; until the series ended in a lumbar region somewhat more abruptly than at its beginning. The groups were largest between the sixth and tenth dorsal vertebræ ; and this part presented the appearance of ribbon with a symmetrically dentate borders, each pair of dentations corresponding to a vertebra. Subsequent investigation showed that each dental projection corresponded to an arch of a vetebra. Here and there the dentations were prolonged on the lateral, and partly on the anterior, surface of the dura mater ; but Dr. Heschl never found them forming complete rings. Subsequently to making the observation above described (in November, 1880), Professor Heschl has had examinations of the spinal meninges made in a number of subjects of both sexes, of ages varying from twenty-one to ninety-three. He finds that no extensive calcareous change of the kind described is to be met with before the sixtieth year, while a few limited and imperfectly defined spots may be observed before that age. The change is most conspicuously marked between the ages of sixty-five and seventy-five; beyond this, he has as yet met with only one case, in a person aged upwards of ninety. Microscopic examination of the spots showed an assemblage of minute points, dark, or with sharp dark outlines, in many places producing complete opacity ; there was also the ordinary network of fibres of connective tissue. It was further found that, while the epithelioid lining and the innermost layer of dura mater were unaffected, it was the inner third or inner half of the membrane which contained the calcareous granules, both in and between the fibres. A careful chemical examination of the deposit was made by Professor Ludwig. On analysis, it was found to have the same composition as bone-earth ; *i. e.*, to be composed of three molecules of phosphate with one of carbonate of lime ($CaCO_3$ $+3Ca_3P_2O_8$). In the deposits in the dura mater, the lime was replaced to a small amount by magnesia. From a consideration of the conditions in which the calcareous deposit was found in the several subjects examined, Professor

Heschl concludes that it is a senile change, and not necessarily connected with any pathological condition of the nervous centres; and that hence it can only be called "pathological" so far as the term is applied to other changes incident to old age. It is, he says, remarkable that it has been overlooked, or at least not noticed in their writings, by such eminent anatomists and pathologists as Morgagni, Voigtel, Meckel, Andral, Cruveilhier, Rokitansky, Förster, R. Mayer, Birch-Hirschfeld, Schwann, Henle, Vogel, Kölliker, Key and Retzius, Frey, Cornil, Rindfleisch, or by any other author to whose works he has access.—*British Medical Journal*, March 5, 1881.

Rare Form of Intraventricular Communication.

At a recent meeting of the Vienna "Medizinisch Doktoren-Collegium," Dr. CHIARI described a rare form of communication between the ventricles of the heart, which he found in a female child aged one year, who had died of tuberculosis. During life, there were observed enlargement of the area of cardiac dulness, systolic and diastolic murmur over the origin of the pulmonary artery, and occasional cyanosis. At the necropsy, the right half of the heart was found to be in a state of excentric hypertrophy; the orifice of the pulmonary artery was narrowed; the pulmonary valves were contracted, and partially adherent. The ventricular septum presented the usual arrangement of trabeculæ, but the intratrabecular spaces appeared unusually deep; and, on closer examination, it was found that, in several of them, there was a direct communication between the ventricles. Altogether, five such orifices were found, the largest being about one-ninth of an inch wide; all were lined with a delicate endocardium. Dr. Chiari believed that this defect was to be regarded as due to arrest of development, the intratrabecular apertures which exist in the septum in embryonic life not having become filled up. Hitherto, but little reference has been made to this kind of malformation.—*British Medical Journal*, March 5, 1881.

The Cremaster considered as an Æsthesiometer.

The researches of Dr. JOSE ARMANGUE, to ascertain whether the cremaster could furnish an index of sensibility, have led him to the following conclusions (*El Siglo Medico*, No. 1401, Oct. 31, 1880, p. 698). 1. The maximum contraction of the cremaster is obtained upon excitation of the skin over Scarpa's triangle, as it has been already noticed by Dr. Esquierdo. 2. The other regions, according to the intensity of the reaction, are—the remainder of the thigh, excepting its external part, the anterior region of the abdomen, the internal of the legs, the external of the thigh, and the posterior of the thorax. 3. Excitation of the upper extremities, the face, the feet, and the external region of the leg, determines very feeble contraction of the cremaster. 4. Both sides of the scrotum are drawn up upon excitation of those parts which induce a strong cremasteric contraction, but the retraction is always greater on the side corresponding to that of the part excited. The half of the scrotum corresponding to the side of the local excitation only contracts when the irritated cutaneous part acts slightly on the cremaster. 5. The contraction is not absolutely equal upon excitation of homologous points, but the difference is really so insignificant, that it may be ascribed to the difference of sensibility between the halves of the body. As a general rule, the testicle which hangs down lower always exhibits the greater contraction. 6. The contraction is proportionate to the strength of the excitation, in confirmation of Paget's law, that the degree of reflex action corresponds with that of the sensations which originate them. 7. The contraction varies with the nature of the excitation, being slight when the skin is tapped with the end of the fingers, very remarkable when the skin is scratched with the nails, and reaching its maximum when the person is tickled. Tickling, however, may easily lead us into error, as it causes laughing, which by itself elicits energetic contractions of the scrotum. 8. The contraction of the cremaster has never failed to be produced upon excitation of the proper points in sound individuals. The same may be stated in reference to the irritation of normally sensible regions of the skin in individuals with anæsthesia. 9. Some persons exhibit in their normal condition little cremasteric contraction ; they always submitted, however, to the above laws, though less intensely. This individual change in the intensity of the cremasteric contraction prevents its serving as a guide to estimate the loss of sensibility symmetrically affecting both sides of the body ; since, unless acquainted with the normal antecedents of the case, we cannot judge whether the diminished contraction results from loss of sensibility, or from congenital absence of reflex excitability. 10. This method may be applied to recognize the absolute loss of sensibility ; for then, as it follows from the preceding remarks, there will be no contraction whatever of the cremaster, which, on the contrary, will always be more or less manifest whenever sensibility is not impaired. 11. This method may be again applied to surgical anæsthesia, and may be perhaps substituted, in regard of simplicity and reliability, for the other æsthesiometers (Schiff has given this name to the pupil, and Ludwig to the arterial tension) 12. This means is superior to the usual æsthesiometers, the model of which is Weber's compasses, because it does not require for its application conditions which are not constantly met with in every patient. The great advantage of the organic æsthesiometer is that it does not require any active co-operation of the patient ; for, when once we interrogate the body, the response comes of itself, not subject to the will, intelligence, and other psychical and emotional conditions of the patient. 13. This method, finally, answers to special indications, and is not free from important inconveniences. Some of them may be, however, avoided by practice and careful application ; but the method will always present two inevitable defects, namely, that it cannot be applied to the extreme parts of the body, nor to females.—*London Med. Record*, March 15, 1881.

Materia Medica and Therapeutics.

Physiological Properties of Thalictrin.

M. Doassans, in an inaugural thesis published in Paris, and abstracted in the *Revue Scientifique*, has given some very interesting particulars in regard to the action of the essential principle of a plant rarely found in the Pyrenees, named the Thalictrum macrocarpum, belonging to the Ranunculaceæ. The root of this plant contains two substances, which have been isolated. One is an alkaloid, to which M. Doassans has given the name of thalictrin, and which proves to be, although as yet he has only been able to obtain it in too small quantities to permit its composition to be determined, a crystallizable substance, capable of combining with acids to form crystallizable salts. The other substance is a yellow colouring matter, which apparently confers the yellow tint characteristic of the fresh section of the root. On treatment of the root with successive portions of alcohol, and with water acidulated with hydrochloric acid, this yellow substance can be obtained in a state of purity, and has been christened *macrocarpin*. Macrocarpin is neither an alkaloid nor a glycoside, but a substance which chemically resembles beberin, from which, however, it differs in some particulars; it has no therapeutic action.

Thalictrin, on the contrary, has well-defined and powerful physiological properties. If a certain quantity of the aqueous extract be subcutaneously injected into a frog a local action is immediately observed, the contractile power of the muscles becoming impaired. After a short interval the muscles contract, and the limb which has been injected becomes hard and rigid. Injected beneath the skin of a dog, it causes sharp pain, and sometimes, owing to its irritating local action, the formation of an abscess. A dose of from two to three centigrammes proves fatal to a frog in the course of three or four hours, and about ten times the quantity of the salts of thalictrin is required to produce the same effect. A dog is killed with quantities varying from two to four grammes when subcutaneously injected, but its toxic influence is much less when swallowed. The principal symptoms observed are general weakening of all the functions governed by the nervous system. The arterial pressure is lowered to an extreme degree, which is dependent, not on dilatation of the capillaries, but upon great diminution of the force of the cardiac impulses. The pulse becomes more frequent. The respiratory acts are also increased in number yet no true asphyxia is perceptible, for the arterial blood remains red, and the relative amount of oxygen it contains is augmented rather than diminished. Indisposition to perform voluntary movements is observed, but the general sensibility is not generally much impaired. The nerves preserve their action on the muscles to the end of life, and the pneumogastrics continue to act upon the heart. The muscles preserve their irritability. Death appears to follow as the result of progressive weakness of the heart, respiration continuing frequently some time after the heart has ceased to beat, which shows that the centres presiding over the respiratory movements are not so profoundly affected as those which govern the cardiac movements.—*Lancet*, March 26, 1881.

The Spray Question.

As to whether the spray is or is not a necessary part of the Listerian method, is a question which at the present time is much discussed, especially in Germany. There are two points of view from which this question has been looked at. First, does the spray really render inert the causes of fermentation which we know to be present in the atmosphere? and secondly, whether it does so, or no, is it necessary, or may it not be replaced by some more convenient means?

Last year Stimson[1] and others published a series of experiments which in their opinion showed that the spray was not effectual in destroying all living particles in the atmosphere. In Stimson's experiments, however, by sweeping the floor of the rooms in which the experiments were carried on, or in some other way, the grosser particles of dust were raised, and mention is specially made of these large masses. On the other hand, experiments have been performed, as for instance, by Cheyne, which show, that acting in the ordinary air of rooms or wards the spray is apparently effectual in destroying all traces of life floating in the ordinary but little disturbed atmosphere. From this point of view, it is simply a question of size of the particles which the spray meets with. If these are minute and but little compact, they will be disinfected. If they are large and dense, as will be the case if the floor be swept during or immediately before the experiment, one could not expect the spray to soak through them sufficiently during their transit. There is another way, however, in which the spray may act on these larger particles, viz., by bedewing the surface of the wound, and thus keeping up the action on the dust which began during its transit through the spray. In fact, the particle of dust already moistened, while passing through the

[1] Amer. Journal of the Medical Sciences, Jan. 1880, p. 83.

spray, falls into a thin layer of carbolic lotion and thus disinfection is completed. As a rule, however, particles of dust which are small enough and light enough to float about in the atmosphere, such particles as are present in ordinary rooms or wards will, as far as we can judge, be acted on directly in a sufficient manner by the spray, for they will not fall straight through it, but will be carried along with it after being moistened with carbolic acid before reaching the wound.

Seeing, then, that the spray is really of use in one or other of the ways, just indicated, the second question arises as to whether it is necessary, or whether some other mode of manipulation might not be more conveniently substituted for it. That the spray is not by any means absolutely essential for antiseptic work, and that aseptic results may be obtained without its use, is at once evident from the experience of Mr. Lister himself   For it must not be forgot, that it was only after several years' practice of antiseptic surgery that Mr. Lister adopted the spray, and that before that time he had been performing operations only justifiable when the causes of fermentation can be excluded from wounds.   He only adopted the spray as a more convenient and certain mode of obtaining the same results which he had previously got.   Before the spray period, however, he had used various precautions, such as irrigation of the wounds with carbolic lotion or carbolic oil, etc.

Mr. Lister's original method has of late been revived and advocated in Germany, more especially by Prof. Trendelenburg.   For several years he has given up the use of the spray in his practice, and resorts instead to frequent irrigation of the wound with the lotion.   When he has concluded the operation, he washes out the wound thoroughly with carbolic lotion, and after stitching it up, he frequently injects it by means of a syringe.   A similar method has been practised by von Bruns and advocated by Mikulicz.   The results obtained in this way are, as is only to be expected, very excellent; but we doubt whether we have here a better or a more convenient method than by the use of the spray itself; indeed there are two serious objections to it.   In the first place, as Wernich has pointed out, the element of certainty with regard to the result is very much diminished, for one can never be sure that every particle of dust which has fallen on the wound during an operation is thoroughly acted on by the carbolic acid at the end, and it is as likely as not to happen, that the particle of dust which escapes this action is a living particle, and may set up fermentation in the wound.   And then, in the second place, this free application of carbolic acid is by no means a desirable thing, for by it the tissues are unnecessarily injured and irritated, while the chance of an inconvenient absorption of the acid, and consequent carbolic poisoning is very much increased.   On the other hand, the spray is really not the inconvenience which some make it out to be; it requires no extra assistant; it does not obscure the field of vision; it does not irritate the wound so much as the other method, while at the same time it adds a considerable element of certainty to the result. The form which this discussion is apt to take is a useless one, the fact being, as we have attempted to show, that, in the present state of science, if the spray is dispensed with, some other means ought to be adopted in its stead.

Whether the spray remains the best means of attaining the wished for result, purification of the air, or whether it be replaced by some other more convenient method, does not affect in the least the truth of the great principles of antiseptic surgery as enunciated and taught by Mr. Lister.—*British Med. Journal*, Jan. 29, 1881.

———

On Five Cases of Transfusion of Blood into the Peritoneal Cavity.

The cases reported by Von Kaczorowski (*Wiener Mediz. Woch.*, No. 46) were one of each of the following: Puerperal fever, great anæmia with hysteria, phthisis, marked anæmia in a woman with fungous cervical ulcers and bronchitis, and a case of typhus fever in a female drunkard. In each of these cases, transfusion into the peritoneal cavity, according to Ponfick's method, previously described in these columns, benefited the patient, and in no case did unpleasant complications arise. One of the manual advantages of this simple mode of transfusion seems to be that little surgical dexterity is required for its performance, while it does not appear to have the inherent risks of the venous method. With antiseptic precautions, a trocar is passed through the abdominal wall in the linea alba, and, by means of a tube provided with a glass funnel, the defibrinated blood is poured through the canula into the abdomen. The researches of Bizzozero and Golgi, reported in the *London Med. Record*, have demonstrated the sound physiological basis of "peritoneal transfusion."—*London Medical Record*, March 15, 1881.

Medicine.

On the Treatment of Fever in Children.

In order to diminish fever, M. STEFFEN (*Jahr. fur kinder.*, N. S., Band xv, Heft 3 and 4), has made comparative experiments on the effect of cold baths and salicylate of soda. In all, 148 cases of abdominal typhus (enteric fever) and 30 of exanthematous typhus were treated. Of typhus abdominalis, 48 cases were treated with baths. The latter had at first a temperature of 15 to 20 deg. R. (65.75 to 77 deg. Fah.) ; but, as the patients could not bear them well, the temperature was in most cases raised to 28′ deg. R. (95 Fah.), and was cooled down to 20 deg. R. In some cases of severe fever, sulphate of quinine, in doses of half a gramme (7½ grains), was given in the evening. Several tables are given showing the age of the patient, the day of disappearance of the fever, and the number of baths used in each case. The effect of the baths on the temperature, pulse, and respiration is described minutely. Out of forty-eight cases five proved fatal. The author is of opinion that the treatment with cold baths promotes the occurrence of inflammatory processes in the respiratory organs. Contra-indications against the applications of baths, are the frequent reluctance of patients to take them, and collapse, often relieved only with difficulty. Salicylate of soda was employed only when the temperature was above 39.0 deg. C. (102.2 Fah.). In children of very early age, half a gramme or less was given ; to older ones, as a rule, one gramme ; rarely two grammes. The tables show here, in the place of baths, the doses of salicylate of soda. Whilst the temperature sank in the baths, on an average, from 0.6 deg to 1.5 deg. (Cent.), the differences in the majority of cases are here marked about 2.0 deg. (Cent.). It is characteristic of salicylate of soda, that the effect is not so sudden as with cold baths. The highest point in the difference before and after the remedy occurred only after from four to seven hours. On the other hand, the reduction in the temperature lasted longer than in cold baths, and rose then gradually. In these, as well as in the first forty-eight cases, the sudden cessation of fever differs from what was expected. The conditions of pulse and respiration were the same as with treatment with water. Out of 100 patients, six died. The following secondary effects of the use of salicylate of soda were not of evil consequence, and disappeared soon after the employment of the medicine ceased : dryness and burning in the mouth (the medicine should, therefore, be diluted in at least half a glassful of sugared water), vomiting, ringing in the ears, and difficulty in hearing, delirium, more or less profuse sweating, erythema of the hands and feet, transudation into the subcutaneous cellular tissue, in one case into the serous cavities, sudden collapse, which, however, can be avoided by precaution (too large doses should not be given at too short intervals, and the remedy should not be applied too long). The author has not observed an irritated state of the mucous membrane, but increased diuresis. Twenty cases of exanthematic typhus were treated with cold baths, six with salicylate of soda. The results did not differ from the above.—*London Med. Record*, March 15, 1888.

———

Dengue in Egypt.

Dr. MACKIE, Surgeon to her Britannic Majesty's Consulate, sends to the *British Medical Journal*, March 5, 1881, an interesting account of the epidemic of dengue which has prevailed recently in Egypt. It seems first to have appeared in that country in 1877, when an outbreak occurred in Ismailia. In that year, so many inhabitants of the town were attacked, that the tribunals and commercial offices were temporarily closed. It occurred again in Ismailia in the autumn of 1878 and 1879, and also to a slight extent in the autumn of 1880. The disease subsequently invaded every town and village from Alexandria to those situated in Upper Egypt. It visited Alexandria in the beginning of October; and it was in this town that Dr. Mackie and Dr. Murison had the opportunity of observing it.

Dr. Mackie tells us that the disease commences, in mild cases, with slight pains and malaise; in severe cases, with slight shivering, followed by high fever, severe pain in the head, redness, smarting, and suffusion of the eyes. The most characteristic symptom, however, is pain in the back and in the muscles and joints of the limbs. With these symptoms, the temperature of the body is increased to 104° and 105° Fahr. Dr. Mackie noticed that, in comparison with the increase of temperature, the pulse is slow, a temperature of 104° often being accompanied by a pulse of 84 or 90, although it may range between 84 and 130. The pain is special in character, and differs from that of rheumatism or neuralgia. Dr. Mackie compares it to what might be produced by a red-hot iron applied to the affected joint. The tongue is coated with white or yellow fur, and the bowels are constipated. The urine is high coloured, sometimes albuminous, rarely bloody. The skin is hot, and usually dry; the face flushed, and the throat sometimes dry, congested, and painful. In cases of ordinary severity, the fever declines about the third day, and a rash, sometimes resembling that of measles, but more frequently that of scarlatina, appears on the neck, upper part of chest, large joints, and sometimes extends over the whole body. The rash may, however, appear earlier, whilst its duration is usually limited to four or five days; it is not followed by desquamation, as in scarlatina, but, where it is well developed, is occasionally followed by the shedding of fine furfuraceous scales. Convalescence is very slow, the patient remaining weak and prostrate, often troubled with sleeplessness. Children suffer less severely than adults, and usually have a rash which more resembles measles. They convalesce more rapidly than adults. In childhood, the attack is often ushered in by convulsions; whilst, at a later age, a mild delirium is often an early symptom. Although adults suffer from confusion of ideas, and see strange people, birds, insects, etc., in their room, they are usually conscious that these figures are delusions. In mild cases, the symptoms are much less marked, and the patient is able to continue to attend to his duties, although he has much difficulty in so doing. The rash, also, is a much less prominent feature, but, in Dr. Mackie's experience, is never altogether absent. The disease is undoubtedly contagious; if one member of a family is attacked, the whole household are almost certain to suffer.

With regard to treatment Dr. Mackie and Dr. Murison both found that the administration, at the commencement of the disease, of two or three half-drachm doses of salicylate of soda gave immediate relief to the pain, and reduced the temperature. During convalescence, beef-tea and wine for food, with suitable treatment for special symptoms, such as sleeplessness, have been found sufficient. Quinine, in Dr. Mackie's hands, has not proved successful as a remedy. Fortunately, the disease never kills; although one attack will not always protect a patient from subsequent ones, it does not leave him permanently damaged, troublesome boils being the worst sequelæ observed by Dr. Mackie.

—

Catarrhal Diphtheria.

MARX, who has, under the superintendence of Professor Oertel, studied a series of these cases, defines catarrhal diphtheria (*Archiv für Klin. Med.*, Band xxvii., Heft 1, 2) as that form in which there is only superficial and limited diphtheritic membrane combined with simple catarrh of the mucous membrane, slight constitutional symptoms, inconsiderable glandular swelling, and limitation of the disease to the throat. That it is a true diphtheria, he considers, is shown (1) by its clinical character; (2) by its not unfrequently passing into the severer forms; (3) by its infective power; and, lastly (4), by its microscopic pathology. The disease begins with slight fever, malaise, and pain in swallowing. The mucous membrane of the throat at some part, generally the tonsil, is swollen, red, and has on it one or more grayish spots like boar-frost. These spots are superficial, limited, and disappear in two to three days, rarely lasting six days; unless, as sometimes occurs, the disease passes into the severe form with thick and spreading membrane. Microscopically these spots are found to consist of colonies of micrococci, which pass through the comparatively unaltered superficial epithelial layers into the deeper layers where the cells are swollen up and contain large nuclei. After twenty-four hours, pus forms in the deeper layers, and the superficial layers are thrown off. Catarrhal diphtheria differs from the severe form in the absence of a fibrinous exudation between the epithelium, and from simple catarrh of the mucous membrane by the presence of micrococci in place of the numerous organisms in catarrhal muco-purulent secretion, such as leptothrix buccalis, oïdium albicans, etc. In the treatment of this affection, the author recommends (1) immediate isolation of the case, notwithstanding apparent mildness; (2) frequent inhalations of steam; and (3) disinfection of the mouth with gargles, etc. Astringents ought to be avoided as checking the separation of the membrane, which is furthered by a rapid formation of pus under the influence of warm inhalations.—*London Medical Record*, March 15, 1881.

—

On an Organism in Diphtheritic Membranes.

M. TALAMON communicated last month to the Société Anatomique a description of an organism which he considers to be the determining cause of diphtheria. His papers appear *in Extenso* in the *Progrès Médical* for February 12th. He obtained, by the cultivation of false membranes taken from eight undoubted cases of the disease, a fungus which consisted of long-jointed mycelial rods, and spores of two kinds: the one oval or round, and giving rise, by a process of gradual elongation, to the mycelium; the others rectangular, and showing, after a short time, minute brilliant specks in their interior, about the size of an ordinary micrococcus. These rectangular bodies he considers to be conidia; and the micrococcus-like specks which subsequently develop in them, are, he thinks, the "veritable germs of the fungus."

Rabbits, guinea-pigs, frogs, and pigeons inoculated with the fluid in which this fungus had been cultivated, all, with two exceptions, died ; and, in all cases, he obtained from some of the fluids of the body the conidia considered to be characteristic. One rabbit died with an enormous swelling of the throat, comparable to the œdema which occurs in some cases of diphtheria. In four pigeons he succeeded in producing false membranes ; the inoculation, effected by scraping the mucous surface with a bistoury, and then dabbing the bared surface with the fluid in which the fungus had been cultivated, was followed by the appearance of a false membrane, which covered the inner surface of the cheeks, the tongue, the velum palati, and the upper part of the pharynx ; this membrane consisted, as in the case of membranes obtained from man, of epithelial cells, fat-granules, micrococci, bacteria, and yielded, on cultivation, the characteristic organism. In the case of the frogs, the stomach was the organ which underwent a diphtheritic inflammation. Three frogs were inoculated, and died in from eight to twelve days, their tissues "stuffed" with the organism. A fourth was then placed in the water in which the other three had lived and died ; after ten days, he also succumbed ; and, on examination, the stomach was found intensely inflamed, and covered with false membranes, which were also seen on the peritoneum.

The author points out that, in this reproduction of false membranes, his experiments differ from that of Letzerich and Klebs, who have also described organisms as existing in diphtheritic membranes : but the fluid obtained by cultivation by these observers, though fatal to rabbits, did not produce false membranes, and killed with such rapidity, that the deaths are, with much probability, attributed to septicæmia. Undoubtedly, this reproduction of false membranes, by inoculating birds with material obtained by cultivation of diphtheritic membranes, is of great interest, and lends a definiteness to the results of M. Talamon which has been wanting in the case of other observers ; knowing, however, the difficulties which surround the mode of investigation adopted, and, unfortunately, it appears to be the only one at our disposal, we shall hesitate to accept his results in their entirety. The whole subject of diphtheria, and its relation to other forms of angina, is one which urgently calls for elucidation ; and we shall await with interest the further facts promised to us by M. Talamon at the conclusion of his labors.—*British Med. Journal*, March 5, 1871.

On a Peculiar Form of Rheumatic Fever in Childhood.

Dr. HIRSCHSPRUNG (*Hospitals-Tidende*, series 2, Band vii.) comments on the peculiarities of rheumatic fever in children, and refers to the form of the disease to which attention was first called by Meynet, which is characterized by more or less extensive affection of the sheaths of the tendons, and of the fibrous tissue. He has observed three cases. The rheumatic fever in these cases was not very intense, but was prolonged. Relapse occurs in most of the cases, and the cardiac symptoms are severe. At a varying time in the disease, swellings of various sizes, and in various numbers, appear in the tendons and their sheaths, or in parts where portions of bone lie close under the skin, as the patella, the malleoli, the spinous processes, or the skull. They are as hard as cartilage or bone. They often disappear spontaneously. In very few cases is there any remarkable tenderness or pain in the part, and only exceptionally a slight redness of the skin. The fever does not seem to have any definite relation to the outbreak, and it cannot be decided whether the deposits are confined to the region of the affected limb. In one of the author's cases, the child died of heart disease, and the necropsy showed that the nodules, which appeared to proceed from the tendons, might be regarded as consisting of a new growth of connective tissue, most like the result of chronic inflammation, with some tendency to necrobiosis.—*London Med. Record*, March 15, 1881.

Treatment of Bronchitis and Pleurisy by Pilocarpin.

M. Vulpian having arrived at the conclusion that catarrhal inflammation of the respiratory tubes, and inflammation of the serous membranes in their first stage, are those in which jaborandi or its alkaloid pilocarpin have the most incontestable use, M. TAULEIGNE states, in his graduation thesis on the subject, that he has employed them in a series of cases, of which he relates fifteen. The effect of jaborandi or pilocarpin is most prompt, and its success most evident, at the out-set of the disease. A single infusion of four grammes (one drachm) of leaves of jaborandi is often enough to get rid of the affection ; and M. Vulpian cites a case of well-marked pleurisy in a child, aged ten years, which, treated from the out-set, yielded to the action of pilocarpin in two days. Much less is to be expected from its use in long-standing cases. The author relates from his observation of pleuritic effusion without fever or inflammation in which jaborandi has given good results, one case in which considerable effusion had for a month resisted the use of tincture of iodine, eight large blisters, and diuretics, and yielded in seven days to two doses of jaborandi. The fluid once absorbed, and pleuritic rubbing having being noted, jaborandi becomes useless. Recourse must then be had to tonics, and the application of tincture of iodine. Pilocarpin is indicated in the various forms of bronchitis. The author relates a remarkable case of chronic bronchitis, which had persisted during four years, with continued cough, difficulty of breath-ing, and suffocation, which recovered after the administration of two draughts containing four centigrammes of nitrate of pilocarpin. As to the mode of admin-istration he recommends the hypodermic injection of the nitrate of pilocarpin, in doses of one centigramme. The patient should be fasting, without which the medicine is apt to provoke nausea and vomiting, as soon as sweating is estab-lished. In constipated subjects it acts badly, and it is necessary to give a pre-liminary purge.—*London Med. Record*, March 15, 1881.

The Treatment of Pneumonic Fever (Acute Lobar Pneumonia) by the Employment of the Wet-Sheet.

Dr. AUSTIN FLINT, in a recent clinic (*Gaillard's Medical Journal*, March, 1881), presented three cases of pneumonic fever, treated antipyretically by means of the wet-sheet, no other active measures of treatment having been em-ployed. The favourable course of the disease under this treatment, in these cases, was highly gratifying. Dr. Flint said, "Inasmuch as these cases are but a small proportion of those which have been treated in my wards during the session, you may ask why the treatment has been thus limited. The treatment is, as yet, novel in this country. In relating the first two cases at a meeting of a medical society of which I am member, doubt was expressed by other members as regards a favourable influence produced by the treatment, together with distrust of its propriety and safety. I was not without apprehensions, in the first place, in respect of the treatment itself, and, in the second place, as taking the place of other therapeutical measures, notwithstanding the strong testimony of some Ger-man writers in behalf of the efficacy of cold baths in this disease. These con-siderations led to a careful selection of cases. The cases selected were those in which the disease was in an early stage, the patients apparently robust, the pyrexia considerable or high, and no complications existing. I am by no means sure that the treatment might not have been employed in other cases with advantage, but it was thought best to select cases in which there was the least likelihood of harm were the effect not satisfactory."

The plan of treatment was as follows : The directions were to employ the wet-sheet whenever the axillary temperature exceeded 103° Fahr. The patient was wrapped in a sheet saturated with water at a temperature of about 80° Fahr., the bed being protected by an India-rubber covering. Sprinkling with water of about the same temperature was repeated every fifteen or twenty minutes. If the patient complained of chilliness, he was covered with a light woollen blanket, which was removed when the chilly sensation had disappeared. In none of the cases was the blanket used much of the time while the patient was wrapped in the wet-sheet. The patient remained in the sheet until the temperature in the mouth fell to 102° or lower, care being taken to watch the pulse and other symptoms. When the temperature was reduced, the wet-sheet was removed, and resumed if the temperature again exceeded 103° Fahr.

The first case entered the hospital on the third day after the attack. On the second day after his entrance the wet-sheet was employed thrice. He remained in the sheet the first time, two hours and forty-five minutes; the second time, an hour and a half, and the third time an hour and ten minutes. On the second day the wet-sheet was employed once, and continued for one hour. On the third day, the wet-sheet was not employed, the temperature not rising above 103°. On the fourth day, the wet-sheet was employed once, and continued for an hour. There was complete defervescence on the fifth day, and no return of the fever afterward. Dating from the attack to the cessation of fever, the duration of the disease was seven days. The patient had no treatment prior to his admission into the hospital. The treatment in the hospital, in addition to the employment of the wet-sheet, consisted of carbonate of ammonia in moderate doses, whiskey given very moderately, and a little morphia. The patient was up and dressed five days after the date of the defervescence. There were no sequels, and the patient was discharged well.

The second case entered hospital seven days after the date of the attack. She had no medical treatment prior to her entrance. The wet-sheet was employed on the second day after her admission, and continued for six hours. Complete defervescence took place on the third day. Recovery followed without any drawbacks. Both lobes of the left lung were involved in this case. The invasion of the second lobe, probably, was about the time of her admission into hospital.

The third case entered hospital three days after he was obliged to give up work. On the day of his entrance the wet-sheet was employed, and continued for ten hours. The wet-sheet was employed on the second day after his admission, and continued for five hours. Defervescence took place on this day. The duration of the fever was five days, dating from the time he was obliged to give up work, and seven days from the occurrence of chills and pain in the chest.

Dr. Flint said the histories of these cases as bearing upon the treatment employed, were of considerable interest. They certainly show that in cases like those which were selected, the treatment is not hurtful. More than this, they render probable the inference that the disease was controlled and brought speedily to a favourable termination by the treatment. They also go to show that the disease is essentially a fever, and that treatment is to be directed to it as such, and not as a purely local pulmonary affection. It remains to be determined by further observations how often and to what extent this method of treatment has a curative efficacy. It is also an important object of clinical study to ascertain the circumstances which render the treatment applicable to cases of pneumonic fever, and, on the other hand, the circumstances which may contra-indicate its employment in this disease.

To this series Dr. Flint adds a supplementary case of decided interest in which the pneumonia began with a well-pronounced chill, fever, headache, pain under the left nipple, cough, and a feeling of general prostration. Being without a home, the patient spent the time from Feb. 18th to the morning of the 21st in a lumber yard without food, and with no shelter but a pile of boards. During this time there was a snow-storm of considerable severity, and the temperature fell as low as 10° Fahr. On admission there was a dusky redness of the face, and the expression was anxious ; pulse 122, respiration 52, temperature 102.25°. He complained of dyspnœa, pain in left side and cough. The expectoration was semi-transparent, adhesive, and had a reddish tint. Increased vocal fremitus, dulness, bronchial breathing, and bronchophony over the left lung.

Treatment.—Whiskey, ℥ss, Ammoniæ carb., gr. v, every two hours, and a milk diet. Temperature in the afternoon, 104.25° F.

22d. Temperature, A. M., 99°; P. M., 99.25°. Pulse 115 and feeble. Ordered tr. digitalis, gtt. x, every three hours.

23d. Patient improved. All the signs of solidification are yet present, and the crepitant râle is heard behind. Pulse 70 and full. Digitalis discontinued. Respiration 32. Flush had disappeared from the face.

24th. Temperature, A. M., 98.25°; P. M., 98.25°. The physical signs now show beginning resolution. Dulness is less marked, bronchial respiration has given place to broncho-vesicular, bronchophony to increased vocal resonance, and the subcrepitant râle is frequently heard.

25th. Much better. Temperature, A. M., 97.50°. Has a good appetite, takes beef-tea and milk.

28th Patient is up and dressed.

Two inquiries suggest themselves in connection with the history of this case. One is, did the disease end from an intrinsic tendency to recover in spite of the circumstances under which the patient was placed for the first two days of his illness ? It is, of course, absurd to suppose that the disease was arrested by the whiskey and ammonia which were given after his admission into the hospital. The second inquiry is, did the exposure in the open air for three days shorten the duration of the disease by means of an antipyrectic effect ? These inquiries are submitted by Dr. Flint without discussion for the reflection of the reader.

—

The Import of the Sweating of Consumptives.

Dr. ROUSSELOT, of Saint-Die, discusses, in the *Revue Méd. de l' Est,* some of the peculiarities of phthisical sweating, the variable period of the appearance of this symptom, and the point whether the sweating of phthisical persons is to be considered an evil symptom, and one which is to be combated. M. Rousselot believes that, in a certain number of cases, there is a correlation between the sweating and the fever. He remarks, in the first instance, that nothing is more variable than the period of appearance of the sweating in the course of a pulmonary phthisis. There is an active tubercular evolution, and a torpid evolution in some sort passive. In the second case, pulmonary lesion has no influence on the organism. It has not an effective evolution, and it may last for some time without producing fever, and, in consequence, without the procession of symptoms which are ordinarily observed with fever, and particularly in nocturnal sweating. When, on the contrary, there are, from the outset, an active evolution, nocturnal fever, and disordered condition of all these symptoms, then, in general, a hasty appearance of nocturnal sweating may be observed. In this case, the thermometer will render great service in enabling us to study the degrees of morbid combustion. The sweating, which is then very often extremely abundant, allows the elimination of a great quantity of the products of morbid combustion. It may, then, be admitted, according to M. Rousselot, that the sweating affords a derivation favourable to the fever, and does, to some extent, moderate that symptom. If, then, in certain tubercular persons, nocturnal sweating appears, as it were, at the outset of the affection, it is because these individuals have a tuberculous evolution of an active form, and one which tends to a fluxion and precocious fever. In others, on the contrary, the evolution affects a silent, indolent, torpid form, without any recoil on the organism; or, more strictly, there are tubercles in the lung, but no tuberculous evolution, and the subject is not phthisical.—*British Med. Journal*, Jan. 22, 1881.

Temporary Aortic Insufficiency and Triple Aortic Second Sound.

Whether there are actual cases of temporary insufficiency of the valves of the heart caused by abnormal widening of the apertures or by disturbance of the closing mechanism (relative and functional insufficiency) has been much disputed. Although denied by competent authorities, there seems good reason to believe that relative insufficiency is not at all an uncommon condition of the tricuspid valve. Last winter, Dr. Heitler of Vienna, in an address delivered before the Medical Society of Vienna, recorded a number of cases in which he had diagnosed relative insufficiency of the mitral valve, mostly cases of Bright's disease and anæmia which he had had under prolonged observation, and in which he had had an opportunity post mortem of verifying his diagnosis. For the mitral valve the diagnosis of relative and functional insufficiency must probably in all cases remain uncertain, owing to the difficulty of excluding hæmic murmurs. With the aortic valve it is not so; and Professor DRASCHE, of Vienna, in a recent number of the *Wiener Med. Wochenschrift*, records two cases interesting in themselves and of considerable importance in relation to this question.

The first case was that of a silk weaver, fifty-five years of age, who first came under observation in June, 1879, during which month he was treated in hospital for simple mitral insufficiency. Four months later he appeared again at the hospital and was admitted. For several years, without any known cause or preceding illness, he had been affected with cough and dyspnœa, which symptoms in November, 1878, increased very much in severity, and were several times accompanied by hæmoptysis. When admitted in October, 1879, he also complained of palpitation on exertion, and of symptoms pointing to gastric disturbance. On examination the lungs gave normal resonance, here and there mucous râles, and a little crepitation, with a slight purulent expectoration tinged with blood. The liver-dulness extended three fingers' breadth below the cartilages of the ribs. The heart's impulse was felt to the left of the normal position; and the heart on percussion showed considerable enlargement in the transverse direction, very little in the longitudinal. Over the apex was heard a harsh diffused systolic bruit, with somewhat muffled second sound. The second pulmonary sound was strongly accentuated. Over the aorta both sounds were normal, the close of the second sound, if anything, slightly marked. Pulse small, but regular; temperature normal. The diagnosis naturally was mitral insufficiency. Repeated examinations during several weeks showed no essential difference in the above physical signs. The patient gradually improved, and was allowed gentle exercise in the ward. One day the patient was required for a clinical demonstration in a distant ward, to reach which he had to cross several courtyards and ascend several flights of steps. This exertion caused severe palpitation, and on examination an aortic diastolic bruit was heard in addition to the mitral systolic, the case being therefore pronounced to be one of insufficiency of the mitral and aortic valves. The patient now returned to bed, and next day the most thorough examination could detect only the mitral systolic bruit. Soon after, however, the patient had had a walk immediately before the visit, and now, on examination, the physical signs were quite different. First, the heart's impulse was somewhat stronger and broader, and over the third left costal cartilage a fine, short, localized thrill was felt during diastole. At the same spot was heard a short diastolic sound, tailing off into the characteristic blowing bruit of aortic insufficiency. The systolic apex bruit was now of a rougher character, the diastolic sound more muffled, and the radial pulse larger and fuller. The thrill and bruit could be readily produced by exertion on the part of the patient, accompanying three or four beats, intermitting two or three, and disappearing entirely after rest in bed. The diagnosis of temporary aortic insufficiency was therefore considered justified.

The second case has both a clinical interest as bearing on the last, and also a physiological interest in relation to the production of the heart-sounds. The patient was a locksmith, aged twenty-nine, with phthisis of both lungs and Bright's disease. During the nine days he was in hospital the patient suffered greatly from dyspnœa, dropsy, and the other usual symptoms of phthisis and Bright's disease. Percussion showed the heart considerably enlarged in the transverse direction. Its action was rapid but regular, and over the apex were heard two normal but weak sounds. Over the aorta were heard with some difficulty a muffled first sound, and a reduplicated diastolic sound. With the breath held back, the second sound was heard to be replaced by three distinct short sounds. Although repeatedly examined for, no diastolic bruit was at any time heard. The post-mortem examination showed phthisis of both lungs and chronic desquamative nephritis. The right ventricle of the heart was hypertrophied by a half, and the intima aortæ and a few papillary muscles were slightly fatty. The mitral and aortic valves were in no way thickened, and under the water test the latter was found competent. The semilunar valves of the aorta were, however, peculiar, having a step-like arrangement, the posterior valve being at the normal level, the left somewhat lower, and the right lowest of all. They were likewise of unequal breadth and depth, and slightly united at their commissures.

These conditions Professor Drasche considers explain the threefold second sound, the semilunar valves being distended in order with a short but distinct interval. Apparently they were perfectly competent during life, but we can very readily understand how a disturbance of the heart's action—e. g., from an obstruction to the circulation—would influence them, and as this obstruction may be temporary, so might the insufficiency produced be temporary, not necessarily leading to hypertrophy. Perhaps in the first case similar differences of position, size, and depth of the valves existed, combined, very possibly, considering the later age of the patient, with thickening and shrinking of the valves such as was probably present in the mitral valve. While admitting that the above is a possible or even probable explanation of the reduplication of the second aortic sound in this case, we would add the comment that such reduplications have, as Walshe points out, very generally little diagnostic significance. They may be produced by various causes—e. g., a deep inspiration—and appear to originate from a want of synchronism in the contraction of the two sides of the heart. Why should the second sound in this case have been single at the apex? Professor Drasche says nothing of any difference between the three sounds, to explain one being heard rather than the two others, and we cannot here give Flint's explanation for the singleness in those cases of want of synchronism referred to above—viz., that the weaker pulmonary sound is not transmitted.—*Med. Times and Gazette,* March 5, 1881.

Extract of Calabar Bean in Atony of the Intestines.

From experiments on animals, which showed powerful action of the muscular coat of the intestine under this drug, SCHAEFER (*Berl. Klin. Woch.,* No. 51) has prescribed it with excellent results in five cases of obstinate intestinal atony with constipation and flatulence. The dose was about 1.45th of a grain in glycerine, three times daily.—*London Med. Record*, March 15, 1881.

—

Intestinal Obstruction by Large Biliary Calculus.

M. Duménil presented to the Medical Society of Rouen a biliary calculus of great size, which had given rise to intestinal obstruction. A patient, aged 46, was seized on the night of the 19th and 20th July, with violent abdominal pain and biliary vomiting. The circumstances of the intestinal obstruction continued in spite of treatment for six days, when the object which had given rise to the occlusion was expelled, and health was restored. This body consisted of three biliary calculi; one large and two much smaller, but connected together in the shape of a stirrup by fecal matter and detritus, with intestinal mucus: prolonged washing separated the parts. M. Duménil discusses how this enormous biliary calculus made its way into the intestine; he cannot admit that it was by traversing the ductus choledochus, but attributes it to ulceration of the gall-bladder or biliary canals. This fact is interesting in the view of the symptoms of obstruction to which it gave rise, and may be remembered in connection with a case of intestinal obstruction. The form and condition of the calculus proved that it had remained for a long time in the gall-bladder, and its passage into the intestine showed that old serous adhesions must have existed between the gall-bladder and the corresponding part of the intestine.—*London Med. Record*, March 15, 1881.

—

The Pathology of Diabetic Coma.

Von Jaksch (*Prager Med. Wochenschrift*, 1880, Nos. 20 and 21) reports a case of diabetic coma in a boy aged 13. The nervous symptoms supervened three weeks after the appearance of the diabetes was recognized; and the boy died in four days, with a rectal temperature of 33.3° Cent. (91.9 Fahr.). The blood examined during life showed destruction of the red blood-corpuscles, but no fat drops. The urine gave a strong acetone reaction with ferric chloride. He also describes a case of acetonæmia in a boy who was not the subject of glycosuria, and who recovered completely after free purgation.—*British Med. Journal*, Jan. 22, 1881.

—

Cases of Diabetes treated with Salicylic Acid.

Dr. Latham had been led to try salicylic acid in cases of diabetes, from theoretical considerations, arising out of a hypothesis as to the curative action of the same drug in acute rheumatism. He contended that the substance cured acute rheumatism by entering into chemical combination with the antecedents of the *materies morbi*, which was probably lactic acid. The glucose of diabetes might have a common origin with the former, and the administration of salicylic acid might be equally serviceable in preventing its formation. He tried it in six cases of diabetes with very varying success, but still with such results as seemed to warrant further trial and investigation. In one case, the sugar had entirely disappeared. The patient, a married woman, aged 53, had, in June last, great thirst and polyuria, passing seven to eight quarts in twenty-four hours. The specific gravity was 1042, and the amount of sugar was large. The symptoms had begun two months before. Under a regulated diet, she improved much; but on December 2d, when the salicylic acid was tried, she was still passing three pints of urine during the night, of specific gravity 1025, and containing a quantity of sugar. Fifteen grains of salicylic acid were given three times a day, and distinct improvement immediately followed. The sugar gradually disappeared, till on December 22d, the specific gravity being 1017, there was no trace of sugar, but under the microscope, crystals of oxalate of lime and of uric acid. On December 28th, she was suffering from rheumatic pains in the joints. She had experienced the same for the first time in her life a few months before the diabetes was discovered. In another case, the sugar disappeared from the urine after salicylic acid was administered; but the patient meanwhile had swelling and suppuration of the parotid gland and surrounding tissues, of which he died. In a third case, the results were ambiguous. Three other cases are at present in the hospital under treatment. Dr. Latham has not ventured in any of the cases to try the enormous doses of fourteen to sixteen grammes daily which had been given in Germany (in the Medical Clinique at Kiel; see *Berliner Klinische Wochenschrift*, 1877). In the above cases, even sixty grains a day had been sufficient to produce some of the physiological effects of the drug. He thought the remedy was of use in diabetes; but in what cases, or under what limitations, must be matter for further investigation.—*British Med. Journal*, Feb. 19, 1881.

—

On Morbid Sweating.

M. Bouveret, in an excellent thesis on this subject (*Jour. de Méd.*, Jan. 1881), mentions some remarkable and important cases of ephidrosis or local sweating. Sweating of the legs is mentioned by Verneuil as a frequent sign of deep-seated varices: there is a notable and habitual increase of the sweat, which is often accompanied by itching, eczema, and erythema. The fact is important to note in the obscure diagnosis of deep varicose veins.

Another singular example of local sweating is parotidean ephidrosis; it occupies the region of the parotid gland, sometimes extending over the neighbouring parts, and even over a considerable portion of the face. It is not continuous, but generally intermittent, and only appears during mastication. It follows injury, such as a wound or opened abscess of the parotid gland. The duct of Steno is most often closed, but the phenomenon is not due to a transudation of the saliva, as one would suppose: it is really a local sweating of reflex origin. Facial ephidrosis is also commonly reflex, and due to excitation of the nerves of taste. The excessive secretion sometimes extends over the entire face, sometimes it remains unilateral; it has been observed exactly limited to the region of the face supplied by the supreme maxillary branch of the trigeminal nerve.

Von Graefe has seen four cases of palpebral ephidrosis. The skin of the eyelid presented well-marked hyperæmia, and, on examination by a lens, during effort or emotion, a clear fluid could be seen to escape from a multitude of little orifices. Ephidrosis may occupy one entire side of the body.

Habitual general sweating may show itself in variable and ill understood etiological conditions. One of the most interesting is that of the menopause, which M. Liégeois has studied very completely. It is well known that, at the menopause, women are subject to flushes of heat and sweating; but what is less known is, that these sweats, though independent of any other affection, may become morbid. It may not be the case always of women who no longer menstruate; the hyperidrosis may come earlier, and appear when the near approach of the menopause announces itself by certain irregularities of menstruation. It is not always a passing symptom; M. Liégeois cites several cases where women were affected by it for several years; he was able, however, in most cases, to check it by the use of atropine. In most of these patients the hyperidrosis appeared especially towards the end of the night. M. Liégeois advises the administration of atropin some hours before the expected return of the sweating. Half a milligramme is a sufficient dose; it is well to continue the medicine several days after the cure.

Besides these forms of morbid sweating, M. Bouveret has studied those which are characterized by a peculiar colour. Chromidrosis, for example, or blue sweat, so rare that its existence has been denied by many authors, is affirmed as a scientific fact. Like sweating of blood, this singular alteration of the sweat appears most often among that set of symptoms which characterizes hysteria. Violent moral emotion is frequently the occasional cause of it; the eyelid is nearly always first attacked, and most often the lower one; blue sweat may, however, appear in other regions, the feet, the axillæ, the epigastrium, forehead, cheeks; the ears are always spared. Sometimes the blue colouration extends over large surfaces; sometimes it is developed on little patches of the integument. The colour varies from blue to black, passing sometimes to deep violet. The abnormal secretion proceeds by successive attacks, returning at variable intervals, generally preceded, as in the first attack, by disorders of menstruation, and by local derangements of the circulation or of sensibility. The colouring matter which gives the special aspect to this secretion is analogous to indigo, and its secretion seems to be produced under the influence of a vaso-motor disturbance. The same is true of hæmatidrosis, a phenomenon very much discussed, and of which the labours of M. Parrot especially have clearly shown the nature.

The sweating of blood, which shows itself nearly always in hysterical women, may occupy very variable extents of the integument, sometimes oozing out in droplets, sometimes in the form of filiform jets; the liquid is composed of blood containing all its elements. It is intermittent, proceeding by steps, coincident with painful eruptions of the skin. These hemorrhages are never alarming from their abundance; moreover, the fluxes of blood in hysteria often enjoy the singular privilege of not compromising the health or the life by reason of their quantity; for the hæmatidrosis should be regarded as a sort of hemorrhagic hysteria, all the more so as it accompanies, in many cases, hemorrhages of the stomach, of the uterus, of the bronchia, of which the neuropathic nature cannot be doubted; its existence, on the contrary, is doubtful except in hysteria.

The remarkable and nearly constant effects of atropin, administered according to the method of Sydney Ringer (attributed by M. Bouveret, *more Gallico*, to M. Vulpian), are clearly demonstrated. In a good many diseases, far from respecting profuse sweats as a useful symptom, on the contrary, it is desirable we should combat them; this is especially the case in acute articular rheumatism, where the abundant sweats may be suppressed without inconvenience.—*Lond. Med. Record*, March 15, 1881.

—

Cure of Lichen Ruber by Hypodermic Injections of Arsenic.

In the *Berl. Klin. Woch.* of 13th Dec. 1880, Herr KOEBNER records the history of a well-characterized case of lichen ruber exudativus treated by hypodermic arsenical injections, with a favourable result. Regarding this disease, often mistaken for eczema, and attended by progressive wasting, Hebra pronounced the opinion that when extensive it is invariably fatal, and that treatment is unavailing. Of late years, the prognosis has not appeared so hopeless, if heroic doses of arsenic be administered. Dr. Koebner thus describes his case. The patient, a carpenter, aged 39, observed in May, 1879, a red, itchy patch on the right shin; five months later, a similar patch on the left shin, then on the back, whence the trouble spread to his whole trunk, depriving him of sleep and strength. For two months he had been taking five to eight drops of Fowler's solution daily. When seen by Koebner his whole body, from the neck downwards, was studded with innumerable dark red papules, somewhat glistening, and here and there umbilicated on their apices, occasionally covered with a fine scale, and conical in shape. They formed a sheet of eruption, discreet at parts, but mostly confluent, unmarked by any appearances of vesiculation or pustulation, and reaching down to the knees on the one hand, and the wrists on the other hand. The back was worse than the belly, and the extensor aspects of the limbs were worse than the flexor aspects. Thick infiltrated scaly patches of skin existed here and there on the most affected situations, and the penis showed a few papules. The legs were free. The patient was much troubled with scratching, a process he continued even while being examined. He was thin, wasted, and weak, but still perspired normally. All the viscera were healthy, but he showed the marks of a cured periorbital necrosis, as well as of white swelling of the left elbow joint, which was now ankylosed. The pulse and temperature were normal; there was nothing special in his previous history. He was treated by daily injections of Fowler's solution, diluted to one-third of its strength with water, the dose varying from about three to six minims of the Fowler's solution, with immediate relief to the itching. Its administration by the mouth in doses of from ten to fourteen drops a day, tried for convenience' sake, proved a failure, and the endermic applications had to be resumed. These were repeated in like doses, at first daily, then at longer intervals; and by the whole treatment, which lasted two months, the patient obtained rapid improvement, ending in complete cure. Three months later, there was no return of the disease; traces of which remained only in the form of white scars.—*London Med. Record*, March 15, 1881.

Surgery.

Gastrostomy in Cases of Stricture of the Œsophagus.

Dr. T. F. PREWITT, Professor of Clinical Surgery in the Missouri Medical College, records (*St. Louis Courier of Medicine*, March, 1881) a case of stricture of œsophagus (either cancerous or syphilitic) in which he performed gastrostomy when *in extremis*, with an unfavourable result. Dr. Prewitt tabulates fifty-nine cases of the operation and from their study deduces the following propositions:—

1st. All attempts at dilatation fail in a large proportion of cases of stricture of the œsophagus.

2d. In very few of the cases does dilatation prove beneficial, and in a still smaller number curative.

3d. In malignant and ulcerative conditions catheterization is fraught with danger, and is *absolutely contra-indicated*.

4th. In cicatricial stricture it is permissible to attempt dilatation with soft, flexible instruments, incapable of perforating the œsophageal walls.

5th. In cases of cicatricial stricture which have failed to yield to reasonable efforts at dilatation and in which the emaciation is progressive and starvation threatens, and in all cases of malignant and ulcerative stricture, as soon as solids cannot be swallowed, gastrostomy should be performed.

Serious mishap after Gastrostomy.

Dr. P. KRASKE reports (*Cent. für Chir.*, No. 3, 1881) a case in which after gastrostomy had been performed by Professor VOLKMANN, for advanced cancerous disease of the œsophagus, the patient, a man, aged 48, died on the second day in a state of coma. In the operation, which was performed under the car-

bolic acid spray, the stomach, found to be not·quite empty, was fixed to the
edges of the external wound by a dozen silken sutures, some of which were passed
through the whole thickness of the anterior wall of the viscus.   No further steps
were then taken, save covering the wound with antiseptic dressing, as it was proposed to open the stomach at a later period. ᐟ At the *post-mortem* examination,
the condition of the wound was proved to be very good ; but, on the anterior wall
of the stomach, near the pylorus, and also on the left lobe of the liver, was observed a thin layer of loosely adherent exudation of a dirty-brown colour, which,
on microscopical examination, was proved to contain gastric contents, namely,
vegetable cells and *débris* of distinctly striated muscular fibre.   The peritonitis
had not extended to any other part of the abdominal cavity.

In his remarks on this case, Dr. Kraske states that the peritonitis which,
though limited, was the cause of death, had been set up through the discharge
into the peritoneal cavity of a portion of the contents of the stomach.   Apart from
the fact that the appearance of the wound, and the condition of the peritoneum
in its immediate neighbourhood, forbade any supposition of the peritonitis having
been the result of an infection at the time of the operation, certain constituents
were found in the inflammatory exudation, as to the nature and origin of which
not the least doubt could be entertained.   These constituents had certainly been
discharged from the interior of the stomach ; and, as the wall of this viscus had
not been incised, they must have passed through the punctures occupied by the
sutures.   This case, then, demonstrates that it is possible, after an incomplete
gastrostomy, for the contents of the stomach to be discharged through the small
perforations made by the sutures.   This result, it is stated, is not surprising.   The
stomach, when dragged forwards and retained in an abnormal position, has
naturally a great tendency to sink backwards ; and the margins of the small punctured wounds may be thus stretched and torn so as to permit during coughing or
vomiting the free passage of gastric contents into the peritoneal cavity.   This
accident, it is evident, is the more likely to occur when the stomach is well filled,
but still cannot be effectually guarded against by operating on a stomach with
but scanty contents.

Dr. Kraske, in considering whether and how this accident could have been
prevented, states that it occurs at once to the surgeon that the wall of the stomach might have been transfixed through its external and middle coats only, the
mucous layer being left intact.   It has been proved, however, that this is not
a safe course, since the stomach, in the course of a very few hours after the operation, tears itself away from the sutures, and falls backwards to its normal position.   The danger of discharge of the gastric contents might be certainly prevented by rejecting sutures, and by attempting by some other means to keep the
anterior wall of the stomach in sufficiently prolonged contact with the external
wound for the establishing of firm adhesions.   How such a plan, which, as is
well known, has been carried out by Volkmann with much success in the treatment of hydatid cyst of the liver, is to be applied to so movable an organ as the
stomach, is a question that has yet to be settled.

It is next considered whether, with the object of preventing extrusion of the
gastric contents along the sutures, gastrostomy ought not to be always performed
in one stage.   There can be very little doubt that this accident might be prevented by at once incising the stomach after it has been fixed by sutures, and by
washing out its interior.   Dr. Kraske does not give any decided opinion as to the
necessity of giving up in future the operation of gastrostomy in two stages ; but to
those who practise the single operation, he recommends that the wall of the
stomach be transfixed by two sets of sutures, the first involving the serous and

muscular layers only, and the second, applied after the viscus has been incised and opened, involving also the mucous coat.—*London Med. Record*, March 15, 1881.

On Colotomy.

In an article in the *Hospitals-Tidende*, series 2, Band vii., Dr. C. STUDS-GAARD examines the merits of the two operations—anterior colotomy or laparocolotomy, and posterior or lumbar colotomy. He gives the preference to the former (Littré's method), especially since the use of antiseptics has materially diminished the danger of opening the abdominal cavity. Costallat's advice to perform the operation in two stages—the bowel being first opened some days after the incision is made, in order that the edges of the incision in the abdomen may granulate before they come into contact with the fecal matter, and that the risk of diffuse inflammation may be diminished—he regards as rational, provided that the urgency of the symptoms of ileus do not demand immediate relief, in which case he considers it quite superfluous to open the bowel with the cautery instead of the knife. Cauterization of the wound with a 10 per cent. solution of chloride of zinc is sufficient to obviate infection, the more so as it is only in exceptional cases that fecal matter passes in the first days. The incision in the intestine should be $1\frac{1}{4}$ inches long ; not smaller, in order to give room for the passage of feces ; nor, if possible, larger, lest prolapse of the mucous membrane of the bowel should occur. The size, however, which should be given to the opening in the bowel must in some measure depend on the indications for the operation. In cases where it is difficult to be certain that the function of the fistula will be permanent, Dr. Studsgaard has modified the application of sutures to the intestine. The lowest sutures are introduced into the intestine in such a way, that a great part in front lies free between two corresponding sutures, while the posterior ones are passed through the bowel closer to one another in the neighbourhood of the mesentery ; in this way, a kind of spur is left at the lower angle, which will obstruct the passage of feces into the rectum. Dr. Studsgaard finally relates seven cures of anterior colotomy performed by him in the Communal Hospital of Copenhagen. Of the patients, two died in the hospital and five were discharged, one of whom died six months afterwards of metastatic cancer.— *London Med. Record*, March 15, 1881.

Healing up, under Antiseptic Precautions, of Fresh and Dead Tissues in Serous Cavities, and the Subsequent Fate of these Tissues.

Starting from the observation that foreign bodies and ligatured portions of tissue, *e. g.*, the returned pedicle in ovariotomies, may without injury to the patient be left in the body, ROSENBERGER (*Archiv für Klin. Chir.*, Band xxv. Heft 4) has performed certain experiments with living material, mostly pieces of muscle, but also whole organs (the kidney). The results of these experiments are as follows. With antiseptic precautions, pieces of living tissue heal up in the serous cavities of animals, either quite without, or with only the very slightest reaction. After a time, these pieces disappear without leaving a trace. The tissue need not be from the same animal—need not even be from the same species of animal. The process is not one of digestion, but commences with the encapsuling of the tissue on the third or fourth day. From the capsule, cells wander into the inclosed tissue and break it up. A rarer method is for the piece of tissue, after five or six days, without having caused any irritation in the peritoneal cavity, to have still little or no union with its surroundings ; the capsule becomes firmer, receives a capillary network, and the tissue thus nourished, lives on. This method occurred only in the case of animals of the same species. A third method is precisely the same as the last, with the exception that, in the centre of the piece, probably owing to insufficient nourishment, a pus-cavity is found.—*London Med. Record*, March 15, 1881.

Amputation of the Breast by a Bloodless Method.

In No. 30 of *Centralb. für Chir.*, 1880, Leisrink has mentioned a screw-compressor, which he has used twice in removing the breast, to make the operation quite bloodless. This apparatus consists of a flattened U-shaped iron, the vertically standing arms of which are placed in the holes of a straight iron staff. The latter, as soon as the female screws are applied to the vertical arms and screwed, presses the base of the breast against the horizontal bar of the apparatus, making the breast free from blood. SZUMAN recommends (*Ibid.* No. 40) a process to make the amputation bloodless, which can be used not only with a pendulous breast, but with any other. He operated on a medullary sarcoma of the breast with a broad and flabby base, in the following manner. The base of the breast was pierced close to the thorax three times by means of a long straight needle, which was armed with a double and very strong silk thread; the threads were then fastened in such a manner that the base of the breast was divided into four parts, constricted by ligatures, and thus made free from blood. Above the ligatures, the tumour was removed, the veins tied, and the wound sewed together. Complete union by first intention was obtained.—*London Med. Record*, March 15, 1881.

Chlorate of Potash in acute Blennorrhagia.

Dr. GAMIR (*El Siglo Medico*, October, 1880), of Havana, reports four cases of acute gonorrhœa, which he treated with chlorate of potash. The average duration of treatment was ten days in each case, and the salt was prescribed in doses of from 10 to 20 grammes daily.—*London Med. Record*, March 15, 1881.

Trephining of the Ilium.

Dr. G. FISCHER, of Hanover, has recently reported (*Deutsche Zeitschrift für Chirurgie*, Band xiii., Heft 506) a case of large psoas abscess from spinal disease, in which an opening made below Poupart's ligament had not been sufficient for a free discharge of the pus. As fluctuation could not be felt in the lumbar region, and the extremity of a long probe passed into the cavity of the abscess could not be felt under the skin, Dr. Fischer, in order to make a free counter-opening, trephined the ilium. The soft parts having been divided near the postero-superior angle of the bone, the ilium was perforated, and pus at once flowed through the opening. There was very slight reaction after this operation. The patient, whose condition was weak for a time, died ten weeks later from tuberculosis.

Two other cases of trephining of the ilium have since been published by Dr. M. RIEDEL, of Göttingen (*Centralblatt für Chirurgie*, No. 52, 1880).

A boy, aged 16 years, came under treatment in October, 1877, in a very exhausted condition, and with an open abscess of long standing at the back of the thigh. On examination, whilst the patient was under the influence of chloroform, a long probe was passed first upwards and forwards to the upper third of the front of the thigh, and then upwards under Poupart's ligament, and along the inner surface of the ilium, until it grated against a bare and rough osseous surface at a distance of about two inches and a quarter from the postero-superior spine.

As the spine and the sacro-iliac articulation seemed to be quite healthy, this patch of bare bone was regarded as the starting-point of the abscess. The ilium was trephined at this point, and vent given to some very putrid pus. Erosion of bone was found on the inner surface of the bone, but not any sequestrum. The sacro-iliac joint was found to be quite healthy, but a small fistula was observed leading upwards to the spine. The patient made a very slow recovery after this operation. After a treatment of nearly two years' duration, the patient was discharged as convalescent. The back was then straight, but there existed several open and scantily secreting fistulæ. When seen again a year later, and after he had been working in a factory, the patient presented a well-marked spinal curvature in the lumbar region. The numerous fistulæ at this time had almost all closed.

The subject of the second case—a boy, aged 15—was admitted into the Göttingen Surgical Clinic on June 14, 1880. He had fallen on the left hip about eight weeks previously, and a few days later he became feverish, and began to suffer pain at the seat of injury. When first seen by Dr. Riedel, the thigh was flexed on the pelvis at an angle of 50 deg., and some swelling could be observed in front of the hip. Two months later, in consequence of fluctuation having been made out, an incision was made into this swelling, at a point just below the antero-inferior spine of the ilium. Through this opening the finger could be passed into a cavity on the inner surface of the ilium, which cavity was surrounded by newly-formed bone, and contained a small sequestrum. After unsuccessful attempts to drain the abscess by an anterior opening by the side of the rectus muscle, and a posterior opening made through the muscles on the outer side of the thigh, the ilium was trephined at the seat of the disease. This operation was followed by a free discharge of pus, and subsequently by recovery of the patient

This operation, Dr. Riedel states, is not attended with difficulty. Severe hemorrhage may be avoided by tearing through, instead of incising, the subcutaneous soft parts, and there is but slight reaction after the proceeding. The propriety of Dr. Fischer's indication for this operation is questioned by Dr. Riedel. The former surgeon would trephine the ilium, in order to obtain the best possible outlet for the purulent contents of a pelvic abscess. But when such abscess is due to vertebral disease, the best situation for a counter-opening, or an opening for drainage, is just above the crest of the ilium. In order to make an incision into the abscess in this region without any danger, the surgeon need not insist on fluctuation, but should cut down on the end of a long probe introduced, *not* below Poupart's ligament, but through a puncture made above this structure, near the antero-superior spine, the probe being then carried backwards and outwards until it can be felt under the skin of the back of the patient. The danger of wounding the peritoneum, in case of no abscess existing in the lumbar region, is not very great, provided the sound be introduced carefully. An incision made above the crest of the ilium at its posterior portion is regarded by Dr. Riedel as the best means of draining a pelvic abscess consequent on vertebral disease, and far preferable to a perforation in the ilium. Trephining of the ilium, it is held, is indicated in cases of abscess dependent on disease either of the inner surface of this bone, or of the soft parts contained within the pelvis. In such cases, the operation not only affords a free outlet for pus, but it exposes to direct attack the seat of the primary disease.—*London Medical Record*, March 15, 1881.

—

Pulsating Encephaloid mistaken for Aneurism; Ligature of Right Common Carotid Artery.

Surgeon M. D. MORIARTY reports (*Indian Med. Gazette*, Feb. 1, 1881) the case of a man, aged 45, who applied to him, Feb. 5, 1880, with the following history. About sixteen years before he noticed a pulsating tumour of the size of a small walnut, seated immediately below his right ear, which caused him no great inconvenience. About two months ago the tumour became painful and began to increase in size, and the right side of his face became paralyzed.

On examination a tumour, the size of a small orange, was found to occupy the right parotid region; it extended upwards in front of the ear to about the level of the temporo-maxillary articulation, and behind the ear to a similar level; its lower border was about half an inch above the level of the upper border of the thyroid cartilage. The lower part of the ear was bulged upwards, the external auditory meatus being almost closed. The tumour was more or less globular, with a slight irregularity in the shape of a little prominence at its lower posterior part. On the upper and back part of the tumour were two small blue veins; the skin over the tumour was somewhat congested, especially posteriorly, but was freely movable. The tumour was more or less movable from side to side, its base however appeared to be fixed; it pulsated, the pulsation being systolic and distensile, and on auscultation a well-marked bruit was heard. To the feel the tumour was rather tense, but apparently fluid, the posterior part being perhaps a shade less tense than the rest of it; pressure on it somewhat diminished its size. The right common carotid beat more vigorously than its fellow of the opposite side. Occlusion of it diminished the size of the tumour and completely arrested its pulsation. (No note was made as to whether the consistency of the tumour was also altered, but it must have been to some extent). When the artery was let go the blood entered the tumour with a soft distensile pulsation, and the tumour returned to its original state. Above the tumour the right temporal artery beat more feebly and a little later than the left. Pressure on the tumour, especially in front of the antitragus, caused pain. There was complete right facial hemiplegia; the uvula was straight; the right side of the throat including the tonsil bulged considerably inwards; the tonsil was hypertrophied, and pulsated, the sensation of fluid from within the throat was not however very marked; there was no marked interference with respiration or deglutition; the heart and large vessels appeared to be healthy; the patient never had syphilis, and had only once or twice in his life tasted spirits; the lymphatics in the neck were apparently healthy.

The diagnosis was aneurism, probably of the internal carotid.

On 18th February Mr. Moriarty ligatured the right common carotid just above where it is crossed by the omo-hyoid muscle; and all pulsation in the tumour ceased. On 28th of Feb., slight pulsation was observed in the tumour which had never hardened as a consolidating aneurism should.

The patient kept in pretty fair health up to October, then the symptoms of malignant disease became unmistakable,—rapid growth, implication of the skin, fungation, severe pain, occasional hemorrhages, glandular implication, fetor, emaciation. He died on 30th November.

On examination of the body next day, the disease was found to be encephaloid of the parotid gland. Peripherally, to a depth of about half an inch, the tumour looked like congested cerebellum; centrally it was like boiled udder (Erichsen); the external carotid was lengthened, it ran at first superficial to the tumour, but afterwards sank into it. The tumour extended very deeply, the pinna was quite separated from the external auditory meatus, and the bone all round the latter was eaten away and covered with a horribly fœtid slough. The tumour extended almost to the jugular fossa, it encircled the internal carotid for a small part of its jugular course; lower down it touched the transverse process of the atlas.

In this case most of the symptoms of aneurism were present, but were deficient in quality, especially was this true of the pulsation which was not quite
what the thump of an aneurism should be.

[The difficulties of diagnosis in cases like the above are oftentimes very great,
and in this connection a series of very excellent papers on this subject by Dr.
Stephen Smith, of New York, in the *American Journal of the Medical Sciences*
for April and Oct. 1873, and Jan. 1874, may be read with interest.—ED.]

On the Ox Aorta Ligature, and on the Variability of Catgut.

Mr. RICHARD BARWELL read, at a recent meeting of the Royal Medical and
Chirurgical Society (*Lancet*, March 12, 1881), a paper on his experience with
the ox aorta ligature and on the variability of catgut. The object of a paper
which Mr. Barwell read two years ago was, first, to point out the cases of aortic
aneurism which might be benefited by deligation of the right carotid and subclavian; secondly, to show the advisability of leaving all the coats of arteries
tied in continuity intact; thirdly, to introduce a flat ligature to carry out this
object. The experience, necessarily small, which he could then adduce he now
supplements by two additional cases of aortic aneurism treated by tying the
above-named vessels with the ox aorta ligature; thus there are three in all. 1.
His own case; lived sixteen months in fair health and comfort. 2. A case of
Dr. Lediard (now of Carlisle); lived ten months. 3. A case by Dr. Wyeth of
New York; now alive and in good health. Besides these Mr. Barwell reports
a case in which he tied for aortic aneurism the vessels on the left side of the neck.
The operation failed to prolong, but he does not know that it shortened, life. The
patient survived thirty hours. The parts of his first case, and of Dr. Lediard's
case (by the kind permission of Dr. Hopkins), were exhibited, as were also
certain specimens removed from the last case. The arteries of the first were injected; the carotid ligature was *ab origine* tied too loose. It was the first artery
Mr. B. had tied with the ox aorta, and he attributed the almost immediate return
of temporal pulse wrongly to free collateral circulation. The loop of ligature
probably remains on the vessel. The subclavian is quite closed, and, being slit
lengthwise, shows the tunics entire. Collateral circulation is well established.
Of the second case Dr. Lediard writes: The aneurism is filled with very firm
clot. Nothing could have been more satisfactory than the action of your ligature
in this case. The vessels were entirely occluded, there being no trace of the
bands seen, but a firm clot above and below the seat of constriction, such as is
usual in vessels tied in continuity. The parts from the last case are the subclavian, showing where tied no injury to any of the coats—the severed ligature
from that artery; the other ligature with the knot entire, and showing no tendency to loosen. Four other vessels have been tied with this ligature—two iliacs
(Mr. Holmes and Mr. Johnson Smith), two femorals (Mr. Bellamy and Mr. Barwell); in these four cases the aneurisms did perfectly well, the wounds healed at
once, and nothing more was seen of the ligature.

The twelve deligations are more than sufficient to show that the ox aorta ligature becomes absorbed with sufficient slowness to be perfectly reliable in tying
vessels in continuity. They show this with the more force because this material
is not prepared, the ligatures are cut from the fresh aorta and dried, hence they
are uniform. What has happened with those that have been employed will happen with all. This power of becoming gradually absorbed is common to all the
soft connective tissues, provided they are perfectly fresh—*i. e.*, not decomposed.
The submucous tissue of sheep's intestine, of which catgut is made, would, if it
were dried while fresh, act like other soft connective tissues, with no need what-

ever for after preparation. But in the manufacture of catgut this structure is separated from the rest by processes of scraping, a procedure which would be impossible unless the intestine were to some extent decomposed. The various modes of preparing catgut into ligatures are devices for getting rid of the results of this decomposition. Catgut sutures, more easily watched than ligatures, dissolve in very various periods, though prepared in identically the same way. One of the chromic acid processes gives cords, dissolving some in nine, some in nineteen days. The usual (old) method has supplied Mr. B. with sutures, some of which have dissolved in forty-eight hours, some remained persistent, and had to be cut away on the fourteenth day. This results from the various degrees of decomposition in the catgut itself; it cannot happen with tissues that are fresh and require no after-elaboration. When a piece of catgut is buried deep round a large vessel, we cannot be more sure of its behaviour than we can predict the duration of the sutures; nor can we deduce from the good behaviour of certain such ligatures that the particular piece supplied us will act properly. For tying large vessels near the heart, or lying deep, a material whose action is more uniform, which is therefore more reliable, is essential.

Mr. LISTER said it was interesting to learn that the tissue of the aorta resisted absorption for so long a time. He disputed the statement that the preparation of catgut by scraping was due to putrefaction. On the contrary, the fresher the intestine the better the quality of catgut. The rapidity of absorption of improperly prepared catgut was not due to the state of putrefaction, but to the difference between cellular tissue and aortic tissue. Unlike Mr. Barwell, he had found old catgut less readily absorbed than new catgut; but by the new mode of preparation he had described both kinds were brought to the same level in this respect. Speaking of the desirability of dividing the inner and middle coats of an artery tied in continuity, he said that in one of his early experiments (using a ligature of a strip of ox's peritoneum) he had tied the carotid of a calf without dividing the middle coat; but this did not prove that the division of the inner and middle coats was not essential. Indeed, general experience went to show the desirability of such division—incomplete ligature or insufficient injury to the coats being followed by a tendency to the opening up of the vessels. He always applied the catgut ligature so as to divide the inner and middle coats; although whether this was absolutely necessary when the catgut was of the best form— (i. e., not too readily absorbed), he was not prepared to say. Referring to the case recently related by Mr. Treves, where the opening up of the carotid artery after antiseptic ligature was ascribed to the rapid healing of the wound, the subclavian in the same case being perfectly occluded, and the wound not antiseptic, Mr. Lister showed a specimen where the external iliac had been tied for femoral aneurism. An antiseptic silk ligature was used, and the wound followed an antiseptic course. The external iliac artery was wholly occluded. A small knot of silk remained, and a minute abscess occurred at the seat of ligature. Death took place one year after ligature. Here was evidence of extensive obliteration following the application of an antiseptic ligature. On the other hand, secondary hemorrhage from the distal side followed sometimes on the use of ordinary ligatures, from absence of coagulation; and such cases proved that suppuration around the vessel did not invariably lead to obstruction. That failures in occlusion might follow the use of catgut, when not of proper quality, he was fully aware. Such failures were recorded, but the multitude of successful cases were not. He felt sure that if all the cases were reckoned in which the catgut ligature was applied to arteries in their continuity with strict antiseptic treatment, the results would compare very favourably with other methods of ligature. But if surgeons use the catgut ligature and allow the wounds to putrefy, good results could hardly be hoped for. Such cases as those recorded by Mr. Bryant were due to the lucky chance that union by first intention took place in the deep parts of the wound, thus preventing putrefaction around the ligature. He ventured to think that surgeons who undertake such operations are bound to take measures to avoid putrefaction. At the Cambridge meeting of the British Medical Association he adduced a long series of cases in which no putrefaction occurred, and since then he had had many more cases without putrefaction in a single instance. He did not state this in a spirit of boasting, but simply as a matter of duty. His cases at King's College Hospital were not dressed by himself, but by the house-surgeon and dresser, to whom the praise was due. Surely if such results can be obtained it was worth while to master the simple measures of preventing putrefaction. By the use of such measures the two great dangers to ligature of arteries in their continuity—viz., secondary hemorrhage and diffuse suppuration—may be avoided, and these were objects deserving the best attention.

Mr. TREVES said that in the case he had reported where the carotid after antiseptic ligature became partially reopened, the catgut was of good quality and the coats divided. The small abscess at the seat of ligature in Mr. Lister's case of iliac ligature was hardly consistent with an absence of inflammatory reaction. With regard to the mode of tying arteries alluded to by Mr. Barwell, he had found by experiment that it was almost impossible to divide the inner and middle coats when a double hitch was made in the ligature before tightening it.

Mr. LISTER pointed out that the abscess referred to was of very minute size, and could not have produced any inflammatory action around the vessel.

Mr. HEATH remarked that in one of Mr. Barwell's specimens the carotid artery which had been ligatured was quite pervious, and showed no trace at all of any ligature. The subclavian in the same specimen was completely obliterated. Was there division of its internal and middle coats? He doubted if the surgeon could so graduate the force he applied as not to cut through the inner and middle coats.

Mr. BARWELL, in reply, said that much depended on the mode in which the ligature was tied. He had found that, owing to the roughness of catgut, it was difficult to tell from the sense of resistance whether the artery was being sufficiently pressed on or not. The carotid artery in the specimen alluded to by Mr. Heath had been incompletely tied. The condition of the coats of the subclavian was not ascertained in that specimen; but in another the internal and middle coats were not divided. By means of flat ligatures it was hardly possible to tie the vessel so tightly as to divide the inner and middle coats. He had been struck with the fact that the recorded cases of ligature of the largest vessels were fatal from secondary hemorrhage, and it struck him that this would be obviated by keeping the artery entire. He did not at all suppose that this could only be done by means of the ox aorta ligatures. Mr. Pollock last year tied the subclavian and carotid successfully, using ligatures of kangaroo tendon. Professor Wyeth had used ligatures of the whole thickness of the aorta. Why should not catgut act in the same way? He certainly thought the preparation of catgut was attended by putrefaction, and had attributed its unreliability largely to this. One surgeon used chromic acid many times the strength of that used by Mr. Lister to make the catgut reliable. In the old methods of preparation Mr. Lister had got perfectly reliable ligatures; but in one case where he had supplied Mr. Pemberton with such a ligature a large abscess formed, and the ligature came away. In a case of double popliteal aneurism Mr. Bellamy tied one femoral with the aortic ligature, and with good result. The same operation performed on the opposite leg with the chromic catgut ligature supplied by Mr. Lister was followed by the formation of a sinus leading down to the ligature, the rest of the wound healing by first intention. These different modes of preparing catgut ligatures may suit one or other form of catgut, but not all, and therefore he said the catgut ligature was not a reliable one. Nor did experiments in blood serum touch the point, for the experiments should be made in the living body in the midst of the tissues.

Midwifery and Gynæcology.

The Treatment of Extra-Uterine Gestation.

At a late meeting of the Medical Society of the County of New York, Dr. WILLIAM T. LUSK read a paper on the above subject. In commencing he alluded to the fact that extra-uterine pregnancy was a condition which existed much more frequently than was formerly supposed to be the case, and stated that for its present knowledge of the subject the profession was greatly indebted, first to the late Dr. John S. Parry, of Philadelphia, and, secondly, to Prof. T. Gaillard Thomas. As cases of this kind were now known to be comparatively common, the question of treatment, therefore, assumed a high degree of importance.

The natural termination of tubal and interstitial pregnancy was by rupture of the sac, hemorrhage, peritonitis, and death ; although there was a certain number of spontaneous recoveries on record, either through the mummification of the fœtus or the formation of a fistulous tract through which it was gradually discharged in small portions. In ovarian and abdominal pregnancies the death of the fœtus might take place either prematurely or at full term, and in the majority of cases it resulted in suppuration, which was almost sure to be followed by peritonitis and the death of the mother. Occasionally, however, the latter survived, and a fistulous opening was established into the vagina or rectum, or through the external abdominal walls, by means of which elimination took place. But this process of elimination was ordinarily a very slow one, and in the greater number of instances the patient required active interference on the part of the medical attendant, or else death would eventually ensue from blood-poisoning or exhaustion. Again, in a certain proportion of cases the fœtus after its death became coated with a bony or earthy crust, and remained as a comparatively innocuous tumour during the rest of the woman's life. Its presence under such circumstances did not prevent the occurrence of pregnancy subsequently.

The treatment of extra-uterine gestation, Dr. Lusk continued, varied according to the stage of pregnancy. In cases of early gestation the indication was plainly to destroy the life of the fœtus, and in order to accomplish this without injury to the mother a number of methods had been suggested and practised. One of the most simple was the puncture of the sac, and this could usually be easily effected by means of a trocar introduced through the walls of the vagina or rectum. It was true that a number of recoveries were on record in cases where this plan was adopted, but the results, as a rule, were unfavourable. The second method mentioned was that of injecting poisonous solutions into the sac by means of the hypodermic syringe. The first used was one-fifth of a grain of sulphate of atropia in a small quantity of water; but Friedereich had substituted the fifth of a grain of morphia for this, and had reported two successful cases under its use.

The third method was that resorted to by Thomas, namely, the use of the galvano-cautery. One case barely escaped resulting fatally in his hands, however, and in the latest edition of his work on diseases of women (which contained a chapter on extra-uterine pregnancy) he recommended Paquelin's cautery. It was to be employed only after the pregnancy had given rise to symptoms of trouble. The fourth and last method considered was the use of the faradic current. It was to be kept up from five to ten minutes through the seat of the product of conception, and repeated from time to time, if necessary, for one or two weeks, until the shrinkage of the tumour left no doubt that the passage of the current had produced the desired effect. Dr. Lusk then related in detail the history of a very interesting case in which he had called Dr. Thomas in consultation, and in which the faradic current had been employed with complete success. The use of the faradic current, in this connection, he continued, the profession owed to Dr. James G. Allen, of Philadelphia, who reported two cases successfully treated by it in 1872. This method, Dr. Lusk considered, offered a much better chance of recovery than any other, and one great advantage of it was that it was accompanied by no drawbacks. So far as he knew, it had now been resorted to in nine cases, and in every one of them the result had been successful. When it was remembered that in one hundred and fifty cases collected by Hume there were only seventeen recoveries, the advance that had been made could be better appreciated. The subsequent treatment was that for peritonitis.

The second class of cases was that in which gestation was in an advanced stage and the fœtus was still living. Here symptoms of exhaustion finally came on, and the patient was in great danger. Laparotomy in such cases, Dr. Lusk thought, ought to enjoy the highest confidence of the surgeon, provided its performance did not increase the jeopardy of the mother. Parry had reported twenty cases of primary operations, with eight children and six mothers saved ; but after a careful study of these cases he had found that five out of six of the maternal recoveries ought really to be stricken out. The great and unavoidable danger in such operations was the difficulty or impossibility of removing the placenta.

Finally he considered the class of cases in which gestation was prolonged after the death of the fœtus. Under these circumstances it was a well-established rule not to operate during the continuance of labour-pains. The fœtus might at length become converted into a hard, innocuous mass, as mentioned at the outset ; but this was the exception, and not the rule. Most commonly it underwent maceration, and the patient sooner or later began to suffer from exhaustion and symptoms of septicæmia. In some cases a fistulous opening was formed into the vagina, into the rectum, through the abdominal walls, or even into the bladder. Under such circumstances the treatment consisted in the enlargement of the fistulous tract, and the extraction of the fœtus piece-meal through it.

Secondary laparotomy was a justifiable operation, and out of thirty-three cases reported there had been nineteen recoveries. Of the two great dangers of the primary operation, hemorrhage and septicæmia, the first was very greatly diminished by the death of the fœtus and the changes ensuing upon it, and the second could be avoided to a considerable extent by the judicious use of the antiseptic precautions now at the surgeon's command. When circumstances permitted, therefore, it was advisable to delay operative procedures until obliteration of the maternal vessels had taken place. Whenever the operation was demanded by the condition of the patient, however, antiseptic surgery offered a fair chance of success.

The paper being before the society for discussion, Dr. JACOBI remarked that he had had but one case of extra-uterine pregnancy in his own practice. This occurred some time ago, and he had not treated it by the method so highly recommended by Dr. Lusk, although he was happy to say that the result had been a favourable one. The patient was probably at the beginning of the third month of gestation, and he had punctured the sac through the vaginal walls. He had also made a second puncture two days afterward. Half a year later, when he examined the patient, he had found a hard substance to the left of the uterus which to the touch reminded him of cicatricial tissue in any other part. Even to this day, although it was seventeen years since the operation, the fundus of the uterus was drawn over to the left by means of the contraction that had resulted, while the cervix pointed decidedly toward the right. With his present knowledge of the subject, and especially after listening to the results mentioned by Dr. Lusk in his paper, he would undoubtedly employ the treatment by the faradic current if he were to meet with another similar case.

Dr. ROCKWELL stated that he had successfully employed electricity in the treatment of three cases. The first was that of Dr. McBurney, which had been alluded to by Dr. Lusk, and which, having been published in full in the *New York Medical Journal*, was well known to the profession at large. The correctness of the diagnosis had been disputed in some quarters, but he did not propose to discuss this point. The second case was that of Dr. Billington, also mentioned in the paper of the evening, and the third he had seen quite recently. Dr. Lusk had spoken particularly of the use of the faradic current, but it seemed to him that the galvanic current would prove the most efficient in destroying the fœtus. In Dr. McBurney's case this was employed, and two applications were made. Before it was resorted to Dr. Thomas, who was one of the consultants, asked him if he could kill the fœtus in this way without doing injury to the mother, and he replied that he thought he undoubtedly could. The result, as was well known, was entirely satisfactory. In Dr. Billington's case he had made but a single application of electricity, and did not know how many had been made subsequently. In the third case there had been but one application—of the galvanic current—altogether, and the recovery had been as successful as in the other instances. These three cases constituted all his experience in regard to this interesting subject, but they at all events went a considerable distance towards settling the point that the fœtus might be destroyed without injury or danger to the mother.

Dr. BILLINGTON said that in his case a positive diagnosis was made by Dr. Thomas, whom he called in consultation, and that he had made four applications after the first one by Dr. Rockwell. The first three times he employed fourteen or fifteen cells, but the last time he used the full strength of the battery, thirty-six cells.

Dr. MUNDÉ had seen three cases of extra-uterine gestation altogether. The first was in the service of Scanzoni, and was fatal. It was a case of ventral pregnancy, and the patient went beyond full term. The second occurred in Braun's clinic. The pregnancy had originally been either interstitial or tubal, and the fœtus at length escaped into the abdominal cavity. The woman was in a very cachectic condition, and it was decided to wait till her death before operating for the purpose of saving the child's life. As soon as she expired laparotomy was performed, but the child which weighed nine pounds, was asphyxiated. The third case occurred in his own practice, and the circumstances were peculiar, the fœtus escaping through the uterine canal, as in Dr. McBurney's case. Before he met with it he had been disposed to doubt the accuracy of the diagnosis in the latter, as he could not understand how the fœtus could pass through the undilated uterine canal. Now, however, he was quite willing to take back all that he had said upon this point, for the case in his own experience had completely convinced him that such a thing was quite possible. In this case he had sounded the uterus with the probe and found it empty, and yet twenty-four hours afterward he found the uterine cavity occupied by the fœtal mass, while the tumour which had previously existed above the uterus had entirely disappeared. In this instance bi-manual examination was unusually easy, and there could be no doubt whatever of this latter fact.

It seemed to him that Dr. Rockwell was correct in his view that the galvanic was to be preferred to the faradic current in these cases. There were two reasons that occurred to him why the galvanic was preferable. First, the faradic current had the effect of causing a contraction of the muscular fibres of the tube, and, secondly, while the faradic current might kill the foetus by the shock it produced, the galvanic had the additional advantage of decomposing the amniotic fluid.

In Dr. McBurney's case Dr. Emmet had made a suggestion, which he thought might prove of service in a certain proportion of instances. "Why not dilate the uterine cavity," said he, "and extract the foetus in this way?" This might, perhaps, be a bold and difficult procedure, but, in the hands of an operator as skilful as Dr. Emmet, could no doubt be successfully accomplished in some cases of tubal or interstitial pregnancy. When rupture of the tube had taken place, he believed it to be quite justifiable to perform laparotomy, as proposed by Kiwisch, and, with all the resources of modern surgery now at one's command, he thought that the prospect of success would be as good as in many bad cases of ovariotomy.

In concluding the discussion, Dr. Lusk remarked that the galvanic current had been proposed in the treatment of extra-uterine pregnancy as early as 1857. At first its introduction in this field of surgery was hailed with great enthusiasm; but afterwards the plan was abandoned because the operators found that they did not obtain as good results from it as from simple puncture of the sac. It was after the use of the galvanic current had been given up that Dr. Allen resorted to the faradic current, and up to the present time (as he had mentioned in the paper) nine cases had been reported in which it had been successfully employed without the occurrence of a single bad symptom. Or, leaving out Dr. McBurney's case, in which he had been under the impression that the faradic current had been used, until corrected by Dr. Rockwell, this evening, there would be eight successful cases on record.—*Boston Medical and Surgical Journal*, March 17, 1881.

—

On the Determination of the Indications for Gastrotomy in Cases of Extra-Uterine Foetation.

Dr. C. Litzmann, in a paper on this subject (*Archiv für Gynäkalogie*, Bd. xvi. p. 323), grounds his observations on two cases of the kind on which he operated on successive days, and on an analysis of forty-three cases extracted from various sources.

The cases were: I. Mrs. P., a healthy, well-built woman, aged 25, pregnant for the second time. After her first confinement she had a pelvic inflammatory attack. She came under observation in the ninth month, and had had during her whole pregnancy repeated attacks of abdominal pain, and twice in the early months hemorrhage from the vagina. The urine contained albumen. Passing from the right side of the abdomen above, to the left side of the pelvis below, was a large, oval, completely-fixed tumour, over which the abdominal wall was partially movable, and in which, at its upper part could be felt a child's head. To the left, and about the height of the umbilicus, could be felt the enlarged uterus, which was slightly movable on the mass. The heart-sounds were audible on the right side and high up. Per vaginam, the lower part of the swelling could be felt projecting into the roof; to the right side and to the left, and higher up, lay the os uteri. The uterus was movable, the swelling was not. A right tubo-uterine pregnancy was diagnosed. Gastrotomy, with antiseptic precautions, was performed, and the placenta was not interfered with. There was only slight bleeding. The child weighed five and a half pounds, was greatly deformed from pressure, and died almost immediately. There was hardly any liquor amnii. A drainage-tube was passed into the cavity, through which it was washed out once or twice daily with carbolic water. On the thirteenth day this washing out caused profuse hemorrhage, which was stopped by compression. Two similar bleedings occurred on the two subsequent days. On the seventeenth day the placenta was removed without much hemorrhage taking place, and on the eighteenth the patient died. The pregnancy was found to be tubal, not inter-stitial.

Case II., aged 35, pregnant for the seventh time; presented the ordinary history of extra-uterine pregnancy. On examination, the apparently empty uterus was felt pressed backwards by a large, round, fluctuating tumour, in which could be felt the small parts of a child, and over which could be heard the fœtal heart. At the end of the thirty-second week the fœtal movements ceased to be felt, and at the same time the heart-sounds became inaudible. Five days afterwards the breasts swelled, and a mass, probably decidual, was expelled from the vagina. A fortnight later small quantities of very fetid matter came away from the vagina in gushes. Menstruation came on seventeen days after the death of the child. Nine weeks later gastrotomy was performed, and the fœtus removed, along with the placenta and the greater part of the membranes. Though the placenta was cut into by the incision, there was no serious bleeding. The operation was conducted antiseptically, and recovery was uninterrupted.

After contrasting these two cases, the author reproduces from various sources, German, American, and English, accounts of forty-three cases of extra-uterine pregnancy where gastrotomy was performed, and divides them into cases operated on during the life of the child, and cases operated on after its death. He, however, excludes from the reckoning all those cases where a single abdominal incision was made to evacuate an abscess which had formed in the sac. In ten cases of the former class there were nine deaths and one recovery, while in thirty-three of the latter the deaths were fourteen and the recoveries nineteen. After a full analysis of these cases he comes to the conclusion that the dangers of hemorrhage, either during the operation or on the subsequent separation of the placenta, are, in general, too great to warrant gastrotomy during the life of the child, which, moreover, in consequence of compression within its sac, is usually so much deformed and so imperfectly developed as to be unable to live. Accordingly, except in those cases in which the size of the sac and of the living fœtus contained in it are such as render it nearly certain that the child is large, well-formed, and likely to be-viable, Litzmann maintains that the proper course is to wait for a sufficient length of time after its death to allow of complete thrombosis and obliteration of the placental circulation before interfering. He does not attempt to define the period necessary to wait until the circulation is closed, but thinks it ought to be a good few weeks. In his own case the operation was performed eleven weeks after the death of the child.—*Edinburgh Med. Journal,* Jan. 1881.

—

Vesico-Vaginal Fistula treated by the formation of a Recto-Vaginal Fistula and Closure of the Vagina.

Complete occlusion of the vagina has long been looked upon as the *dernier ressort* in cases of vesico-vaginal fistula in which, either from their size, or the unhealthiness of the tissues bounding them, restoration of the vaginal wall to its integrity seemed hopeless. But the data from which to judge as to the effect of the urine upon parts not adapted to contain it, and as to what is the way to get the best artificial reservoir, are as yet scanty. A case by Dr. GEZA ANTAL, published in the *Archiv fur Gynäkologie*, gives us some information on this head. His case was one in which the loss of tissue was so great that closure of the fistula was thought out of the question. His first thought was to close the vagina in its lower third, letting the urine and menstrual fluid be passed per urethram. But repeated operations for this purpose all ended in failure. Then it occurred to him to unite the labia, first making a recto-vaginal fistula; thus making the rectum a common cloaca, and trusting to the rectal sphincter to retain both kinds of excreta. This he did. While the patient was under surgical treatment, the bladder was washed out with ½ per cent. solution of carbolic acid. The operation was successful. The result has been that the patient now passes urine per rectum at intervals of from two to two and a half hours. During these intervals she does not complain of any discomfort. Menstruation is regular, the blood escaping without hindrance. Several months after the operation no change could be discovered with the speculum in the rectal mucous membrane. The favourable results above described had lasted, when the author wrote, for seven months after the operation.—*Med. Times and Gaz.*, March 12, 1881.

—

Extirpation of Uterus and Ovaries.

At a late meeting of the Obstetrical Society of London Dr. THOMAS CHAMBERS (*Lancet*, Feb. 5, 1881), read a paper on "Complete Extirpation of the Uterus with both Ovaries, weighing ten pounds; recovery." Jane S——, aged forty-three, was admitted into the Chelsea Hospital for Women on May 24th, 1880. In 1870 she first noticed a lump in her right groin, which grew slowly for five years. After this menorrhagia commenced, and gradually increased. Pain and hemorrhage were excessive, and she eventually became too weak to attend as an out-patient, and was remarkably emaciated. The tumour was freely movable from side to side, and was very soft and doughy, but without fluctuation. The pelvic cavity was unoccupied, the vagina drawn up into a cone, with the os and cervix, both small, in the centre. There was a periodical discharge of watery fluid through the vagina. Hence a diagnosis of fibro-cystic tumour was made. Medical treatment having proved of no avail, extirpation of the uterus was proposed to the patient, and she decided in favour of the operation. It was performed on June 2d. The abdominal incision was extended to eleven inches. The broad ligaments were tied with silk at each side, a parallel clamp placed above the ligatures, and the uterus cut away. After a few minutes arterial hemorrhage occurred from a large vessel, which was at once secured. The cervix was then transfixed by a double ligature, the clamp removed, the ligatures tightened, and the stumps replaced. By the twenty-first day the patient was convalescent, a free discharge of offensive matter from the vagina having taken place suddenly on the fourteenth day. The tumour proved to be a lobulated white fibroid, not fibro-cystic, and contained very large vessels.

' Dr. HEYWOOD SMITH thought that the term hysterectomy should be limited to amputation of the uterus. He considered oöphorectomy safer than removal of the uterus when life was threatened by flooding and pain.

Dr. ROUTH had some years ago tabulated a number of fibro-cystic tumours as compared with pure fibroids of the uterus, and had found that in fibro-cystic disease menorrhagia was rare.

The Therapeutics of Ovarian Compression.

M. Bourneville (*Le Progrés Médical*, No. 2, 1881) records the following case. He was called to see a young married lady, aged 22, who had suffered from hysteria for some years, but latterly the attack had been of daily occurrence. After one of these, which occurred on December 21, she became paralyzed on the right side, with hemianæsthesia of the same side. During the night of the 30th, spasmodic contraction of the lower jaw supervened. On December 31st, M. Bourneville found the following symptoms: Right hemiplegia and hemianæsthesia, with stiffness of the joint; double ovarian hyperæsthesia; contraction of the jaw. After practising ovarian compression for some minutes, the spasm of the jaw relaxed, and the patient could put out her tongue; but, when the compression ceased, the spasm reappeared. After a short interval, he again compressed the right ovarian region, with a similar result; and, when compelled to desist, from fatigue, he discovered that the spasm of the jaw did not recur, that sensibility returned to the right side, and that the patient could move her right arm and leg. A further compression resulted in the complete disappearance of all the symptoms, so that the patient got up and walked. M. Bourneville remarks that such astonishing results may be obtained, if the medical attendant will employ ovarian compression for a sufficient length of time, and repeat it frequently at short intervals.—*British Medical Journal*, March 5, 1881.

Medical Jurisprudence and Toxicology.

Poisoning by Atropia successfully treated by Hypodermic Injection of Pilocarpin.

Professor Purjesz relates in the *Pester Med.-Chir. Presse*, Nos. 15, 17, and 18, 1880, the case of a hospital patient, aged 19, under treatment for aortic insufficiency and keratoiritis, who drank with suicidal intent the contents of a bottle of solution of atropin which was used for dropping in his eye. The quantity of atropin taken was about nine-tenths of a grain. The pupils were dilated to the maximum, the face was pale; respirations frequent, 40 to 50 in the minute; pulse 140 to 150. The patient was perfectly unconscious; sensibility was not lost. Relying on the observation by Luchsinger of the physiological antagonism between atropin and pilocarpin, Dr. Purjesz injected in succession six syringefuls of a one per cent. solution of pilocarpin (about 0.9 grain in each); and repeated the injection at intervals from five to eight minutes. After the tenth injection, the patient began to speak; the pupils were distinctly narrower; and, as the secretion of saliva and sweat had not yet appeared, another injection of nine-tenths of a grain of pilocarpin was made. After this dose, the patient gave rational answers; the pulse fell to 80; the pupils regained their normal size, but reacted rather slowly to light; the respiratory movements became normal, the skin moist, and all the symptoms of poisoning by atropin disappeared.—*British Med. Journal*, Feb. 26, 1881.

Localization of Strychnia.

Husemann, Dragendorff, and other chemists have advised, in cases of poisoning, that chemists in looking for strychnia should especially direct their researches to the liver. Dragendorff alleges that he has never been able to isolate the alkaloid from the brain, even when the whole organ has been used for the chemical examination. He further states that Gay has isolated strychnia from some special parts of the nervous system, as for example, the medulla oblongata, and the pons Varolii, and that he has himself succeeded in extracting it from the medulla oblongata in cases of poisoning. LAJOUX and GRANDRAL have published their results from analysis of the brain of a person who died from the effects of 2.35 grammes of tincture of nux vomica, corresponding to only 0.0036 gramme (.0525 grain) of strychnia. Three-fourths of this were employed subcutaneously, and the rest was administered by the mouth. Although the quantity was very small, yet strychnia was found throughout the brain, and gave its characteristic reaction. If this observation be correct, chemists will do well to examine the brain in cases of suspected strychnia poisoning, as well as the other organs.— *British Med. Journal*, Feb. 12, 1881.

—

Poisoning by Glycine.

Dr. LÉONFFRE, Physician of the Orphan Asylum at Rocca, relates in the *Lyon Médical* cases of poisoning which he has observed in several orphans of the institution. These young children had been chewing fragments of roots of glycine instead of Spanish liquorice. At the outset, they complained of a gastralgic pain; the face became congested, and the cheeks reddened; but this reddening was very transient, and gave way to paleness as soon as the children felt nauseated. A few minutes afterwards, vomiting commenced, consisting first of alimentary matters, then of bile and mucus. The patients then complained of a great feeling of uneasiness; the face was pale and pinched; the eyes sunken, and surrounded by blue lines; the pupils were largely dilated; the skin, and especially the extremities, cold; muscular weakness was very marked; and the patients complained of feeling their legs bend under them. Among those who were most ill, an irresistible tendency to sleep was observed. The children complained of chill; the pulse remained at 80, very weak; and in two cases the voice was imperceptible. The capillary circulation was defective; and in two patients, whose pulse was hardly perceptible, the extremities were reddened, and the face, as well as the skin of the trunk, marbled with blue lines. The respiration was normal, and rather slackened than obstructed. There was neither delirium nor convulsion. The intellectual faculties were intact, except for the torpor. The secretions were not disturbed, the skin not presenting that appearance of sweating which is met with in analogous conditions. The action of the glycine on the intestinal tube was not marked in any of the eighteen cases, except in one girl, who was purged eleven times. The accidents observed were rapidly counteracted by the administration of hot tea and coffee, and the application of hot water bottles. In one case only, energetic friction was necessary to combat collapse and the tendency to sleep. Dilatation of the pupil was the earliest and most constant of all the symptoms. The quantity of glycine chewed by each child must have varied from one to six *grammes* (fifteen to ninety grains). Thus it seems that glycine possesses marked toxic properties, and that it acts like tobacco. This action of glycine was unknown to Dr. Léonffre, and he has not found it mentioned anywhere.—*British Med. Journal*, Jan. 1, 1881.

MEDICAL NEWS.

IMPURE ICE AS A CAUSE OF INTESTINAL DISEASE.

That period of the year, when ice (which is now used by all classes to an extent entitling it to rank as a *necessity* instead of, as formerly, a *luxury* of life) is employed in various beverages to the amount of millions of pounds, cannot delay much longer, so that a few words of caution in regard to the purity of this article will be seasonable.

It is popularly believed that water frees itself from dangerous organic matter, as it does from some saline contaminations, during the process of freezing, and also that the vegetable or animal germs of typhoid and other zymotic fevers are killed, or at least sterilized by congelation of water in which they exist. Both of these ideas, however, are unquestionably erroneous, as has been repeatedly proved by various experiments which ignorant hotel-keepers try, without the least intending it, upon their guests on a scale which would make the boldest vivisector stand aghast before the suffering inflicted, even if it were only upon the brutes which form the subjects of his researches.

Such was notably the case in an epidemic of intestinal disorder which occurred at Rye Beach, N. H., a few years since, of which an excellent account was published in the Report of the Massachusetts Health Board for 1876, by Dr. A. H. Nichols, who attended most of the persons suffering from the malady. It appears that early in the season a mild form of gastro-intestinal disturbance made its appearance among the guests of a particular hotel at this watering-place. The symptoms were, in general, giddiness, nausea, or vomiting, diarrhœa, and severe abdominal pain, accompanied by fever, loss of appetite, and mental depression. The disorder was at first attributed to the well-water of the place, which is strongly impregnated with sulphate and carbonate of lime and magnesia, but the peculiar grouping of the patients almost exclusively among the sojourners at a single hotel, accommodating about three hundred, whilst occupants of another hotel and of neighbouring cottages, to the number of about seven hundred persons, were free from illness, strongly indicated some specific local origin. The well-water was almost immediately suspected of sewage contamination, but, on inquiry, it was found that the wells were all sunk in an elevated ridge safely removed from drains, cesspools, and other sources of pollution. Moreover, it was also ascertained that in some cases the individuals affected, being suspicious of the water, had limited themselves to other beverages; but, as afterwards transpired, had not hesitated to use ice, either melted or otherwise. The drainage system of the establishment, which had recently been put in complete order, was found almost faultless, and the milk-supply of unquestionable purity ; but, on the attention of the examining physician being directed to the stock of ice used in the hotel, conclusive proof of its dangerous quality was promptly obtained. A resident of the place stated that, on testing a portion of the ice the previous winter, he had experienced nausea and distress for the remainder of the day. Two gentlemen having taken a quantity of ice with them upon an excursion, during which they drank the water formed from it, were made violently ill. Both the house in which the ice was stored and the water from the melted ice gave off a decidedly disagreeable, or even offensive, odour. Finally, a visit to the pond from which the ice had been gathered disclosed the fact that much of its water was dark-coloured, foul, and highly contaminated with filthy marsh mud and decomposing sawdust. Chemical analyses showed that both it and the suspected ice contained a large excess of organic and volatile impurities, including .04 of a grain per gallon of albuminoid ammonia. The crucial test, however, of injurious quality pertaining to this ice was afforded by its disuse in the hotel, coincident with which was noticed an abrupt amelioration of the symptoms in all who had previously been ill, and the entire absence, so far as known, of any new cases. The ice was partaken of during a period of six weeks by about five hundred persons. Of these, the majority escaped without injury ; a large number suffered slight or temporary attacks of illness ; and twenty-six adults manifested grave, continued, and characteristic symptoms.

The Connecticut State Board of Health (Report for 1879) informs us that, in several instances, attention has been drawn to sewage-contaminated ponds with ice-houses upon their borders, and that several isolated cases of enteric disease, and one death, from the free use of ice polluted by sewage, have been recorded in that State during the year.

The curious natural experiment of the United States vessel " Plymouth," an elaborate report of which was reviewed in the *American Journal of the Medical Sciences* for Jan. 1881, shows conclusively that the germs of yellow fever are not infallibly destroyed by a freezing, probably not by a zero temperature. Without venturing on any of the unsound reasoning from analogy, too common among medical theorists, this fact alone is sufficient to warn us of the possible danger that the poisons of enteric fever and other zymotic affections are not destroyed by the congelation of the water in which they float, even without the direct and positive testimony such as that given above that impure ice, especially when gathered from ponds polluted by sewage, may constitute a prolific cause of disease.

Resection of the Stomach.—The health of the patient on whom Professor BILL-ROTH performed the operation of removal of a carcinomatous portion of the stomach (see last number of *Medical News and Abstract*, page 232), is satisfactory. The wound is perfectly healed, and the sutures were removed at the end of last week. The patient takes milk and wine, only complaining of constipation, which is relieved by enemata, and of a bedsore on the sacrum, which was caused by her depressed condition. All experiments with semifluid food have failed, and the nourishment has been confined to milk.—*British Medical Journal*, March 5, 1881.

Under date of April 2, we learn that the patient has returned home apparently well, and able to take solid food. Dr. Billroth has since performed the operation twice. The second patient survived eight days. The third, on whom he operated on the 12th of March, for a considerable cancerous tumour, died in twelve hours. The facility of the operation, the absence of peritoneal reaction, and the holding power of the sutures, were apparent in all the three cases.

—

Health of New York.—Smallpox has increased considerably during March, the number of cases being more than double that reported for February. Scarlet fever and diphtheria have decreased, while typhoid fever and measles have increased. Considerable alarm has been created by the appearance of typhus fever, which has not prevailed in the city for a number of years. The first cases were found in a densely crowded lodging-house, at the corner of Prince and Marion Streets, where four hundred lodgers were nightly sheltered. These cases were at once removed to special pavilions on Blackwell's Island, and the premises thoroughly disinfected by the Health Board. During the first week of the endemic 41 cases were reported. During the second week only 5 cases were discovered, but the number rose to 45 in the third week (ending April 10). The type of the disease has been comparatively mild, although many cases have terminated fatally. On April 4th there were 99 cases of variola and 51 of typhus at the Riverside Hospital. On April 14th there were 119 of variola and 90 of typhus fever.

The medical profession of New York has shared the lively and unabated popular interest on the subject of street cleaning. The April number of the *Medical News and Abstract* contained the resolutions adopted by the Academy of Medicine having reference to the causes for the present increased malignity of disease, and the alarmingly high rate of mortality in the city. These resolutions were presented to the Citizens' mass-meeting held on March 18th. A committee of twenty-one, appointed at that meeting, to devise measures for securing a rapid and thorough cleansing of the streets, prepared and presented to the Legislature a bill removing control of the Street Cleaning Bureau from the Police Board and conferring it upon the Mayor, with power to nominate a superintendent of the work. The bill was passed by the Senate on March 30, but rejected on April 8 by the Assembly, which body adopted a substitute, intended to reserve the patronage to the dominant party, giving the Board of Health power to confirm the Mayor's nominee for superintendent. A second indignation mass-meeting was held April 12, and resolutions condemning the action of the Assembly in rejecting the bill of the committee of twenty-one, and urging its immediate reconsideration and adoption, were unanimously passed. A large and enthusiastic mass-meeting of physicians in favour of the Citizens' street cleaning bill was also held on April 13, at Chickering Hall. Dr. Willard Parker presided, and addresses were delivered by Drs. Barker, Dalton, Sayre, Loomis, and other eminent medical men. Resolutions were adopted protesting against the rejection of the Citizens' bill by the Assembly, and demanding that the representatives of the city in the Assembly reverse their action, and endeavour to secure the passage of the bill. A committee of five were appointed to present the resolutions to the Governor of the State, the President of the Senate, and the Speaker of the Assembly.

—

Medical Experts.—A trial took place recently in the Common Pleas Court of Montgomery County, Ohio, which afforded an incident of some interest to the profession. It was a suit for damages alleged to have been inflicted by one woman on another while scuffling in a playful way. Expert testimony was called as to injuries to the shoulder-joint and arm, and it was proposed that a personal examination be made of the plaintiff and an opinion given as to the condition of the parts. Dr. Reeve, of Dayton, being on the stand, demurred to this and appealed to the Court, urging the injustice of a medical witness being compelled to make such an examination without compensation, and declining to make it unless under direct order of the Court. Judge Elliott in reply fully and freely recognized the fact, that a professional man's education was his capital and ought not to be called upon without recompense. The attorneys also openly deplored the injustice of the law in such cases, and admitted that a reform was much needed. Finally, the party interested agreed to pay a fee, and the trial proceeded.

There is no doubt that Dr. Reeve's example might often be followed to advantage. The Courts would, we believe, generally recognize the injustice of the proceeding, and one so widely different from that pursued toward lawyers in similar circumstances, as was pertinently urged by Dr. Reeve.—*Cincinnati Lancet and Clinic*, March 12, 1881.

—

Revision of the German Pharmacopœia.—The revision of the German Pharmacopœia began on October 15th, on which day the commission appointed for the purpose commenced a series of sittings, presided over by Dr. STRUCK, for the purpose of making preliminary arrangements, and concluded their work on the 25th of the same month. A further meeting of the committee will be held, probably next Easter, for the final revision of the text; meantime the editing is entrusted to the chemists and pharmaceutists of the commission, with the addition, as medical experts, of Professors Ziemssen, Gerhardt, and Eulenberg. The composition of the commission is very comprehensive, and is considered in Germany to be very happy, including the representatives of all those who are interested in the work—physicians, public medical officers, clinicists, pharmacologists, chemists, and apothecaries. We quote it here because it is interesting as compared with that of the British Pharmacopœia Committee. The new pharmacopœia, unlike the old Prussian, Austrian, and Swiss Pharmacopœias, will be published in the German language, including the heading of each article, to which, however, the Latin titles will be added. The title of the new edition will be *Arzneibuch des Deutschen Reiches*. Only two voices were raised, it is said, against this resolution; those, it is believed, of Flükiger and Poleck, who considered it might be inconvenient not to have the pharmacopœia in the international Latin tongue, especially in reference to the possibly approaching international pharmacopœia. This was overruled, however, on the ground that such an international pharmacopœia is still far distant; and that, even if it should be published, it will certainly very rapidly be translated into the language of each country; just as all Latin pharmacopœias have always had alongside of them translated pharmacopœias of much greater popularity. The commission has treated the question of striking out unnecessary drugs and preparations in a very radical fashion. It is said that, of 797 articles in the German Pharmacopœia, no fewer than 370—that is to say, nearly a half—are eliminated by this commission. Among them are acetum colchici, aconitin, ammonium carbonicum, pyro-oleosum, valerianates of bismuth and of quinine, bromine, prepared shells, elemi, dry and inspissated ox-gall, several preparations of iron, kino, logwood, mastich, acetate of morphia, santonate of soda, oxymel of colchicum and of squills, guaiacum and scammony resins, lactate and valerianate of zinc, etc.; as well as about half of the hitherto officinal distilled waters, plasters, extracts, ethereal oils, tinctures, and ointments. They are proceeding much more cautiously in adding new agents to the pharmacopœia. They have added salicylic acid, nitrite of amyl, apomorphin, physostigmin, jaborandi, and pilocarpin; on the other hand, they have rejected condurango, coto bark, quebracho bark, leaves of eucalyptus and the preparations thereof, araroba and chrysophanic acid, butyl-chloral, bromide of camphor, gelsemium, etc. In the matter of antiseptic dressing, materials have been added, as concentrated carbolic solution, and carbolic water prescriptions formulated for absorbent cotton-wool; catgut in three strengths, gutta-percha paper, thymol, and acetate of alumina. The constitution of this committee appears to have enabled it to set to work with great vigour, and get through it with rapidity.—*British Medical Journal*, Jan. 15, 1881.

The Medical Law of New York.—The Act of 1880 provides that no person shall "practise physic or surgery within the State unless he is twenty-one years of age, and either has been heretofore authorized so to do pursuant to the laws in force at the time of his authorization, or is hereafter authorized so to do," either by a license from the regents of the University of the State of New York, a diploma of an incorporated medical college within the State, or a diploma of a similar institution without the State, provided it be endorsed as approved by some proper medical faculty of the State. But every physician and surgeon, with the exception of practitioners of ten years' standing and a few others, must register in the office of the clerk of the county where he is practising, or, if hereafter authorized, intends to practise, his name, residence, place of birth, together with his authority to practise, to all of which he must subscribe. He also must make affidavit as to the manner of his license or authority, the date of the same and by whom granted, which, if wilfully false, shall subject the affiant to conviction and punishment for perjury. Any one who violates either of these provisions or the one in regard to practising, or who shall practise under cover of a diploma illegally obtained, shall be deemed to be guilty of a misdemeanor, and on conviction shall be fined not less than fifty dollars nor more than two hundred dollars for the first offence, and for a subsequent offence he shall be fined not less than one hundred dollars nor more than five hundred dollars, or imprisoned not less than thirty days, or both.—*Popular Science Monthly*, April, 1881.

Cremation in the United States.—According to the *Popular Science Monthly*, April, 1881, steps have been taken in New York to provide the necessary organizations to furnish facilities for cremation. A draft of a charter has been approved by the persons concerned in the movement, for the formation of "the United States Cremation Company (limited)," with a capital of fifty thousand dollars, whose peculiar object shall be "to cremate the human dead in the quickest, best, and most economical manner." A plan has also been adopted for the formation of the "New York Cremation Society," as an association distinct from the purely business enterprise, having for its object "to disseminate sound and enlightened views respecting incineration as preferable to burial, and to advance the public good by offering facilities for cremation."

Fracture of both Clavicles Simultaneously.—In the *Gazzetta Med. Lombardia,* Jan. 8, an abstract is given of a case in which both clavicles were simultaneously fractured—this being so rare an occurrence that Malgaigne only met with it once in 2358 cases of fracture of the clavicle; and Gurlt, in his great work on Fractures, states that he has only been able to meet with fifteen recorded eases. Sayre's apparatus was employed, and the patient was perfectly cured in thirty days, no trace of deformity being visible.—*Med. Times and Gazette,* Jan. 29, 1881.

The Columbian Institute.—A medical institution called the Columbian Institute has been recently incorporated in New York City. The object of the institute is to provide an establishment at which patients may, if they desire, be treated by their own physicians. The institute will chiefly devote itself to the treatment of chronic diseases.

Training Schools for Nurses.—A training school for nurses has been established in connection with the Brooklyn City Hospital. It is conducted upon the same plan as the New York training school connected with Bellevue Hospital. The report of the latter school for 1880 states that sixty-three nurses are now in the institution. The school has been in operation since 1873, and has graduated one hundred and twenty nurses. The demand for training school nurses in private families far exceeds the supply. Two graduates are about to establish a training school in connection with the Cook County Hospital, Chicago.

Inspection of Plumbing.—A bill requiring the plumbers of New York and Brooklyn to register their names, and giving the Board of Health supervision over all new plumbing has been presented to the New York Legislature. The bill was framed by the Society for Sanitary Reform.

International Medical Congress, London, 1881.—The following subjects are proposed for discussion in Section III. (*Pathology and Morbid Anatomy*): 1. The relations of minute organisms to certain specific diseases, such as relapsing fever, ague, and malignant pustule [anthrax]. 2. The relations of minute organisms to unhealthy processes arising in wounds, and to inflammation in general. 3. Tubercle: (*a*) Its histological characters. (*b*) Its relation to inflammatory processes in different organs, such as the lungs, lymphatic glands, bones, and joints. 4. The origin of cancer and sarcoma, and their relation to the normal tissues in which they arise. 5. Diseases of the kidneys: (*a*) The morbid histology of the different forms of Bright's disease. (*b*) The relation of renal disease to disturbances of the general circulation, and to alterations in the heart and bloodvessels. 6. Recent researches in the morbid anatomy of the brain and spinal cord.

For the pleasure of the members of the Congress the Reception Committee are arranging a series of entertainments and excursions during the week of the Congress, of a most attractive character. On Tuesday, Aug. 2d, an informal reception will be held in the afternoon, at the Royal College of Physicians, which occasion, it is thought, will afford an excellent opportunity for introductions. On the evening of Wednesday, the English members will entertain their foreign *confrères* at a *conversazione* at the South Kensington Museum. Entertainments will also be given on Thursday and Friday; but up to this time their nature has not been definitely fixed upon. On Saturday, August 6th, there will be no business meetings later than 1 P. M.; and excursions will be made to various places of interest in the neighbourhood of London. On this day the Harvey Memorial Committee purpose that the statue of Harvey shall be unveiled at Folkestone. A special train by the Southeastern Railway will take between one and two hundred members of the Congress, with other distinguished persons, to Folkestone, free of cost, where they will be received by a deputation of local magnates, and conducted to the statue which will be unveiled. After the completion of the ceremony, the mayor and corporation will entertain their visitors at a banquet in the town-hall. This visit will afford an excellent opportunity of seeing an English watering-place at its best. On the same day, a charming excursion has been planned by Dr. Langdon Down, who has generously invited five hundred members of the Congress to a garden party at Normansfield, Hampton Wick. Dr. Down will meet his visitors at Teddington station, and will guide them through Bushy Park to Hampton Court Palace. The party will then proceed by water to Normansfield, where a select party of Dr Down's friends will meet them. On the same day Sir Joseph Hooker will receive a number of members at Kew Gardens. On Sunday special services will be held in St. Paul's Cathedral and Westminster Abbey, at which Canon Liddon and Dean Stanley will respectively officiate. The Royal College of Surgeons has signified its intention of entertaining the *Congress* at a *conversazione*.

A temporary museum will be opened during the sessions of the Congress in the rooms of the Geological Society for the exhibition of living examples of certain rare diseases, microscopic specimens, and objects of novelty or rarity having reference to the processes of disease or the results of injury.

———

Prescribing over the Counter.—The Medical Association of the District of Columbia held a meeting April 5th to consider the question of certain abuses by druggists in prescribing over the counter, and in the unwarrantable renewal of prescriptions. They adopted the following resolutions:—

Whereas, It has come to the knowledge of the Medical Association of the District of Columbia, through information of several of its members, that a number of druggists of this city are in the habit of prescribing for and taking charge of cases of sickness; and

Whereas, The diagnosis and treatment of disease belongs to the province of a distinct profession, and as a pharmaceutical education does not qualify the pharmacist for these responsible offices, and

Whereas, The renewal of certain prescriptions merely at the request of the patient or other person who may be ignorant of the evil results attending the continued use of a medicine ordered for the occasion only, may work serious injury to the patient, therefore be it

Resolved, That the public welfare, as well as the best interests of both the profession of medicine and that of pharmacy, are opposed to druggists usurping the functions of the physician by prescribing or giving medical advice.

Resolved, That when the physician shall consider it desirable that a prescription should not be renewed, he will write on it "not to be renewed," and that prescriptions so marked should not be renewed by the pharmacist without order of the profession.

Resolved, That members of this Association will withhold their support and patronage from such druggists as thus fail in their duty to their own profession, or disregard the directions of the physicians in reference to renewals.

Resolved, That the interests of the medical profession are safe in the hands of reputable pharmacists, who govern themselves according to the code of ethics of the College of Pharmacy of the District of Columbia.

Resolved, That professional courtesy between physicians and pharmacists, demands that a due regard be shown towards each other in all matters pertaining to prescriptions, that neither may be unduly reflected upon nor compromised.

—

A Triumph of Dentistry.—At the last meeting of the Medical Society at Strasburg, reported in the *Medical Gazette* of Strasburg, Dr. JULES BŒCKEL presented, in the name of M. Sauval, dentist, a lady for whom the latter had extracted a small molar tooth for dental caries, with violent pain ; and, having found it slightly carious to the bottom of its root, he sawed off the points of the root, filled it with gold carefully throughout the carious channel, and then reimplanted the tooth. The lady was free from all her pain ; the tooth re-established itself solidly in the mouth ; and, at the date at which she appeared at the Society (three weeks after the operation), the tooth served for mastication as well as her other teeth. This is certainly a remarkable example of what is technically described as dental autoprothesis with aurification.—*British Medical Journal*, Jan. 29, 1881.

—

Endowment of Presbyterian Hospital, New York.—An effort is being made by the officers of the Presbyterian Hospital, N. Y., to secure an endowment fund for that institution. One of the directors has promised to give $60,000, provided $100,000 be contributed by others.

—

A Swindler preying upon the Doctors.—An impostor personating Dr. Geddings, of Charleston, S. C., has recently swindled a number of the leading physicians of New York. He states that his funds have been exhausted, and he has obtained considerable sums from his victims for the ostensible purpose of returning home.

—

Graduates in Medicine in 1881 *(continued from p. 248).*

Columbus (O.) Medical College,	63
Cleveland Medical College,	51
Starling Medical College (Columbus, O.),	36
Missouri Medical College (St. Louis),	119
St. Louis Medical College,	43
College of Physicians and Surgeons (St. Joseph, Mo.),	14
Detroit Medical College,	27
Memphis Hospital Medical College,	18
Chicago Medical College,	45
Albany Medical College,	58
Columbian University (Washington, D. C.),	5
University of Georgetown (D. C.),	5

We are requested to state that in addition to the 110 graduates at the March commencement of the University of Pennsylvania, there were 5 graduates at the preceding commencement in June, making a total for the year of 115.

The New York Smells.—The Committee of the State Board of Health has, during the past month, prosecuted its investigations into the source of the offensive odours emanating from Hunter's Point, Brooklyn, and has visited the factories suspected of producing the odours. A bill has been prepared which provides for the abolishment of the Hunter's Point nuisances.

Sanitary Convention.—A very successful Sanitary Convention was held at Battle Creek, Mich., March 29 and 30, under the auspices of the State Board of Health. A number of excellent papers were read, and there was an instructive exhibition of sanitary apparatus and appliances.

Scarlet Fever in Charleston, S. C.—For some weeks a serious type of scarlet fever has prevailed among the children of Charleston. During March there were twenty deaths. The first case was reported on the 1st of January, and the first death occurred on the 1st of March. The death rate has increased, and there has been no diminution in the number of cases. It is estimated that there have been nearly two hundred cases. In some instances the attacks have been very severe, and in one case death resulted in sixteen hours after the first symptoms of the disease appeared.

The fever has so far been mostly confined to the white children, not more than one case in ten of the whole number reported having occurred among the coloured people.

A Congress of Laryngology is announced for September, 1882, in Paris. The members of the organizing committee are MM. Fournier, Gouguenheim, and Krishaber.

Influence of the Antiseptic Method on Medical Jurisprudence.—In a lecture at the close of his last session, Professor NUSSBAUM (*Wiener Medic. Presse,* Nos. 21–23, 1880), discusses the consequences following to medical jurisprudence from the revolution in surgical opinion caused by the antiseptic method. So strong an adherent is he of this method, that he would extend the statute of the German penal code, dealing with bodily injuries and damage to health through negligence or malapraxis, to such a case as a surgeon examining a wound with a finger not disinfected according to the strictest antiseptic principles. He considers, also, that the duty of carrying out these principles excuses the medical man from making, in a medico-legal case, that thorough and searching examination of a wound formerly required.—*British Medical Journal,* Jan. 8, 1881.

Sea-side Nursery.—St. John's Guild, of New York, is about to erect a seaside nursery at Cedar Grove, Staten Island. The object of the nursery is to receive from the Floating Hospital of the Guild such children as are in need of a prolonged sojourn in the bracing sea air. The nursery will be ready for occupation in June.

Private Gynæcological Hospital.—Dr. T. GAILLARD THOMAS, of New York, has recently built a private hospital, for the treatment of women's diseases, at the corner of Lexington Avenue and Fifty-second Street, New York. The resident physician is Dr. Jas. B. Hunter.

Physicians' Mutual Aid Association of New York.—The twelfth annual report of the Board of Directors of the New York Physicians' Mutual Aid Association states that the Society is prospering. The funds have been increased from $3000 to about $6000. The number of members is 350.

—

Kentucky State Medical Society.—This society met in twenty-sixth annual session at Covington, on April 5, 6, and 7. Dr. L. B. Todd, of Lexington, President in the chair. A number of papers were read. The following officers were elected for the ensuing year. President, J. W. Holland, M.D., of Louisville; Vice-Presidents, Drs. Charles Munn, of Nicholasville, and C. H. Thomas, of Covington; Secretary, Dr. L. S. McMurtrie, of Danville. The next meeting will be held at Louisville, on the first Wednesday in April, 1882.

—

University of Pennsylvania.—Dr. Charles K. Mills has been appointed Lecturer on Mental Diseases. This course of lectures will be supplemented by clinical instruction at the Philadelphia Hospital, the Pennsylvania Training Institututution for Feeble-Minded Children, and the State Hospital for the Insane at Norristown.

—

University of Maryland.—Professor L. McLane Tiffany has been elected to the chair of Surgery in this institution, rendered vacant by the resignation of Prof. Christopher Johnston. Dr. I. E. Atkinson has also been elected Professor of Pathology and Clinical Professor of Dermatology.

—

Munificent Gifts.—Col. Thomas A. Scott, of this city, has given $50,000 to the Jefferson Medical College, $50,000 to the University of Pennsylvania, and $30,000 to the Philadelphia Orthopædic Hospital and Infirmary for Nervous Diseases. The Hospital of the University of Pennsylvania has just received a bequest of $10,000, the income of which is to be applied to the support of free beds for cases of recent accidents.

—

West Virginia State Board of Health.—The Legislature of West Virginia has just passed a bill establishing a State board of health with power to appoint a local board in each county, and regulating the practice of medicine.

—

Night Medical Service.—A bill to establish a night medical service in Brooklyn has been favourably reported by the Committee on Public Health. The New York night medical service responded to forty-one calls for assistance in January, and to sixty calls in February.

—

Epidemic among Horses.—A new equine epidemic, characterized by the simultaneous occurrence of symptoms resembling those of glanders and of spinal meningitis has prevailed in the stables of several New York horse-car companies during the last few weeks. It is rarely fatal.

—

Prize Awarded to Mr. Lister.—At the meeting of the Academy of Sciences in Paris on March 12th, the Bondet prize of 6000 francs ($1200) was awarded Professor Lister, for his application of M. Pasteur's researches to the improvement of the art of healing.

Meetings of National and State Medical Societies will be held during the month of May as follows :—

American Medical Association at Richmond, Va., on Tuesday, May 3.

American Laryngological Association, at Philadelphia, on Tuesday, May 10.

State Medical Society of Arkansas, at Little Rock, on Wednesday, May 4.

Iowa State Medical Society, at Dubuque, on Wednesday, May 25.

State Medical Society of Kansas, at Topeka, on Tuesday, May 10.

Medical Association of the State of Missouri, at Mexico, on Tuesday, May 17.

Medical Society of North Carolina, at Asheville, on Tuesday, May 31.

Pennsylvania State Medical Society, at Lancaster, on Wednesday, May 11.

—

Guy's Hospital.—The nursing question at Guy's is virtually ended by the adoption of a series of new regulations for the nurses, which have been submitted to and approved by the medical officers, and which we are glad to learn concede all for which they had contended. Under the new regulations the nurses are placed under the direction of the medical officers.

— -

Library of the New York Academy of Medicine.—Dr. Fordyce Barker, President of the Academy, has intimated his generous intention of giving to the Academy a collection of books, which he is seeking to make as complete as possible, in the department of obstetrics and gynæcology.

—

A Good Example for Hospital Managers.—A wise and proper recognition of the medical staff has lately been shown in the government of St. Bartholomew's Hospital, London, by the election of four members of the staff as members of the Board of Governors. We commend the example to the governing boards of all hospitals.

—

Banquet to an American Consul.—In the beginning of March a banquet was given by many of the leading citizens of Bristol, England, to the Hon. Theodore Canisius, M.D., who, after six years' residence there as United States Consul, was about to leave the city. At the conclusion of the banquet an address was presented to Dr. Canisius, signed by the Mayor of Bristol and several of its more influential inhabitants.

—

Another Literary Piracy.

A few months ago we were constrained to expose the piracy by a London publishing house of Dr. Keen's " American Health Primer" series, and now we are under the similar necessity of calling attention to another piracy which is, if possible, even more disgraceful, inasmuch as it not only appropriates the work of an American author, but also publishes it under the name of a young London physician.

About a year and a half ago Dr. George R. Cutter, of New York, as "the result of many years of industrious research," published a very useful " Dictionary of the German Terms used in Medicine," which was favourably received by the profession. Mr. H. K. Lewis, of London, has just issued a " German-English Dictionary of Words and Terms used in Medicine," by Fancourt Barnes, Physician to the British Lying-in Hospital. In a letter to the *Medical Record* Dr. Cutter says of it, "After a careful examination I find that Dr. Barnes has copied nearly every one of my words, with their definitions; the latter in the same sequence and with the same punctuation. The few typographical and other errors which escaped correction in the first edition and remained in my plates have, in nearly every instance, been so faithfully copied as to appear ludicrous, were it not for the fact that this alone affords sufficient proof of a shameless piracy. . . . In short there is not a page in his book which does not reveal the fact that he has stolen my whole work, adding a very few medical words and a number of chemical and zoological terms which may be found in the ordinary German dictionaries. I do not find more than a score of my words omitted, and the two books contain the same number of pages."

OBITUARY RECORD.—Died at Philadelphia on the 31st of March, in the 75th year of his age, ISAAC RAY, M.D., LL.D., formerly superintendent of the Butler Hospital for the Insane, Providence, Conn. Dr. Ray was widely known as an eminent authority in all matters relating to insanity, and his writings are held in the highest esteem. He was born at Beverly, Mass., in 1807, graduated in Bowdoin College, and commenced the practice of medicine in 1827. He was one of the originators of the Association of Medical Superintendents of American Institutions for the Insane and was its President from 1855 to 1859. A biographical sketch of Dr. Ray will appear in the next number of the *American Journal of the Medical Sciences*, to which journal he was a frequent contributor.

—— At Louisville on April 2d, aged 42 years, RICHARD OSWALD COWLING, M.D., Editor of the *Louisville Medical News*, and Professor of Surgery in the University of Louisville.

Dr. Cowling was prominent among Kentucky's most eminent surgeons, gifted citizens, and beloved sons. His personal traits are thus described in a minute adopted by the Medical Faculty of the University of Louisville: "As a teacher, Dr. Cowling was comprehensive, luminous, and exact; as an operator, bold but cautious, daring but prudent; as a man, dignified, upright, generous, brave, with a child's simplicity of ways and disposition. A scholar of rare attainments; a thinker original, logical, sustained; a writer incisive, varied; a successful author, he added to the fame of the University which he entered as a pupil and where in time he rose to the rank of professor, a position which he in every way adorned.

At a meeting of the physicians of Louisville, held April 4th, the following resolutions were adopted.

Whereas, Providence has removed by death Dr. Richard O. Cowling, a valued and distinguished member of the medical profession of this city, and a man known and appreciated by this community; therefore

Resolved, That in the death of Dr. Cowling the profession has lost a member of gifted and brilliant qualities, of rare social virtues, and goodness of heart.

Resolved, That in all the relations of life he has shown himself a man of generous nature, a sincere friend, a faithful husband, and an indulgent father.

Resolved, That we tender to his family—father, mother, sister, brothers, widow, and children—our condolence for the loss they have sustained by his death, and that a copy of these resolutions be transmitted to them by the officers of this meeting as indicative of our sorrow for them in this hour of sudden affliction.

To Readers and Correspondents.—The Editor will be happy to receive early intelligence of local events of general medical interest, or which it is desirable to bring to the notice of the profession. Local papers containing reports or news items should be marked.

CONTENTS OF NUMBER 462.

JUNE, 1881.

CLINICS.

VOL. XXXIX.—21

MEDICAL NEWS.

THE

MEDICAL NEWS AND ABSTRACT.

VOL. XXXIX. No. 6.   JUNE, 1881.   WHOLE No. 462.

CLINICS.

Clinical Lectures.

ON THE TREATMENT OF TYPHOID FEVER.

AN ADDRESS DELIVERED BEFORE THE KENTUCKY STATE MEDICAL SOCIETY,
APRIL 8, 1881.

BY L. S. McMURTRY, A.M., M.D.,
OF DANVILLE, KENTUCKY.

MR. PRESIDENT AND GENTLEMEN: In discussing the subject of the treatment of typhoid fever, I can lay no claim to your attention from novelty of views or of practice, but only from the intrinsic importance of the subject. It is a well-known fact that in the rural districts of our State, epidemics of this disease are so rare of late years that one is almost justified in the assertion that epidemic typhoid fever in this locality is extinct. Twenty years ago the disease prevailed in epidemic form throughout the villages and farming districts of this State almost every season with frightful severity. Now we rarely encounter typhoid fever except in isolated cases in which the disease was contracted elsewhere and brought home in the formative stage. It may be assumed upon the highest authority that typhoid fever is never of spontaneous origin, that the disease is produced by a specific poison, and that this poison always comes from one suffering with this specific fever. It is a well-known fact that the most common medium of communication and dissemination of the disease is drinking water. Formerly wells with free sub-soil communication were the sources of drinking water. Now cisterns are the almost universal sources of water supply in Kentucky. The geological formation is admirably adapted to the construction of cisterns, and the cemented cisterns of this State are practically sealed bottles into which water pours through filters. That to this improved supply of drinking water, together with the care given by modern physicians to the disposal and disinfection of the dejections of typhoid patients, is due the immunity in this region from epidemics of typhoid fever, there seems to be no reasonable doubt.

Nevertheless there is scarcely a year that passes that every general practitioner among us is not called upon to treat several cases of typhoid fever. The natural history is of such long duration, and the balance between life and death so evenly poised, that the management of this malady must at all times command most careful and thoughtful attention.

The unsettled state of professional opinion as to the management of the disease is indicated by the diversity of views and practice among those best qualified by clinical experience to judge of the efficacy of the several plans of treatment. And it must be observed that the two methods of treatment most prominently advocated at the present time are in their essentials and details so diametrically opposed to each other, that one is compelled to decide between the two, and adopt a method of practice either somewhat heroic or altogether expectant. The care of several cases of typhoid during the past summer and autumn has directed my attention particularly to the consideration of the methods of treatment now before the profession, and has for the time at least invested the subject with peculiar interest.

The publication in this country of Niemeyer's work on the "Practice of Medicine," and more recently of Ziemssen's "Cyclopædia," has brought authoritatively to the attention of American physicians the method of treatment known among us as the German method. This treatment is based upon the existence of specific remedies for the disease, the remedies to which such power is attributed being calomel and iodine. In the early stage of the disease, when in the majority of cases treatment is instituted, calomel is according to this method to be administered in doses of half a scruple, and the remedy repeated in similar doses four times in twenty-four hours. Iodine is also to be given in the form of Lugol's solution or iodide of potassium, so that from a scruple to a drachm of the latter is given in twenty-four hours. According to this method calomel is administered daily, or on alternate days during the first week; and the iodine is continued over two weeks, or until the beginning of convalescence. Beyond the use of these remedies the main feature of this method of treatment is depressing the temperature by active measures. It is assumed that the greatest danger to the patient lies in the injury done the tissues by the fever heat. It is claimed that the danger is in the parenchymatous degeneration which results from a high and prolonged elevation of temperature. The remedies resorted to for reducing temperature in this disease are hydrotherapy, quinia, and digitalis. The cold bath alone may be applied and repeated until the temperature is reduced, or quinia may be administered in scruple doses every four hours until this result is obtained, or the cold bath, quinia and digitalis, all in conjunction may be resorted to for the desired result. This so-called specific method is advocated in one of the most recent and best of our American books on practical medicine,[1] while the antipyretic measures mentioned are advocated in whole or in part by various authorities in Great Britain and America. The Croonian Lectures for 1880[2] are essentially devoted to the advocacy of treating this disease by the fearless exhibition of the antipyretic method particularly as to cold baths.

There are two methods of estimating the efficacy of various plans of treating a given disease, consisting of the analysis of results from the numerical record of cases; and the testimony of individuals based on pathological study together with clinical experience. In the former, the statistical method, the circumstances of the patient, accuracy in diagnosis, and skill in treatment, are such variable elements as to greatly impair the reliability of the deductions made. A careful investigation of the etiology

---

[1] The Practice of Medicine, by Roberts Bartholow, M.A., M.D., p. 701.
[2] On Some Points in the Pathology and Treatment of Typhoid Fever, by Wm. Cayley, M.D., F.R.C.P. London, 1880.

and pathology of the disease, aided by clinical observation, must at last be the guide to individual views and practice.

Until the mechanism of fever is accurately determined, and it is demonstrated that elevation of temperature produces effects alike or uniform in character, the antipyretic treatment of fevers is without a secure foundation in theory, and until the results of this method are more eminently superior it will not be generally adopted in practice. At a recent meeting of the Metropolitan Counties Branch of the British Medical Association, the utility of cold baths in treating typhoid fever was quite thoroughly discussed. It was demonstrated that this method of treatment is not in general favour, and that it is by no means an established therapeutic measure in England. In America it has not met with favour, and occupies a very questionable place in practical therapeutics. Indeed, the more conservative methods of treating the disease are gaining in favour and confidence both in this country and Great Britain.

There are certain established facts in the etiology and pathology of typhoid fever which furnish the only trustworthy guides to the management of the disease. The most important of these are that the disease results from the introduction into the system of a specific poison; that when the poison is once lodged in the system all the stages of the disease are inevitable and must be encountered before the patient can be well; that the natural history of the disease extends over a period of twenty-eight or thirty days and cannot be abbreviated; and that there are no known drugs or remedial measures by which the disease can be aborted, cut short, or cured. These facts being firmly established, that treatment is the best which looks to conserving the patient's strength, avoiding special complications and dangers, and keeping the patient alive until convalescence is reached.

At the onset of an attack of typhoid fever the patient must be protected from his own imprudence. He will almost invariably think that he is suffering from a cold or disordered digestion (biliousness), and will endeavour to throw off the headache and malaise by purgative medicines and exercise. As soon as the diagnosis is made, and in this the thermometer will furnish the best aid, the patient should be put to bed and given attention at once. The management of the case from this time may be considered under the following heads: (1) The Surroundings of the Patient; (2) Diet; (3) Medicines; (4) The Use of Stimulants; (5) The Use of Antipyretics. One who has seen much of typhoid fever cannot but feel the importance of minute details in its management. The course over which the patient must run presents so many dangers, and, at best, the balance is so evenly struck between a favourable and fatal issue, that an apparently trivial factor may determine the result. Hence the hygienic surroundings and psychological status of the patient become matters of serious import.

In the management of a case of typhoid fever the arrangement of the sick-room and surroundings of the patient are matters of the greatest importance, and must receive the personal attention of the physician. The room should be well ventilated, the light subdued, visitors excluded, and quietude maintained. During the first week of the disease the febrile action is high, and frontal headache and sleeplessness are the prominent symptoms. All causes of irritation must be obviated, and rest must be encouraged in every possible way. The surface of the body should be frequently sponged, and the bed and body linen changed every day. It is an excellent plan to also change the bed of the patient. During the hot

weather of last August I managed to restoration a case of the disease of
more than average severity, in which the patient frequently occupied three
beds in the course of twenty-four hours; the bed being rolled to the cool
portion of a large hall in the morning, changing to the opposite side in the
afternoon, and the patient changed to a fresh cool bed at convenient intervals.   The services of a properly qualified nurse are of inestimable importance in the management of this disease.

The diet of typhoid patients requires the closest attention, and demands
the utmost care and judgment.   The specific lesions of the disease being
in the alimentary canal, errors in diet produce injurious results which are
immediate.   The Peyerian patches and the solitary glands in the lower
part of the small intestine are always the seat of important pathological
changes in typhoid fever.   During the first week of the disease the mucous
membrane in the vicinity of the ileo-cæcal valve and surrounding these
glands is hyperæmic and swollen.   The glands become more elevated, and
their surface assumes a dark-reddish colour ; when in the second week by
active cell development and multiplication the agminated and solitary
glands are swollen, and the adjoining mucous membrane infiltrated with
cells.   By the end of the second week the ulcerative process is well advanced, and the typhoid ulcer is formed.   Usually the sloughing and
removal of the necrotic tissue take place during the third week of the
disease.   The loss of substance may extend to the deeper layer of the
mucous membrane, or it may involve the muscular coat to a greater or
less extent, and may extend to perforation of the intestinal wall.   During
the fourth week granulation of the ulcerated surfaces begins, and, under
favourable circumstances, this process advances to cicatrization.   With a
knowledge of these lesions before us, it is evident that the food should be
easy of digestion and unirritating to the bowel.   The enfeeblement of the
digestive and assimilative powers resulting from these glandular changes,
renders the digestion of solid food impossible, while the arrest of the salivary, and probably the pancreatic, secretion which obtains, likewise excludes starchy materials from the diet.   The article of diet most efficient
and capable in repairing the rapid waste of tissue which characterizes the
disease is milk.   We not only have in this article the essential elements
of nutrition, but they are in the form and condition to be most readily and
easily assimilated.   If the stomach is irritable, lime-water may be added
to the milk.   Chicken broth, beef-tea, eggs, meat essences, and arrowroot
are among the articles in common use, but all are inferior to milk.   It is
a common observation that persons who object to milk in health find it
acceptable in this disease.   Beef-tea and meat essences are not well tolerated by a healthy stomach, and hence are not suitable articles of diet for
typhoid fever patients.   Milk is *the article* of diet in typhoid fever, and
should be given, according to the circumstances of the case, in small quantities every two, three, or four hours, so that three or four pints are taken in
twenty-four hours.   With the advent of convalescence comes an appetite
which develops into a lust for food.   Relapses at this stage of the disease are frequent, and it should be remembered that intestinal irritation,
diarrhœa, hemorrhage, and perforation may be induced by imprudence in
diet during convalescence.   Cream and the white of eggs may be added
to the milk at this time, and when convalescence is well advanced bread
and milk, and soup may be taken, afterwards allowing meats.   The patient
should have cold water freely throughout the disease.

I know of no intelligent physician familiar with the pathological character and clinical history of typhoid fever, who believes that there is any specific remedy for this disease. Indeed it is generally conceded that we have no antidote for the typhoid poison; that there is no remedy which will cut short or abort its course; and all that lies within our power is to treat the symptoms as they arise. In cases of average severity it often happens that no medicines are required for their successful management. During the past summer I managed to recovery a case of typhoid, the patient being a robust young man, in which two small doses of chloral during the first week, and a bottle of white wine during convalescence, formed the sum total of all medicines used. Although we can neither neutralize nor eliminate the typhoid poison, yet we can in most cases control and relieve its most distressing and dangerous symptoms. Of these symptoms, diarrhœa is one of the most frequent, troublesome and dangerous. There are even now physicians eminent in the profession, who believe that the specific poison of the disease is eliminated by the bowels, and hence would encourage the diarrhœa by laxatives, and excite it by appropriate remedies if absent. As already described, the lesions of this disease impinge directly upon the alimentary canal, and the inflammation of the intestinal mucous membrane readily accounts for the intestinal catarrh. During the early period of the disease, the diarrhœa is not accompanied with much danger; but later in the disease, the increased peristalsis is an immediate danger to the diseased intestine. When brought on artificially, or when laxatives are used to relieve the constipation which is sometimes present, it is usually controlled only with great difficulty. For the control of this diarrhœa opium is the great remedy.

It must be borne in mind that our principal purpose in treating this condition, is to control the peristalsis of the bowel, rather than to check an increased discharge. Hence the indications for opium greatly exceed those for astringents.

As is well known, the large intestine may be torpid, and constipation result, while the small intestine is actively discharging its contents through the ileo-cæcal valve. This condition is indicated by constipation, with gurgling and griping over the small intestines. This state of the bowels, which apparently is the opposite one to diarrhœa, is best relieved by opium. It is a very rare combination of symptoms which will justify the use of cathartics in this disease. After the first week, should constipation demand attention, a simple enema will furnish the safest relief.

The use of antipyretic remedies—quinia and digitalis—has already been mentioned in detail. To these antipyretic remedies, the salicylate of soda has recently been added. Dr. Henry Tomkins, of Manchester, has recently set forth the value of this article as an antipyretic agent in typhoid fever; and since it is a powerful germicide, he gives it the first place in the list.[1] He administers the remedy in doses of fifteen or twenty grains every two hours, and usually finds six doses sufficient to bring the temperature within a safe range. Quinia in large and frequently repeated doses occupies a very favoured position as an antipyretic in the estimation of American physicians. The great objection to the use of these remedies is that the doses necessary for the antipyretic effect are so large as to be taken with extreme loathing on the part of the patient, and often materially interfere with nutrition by producing disturbances of the stomach.

Hemorrhage from the ulcerated surfaces of the bowel in typhoid fever

---

[1] *Vide* Lancet, March 12, 1881, p. 409.

is always an alarming symptom. It is by no means of infrequent occurrence. For the control of this condition opium is the one reliable remedy.
The object is to place the bowel at rest, and it is doubtful if ergot, tannic
acid, acetate of lead, or perchloride of iron, have the power to even give
material aid to the control of this condition. If possible the exhibition of
opium should be limited to enemata. Ice-cold drinks may be given freely
and an ice-bag applied over the region of the ileum.

There is good authority for the statement that perforation of the bowel
is always fatal. This accident is quickly followed by peritonitis, and the
indications are to give opium freely and continuously.

Tympanites is often a very troublesome symptom in this disease. In
all cases there is some distension by flatus, but frequently the accumulation
of gas is so great as to interfere with the play of the diaphragm. This
paralyzed condition of the bowel is the result of the intestinal ulceration.
For the relief of this condition, turpentine has long been the standard
remedy. It is administered internally, and applied to the abdomen in the
form of stupes. To my mind the method of its action is not clear, and
though familiar with its application for the relief of tympanites, I have
never seen convincing evidence of its efficacy. Charcoal administered in
small and frequently repeated doses is a more efficient remedy. Wishing,
however, to do everything for the relief of a troublesome symptom, and
knowing the confidence placed in turpentine for control of this condition
by eminent practitioners, I would apply turpentine stupes over the abdomen when the tympanites becomes excessive and troublesome. The use of
a cathartic at the beginning of the treatment, and the exhibition of calomel after the German method, beget intestinal commotion, increase the
extent of the lesions, favour diarrhœa and intestinal and peritoneal complications. The indications for rest and preservation of the functions of
the stomach should never be lost sight of throughout the management of
the disease.

Respecting no single point is nicer discrimination required than the exhibition of alcohol in the treatment of this disease. Probably there is no
one article capable of such great and good results when used in the proper
time and emergency in typhoid fever, which has been so much abused.
It must be remembered that the condition of a typhoid fever patient during
the third and fourth week is very different from that of the earlier days
of the disease. When about the beginning of the third week we find an
irregular, rapid, and feeble pulse, accompanied with coolness of the surface
and extremities, together with great exhaustion, we recognize this array of
symptoms as indicating a failure of the power of the heart. This condition results not only from enfeebled muscular power, but also from altered
and disturbed nerve influence. Together with these symptoms are often
found a dry brownish tongue, tremor, and varying degrees of mental disturbance. For the relief of this condition alcohol is the remedy. Just
at this stage is often the critical point in the disease, and the exhibition
of alcohol may safely tide the patient over. When the use of stimulants
is instituted the patient must be watched closely and examined every few
hours. If the pulse becomes more distinct and regular; if the delirium is less
active ; the temperature lower ; and the patient more in his right mind, we
may be assured that the desired effect is being obtained. If, however, these
symptoms are aggravated, the stimulants must be at once discontinued.
When once instituted, stimulants must be given with regularity at fixed
intervals. It must be kept in mind that stimulants may produce much

harm if given at the wrong period and in excessive quantity. It is rare that more than from four to eight ounces of whiskey or brandy are required in twenty-four hours. For the management of the greater number of cases of the disease, alcohol is not essentially required. The following words upon this point by Sir William Jenner, are full of wisdom : " For the last thirty years I have made it the rule of my practice in the treatment of typhoid fever, to abstain from giving alcohol if, in the case before me, I *doubted* the wisdom of giving it ; when in doubt I do not give alcohol in typhoid fever, and when there is a question in my mind of a larger or smaller dose, I, as a rule, prescribe the smaller."[1]

Elevation of temperature is an essential part of the natural and uncomplicated history of typhoid fever. But when the temperature reaches 105° or 105.5°, and is disposed to advance or be continuous, we know that unless lowered the death of the patient will surely and speedily follow. Hence the theoretical ground for the antipyretic treatment of this disease has to this extent a foundation. I have already referred in detail to the antipyretics which are in use. There are many and serious obstacles to the general adoption of cold baths in practice. Indeed, in private practice, deprived of the conveniences and discipline of a hospital, together with the prejudice of the laity, it is almost impossible to carry out this treatment in all its details. But there are more serious obstacles to the general adoption of this method. There are strong indications that relapses are more frequent after this treatment, and that serious pulmonary lesions are caused by the baths. In the sulphate of quinia, exhibited in large doses, we have a reliable and efficient remedy for reducing temperature. This remedy, assisted by sponging the body with tepid water and the application of cold to the head and abdomen by means of the rubber tubing cap and ice-bags, will avert the danger of a high temperature when this is possible. Indeed, Liebermeister declares that, if compelled to choose between the use of cold water and quinia to reduce temperature in this disease, he would prefer the latter.[2]

I cannot better conclude the consideration of this important subject than to quote the expressions of two renowned and skilful practitioners. In a masterly address on the treatment of typhoid fever by Sir William Jenner, to which I have already referred, the following statement occurs :—

" While admitting without reserve that heroic measures, fearlessly but judiciously employed, will save life when less potent means are useless, the physician whose experience reaches over many years will, on looking back, discover that year by year he has seen fewer cases requiring heroic remedies, and more cases in which the unaided powers of nature alone suffice for effecting cure ; that year by year he has learned to regard with greater diffidence his own powers, and to trust with greater confidence in those of nature."

The following is the language of Dr. John Syer Bristowe, the Senior Physician to St. Thomas's, London :—[3]

" Let me state briefly the treatment to which I should like to be subjected if ever, unfortunately, I should become affected with enteric fever : I should like to be placed in a cool well-ventilated room, and covered lightly with bed-clothes ; to have a skilful and attentive nurse to look after me ; to be fed solely with cold milk, unless vomiting should demand the addition to the milk of medicines calculated to allay vomiting. If diarrhœa became troublesome, or ever there was

[1] Medical News and Abstract, March, 1880, p. 156.
[2] Ziemssen's Cyclopædia, vol. i. p. 216.
[3] British Medical Journal, Nov. 27, 1880, p. 841.

much pain or tenderness in the cæcal region and in the bowels, I should like to be treated, not with laxatives, but with opium, given either by the mouth or by the rectum. If constipation were present, I should, except in the first week, like to have enemata only employed for its relief. In the event of intestinal hemorrhage coming on, I should like to have ice to suck or ice-cold fluids to drink, cold compresses to the belly, and cold injections into the bowel; and though I am sceptical as to their efficacy, I should still choose to have astringents, and more especially lead, given to me at short intervals. If perforation should take place, let me have large and repeated doses of opium. Stimulants I should prefer to be without early in the disease; later, however, and during convalescence, I should like to have them in moderation. As to cold baths, I would rather not have them; but I would, nevertheless, leave it to my physician to exercise his discretion in the matter. I would leave it also to him to decide, according to circumstances, whether alcohol should be administered to me in large quantities; I would prefer not to be treated at a temperance hospital."

ON A PUNCTURED WOUND OF THE SKULL.

A Clinical Lecture.

By J. W. HULKE, M.D.,
Surgeon to, and Lecturer on Surgery at, the Middlesex Hospital.

GENTLEMEN: Trephining in wounds of the skull, formerly so frequent, has now become so infrequent that most of you during the whole three years of your studentship will probably not see it done more than once or twice, and possibly not at all. It happens, however, that there are now in the wards two patients whom I have recently trephined, and to the case of one of these I now ask your attention.

The record by my dresser, Mr. Ed. Davis, is in effect as follows:—

Late in the afternoon of January 7 last a little flaxen-haired girl was taken into Bird ward suffering from the effects of a wound of the head. The child was quite conscious. She was remarkably quick and intelligent for her age, and she answered readily and pertinently questions put to her. Her face, very pale, was distorted by frequent spasms, which chiefly affected the mouth and the eyelids; both sides of the face appeared to be equally convulsed.

In the middle of the right parietal region was a small festering scalp-wound, through which the House-Surgeon had just before detected with a probe that the underlying bone was irregular as if broken, and slightly displaced.

The account given by the child's mother (which we had afterwards reason to think false) was that eleven days previously she had fallen off a low stool and cut her head by striking it against a fender. This stunned her for a little while, but she soon came to, and when the bleeding, which was inconsiderable, had ceased, the mother covered the cut with a piece of sticking-plaster. For two days the hair about the cut was wet with a watery oozing, and as the child seemed less lively than usual, on the third morning she was brought to the hospital surgery, where the junior House-Surgeon saw her. He found the cut had festered, and on taking off the plaster a couple of drops of pus escaped. Thinking it merely a superficial cut, it did not appear to him necessary to have the child admitted. Light Goulard-water dressing was put on, and the mother was told to bring her daily, which she did. Nothing unusual was noticed until the eleventh day after the accident, when at 4 P. M. the child had a fit, in which her left side "worked" more than her right; and when the fit was over she appeared to be in a deep sleep. In great alarm the mother ran with her to the hospital, and, the gravity of the case being apparent, she was instantly admitted. Her state at this time has just been told to you.

Throughout the evening her face was often convulsed, and at 11.30 P. M. a little difference of expression was first observed, suggestive of a slight degree of facial palsy. The child was also now noticed to take hold of anything offered to her exclusively with the right hand, and when trying to sit up in bed she supported herself with this arm only, suggesting a slight degree of hemiplegia of the left arm.

At 1 A. M. on January 8, facial palsy had become unmistakably marked, though not complete, and no doubt could be felt of the palsy of the left arm and hand; with the right hand she grasped strongly and with precision, whilst the grasp of the left hand was feeble and faltering.

One hour later, at 2 A. M., the scalp was turned back from the bone at the wound, which exposed a small grayish button, apparently a puriformly softening clot; and when this was detached, a circular hole in the parietal bone came into view. It was as sharply cut as if it had been cut with a punch. The pericranium around the margin of the hole for the breadth of about two inches was detached, swollen, and grayish. The parietal bone (the child being so young—four years and a half) was found to be so thin and elastic that it did not offer enough resistance to enable the teeth of the trephine to bite; the hole was therefore enlarged with a cutting forceps, and whilst this was being done a little pus welled up from beneath the bone. The grayish button had a stalk which passed through a sloughy ragged hole in the dura mater. Exploring with a probe very cautiously through this hole for any splinters which might have been thrust in through the membranes, at the depth of about three-quarters of an inch from the surface something hard was felt, and withdrawn with a slender forceps. It proved to be two pieces of detached bone with hairs entangled around them. A little boric lint-charpie was now laid lightly on the wound, and fixed with a gauze capeline.

The temperature before the operation unfortunately was not recorded. During the first six hours afterwards it was subnormal, as these figures show—at 3 A. M., 98.2°; 4 A. M., 97.6°; 5 A. M., 97.2°; 6 A. M., 96.8°; 7 A. M., 98 4°; 8 A. M., 97.0° Fahr.

At 10 A. M. the temperature was rising, and the pulse 112. The child was quiet. The palsy of the face and left arm continued, and slight palsy of the left leg was noticed.

At 11.30 A. M. the axillary temperature had risen to 101.6° Fahr. The hair was now clipped short and an ice-cap put on. This seemed to soothe the child. At 4 P. M. the temperature had fallen to 99.6°, and at 9 P. M. a further fall of .6° was noted. At midday, after taking some beef-tea, she vomited, and again several times in the course of the afternoon.

January 9.—Temperature at 1 A. M. 99°, and at 9 A. M. 98°. No vomiting since yesterday evening. Inclined to sleep. On dressing the wound the charpie was found wet with pus. At 9 P. M., temperature 98.4°, pulse 100. Once sick.

10th.—8.30 A. M., temperature 98.4°. Fretful through night, and twice sick. Left pupil perhaps slightly larger than the right. The facial palsy seems not quite so marked. 10.30 P. M., temperature 96°.

11th.—4.30 A. M., temperature 96.6°; 11 A. M., temperature 97.6°, pulse 100. A rather restless night. Bladder not emptied since yesterday. Several ounces of urine withdrawn with catheter. 6 P. M., drowsy; temperature 97°.

12th.—She moves her left arm better. Temperature at 5 A. M., 98°; at 10.30 A. M., 96.4°, pulse 78; at 7.30 P. M., temperature 97.4°. Has voided urine.

In the afternoon hungry; asked for and ate with relish a slice of bread-and-butter.

13th.—A small hernial button projects through the opening in the bone.

It would be wearisome, and it is not necessary, to continue reading the daily reports from this date. The hernia rose above the level of the scalp, and attained the size of a small nut. It then shrank and disappeared. On the 18th the facial palsy was gone; she was sitting up in bed, playing with toys and prattling merrily at the midday visit. The temperature, however, was still subnormal—it ranged between 98° and 97°, and averaged 97.3°—the normal, 98.5°, not being attained until the 26th. . At this date the wound was clean and granulating, and had contracted to about one-half. The left arm was still very feeble; it was colder than the right, and its surface, including the hand, was bluish and mottled; its circulation was manifestly weak.

February 9.—Slight contraction of the fingers of the left hand has occurred; the palsy and feebleness of circulation in the limb continue little changed.

26th.—The mottling of surface and coldness of the limb are less marked, the grasp is also stronger, and the palsy of the leg has disappeared.

On March 10 and 27 two small exfoliations came away. After this the wound quickly closed, and on May 10 the scar appeared thoroughly sound; it was, however, thin, and pulsated very perceptibly. She may now be considered convalescent. Every trace of palsy is gone. But, knowing her to have an unhappy home, she is detained still, in order to keep her under observation.

I have given the details of this case at some length because of its importance. The points to which I would particularly ask your attention are, the duty of thoroughly examining every fresh head-injury, the nature of the wound, the date when cerebral symptoms were first noticed, the one-sidedness of the symptoms, the nature of the intracranial disorder denoted by the latter, the value of a true recognition of the association of these symptoms with abscess, the increase of the palsy immediately after the operation, the initial rise of temperature, the fall of temperature on using the ice-cap, the long-continued subnormal temperature, and the hernia cerebri. It will be convenient to take these *seriatim*.

The importance of examining every head-wound when first seen. Had this been done, the fracture—since it was compound, and not a mere crack without irregularity of surface—could not have been overlooked. The omission is very pardonable, for the child was not brought to the surgery till the third morning after the accident, and the absence of symptoms misled. There was not anything in the child's condition to arouse suspicion of a grave injury, and the wound was therefore supposed to involve the scalp only.

The nature of the injury. A punctured wound. Such wounds are, as is well known, often complicated with the impaction of splinters and foreign substances, and are on this account more dangerous than other forms of wounds. (I have mentioned that the mother's account of the way in which the injury was received appeared improbable. An anonymous letter afterwards received, purporting to be written by a neighbour, said that the child's drunken father in a passion threw a small poker at it, and that this stuck in her head.) A wound of this kind ought, therefore, always to be very carefully explored, in order that any splinters, etc., driven through the membranes into the brain may be extracted before the onset of inflammation, since their extraction may avert this.

The late date at which the symptoms of grave encephalic disorder manifested themselves. Eleven days passed between the date of the wound .and the fit. Such late appearance of symptoms of grave cerebral disturbance is by no means unusual even in compound fractures of the skull, whilst it is the rule in simple fractures and in severe bruises with or without external wound, when the ence-phalic disorder is localized and not diffuse.

Very early in professional life I was taught this by two cases of compound frac-ture of the vault of the skull by a glancing rifle-bullet, which came under my observation in the Crimean campaign. In one of these cases the parietal bone was shattered and driven in upon the superior longitudinal sinus and brain in which an abscess formed under the fracture. Yet here no grave symptoms were present till after the sloughs had fallen and the wounds had nearly closed. Both men, who had been supposed to have only scalp-wounds, were meanwhile up and about. A woman some years ago admitted into Bird ward furnished an apt ex-ample of this late development of symptoms of cerebral disorder. She had been struck in a fray with a brickbat on the right temple, thought little of the cut, drank hard, and went about as usual until a month afterwards, when she fell un-conscious, and had convulsions restricted to the left limbs. In the anterior lobe of the right cerebral hemisphere was a large abscess, which was evacuated by trephining.

The kind of symptoms. One-sided spasm and palsy; hemiplegia supervening, not directly, but after an interval, has been thought to be pathognomonic of dif-fuse inflammation of arachnoid. In the case of our little child, and also in the other cases to which I have just referred, one-sided spasm and palsy, appearing late, were associated with localized and not diffuse inflammation, with cerebral abscess and not diffuse meningitis; and I think this is the rule.

The importance of recognizing the association of intracranial abscess with late cerebral symptoms is evident, since trephining may evacuate an abscess and save the patient's life, whilst in diffuse meningitis trephining is useless.

The increase of the palsy after the operation makes it probable that the hemi-plegia was not the direct consequence of pressure (which, in presence of an open-ing freely communicating with the external surface, could not have been great), but to inhibition of function through nutritional disturbance of brain-tissue around the inflammatory focus, a temporary increase of the local inflammation being pro-voked by the fresh injury unavoidably inflicted in trephining. The rise of tem-perature some hours later is favourable to this construction.

The fall of temperature upon the use of the ice-cap. I cannot too strongly impress on you the value of this way of applying cold to the head. I have the strong conviction that I have seen patients with fractures of the skull recover, who but for it would most probably have perished from consecutive intracranial inflammation.

The subnormal temperature observed, lasting during several days, is not un-usual in these cases. It occurred also in a case of cerebral abscess successfully trephined in a boy in Percy ward two years ago.

The hernia. Probably this consisted mainly of granulation-tissue and inflam-matory products. It was in the main a false hernia cerebri, with little admixture of brain-tissue. No pressure was made on it, and no escharotics were applied to it. It appeared to be maintained by the irritation of the necrosed bone, and to subside on the exfoliation of this.

The child appears to be now quite well, but can we confidently expect she will continue so? May no ulterior consequences ensue? We cannot affirm this. On the contrary, epilepsy not infrequently attacks the subjects of such injuries months afterwards, when they seem to have thoroughly recovered and to be in perfect health.

At the date of publication she continues perfectly well.—*Med. Times and Gaz.*, April 23, 1881.

Hospital Notes.

Atony of the Bladder; Recovery.

J. L., labourer, aged 57, with marked arcus senilis, was admitted into Mr. PEARCE GOULD'S ward at the Westminster Hospital, on August 10, 1880, suffering from retention of urine. He had always enjoyed good health until twelve months before, when he found difficulty in passing his urine. This gradually increased until the night before admission, when after a hard day's work he was unable to pass a drop. The "difficulty" he noticed was a slow, feeble stream, and inability to empty his bladder, with frequency of call to micturate.

On admission the distended bladder formed a prominent tumour in the hypogastrium, reaching almost up to the umbilicus. The prostate felt from the rectum was hard and moderately enlarged. Mr. Gould passed without any difficulty an olive-headed catheter, No. 10, English scale, and drew off rather more than four pints of clear, acid, healthy-looking urine. The urine flowed slowly, falling vertically from the end of the catheter. The influence of respiration on the stream was evident. After the escape of about a pint the flow ceased, and the rest was forced out by the hand above the pubes, and when the pressure was relaxed air was heard to be sucked in through the catheter. The man was kept in bed on full diet, and his bladder was emptied by catheter night and morning. On Aug. 15 a mixture containing five minims of tincture of nux vomica was ordered to be given three times a day. The catheter was always carefully washed in carbolic lotion—5 per cent.—before being used, and lubricated with carbolic oil— 10 per cent. This appeared to cause some irritation of the meatus, and vaseline was substituted for the oil, and the irritation quickly passed away. There was no sign of any vesical irritation; the urine remained clear, acid, free from mucus and albumen, and the bladder gradually regained its expulsive power. Thus on Aug. 15, the patient could pass 4 oz. of urine by his own efforts, and on Aug. 17 this had increased to 10 oz., and thus he improved until on his discharge on Sept. 15, there was only half an ounce of "residual urine" to be drawn off.

Remarks.—This case is an example of the extreme degree of atony of the bladder with complete retention of the urine, not unfrequently met with in connection with chronic prostatic enlargement. The daily use of the catheter has long been recognized as the proper mode of treatment for such a condition, but the occurrence of decomposition of the urine with subsequent chronic cystitis have too often prevented the attainment of a perfect result. The case illustrates one application of antiseptic surgery to urinary surgery, and its value in preventing the decomposition of the urine can hardly be overrated. The result of the daily emptying of the bladder in leading to a gradual and almost perfect recovery of the bladder's power, throws considerable light on the way in which this atony of the bladder is originally produced. For it is clear that it is not by obstruction to the outflow of urine with retention and stretching of the muscular coat of the bladder, nor is it from any local action of decomposed urine; but rather, it seems, from a small primary "residue" of urine. A few drachms which the bladder cannot evacuate have a paralyzing influence upon the bladder muscle, which leads to the retention of a greater amount of urine; this, again, to further diminution of expulsive power, and so on until the stage of complete retention and atony is reached. The history of such cases before they come under treatment, as well as the results of catheterism, bear out this view. The symptoms often arising from a very small quantity of "residual urine" and the importance of its relief have been laid stress upon by Sir H. Thompson. The patient's condition (March 2) remains as on the date of his discharge; he continues to draw off the few drachms of "residual urine" every night. The quantity has not increased since he left the

MONTHLY ABSTRACT.

Anatomy and Physiology.

A Case of Movable Liver.

In the *Wiener Med. Blätt.* is recorded an observation accidentally made on a physician by Dr. CHVOSTEK. There were no symptoms whatever of anything wrong in the abdomen, and there was no history of violence or of any occurrence that threw light upon the condition. When the man stood up, the upper and posterior border of the liver was felt to come forward from under the margin of the thorax, and to be six centimetres and a half below the tip of the xiphoid cartilage in the right parasternal line, and one centimetre below that point in the left parasternal line. The left end of the liver was plainly felt through the abdominal wall, and from it the anterior, or rather the lower edge of the liver could be traced arching down to the right, being in the middle line fifteen centimetres below the xiphoid process, and in the right nipple and axillary lines respectively seven and one-and-a-half to two centimetres below the edge of the thorax. The liver did not markedly descend on taking a deep inspiration. In the horizontal posture it could be replaced under the ribs to a considerable extent. In lying on one side the organ fell to some extent towards the dependent side. The lower edge of the suspensory ligament could be felt tightly stretched, but this produced no pain, and so completely absent were all symptoms that the condition was only discovered accidentally.—*Lancet*, March 12, 1881.

The Source of the Liquor Amnii.

Our knowledge concering the source of the liquor amnii is somewhat uncertain, and two theories are held with regard to it. The first is that it is the product of the secretion or transudation from the maternal vessels in the uterus; the other, that it is the product of the secretions of the foetus. Accurate knowledge upon this subject is of very great importance, for its elucidation lies at the foundation of the pathology of some of the diseases of pregnancy and intra-uterine life, and involves the whole question of the activity of the kidneys in the foetal state. Experiments have been made upon pregnant animals with a view to solving the problem, and the most recent are those conducted by WIENER in Breslau, the results of which are published in a paper in the *Archiv für Gynäkologie*.

Two or three kinds of experiments have been performed. In the first, a solution of sulph-indigotate of soda was introduced into the jugular vein of rabbits in an advanced state of pregnancy, and the animals killed at intervals ranging from a quarter of an hour to two hours and a half after the injection was made. It was then found that the liquor amnii in all the cases contained the colouring material used, its presence being proved by the microscope. In none of the cases was the colouring material found in the organs of the foetus, with the exception of the stomach and intestines, into which it had obtained admission by the process of swallowing; none appeared to have passed by the foetal kidneys. The quantity of the material found in the liquor amnii was small, and this appeared to be due to its elimination by the maternal kidneys. To obviate this the kidneys were extirpated before the injection was made, and in cases thus treated a large quantity of it passed into the amniotic fluid. When animals in the early stage of pregnancy were similarly treated, hardly a trace of colouring matter was found in the liquor amnii. To decide what part the fœtus plays in the production of the liquor amnii, the colouring material was introduced into the body of the fœtus. A quantity of the coloured solution was injected into the amniotic sac and the fœtus made to swallow, but it was found that the material did not in this way enter the blood of the fœtus. It was then injected under the skin of the back of the fœtus. On subsequent examination, the colouring material was found in the kidneys of the fœtus in precisely the same situation as it was found in those of the mothers in the first series of experiments. It was traced there as soon as twenty-five minutes after the injection, and in one case a drop of coloured urine was discovered in the bladder. In these experiments, moreover, the liquor amnii was coloured blue.

From these data Wiener argues that the fœtal kidneys are not only active during fœtal life, but that they secrete rapidly, and are the chief source of the liquor amnii. He maintains, moreover, that during early life the fluid comes exclusively from the embryo until the fœtal membranes come into intimate contact with the maternal tissues, and the placenta is formed. At first the fluid is derived from the cutaneous vessels of the fœtus, afterwards from the Wolffian body, and later from the kidneys. After the membranes have come into intimate connection with the uterus, a portion of the fluid comes from the maternal vessels. Wiener explains the varying results of chemical analysis of the liquor amnii, and the occasional absence of urea in it, by the statement that the urea in it continuously undergoes decomposition or diffusion into the maternal blood.

Besides the experiments referred to, other evidence bearing upon the question is brought forward and discussed, especially that furnished by cases in which occlusion of the urinary passages had occurred during fœtal life. In these cases considerable quantities of urine have been found behind the occlusion, the secretion of which, according to Fehling, is pathological. This opinion of Fehling is, in our opinion, successfully controverted by Wiener. It cannot be questioned after the evidence brought forward, that both the maternal vessels of the uterus and the secreting organs of the fœtus contribute to the production of the amniotic fluid, but the proportion the contributions of each bear to one another cannot be regarded as finally settled. The evidence adduced by Wiener in favour of the fœtal kidneys being the chief source, although indirect in its characters, goes far to prove his view; but until further and more conclusive evidence is adduced we cannot go beyond the statement that the liquor amnii is the joint product of the vessels of the uterus and of the fœtal kidneys.—*Lancet*, March 12, 1881.

Materia Medica and Therapeutics.

Chaulmugra Oil.

Chaulmugra oil is obtained from the seeds of *Gynocardia odorata*, a large tree, much branched, with ash-gray globular fruit, some three or four inches in diameter. It is a native of Pegu, Tenasserim, and other parts of the Malayan peninsula, whence it extends into India, being found in Assam, Khasia, and Sikkim, but not in the central or western parts. The seeds (*Gynocardiæ semina*) are officinal in the *Indian Pharmacopœia*, and are popularly known as chaulmugra, chaulmogra, or chaulmoogra seeds. The oil expressed from these seeds has been known for centuries to the Fakirs of India, by whom it is largely used in the treatment of leprosy, and skin diseases generally. There is evidence to show that it has been employed by the aboriginal tribes in certain parts of India from the remotest times.

At the ordinary temperature, the oil is solid, has a light-brown colour, and a decidedly disagreeable taste and smell. It may be readily melted by placing the bottle in hot water, or allowing it to stand for a few minutes in front of the fire. It has been analyzed, and is found to consist of palmitic, gynocardic, hypogæic, and coccinic acids. The palmitic constitutes sixty-three per cent.; but the gynocardic acid, which is found in a much smaller proportion, is probably the active ingredient. The oil is given internally, and is also used as an external application. It is most conveniently administered in empty capsules, or in *perles;* but many patients take it well in milk, cod-liver oil, or almond-oil. The usual dose is from five to fifteen minims. It is best to begin with a small dose, say two or three minims, three or four times a day, gradually increasing the quantity as the patient becomes accustomed to it. Dr. Murrell, as the result of a large number of observations, found that, when administered in milk or cod-liver oil, ten minims very frequently upset the stomach, giving rise to nausea and vomiting, and not unfrequently diarrhœa. The chaulmugra oil *perles* contain four minims each, and most patients will take from one to four of these at a dose. When it is desirable to vary the dose frequently, the empty gelatine-capsules will be found useful. It is almost essential that some such special mode of administration should be adopted, as few patients like the taste of the oil, or will consent to take it by itself for any length of time. It must always be given after meals.

Chaulmugra oil has long been used in India in the treatment of leprosy, and has acquired a high reputation as a remedy for that disease. From the comparative rarity of true leprosy in England, much difficulty has been experienced in collecting a sufficient number of cases in which to try its effects. This difficulty is increased by the fact that, in temperate climates, the disease often exhibits long periods of comparative rest or subsidence, quite apart from any special treatment. Dr. Robert Liveing has published a record of six cases of elephantiasis. Græcorum, in which he was able to give the chaulmugra a long and continuous trial. He found that all six cases were decidedly benefited by the treatment, and the patients themselves were strongly impressed with the belief that they had decidedly improved under its internal use as a medicine. Mr. Wyndham Cottle has also published two cases in which equally good results were obtained. The oil was here given either as a mixture suspended in gum, or in the form of emulsion. Unusually large quantities were administered, the dose being gradually increased to as much as a drachm three times a day. Moreover, an ointment, consisting of twenty grains of chaulmugra oil to the ounce of lard, was applied freely to the skin. Quite recently, Dr. David Young of Florence has published a more extensive series of cases in which most striking results were obtained. The forms of the disease noted were : macular leprosy, four; anæsthetic leprosy, twenty-three; tubercular leprosy, fifteen; and mixed cases, eleven. The patients were all adults, the proportion of males to females being about three to one. The treatment consisted in the internal administration of doses varying from five to twenty drops, three times a day, commencing with the smaller quantity, and gradually increasing it until the latter was reached. Externally, a liniment, composed of an ounce of the oil, mixed with a drachm of rectified spirit, was applied to the diseased surface. Dr. Young found that, in the macular and in the early stage of the anæsthetic forms of leprosy, the chaulmugra was of decided value. The good results appeared earlier when the powdered seeds were given in addition to the oil. A liberal milk-diet was found to be a valuable auxiliary. Several of the cases were complicated with bronchial affec-

tions, which were markedly benefited during the treatment, all the patients gain.
ing flesh rapidly.

In many skin diseases, the chaulmugra oil treatment proves beneficial. It has
been tried with success in psoriasis, lupus, and obstinate cases of scabies and
ringworm.

Chaulmugra oil was originally introduced as "a specific for consumption;"
but there is certainly as yet no evidence to show that it deserves this distinctive
title. Dr. Burney Yeo has reported nine cases of phthisis in which it was given
internally with little or no benefit. He considers that it gives no promise of help
in well marked cases where the disease has reached the stage of infiltration and
softening of any considerable portion of the lung. Dr. Murrell, as the result of
a series of observations extending over two years and a half, arrives at a some.
what different conclusion. In thirty-one of his cases, the chaulmugra oil was
given in milk, in doses ranging from three to ten minims, four times a day ; and,
in twenty-four of these, decided benefit was experienced. The chaulmugra
seemed to act, first, as an expectorant ; then the cough became less troublesome ;
and, finally, a gradual improvement took place in the general symptoms. The
best results were obtained when, in addition to the internal administration, from
two to four ounces were rubbed into the chest weekly for two or three months.
The inunction never upsets the stomach or gives rise to unpleasant symptoms.
The smell is not very agreeable, but is readily covered by using a little violet.
powder. The oil may be employed alone or simply as an adjunct to other treat.
ment.

It is found that children, as a rule, take the chaulmugra without difficulty ; and
its internal administration, combined with inunction, has been employed with
benefit in scrofula and in cases of marasmus.

In chronic rheumatism and in rheumatic gout, it is most useful. A patient,
recording his own experience, says : "A month since, I was suddenly seized
with a severe attack of rheumatism ; and so acute was the pain, that, for two
days and nights, I could not sleep, and the swelling of my hands made me quite
helpless. I could neither dress nor feed myself. Having had a sharp attack of
rheumatic fever about twenty years ago, I was very much afraid that I was again
to be laid aside from business ; and you, I fear, will hardly believe that, within
three hours of the application of the oil, the use of my hands was restored to
me ; and that, from that day to this, I have had no return of the pain." Non-
professional testimony is not, as a rule, very trustworthy, but there are occasions
when it cannot be ignored. For stiff joints, sprains, and bruises, both in men
and horses, the oil is said to be equally efficacious.

For neuralgia and sciatica, the chaulmugra oil is generally mixed with camphor
and chloroform, or with an equal weight of a saturated solution of menthol in
chloroform, and then rubbed in over the painful part.—*British Med. Journal*,
March 26, 1881.

—

Therapeutic Use of Pilocarpin.

That jaborandi, or, rather, its alkaloids, are likely to come into more general
use as powerful therapeutic agents, appears to be indicated by the numerous notices of their employment which have recently appeared in the periodical literature of Europe and America. Within the last year, the use of pilocarpin has
been advocated by more than one writer—notably, by Dr. Berkart—and it may,
therefore, be of some service to our readers to consider certain of the facts in
regard to its action which have been recently brought to light.

In August last, HARNACK and MEYER published (*Arch. für Exper. Path.*, etc., vol. xii. p. 366) the results of observations which they had made in Professor Schmiedeberg's laboratory in Strassburg on jaborandi and its alkaloids. They found that the jaborandi leaves contained not only the alkaloid pilocarpin, but also another similar body, which they named jaborin, which was, to a great extent, antagonistic to pilocarpin in its action. This second alkaloid they found to be present in all ordinary specimens of pilocarpin; and to the presence of this adulteration they ascribed the somewhat contradictory results obtained by former observers. The pure pilocarpin causes, in warm-blooded animals, at first irritation of the terminations of the vagus in the heart, and, indirectly, of the vaso-motor centres; and, later, and in larger doses, paralysis of these terminations and centres. In spite of the paralysis of the vagus, the pulse becomes slower and slower. In regard to its action on the heart and bloodvessels, it closely resembles nicotin. Pre-eminently may pilocarpin be characterized as a drug which causes increased glandular secretion. It acts most energetically upon the salivary, sweat, mucous, and lachrymal glands; and that this increased secretion is not caused by the vaso-motor paralysis, of which we have spoken, is shown by the fact that that paralysis comes much later than the outpouring of the secretion, which is the first symptom of the action of pilocarpin. This result is probably due to an irritation of the nervous apparatus governing the gland. To the other actions of pilocarpin—on the pupil, the intestine, the uterus, etc.—we need not here refer.

The greatest value of pilocarpin appears to consist in its power of causing rapid elimination of effete material in cases of scarlatinal nephritis. It has been frequently administered in such cases, and with much benefit; and it appears likely that, if it be given with proper precaution, and with a due appreciation of certain dangers which surround its use, it may frequently be the means of saving life. What these dangers are has been lately very carefully pointed out by Dr. Seemann of Berlin (*Zeitsch. für Klin. Med.*, 1881, vol. ii. p. 552), and they demand the consideration of every intelligent physician. That œdema and uræmic phenomena, in cases of scarlatinal nephritis, are neither proportionate to one another nor to the quantity of urine passed, can readily be observed. In some instances, uræmia occurs when a normal quantity of urine is excreted, while in others no uræmic symptoms follow several days of anuria. In the former cases, the urine contains little urea, and in the latter the urea passes from the blood into the œdemic fluid, and hence becomes harmless for the time. When, however, at the beginning of convalescence, the excrementitious materials pass back into the blood, uræmia may come on; and obviously, the more rapidly they pass back the more danger is there. In virtue of its power of producing prompt and energetic increase of the sweat, salivary, and other glandular secretions, pilocarpin causes a very rapid reabsorption of the transudation, and, therefore, its administration may give rise to uræmic phenomena, which, though transient, may be highly dangerous. Seemann instances one case, in which this untoward result followed the administration of pilocarpin. Ohms (*Petersburg Med. Woch.*, 1878, No. 6), as well as Seemann, has observed that pilocarpin may cause, not merely dilatation of the small arteries, but even rupture of these vessels, and consequent hemorrhage; and if we recollect that the child affected with scarlatinal nephritis lies on his back, too weak to cough up the rapidly augmenting mucus which the pilocarpin calls forth, it will be seen that the circumstances of the case may predispose to catarrhal pneumonia to a dangerous degree. Seemann gives the following indications for the use of pilocarpin in such cases of nephritis:—

" 1. Muriate of pilocarpin is useful in cases of scarlatinal nephritis, and may often save life when other remedies fail; but it must not be resorted to except in very serious cases. 2. When, after its successful administration, the œdema begins to lessen, cure should be left to nature and to other remedies, because renewed doses of pilocarpin may cause too rapid absorption of the transudation, and may thus lead to uræmia. 3. After each dose of pilocarpin, the state of the respiratory organs must be carefully watched; if the bronchial mucus be not satisfactorily expectorated, or if the slightest indication of pneumonia show itself, further doses of the drug must not be given."

We believe that, if such indications be borne in mind, pilocarpin may be used safely and with great success in cases of scarlatinal nephritis which are otherwise hopeless; but the preparation used must be obtained from a thoroughly trustworthy source, and must be free from the jaborin which most specimens are said to contain, and which materially modifies the action of the drug.—*London Med. Record*, March 15, 1881.

Medicine.

Pathology of Atheroma.

The theory of the origin of atheroma, to which Virchow has given currency, regards it as of inflammatory origin, and has been conveyed into modern pathology by the help of the name "endarteritis deformans." This designation, although not unassailable, has been widely accepted on account of the apt expression which it gives to the conspicuous characters of the morbid change. The same theory of initial inflammation has been, in effect, adopted by Lancereaux, while Cornil and Ranvier do not admit any other element in the morbid process than simple degeneration.

The latter view is regarded as the more probable by the writer of a recent memoir in the Paris *Revue de Médicine*, M. HIPPOLYTE MARTIN, who has endeavoured to ascertain the pathological origin of the degeneration, and believes that he has found it in a lesion of the nutritive arteries of the walls of the vessels, to which the visible degeneration is simply secondary. In the early stage of the affection the cells of the connective tissue of the vessels may be found notably increased in number, and the middle and internal coats are increased in thickness; these changes cannot be regarded as the result of any irritation by the globules of fat which may be found sparsely scattered through the wall. If the minute vessels which ramify in the external coat before penetrating the middle layer are examined, they are found to be healthy, with the exception of those which correspond to the spot of atheroma. Here, however, the nutritive artery of the degenerated region presents a striking proliferative endarteritis, which, in the case of extreme degeneration of the atheromatous patch, amounts to almost complete obliteration of the minute vessel, so that very little blood can circulate through it. This lesion is never absent, although considerable care may be necessary to find it. The change is only found in the vessel going to the diseased spot; other arteries, although closely adjacent, may be perfectly healthy. But it may be held that in the old, in whom generalized arterial disease is common, the affections of the arteries and of the nutritive vessels may be due to the same cause, and do not stand in any causal relation. In contravention of this objection, M. Martin describes the case of a lad, nine years of age, who died of diphtheria. At the autopsy two atheromatous spots were found in the commencement of the aorta, above the sigmoid valves. They were well marked, about a square centimetre in extent. All the other vessels were healthy. Sections at the position of the atheromatous patches showed, in the middle of healthy tissue of the outer, and even of the middle coat, a perfect example of endarteritis of the nutritive vessels, one of which was almost obliterated. Moreover, it was evident from the histological characters of the two that the affection of the nutritive artery was of older date than that of the inner coat of the aorta.

This lesion in the vasa vasorum appears to commence in their inner coat, the nutritive supply to which is always the most difficult, but at a later stage the middle coat is also affected, and its muscular fibres may be observed to undergo a fatty degeneration. This alteration is regarded as inflammatory in nature, the result of some, at present unknown, cause. The facts Martin has ascertained are of much interest and importance, but they only put the origin of the disease farther back, and farther into the region of pathological mystery. It is conceivable that mechanical strain and other causes may determine the occurrence of a degenerative inflammation beginning in the wall of the strained vessel, but the cause of the affection of the vasa vasorum is entirely unknown. The changes in the larger artery may be due to the disease of the minute vessels, but what is to explain the latter lesion? And if we admit it to be a primary endarteritis, may not the disease of the wall of the larger vessel be in many instances of the same nature?—*Lancet*, March 26, 1881.

Inoculation with Hydrophobic and other Saliva.

Prof. PASTEUR some time since announced to the Academy of Medicine that, in the blood of some rabbits which he had rapidly killed by inoculating them with some of the virus from a child suffering from hydrophobia, he had found a new *microbe*, which he evidently regarded as the microscopic being to which were due the specific properties of the hydrophobic virus. As in several other of his discoveries, his conclusion seems to have been a somewhat hasty one, for in a subsequent communication to the Academy (*L' Union Méd.*, March 24) he announces that in same experiments performed with the saliva of children dying of broncho-pneumonia he had produced exactly the same results. He therefore had to abandon his supposition that the *microbe* in question was specially connected with rabies; but, far from regarding this result as unfavourable to his doctrine as to the parasitic origin of virulent diseases, he considers that the detection of the *microbe* in the saliva of children dying from ordinary diseases opens up a new horizon to the doctrine of the parasitic origin of diseases, removing it from the restricted circle within which it has hitherto been confined, to the wider field of general pathology.

Prof. VULPIAN has recently addressed a note to the Académie de Médecine (*L' Union Méd.*, March 31), stating that he had injected under the skin of some rabbits saliva collected at the moment from persons in perfectly good health, and that the injection caused the death of the rabbits within forty-eight hours. Their blood was found filled with *microbes*, including the special one found by Prof. Pasteur after inoculating with the saliva taken from a hydrophobic patient. A drop of this blood diluted in ten grammes of distilled water, and injected under the skin of other rabbits, caused likewise the deaths of these animals, their blood also being found filled with *microbes*. These singular results, the interpretation of which is not very easy, are accompanied by another no less singular in not being constant. Other rabbits placed under identical conditions, and inoculated with the same saliva, did not experience the slightest inconvenience. It would certainly seem that experimental microbiology is scarcely yet on the way of becoming a clear or easy science in spite of the *fiat lux* of Prof. Pasteur.—*Med. Times and Gazette*, April 2 and 16, 1881.

Arsenic in Pseudoleukœmia.

Dr. F. W. WARFYINGE relates in *Hygeia* for 1880 (*Nord. Med. Arkiv*, Band xii. Häft 4) four cases of pseudoleukæmia, principally with the object of showing that treatment by arsenic has a decidedly favourable effect. The first patient, a man aged 56, had enlarged lymphatic glands in the neck, groins, and axillæ, varying in size from a walnut to a hazel-nut; splenic dulness was 11 centimetres (4.3 inches) long by 10 centimetres (4 inches) wide. There were 3,220,000 red blood-corpuscles in a cubic millimetre; the white corpuscles were in the proportion of 1 to 140 red. Solution of arsenite of potash was given in two-drop doses twice daily; it was not tolerated at first, but, after a catarrh of the digestive and respiratory organs had disappeared, it was again taken without any inconvenience. Under the use of this medicine, a marked improvement showed itself; the lymphatic glands and the spleen diminished, and, after the arsenic had been taken (always in the dose above mentioned) for five weeks, the spleen had regained its normal size, and only slight traces of the enlargement of the glands remained. After apparent recovery, the disease returned, and the patient died a month afterwards. The second patient was a woman aged 62, with enormous lymphatic swellings in the neck, groins, and axillæ, and splenic dulness 9 centimetres in breadth. There were 3,700,000 red corpuscles in a cubic centimetre, and 1 white to 450 red. Four drops of liquor arsenicalis were given twice daily, and injections of arsenic (first 4, afterwards 9 drops a day) were made into one or other of the axillary glands. After twenty-five injections, the mass of glands was reduced from the size of a fist to a mass one inch in diameter. The patient died in an attack of asphyxia. At the necropsy, many lymphatic glands, varying in size from a hazel-nut to a walnut, were found in the anterior mediastinum. The cervical and retroperitoneal glands were swollen; the spleen was 15 centimetres long, and 9 centimetres broad. The ribs and sternum were very brittle; a gray-red mass escaped from the broken surfaces. The marrow of the femora presented the same appearance. In the third case, a woman aged 27 had a mass of enlarged glands, varying in size from a walnut to a hazel-nut, lying on the left side of the neck, and extending from the angle of the lower jaw into the subclavicular and axillary regions. In the groins and axillæ the swellings were somewhat smaller. There was nothing abnormal in the internal organs. The number of red corpuscles in a cubic millimetre was 3,700,000; and there was 1 white corpuscle to 250 red. Under the use of arsenic, reduction in the size of the lymphatic glands proceeded slowly but steadily, so that their size was considerably diminished. The fourth case was that of a boy, aged 8, with considerable enlargement of the cervical, axillary, and inguinal glands. The internal organs were healthy. There were 4,370,000 red blood-corpuscles in a cubic millimetre, and 1 white corpuscle to 190 red. Four drops of liquor arsenicalis were given twice daily, from July 18th to December 17th, with two short intervals. The lymphatic swellings diminished gradually, and the patient's appearance became more healthy.—*London Med. Record*, March 15, 1881.

———

Pathology of Diphtheria.

The pathological relations of diphtheria and the discovery of a micrococcal organism in the false membrane have made it almost certain that the morbid poison which gives rise to the disease is a parasitic organism. The observations to which we lately called attention that bacilli were to be found during life in the urine of patients suffering from the disease, and after death in the kidneys, constitute another step in the demonstration. From a communication to the Paris Société Anatomique we learn that a French "interne," M. TALAMON, has succeeded in cultivating the organisms from eight cases. In the condition of complete development they presented a characteristic mycelium and spores. The former are tubes with partitions, at intervals, from two to five thousandths of a millimetre in length. These, under favourable circumstances, elongate and bifurcate, the bifurcations being characteristic in consequence of their incurved branches, like the sides of a lyre. In other conditions the mycelia do not become elongated, although they multiply so as rapidly to cover the surface of the cultivation liquid; they remain short and assume irregular forms, and give rise to numerous straight rods.

The spores are of two kinds, round or oval, which may be termed the spores of germination, and rectangular spores or conidia. The latter characterize the species. They form small rectangles of various sizes, their length being sometimes fifteen thousandths of a millimetre. They may be isolated or united in festoons or zigzag chains. At first homogeneous, they soon become filled with small round granules, highly refracting, and of the size of ordinary micrococci. The round or oval spores are those which, by their elongation, constitute the mycelium. They appear as clear points, from three to five thousandths of a millimetre in diameter, in the middle of a mass of granular material.

M. Talamon has inoculated this organism into the mucous membrane of the mouth or nose, or has given it with the food, in six rabbits, two guinea-pigs, four frogs, a fowl, and four pigeons. The rabbits died at the end of six, eight, ten, and eighteen days. That which died soonest presented an enormous swelling of the neck resembling the œdema of the neck in diphtheria, and due to a serous infiltration of the connective tissue, and the culture of this serosity showed the same organism with the characteristic conidia. The rabbit which died at the end of eighteen days presented a bilateral fibrinous pleurisy, with effusion. The effusion and pleuritic membrane also yielded, on culture, the organism which had been inoculated; and it could be recognized, either by simple microscopical examination or by culture, in most cases in the liquid contained in the pericardial and peritoneal cavities, and often in the kidneys. The organism was never obtained by cultivation of the blood contained in the heart. The liquid either remained clear or presented only ordinary bacteria.

In the four pigeons M. Talamon succeeded in producing characteristic false membranes. He first scratched the mucous membrane of the mouth with a bistoury, and then placed some of the cultivated organism in the interior of the mouth. At the end of twenty-four hours a thick membrane lined both sides of the mouth, the tongue, the false palate, and the back of the pharynx. It was yellowish-white in colour, and was formed, like the diphtheritic membrane in man, by epithelial cells, fat, micrococci, and bacteria. There were very few of the rectangular conidia, but these were abundantly obtained from the membrane by cultivation. Two of the pigeons died at the end of three days. In one the entrance to the larynx was covered by false membranes, and the trachea was full of a thick mucus from which the organism was obtained by cultivation, as also from the pericardial and peritoneal liquids, but not from the blood. The third pigeon remained ill for eight days, and then the false membranes became separated and the animal recovered. At this point, unfortunately, the experiments have been for the present arrested. They were carried on in the laboratory of the Hôtel Dieu, and some of the physicians, fearing lest some of the organisms might contaminate the patients, stopped the observations. We are promised a resumption of the inquiry at an early period. The facts ascertained are of the greatest importance, and seem to open out an entirely new field of investigation as to the etiology of the disease, since M. Talamon hints that he possesses a clue as to the source from which the organism is derived in the case of human infection.—*Lancet*, April 9, 1881.

—

Treatment of Diphtheria with Muriate of Pilocarpin.

LAX (*Aertz. Intel. Blatt.* 1881, No. 43), following Guttmann, has employed muriate of pilocarpin in a small epidemic of diphtheria, and has obtained results so far beyond his most favourable anticipation, that he thinks himself obliged to recommend it most earnestly for wider use. Between September 24 and November 17, he treated for diphtheria sixteen children of various ages, from one to sixteen years. The first six children were treated by pencilling with a four per cent. solution of nitrate of silver, and a solution of chlorate of potash as a gargle. To two quite young children, a mixture of chlorate of potash was given. Of the six children, four recovered quickly, while two, whose cases were very severe, died. In the last ten cases occurring after October 5, Lax employed exclusively the muriate of pilocarpin. Six of these were very severe, and in two of them death was expected every night. Nevertheless, all these children treated with pilocarpin entirely recovered. An increased secretion of mucus and saliva occurred, and great masses of diphtheritic effusion were expelled from the mouth as well as the nose. The breathing became freer, *râles* ceased to be heard, the fever passed away, and the appetite recovered. The children generally recovered in from three to five days. Labial herpes indicated the favourable processes in all cases. On the third day already all trace of the deposit on the soft palate and tonsils was removed. According to the age, Lax prescribed two to four centigrammes of muriate of pilocarpin, 60 to 80 centigrammes of pepsin, with two to three drops of hydrochloric acid in 70 grammes distilled water, giving every hour from one teaspoonful to one tablespoonful. In addition, Tokay wine was given hourly (a teaspoonful to a tablespoonful), and warm packs were applied to the neck.—*London Med. Record*, March 15, 1881.

—

Diabetes associated with Disease of the Pancreas.

In 1877 M. LANCEREAUX read a note at the Académie, in which he demonstrated the existence of a form of diabetes mellitus, found in conjunction with pancreatic lesions. This, he alleged, constituted a special and distinctive variety of diabetes, characterized by a *début brusque*, considerable emaciation, with polydipsia and polyphagia, by peculiar alvine evacuations, and especially by a very rapid evolution. The study of Lancereaux has been made the basis of further investigations by M. DEPIERRE (*Jour. de Méd. et de Chir. Pratiques*, Dec. 1880), which have led to the discovery of new facts in this connection. Various kinds of pancreatic alterations may be regarded as leading to this kind of diabetes. They may be primary lesions, or they may be the secondary result of the presence of calculi, or else they may be caused by compression of the ducts by neoplasms. In all such cases, there appeared to be a complete abolition of the pancreatic function. This suppression of a digestive function is revealed by special symptoms, thus constituting a variety of diabetes (called by the author "emaciating diabetes") which differs greatly in its clinical aspects from ordinary polyuria. In the latter disease there is said to be, as a rule, an initial stage of obesity, or at least of apparent health, thus rendering the progress of the malady slow and insidious. In pancreatic diabetes, on the other hand, we notice along with the absence of *embonpoint* a quite sudden explosion of symptoms. These ordinarily consist of grave intestinal manifestations, vertigo, vomiting, and jaundice. These symptoms after a while indeed disappear, but they leave the patients in a condition of profound debility. Soon the essential symptoms of the disease put in their appearance. Sometimes, indeed, they occur from the very beginning, without any previous indications of morbid changes. They are polydipsia, polyphagia, polyuria, and autophagia (the latter probably meaning tissue-waste and emaciation). This combination of symptoms is rapidly established, reaching an acme in a few weeks or months, and it is this very point which appears to afford pathognomonic indication of the existence of this variety of diabetes. The habitual presence of diarrhœa is also noted. Sugar is voided in great abundance with the urine. Pulmonary phthisis is also a frequent complication. Emaciation is rapid. In a few months the patients lose successively their physical, intellectual, and genital powers. Then complete prostration and profound marasmus set in, to which there is superadded hectic fever, with the symptoms of consumption. The average duration of the sickness is about twenty months, though it may end in half a year, or last even three years. Greasy or creamy stools may afford a clue to the establishment of the diagnosis of pancreatic diabetes, but it must be remembered that they occur also in other affections of that organ. Another point which must be considered is the deficient digestion of nitrogenized substances in atrophic conditions of the pancreas. Thus, pieces of undigested muscle found in the stools of patients may awaken a suspicion of this disease. Besides the ordinary treatment of diabetes mellitus, the administration of pancreatine suggests itself as affording a possibility of artificially supplying the lacking aids to digestion.—*London Med. Record*, April 15, 1881.

Medical Ophthalmoscopy.

In the *Berliner Klinische Wochenschrift* (Nos. 1 and 2, 1881) Dr. LITTEN gives an account of certain clinically interesting changes in the fundus of the eye.

1. In *General Anœmia.*—The fundus is bright red; the disk pale and sharply defined, becoming ultimately quite white, but without the bluish tint of atrophy. The arteries and veins are small, the central streak indistinct. Less characteristic, though more striking, are hemorrhages and white or grayish-white spots on the retina. Later the symptoms of neuritis or neuro-retinitis occasionally appear —the radial streaked clouding first of the disk, then of the retina, with the development of a white border to the vessels. Examining such retinæ microscopically, Dr. Litten observes a general cell-infiltration of the retina, and an inflammatory exudation of pus corpuscles ensheathing the vessels, these changes not proceeding in anæmia to the alterations in the interstitial tissue characteristic of chronic retinitis. The neuritis is sharply intra-ocular, and consists in cell infiltration and hypertrophic nerve-fibres. The white patches consist sometimes exclusively of white blood-corpuscles, with occasionally hypertrophic nerve-fibres, but never, he finds, exclusively of the latter. The power of vision is very little affected by the hemorrhages or the white patches unless actually in the central part of the retina. No one of these changes, he finds, is characteristic of particular forms of anæmia. Hemorrhages are in no way characteristic of pernicious anæmia, and, except as showing that the anæmia has reached a high grade, in no way justify an unfavourable prognosis. These hemorrhages and white patches he believes are, in general, of much commoner occurrence than is usually supposed. For example, he has met with them very frequently in cases of carcinoma uteri, more especially in fat, flabby females with cardiac symptoms like those produced in anæmia. Neuritis and neuro-retinitis are, in Dr. Litten's experience, more common after great loss of blood than in chronic anæmia, coming on generally in the first or second week after the loss, and leading frequently to atrophy.

2. In *General Venous Congestion.*—The fundus is here dark or even blackish-red, the disk also dark red. The vessels are gorged and tortuous, the tortuosities rising occasionally out of the plane of the fundus. With these differences from anæmia, there occur the same hemorrhages, white patches, and inflammations of the retina and optic nerve. The hemorrhages accompany the veins, and are not unfrequently in the periphery, where they may be readily overlooked. The white patches are rarer than in anæmia; inflammation, with marked swelling of the disk, more common. This inflammation he considers must depend on some other cause than simple anæmia or simple congestion, as he has in numerous experiments produced these conditions without being able to cause inflammation. The above changes he has observed most frequently in the general venous congestion of chronic bronchitis and emphysema, and in two such cases with marked cyanosis he saw in the periphery peculiar coin-like hemorrhages which we do not remember having seen described. They were of various sizes, with sharply defined edges, mostly in relation with the veins, hanging on them like berries on a stalk. In one of these patients a second and fatal attack showed hemorrhages of the same peculiar character, lying chiefly in the outer retinal layers.

3. *Case of Poisoning with a Mixture of Nitro-benzol and Aniline.*—The patient was admitted in the deepest coma, which lasted forty-eight hours. The skin and mucous membranes, in place of the usual blue or grayish-blue of pure nitro-benzol poisoning, had a deep violet colour. The fundus was of an intense violet colour, with a few slight hemorrhages, the vessels as if filled with ink. There was no affection of sight, either as to sharpness or perception of colour. Whether the blue colour in pure nitro-benzol poisoning result from reduction of the nitro-benzol to aniline, or, as seems more probable, from deficient absorption of oxygen, there appears good reason to suppose that the violet colour in this case resulted from the aniline mixed with the nitro-benzol.

4. *Apoplexy of the Brain and Retina from miliary aneurisms.*—The patient was struck down suddenly with left hemiplegia and the usual partial facial paralysis of the same side. The ophthalmoscope showed numerous and extensive hemorrhages, completely hiding the fundus. The post-mortem examination disclosed numerous subarachnoid and intra-cerebral hemorrhages, with aneurismal dilatations of the vertebral and middle cerebral arteries. The retina was suspected to be similarly affected, and on examination was found to be so, but owing to the diseased vessels lying everywhere amid the hemorrhages, no accurate examination of their coats could be made. What could be seen was sudden dilatation of the calibre of the vessels, which had ruptured at the same time as those in the brain from some sudden increase of the already high arterial pressure.—*Med. Times and Gazette*, March 19, 1881.

—

Nerve-stretching in Locomotor Ataxia.

The operation of nerve-stretching as a means of treating locomotor ataxy was introduced, it will be remembered, by Dr. LANGENBUCH, who recorded a startling improvement in a case so treated, the intense pains and considerable ataxy having almost entirely disappeared after the operation, and the diminished sensibility having returned to the normal. Symptoms of similar character and of marked degree persisted in the upper limbs, and, indeed, appeared to have become more intense. Hence it was decided, three months later, to stretch also the nerves of the arms. While the patient was under the influence of chloroform an epileptic fit occurred and he died. The spinal cord from this important case was given for microscopical examination to Professor WESTPHAL, who has just published the results in the *Berlin. Klin. Wochenschrift.* The cord was seriously crushed at certain places, probably in the process of removal. Other parts, however, were in good condition for examination, especially the lumbar enlargement, the upper part of the cervical region, and small parts of the dorsal region. These parts showed nowhere the clear tracts which indicate the presence of sclerosis in hardened cords. Microscopical examination in glycerine showed no granule corpuscles nor the translucent appearance which indicates degeneration. After tinting, the posterior columns were found intact throughout, without a trace of sclerosis or of atrophy of the nerve-tubules. The periphery of the posterior columns, in which a slightly paler colour had been noted with the naked eye, tinted more deeply than the rest, and here the regular arrangement of the nerve-fibres was wanting, and the condition showed clearly that this appearance had only arisen from an injury during the removal of the cord. Sections from the dorsal region and the upper cervical region showed also a perfectly normal white substance, nowhere any trace of sclerosis or of atrophy. No abnormal changes were found in the gray substance, and the nerve-fibres of the anterior and posterior roots exhibited also no trace of atrophy.

It is certain from these facts that the case was not one of posterior sclerosis. Can we (Westphal asks) from these facts draw the inference that in a certain stage of tabes the disease may exist as a neurosis without structural changes, and that the degeneration of the posterior columns represents a later and consecutive change which has nothing to do with the special symptoms, in accordance with the older view held by Trousseau? This conclusion seems incompatible with the fact that in all cases examined hitherto, without a single exception, structural changes in the posterior columns have been found. Moreover, the case of Dr. Langenbuch does not, he urges, point to such a conclusion. The clinical history has only been very briefly recorded, but the facts as stated are altogether peculiar. The affection had been of very rapid development; although the symptoms were advanced, they had only existed for a few months, and the arms were considerably affected a few months later. The case thus resembles those of so-called "acute ataxy," such as occur spontaneously or after acute febrile diseases, and which have a course altogether different from that of ordinary tabes, often ending in complete recovery. The nature of these cases is unknown.

Langenbuch was inclined to regard his case as one of a primary affection of the peripheral nerves, but, unfortunately, the large nerve trunks could not be removed at the post-mortem examination. It is, however, noteworthy that at the operation the left sciatic was seen to be "reddish and somewhat swollen."

In publishing these facts, Westphal does not desire to discountenance the operation in other cases in which the existence of a spinal lesion is undoubted, since, as he rightly points out, experience rather than theory must be our guide; but he strongly urges, and with reason, the great importance of a thorough and skilled examination of the nerve symptoms in all cases before the operation, that we may know whether the cases so treated are to be regarded as examples of true posterior sclerosis or not.—*Lancet*, March 26, 1881.

On the Disappearance and the Localization of the Knee Reflex.

The value of this reflex, as a means of diagnosis in diseases of the spinal cord, was first established by Professor Westphal, of Berlin, who designated it the "knee phenomenon." The term commonly employed—"patellar tendon reflex" —is objectionable, as involving the idea that it is a simple reflex process connected solely with the patellar tendon. A much better name is that given to it by Dr. Hughlings-Jackson—the "knee-jerk." It consists, as is well known, in the contraction of the quadriceps extensor cruris following, in health, a blow on the

patellar tendon. Westphal believes that it is no simple reflex action, but a complex phenomenon, depending primarily on the muscular tone of the quadriceps
extensor, and secondarily on a reflex. In typically developed cases of gr^a_y
degeneration of the posterior columns of the spinal cord (tabes dorsalis or
locomotor ataxy) this reflex is absent, its disappearance is one of the earliest
symptoms of this degeneration, frequently preceding the disturbances of sensation
and motion that mark the full development of the disease. Its disappearance
implies disease of the reflex track, or, excluding the nerves and their roots, it
implies disease in the lumbar enlargement of the spinal cord. Professor WEST-
PHAL, in an address to the Medical Society of Berlin, has sought to answer the
further questions—(1) In those cases where the disappearance of the knee reflex
forms the first symptom of tabes, is there already anatomical change in the lumbar
posterior columns? and (2) If so, where; that is, in the postero-external column
(root-zone of Charcot) or in the postero-median column? An answer to these
questions need not be looked for in cases where the fully developed disease has
caused death, but Professor Westphal thinks the following case throws some
light upon them: In March, 1877, a male patient aged thirty-two, was admitted into Charité suffering from mental aberration. His family history showed a
strong tendency to psychical and nervous disease. A year before the above date
the patient complained of weakness of sight, but ophthalmoscopic examination
gave a negative result. Six months thereafter he became completely blind, and
optic atrophy was now found. The mental disease for which he was admitted
appeared in a marked form eight days before admission. His blindness was very
nearly total on both sides—the pupils insensitive to light, but reacting on accommodation; his articulation was slightly affected; but with these exceptions there
was no alteration in the nervous system. Sensation and motion were perfect,
and his gait was the normal walk of the blind. The knee reflex on both sides
was normal. His mental aberration consisted in moderate intellectual weakness
with delusions. In June, 1878, the delusions had all disappeared, the intellectual weakness alone remaining. Next he became hypochondriacal, and his
articulation was more affected. Ultimately he spoke nothing, became uncleanly
in his habits, and refused nourishment. In 1879 he was again in the condition
of simple intellectual weakness. During all this time there was no change in
sensation or motion. The knee reflex was proved from time to time, and failed for
the first time in October, 1879, in the right leg, that of the left being still weakly
present. In December, 1879, diarrhœa with bloody stools appeared; and in January, 1880, the patient died with fever, delirium, and tremor of the limbs. Five days
before death the knee reflex failed in the left limb also. The post-mortem examination showed slight membranous exudation on the surface of the dura mater,
cloudiness but no adhesion of the pia mater, and atrophy of the optic nerves and
tracts. To the naked eye the spinal cord appeared normal, but hardened in
bichromate of potash, it showed degeneration of the postero-external columns,
and in a less degree of the posterior parts of the lateral columns. The degeneration
was most extensive at the lower part of the cord, gradually diminishing upwards,
and nowhere affecting the postero-median column. It showed microscopically,
numerous "granule corpuscles," considerable disappearance of medullated
nerves, and thickening of interstitial tissue; not, however, the complete atrophy
of fully developed gray degeneration. The gray substance and posterior roots
were normal. Professor Westphal considers himself justified in arguing that the
degeneration of the postero-external column produced failure of the knee reflex.
The degeneration in the lateral column could not be the cause, for (1) frequently
in tabes, when the knee reflex fails entirely, the lateral columns are quite normal,
and (2) the lateral columns have been found diseased to the lumbar enlargement,

without the slightest decrease of the knee reflex. The argument, he remarks, is supported by the following facts : (1) the almost constant failure of the knee reflex in tabes dorsalis, combined with the almost constant occurrence of degeneration of the postero-external column as its first change; and (2) the occurrence of complicated cases of spinal disease, where the knee reflex is retained, and where also uniformly the postero-external column is healthy.

Professor Westphal then proceeds to discuss certain fallacies with regard to the knee reflex. He points out that although many authors have given cases of developed tabes with the knee reflex retained, no case has been published where the ordinary symptoms of tabes were present, with the exception of the absence of the knee reflex, and where the post-mortem examination has shown gray degeneration of the posterior columns to the lumbar enlargement. Numerous cases, he says, of disseminated gray degeneration with muscular spasm and even foot clonus have been brought to him as tabes dorsalis. With regard to the 1.56 per cent. of healthy individuals in whom, according to Berger, the knee reflex fails, Professor Westphal says he never met with a case of failure in an undoubtedly healthy person, but he points out that the reflex is difficult to produce (1) in those who have short, thick legs, or (2) short patellar tendons not furnishing length sufficient for the necessary vibration; and (3) the reflex will be absent where the muscular tone of the quadriceps extensor is absent, e. g., in extensive acute disease of the gray matter of the cord, etc. The absence of the knee reflex in a seemingly healthy individual, Professor Westphal would consider a sign of latent tabes, which may remain undeveloped for years, or, since the disease is not necessarily and absolutely progressive, may never be developed. Naturally, the gradual disappearance of the phenomenon if observed has a much higher diagnostic worth than the simple discovery of its absence. The knee reflex, Professor Westphal remarks, ought to be proved in all obscure cases of nervous disease—e. g., in hypochondria. He has met with several cases of hypochondria with no spinal disease, and the knee reflex retained, where tabes dorsalis has developed itself later.

What was the nature of the case discussed above ? The lightning pains of tabes and the disturbance of sensation and motion all failed here. The degeneration in the posterior parts of the lateral columns occupied the position of the "crossed pyramidal tracts"—i. e., of the fibres which cross at the anterior pyramids. The disease could not be followed into the pyramids, and this, along with the fact that no centre of disease was found in the cerebrum, shows that it was not a case of secondary descending degeneration, but a primary degeneration of the above-mentioned system of fibres. Whether the degeneration of the postero-external columns is also a "system disease"—i. e., a disease of a column of functionally equivalent nerve-fibres—is a much more difficult question, chiefly because the results of development and pathology are not yet at one in the differentiation of the two parts of the posterior column. The localization of the knee reflex, however, in the postero-external column seems thoroughly justified. Disease of that column appears on reaching a certain intensity to destroy the tone of the quadriceps extensor, and thereby the knee reflex, giving us a means of most accurate (or even, as Professor Westphal says, elegant) diagnosis in diseases of the spinal cord.—*Med. Times and Gaz.*, March 12, 1881.

—

On Spastic Spinal Paralysis.

In an article in the *Hospitals-Tidende*, series 2, Band vii. Dr. A. FRIEDENREICH gives a short sketch of the history and symptomatology of this form of disease, and discusses the question, how far it is in itself a disease, and whether it has a constant course, and a constant pathological basis. He refers to the cases of spastic spinal paralysis with a more or less acute course described by others, especially Veldens and Hench, and relates a case of similar nature which had come under his own observation.

A man aged 39 presented in as marked a form as possible the muscular rigidity, the spastic gait, and the enormously increased tendon-reflexes, characteristic of spastic spinal paralysis. The disease had probably been caused by the influence of alternations of heat and cold ; it began with symptoms which were referred to rheumatic fever, and had apparently reached its culminating point when the patient was admitted into the Communal Hospital at Copenhagen. The duration of the illness was about three months and a half, and ended in almost complete recovery. The author then notices the literature treating of the transitional forms between spastic spinal paralysis and other forms of chronic myelitis, and finally speaks of the pathology of the disease. After noticing the *post-mortem* appearances described by Stofella, Westphal, and Charcot, he describes the following case :—

The patient was a man aged 31, who had been somewhat imbecile from infancy. His illness began about half a year before he came under observation, and he presented in the most distinct form the motor disturbances characteristic of the disease. He died about a year and a half after the commencement of his illness. The spinal cord was everywhere softened, being in some parts almost fluid. On minute examination, numerous portions were found, varying from microscopic smallness to the size of a pea, while the tissue was completely broken down and reduced to detritus, while at the circumference of the completely destroyed portions there were generally found parts of which the structure was still recognizable, while networks of the neuroglia were found, if not destroyed, to be filled with an amorphous more or less granular mass, coloured in various shades by carmine, and having scattered roundish nuclei ; in other parts there was a quite amorphous exudation, which was coloured rather strongly by carmine, and contained similar nuclei. There was also found, diffused over nearly the whole mass of the spinal cord, but in very varying degrees in different parts, hypertrophy of the interstitial tissue, while the nerve-fibres were partly thrust asunder, and showed here and there distinct swellings, especially of the axis-cylinders. There was no indication of a systematic diffusion of the interstitial changes. The gray substance, especially in the cervical region, showed very scanty ganglion-cells, there being often only a single one in a section of the whole anterior cornua, while the cells of the posterior cornua were on the whole better preserved. Of the existing cells, some were rather small and highly pigmented, while others were of normal size, but very pale, and having an abnormal tendency to a globular shape. The central canal was obliterated throughout ; the pia mater was thickened, and very adherent in some parts.

Dr. Friedenreich believes that he is justified in drawing the following conclusions : 1. Spastic spinal paralysis is not an independent disease, but a congeries of symptoms which may occur in various affections of the spinal cord. 2. The phenomena depend on an increase of the tendon-reflexes, in combination with partial preservation of voluntary motor power. 3. Where the phenomena of spastic spinal paralysis occur, they may indicate sclerosis of the lateral columns ; but, in the present state of science, they do not prove it. Still less can they prove the existence of an exclusive or only transient affection of the lateral structures of the pyramid.—*London Medical Record*, March 15, 1881.

Œdema of the Right Arytenoid Cartilage.

Dr. E. MARTET (*Annales des Malad. de l'Oreille, du Larynx, etc.*, Dec. 1880) relates the case of a sergeant-major who, with a history of great hoarseness and dysphagia of three days' duration, presented a round swelling of the right arytenoid eminence, of the dimensions of a medium-sized grape. Its mucous membrane was stretched, shining, and of a grayish colour. The epiglottis was red and slightly swollen, the remainder of the larynx being normal. The œdematous part was twice touched with a solution of chromic acid (1 in 4), and in three days recovered its normal appearance, the hoarseness and dyspnœa having completely disappeared. The etiology of the affection appears to have been the excessive use of the voice whilst commanding, and the effect of damp cold, in a person of drinking habits. The author also mentions a case of syphilis of the larnyx, accompanied by œdema of the glottis threatening asphyxia, in which the latter symptom was successfully relieved by applications of chromic acid.—*Lond. Med. Record*, April 15, 1881.

Uræmic Dyspnœa.

M. G. SÉE (*Le Practicien*) has published notes of the case of a young woman attacked by urgent dyspnœa, with great oppression and cyanosis. There were a faint systolic apex-murmur, and a few râles over the lungs posteriorly, but nothing sufficient to account for the symptoms. The urine was very albuminous. There was no œdema. She died in a few days. The kidneys were large and red. Mr. Sée lays down the rule that, when a person is attacked with dyspnœa without obvious cause in the thoracic organs, the urine should be examined for albumen. He relates two other cases, in which the dyspnœa simulated spasmodic asthma, and was not readily diagnosed on that account.—*Lond. Med. Record*, April 15, 1881.

Treatment of Pleurisy in Children.

Dr. J. LEWIS SMITH, in a paper upon this subject (*Med. Record*, April 9, 1881), speaks of the treatment appropriate to each of the three stages :—

1. The stage which precedes the effusion ; 2. The stage of effusion ; and 3. The stage of absorption and convalescence.

In the beginning of the disease measures should be adopted which are appropriate for reducing inflammation and limiting exudation. The abstraction of blood in idiopathic pleurisy may be beneficial if judiciously employed, but only one or two or three leeches should be employed in a robust child two, three, or four years old. As a rule, the loss of blood is injurious in all cases of secondary pleurisy, such as follows scarlet fever, etc., and also if the quantity of effusion is great. Emollient and simply irritating poultices are serviceable in the first stage, and he recommends a mixture of *one* part of mustard to *sixteen* of linseed. It should be made very wet, spread thin, applied over the chest in front and behind, covered with oil-silk, and changed twice in twenty-four hours. For children under six or seven months of age, rubbing the chest with camphorated oil, and applying a simple poultice, may be sufficient.

Blistering at this early stage of the disease should not be employed, as it increases the inflammation, and Dr. Smith has seen a case which terminated fatally, in which there was found an increased area of inflammation, corresponding exactly in situation, size, and shape to a blister that had been applied.

The indications for the use of internal remedies in the first stage are to diminish the frequency of the pulse, relieve the pain, and allay the cough.

To a child *three* years old the tincture of aconite may be given in doses of half a drop, and for a child *six* years old in doses of *one* drop, every three hours for two or three days. In the first stage of primary pleurisy the cardiac sedatives may be used ; but digitalis is a safer and better remedy in all other cases, and it also can be used in the second stage.

To a child *two* years old the tincture of digitalis may be given in doses of *one drop every three hours*, and to a child five years old *two* drops with the same interval. An opiate is ordinarily required : Dover's powder, one to three grains, every three hours. Hyoscyamus may be used to relieve the pain and cough ; digitalis may be combined with an opiate ; and morphine and aconite may be combined.

In secondary pleurisy digitalis is preferable to aconite.

In the *second* stage, unless the effusion is small, measures designed to remove it are required. The propriety of using blisters in this stage is very doubtful.

A relaxed condition of the bowels favours absorption of serous effusion. Diaphoretics do not aid much in the removal of the fluid. Pilocarpine produces a depressing effect which renders it unsafe.

Diuretics and tonics are beneficial. Digitalis, with the acetate of potash, is very serviceable.

℞. Infus. digitalis ℥iv ; potass. acetat. ℨj.—M. S. Teaspoonful every three hours, to a child four or five years old.

Bitter tonics are especially useful in this stage, and the acetate of potash may be combined with a decoction of cinchona, with good results. A full amount of nutriment should be taken, with but little fluid. Of course, the suggestion to use a dry diet and diminish the quantity of drink is not applicable to young children. If the appetite and the general health are good, and there are no symptoms due to the presence of the fluid, but little medication is necessary. If there are such symptoms and the fluid does not disappear, the question of surgical interference arises, and the indications for it are the following :—

First.—Oppressed breathing due to the liquid present, whether it be serofibrinous, purulent, or hemorrhagic.

Second.—If there be flat percussion note over the entire affected side, with displacement of the heart, even if there be no dyspnœa, for the latter may occur suddenly.

Third.—Moderate effusion, without material decrease in quantity by absorption after some weeks of treatment. There is danger that catarrhal pneumonia terminating in cheesy pneumonia and tuberculosis may occur in portions of the compressed lung. Besides, the longer the lung is compressed, the slower will it return to normal expansion after the pressure has been removed.

Fourth.—A moderate quantity of fluid co-existing with disease of the opposite lung, or of the lung of the affected side.

Fifth.—Extension of the inflammation to the pericardium. Pericarditis as an extension of the inflammation is not infrequent.

Sixth.—The existence of valvular lesion of the heart.

Seventh.—The presence of pus ; empyema.

The operation of thoracentesis should be performed in the eighth intercostal space, on a line perpendicular with the angle of the scapula. The admission of air to the pleural cavity should be carefully avoided. The thickness of the thoracic wall is about half an inch ; in emaciated children it is less. Introduction of the canula to the depth of *one inch* is sufficient to pass beyond the exudation and allow the liquid to flow through the canula. The sharp needle should not be used. Washing out the pleural cavity is unnecessary ; it is injurious rather than beneficial, except in cases in which the pus is offensive. To empty the pleural cavity and approximate the pleural surfaces is the indication. Dr. Smith thinks there will be a reaction against the removal of a portion of the ribs in cases of empyema.

Idiopathic Enlargement of the Heart.

Under the term enlargement of the heart are generally included three anatomical conditions: first, where the cardiac cavities are increased and the cardiac walls thickened in direct ratio—simple enlargement; second, where the cavities are increased and the walls thickened, but the cavities in higher degree—excentric or dilated enlargement; and, third, where the cavities are actually diminished by the thickening of the walls of the heart—concentric enlargement. Doubt has been thrown on the existence of this last class of cases; and, in some recent remarks on the subject, Professor FRÄNTZEL, of Berlin (*Berl. Klin. Woch.*, Feb. 1881), protests against the terms excentric and concentric cardiac hypertrophy. His distinction of idiopathic enlargement of the heart into dilatation *with* and dilatation *without* hypertrophy is undoubtedly the expression of a difference of first importance clinically. Hypertrophy, speaking broadly, means life; its absence indicates impending death. The conditions of its development are chiefly the vigour of the patient and the gradual development of the resistance producing the enlargement. For the left ventricle, its presence is shown by high tension of the radial arteries, abnormally resistant heart's impulse, and marked or ringing second sound in the aorta; while, for the right ventricle, the only sign is marked or ringing second sound in the pulmonary artery. As to the percussion of the heart, Dr. Fräntzel emphasizes that it is not simply what we find, but the interpretation thereof, that is important. The actual projection outline of the heart, he believes, it is impossible to discover; but should the percussion note over the body of the sternum be duller than over the manubrium, he considers we may diagnose cardiac enlargement to the right, that is, in general, dilatation of the right ventricle. A dulness extending beyond the usual triangle of cardiac dulness indicates, in the absence of disease of the neighbouring organs, an affection of the heart, either fluid in the pericardium or dilatation of a cardiac cavity, according to the position and shape of the dulness. The obverse of this, however, is by no means invariably true. A dulness not extending beyond the above-mentioned triangle is in no way a sure indication of the absence of dilatation. A heart's dulness of normal dimensions in a *wide* thorax, according to Dr. Fräntzel, indicates dilatation; and again, in the barrel-shaped chest, where no heart's dulness ought to be found, the presence of dulness at all indicates a most pronounced dilatation. Such a diagnosis made some time before death may be contradicted, Dr. Fräntzel says, by the necropsy, but this he holds to show simply that dilatation, like hypertrophy, may regress on the causes ceasing to act.

In enumerating the causes of idiopathic enlargement of the heart, Dr. Fräntzel makes special mention of those cases of a single great bodily exertion which, by acute distension of the left ventricle, may cause irreparable cardiac debility, leading to rapid death. This, we may presume, he has observed mostly in persons well on in years. A rush to catch a train may cut half a score of years or more off a comparatively healthy man's life. In discussing obstructions to the circulation in the lungs and kidneys as causes of cardiac enlargement, he seeks to explain the enlargement of the left ventricle in kidney-disease by the obstruction to the renal circulation. He ignores apparently the frequent want of concomitancy between the amount of cardiac enlargement and the degree of renal disease, and refuses the more modern explanation which regards both diseases as local manifestations of a common disease, in all probability acting and reacting on one another. With regard to the large class of cases in which cardiac enlargement is attributed to arterial sclerosis, Dr. Fräntzel agrees with Traube in considering both the arterial sclerosis and the cardiac enlargement to be the results of a common cause, namely, high systemic tension, produced either by gluttony and

drunkenness, or by hard labour. Both classes, he says, benefit much by purgatives, combined in the former with opium, in the latter with absolute rest.—
London Medical Record, April 15, 1881.

Pulsus Bigeminus.

Dr. FRANZ RIEGEL (*Deutsches Archiv für Klin. Med.*, Feb. 1881) contributes a careful study of two such cases, with numerous graphic tracings. The one
case had a systolic, mitral, and tricuspid murmur, with 80 apex-beats per minute,
80 visible undulations of the jugular veins, and 40 radial pulsations. Two apex-
beats and jugular undulations were close together, and corresponded to one radial
pulsation. The other case had no venous undulation, and had 88 heart-beats,
with 44 radial pulsations. These cases, then, were similar to those described by
Leyden and others, as instances of independent contraction of one ventricle without the other—the right contracting twice for one systole of the left. But the
author shows from sphygmographic evidence that each radial pulsation is followed
by a faint wave, imperceptible to touch, and synchronous with the second of the
redoubled cardiac impulses. He, therefore, holds that such cases have been
erroneously apprehended, and that both ventricles simultaneously contract,
although the second is fainter than the first of the double heart-beats, and does
not send out a wave strong enough to reach the wrist.—*London Medical Record*,
April 15, 1881.

Treatment of Vomiting in Phthisical Patients.

M. FERRAND, physician to the Hospital Laennec, sums up as follows, in
L' Union Médicale, the principal indications presented in the vomitings of consumptive patients. The forms of vomiting are : 1. the mechanical vomiting resulting from the excitation of the respiratory nerves, which is sometimes combined
with a certain degree of pharyngeal or gastric irritation; 2. gastric vomiting properly so-called; central and bulbar vomiting. These varieties of vomiting differ,
not only in their mechanism, but also in their period of appearance, and in the
nature of the vomited matters, etc. The mechanical vomiting of phthisical persons, which may be called direct vomiting, occurs at the outset of the disease. It
brings up substances which are in a large measure alimentary. The first indication in this case is to calm the cough. This, however, is more easily said than
done. Emollients, alkaline, and soothing gargles should be employed. When
the irritation of the pharnyx is deep-seated, modifying astringents (alum, tannin,
confection of roses, etc.) should be resorted to, and even such remedies as tincture of iodine, nitrate of silver, or ammonia. What are most often employed are
the narcotics, the fumes of belladonna, datura, and then anæsthetics and antispas-
modies. In this contingency, M. Woillez recommends touching the pharynx
with a solution containing one-sixth of bromide of potassium. Gastric vomiting
is the most common of digestive disorders in phthisis. It occurs in three-fifths of
patients, according to Andral, and in four-fifths, according to Louis. It is the
vomiting of the middle period of the disease. These matters are not purely alimentary; they are substances more or less changed by the digestion and fluid.
They include also mucus and bile. There are four varieties of gastric vomiting.
1. Vomiting from apepsia. For this, bitter and tonic digestives are to be employed, or, in case of need, an emetic; in default of the latter, chloral, and chloroform in preference to ether ; and diastase, because of its peptic qualities, may
render real service in these cases. 2. Vomiting from 'hypercrinia,' observed
especially in cachectic patients, is combated by absorbents (magnesia, charcoal)
or astringent powders (rhatany, calumba). Powdered opium renders great ser-

vice in these conditions. 3. The vomiting from convulsive gastralgia demands the administration of narcotics (opium, chloral, ether). The application of ether-spray to the epigastric region and the back has given good results. 4. Vomiting by gastric irritation. Here the diet must be regulated, the meals must be given at fixed times, and milk-diet prescribed. Alkaline remedies and iodide of potassium in small doses should be given. Opiate blisters should be applied, and in case of failure, revulsive agents (tincture of iodine and blisters) should be used without fear. Central or bulbar vomiting may occur at the outset of the tuberculosis, but usually at an advanced stage. It may be symptomatic of an encephalic irritation, or the effect of bulbar anæmia. The vomited matters consist mostly of mucus and bile. The therapeutic agents at the disposal of the physician are first chloral; then chloroform, opium, and morphia, as well as bromide of potassium, in doses of 1 to 2 grammes (15 to 30 grains) at meal times.—*Lond. Med. Record*, April 15, 1881.

———

Treatment of Dysentery with Enemata of Cold Water and finely crushed Ice.

After trying various methods of treatment, MICHAILOW (*Mediz. Obosr.*, vol. xiv. Aug. 1880) has ended at last with the method of enemata of cold water and finely crushed ice, which, he says, has not failed him in a single case for four years. It proved especially successful in the cases of his own children. A short description of two cases follows. Quinine, in the form of Botkin's cholera drops, was administered internally in all cases. (Compound tincture of quinine, Hoffmann's anodyne spirit, of each half an ounce; hydro-chlorate of quinine, one scruple; dilute hydrochloric acid, half a drachm; tincture of opium, half a drachm; peppermint-oil, fifteen drops.) The diet consisted of *bouillon*, milk, and eggs; the drink was cold water and red wine. The enemata were made in the following manner: Ice was crushed to paste; from this mass of ice two glasses were taken for grown-up men for every enema; for children, according to age, beginning with half a glassful, and so on. Water was then added while the ice floated. It was then poured into a glass funnel connected with a long tube. This funnel, fixed on a stand, remained near the sick bed; in other words, the apparatus remained in action until the mass of ice melted and flowed slowly into the rectum, which process lasted about one or one and a half hours. The enemata were employed every two hours, then every three and four hours; finally, twice or three times daily. The author succeeded in all cases in curing the disease in eight or ten days.—*London Med. Record*, March 15, 1881.

———

On the Hygienic Treatment of Biliary Calculi.

Professor BOUCHARDAT, who is the leading authority in France on medical dietetics, recommends (*Bull de Thér.*, Aug. 1880), for the treatment of biliary calculi, that the patient should abstain from bread, cereals, eggs, and nitrogenous food in excess; sorrel, tomatoes, strong liquors, shell fish, and cheese; that he should eat ordinary vegetables, preferring those rich in potash to those which are rich in soda. He should also employ an indirect alkaline treatment in the form of malates and citrates, as they are contained in fruits, and drink light red wine diluted with water. He should keep the bowels free by taking every morning a teaspoonful of tartrate of potash and soda and sulphate of soda in equal parts. He should take moderate exercise. The action of the skin should be stimulated by washing, frequent friction, and shampooing by the hand moistened with a few drops of perfumed oil. Every week from one to three baths should be taken, each bath containing 100 grammes of carbonate of potash, 2 grammes of essence of lavender, and 5 grammes of tincture of benzoin, followed by lengthened friction and shampooing. With the object of the expulsion of the calculi, the patient should take, night·and morning, one to three *perles* of essence of turpentine, and one or two *perles* of ether. They may be taken with the meals, but in preference between them. To prevent the formation of calculi, the patient should take for ten days, night and morning, before each repast, a pill containing one decigramme (1½ grain) of tartrate of potash and lithia ; for ten subsequent days he should take full doses of acetate of potash, with a light aperient night and morning ; for ten subsequent days, every day a pint and a half of water containing tartrate of potash and soda. During the spring, on rising in the morning, he should take, for a month, 120 grammes of the juice of lettuce, chicory, and dandelion, equal parts, with five grammes of acetate of potash. He should spend a season at Pougues, Vals, or Vichy.—*London Medical Record*, March 15, 1881.

Treatment of Psoriasis by Baths of Sublimate.

Having to deal with a case of obstinate psoriasis which defied all their efforts for four months, Dr. Voss and Dr. SPERK (*Gaz. Med. Chir. de Pesth*) hit upon the plan of trying baths of sublimate only. The result may be truly designated as wonderful. After a series of fourteen baths, the skin lost its reddish colour, the epidermis desquamated in large lamellæ, the integuments finally, which were thickened and infiltrated, became supple and elastic. However, during the course of treatment, there were fresh eruptions, but the new patches were less injected, and covered with thinner epidermic scales. Scratching did not bring on any sanguineous exudation. Forty-six baths completed the cure. So remarkable and unexpected a result encouraged Dr. Voss to persevere in the same path ; four other cases of inveterate psoriasis treated in the same way obtained a good result in a comparatively short time. The first patient took thirty-two baths, the second forty, and the third forty-eight, and at the time when this report was written, a fourth patient had greatly improved, but was not completely cured. As far as possible the baths were given daily ; the water was at a temperature of 27–29 deg., and the patient was required to remain in them from thirty to forty minutes. Dr. Voss has never observed the symptoms which are easily caused by mercurial preparations, such as salivation, swelling of the gums, etc. The advantages of this new treatment may be described under the three heads of (1) rapidity ; (2) facility of administration, as baths require but a very short time, and the patient is not obliged to interrupt his daily occupations ; and (3) cleanliness. The patient is also able to dispense with topical applications of all sorts, which generally exhale a more or less unpleasant odour.—*London Med. Record*, April 15, 1881.

Surgery.

Multiple Cutaneous Gangrene.

In 1878, Professor Simon first called attention to this comparatively rare disease, which for the most part affects children of various ages, and has a malignant character. Dr. EICHHOFF (*Deutsch. Med. Woch.*, Aug. 21, 1880) recently observed a case of this kind at the Breslau clinic for cutaneous and syphilitic diseases. The child, aged 3, was first seen in April, and was then suffering from extensive eczema of the face, breast, and back. Constitutional symptoms were not marked at this time, and the eczema rapidly yielded to appropriate treatment. In May the child was again brought to the clinic, when its general health was found to be much depreciated. The back had been covered with dark-red patches, the largest about the size of a millet-seed. Vesicles soon appeared above these patches, but they rapidly collapsed, leaving ulcers, which soon became gangrenous. The sloughing extended deeply down into the subcutaneous connective tissue. Local and constitutional treatment caused these sloughing ulcers to heal, with cicatrices resembling those of variola. Some time after this a corneal ulcer developed, and, simultaneously with its appearance, the head became affected with gangrenous ulcers. The latter slowly healed, leaving deep cicatrices. A second exacerbation occurred in June, and again a corneal ulcer was one of the complications. The ointment, applied locally, consisted of 15 parts each of camphor and myrrh, with 100 parts of vaseline. The pathogenesis of this affection was said to resemble that of ordinary bed-sores. The appearance of the corneal ulcers was explained by the depreciation of the child's general health and insufficient *vis à tergo.—London Medical Record*, March 15, 1881.

Tar, Soot, and Tobacco Cancer.

The workman in coal-tar and paraffin manufactories suffer very frequently from acute and chronic inflammations of the skin. Volkmann has already described several cases, in which true epithelial cancer was developed from these chronic inflammations, and TILLMANNS (*Deutsche Zeitschr. für Chir.*, Band xiii. Heft 5 and 6) now adds another, ending fatally after numerous operations. This form of cancer, and also chimney-sweepers' cancer, and epithelial cancer of the lip and tongue in inveterate smokers, the author attributes to irritation by the products of imperfect combustion ; not, however, saying that this is the actual cause, but simply that it is the exciting cause in those disposed to the development of cancer.—*London Med. Record*, April 15, 1881.

Secondary Suture of Nerves.

Among the advances in nerve pathology and therapeutics of the last few years, not the least interesting and important have been the practice and results of surgical interference. The operation of nerve-stretching has established itself as a recognized proceeding, and recent experience is rapidly extending its sphere of usefulness, although its *rationale* is involved in considerable obscurity. The primary suture of divided nerves has been practised for several years, and many recorded and unrecorded cases testify to its value. Quite lately, however, the secondary suture of nerves has been practised, and although not with uniform success, yet with most encouraging and, we may add, surprising results. The best test cases are those of union of severed motor nerves, for the return of sensation in parts supplied by a divided and then sutured nerve is open to another explanation than that the nerve trunk has again become capable of conducting sensory impressions. For this reason a case of Langenbeck's, of secondary suture of the musculo-spiral nerve, is very valuable. The patient, a labourer, thirty-one years of age, received a severe contusion of the outer side of the right arm below the middle, which was attended with paralysis of the extensor muscles of the forearm and hand. An abscess subsequently formed and was opened. Two-and-a-half months after the injury, as the paralysis continued, Langenbeck cut down upon the divided nerve, freed its ends, which he found lying two centimetres and a half apart, and united them by a catgut suture. Although there was considerable tension, healing took place by first intention, and nineteen days afterwards the extensors reacted to the induced current, and after a month and a half considerable active extension movements were possible. Mr. Hulke has brought forward at the Clinical Society a case. in which he had united the cut ends of the median nerve nearly six weeks after the injury, and another case in which he practised a similar operation on the ulnar nerve fifteen weeks after division, and in each instance there was distinct evidence of restoration of function. Esmarch and Létiévant have each had a case of suture of the musculo-spiral nerve, the former successful. These and other like cases afford great encouragement not only to unite by suture the cut ends of nerves in recent wounds, but, where necessary, after cicatrization is complete.—*Lancet*, March 19, 1881.

—

Suture of Nerves and Tendons.

The case communicated by KRAUSSOLD (*Central. für Chir.*, 1880, No. 47) is of some interest, as showing to what an extent suture of these structures may be employed with benefit. A female patient, melancholic and suicidal, had made a transverse cut on the palmar surface of both forearms, an inch and a half above the left wrist-joint, and two inches and a half above the right. On the left side, the radial and ulnar arteries were divided ; the radial and ulnar nerves completely, the median nerve more than three-fourths; also the tendons of the flexor sublimis digitorum entirely, and those of the flexor profundus digitorum partly. On the right side, the radial, ulnar, and interosseous arteries were divided, the radial and median nerves completely, the ulnar nerve two-thirds, also the tendons of the flexor profundus and sublimis, and of the flexor longus pollicis. Both ends of the arteries were ligatured, and the nerves and tendons brought together with sutures. Three weeks after the injury, sensibility was perfectly normal and active, and passive movements were all possible, although still slow and weak. A small defined spot on the ball of the little finger became gangrenous, but otherwise there was no fever or reaction.—*London Med. Record*, April 15, 1881.

—

Unilateral Injury of the Spinal Cord.

The patient in this case, reported by SCHULZ (*Cent. für Nerven.*, 1880, No. 15), a male, aged 29 years, received a stab in the back between the spines of the fifth and sixth dorsal vertebræ, a little to the right of the middle line, and about two inches in depth. Soon afterwards there appeared paresis and hyperæsthesia of the right lower limb, anæsthesia (with intact motive power) of the left lower limb, involuntary passage of feces, and retention of urine. Half a year later, the right lower limb showed paresis, with laboured but not ataxic movement. It was also thinner than the left, but presented no difference in colour or temperature. The left limb showed also no ataxy. The muscular sense of the left limb was normal, that of the right diminished. On the right side the skin was hyperæsthetic as high as the seventh dorsal vertebra ; above this, as high as the sixth, it was anæsthetic. The sensations of tickling, touch, and pain were all increased on the right ; the sensation of temperature was normal. For electric currents, the skin on the right side, both limb and trunk, was very sensitive ; while, on the left side, it was normal, or even diminished   The left side showed no actual anæsthesia, but a marked analgesia ; and, corresponding to the anæsthetic zone of the right side at the sixth dorsal vertebra, was a zone of hyperæsthesia. The tendon-reflexes were normal on the left side, much increased on right. The electric irritability of the nerves and muscles was alike on both sides. —*London Med. Record*, April 15, 1881.

Syphilitic Disease of the Spine.

In the current number of the *Annales de Dermatologie et de Syphiligraphie*, M. FOURNIER reports at great length a very interesting case of Pott's disease caused by syphilis. The patient, a coachman, aged 56, was admitted into the Hôpital St. Louis in July, 1876. The man had had venereal disease in his youth, but no clear history of syphilis could be obtained. He stated that his health had always been good until a few months before admission, when he gradually lost his appetite, and began to suffer from pain in the loins, which afterwards extended to the legs. M. Fournier could not find anything wrong with the spine, but the patient had well-marked syphilitic disease of the testis, gummata of the skin, etc. The testis and the gummata were much benefited by antisyphilitic treatment, but the general health declined, ascites and pleural effusion appeared, and the man died about three months after admission. At the post-mortem examination, ample evidence of syphilis was found in various parts of the body, as well as the following condition of the spine. Antero-posterior section showed the bodies of the third and fourth lumbar vertebræ, in their posterior half, to be infiltrated by a yellow cheesy material. The posterior three-fourths of the intervertebral substance was also destroyed, a cavity containing purulent fluid being left. The intervertebral substance between the fourth and fifth vertebræ was softened, and infiltrated with pus in its posterior half; and there was a cavity in the body of the third lumbar vertebra. Under the microscope, the third, fourth, and fifth lumbar vertebræ presented the typical appearances of condensing osteitis, with purulent and caseous infiltration, exactly as is seen in gummy osteomata. There was also double psoas abscess. The further examination was carried out by M. Hayem, who found a gumma on the fourth lumbar nerve at the point where it left the foramen. In this situation there was also another gummy growth, which appeared to have originated in the periosteum of the corresponding vertebra. Above the gumma the nerve was affected by interstitial neuritis, and there was partial atrophy of the nerve-tubules. The third and fifth lumbar nerves presented only appearances due to irritation and pressure, without decided alteration of the nerve-elements.—*British Med. Journal*, April 2, 1881.

Transparent Cysts of the Eyelids.

From a careful examination of the transparent cysts which are often found on the free edge of the eyelids, Dr. DESFOSSES (*Archives d'Ophthalmologie*, Dec. 1880) believes them to be formed from modified sudoriparous glands. He is led to this opinion by the form and arrangement of their epithelium, the presence of a layer of unstriped muscle, and their deep attachments, which seem incompatible with an origin from sebaceous glands. The author's paper is illustrated with some well-executed woodcuts of microscopical preparations.—*London Medical Record*, April 15, 1881.

Fatty Degeneration of the Cornea.

Dr. CUIGNET, of Lille (*Recueil d'Ophthalmologie*, Nov. 1880), describes a form of parenchymatous fatty keratitis, which, he believes, has hitherto escaped the notice of ophthalmologists. He narrates six cases of this affection, which he first noticed in Algiers, but subsequently recognized in Europe. It consists of white calcareous-looking patches on the cornea, which at times, however, may be yellow or gray, and present a smooth lustrous appearance. Their usual seat is the centre of the cornea, over which they gradually extend transversely. They commence by a small granular patch, which becomes gradually larger by the aggregation of neighbouring patches. Their seat is directly under the epithelium in the substance of the cornea propria, within which they slowly increase in size and thickness. The first formed patch is generally the most superficial; those formed later both lie deeper and have a different tint. Vessels, which have their origin in either the external or the internal *cul-de-sac* of the conjunctiva, penetrate these patches, and at times give them a dark red pannus-like appearance. Together with these corneal changes there exist, as a rule, alterations in the ocular, palpebral, and ciliary conjunctiva. The affection is, as a rule, chronic; in one case, however, the author saw it assume decidedly acute symptoms. The most constant and best marked symptom is the impairment of vision, which, if the fatty patch occupy the whole of the pupil, may lead to complete obscuration, the patient having merely perception of light. The seat of the lesions is characteristic, being always near the centre of the cornea, and at a greater or less depth below the epithelium in the cornea proper. It is probable that the disease is incurable, either by treatment or by time, as the author has as yet met with no case in which the deposited matter has been reabsorbed. It remains permanent and innocuous, though in one case iritis was noticed as a complication; and it is probable that other complications, such as a glaucomatous condition, iridochoroiditis, etc., might supervene. Microscopically, the disease consists of a number of minute fatty particles mixed in some cases with crystals of cholestearine, which are gradually and progressively formed in the corneal tissue. Pathologically, it may be compared with the changes which take place within the arteries, and which lead eventually to endarteritis and atheroma. Etiologically, it is probably a manifestation of the strumous diathesis, provoked more immediately by changes in the conjunctiva, which affect the nutrition of the cornea. The differential diagnosis of this affection lies between (1) calcareous or metallic deposits; (2) cretaceous keratitis; (3) and plastic parenchymatous keratitis. The appearance, history, and course, will generally enable it to be recognized. The prognosis is unfavourable, and direct treatment is of little avail. Any causes of irritation in the conjunctiva, lachrymal passages, cilia, etc., should be removed: and if the opacity be over the pupil, iridectomy might be performed, and the opacity itself subsequently tattooed.—*London Med. Record*, April 15, 1881.

—

The Pathology of Glaucoma.

At the present time a point has been reached in the discussion of the question of the pathology of glaucoma at which it is worth while to summarize the facts accumulated, and to estimate the value of the theories which have been based upon them.

Glaucoma, whether primary or secondary, and however caused, is the generic name for a state of increased tension of the eyeball, due to excess of the intraocular fluids.

The older writers of the present generation—Donders, Bowman, and Graefe—contented themselves with the explanation that the condition was due to increased secretion of the intraocular fluids, occurring under certain conditions of vascular turgescence.

In 1876 Max Knies announced the discovery that the angle of the anterior chamber is almost invariably found closed in glaucomatous eyes; a fact which derived its significance from the observations of Leber, that the aqueous humour escapes normally by that channel. Max Knies attributed the closure to primary inflammation in the part.

These observations were mainly confirmed by Adolph Weber, who, however, regarded the cause of the closure to be the swelling of the ciliary processes.

Mr. Priestley Smith made an important contribution to the question by establishing, by careful experiments upon the fresh dead eyes of pigs and human subjects, that a very slight excess of pressure in the posterior chamber suffices to drive the ciliary processes forward against the periphery of the iris, and to close the angle of the anterior chamber ; he also showed that the fluid of the posterior chamber passes by osmosis through the suspensory ligament, where it stretches between the lens and the ciliary processes, and escapes with the aqueous by the angle of the anterior chamber. It therefore follows that, in the absence of any local obstruction by new growths, inflammatory exudations, hemorrhage, etc., glaucoma may be mechanically caused by any increase of pressure in the posterior chamber.

Mr. Priestley Smith points out that this increase of pressure in the posterior chamber would be produced by any cause tending to diminish the "circumlental space" through which the fluid from the posterior chamber has to pass ; and he suggests that this might be effected either by swelling of the ciliary processes alone, or by an increase in the diameter of the lens, or by a combination of these two factors. He has shown, by careful measurements of a series of lenses at various ages, that the diameter increases with the age ; and the diameters of the lenses from three cases of primary glaucoma are given to show that they exceed the largest of the healthy series.

Dr. Brailey has contributed several papers to the pathology of glaucoma. He has drawn particular attention to the atrophy of the ciliary muscle, which in health has probably a regulating action over the blood-supply to the ciliary processes ; he has also shown that the bloodvessels in the ciliary region are dilated and thin-walled. He attributes glaucoma to (1) increased inflow, due to "a visibly increased blood-supply, and sometimes to inflammation, especially of the ciliary body and iris ;" and (2) to obstructed outflow, due to obstruction "in the region of the ligamentum pectinatum, or in some few to the exits from the perichoroidal space ;" and to this not very clear statement he adds, "obstruction at the entrance of Schlemm's canal is ascribed, in most cases, to valvular action of the iris, induced either by its position or by the condition of it and the ciliary body."

After a careful consideration of the evidence, we think the following facts may be taken as proved : 1. The intra-ocular fluid has its sole channel of escape by the angle of the anterior chamber ; 2. There is a normal current of fluid from the vitreous to the aqueous chambers through the suspensory ligament ; 3. A very slight excess of pressure in the posterior chamber causes obstruction to the outflow of fluid by compressing the ciliary processes against the iris, so as to close the angle of the anterior chamber ; 4. The angle of the anterior chamber in glaucoma is almost invariably found closed, or traces of its former closure may be observed ; 5. The ciliary muscle is frequently atrophied ; 6. The bloodvessels of the ciliary region are frequently dilated.

From these facts, we are warranted in concluding that the efficient cause of glaucoma is obstruction to the angle of the anterior chamber, which may be effected by the pressure of new growths, inflammatory exudations, hemorrhage, etc., or by the mechanical action of excess of pressure in the posterior chamber. Increased pressure in the posterior chamber is caused by increased blood-supply, occurring under conditions favouring vascular turgescence, and promoted by dilatation of the vessels and atrophy of the ciliary muscle. Additional observations are wanting to confirm the view that an increase in the diameter of the lens plays an important part in the causation of glaucoma ; so far as Mr. Priestley Smith's researches have been carried, there is nothing to contradict the hypothesis ; but the number of cases hitherto examined is too small to permit of his conclusions being accepted at present. Should further investigations confirm the view, the existence of an all-important predisposing factor will have been established.— *British Med. Journal*, March 15, 1881.

—

Tracheotomy for Diphtheria in Children.

In the recently published report of the Bethany Hospital in Berlin (*Langenbeck's Archiv für Klinische Chirurgie*, vol. xxv. page 815, November, 1880), Dr. Körte, the author, gives the result of the tracheotomy operations during the year 1878. The number was unusually large, even for Berlin, and the disease was of a severe and dangerous form, especially during the latter half of the year. Thus, during the first six months there were 56 operations, with 30.3 per cent. of successful cases, while during the second six months there were 93 operations, with only 18.2 per cent. of successes. The disease was at its worst during the months of October, November, and December, during which period 62 operations were performed, of which only 12.9 per cent. recovered. The children, when admitted into hospital, were mostly very ill, presenting the ominous swelling of the submaxillary glands, slowed respiration, livid aspect, and other appearances of a serious diphtheritic intoxication. The disease was in many cases complicated by scarlet fever or measles. In the latter half of the year comparatively often some of the children presented an eruption like measles; but further observation showed that it was not measles, but rather a purplish rash, which quickly disappeared, was not infectious, and exercised no unfavourable influence on the diphtheria.

No marked differences between croup and diphtheria were remarked in the cases; the two were regarded as different stages of the same disease, and ran one into the other in the most varied manner.

Of the 149 cases, 34 (or 22.8 per cent.) recovered. The greatest mortality ocenrred among the children under three years of age. There were no cases under one year of age; 29 cases during the second year of life, with 3 recoveries; 27 in the third year, also with 3 recoveries. The percentage of recoveries gradually improved with the increasing age of the *opérés*.

The chief indication for the operation was the dyspnœa, and it was carried out without any regard to age; and was only withheld when extensive lung-disease precluded almost necessarily a successful issue. In the generality of the cases the operation had to be performed at once, owing to the very serious condition of the patients when first seen. For the most part, the trachea was opened below the thyroid isthmus. The after-treatment consisted in inhalations every two or three hours. The trachea was swabbed out with solutions of lactic acid, common salt or alum; and during the three months when the mortality was so high many other substances were tried, such as carbolic acid or thymol solution, etc., without any good results. No local treatment of the trachea was undertaken except swabbing, sucking out the membrane, and keeping the canula clean. As regards other local treatment, the author thinks it is unavailing, or of " extremely small value." The experience of former years teaches that the success after tracheotomy depends less on the treatment than on the nature of the epidemic itself. Thus, in 1877, under an exactly similar mode of treatment, in 89 operations there were 40.4 per cent. of successful cases.

Of the 115 deaths, 79 occurred within the first three days after operation; they were mostly due to descending bronchitis, and in a few cases to collapse. The remaining deaths occurred after more than three days, and were then brought about either by broncho-pneumonia or diphtheria of external parts.

The actual percentage of recoveries in relation to age was as follows: Under two years of age, 10.3 per cent.; under three years, 11.1; under four years, 23.6; under five years, 27.2; under six years, 38.4; under seven years, 30.0; under eight years, 66.6; under nine years, 50.0; under ten years, 33.3 per cent. Twice the operation was performed on adults for this disease; both died of descending diphtheritis.—*Med. Times and Gazette*, April 9, 1881.

Inoculation of Syphilis by Razors.

M. DESPRÉS (*Journal des Connaissances Méd.*, No. 49, 1880) has lately observed two cases of syphilis, in which the initial lesion was on the face, and in which contagion was supposed to have occurred during shaving. Case 1. D., aged 54, of sober habits, having never had any venereal disease, was shaved by a barber on July 11, 1880. On leaving the shop, the man noticed that he had three cuts on his chin. On the 14th he was again shaved, and the sore places bled during the operation. On July 25, the patient (having had nothing to do with women for ten weeks) noticed some swelling about the site of each cut, and applied a poultice. On September 1, he came under the care of M. Després, having been sent to him as a case of cancer. There were at that time three ulcers on the chin, surrounded by some red and rather hard papules. The ulcers were not painful. There was a hard gland beneath the jaw, but no further signs of syphilis about the body. On September 15 a general papular syphilide appeared, and was followed by mucous patches, etc. The second case was that of a man, aged 22, who came to Paris in May, 1880, having had no sexual intercourse for about two months. There was no history of any venereal disease. During his stay in Paris he was shaved by a barber every other day, but did not remember having been cut by the razor. About July 12, a little scab appeared in the furrow between the chin and upper lip. Beneath the scab was a sore with hard borders, and soon afterwards the patient noticed a lump beneath the chin. About August 10 M. Després saw the man, and diagnosed syphilis. On August 19 roseola appeared, and shortly afterwards mucous patches of the throat and anus.—*London Med. Record*, April 15, 1881.

Destruction of the Chancre as an Abortive Measure in Syphilis.

M. HENRI LELOIR, in a long and valuable paper (*Annales de Derm. et de Syphil.*, No. 1, 1880, p. 69) reviews and criticizes very fully the different experiments that have been made on the excision and destruction by other means of the initial lesion of syphilis with the view of preventing further development of the disease. The author also adds a very complete bibliography of the subject. The oft-quoted experiments of Auspitz and Unna. Kölliker, and others, are noticed, and their weak points are well brought out; the result being to show how little evidence there is, up to the present time, that general syphilis can be prevented, or even rendered milder in its course, by the destruction of the initial manifestation. M. Leloir concludes his paper with a brief account of a personal interview which he had with Ricord on the subject. This portion of the paper is particularly interesting, as it gives M. Ricord's matured opinion, and shows how entirely he has abandoned his former conviction, viz., that the destruction of the primary sore, within a short period of its existence, could prevent the sequence of general syphilis. Ricord now says " that he has completely abandoned the practice of cauterizing or of excising infecting chancres; that he considers the destruction of the infecting chancre to be absolutely useless at any period; as soon as it appears, before its appearance even, syphilis exists. If the penis were amputated on the appearance of the infecting chancre, syphilis would none the less be produced."—*London Med. Record*, April 15, 1881.

Treatment of Orchitis.

Dr. SABADINI, of Constantinople, following the plan of treatment advocated by Dr. Bourdeaux (*Gaz. des Hôp.*, 1881, No. 18), applied an ointment com- posed of one part of iodoform and ten parts of vaseline, with success in a case of gonorrhœal orchitis. The pain rapidly ceased, and the swelling disappeared in eight days.—*London Med. Record*, April 15, 1881.

—

Innominate Aneurism treated by Simultaneous Distal Ligature of the Carotid and Subclavian Arteries, with remarks on the behaviour of a Tendon Ligature.

At a recent meeting of the Royal Medical and Chirurgical Society (*Lancet*, March 26, 1881) a paper was read on a "Case of Innominate Aneurism treated by simultaneous distal ligature of the carotid and subclavian arteries, with re- marks on the behaviour of a tendon ligature," by Mr. C. T. DENT. The chief object of this paper is to describe the changes observed in an artery tied with a tendon ligature. The parts were examined ten days after death.

The history of the case was as follows: S. L., an engineer, aged thirty-seven, was admitted with an aneurism of the innominate artery, the first symptoms of which had been noticed about twelve months previously. He improved at first under rest and iodide of potassium, but then as the growth increased the carotid and subclavian arteries were ligatured subcutaneously by Mr. Pollock. For the carotid artery catgut was employed as well as the tendon ligature; the subclavian was secured with a flat tendon ligature only. Both arteries were healthy. The aneurism improved, but the patient had at times very severe attacks of dyspnœa, and died ten days after the operation. A large ulcerated opening was found in the trachea, which did not communicate with the cavity of the aneurism. The carotid artery was dissected out and examined; the following points were ob- served: A very moderate amount of lymph was effused about the tied artery, though sufficient to bury the knot of the ligature. Well-formed clots were found in the proximal and distal ends of the completely obliterated vessel. No trace of the catgut ligature could be found. Much of the tendon ligature, where not in contact with the artery, was unaltered. The external coat of the artery was not ulcerated. This the author ascribes partly to the fact that tendon, like other animal ligatures, is capable of slight softening and swelling, and partly to the fact that new bloodvessels are early developed in parts lying close to the artery. The inner coats of the artery were ruptured. The tendon ligature, in many of the sections, was in most close connection with the artery, and in these places was infiltrated with small round granulated cells, which in places split up the fibrous material into longitudinal bands. Some of the cells seem to be more elongated than in others. In connection with these cells, and formed by them, were seen new bloodvessels. Here and there it appeared possible in the sections to trace bloodvessels passing across the line of connection, extending into the artery on the one hand, and into the tendon on the other. In conclusion, the author states that though he did not share in the objection urged against catgut ligature, still it seemed that tendon might furnish an animal material which would require less preparation than the carbolic or chromic catgut ligature, and which would prob- ably be more constant in its behaviour.

Mr. BRYANT said the question of the use of flat ligatures involved the import- ant principle whether it were necessary for permanent occlusion that the inner and middle coats should be divided, the point established by Dr. Jones; and he had himself some years ago come to the same conclusion that permanent occlusion could only be thus obtained. The flat ligature, which only compressed the vessel, would cause simply a temporary occlusion, long enough in some cases to allow of coagulation in an aneurism, but not in the other more difficult cases where ligature had to be resorted to. He compared the action of the flat ligature to that of acupressure, which had been almost abandoned because (in the case of severed arteries) it was frequently followed by secondary hemorrhage, the vessel not being occluded long enough to allow of permanent clotting. Hence those cases of aneurism which could not be cured by other means of compression were not suitable for the application of the flat ligature. A similar mode of temporary obstruction was devised by Mr. Dix of Hull some years ago, consisting in a wire loop placed round the artery and secured over a piece of cork. He thought much evidence was required before the fact of organization of an animal ligature could be admitted. He had examined six or seven weeks after ligature by carbolized or non-carbolized catgut, and although he had seen new vessels around the material he could not believe they had been formed at its expense.

Mr. SAVORY thought it strange if dead matter could be converted directly into living tissue. Several years ago it had been shown that masses of dead tissue introduced into the living tissues became infiltrated with leucocytes; but the inference was that the leucocytes had proceeded from the irritated living tissues, and had absorbed the dead material. In Mr. Dent's case new vessels appear to have formed in the dead substances. The same criticism was applicable to the subject of organization of blood-clot about which so much had been heard lately. John Hunter studied it, and some of his specimens were in the College of Surgeons' Museum; but in his case he dealt with living and not dead clots. It was different in the case of large masses of blood-clot in wounds, masses which must be inert and act as foreign matter; which could not organize, but which might be replaced by new tissue proceeding from the living parts around. If an animal ligature could organize it would be important to know from what source it was prepared, and whether it was old or recent.

Mr. HOLMES, from his own limited experience, had arrived at a different conclusion about the efficacy of animal ligatures to that of Mr. Bryant. He fancied Mr. Barwell had slightly exaggerated the difference in the action of a ligature of flat shape as compared with a round one; for he (Mr. Holmes) had been able on the dead subject to divide the internal and middle coats partially or completely by means of the flat ligature when tied sharply. In the two cases in which he had tried Mr. Barwell's ox-aorta ligature the vessel was permanently occluded, one was a case where he had tied the iliac for rapidly enlarging iliac aneurism with good result; the patient was long under observation (requiring two amputations before his discharge), but the aneurism remained perfectly occluded. In another case, where the patient died in consequence of a debauch two weeks after operation the ligature was found firmly attached to the artery, which was quite closed. In a third case, where two arteries had been tied, they were found occluded by a diaphragm, as in Mr. Treves's case, the ligatures having disappeared. The evidence, so far as it goes, is in favour of the permanence of these ligatures, and that an artery may be safely occluded whether the material used be oxen aorta or tendon. It had been explained that the ligatures did not themselves become organized, but that they disappeared, and were replaced by a ring of fibrous tissue. That such a replacement was not peculiar to healing under antiseptics was shown by this case of Mr. Pollock's and Mr. Dent's, where no antiseptics were used. It seems that these animal ligatures may be invaded by leucocytes and caused to disappear, new tissue taking their place; and this is now allowed by Professor Lister to be what is meant by "organization" of the ligatures. So also in the case of blood-clot, the actual organizing elements and new vessels being supplied from the surrounding tissues, the walls of the arteries, etc., surrounding the clot. It is quite possible that an animal ligature may excite this formative influence, and its results could not be compared with the effect produced by acupressure.

Mr. BARWELL was not sure that inert matter would not take on vital properties again, and thought that skin-grafting was an instance in point. In a recent case of a large burn, where the "grafts" did not take on the granulating surface, he had found that minute portions of the inner coat of the ox's aorta placed on the surface became converted into a distinct epidermis, others of them melting down into pus. He reminded Mr. Bryant that at the last meeting of the Society he had recorded twelve cases in which perfect occlusion had followed the use of the oxen ligature, and had been able to show the specimens from two of these cases; so that the flat ligature in no way resembled acupressure in its effects. The question as to the need for the division of the inner and middle coats was different now than when Dr. Jones wrote, for at that time ligatures were used which subsequently came away by ulcerating through the outer coats. Now, however, we have ligatures which can be left on the vessels, and which do close arteries permanently. It was essential that the animal ligature, whether tendon or not, should be used first, or should have been dried when fresh, for if putrefaction take place in it its characters are altered and its efficacy impaired.

Dr. B. O'CONNOR said that a short time ago he examined microscopically a mass of lymph lodged at the inner end of a drainage-tube, which had been removed by Mr. Lister. This lymph, which was not in contact with living tissue, contained distinctly small vascular branches. In reply to Mr. Page, he added that the drainage-tube had been *in situ* about four days.

Mr. DENT, in reply, said that the discussion showed that questions were still unsettled which had been thought to be determined by Dr. Jones. He mentioned that in one of Dr. Jones's experiments a septum was formed in the artery precisely like that lately described by Mr. Treves in a vessel tied by the carbolized catgut ligature. In the present case there was microscopical evidence that the inner coat had been ruptured, and that the artery was permanently occluded. In the subclavian artery, where only a tendon ligature was applied, the clots were not so large and well-formed as in the carotid, where two ligatures, one tendon and the other catgut, had been used. As to "organization," one of the specimens showed vascularizing lymph between the two occluded ends of the artery, at a distance from the tendon ligature; and he believed the view taken by Mr. Savory and Mr. Holmes was probably the true one. Mr. Stirling, who had brought these kangaroo tendon ligatures from Australia, had selected them because of the readiness with which they were prepared. Ligatures of whale tendon had also been suggested. Mr. Dent had used them as sutures, and found them too thin and too readily dissolved in the tissues. There was no reason why the same material should not be used as a round rather than a flat ligature; the great advantage claimed for it over catgut being the time it remains unabsorbed.

Treatment of Lupus by Scraping with Volkmann's Sharp Spoon.

The employment of Volkmann's sharp spoon for the treatment of lupus is likely to meet with more and more general acceptance. It presents several advantages over the older methods of dealing with these painful cases, which indeed are for the most part so unsatisfactory, that surgeons are often tempted to abstain altogether from interference of any kind. The principal merits claimed for this way of treating the disease are, in the first place, its extreme simplicity, and in the second, that it is possible to tell with great accuracy when the limits of the affected parts have been reached. A tolerably sharp spoon should be used, with a short strong handle, and the affected surface should be scraped until all the soft tissue has been completely removed. Nothing is more easy than to tell when healthy structures have been reached, by the sense of resistance they offer; and, unless an unreasonable amount of force be employed, these cannot be materially injured. If an extensive surface has to be scraped, an assistant is necessary, as considerable capillary hemorrhage frequently occurs.

The following method of procedure, according to Mr. RICKMAN J. GODLEE, (*Med. Times and Gazette*, March 19, 1881) will be found effective in checking the bleeding. Several strips of lint having previously been prepared, the surgeon rapidly scrapes a patch, not larger than can easily be controlled by a dossil of lint of a suitable size; this is firmly pressed upon the raw surface, and then another is dealt with in the same way, and a second piece of lint is applied. The process is then repeated until the whole of the affected part has been rendered raw. The pieces of lint are then, one after the other, removed, and if the bleeding has not completely stopped it will be found that a little iodoform powder dusted on the spot quickly arrests it in most cases; but if this should not be the case it is only necessary to continue the pressure for a few minutes longer. A very comfortable and satisfactory dressing for the after-treatment is an ointment formed of iodoform, eucalyptus oil, and vaseline, in the following proportions:—Iodoform, gr. xx.; eucalyptus oil, ʒj.; vaseline, ʒj. This preparation, it may be mentioned, is a very useful one in many forms of ulceration accompanied by a fetid discharge. It is powerfully antiseptic, and at the same time extremely bland, so that it allows healing to go on rapidly beneath it. The ointment may be spread conveniently on thin rag, which adapts itself readily to the inequalities of the face, or, if a larger supply be advisable, it may be put upon the surface of a piece of lint. In all the instances described by Mr. Godlee, the same method of treatment was pursued; besides presenting several features of some little interest, they serve to show how rapidly severe cases of lupus may be, if not cured, at least very much relieved for a considerable length of time, and the disease held very much in check. Some of them also illustrate the fact that when the morbid condition appears to be quiescent, plastic operations may be undertaken without fear that the lupus ulceration will affect the flaps or interfere with their union.

Midwifery and Gynæcology.

Myxoma Fibrosum and Cystic Disease of the Placenta.

Dr. C. BREUS contributes to the *Wiener Medizinische Wochenschrift*, an interesting communication on the former of the above rare conditions. Myxomatous growths are among the commonest of pathological changes which affect the chorion and placenta. They occur in three forms: the *myxoma papillare multiplex*, which is the disease so long known under the name of the "hydatid mole;" another form, in which the morbid change is diffused in a flat, jelly-like layer; and the form which he here more particularly describes—myxoma fibrosum. The name was given to the disease by Virchow. Dr. Breus has seen two cases; he has examined two other specimens put up by Rokitansky; and he refers also to cases described by Clarke, Hildebrandt, and Hodgen. From these sources he gives the following points as being what can be at present stated concerning the disease. It forms tumours which may reach a considerable size—as big as the fist—which are either single or few in number, surrounded by healthy placental tissue, the boundary between the normal placental structure and the tumour being quite distinct. The tumours have often a kind of capsule of connective tissue, and are sometimes stalked, the pedicle consisting mainly of bloodvessels. The surface is uneven or ragged. On section, they have a fleshy, grayish-red appearance, and from their aspect have been repeatedly described as sarcoma. They are elastic in consistence. Microscopic examination shows them to consist of myxomatous tissue richly supplied with bloodvessels, and which is divided into small lobules by thick bands of connective tissue.

As to their causation nothing is known. Hildebrandt supposes them due to localized disturbances of the placental circulation. Dr. Breus is unable to accept this view, because he thinks that in an organ the circulatory system of which is so complex as that of the placenta, such disturbances must be very frequent, and the lesions so. produced must be far commoner than is myxomatous change. These tumours do not exert any prejudicial influence on the course of labour, the most that can be said being that it is possible they may determine its premature commencement. They do not interfere with the life or development of the fœtus. During the detachment of the placenta they not unfrequently get separated from it, and so expelled separately. Should the placenta be adherent, the presence of such a tumour might surprise and puzzle the accoucheur who had to remove the placenta.

. We may, in commenting upon this subject, call attention to the researches of FENOMENOW (*Archiv für Gynäkologie*) in the same field. He has minutely examined two placentæ, in which the most conspicuous morbid change was the presence of cysts. In one of them the whole fœtal surface was studded with cysts, in size from that of a hemp-seed to a hazel-nut, with bright, translucent contents. The cysts were about twenty in number, and were irregularly arranged. In the other case there was one pediculated cyst as big as a large orange, projecting from the fœtal surface; and beside this, that surface presented several solid nodules, some as big as a pigeon's egg. These nodules, examined microscopically, showed a structure like that in Dr. Breus's case—myxoma fibrosum. Before discussing the origin of the cysts in his two cases, Dr. Fenomenow gives some account of the literature of the subject. The kinds of placental cysts that have been described are—(1) gelatinous cysts, seated between the chorion and amnion, the credit of recognizing which is due to Millet ; (2) perivascular cysts ; (3) blood-cysts, springing from the placental sinuses, which have been described by Bustamonte ; (4) cysts of the villi themselves, the results of degeneration ; (5) hemorrhagic or apoplectic cysts—names given by Hegar and Mayer and by Hennig, respectively ; (6) amnion-cysts, arising, according to Ahlfeld, from adhesions between the two layers of the amnion ; and (7) colloid cysts described by Grazeansky. It is of course quite possible that some or all of these theories may be wrong; but the subject has been so little investigated, that whatever errors there may be in the observations, or the interpretations thereof, by the workers quoted, have not yet been corrected. Meantime, we must accept these statements as expressing all that we at present know, and as provisionally true. Dr. Fenomenow carefully considers the origin of the cysts in his own cases. In the first case he believes the cysts not to have been formed out of pre-existing cavities or canals, but to have originated in irritative processes in the tissue of the villi, leading to adhesion at places of the villi to one another, and the formation of closed cavities between them ; then fluid had accumulated in these cavities, and distended them into conspicuous cysts. The cysts are therefore heterologous. As to the reason of the supposed irritative process, he can say nothing. The collection of fluid in the second case he attributes to mucous degeneration of the placental tissue, together with extravasation, the rèsult of vascular degeneration. He can offer no suggestion as to the cause of this pathological process. We may add that lithographic plates illustrate Dr. Fenomenow's paper and increase its value.—*Med. Times and Gazette*, April 9, 1881.

<hr>

Tupelo Tents for Dilating the Uterus.

A recent clinical lecture of Volkmann's collection, by Dr. LEOPOLD LANDAU (*Sammlung Klinischer Vorträge*, No. 187), is devoted to the consideration of the methods of dilating the cervix uteri. That which will be most novel to English readers is his strong recommendation of the tupelo tent. Sponge and laminaria tents are of course well known here; and of the later methods of rapid dilatation introduced by Fritsch and by Schroeder, Dr. Landau expresses disapproval. Tupelo tents are made from the root and stem of the *Nyssa aquatica*. Dr. Landau says that they expand more uniformly than laminaria tents, and that their co-efficient of expansion is somewhat greater than that of any other tent. In expanding they produce the same softening and infiltration of the uterine tissue as other tents. They are almost entirely free from any tendency to produce septic infection, and therefore antiseptic precautions need not be rigidly carried out when these tents are used. To effect dilatation, when one tent has been put in, it may be removed in three or four hours, when it will have expanded enough to allow a larger tent, or more than one, to be inserted. In this way the cavity of the uterus may be made accessible to the finger within twenty-four hours. Dr. Landau has used these tents in this manner for two years, and has never seen any disadvantageous result from their use.—*Med. Times and Gazette*, March 19, 1881.

<hr>

Medical Jurisprudence and Toxicology.

On a Probable Cause of Lead Colic.

At a late meeting of the Royal Medical and Chirurgical Society (*Lancet*, March 12, 1881), Dr. C. HILTON FAGGE read a paper upon this subject. After referring to the fact that in certain observations on the nature of the lead line in the gums, published in the fifty-ninth volume of the Transactions, he had been anticipated by a French physician, M. Cras; the author remarked that both he and M. Cras had on theoretical grounds suggested that it was almost certain that sulphide of lead must be formed in the intestinal mucous membrane of persons exposed to the action of the metal, by the reaction of the sulphuretted hydrogen of the intestinal gases upon a soluble combination of lead circulating in the capillaries. The author had since had few opportunities of examining the bowel in patients who had had symptoms of lead-poisoning. In two instances the results were negative. In the other two instances a marked and extensive blackening of the interior of the bowel was observed. Dr. Stevenson was kind enough to make analysis of the discoloured contents of intestine, and to compare them with analysis of healthy pieces of intestine from the same patients, and he proved that there was an excess of lead in the blackened part, amounting in one case to as much as 320 times the quantity present in the non-coloured part.

Dr. DOUGLAS POWELL asked whether any microscopical examination of the intestine was made, as the precise seat of the deposition of lead might explain whether it occurred by direct action of the sulphuretted hydrogen on the lead in the bowels, or on the lead on the way to being eliminated by the large intestine after its absorption higher up. The treatment of lead colic by iodide of potassium was generally followed up by purgatives, in the view that the lead is so eliminated.

Dr. R. THOMPSON said it was important to remember there were two ways in which the intestine might be blackened by lead. It may be that the metal is deposited in the mucous membrane from the blood, and converted into the sulphide by the intestinal gases, or that, like bismuth, it is acted upon by these gases before absorption. He had found in those who took bismuth that the mucous membrane of the large intestine was blackened by the sulphide of bismuth, which by means of chromic acid could be converted into the yellow chromate. He referred to Dr. de Mussy's observations on the Claremont cases treated by alkaline sulphide baths. The skin was blackened—a condition which Dr. Thompson had found in another case similarly treated to be due to the deposit of sulphide of copper, from the action of the solution in the metal of the bath.

Dr. POWELL added that Dr. Fagge's views as to the cause of the blue line on the gums were confirmed in a very marked case of lead paralysis without any such blue line being present. This absence of the blue line was associated in the case with a complete freedom from tartar on the teeth. It was well known also that no blue line appears on edentulous gums.

Dr. CAVAFY asked Dr. Fagge whether he regarded the deposition of the sulphide of lead in the intestine as the cause of lead colic, and, if so, did he think it acted on the nerves of the intestines. *Prima facie* there was no reason, if this were the case, why the deposition of the salt on the gum should not give rise to toothache.

Dr. A. W. BARCLAY pointed out that lead was undoubtedly absorbed into the blood, and its action was not merely local like that of bismuth. Was the lead only partially absorbed, or was it eliminated again into the alimentary canal, as Dr. Powell stated. The presence of the discoloration in the large intestine was due to the larger amount of sulphuretted hydrogen in that portion of the bowel. He presumed that lead colic had its seat in the small intestine, so that it could not be attributed to the existence of the deposit.

Dr. FAGGE, in reply, said that a microscopical examination was made in the first case, and showed the black granules to be deposited around the capillaries of the villi, just as on the gums. Dr. Thompson's remarks as to the discoloration of the intestine from bismuth were suggestive. Bismuth blackened the tongue, and Brinton suggested that it also produced a blue line on the gums, but this Dr. Fagge had not been able to confirm. The lead line was due to the deposition of the metal in the tissue of the gums, and its conversion into sulphide by the tartar. It was by following out the line of inquiry thus suggested that he had sought for discoloration of the intestinal mucous membrane, where a much greater amount of sulphuretted hydrogen would be in operation than in the gums. There was no reason to suppose that any large quantity of lead would escape absorption. He did not adduce the fact of deposition as explanatory of lead colic, which, however, had, he thought, its seat in the large intestine.

MEDICAL NEWS.

The Law of Copyright as Applied to Oral Lectures.

In the early days of the *Lancet* its enterprise among other forms took the shape of reporting the lectures of the eminent London teachers, whether they were willing or no, and in some cases even notwithstanding the express prohibition of some of them. Sir Astley Cooper even went so far as to lecture in the dark in the illusory expectation of thereby preventing reports being made. At last in 1824, having failed in every other way, Mr. Abernethy determined to invoke the aid of the law in the maintenance of his ownership of his lectures, and he sought to restrain by injunction the publication of his oral lectures delivered at St. Bartholomew's Hospital, on the ground of his absolute right of property in his lectures and his right to reap the pecuniary profits of his own ingenuity and labour. In granting the injunction the Lord Chancellor (Lord Eldon) expressed himself as " clearly of the opinion that when persons were admitted, as pupils or otherwise, to hear these lectures, although they were orally delivered, and although the parties might go to the extent, if they were able to do so, of putting down the whole by means of short-hand, yet they could only do that for the purposes of their own information, and could not publish for profit that which they had not obtained the right of selling." The *Lancet* immediately appealed, and announced that the contest had not been terminated and should not be until the highest tribunal in the country (the House of Lords) had decreed that the publication of these lectures was illegal.

In the next stage of legal proceedings it was stated to the Court of Chancery by the counsel for the *Lancet* that he was now given to understand that the motion for the dissolution of the injunction was not intended to be opposed and he therefore submitted that he was entitled to have the injunction dissolved, and it was so ordered. In commenting on this " triumph" by default, the *Lancet* says, " We do not claim the right of publishing the lectures of any individuals, except those who by an infamous by-law have procured for themselves a monopoly of lecturing to students in surgery,"—alluding to a law of the Court of Examiners, by which attendance upon lectures at certain hospitals (St. Bartholomew's among the number) was requisite to obtain a license to practise, and by which it was claimed Mr. Abernethy became a "public functionary for a public purpose."

Such is the history in brief of one of the most famous law suits in the history of medical journalism, and as the injunction on the *Lancet* was finally dissolved by Mr. Abernethy's failure to continue the litigation, it is easy to understand how in recent times it has become a common belief among the ill-informed that the law upheld the *Lancet*, and that an author had no legal rights over his oral lectures which a journal was bound to respect ; indeed, not long since one of our contemporaries gave editorial notice to very much this effect.

In this country the decisions of our courts have been in conformity with that of Lord Eldon in the *Lancet* case, and while a lecturer cannot lay claim to any vested right in the ideas he communicates, the law holds that the words and sentences in which they are clothed belong to him. Mr. Justice McLean has decided that " lectures, oral or written, cannot be published without the consent of the author, though taken down when delivered ; the person taking them down has a right to their use, but he may not print them," and that " any use of such lectures which should operate injuriously to the lecturer would be a fraud upon him for which the law would give him redress." And Mr. Justice Van Brunt has decided that " the delivery of a lecture to a public audience does not work a forfeiture of the common law right of property in a lecture."

Attention has been recently called to the law of copyright as applied to oral lectures by a suit which was brought by Messrs. G. P. Putnam's Sons, of New York, against Dr. Leo T. Meyer, to restrain him from selling his report of the anatomical lectures of Dr. Darling, they having published the lectures by arrangement with Dr. Darling. A few weeks ago Mr. Justice Van Voorst, of the New York Supreme Court, in granting the injunction, emphatically declared that the point " that lecturers may interdict the publication of their lectures has been distinctly decided."

So much for the law of the subject—of the morals it seems superfluous to speak—and it affords us no little satisfaction to say that the MEDICAL NEWS AND ABSTRACT has always acted in accordance with the only view which has over and again received judicial sanction, and that the clinical lectures which have appeared in our columns have always been authorized publications made by, or with the express permission of, their authors, and have been revised by them, and the right of ownership acknowledged by the tender of pecuniary compensation.

The decision in the case of Putnam *v.* Meyer will be gladly received by the many clinical lecturers in our hospitals and medical colleges, and will stimulate them to speedily put a stop to the unauthorized publications of their lectures which, owing to the frequent gross inaccuracies they contain, have proved as great a fraud upon the reader as they were upon the rights and reputation of the author.

AMERICAN MEDICAL ASSOCIATION.

The Thirty-second Annual Meeting of the Association was well attended, and the proceedings were harmonious. The President's address and the addresses of the chairmen of Sections were carefully prepared, were worthy of the occasion, and were well received. In the Sections the papers were meagre, notwithstanding the efforts of the chairmen to procure valuable contributions, and elicited no notable discussions. In the business sessions, interest centred around the amendment of the Code of Ethics, and the proposition to substitute a weekly medical journal for the annual volume of Transactions. Dr. Billings's substitute for the amendment to the Code was a happy conception, which to a large extent met the arguments of both sides, and at the same time filled the requirements of the case as fully as was probably practicable under any proposition. The action of the Association in relegating for further consideration the question of publishing a weekly journal was at least prudent. The publication of such a periodical involves a much larger annual outlay than it was apparent the Association had at its command, and therefore, with more wisdom than such large bodies usually display in business matters, it wisely deferred action until it had received more accurate information upon which to form a sound judgment than the committee had been able to lay before it. The selection of a President for the ensuing year was happy, and was a proper recognition of the value of Dr. Woodward's labours, as well as those of the Army Medical Staff, in behalf of medical science.

During the sessions of the Association the *Virginia Medical Monthly* issued a daily edition, giving a full and accurate report of the proceedings of the day before. To it we are indebted for aid in the preparation of our report of the proceedings of the Association.

To the local committee of arrangements much credit is due for the careful and painstaking way in which they successfully managed the details of the business and pleasure of the Association. The well-known reputation for hospitality which Richmond has always enjoyed was more than maintained, and this year's meeting will long be memorable to those who participated in it for the unbounded hospitality, both public and private, which was extended to the delegates by the physicians and citizens of Richmond.

—

Proceedings of the American Medical Association, Richmond, Va., May 3, 4, 5, and 6, 1881.—The American Medical Association convened in thirty-second annual session at Mozart Hall, in the city of Richmond, Va., on Tuesday, May 3d, at 11 A. M., John T. Hodgen, M.D., of St. Louis, President, in the chair. The session was opened with prayer by the Rt. Rev. Bishop Keane, and the Association was welcomed to Richmond by Dr. Frank Cunningham, of Richmond, Chairman of the Committee of Arrangements, and by the Hon. F. W. M. Holliday, Governor of Virginia. The President then delivered his Annual

Address, which was an earnest and able advocacy of conservative surgery, and was received by the Association with marked evidence of approval.

Section I. (*Practice of Medicine*, Dr. William Pepper, of Philadelphia, Chairman.) In a paper upon "Bloodletting as a Therapeutic Measure in Pneumonia," Dr. W. C. Wile, of Sandy Hook, Conn., advocated the free use of the lancet, in which he was supported by Drs. N. S Davis, of Chicago; Post, of New York; Quimby, of Jersey City; Whitney, of New York; and S.·D. Gross, of Philadelphia. Drs. J. J. Lynch, of Baltimore; Whittaker, of Cincinnati; Octerlony, of Louisville; and Lester, of Detroit, took opposite ground.

Section II. (*Obstetrics and Diseases of Women*, Dr. James R. Chadwick, ot Boston, Chairman.) Dr. Paul F. Mundé, of New York, made some "Practical Remarks on the Use of Pessaries," and the subject was discussed by Drs. Beverly Cole, of San Francisco; Albert H. Smith, of Philadelphia; H. P. C. Wilson, of Baltimore; Maughs, of St. Louis; and Quimby, of Jersey City. Dr. Wilson dwelt upon the importance of ascertaining whether the uterus can be lifted up before introducing any pessary, and expressed his disapproval of stem pessaries.

Section III. (*Surgery*, Dr. Hunter McGuire, of Richmond, Chairman.) Dr. J. H. Warren, of Boston, read a paper "On the Use of Various New Surgical Instruments;" and Dr. Wm. A. Byrd, of Quincy, Ill., reported "A Case of Ulceration and Perforation of the Appendix Vermiformis, with Remarks upon Abdominal Section in cases of Perforation of the Bowel," in which he advocated operative interference in inflammatory affections around the cæcum. Dr. J. E. Reeves, of Wheeling, presented from Dr. B. W. Allen, of Wheeling, a report of a case of nephritic calculus weighing 480 grains, which had caused a pyonephrosis with a large fluctuating tumour on the hypochondrium. By aspiration 18 pounds of sero-purulent fluid were evacuated, with temporary relief. The patient died, and on autopsy the left kidney was found to have been converted into a sac, 15 inches long, 12 inches wide, and 6 inches deep, containing ten pounds of purulent fluid, together with the above-mentioned calculus.

Section IV. (*State Medicine*.) In the absence of the chairman, Dr. J. S. Reeve, of Wisconsin, this section adjourned.

Section V. (*Ophthalmology, Otology, and Laryngology*, Dr. D. S. Reynolds, of Kentucky, Chairman.) Dr. G. T. Stevens, of Albany, described a "Registering Perimeter." Dr. W. C. Jarvis read a paper on "Nasal Catarrh, with Hypertrophy," and advised the removal of the hypertrophied tissue by the écraseur, and in the case of sessile growths with the aid of transfixion needles. Dr. J. J. Chisolm, of Baltimore, read a paper on the "Treatment of Conical Cornea," in which he advocated puncture of the cornea with a red-hot needle, as advised by some French surgeons.

Section VI. (*Diseases of Children*, Dr. A. Jacobi, of New York, Chairman.) "The Importance of Physical Measurements in Children" was the title of a paper by Dr. H. P. Bowditch, of Boston. He said that it seemed probable that the accurate determination of the normal rate of growth in children will not only throw light upon the nature of the diseases to which childhood is subject, but will also guide us in the application of therapeutic measures. Dr. Bowditch exhibited a chart representing the case of a child, between two and three years old, in which careful and systematic weekly weighing showed, first, the approach, by some weeks, of a chronic disturbance of nutrition, represented by enlarged cervical glands and clay-coloured stools; and, second, after recovery, the approach of an attack of measles, the "danger signal" of progressive loss of weight preceding the eruption by at least a week.

Dr. Lee, of Baltimore, remarked that he had paid especial attention to this subject, and had noticed that a female child could lose more in proportion to its weight, without detriment to its health, than a male child of the same age. He also said that if the loss of weight preceding an eruptive disease was excessive, the case was so much more grave in its prognosis, and that this loss of weight preceded this eruption by from four to five days.

Dr. Busey, of Washington, read a paper on "The Relation of Meterological Conditions to the Diarrhœal Diseases of Children;" and Dr. James C. White, of Boston, forwarded a paper entitled "Some of the Causes of Infantile Eczema, and the Importance of Mechanical Restraint in its Treatment." He described the many and varied external influences which immediately affect the skin of the new-born, as being a common cause of eczema, and laid especial stress on the fact that heat was the more usual cause of the disease than cold. These external influences, however, furnish but a small proportion of all the cases of the disease which occur at this period of life, although by far the great part of those concerning the etiology of which we have any posititive knowledge. During the last twelve years he had treated at the Massachusetts General Hospital 5000 cases of eczema, of which 1770 occurred in children of ten years of age and under, and of which the largest proportion, viz., 569 cases, was in the first year of life. Eliminating the operation of the causes directly acting upon the skin from without, above mentioned, and a few other extraneous agencies, the parasitic chiefly, Dr. White did not hesitate to say that he knew nothing whatever of the causes of the disease in the remainder; also, that as far as his experience went, eczema affected all classes of society alike, occurred at all seasons of the year, came in children of all degrees of health, in the perfectly sound as frequently as in the feeble; that it had no necessary connection with any other disease of childhood; that it showed itself in an equal proportion in bottle babies and those reared at the breast, and was independent of diet; also, that if there were other assigned causes, he would here say that his observation gave him no justification for believing any of them.

After speaking of the extreme suffering which the little patients undergo, Dr. White said that the prime factor of the treatment was the prevention of scratching, and he advocated controlling the child's movements by a system of swathing in a pillow-case, by which the same chances of success in the therapeutics of infantile eczema is given, as exist in the adult. He said that when the strait-jacket treatment is carried out, the child soon becomes used to the confinement, and a wonderful improvement takes place in the disease.

Dr. L. Duncan Bulkley, of New York, believed that Dr. White had laid far too much stress upon local causes, and had ignored entirely the influence of internal, general, dietary, and hygienic causes. Internal treatment he believed to be to a certain degree absolutely necessary, and without it physical restraint would be comparatively ineffective. He advocated the internal use of small purgative doses of calomel every other day, and a mild alkali, as acetate of potassa in liquor ammoniæ acetatis, with a little nitre, and perhaps aconite. As regards mechanical restraint, if the itching is relieved, it is not required; and if it is not relieved, such confinement is torture beyond description. Diachylon ointment Dr. Bulkley believed to be very inefficient in arresting itching. Tar in some form was far more efficacious; indeed, he had little to desire in the way of an application to infantile eczema beyond the following ointment: R. Unguenti picis, ℥j; zinc oxid, ℥ij; unguenti aquæ rosæ, ℥iij. Mix. This should be very carefully prepared and very thoroughly and abundantly applied. If it appears stimulating, less of the tar ointment may be used. He laid great stress upon employing the rose ointment and not simple cerate, or lard, or vaseline, or petroleum. The ointment should be made of a consistency to spread easily and yet not to all melt away after application.

Dr. Bulkley was very positive in the directions given in regard to the use of water to eczematous surfaces in children: they were only to be washed according to direction, and that very rarely, often only at intervals of several days; moreover, it was all important that the protective ointment should be replaced *immediately* after the surface is dried, and renewed sufficiently often to keep the parts completely protected, even twenty or more times the first day. On covered parts the ointment may be thickly spread on the woolly side of sheet lint and bound on. Among the hundreds of cases he had never covered the face with a mask, and had rarely been obliged to restrain the infant much after the first day or so. The only restraint he had ever practised, was putting on muslin mittens, tied around the waist, and then tapes from these passed behind the back or beneath one leg.

Dr. D. H. Goodwillie, of New York, read a paper on "Thumb-sucking."

Second Day. General meeting. The Committee on Nominations was announced, and the Association then proceeded to the consideration of the proposed Amendment to the Code of Ethics, Art. I., paragraph 1st, by adding "and hence it is considered derogatory to the interests of the public and honour of the profession, for any physician or teacher to aid in any way the medical teaching or graduation of persons knowing them to be supporters and intended practitioners of some irregular and exclusive system of medicine."

Dr. Marcy, of Massachusetts, moved to lay the amendment on the table. Lost. Dr. E. S. Dunster, of the University of Michigan, then addressed the Association in a speech carefully prepared, in opposition to the amendment. Dr. N. S. Davis, of Chicago, moved that the amendment be made the special order after the addresses on Thursday. Dr. Howard, of Maryland, moved as a substitute, that the matter be indefinitely postponed. The substitute was lost, and the motion of Dr. Davis adopted.

Dr. William Pepper, of Philadelphia, delivered the Address in Medicine which was devoted to the consideration of the great importance of local lesions, and especially catarrhal inflammation of mucous membranes, as forming the essential cause of many apparently obscure diseases, and also as adding greatly to the danger of many diseases which are now regarded as due exclusively to the presence of some specific poison in the blood.

Dr. James R. Chadwick, of Boston, delivered the Address on Obstetrics and Gynæcology, in which he directed attention to a statistical consideration of the literature of his specialty during the past five years.

Dr. John H. Packard, of Philadelphia, from the Committee on Journalizing Transactions, presented an elaborate and carefully prepared report upon the subject which closed with the proposal of the following resolution.

Resolved, That the President be authorized to appoint a committee of five to digest and report in detail as soon as practicable upon the time, place, and terms of the publication of such a journal, to elect an editor, fix his salary, and to arrange all other necessary details.

Dr. N. S. Davis, of Chicago, moved to strike out so much of the resolution as related to the election of an editor. Adopted.

Dr. Marcy, of Mass., moved that as many of the previous committee as were present at the meeting, be members of the new committee. Adopted.

Dr. Toner, of Washington, moved to add the Secretary and Treasurer to the Committee. Adopted.

Dr. Toner, of Washington, offered a resolution instructing the Secretary to publish with the forthcoming report of the Transactions of the Association an index of all the previous volumes. Adopted.

Dr. Toner presented the report of the Committee on Necrology.

Section I. (*Practice of Medicine.*) Dr. D. W. Prentiss. of Washington, presented a paper entitled " Is croupous pneumonia a zymotic disease ?" and Dr. W. C. Dabney, of Charlottesville, Va., a paper on the " Nature and Treatment of Pneumonia." Dr. L. Duncan Bulkley, of New York, read an elaborate paper on " The Diet and Hygiene of Eczema."

Section II. (*Obstetrics and Diseases of Women.*) Dr. H. P. C. Wilson, of Baltimore, exhibited some instruments, which gave rise to a spirited discussion upon instrumental interference. He showed some dilators by the use of which he is enabled to dispense with the use of tents. Dr. Albert H. Smith, of Philadelphia, expressed a preference for the tents: he said, the instruments make small lesions about the cervical canal, hence the dangers of septicæmia in careless hands. The tents, he thinks, are safer, if not withdrawn before the end of forty-eight hours instead of twenty-four, as is usually done. The tents ought to be cylindrical (not conical), and should be rubbed over with moist soap and dipped in a solution of salicylic acid before being introduced.

Section III. (*Surgery and Anatomy.*) Dr. C. F. Stillman. of New York, described some " new mechanical appliances," and Dr. Alfred C. Post, of New York, read a paper on " Plastic Operations on the Face." Dr. D. H. Goodwillie, of New York, also read a paper on the " Treatment of Arthritis of the Temporo-maxillary Articulation," by means of an apparatus to relieve the joint of pressure on the inflamed articular surfaces. It is made as follows : an impression of the teeth of either jaw is taken and an interdental splint made, the posterior part of which is raised a little for the purpose of a fulcrum, on which the back tooth of the opposite jaw rests. Another impression is taken of the chin, and a rubber splint is made to fit it. A skull-cap is next made to fit the head closely, with elastic bands on each side passing down from it and fastened to the chin-splint. The interdental splint is placed in position in the mouth, and the back teeth of the jaw closed on the fulcrum of the interdental splint ; then, when pressure is made on the chin by tightening the elastic bands connecting the skull-cap with the chin-splint, the joint is relieved from pressure. Dr. Goodwillie reported some successful cases thus treated.

Dr. B. A. Watson, of Jersey City, N. J., read an elaborate paper, the title of which was " An Experimental and Clinical Inquiry into the Etiology and Distinctive Peculiarities of Traumatic Fever.".

Section IV. (*State Medicine.*) In the absence of the Chairman, Dr. J. S. Billings, U. S. A., was elected chairman *pro tem.*

Dr. J. L. Cabell, of the University of Virginia, read an interesting paper on " The National Board of Health and the International Sanitary Conference of 1881." He reported that there was good reason for hoping that an international agreement may be arrived at between the States most frequently threatened with epidemic invasions. And, aside from this, the degree of attention which as a result of the deliberations of the Conference has been given to the subject of . maritime sanitary police, cannot be without fruit in securing greater cleanliness, better ventilation of ships sailing on the high seas ; and in general, an improved sanitary condition of these important instruments of commerce, which become so often the carriers of the most deadly contagion, from the failure to use such precautions as sanitary science suggested, and as it is hoped will now be enforced among the maritime powers of the world.

Dr. C. F. Folsom, of Boston, read a paper on the " relation of the State to the insane." He argued in favor of the establishment of State Lunacy Boards. Among the points made were, first of all, that a lunacy board should embrace men with a thorough knowledge of insanity and its treatment. The chief duties of this board should be to secure proper care for the insane in private dwellings, where they are very much liable to neglect. Secondly, they should examine the commitment papers, and otherwise looking into the cases, so as to be able to tell whether the lunatic should be retained for care or be discharged.

Section V. (*Ophthalmology, Otology, and Laryngology.*) Dr. Carl Seiler, of Philadelphia, read a paper upon "Syphilitic Laryngitis," and Dr. Chisolm one on a form of tinnitus induced by a rhythmical contraction of the tensor tympani muscle. Dr. Eugene Smith, of Detroit, presented a report of a successful operation for blepharoplasty, in which the graft was taken from the arm without any pedicle.

Section VI. (*Diseases of Children.*) Dr. R. J. Nunn, of Savannah, forwarded a paper on the "Treatment of Diphtheria." Dr. E. H. Bradford presented an article on "resection of the tarsus in severe congenital club-foot."

Third Day. General meeting. On motion of Dr. S. D. Gross, of Philadelphia, the By-laws were amended so as to establish an additional section to be known as the Section of Dentistry. A motion to suspend the rules so that the section might be organized immediately was objected to, and therefore could not be considered.

The President announced as the Committee on Journalizing the Transactions, Drs. J. H. Packard, N. S. Davis, J. S. Billings, L. A. Sayre, and R. B. Cole, with the Treasurer and Secretary.

Dr. Hunter McGuire, of Richmond, delivered the address in surgery, and chose for his subject "operative interference in gunshot wounds of the peritoneum," which he advocated as exchanging an almost certain prospect of death for at least a good chance of recovery. He urged operative interference in gunshot penetrating wounds of the peritoneum with intestinal injury, in penetrating wounds of the peritoneum with any visceral lesion, and in similar cases without visceral injury. The wounds in the abdominal walls should be enlarged, or the linea alba opened freely enough to allow a thorough inspection of the injured parts. Hemorrhage should be arrested. If intestinal wounds exist, they should be closed with animal ligatures, trimming their edges first if they are lacerated and ragged. Blood and all other extraneous matter should be carefully removed, and then provision made for drainage. If the wound of entrance is dependent, drainage may be secured by keeping this open. If the wound is a perforating one, and the aperture of exit dependent, the patency of this should be maintained, and, if necessary, a drainage tube of glass or other material introduced. If there is no wound of exit, and the wound of entrance is not dependent, then a dependent counter-opening should be made and kept open with a drainage tube. If it is urged that the means suggested are desperate, it can be said in reply that the evil is desperate enough to justify the means.

In the absence of the address of the chairman of the Section on State Medicine, Dr. J. S. Billings, U. S. A., occupied the allotted time with some interesting remarks on some of the results of the tenth census as regards mortality statistics.

Dr. N. S. Davis, of Chicago, from the Committee on Clinical Observations and Records, presented an elaborate report in which the appointment of a standing committee was recommended. The report was accepted and the recommendation adopted.

The Committee on Nominations presented the following report : *For President,* Dr. J. J. Woodward, U. S. A. *For Vice-Presidents,* Dr. P. O. Hooper, Ark. ; L. Conner, Mich. ; Eugene Gressom, North Carolina ; and Hunter McGuire, Virginia. *Secretary,* Dr. Wm. B. Atkinson, Penn. *Treasurer,* Dr. R. J. Dunglison, Penn. *Librarian,* Dr. Wm. Lee, Washington, D. C. *To fill vacancies in Judicial Council,* Drs. S. N. Benham, Penn. ; J. M. Toner, Washington ; D. A. Linthecum, Ark. ; William Brodie, Mich. ; H. D. Holton, Vermont ; A. B. Sloan, Missouri ; and R. B. Cole, Cal.

St. Paul, Minn., was selected as the place for the next meeting; and Dr. Stone was appointed chairman of the Local Committee of Arrangements.

Dr. Billings, U. S. A., moved the adoption of the report of the committee; and paid a high compliment to Dr. Woodward, the nominee for President, and thanked the committee, in behalf of the Medical Staff of the Army, for the high compliment paid it in the selection of one of its most honoured members for the highest position in the gift of the Association.

The report of the committee was unanimously adopted.

The next order of business was the further consideration of the amendment to the Code of Ethics. Dr. N. S. Davis, of Chicago, made an able and elaborate argument in reply to Dr. Dunster and in favour of the amendment, and Drs. Martin of Mass., and Dunster, of Mich., spoke against it. Dr. Marcy, of Mass., moved to lay the amendment on the table, defeated; and the further consideration of the amendment was postponed until Friday.

The next business was the consideration of the following amendment to By-laws, offered by Dr. J. M. Keller, of Arkansas:—

"In the election of officers and appointment of committees by this Association and its President, they shall be confined to members and delegates present at the meeting, except in the Committees of Arrangements, Climatology, and Credentials." The amendment was adopted.

Section I. (*Practice of Medicine*). Dr. Whittaker, of Cincinnati, read a paper on the "treatment of diphtheria," and advanced the view that diphtheria was first a local and afterwards a general disease, and that it is only when the epithelial barrier is broken down that the blood and the body become infected. He contended that, although he could not kill the germs of the disease in the throat, he could so condense its mucous membrane as to make it a dam to the influx of disease, and to this end he recommended the persulphate of iron in full strength, applied well up behind the velum palati.

Dr. I. E. Atkinson, of Baltimore, read an exceedingly valuable and interesting paper on the "production of albuminuria by use of iodide of potassium in syphilitic disease," and Dr. Henry A. Martin, of Boston, a paper on "variola vaccinæ and variola equinæ in Massachusetts."

Section II. (*Obstetrics and Diseases of Women.*) Dr. Jos. Tabor Johnson, of Washington, read a paper on the "diagnosis of pregnancy in early months," and Dr. Mundé, of New York, exhibited a curette for removal of adherent placenta after abortion.

Section III. (*Surgery.*) Dr. Charles A. Leale, of New York, presented a paper on "facial carbuncle, and its treatment," in which he recommended free incision and the thorough application of pure nitric acid.

Section IV. (*State Medicine.*) No meeting.

Section V. (*Ophthalmology, Otology, and Laryngology.*) The afternoon was occupied by a general discussion of the subject of astigmatism.

Section VI. (*Diseases of Children.*) Dr. Clarence J. Blake, of Boston, presented a paper on "middle ear disease in children in the course of the acute exanthemata." Dr. A. Jacobi, of New York, Chairman of the Section then delivered his address.

Fourth Day. General Meeting. The President announced the following as the "Committee on Clinical Observations and Records," Drs. N. S. Davis, of Chicago; J. M. Toner, of Washington; H. O. Marcy, of Boston; W. H. Geddings, of Aiken; and S. M. Bemiss, of New Orleans.

The Association resumed the consideration of the amendment to the Code of Ethics, and Dr. J. S. Billings, U. S. A., offered the following substitute:—

"It is not in accord with the interest of the public or the honour of the profession that any physician or medical teacher should examine or sign diplomas or certificates of proficiency for, or otherwise be especially concerned with, the graduation of persons whom they have good reason to believe intend to support and practice any exclusive and irregular system of medicine." The previous question was moved, and the substitute was adopted.

The Committee on Nominations presented the following additional report :—

Section on Practice of Medicine—Chairman, Dr. J. A. Octerlony, Kentucky.

Section on Surgery and Anatomy—Chairman, Dr. J. C. Hughes, Iowa.

Section on Obstetrics—Chairman, Dr. H. O. Marcy, Massachusetts.

Section on Medical Jurisprudence and State Medicine—Chairman, A. L. Gihon, Washington, D. C.

Ophthalmology, Otology, and Laryngology—Chairman, Dr. D. B. St. John Roosa, New York.

Diseases of Children—Chairman, Dr. S. C. Busey, of Washington.

Dentistry—Chairman, Dr. D. H. Goodwillie, of New York.

On motion of Dr. Grissom, of N. C., a honorarium of $1000 was voted to the Permanent Secretary.

Dr. Goodwillie, of New York, offered an amendment to the Constitution, enabling permanent members to vote. Laid over for one year.

Dr. D. S. Reynolds delivered the address on Ophthalmology, etc.

The report of the Treasurer showed a balance of $2,208.40.

The report of the Committee on Publication was presented.

The Librarian reported that 273 titles had been added to the library during the year, and asked for an appropriation of $200 for current expenses, and that an appropriation of $50 be made in aid of the publication of the index medicus. Accepted, and appropriations passed.

The Convention unanimously adopted the following:—

Resolved, That the thanks of this Association are hereby tendered to the Committee of Arrangements of this Association for the faithful attention they have given to their duties and requirements; to the medical profession and citizens of Richmond for their hospitality and endeavours to make the time spent by us while here pleasant and agreeable; to Drs. McCaw and McGuire for the elegant special entertainment given by them at the Westmoreland Club; to Mr. McClure, Superintendent of the Telephone Company, for special facilities given the Committee of Arrangements and the Association; to Vice-President Parsons, of the Richmond and Allegheny Railroad, for his kind invitation for a free ride on his road to show us the interior of the State of Virginia; to Mr. Powell, manager of the Richmond Theatre; to the managers of the Mozart Association, and all others who have contributed to our pleasure and comfort; to the press, and especially their reporters, in giving such a full *résumé* of the proceedings in the daily papers; to the railroad companies generally who have so liberally reduced the rates of transportation for our benefit and any other modes of conveyance that have so contributed; to Mr. Valentine for his kind invitation to his studio.

Be it Especially Resolved, That our thanks are particularly due to the ladies of Richmond for attention and kind interest in making our sojourn so very pleasant and agreeable.

The Association then adjourned to meet at St. Paul on the first Tuesday in June, 1882.

The Association was entertained on Tuesday evening by Dr. and Mrs. McCaw and Dr. and Mrs. Hunter McGuire at a very handsome reception at the Westmoreland Club; on Wednesday evening by an operatic performance (The

Doctor of Alcantara), tendered by the physicians of Richmond; on Thursday evening by the citizens of Richmond at a promenade concert at the Richmond Theatre; and on Friday afternoon by an excursion along the valley of the James River, by the Richmond and Allegheny Railroad Company.

—

The American Surgical Association.—The American Surgical Association met at Richmond, May 5th, at the Hall of the House of Delegates. Dr. S. D. Gross, of Philadelphia, presiding, and J. R. Weist, of Indiana, acted as Secretary.

At the request of the President, Dr. Packard, of Philadelphia, read the proposed new Constitution and By-Laws. On motion of Dr. Davis, the Constitution and By-Laws, as read, were unanimously adopted. · Under this Constitution, surgeons known as "specialists" are allowed to become members of the Association. Under the old Constitution, that class of surgeons were excluded.

Drs. Marcy and Martin, of Boston, and Watson, of Jersey City, were recommended for membership.

Dr. Packard, the Treasurer, reported that he had received $925 from members, which, with the interest ($9.25), was deposited to the credit of the Association.

An amendment to the Constitution was adopted, to the effect that all nominations for membership shall lie over until the next regular session.

The Oriental Hotel, Coney Island, New York, was selected as the place for the next annual meeting. The 13th, 14th, and 15th of September was selected as the time.

The Association then adjourned until the above time and place.

The following is the list of officers of the society:—

Samuel D. Gross, M.D., President; Vice-Presidents, Drs. L. A. Dugas, James R. Wood; J. R. Weist, Recording Secretary; W. D. Briggs, Cor. Secretary; John H. Packard, Treasurer.

Council—Drs. Moses Gunn, John T. Hodgen, Hunter McGuire, J. C. Hutchison, Samuel D. Gross, J. R. Weist, and R. A. Kinloch.

—

American Medical College Association.—This body convened at Richmond on May 2, Dr. S. D. Gross, of Philadelphia, President, in the chair. Owing to the absence of a quorum, the Association adjourned from time to time until May 4, when a quorum was finally secured.

On motion of Dr. Bodine, of Louisville, the regular order of business was suspended to enter upon the election of officers. Dr. Gross stated that he would under no circumstances accept a re-election. The following officers were then elected:—

President, Professor J. M. Bodine, of the Medical Department of the University of Louisville, Ky.; Vice-President, Professor W. T. Briggs, of Nashville, Tenn.; Secretary and Treasurer, Professor Leartus Conner, of Detroit, Michigan.

Secretary Conner's report was then presented and received. It shows an increase of two in the active membership of the Association since the last annual meeting. From the reports of the several colleges made to the Secretary, it appears that these institutions had conformed more universally and completely with the requirements of the Association than heretofore, and that everything pertaining to their connection with the body was entirely satisfactory.

The report of the Committee on Medical Colleges showed that sixty-four catalogues of colleges had been examined, and that only sixteen of them had failed to come up to the Association's requirements in the matter of graduation. It also appeared that twenty-two of the colleges had surpassed these requirements in one or more of the three following particulars: First, matriculation examinations; second, nine months' regular attendance; third, the three regular terms required.

After the transaction of some unimportant business, the Association adjourned until 5 P. M.

Upon the assembling of the Association at half-past five o'clock, it was found there was no quorum present. After waiting some time, and a quorum still being needed, the body adjourned, subject to the call of the President.

—

Health of New York.—The city's sanitary condition is far from satisfactory, and the mortality is constantly increasing. During the first four months of 1880 there were 9266 deaths. This year, during the same period, there were 12,420 deaths, and the number for the week ending May 14th was 822. Typhus fever still prevails, although not to so alarming an extent as during the first month of the endemic. This fact may be fairly attributed to the energetic and efficient measures for disinfection and isolation adopted by the health board. During the fourth week of the fever's prevalence, ending April 16, there were 68; in the fifth week, only 4; in the sixth week, 17; and in the seventh week (ending May 1st), 29 cases reported. On May 10th there were 63 cases of typhus, and 156 of variola, at the Riverside Hospital. The Shiloh lodging-house, in which the fever originated, will probably soon be vacated by order of the Health Department. The type of the fever is still mild.

Diphtheria has decreased slightly during April, but measles, scarlet fever, and smallpox have markedly increased, the number of cases of variola being double that for March, and four times that for February. Several cases of variola have been imported by European emigrant steamers, and some cases have been discovered in Brooklyn and Jersey City. There is no truth in the sensational report that several cases of Asiatic cholera had been observed in the city. Some apprehensions having been excited by the apparently impure condition of the Croton water, the Board of Health has promulgated a report to the effect that no injury can result from its use, as it contains no harmful ingredients. The supply of water is, however, inadequate to the increasing demand, caused by the advent of summer, which was announced by the occurrence, on May 10, 11, and 12, of about thirty cases of insolation, several of which were fatal. No progress whatever has been made by the Legislature with reference to the passage of a street-cleaning bill since the last issue of the MEDICAL NEWS AND ABSTRACT. Conference committees were appointed, by the Senate and the Assembly, for the purpose of framing a bill which would be acceptable to their respective houses; but, having failed to effect a compromise, were discharged. New conference committees will now be appointed. The grand jury has indicted the members of the police board for failure to properly clean the streets. The trial before the Mayor of these officials for the same offence has just been completed.

—

Bellevue Hospital.—Important improvements are about to be undertaken at Bellevue Hospital which will materially alter the appearance of its grounds. Mr. Marquand, a philanthropic capitalist, is about to present the hospital with a beautifully finished and appointed pavilion, in token of his appreciation of the care and attention bestowed upon his brother, who has been a recent inmate of the institution. The dimensions of the pavilion, which will be erected at the corner of Twenty-sixth Street and First Avenue, within the hospital inclosure, will be 120 by 130 feet, and the estimated expense of its construction about $20,000. It will be chiefly devoted to the treatment of women and children, but four separate rooms will be fitted up, in a remote portion of the building, for the exclusive use of ovariotomy cases. The new building will consist of red brick and blue stone. The interior, which will be planned in accordance with suggestions from some of the visiting physicians, will be finished in rosewood. The floors will consist of tiles. The bath-rooms and closets will be of the most approved pattern. The unsightly stone wall, now inclosing the grounds upon the corner to be occupied by the new pavilion, will be replaced by an iron railing.

The Commissioners of Charities and Correction are now having erected another new pavilion, at the water's edge, for the treatment of erysipelas cases. Its dimensions will be 90 by 36 feet, and its cost $6000. Its fire-proof walls and partitions will consist of two layers of corrugated sheet-iron, the interval between which will be filled with plaster-of-Paris. This pavilion will accommodate twenty-four patients. A median partition will separate it into male and female departments, which will be thoroughly ventilated and provided with all modern conveniences. The new building will be ready for occupation on June 15th.

A small temporary reception hospital has been constructed at Bellevue Hospital for the detention and isolation of typhus fever cases, presenting themselves at the examining office, until their removal to the typhus pavilions on Blackwell's Island. It is built upon a scow which is anchored at a certain distance from shore. It is a one-storied building, and has separate apartments for males and females. Nurses, provided by the Board of Health, are in attendance, and the hospital steamer calls twice a day to remove patients to Blackwell's Island. The hospital is perfectly ventilated and provided with every convenience. The plan of a floating hospital was adopted in order to prevent the communication of typhus fever to the inmates of Bellevue Hospital.

———

Prosecution of Unqualified Practitioners.—The Medical Society of the County of New York has begun active legal proceedings against illegally registered and unqualified medical practitioners by the arrest of two persons, who are accused of practising medicine without physicians' licenses. The censors of the society have ample evidence against a number of illegally registered practitioners, and propose to prosecute them as soon as the present cases shall have been disposed of.

———

The Street Cleaning Agitation in New York.—At the regular meeting of the Medical Society of the County of New York, held on April 25, 1881, and at that of the Medico-Legal Society, on May 4, 1881, resolutions expressing the sympathy of the respective societies with the citizens' street cleaning bill were unanimously passed, and the presidents and secretaries of the societies were empowered to endorse the resolutions, and to present them to the President of the Senate and the Speaker of the Assembly.

The Council of the New York Academy of Medicine adopted, on April 26, the following resolution : "*Resolved*, That the members of this Council, knowing the filthy streets to be an active cause of disease, and that those of the city of New York are in a disgracefully dirty condition, respectfully urge upon the Legislature of the State of New York, as an efficient means of relief, the passage of the bill in reference to street cleaning known as the ' Citizens' Bill,' now before the Conference Committees.''

———

New York Stenches.—The Committee of the State Board of Health on the stench nuisances at Hunter's Point, Brooklyn, having reported that the complaints in regard to the noisome odours were well founded, and having indicated as the source of the offensive emanations the various factories mentioned in the April No. of THE MEDICAL NEWS AND ABSTRACT, the State Board forwarded an abstract of the report to Governor Cornell. A proclamation was immediately made by the Governor, directing the owners of all the factories designated as sources of offensive effluvia to take measures for the abatement or prevention of the latter before June 1, 1881. In the event of failure on the part of the factory proprietors to comply with this regulation, the district attorneys of Kings and Queens Counties will be directed by the Governor to bring action against the offenders. Authority for this action is furnished by a law passed in 1880 (8th sec. of the 322d chapter of Laws of 1880).

———

The Visiting Staff of Bellevue Hospital.—Dr. T. T. Sabine has resigned his position as visiting surgeon to Bellevue Hospital, and Dr. Chas. McBurney has been appointed his successor.

———

A Night Medical Service in Brooklyn.—Governor Cornell has signed the bill for the establishment of a night medical service in Brooklyn.

———

College of Physicians and Surgeons, New York.—At the annual commencement of the medical department of Columbia College, held on May 13, 120 graduates received their diplomas. A social meeting of the alumni of the college was held in the evening at Delmonico's.

———

Meetings of State Medical Societies :—
Connecticut State Medical Society meets at Hartford, June 22.
Massachusetts Medical Society meets at Boston, June 7.
Michigan State Medical Society meets at Bay City, June 8.
New Hampshire Medical Society meets at Concord, June 21.
Ohio State Medical Society meets at Columbus, June 14.
Wisconsin State Medical Society meets at Milwaukee, June 7.
On the 7th and 8th of June the Massachusetts Society will celebrate their Centennial Anniversary with proper honours, and addresses will be delivered by Drs. Samuel A. Green and J. Collins Warren, of Boston.

———

OBITUARY RECORD.—At Berlin, on the 21st of April, after a short illness, Dr. LUDWIG WALDENBURG, in the forty-third year of his age. Dr. Waldenburg was professor in the University of Berlin, physician to the Charité Hospital, and editor of the *Berliner Klinische Wochenschrift*. He devoted his attention chiefly to diseases of the respiratory organs, on which he has written a comprehensive treatise, and was the inventor of an apparatus for the inspiration of compressed air, which has been much used. Dr. Waldenburg exercised great influence throughout the medical profession in Germany in his position as the acknowledged editor of its most influential medical journal. The *Berliner Klinische Wochenschrift* was always well edited, contained valuable scientific matter, and had an useful influence on those social and political questions in which the medical profession is constantly called upon to pronounce an opinion, and to direct public opinion, and frequently to prepare the way for necessary legislation. His independent character and his discretion lent force to his advocacy, and gave great weight to his judgments.—*British Med. Journal*, April 23, 1881.

——— At New York, on April 30th, aged 58, SALVATORE CARO, M.D., a physician of recognized ability and very enviable reputation. Dr. Caro graduated at the University of Palermo, in 1848, and came to this country in 1852.

CONTENTS OF NUMBER 463.

JULY, 1881.

CLINICS.

MONTHLY ABSTRACT.

MIDWIFERY AND GYNÆCOLOGY.

MEDICAL NEWS.

THE

MEDICAL NEWS AND ABSTRACT.

VOL. XXXIX. No. 7.　　　　JULY, 1881.　　　　WHOLE No. 463.

CLINICS.

Clinical Lectures.

ON ATYPICAL TYPHOID FEVER.

A CLINICAL LECTURE DELIVERED AT THE PHILADELPHIA HOSPITAL,

By JAMES C. WILSON, M.D.,

ATTENDING PHYSICIAN TO THE HOSPITAL.

GENTLEMEN: Your attention is invited this morning to the careful review of a completed case of acute disease. The patient before you, although still in bed and still requiring care, has fairly entered upon convalescence—his sickness is over. Two principal dangers beset his way back to full health: first, the danger of a recrudescence of fever—this we may reasonably hope to avoid by proper management until convalescence is completed; second, a true relapse of the disease, which we can neither foresee nor prevent, being as yet altogether ignorant of the cause of typhoid relapse in particular cases, and much in the dark as to its etiology in general. Typhoid relapse is, however, of comparatively rare occurrence, and we may therefore hope that our patient will also escape this danger. For reasons that will presently appear, I do not fear local trouble from the intestinal lesions in this case.

You have already seen this patient. Two weeks ago I brought him before you. It was the eleventh day of his sickness, and he presented the characteristic phenomena of well-developed typhoid fever of moderate intensity. You will recall his face, listless, apathetic, pale, with a faint flush over the cheek bones; his deafness, and the slow, dull manner of his replies; his tongue pale, coated, and trembling slightly as it was protruded. You will remember that there were a few scattered loud râles heard upon auscultation of the lungs, that there was diarrhœa amounting to three or four loose stools in the twenty-four hours, slight tympany without either tenderness or gurgling, and that there were scattered over the anterior surface of the chest and abdomen some lenticular rose spots which faded upon pressure and at once reappeared upon the removal of the pressure. These spots were first seen on the fifth day after admission, or the ninth of the attack. I was enabled to demonstrate an extended area of splenic dulness. You will readily call to mind the elevated temperature and its range, for it was to these that our joint attention was chiefly directed.

The absolute temperature was not high, and the range between the evening
and morning, the maximum and minimum of the diurnal cycle, was considerable, amounting to a full degree of the Fahrenheit scale during the
first three days the patient had been under observation, and to nearly
three degrees afterward, the evening temperature only once exceeding, by
a fifth of a degree, 103° F. The investigations of Wunderlich long ago
brought to light the fact that, as a rule, in uncomplicated typhoid fever
the temperature during the whole course of the attack rarely exceeds the
maximum attained at the close of the first or the beginning of the second
week (or period). It is further well known that a temperature-range
characterized by considerable morning remissions is much less injurious to
the tissues, even when the evening maxima are relatively higher, than a
continuous or subcontinuous fever. The consideration of these two facts,
together with the absence of symptoms indicating either excessive constitutional action of the fever-poison (zymosis), or extensive or severe local
lesions, led me to predict with some degree of confidence a favourable
course for the attack. The prognosis has proved to have been correct.
The temperature at no period after the evening of the day upon which
you saw the case rose above 103° F. On the contrary, it steadily but
slowly declined until the night of the sixteenth day, when it fell more than
three degrees, from 100.2° to 97°, and it has since that date varied but

little from the normal. The patient no longer presents the symptoms of
typhoid fever. He is pale, but his expression is neither languid nor listless. The flush has disappeared; he hears well, and replies to my questions promptly and with interest. We learn from him that the statements
made by those who brought him to the hospital were in the main correct.
He is a cellar-digger, 40 years of age, married, temperate, and of previous
good health. Whilst at work four days before admission, he was *suddenly*

seized with chills, which recurred several times in the course of the day; there was severe frontal headache and disinclination to take food; at night he had fever and pains in his joints. The next day he was unable to go to work. I desire to call your attention especially to the fact that up to the day of the chills he had felt nothing amiss, but had worked as usual, and thought himself well. From his manner of replying it is clear that he is intelligent and that his memory is good. The râles are no longer heard, the tympany and spots have disappeared, diarrhœa has given place to slight constipation with formed stools, and the area of splenic dulness has diminished. About the thirteenth and fourteenth days there was slight pulmonary hypostasis; epistaxis did not occur, and there was no delirium. Two or three new spots appeared on the fifteenth day. Albuminuria did not occur.

Aside from the moderate severity of the symptoms in this case, in which respect it certainly stands forth in striking contrast to the examples of typhoid fever that are usually shown you in this theatre, your attention at once fixes itself upon three facts in the history, that are not in accord with the picture of the typical disease, as you have found it correctly drawn for you in the text-books, or vividly portrayed in the lecture-room, or have commonly seen it in the clinic, the wards, or in your own practice. These are, first, the abruptness of the onset; second, the short duration of the sickness, defervescence being complete upon the seventeenth day; and third, the comparative abruptness of the defervescence.

Great as are the variations from the ordinary type which this case presents in its origin, its course, and its termination, the symptom-grouping makes it clear beyond all doubt that we have had to do with an example of typhoid fever. This being established, the questions at once arise: To what group of the forms of typhoid is this case to be properly referred? And what are the departures from the common pathological conditions of typhoid fever by which to explain these conspicuous variations from the usual course of the disease?

In order to reply to these questions it is necessary to revert to a convenient nosological arrangement to which the various forms of disease due to the typhoid poison may be referred, and to briefly consider the influences by which the action of the poison is so modified as to produce well-marked and more or less constant variations in its clinical manifestations.

All cases may be referred to one or the other of two comprehensive groups :—

     A. The typical.
     B. The atypical.

A. The typical, or perfect, or common form is too familiar to require in this connection a word of description. Its insidious beginning, its prolonged duration, its gradual defervescence and tardy convalescence are as well known to you as is its unmistakable symptom-grouping. That different cases of such a disease should present variations in the prominence of certain symptoms or groups of symptoms, is quite in accordance with our experience in all diseases both acute and chronic. These variations are due, on the one hand, to differences in the relative degree of intensity of the action of the cause upon the fluids of the body at large, or upon the lymphatic system of the ileum; and, on the other, to differences in individuals as regards bodily constitution, temperament, previous condition of health, and so forth. Notable variations arise also in consequence of the presence of complications. But clearly apparent through all such variations is the conformity to type, which sets forth the nature of the disease and renders the diagnosis a comparatively easy task. It is th's conformity to type that renders subdivisions of this group unnecessary, and the discrimination of such forms as *bilious, nervous, ataxic, adynamic,* or *cerebral, thoracic,* and *abdominal,* not only useless, but positively misleading both in the lecture-room and at the bedside.

It is important to bear in mind that the fever in the typical cases, like that of scarlet fever and of smallpox, is made up of two distinct febrile movements—first, a primary fever, resulting from the infection of the tissues of the body by the specific virus; and later, a secondary, irritative or hectic fever, caused by the localized ulceration in the intestines, the formation of slough, and the resorption of septic materials.

B. The atypical or imperfect forms are much more rare, and present difficulties in their clinical study proportionate to their want of the very conformity to type that renders the investigation of the cases belonging to the first group relatively a simple matter. So great is this want of conformity to type in many of the atypical cases of typhoid fever, that they are not to be recognized by their clinical manifestations, but only in the light of a common etiological relation to well-developed cases occurring in more or less extended (local) epidemics. This statement is true of most epidemic diseases. Side by side with well-developed cases are seen imperfect, slight, or abortive cases manifestly due to the prevalent epidemic influence, but so faintly marked as to be recognizable only in the light of that influence.

The second comprehensive group must, from this point of view, be subdivided into a number of forms, which may be arranged in order, according to the degree of their departure from the typical disease. These forms are :—

    a. Mild typhoid (including walking typhoid).
    b. Abortive typhoid.
    c. Typhoid of childhood (so-called infantile remittent).
    d. Typhoid of the aged.
    e. Cases of febrile intestinal catarrh.
    f. Cases of afebrile intestinal catarrh.

These atypical or imperfect forms constitute, in most epidemics, a large proportion of the cases, and they will be found, I believe, to be much more common where the disease is endemic than has usually been thought, when the attention of physicians is more closely turned to the study of typhoid fever from an etiological as well as from a clinical standpoint. The modifications which characterize such cases are partly due to mild infection, or the smallness of the dose of the fever-producing principle; partly to an imperfect susceptibility on the part of the patient, and partly to differences in the reaction of the organism to the fever-poison and the products of unduly rapid waste at different periods of life.

a. The mild cases present the symptoms of the typical disease modified in respect of intensity, and in particular is this true of the febrile movement, which is of a lower grade. The commencement of the attack is usually gradual; there are prodromes, which pass step by step into the declared disease. Chilly sensations may occur; a decided chill is unusual. There is headache, diarrhœa; the nose may bleed, and the eruption may or may not appear. The temperature may reach upon the fourth or fifth day 104° F., but it rarely exceeds that point, and much more commonly does not attain it. The temperature-range corresponds to that of the typical form, save that upon corresponding days it is a degree or more lower. The duration of this form may be four full weeks; it is perhaps oftener less than this, each of the four periods not exceeding four or five days. The febrile movement corresponds to the primary and the secondary fever of the fully developed disease. The intestinal lesions do not undergo resolution, but go on to sloughing.

The latent, or ambulatory form (*walking typhoid*) belongs to this group. In this form all the symptoms are at first mild; the disease shows itself in general malaise, prostration, and elevation of temperature, yet the sickness extends over three or four weeks, and the intestinal lesion proceeds to sloughing and ulceration. Herein lies the danger of this form of the disease. The patient regards himself as suffering from some slight indisposition, a "cold," or a "bilious attack," and continues to go about in a wretched way, or even, if he be a person of determined will, to attend to his ordinary occupations, and to eat such food as his appetite perm ts, until sudden delirium reveals to his friends the serious character of his illness, a profuse hemorrhage occurs, or, and this is still more common, symptoms of perforation supervene, and are followed, after a few hours, by death.

b. The abortive form appears to be not uncommon in Europe. In this country it is certainly rare. The attack begins abruptly; prodromes are usually of short duration, or they may be absent altogether. The temperature-range is, at first, that of the typical disease, save that it in some instances more rapidly attains its maximum. The invasion is often accompanied by rigors, sometimes by a decided chill. There is usually moderate diarrhœa; tympany, enlargement of the spleen, sometimes epistaxis, and often more or less bronchial catarrh. The characteristic eruption is frequently observed, and transient albuminuria is met with. Some time in the second week or early in the third, the sickness takes a sudden turn, and runs a similar course as regards ordinary typhoid fever, to that which varioloid runs as regards variola.

The defervescence is rapid, often being completed in from twenty-four to seventy-two hours, and is frequently attended by profuse sweating. Convalescence is also rapid. It is in the highest degree probable that in these cases the intestinal lesions undergo resolution, their evolution being arrested short of the ordinary necrotic processes. We, therefore, have to do with the primary fever due to the action of the special poison, and not with the secondary or septic fever due to ulceration and the formation of sloughs. The parallelism between these cases as compared with typical typhoid fever, and varioloid as compared with variola, is complete.

c. The term infantile remittent fever has been applied to typhoid fever as it occurs in children, for the reason that the pyrexia often assumes in them a distinctly remittent type throughout the whole course of the attack. The symptoms and complications are modified by the age of the patient. Children are very susceptible to typhoid.

d. In the advanced periods of life typhoid fever is rare. When it occurs, it runs a modified course. Its onset is insidious, the febrile movement is less intense than at earlier periods of life, and the temperature often falls during convalescence to markedly subnormal ranges. There is especial danger of collapse. Acute delirium is not so common, and diarrhœa is less apt to be urgent. The characteristic eruption is rarely observed.

e. In rare instances a slight disturbance of the functions of the body results from the infection, and gives rise to intestinal catarrh with elevation of temperature so slight and so irregular that it scarcely deserves the name of fever (100.4° F.).

f. Finally it may be stated upon the authority of Liebermeister and Dr. Cayley, that intestinal catarrh occasionally occurs in consequence of typhoid infection, in which there is no elevation of temperature at all.

It is evident that the case which occupies our attention to-day must be referred to the second of the subdivisions of the atypical forms of typhoid fever. The sudden onsent of the attack, the rapid temperature-rise, which nearly attained its maximum upon the evening of the fifth day, the short duration of the whole sickness, and the abrupt fall of the temperature during the night of the sixteenth day, are characteristic of that form of typhoid fever properly called " abortive."

The sudden onset of the attack has been established by a careful cross-examination o˙ the patient and his friends. The fact that the headache, still present when he came under observation, spontaneously ceased four d ys later, and that the eruption was first discovered on the fifth day afte˙ admission, the ninth of the attack, confirm this statement. For, as you well know, the eruption of typhoid usually appears at the close of the first or early in the ˡsecond week, and the headache commonly ceases spontaneously about the tenth day.

The whole course of the attack has probably comprised only the primary fever due to the constitutional action of the typhoid-poison. For some reason unknown to us the intestinal lesions have undergone resolution without sloughing, and our patient has escaped the secondary or septic fever, which in the typical disease overlaps the primary febrile movement at its close, and prolongs the sickness with well-marked remissions and with a gradual defervescence to the end of the third or fourth week. It is for this reason that I do not especially fear trouble from the intestinal lesions during the convalescence in this patient.

The treatment has had no influence whatever in abridging the course of the attack. It has been practically expectant. The patient was kept at rest, not being allowed to rise for any purpose; he was from time to time sponged with cold water, for purposes of cleanliness rather than with any view of acting upon the temperature; his diet was regulated *secundum artem.* Of medicines, he took upon the first day a little calomel, afterwards at short intervals a draught containing compound tincture of cinchona with dilute muriatic acid, flavoured with syrup of orange-peel.

CASE OF INTRAMURAL FIBROID TUMOUR OF THE UTERUS.

A Clinical Lecture delivered at the Middlesex Hospital.

By HENRY MORRIS, M.A., F.R.C.S.,
Surgeon to the Hospital.

GENTLEMEN: Elizabeth B., aged 32, single, an upholsteress, was admitted on October 26, 1880, for complete retention of urine. Her usual medical attendant, Dr. Ayling, sent her to me with a letter to the effect that, on May 20, 1880, he was summoned, and found her suffering great agony from not having micturated for nineteen hours. He introduced the catheter, and drew off over three pints of urine. Next day, catheterization had to be repeated. She then went on for a week before the catheter was next required; then she continued well for three months before she again required help. Of late, it had become necessary to pass the catheter twice daily; and as she had suffered acute pain at times about the pelvis, calculus or some other serious affection of the bladder suggested itself.

On admission, there was complete inability to micturate, so that the catheter had to be used at regular intervals. The urine was acid, of specific gravity 1015, and free from blood and albumen. She was anæmic, of a dark complexion and nervous temperament, with twitchings of the face when spoken to, and an hysterical look and manner. Her general health had been good; but she had had much mental trouble of late, and to this she attributed her illness. When I examined her on October 28th, at 2 P. M., though her urine had been drawn off at 8 A. M., her bladder was distended, and formed a large prominent ovoid abdominal swelling to the right of the middle line, and inclining very obliquely outwards and upwards. In the left iliac fossa there were marked fulness, dulness, and increased resistance, quite distinct from the abdominal tumour formed by the bladder, and suggesting the presence of a solid or tense cystic tumour of rounded outline. A male catheter was easily introduced, and passed a long way before urine began to flow; the catheter took a very oblique course, and it was found possible to introduce it, without resistance, so far into the bladder that the bone ferrule was hidden by the vulva. The bladder being emptied, an examination *per vaginam* was made; but, as a fairly perfect hymen existed, a satisfactory exploration of the pelvis could not be effected without causing pain. It was ascertained, however, that the vagina was markedly inclined to the left, but that its wall was projected on the right side for a short distance upwards, so that the idea of a bifid vagina was for a moment suggested to the mind of the examiner. The uterus was so much drawn up, and to the left side, that at this examination the os and cervix were not felt. The rectum was found flattened by a smooth, round, hard, unyielding tumour in front, which did not feel like the os or enlarged fundus of the uterus. The mass was clearly inclined to the left side, whether examined with the patient on the back or on the side. A simple enema was ordered to be given every morning. Subsequently (October 30th and November 2d) she was seen by Dr. Hall Davis, who found the uterus considerably drawn up, the os being felt as a mere depression close to the upper border of the symphysis pubis; and the uterine sound passed for four and three-quarter inches into the cavity of the uterus.

From October 28th to November 10th, the catheter was not required.

On November 3d, and the following day, she had intense thirst, and the catamenia appeared on the 3d, and lasted till the 7th. In the night of November 6th, she sweated a great deal; and on the afternoon of November 7th, she had nausea, her temperature went up to 102.6°, and she felt considerable pain in the left iliac fossa. These symptoms continued during the night and the next day.

On November 9th, there were the same symptoms, except that the pain in the abdomen was a little more diffused, and there was now tympanites. She also complained greatly of a parching thirst; she had had rigors during the morning and the preceding evening, was very lachrymose in manner, and had an unaccountable and alarming apprehension that she would soon die. For the first time, too, there was on this day a slight purulent discharge from the vagina. Hot fomentations, with opium and turpentine, were continuously applied to the abdomen; opium, in half-grain doses, was given every four hours; and milk-diet and ice to suck were ordered. The enemata had been discontinued.

On November 10th, the catheter had again to be used. The temperature was 99.8°, the pulse 96, and respirations 25. She had had a bad night, owing to frequent retching. There were distension and slight general tenderness of the abdomen, the girth of which was twenty-seven inches.

On November 11th, the patient complained of spasms and tenderness in the abdomen. The tongue was red, dry, and beefy, with prominent papillæ. The temperature was 101.6°, and the pulse 120 ; the respirations were 28 and shallow. The catheter was not required.

On November 12th, she lay with her knees drawn up, complaining of pain in the abdomen, the girth of which was now twenty-nine inches. There was much tympanites, but no marked tenderness on pressure. The tongue was in the same state as on the previous day. She experienced parching thirst, and vomited occasionally. The pulse was 126, not hard, but thready, and very compressible. There was marked muscular tremor, especially of the hands. She was very restless, talkative, and excitable. Towards the latter part of the afternoon, she was troubled with loud hiccough and retching. The temperature was 99.2° in the morning ; 99.6° in the evening During the night, she slept for intervals from 12 to 2 A. M. ; she then awoke, complaining of increased pain and fulness in the abdomen. Fresh fomentations seemed to relieve this ; but about 4 A. M. on the morning of the 13th, she died quietly within a few minutes. Her death was quite unexpected by the nurse, who had been closely watching by her side.

At the *post-mortem* examination, made ten hours after death, Dr. Fowler found recent general peritonitis gluing together the coils of intestine, and in the peritoneal cavity about one pint of turbid fluid, with floating flakes of lymph. The inflammation was most marked about the brim of the pelvis. Recent adhesions bound the structures in the broad ligament to the neighbouring parts on each side. It seemed probable that the peritonitis had commenced at the left ovary, in which were several small collections of pus, one of them communicating directly with a sloughy point, surrounded by a patch of purulent membrane, on the surface of the ovary. The liver and spleen were congested. The right ureter was somewhat distended, as were also the pelvis and calyces of this kidney. The inner surface of the pelvis showed signs of violent and recent inflammation. The surface of the kidney was mottled ; and, on section, the cortex appeared diminished. The left ureter and pelvis were more dilated than the right, and contained purulent-looking urine ; and in the left kidney the inflammation was more extreme, and had extended along the uriniferous tubules. The bladder was pushed up and towards the right iliac fossa ; and, though quite empty, reached one inch above the upper border of the os pubis. Its walls were hypertrophied, and sacculated, and beneath the mucous membrane there were small extravasations, but no appearance of cystitis. The vagina was elongated ; and, owing to the upward traction of the uterus, the vaginal part of the cervix uteri was obliterated, so that the os was a mere slit in the posterior vaginal wall. The uterus and its appendages were displaced upward and to the left by a large tumour, which almost filled the pelvis, and was growing in the right wall of the uterus. The cavity of the uterus was found to measure four and a half inches ; its axis was oblique, being directed upwards and to the left. Both the Fallopian tubes contained pus. The right ovary was healthy ; but the left, though of nearly normal size, was suppurating at various points. The tumour in the right wall of the uterus somewhat resembled the uterus in shape, but far exceeded it in size, and measured six inches in its long diameter and three inches transversely. The uterine tissue was plainly seen on the surface of the tumour, showing it to have been of intramural origin. On section, it had all the characters of uterine fibroids. At the upper part of the uterus, two small fibroid tumours, about as large as chestnuts, were seen sessile upon the peritoneal surface. The left pleura was normal ; but there was recent lymph over the lower half of the right pleura, but no fluid in the pleural cavity.

Remarks.—The first step was to ascertain by vaginal and rectal examination the cause of the displacement of the bladder, and of the intermittent retention of urine; and to connect it, if possible, with the fulness in the left iliac fossa. The next question was as to the character and connections of the tumour, and whether it could be removed, or in any other way dealt with, so as to allow the bladder to resume its place and functions. This was a question of real difficulty in the case. As a rule, I believe it may be assumed that, in the female, a pelvic tumour which pushes the bladder out of the pelvis and to one side of the median line, which causes lateral and upward displacement of the uterus, and is felt *per rectum* as a large mass on the front aspect of the bowel, is, in all probability, either an enlargement of the uterus itself, or of one of the appendages of the uterus. I have seen, however, in one instance, the bladder pushed right out of the pelvis into the abdomen, by a hydatid cyst. In E. B.'s case it was possible to exclude certain other not uncommon forms of pelvic tumours. Thus (1) pelvi-peritonitis (which M. Nonat, as well as Bernutz and Goupil, tell us, have not unfrequently been mistaken for fibroid of the uterus), and (2) pelvic cellulitis were negatived by the absence of any coexisting or previously existing affection of the generative organs, by the absence of all pregnancies or confinements, and by taking into consideration the sudden commencement of her illness, marked by the single symptom, retention of urine. (3) Hæmatocele was excluded by the freedom from all previous catamenial disturbance, of sanguineous discharge, and of febrile symptoms; and by the altered condition of the os and cervix uteri, the increased dimensions of the uterine cavity, and the mode of onset of the illness. (4) Certain morbid states of the uterus itself could be excluded, such as flexion of the womb; because, though these may either cause retention of urine or difficult defecation, the tumour in this case was large enough to flatten the rectum and displace both uterus and bladder, and the uterine sound could be passed, and turned easily in the uterus. (5) Cancer of the body of the uterus sometimes occurs without the os or cervix being affected, at any rate for a long while; in cancer, too, the uterine cavity may be markedly increased, and the uterus itself is commonly fixed, and presses considerably upon the rectum. But cancer was negatived by the entire absence of uterine hemorrhage and of vaginal discharge, by the comparatively unimpaired state of her general health, and by the great displacement of the bladder to one side, and of the uterus to the other—a condition which, so far as my experience goes, is not met with in cancer of the fundus uteri.

Thus the diagnosis was brought down to a question between fibroid of the uterus and ovarian tumour. The reasons for thinking it a fibroid, rather than an ovarian tumour, were the firm hard texture, the absence of any elasticity or fluctuation, the displacement of the uterus in the direction of the tumour, the altered condition of the os and cervix uteri, the enlargement of the cavity of the womb, and the slight degree to which the tumour had risen out of the pelvis. The retention of urine, too, was more in favour of fibroid than of ovarian tumour; for, though ovarian tumours, when retained in the pelvis, have in some instances given rise to retention of urine, dysuria, and other bladder-symptoms, yet there is a great and frequent tendency for fibroids to irritate and mechanically obstruct the bladder. It is even said (West, *Diseases of Women*, p. 289) that retention of urine is occasionally the first symptom of uterine fibroid; and the accuracy of this statement is verified by this case. On the other hand, the elongation of the cavity of the uterus is not at all inconsistent with ovarian tumour, and is commonly stated to be not very unfrequently associated with it.

The reasons for thinking the tumour ovarian, rather than fibroid, were, first and chiefly, the absence of hemorrhage. Hemorrhage being one of the most characteristic signs of fibroid, its absence is of itself sufficient to lead one to suspect the ovary, rather than the uterus, as the seat of the tumour; but this case shows that the most complete immunity from hemorrhage ought not to influence us too strongly against the possibility of fibroid. Secondly, the one-sided situation of the tumour, the high position of the uterus, the smooth and even surface of the tumour as felt *per rectum*, the apparent solitariness of the tumour (fibroids being generally multiple), and perhaps, also, the age of the patient, were also in favour of ovarian tumour.

Nothing could be inferred from the rate of growth of the tumour, since nothing wrong was suspected until the first attack of retention, five months before admission. One means towards a more positive diagnosis was purposely withheld, until after the approaching catamenial period had passed ; and very fortunately, as the case terminated, this was so. I refer to puncturing with the aspirator. This, by yielding a negative result, would have been another factor in favour of fibroid, and would doubtless have clinched the diagnosis.

After thus establishing the non-cystic nature of the tumour, no treatment could have offered any prospect of permanent or real relief. Ergot, which has been found useful in some cases, would have been tried, but one cannot think with much if any good result. Even if an exploratory abdominal section had been ventured upon, the operation must have been abandoned, owing to the firm connections of the tumour, and the way in which it was wedged into the pelvis. The patient, therefore, would have been doomed to a life of misery, had not an acute intercurrent disease mercifully carried her off. .

The attack of peritonitis was, at the outset, quite local, beginning in the left iliac fossa, *i. e.*, the situation of the fulness felt at the time of her admission. From this it spread over the whole abdomen. As the attack followed immediately upon a catamenial period—indeed, commenced before the period was quite over—it was supposed to have been excited by inflammation of the left ovary ; and on the hypothesis that the tumour was ovarian, it was thought that the whole, or a part of the cyst had suppurated (Case by M. Nonat : Bernutz and Goupil, vol. ii. p. 145)—suppuration being indicated by the variable temperature and repeated rigors. Still, on the other hypothesis, it had to be borne in mind that fibroids of the uterus may set up fatal purulent peritonitis without the ovaries, Fallopian tubes, or vagina being affected. (Case by Bernutz and Goupil in *Diseases of Women*, vol. ii. p. 156.)

The immediate cause of the peritonitis was doubtless the extension of inflammation from the ovary, or along the Fallopian tubes to their fimbriated ends ; whilst the cause of the abscess in the ovary (itself a rare condition), and of the suppuration in the Fallopian tubes, as well as of the dilatation of the ureters and the acute inflammation of the kidneys is to be looked for, I think, in the irritation, displacement, and compression exercised upon these various structures by the uterine tumour.—*British Medical Journal*, May 21, 1881.

MONTHLY ABSTRACT.

Anatomy and Physiology.

On the Sense of Light and the Sense of Colour.

Dr. CHARPENTIER details some interesting physiological experiments (*Archives d'Ophthalmologie*, Dec. 1880) on the perception of light as distinct from that of colour. In these researches he used an instrument devised by himself (figured in Wecker's and Landolt's *Ophthalmologie*, tome 1, p. 530), which enabled him to measure exactly the amount of light required to excite respectively luminous or chromatic sensibility in various portions of the retina. He found that all coloured light, however simple in composition, if gradually augmented above zero, first of all produces a sensation of mere luminosity, and only subsequently one of colour. The chromatic sensation is at first ill-defined, and does not become distinct and definite until the light has assumed a certain intensity, which varies with its nature and the portion of retina affected. The luminous sensation is separated from the chromatic by a larger interval, in proportion as the region of the retina affected is distant from the yellow spot. The sensation of white is due to the neutralization of two or more chromatic sensations, owing to which neutralization the sensation of luminosity, which is generally masked, reappears and predominates. A certain quantity of light is lost in overcoming the inertia of the ocular apparatus. This is shown by the fact that, after a sojourn in darkness, a certain minimum intensity of light is required for perception, but this minimum becomes considerably reduced after the retina has been stimulated by previous excitation. On the other hand, the amount of light required to stimulate the chromatic sense remains the same in each case. Chromatic perception is not increased or diminished by the addition of white light; for although in any given case certain coloured rays have been necessarily added, these rays are neutralized by the complementary colour rays existing in white light.—*Lond. Med. Record*, April 15, 1881.

Materia Medica and Therapeutics.

On Blisters.

In a communication to the Société de Thérapeutique, published in the *Revue de Thérapeutique*, p. 152, M. CORNIL states that, when cantharides is administered to an animal—for instance, to a rabbit—either by the mouth or by absorption through the skin, as when a blister is applied, poisoning is produced, characterized by cystitis, nephritis, and inflammatory lesions in the liver and in the lung. In fact, twenty minutes after the cantharides is injected, the following lesions are found in the cavity of a glomerule of the kidney. A large number of white globules are found between the envelope of Miller's capsule and the vascular bundle which composes the Malpighian glomerulus. In addition a granular exudation is found in the uriniferous tubes, which fills and obliterates their calibre. At the end of an hour, the lesions are characterized by the proliferation of the cells, which by mutual pressure become irregularly flattened. There exists, therefore, a true catarrh of the uriniferous tubes. In the bladder the disturbances are nearly of the same kind, but the lesions are superficial ; the irritating principle of the cantharides has acted directly on the internal surface of the bladder. In the lung, the small bronchial tubes are filled with white pus-corpuscles; these lesions, which indicate inflammation of the mucous membrane, are found in all the parenchyma, and are the consequences of the irritating principle, the cantha- ridine, carried into all the organs by the circulation. The same kind of lesion of its mucous membrane is found in the larynx and in the trachea. If a blister be left on sufficiently long, the same lesions are obtained. M. Cornil therefore thinks that large blisters applied to the chest, and left on from fifteen to twenty hours, are more injurious than useful. By this method, not only are cystitis and nephritis brought on, but inflammation of the bronchi and of the pulmonary paren- chyma itself. He has therefore arrived at the conclusion that, in order that blisters should not be injurious, they should not be allowed to remain on more than from three to four hours.—*British Med. Journal*, April 30, 1881.

—

The Action of Tannin on the Animal Body.

Among the oldest known and most frequently employed medicines are to be reckoned the astringents; but pharmacological investigations have been very seldom directed towards them. In a recent paper (Virchow's *Archiv*, Band lxxxi. p. 74), LEWIN furnishes a very exhaustive account of one of the most im- portant of these, namely, tannin. The officinal preparation of this drug being by no means pure, its separation for the observations detailed in this paper was conducted by means of Löwe's method, which is based upon the property of con- centrated solution of common salt to precipitate only tannic acid, and not gallic acid ; the pure tannic acid being subsequently separated from the chloride of so- dium by means of acetic ether. Gallic acid has the property of precipitating albumen and albuminous substances from their solutions. These precipitates, in- soluble in water, dissolve in an excess of albumen or of gelatine solution, in dilute lactic acid, in carbonic acid, and in caustic alkalies. Tannin loses its property of coagulating albuminous bodies, when it is mixed with alkali, to the point of weak alkaline reaction. The alkaline tannate, so produced, has no longer an action upon albumen, but still possesses the characteristic astringent taste of unaltered tannin. The artificial digestion of albumen is not interfered with by the presence of tan- nin, which substance neither acts upon the peptone during its formation, or sub- sequently to that stage of digestion, nor does it precipitate pepsin. This be- haviour is to be ascribed to the presence of free hydrochloric acid.

When a few drops of solution of tannin are added to blood, there forms, at the point of contact of the two fluids, a precipitate of tannin-albuminate, which dis- appears when the fluids are shaken up. If more of the tannin be added, a point is at length reached when the precipitate is no longer redissolved. This point corresponds to the disappearance of the alkaline, and the commencement of the acid reaction. Not only the albumen, but also the colouring matter of the blood, becomes altered on the addition of tannin ; the blood showing, when examined with the spectroscope, the absorption-bands of acid hæmatin.

The antiputrefactive action of tannin was long questioned, since the substance itself in solution, after long keeping, decomposes. But it seems clear that such an action does exist. When a solution is added to putrid blood, the disagreeable odour disappears after a few minutes, and the mixture may be kept in an open vessel, exposed to the air for weeks, without undergoing farther decomposition. This action seems to depend upon the strong chemical affinity of tannin for albu- minous substances, whereby the organisms of putrefaction are themselves seized upon, and their development hindered.

The outward application of tannin to the various tissues alters their physical characters. The connective tissue shrinks together and hardens. The muscles are so affected that their primary and secondary stretching are absolutely less than that of normal muscle; while, when the weight is removed, they return more exactly to their original length. This action upon the muscles takes place in the frog, whether the tannin be injected into the peritoneal cavity, or into the lymph-sac. The cause of this distant astringent action, after the subcutaneous injection of tannin, depends upon two factors: firstly, upon the energetic hygroscopic character of tannin, the abstraction of the water from the tissues rendering their cohesion and elasticity greater; and, secondly, and still more importantly, upon the power of tannin to take up oxygen. The alkaline tannate abstracts oxygen from the tissues, and thereby gives rise to the phenomena pertaining to deficient oxygeneration, which, in the muscles of the frog, correspond exactly with the conditions to which the subcutaneous injection of tannin gives rise.

The absorption of tannin into the body takes place in the following manner: When the solution enters the stomach, it does not affect the peptones present, since they are in a solution of hydrochloric acid; but the fluid unaltered albuminous bodies are changed into a tannate of albumen, provided that there is no excess of dissolved albumen, or of lactic acid. The albuminate of tannin, if it be formed, becomes digested, and the tannin passes into the vessels. As it enters in small quantities, it dissolves in the alkaline blood or lymph, and circulates as a soluble alkaline tannate.

The following are some of the practical suggestions in regard to the administration of tannin, which may be derived from the observations contained in this very able paper: It is to be borne in mind that, when tannin enters the stomach, it forms with albumen precipitates, which, although soluble, require for their solution the presence of certain definite conditions (for example, excess of albumen, of lactic or of hydrochloric acid). If the albuminate of tannin be not soon dissolved, or if the tannin be given in the form of a powder, the solid particles adhere to the gastric walls, and produce extensive irritation of the mucous membrane. This occasions the most uncomfortable sensations, feeling of weight and heat in the epigastrium, loss of appetite, etc. In order to avoid this, the tannin should be given, either as a solution of albuminate of tannin, or as alkaline tannate. In any case, it should not be administered in the form of a powder. A solution of albuminate of tannin can be readily prepared in any concentration, if a solution of albumen be added to tannin dissolved in a little water, and the resulting precipitate redissolved by excess of albumen. Absorption is still more readily accomplished when the drug is given in the form of an alkaline solution, by the addition of sufficient carbonate of soda to render the reaction alkaline. Or, finally, a third rational method of administration consists in precipitating the solution of tannin by means of albumen, and adding sufficient carbonate of soda to dissolve the precipitate.—*London Med. Record*, May 15, 1881.

Medicine.

Tuberculosis and Scrofula.

In a recent communication to the Société Médicale des Hôpitaux de Paris, M. GRANCHER discussed this well worn, but ever interesting subject by the light of recent researches. He considers as primordial the vitreous degeneration, which Virchow attributes to reciprocal pressure of the cells, and Cornil to the primary obliteration of bloodvessels, but which he believes to be produced by a "dystrophy," attacking even the embryonal elements. The caseous nucleus, the giant-cell of tubercle, the lesion of caseous pneumonia, are formed on the same type as the granular. An inflammatory process, accompanied by exudation of fibrin, is developed round the already existing tubercular giant-cell. The microscopic or Köster's tubercle, or the elementary tubercle of Malassez, and the follicular tubercle of Charcot, are essentially characterized by having a giant-cell in the centre, upon which is a vitreous layer of epithelioid cells, and a second layer of embryonal cells. In this anatomico-pathological prototype are two elements, one fibrous and capable of hardening, the other capable of caseation. The characteristic of tuberculosis is a fibro-caseous neoplasm, of a nodular form, tending to become caseous rather than to become hard.

M. Grancher disputed the strange opinion that scrofula is nothing but a local tuberculosis, because the elementary tubercle of Köster is found there; but this never exists there except in an embryonic state; in tuberculosis only, it develops till it arrives at the adult stage, or that of the granulation type. If the giant-cell were sufficient to characterize tubercle, as Schüppel says, then not only scrofula, but even syphilis, and certain sarcomata, would be classed together. Between scrofula and tuberculosis there is only a slight relationship.

In the discussion which followed, M. Féréol remarked that M. Grancher would be more logical in defending the doctrine of the fusion of the two diatheses, as suggested by Friedländer in 1871, and adopted by Charcot in 1877. M. Brissaud, he said, frequently found even the granulation type in strumous deposits. Since scrofulous deposits engender miliary tubercles, why not admit that scrofula engenders tuberculosis? Certainly clinical experience was not opposed to that being the case. Tuberculosis would then be, only, a particular type of scrofula. M. Labbé insisted on the fact that frequently simple inflammations terminate in tubercle, apart from any apparent diathesis, especially after mental emotion, excess, and dyspepsia. M. Cornil has, far from being an unicist, considered that diseases differing in cause and their symptoms can give rise, at a certain period of their evolution, to similar anatomical productions. Tuberculosis is characterized by a constant neoplasm—tuberculosis granulation—of variable aspect according to its period of development, and by the general appearance of the lesions, their seat, and their evolution. Scrofula embraces, on the other hand, a series of very different morbid conditions, to which are added acute or chronic inflammations, of which the oldest tend to caseation, a termination which is also seen in syphilis, in sarcoma, and in chronic pleurisy. M. Grancher had insisted on the pathological anatomy of lupus being similar to that regarded by most as scrofula, in which, however, one finds again the primitive tubercle or tuberculous follicle, never the typical tuberculous granulation; but this last is not found in tuberculosis of the mucous surfaces. The symptoms, course, and evolution suffice to separate lupus from tuberculosis. A single morbid element cannot characterize a disease. Thus, the organism found in diphtheria resembles those of quite different affections; the false membranes of inflamed mucous patches, from which syphilis may be inoculated, are histologically similar to those of croup. M. Damaschino admitted the two diatheses. Scrofula is, as it were, a soil favourable for the growth of tuberculosis equally with other conditions of debility. M. Thaon was an unicist; he admitted the identity of scrofulous and tuberculous glands. Pulmonary tuberculosis, he said, is only scrofula of the lungs; but there is, as it were, an antagonism between the cutaneous or glandular manifestations of scrofula and the manifestations in the lungs. Scrofula, a diathesis of feebleness, attacks the points of least resistance. It is uncommon in the lungs of the mountaineer, fortified by, as M. Thaon said, "gymnastique respiratoire." Tubercle is a special not a specific inflammation, in miliary or voluminous foci, tending to caseation or to fibrous degeneration, and the evolution of which is accompanied by fever. Nothing analogous to this is to be found in tumours, such as sarcoma or carcinoma. M. Labbé pointed out that Laennec regarded tuberculosis as a result of scrofula, the tendency of all debilitating causes, a malady acquired, and not diathetic. Scrofula, a constitutional vice, like all physiological debility, engenders, or at least predisposes to, tuberculosis. Pulmonary inflammation, narrowing of the pulmonary artery, aneurism of the thoracic aorta, and deformity arising from rickets, lung-disease produced by dust, etc., act in the same way. Tuberculosis is not a specific malady; the existence of tubercle gives it, however, a special character. Heredity of tuberculosis is not so undeniable as that of gout. M. Ferrand did not consider tuberculosis as a diathesis; equally with scrofula and with gout, it is a lesion appearing late in certain diatheses, but not special to any one of them. He did not deny, nevertheless, that it may be developed independently of any diathetic or constitutional disease. A scrofulous or a gouty person may become affected with tubercle, but a tuberculous person does not become scrofulous or gouty. Phthisis of scrofulous origin specially affects the mucous surfaces, and undergoes caseation. Consumption, in gouty persons, attacks the serous membranes, and develops into fibrous tissue. Pathological anatomy is not, at present, able to trace any natural affinity between tubercle and syphilis or glanders, any more than between these two last-named diseases. M. Rendu said that he was dualistic in his views, because, in his opinion, the scrofulous tumour does not exist, because the tuberculous follicle does not characterize tuberculosis, and because the giant-cell is not peculiar to tuberculosis. There is nothing characteristic in scrofula, unless it be "torpidity;" it is quite the contrary, however, in tuberculosis, to such an extent as to call to mind an infective, or even a parasitie, disease. This is more especially the case when one considers that it presents, as it were, foci of contagion of epidemic concentration; that its inoculation seems possible; and that it is frequently acquired. Regarding the points of resemblance between scrofula and tubercle, it can only be said that scrofula makes the body a favourable soil for the development of tubercular germs.—*British Med. Journal*, April 23, 1881.

Treatment of Typhoid Fever.

Dr. HALLOPEAU (*L'Union Médical*, March 21) has been making a study of the treatment of typhoid fever by calomel, salicylate of soda, and sulphate of quinine. He has communicated his results to the Société Médicale des Hôpitaux, and his conclusions are as follows: 1. Salicylate of soda and sulphate of quinine generally exercise an appreciable action over the temperature of typhoid fever patients. 2. The action of salicylate of soda is not habitually continuous; at the end of two or three days, even when fresh doses are administered, new rises of the thermometrical curve are observed. As a rule, however, they only attain the initial figures in a temporary manner, and the centre of the thermic oscillations generally remains depressed. 3. Two grammes (31 grains) of salicylate of soda are, as a rule, sufficient to produce an antipyretic action. 4. In doses of 4 grammes and upwards, this drug seems capable of itself producing symptoms, and especially of increasing the dyspnœa, augmenting pulmonary congestion, favouring the tendency to hemorrhage, and sometimes inducing delirium and restlessness. 5. These accidents may be avoided if the salicylate of soda be given in doses of two grammes only, if it be not prescribed for more than three days successively, and if contra-indications be duly observed. 6. These contra-indications are especially thoracic complications, serious cerebral symptoms, and hemorrhage. 7. By prescribing sulphate of quinine and salicylate of soda alternately, the centre of the thermic oscillations is most frequently maintained at a comparatively low figure. The pernicious effects of excessive temperature are thus avoided, and it would seem at the same time that a favourable action is exerted over the course of the disease. In this way, an equally powerful control is obtained over the temperature as with cold baths, without exposing the patients to the same accidents. 8. The antipyretic action of sulphate of quinine is produced even when that of salicylate of soda seems to be exhausted, and *vice versâ*. The therapeutic effect of one is added to that of the other, but not their toxic effects. 9. Cold lotions, cold applications to the abdomen, and cold enemata, may be advantageously employed as accessories at the same time as the antipyretics. 10. In cases when hyperpyrexia persists, notwithstanding this treatment, the daily doses of sulphate of quinine may be increased to one and a half, two, or even three grammes. Four grammes of salicylate of soda may in like manner be given, provided that the dose be repeated not oftener than every second or third day, and that it be ascertained that the medicine is being eliminated by the urine.—*London Med. Record*, April 15, 1881.

——

Gangrene of the Vulva in Typhoid.

Prof. SPILLMANN, of Nancy, terminates an article in the *Archives Générales* of March with the following conclusions: 1. Gangrene of the female genital organs, although rare, nevertheless constitutes one of the most serious complications of typhoid fever. 2. It may be manifested at first in the form of simple œdema, of an inflammation of the vulvo-vaginal glands, or of small superficial eschars confined to the labia. 3. In bad cases the gangrene appears in the humid form, extends over the entire vulva, and may even invade the vagina, the thighs, and the trunk. It often, under these conditions, terminates with symptoms of gangrenous infection. 4. The gangrene may also be confined to the vagina, and then often remains unperceived, and may, at a later period, give rise to stricture of the vagina, with retention of the menstrual discharge. 5. Vulvar gangrene is sometimes induced by a true local infection, and is then propagated by means of erosions or ulcerations of the vulva, or of excretory ducts of the vulvo-vaginal glands. 6. Syphilitic lesions of the vulva seem to easily undergo transformation into gangrenous centres when the patient is attacked by typhoid fever. 7. Gangrene of the vulva is always a serious complication, and in bad cases it proves fatal in two cases out of three. 8. The possibility of such complication should always be borne in mind; and hygienic precautions should always be put in force for all women who become the subjects of typhoid fever. In the adynamic forms of the disease a minute examination (*toilette minutieuse*) should be made daily. 9. Local antiseptic treatment should be put into force from the commencement of the complication. 10. The cicatrization of the wounds should be attentively watched.—*Med. Times and Gazette*, April 23, 1881.

——

Sprue.

There are a multitude of diseases peculiar to tropical and subtropical countries to which the inhabitants are liable, and which foreigners may acquire when exposed to the corresponding morbid causes. There is another class of diseases peculiar to those countries, attacking foreigners, and but seldom, if ever, affecting the natives. One of the latter, known in India and well known in Java, where it goes by the name of sprue, has hitherto received little specific notice from medical writers, though, from its extreme fatality, it deserves careful study and attention. Sprue is defined by Dr. PATRICK MANSON, of Amoy, who has devoted much attention to it, as an extremely chronic and insidious disease peculiar.

to warm climates, the principal symptoms of which are referable (1) to a remitting inflammation of the mucous membrane of the mouth and alimentary canal generally; (2) to diarrhœa and irregular action of the bowels; (3) to anæmia and general atrophy. Great wasting accompanies it, altogether out of proportion to the amount of diarrhœa. The victims have all a withered shrunken appearance. When the disease is of some standing, the patient is feeble, irritable, incapable of much mental effort, and anæmic. It is exceedingly insidious in its onset, and very slow in its progress. Dr. Manson has watched a case for several years. This chronicity is exceedingly characteristic; the patient can seldom say exactly when his disease began, nor, if interrogated from time to time, during its progress, can he say positively he is better or worse. It is only when comparison is made between the condition and weight of the patient at dates widely apart that the gradual and sure progress of the disease can be appreciated. The prognosis in a well-marked case must be grave indeed, unless the sufferer be speedily removed to a colder and more temperate climate. According to Dr. Manson's experience, so long as the patient remains under the conditions in which his disease was acquired, medicine and dietary, although they may do much to mitigate suffering, will not effect a cure; and, after one, two, or three years of suffering, there can be only one termination. As to the cause of sprue, Dr. Manson can only ascribe it to the general unsuitability of the European constitution to tropical climates. It is just possible that some accident to the alimentary canal may act as the immediate and exciting cause, and determine the advent of sprue in those constitutionally prepared by the warm climate and other predisposing influences. Nothing seems to have so powerful an influence in aggravating the disease, and therefore, probably, in inducing it, as long-continued high temperature. In his attempts at cure, Dr. Manson has tried many drugs; but they have one and all disappointed him; and he has come to the conclusion that there is only one remedy for sprue (viz., leaving the country); and that, to be effective, should be tried early in the disease. Is not "sprue," after all, a form of "idiopathic" or "progressive pernicious" anæmia, as described by Dr. Coupland in his lectures now in course of publication in this Journal?—*British Med. Journal*, April 2, 1881.

—

Leukæmia.

Professor W. Leube and Dr. R. Fleischer (Virchow's *Archiv*, Band lxxxiii. Heft 1) publish the case of a strong and healthy woman who developed in four months, after a normal confinement, all the symptoms of rapidly advancing anæmia: diminution of strength and nutrition, vertigo, headache, loss of appetite; at the same time pain and swelling occurred in the left lower extremity, which disappeared only after some time. Five weeks later, examination showed only extreme anæmia, with blowing murmurs over the heart, and a small, easily compressible pulse; no obvious enlargement of liver, spleen, or lymphatic glands. The number of the red corpuscles was notably diminished; that of the white corpuscles was absolutely and relatively greatly increased. The left tibia and tarsus were painful on pressure. The left leg was amputated above the knee for rapidly spreading gangrene. The patient died six days later. The necropsy showed intense anæmia of all the internal organs; advanced degeneration of the heart's muscle; no changes of the liver, spleen, or lymphatic glands; a chronic gastric ulcer. Red hyperplastic marrow was found in the bones, with numerous nucleated red blood-corpuscles (transition forms) and numerous marrow-cells. This lymphoid red process in the marrow has been found by Neumann and others in various cachectic conditions, and is regarded as being the consequence of the anæmia. They conclude that either this process must occasionally and exceptionally give rise to a great development of white corpuscles as in this case, or it must be admitted that the source of the leukæmia cannot always be discovered in the usually recognized blood-forming organs, but that the disease must be regarded as an independent blood disorder.—*London Med. Record*, April 15, 1881.

Epidemic of Sweating Sickness.

M. Jules Rochard has reported (*Le Prog. Méd.*, No. 10) to the Academy of Medicine on the epidemic which occurred in the island of Oléron during the summer of 1880. The disease began in June in the village of Allards, and remained there till the 2d July, during which time there were five deaths. In July a death occurred in a neighbouring village, and became the cause of a new epidemic. The disorder was the sweating sickness, characterized by its sudden onset, special eruption, and grave symptoms. The cases became so numerous that the two doctors on the island were unable to fulfil the requirements of the situation, and two naval surgeons were sent to assist. The disease spread all over the island. No medical man was attacked. The contagion seemed to emanate from the corpses; putrefaction set in very early. The coffins were made very badly, and the products of decomposition probably escaped and contaminated the clothes of those who carried the coffins to the cemeteries; hence the frequency of the disease among these. According to Magnel, the temperature is 41 deg., 42 deg., and 43 deg. Cent. (105.8 deg., 107.6 deg., and 109.4 deg. Fahr.), but in this epidemic such high figures were not noticed. At the commencement it reached 39 deg. Cent. (102.2 deg. Fahr.), and remained at about 37 deg. and 38 deg. Cent. (98.6 deg. and 100.4 deg. Fahr.), while in cases where the sweating was suppressed it reached 41 deg. and 42 deg. Cent. The treatment consisted of ipecacuanha in doses of $1\frac{1}{2}$ grammes (22 grains). Refrigeration gave good results in some cases of high temperature.—*London Med. Record*, April 15, 1881.

Antiseptic Treatment of Diphtheria.

Dr. Weise (*Berlin. Klin. Wochenschrift*, 1881, No. 4) advocates the adoption of the following measures in the treatment of diphtheria. He prescribes a solution of salicylic acid, consisting of one part of salicylic acid and twenty-five parts each of rectified spirit and glycerine. This, although a strong solution, is quite free from danger. The spirit, he explains, is used because, in former cases, benefit was derived from the local application of brandy to the throat; and the glycerine is added to obtain a less irritating solution. If the patient can gargle, the author employs a 1 in 300 salicylic acid gargle. Should the attack be very severe, he prefers a solution of benzoate of soda, 1 in 40, or even stronger. Coincidently with this treatment, he gives Hungarian wines. He pays particular attention to maintaining the patient's strength, and orders nourishment to be taken constantly. in the form in which it can be most readily assimilated. He speaks highly of Rosenthal's extract of meat mixed with yolk of egg, but gives solid food if it can be borne. His directions are somewhat as follows: At one o'clock, paint or gargle the throat with the salicylic acid solution; at half-past one, give a teaspoonful of Hungarian wine; at two, the benzoate of soda; at half-past three, a teaspoonful of Hungarian wine; and, during the next half-hour, more gargling with salicylic acid; the treatment being continued night and day without intermission, except that at night the intervals may be an hour, instead of half an hour. If possible, he employs a special apparatus of his own—a combination of tongue depressor and spray. This, by reaching the back of the tongue, admits a thorough examination with the simultaneous application of an antiseptic. In a few seconds, the whole throat can be washed out with the salicylic acid solution ; and this is very necessary in preventing the spread of the disease. Moreover, by this method, bleeding may be speedily arrested. Sometimes he employs a 5 per cent. solution of carbolic acid as a spray.—*British Med. Journal*, May 7, 1881.

—

Transient Albuminuria.

Albuminuria without structural disease of the kidneys—a symptom of considerable interest and of much practical importance—was the subject of a recent communication by Professor BAMBERGER to the *Vienna Gesellschaft der Aerzte*. "Temporary albuminuria" it is often termed, but he suggests that "hæmatogenic" would be a more accurate term as contrasted with "nephrogenic" due to organic renal disease. This functional albuminuria is often trifling in amount, causing merely opalescence of the urine under the ordinary reagents, but the amount of albumen is sometimes considerable. It may occur in individuals apparently in perfect health, as Ultzmann and Leuhe showed, and their observations have since been amply corroborated. It occurs also in febrile conditions, apparently as a result of the blood state, although standing in no direct relation to the pyrexia. Passive congestion and epileptic attacks also cause it. It is found in the convulsions from strychnine poisoning, but never in the abundant watery urine of hysterical states.

What is the origin of this albuminuria? An answer can be best given to this question by asking another. Why is not albumen always present in the urine, since all capillary vessels allow albumen to pass through their walls, and it would be remarkable if those of the kidney were any exception to the rule. Wittich put forward the theory that the urine which passes through the capillaries of the Malpighian bodies is always albuminous, but that its albumen only serves to nourish the epithelial cells of the urinary tubules, and that the albumen which is not thus used passes back into the circulation. This theory presents the difficulty that it assumes that the epithelium of the kidney is nourished in a different way· from all other epithelium, but it has the support of the pathological fact that when the epithelium is removed from the kidney, albuminuria occurs. And yet, on the other hand, intense fatty degeneration of these cells may exist, as, for instance, in phosphorus poisoning, and no albumen may appear in the urine ; while in cases of transient albuminuria, in which, for instance, albumen appears in the urine after an epileptic fit, it is not conceivable that this explanation will suffice. Rosen has brought forward an experimental objection to Wittich's theory. He placed small fragments of fresh kidney in boiling water, and thus fixed the albumen in the position in which it was produced. In diseased kidneys he found coagulated albumen in the urinary tubules, but he never found it there in healthy organs.

Physiologists assert that albumen is retained in the kidneys on account of the pressure-conditions of the circulation; the pressure is sufficient to lead to the transudation of water and saline substances, but not of albumen. It may be asked, however, How does the pressure here differ from that in other capillary vessels? The size of the renal arteries in proportion to the organ, the structure and arrangement of the capillaries, all point to a high blood-pressure in the kidneys, a condition in which substances only slightly filtrable should readily pass through, albumen among them. Heidenhain goes further, and asserts that nothing of the nature of filtration occurs in the kidney, basing his assertion on the relation which the amount of urea bears to the quantity of urine.

Another explanation which has been given is that the epithelial covering of the smallest renal capillaries keeps back the albumen. Mucous membranes only allow the escape of an albuminous fluid when they are denuded of their epithelium. This theory, however, holds good only for the living kidney; albumen passes out of the kidney after death in spite of the epithelium. Moreover, the epithelium is not equally retentive of all varieties of albumen; egg-albumen, for instance, injected into the vessels rapidly passes out in the urine; serum-albumen does not, while the albumen of red blood-corpuscles, the hæmoglobin, rapidly passes out in the urine if the corpuscles are destroyed.

Runberg has asserted that the amount of albumen which passes through animal membranes varies inversely as the pressure; the lower the pressure the greater the amount of albumen. Hence he believes that when albuminuria is not dependent on structural alterations in the kidneys, it is to be ascribed to the diminution of pressure in the Malpighian glomeruli. He thus accounts for the albuminuria of mechanical congestion of the kidney, in which the blood-pressure in the aortic system is commonly much lowered. The diminished quantity of urine in this condition supports this theory, and also the beneficial influence of digitalis as a remedy for the condition. Febrile albuminuria he ascribes to the same mechanism, the lowered blood-pressure from the enfeebled state of the heart. He has not, however, sufficiently distinguished the influence of the two important factors in the circulation, the pressure and the rapidity of the movement of the blood. In order to ascertain afresh the influence of the first of these factors, Bamberger has performed the experiment of stretching two similar membranes (amnion or pericardium) over cylinders, and allowing equal quantities of albuminous fluid to filter through them, with and without the pressure of a layer of oil poured upon the top. In the first experiment he took some pleuritic fluid, which contained 1·174 albumen. He found that in the cylinder in which the pressure was the greater, the absolute quantity filtered and the absolute amount of albumen were greater, but that in both instances the percentage of albumen in the total filtrate was the same. A second experiment with ascitic fluid containing a large amount of albumen gave similar results. Quite recently Gottschall and Hoppe-Seyler have performed similar experiments, and have obtained the same results. Runberg's theory thus also becomes untenable, and there are other experimental objections to it. When the renal arteries are tied the blood-pressure falls considerably, but the kidneys become congested, and blood and albumen at once appear in the urine. Moreover, in febrile states, the albumen often appears a few days after the commencement of the pyrexia, and while the pulse is still full and bounding. Neither an increase nor a diminution of the blood-pressure will alone account for the transudation of albumen. The only other condition to which it can be referred is the retardation of the blood-current. Albumen is slowly filtrable, and may only pass through when it remains for a comparatively long time in contact with the wall of the vessel. The same relation is seen in inflammation, in which first there is a retardation of the blood current, and then the exudation of an albuminous fluid. This, however, is probably not the only factor. The epithelial cells of the Malpighian glomeruli may lose their function without presenting any anatomical alterations—a hypothesis which can be neither established nor disproved. Another factor is the vaso-motor action, consisting in either paralysis of the vaso-constrictors or irritation of the vaso-dilators. By dilatation of the vessels a retardation of the blood current can readily be produced. In this way the origin of the febrile albuminuria can be readily understood, since vaso-motor disturbances are frequent in that condition, apart from any direct relation to the amount of pyrexia. If the whole nervous system, and therefore also the vaso-motor system of the kidneys, is deranged by an epileptic attack, albuminuria may readily rise in the same way. The same explanation—the hypothesis of a slight vaso-motor disturbance—affords also the most ready explanation of the occasional albuminuria of apparently healthy individuals. At the same time, the possibility of chemical changes in the circulating albumen must not be forgotten. Under some conditions albumen is probably formed which behaves in the same manner as egg-albumen or para-globulin, and, unlike serum-albumen, filters easy, and may thus appear in the urine. This fact, indeed, renders it doubtful whether the phenomena are to be explained at all by the mere physical conditions. We know nothing of the reason why the different kinds of albumen are excreted with various degrees of readiness, and whatever condition is the cause of this difference may also, when deranged, be the source of the temporary albuminuria which still constitutes so great an enigma.—*Lancet*, March 19, 1881.

Menière's Disease.

Dr. EDWARD MENIÈRE has just published a memoir on the disease described by his father in 1861. Menière's disease is constituted by three principal symptoms: 1. The noises or whistlings which precede the crisis; 2. The vertigo, accompanied by nausea and vomiting; 3. Deafness, as a rule incurable. The writer of the memoir details at length the treatment of this disease (*La France Méd.*, p. 239), in which he follows the method proposed by Professor Charcot. The patients take after their meals pills composed of 10 centigrammes of sulphate of quinine and 10 centigrammes of fluid extract of cinchona. He thus commences with 30 centigrammes of sulphate of quinine, and goes progressively up to 70 and 80 centigrammes, and even 1 gramme; then he enjoins absolute abstention from it during a fortnight, three weeks, or even a month, but recommences during the first period of a month, giving 40 centigrammes at first setting off. The effect of the quinine is to diminish and cause the vertigo to disappear, and, on the other hand, to modify the deafness. M. Menière does not pretend to formulate a curative treatment of a disease against which all the resources of therapeutics have hitherto been unavailing, but quinine has, at least, the advantage of calming the most troublesome symptoms.—*London Medical Record*, April 15, 1881.

Paralysis of Hands and Feet from Diseases of Nerves.

Dr. T. GRAINGER STEWART reports (*Edinburgh Med. Journal*, April, 1881) three interesting cases, closely resembling one another, the most important clincal features of which were the coexistence of symptoms referable to the sensory, the motor, and trophic functions of the nerves, the localization of the symptoms in the feet and hands, the intensity being greatest at the most distal points, and the affection corresponding to certain districts of the extremities, and not to the distribution-areas of particular nerves; the symptoms depending on a lesion of the nerves themselves, and in his opinion due to a healing of the axis cylinder. Similar cases have been described by Duménil, of Rouen (*Gazette Hebdomadaire*, 1864 and 1866), Bablon (*Ibid.*, Dec. 1864), Eichhorst (Virchow's *Archiv*, Bd. 69), Eisenlohr (*Centralblatt f. Nervenheilkunde*, 1879), Joffroy (*Archives de Physiologie*, vol. vi. p. 172), and Leyden (*Zeitschrift für Klin. Med.* 1880).

Dr. Stewart finds that "from the facts observed in the cases which I have recorded, taken along with those recorded by others, and with some which, looking back, I now regard as examples of this condition, I find data for drawing up a clinical history of the disease, which seems to me quite distinctive. Its commencement is usually acute and attended by more or less fever. While all the functions of the nerves speedily become affected, it is in connection with the sensory functions that the first changes manifest themselves. Sometimes there is acute pain, but oftener a numbness or peculiar tingling sensation in the affected parts, closely resembling the feeling popularly known as sleeping of the limb—a feeling which is more like this from the circumstance that action of the muscles or pressure upon the skin induces the uneasy or painful sensation commonly known as pins and needles. Along with this there is a distinct diminution of sensibility. Touch is felt indistinctly; two points so far removed from one another as to be distinguished in the healthy conditions are no longer distinguished, and the patient may have the greatest difficulty in localizing the impression which he feels. Sensory impressions are conducted slowly, and at the same time contact is felt painful. These feelings may begin simultaneously in the fingers and in the toes, or may affect first the one and then the other. It seems to be usually in both hands and both feet simultaneously, but not necessarily in an equal degree.

To these sensory changes motor symptoms speedily become superadded. At first there is mere paresis, and affecting the most distal parts; but the paresis spreads up the limb from one group of muscles to another, and as it does so the intensity of the process deepens in the parts first affected. The organic reflexes are very rarely affected, although when the disease spreads upwards it is sometimes found that those connected with the bladder, and perhaps the bowel, are involved. The skin reflexes are modified in proportion to the diminution of sensibility in the parts, being sometimes entirely absent, sometimes absent on slight stimulation, but present even in an exaggerated degree when a strong stimulus is applied. The plantar reflex is often altered, while those higher in the body are natural. The tendon reflex, and especially the patellar tendon reflex, appears to be early and completely lost in these cases. Ankle clonus may be present after the patellar tendon reflex is lost. With regard to voluntary motion, it is found that in some of the muscles it is absolutely lost; in others it is diminished to a greater or less extent. Within a week of the commencement of the seizure it may be found that the patient has no power of flexing or extending the toes and fingers, but retains power of movement of the ankles or the wrist. A week or two later these movements also have become lost, and ere long perhaps the legs and arms in their whole extent are absolutely helpless. There is no special interference with the co-ordinating functions. With regard to the reaction of degeneration, I have not been able to satisfy myself in the cases which I have observed.

The vasomotor and trophic changes manifest themselves most distinctly in the muscles which undergo atrophy—much more rapidly than would be the case in simple motor paralysis. The colour and texture of the skin, also, sometimes change from the normal, patches of congestion or of blueness appearing here and there, and glossiness manifesting itself, especially in the fingers. The nutrition of the nails also becomes altered. In several of the cases I have seen a very distinct degree of œdema not referable to any other than a nervous cause. The intelligence is perfect, and sleep is satisfactory except in so far as it may be disturbed by pain. There is no alteration of the condition of the spine or cranium.

The process may take some weeks, or perhaps months, to arrive at its full development. After a time it appears usually to become arrested, but at first no improvement is manifested. Gradually, however, the patient begins to notice some improvement. His pains or uneasy feelings diminish, sensitiveness to impressions increases, and he begins to feel that his power over the muscles is returning. It is in the upper part of the limb that improvement first sets in. It gradually passes downwards, until at length there is complete recovery. The process may occupy a period of from two to six or more months.

The recovery from such a condition as this seems to be most remarkable. It would appear to one examining the lesion as if it must necessarily permanently destroy the nerve ; and yet we must assume that recovery does actually take place, and that in no inconsiderable proportion of the cases. But what is even more remarkable is, that the process may recur in the same individual and in the same parts time after time. I have met with at least one case in which this apparently occurred three successive times within a few years.

In some cases, probably, the disease extends to involve the cord, and perhaps to pass into myelitis.

The superaddition of any acute disease must be regarded as most formidable where this disease exists. But while recovery occurs in a considerable proportion of cases, it is not the invariable result. In some the process induces permanent atrophy of the nerves, with consequent paralysis. In others extension of the disease may take place, and vital nerves or vital nerve centres becoming affected, death must follow. Further observation will show the proportions in which these various results occur.

I have no doubt that it will occur to many of you that probably in this disease we find the means of explanation of cases which we have regarded vaguely as spinal congestion, slight myelitis, or such like ; and I expect that it will prove that cases of this kind are not very uncommon. I, at least, on looking back, can recall some in which I think I should now find the explanation by reference to this process.

If it be true that in some instances fibres of all kinds in mixed nerves may be thus affected, it seems reasonable to believe that in individual mixed nerves either the motor fibres alone, or the sensory fibres alone, might be the seat of change. And if so, we should expect to find in the former a clinical history closely resembling Landry's acute ascending paralysis ; in the latter, certain forms of neuralgia with loss of sensibility.

It remains for me to mark off the clinical history thus sketched from those proper to some other affections with which, at first sight, it might be confounded. It resembles at first sight and in some respects the Acute Ascending Paralysis to which I have just referred, which was first described in 1859 by Dr. Landry. In it there is paralysis commencing at the distal parts and spreading upwards, sometimes terminating in recovery, sometimes extending to vital centres and so proving fatal. In the cases which do prove fatal no lesion has been found. The disease which I am bringing before you to-night differs from it in that it affects the sensory as well as the motor functions, and exhibits well-marked pathological changes. But the processes may, on further examination, turn out to be related to one another in the way I have just suggested. It also very naturally suggests the form of disease which was described in 1853 by Duchenne under the name of General Spinal Paralysis, and which he afterwards spoke of as Anterior Spinal Paralysis, acute and subacute, in which the lesion was more accurately defined by Charcot and Joffroy, and which has been termed by Kussmaul and Erb, Polio-myelitis anterior, by Westphal, Acute Atrophic Spinal Paralysis of adults, and by Eulenberg, Acute and Subacute Spinal Paralysis of adults. In that disease the lesion is situated in the anterior horns of gray matter, and the clinical features are well defined. Commencing generally acutely with some degree of febrile disturbance, there is developed paresis of the limbs, which rapidly passes into paralysis with speedy wasting of the muscles. It spreads from the legs upwards. The same process may occur in the arms ; it may, indeed, begin in the two places simultaneously, gradually advancing in the trunk as the cord becomes more extensively affected. The process may extend to vital structures and prove fatal, or it may become arrested and complete recovery take place, but throughout the course of the disease there is no affection of the sensory functions. Peripheral Paralysis of the kind we are describing differs from it in that it affects the sensory as well as the motor and trophic functions, and that it is so distinctly ascending in the limb it involves, while pathologically the changes are essentially different; and thus, although one of the most careful and distinguished of living workers in neurology, Professor Leyden of Berlin, draws special attention to the resemblance between them, it is yet clear that they are to be readily distinguished from one another.

There should be little tendency to associate this disease with Acute Transverse Myelitis, a malady in which the whole of the strands of the cord are diseased at the same point, for in that disease it commences to manifest itself at once at all points below the seat of disease, and does not spread upwards, as in our malady; moreover, in myelitis there is a marked tendency to alterations of the organic reflexes, to sloughing of skin, alkalinity of urine, and vesical catarrh, none of which occur in the malady we are considering.

Certain forms of diphtheritic paralysis more or less closely resemble the disease under consideration; but they may be readily distinguished by the fact that there is no history of any throat affection, no tendency to paralysis of laryngeal or pharyngeal muscles, nor is the distribution of the malady at all like what is seen in post-diphtheritic cases. It is interesting to remember in this connection that in some cases of diphtheritic paralysis Charcot and Vulpian have found a distinct lesion of the nerves of the affected parts, and that this has been confirmed by others. 'It will be interesting to ascertain how close the resemblance between them may be.

One of the main points of interest in connection with this disease is the light which it appears fitted to throw upon some obscure questions in nervous pathology; among these I may mention Locomotor Ataxia. You are all aware how frequently that disease is heralded by passing nervous attacks of various kinds, sometimes paralytic, affecting one nerve or some particular branch of a nerve, and generally after a time disappearing, but sometimes persisting. Such paralyses may be best explained by assuming them to be due to this disease. But, again, girdle pains often appear as an early symptom, and may be also quite reasonably referred to such a malady, for the girdle pain is usually associated with hyperæsthesia, and while it sometimes entirely disappears, it sometimes also produces a permanent anæsthesia of the region affected. Another very distressing symptom is that which is known as "lightning pains," which may be due to disease of the sensory fibres; and in cases of locomotor ataxia it must have struck many observers how strangely pain, hyperæsthesia, and anæsthesia may come and go in certain parts in a way that seems scarcely explicable unless on the hypothesis of local nerve change. In regard to the eye changes, the temporary and passing amauroses, and other symptoms connected with special sense, I may refer to some facts recorded by Dr. Althaus.[1] Having referred to the optic neuritis as being well known in association with Locomotor Ataxia, he gives cases in which the olfactory and auditory nerves were the seat of disease, resulting in alteration or destruction of the functions of these nerves.

It is interesting to know that while, from clinical considerations, I was led to this view of these symptoms, Dr. Hamilton has been led in the same direction by

---

. [1] Althaus "On the Pathology of Peripheral Nerve Disease," American Journal of the Medical Sciences, 1879.

his pathological observations. It has, indeed, long been known that atrophy of cranial nerves occurs in the course of locomotor ataxia, but what I have brought before you to-night is fitted to clear up our conceptions on the matter.

Another point of practical interest is the light that this may be fitted to throw on the beneficial effects of nerve-stretching. The demonstration of such changes as these may be followed one day by proof that some allied change exists in the axis cylinder of nerves in the cases which are benefited by nerve-stretching. And taking together what we have said regarding locomotor ataxia and this plan of treatment, the thought will naturally occur that we may herein find the explanation of the marvellous results of nerve-stretching recently described as having occurred in that disease.

With regard to treatment I cannot as yet speak very positively. Certainly strychnia seems injurious in the early stage and beneficial in the later, while ergot of rye seems to be useful in the early periods. It remains to be seen whether nerve-stretching is applicable or not at any stage. Many remedies may be useful for relieving pain—quinine, salicylic acid, salicylate of soda, morphia. During the period of advance the patient should be kept at rest. When the acute stage has passed, friction, electricity, passive and then active exercise, should be carefully tried.

———

Histology of Spinal Paralysis of Children and Progressive Muscular Atrophy.

MM. ROGER and DAMASCHINO (*Revue de Méd.*, Feb. 1881) contribute an exhaustive paper on this subject, and from abundant evidence arrive at the following conclusions. 1. The characteristic alteration in infantile paralysis is a spinal lesion, causing atrophy of nerves and muscles. 2. Its seat is in the anterior part of the gray matter, and it shows itself as softened patches. 3. The softening is of inflammatory origin, and the lesion is, therefore, a myelitis. 4. Progressive muscular atrophy consists essentially in atrophy of the motor-cells, without any patches of inflammatory softening.—*Lond. Med. Record*, April 15, 1881.

———

Iodine as a Specific in Croupous Pneumonia.

Iodine or iodide of potassium is, according to SCHWARZ (*Deutsche Med. Woch.*, Band vii. No. 2, 1881), a specific in simple uncomplicated croupous pneumonia. If given during the first twenty-four to thirty-six hours from the onset of the initial rigor, it will arrest the further progress of the disease. In illustration of this view, ten cases are recorded in which the crisis occurred before the end of the second stage, and in one case at the end of the first day. The following are the formulæ adopted by Schwarz: Tincture of iodine, five drops; water, 120 grammes (4 ounces); one tablespoonful hourly. Iodide of potassium, 1½ grammes (22 grains); simple syrup, 30 grammes (1 ounce); water, 120 grammes (4 ounces); one tablespoonful hourly.—*London Med. Record*, May 15, 1881.

———

Steatosis of the Liver.

Upon this subject, to which Prof. VERNEUIL has frequently alluded, he delivered an interesting clinical lecture, at the Pitié, which is reported in the *Gazette des Hopitaux* (March 3), under the heading "Pathological and Physiological Steatosis of the Liver in Large Suppurations and Pregnancy."

I return, he says, intentionally to the case of a patient about whom I have already spoken to you, and who died six days after I had performed amputation of the thigh. I return to the case because we have found a visceral lesion which I had diagnosed during life, and of which you must take account in deciding the question of operating; indeed, I shall always call your attention to it whenever the opportunity offers itself. This man, whose knee-joint had been opened, and in whom there existed very extensive suppurations, consequent on burns, was condemned beforehand to certain death; and the operation, performed at his reiterated supplication, did him neither good nor harm. Without dwelling on the diseased state of the bloodvessels and the commencing fatty degeneration of the heart found at the autopsy, there is to be noted the fatty degeneration of the liver which is the result of the existence of vast suppurations. Whenever, in fact, you see a patient who has been long in the hospital, a prey to constant and abundant suppuration, seized at a given moment with intense diarrhœa which is not of a renal origin (that is, if no anterior lesion of the kidneys has existed), you may boldly pronounce it of hepatic origin. More than this, if the diarrhœa becomes complicated with œdema of the lower extremities, when there is no disease of the heart or kidneys, this œdematous condition is an additional sign of the hepatic lesion.

I may refer to another patient in the hospital, who is in the same condition as the other, and who in all probability will shortly die. This woman, still strong and vigorous prior to her last confinement, entered the hospital six weeks after that had taken place, with symptoms which were at first considered to be due to phlegmon of the iliac fossa, but which eventually proved to be a deep-seated, ossifluent abscess proceeding from the hip-joint. As in the former case, this woman became pale and wan; she has lost her appetite; both her legs are œdematous; and for some days past she has suffered from an invincible diarrhœa. At the same time the urine exhibits no alteration, and the heart is healthy; and there certainly is here steatosis of the liver, which, on the one hand, is the result of prolonged suppuration, and, on the other, prevents the wound cicatrizing. The patient will finish by sinking from exhaustion. But, in her case, why and how did this steatosis arise? Pregnancy, as is well known, entails a steatosis of the liver which may be termed natural—a physiological steatosis, which disappears with the cause that produced it. This fact is completely recognized and proved by researches made on the females of mammalia; and this normal phenomenon explains the pyogenic tendency of recently delivered women, similar to that of all individuals having a fatty liver. This patient, then, has retained her physiological steatosis—a steatosis which later on became pathological, and which has continued to increase daily since the formation of the abscess, and the suppuration to which this has given rise. This patient will certainly succumb to this fatty degeneration of the liver, whether she dies from exhaustion and famine, or is carried off by some complication supervening at a later period. Such complications in steatosis of the liver most frequently are met with in the serous membranes, which have a great tendency to become implicated, whether it be the pleura or, more probably in this case, the peritoneum.

After recapitulating the phenomena of the two cases in the order of filiation, which is always observed in such, Prof. Verneuil observes that the lesson to be drawn from facts now so well established is to operate as seldom as possible on patients who are subjects of steatosis of the liver, although this is not a formal contra-indication in every case, the exception confirming the rule. Thus, in a case of comminuted fracture of the leg, after every attempt had been made to save the limb in vain, amputation was performed in spite of the well-ascertained existence of steatosis of the liver, which increased proportionally with the suppuration. After the operation, the pus having diminished, the condition of the liver was ameliorated, and the steatosis progressively disappeared as cicatrization advanced.

" Steatosis of the liver thus plays a great part in the results of surgical operations."—*Med. Times and Gaz.*, April 23, 1881.

Surgery.

Treatment of Syphilis by the Subcutaneous Injection of Mercurial Solutions.

M. TERRILLON records (*Bull. et Mém. de la Soc. de Chir.*, 1880, p. 534) the results of experiments made at the Lourcine Hospital with the solution of peptonized mercury recommended by Bamberger. The solution is made as follows : Take a 5 per cent. solution of corrosive sublimate in distilled water, and a solution of chloride of sodium (18 to 20 per cent.) also in distilled water. Dissolve one gramme (15 grains) of flesh peptone in 50 cubic centimetres of distilled water, and filter. To the filtrate add 20 cubic centimetres of the sublimate solution, and afterwards a quantity of the sodium solution (about 15 or 16 cubic centimetres) sufficient to dissolve the precipitate. Pour into a graduated cylindrical vessel, and add distilled water until the whole measures 100 cubic centimetres. Cover the vessel and let it stand for a few days. A whitish flocculent precipitate will form, and must be separated by filtration. The solution will then keep clear for at least three months, and is not precipitated by heat, acids, or alkalies. With this solution M. Terrillon has made 487 injections of 1 cubic centimetre each, containing 1 centigramme (about ⅙th grain) of peptonized mercury ; and 88 injections of about half that quantity. A Pravaz's syringe with vulcanite mounts was used. The dorsal region was preferred for the site of the injection, which was performed slowly, and the diffusion of the solution was assisted by slight kneading with the finger. In no case did abscess occur. The larger dose sometimes caused more or less prolonged pain about the seat of injection ; and in one case, after a large number of injections, partial anæsthesia followed. The smaller dose never caused pain or other inconvenience. Salivation was produced in several cases after four or five injections of 1 centigramme repeated daily ; and examination of the urine some hours after the injection showed the presence of mercury in it. M. Terrillon reserves his report of the therapeutic action of this mode of treatment for a future occasion, as the patients have not yet been sufficiently long under treatment for a trustworthy conclusion to be arrived at.—*London Med. Record*, April 15, 1881.

—

On the Prophylactic Treatment of Ophthalmia Neonatorum.

Profs. CREDÉ, of Leipzig (*Archiv für Gynäkologie*, Bd. xvii. Hft. 1), R. OLSHAUSEN (*Centralblatt für Gynäkologie*, 1881, No. 2), and D. HAUSSMANN, of Berlin (*Ibid.*, No. 4), agree in the necessity of prophylaxis against this disease, in all lying-in institutions, at any rate, but differ somewhat as to details. Credé commenced by treating the eyes of children born of mothers who had a vaginal catarrh, first with 1-60 boracic acid solution, which failed, and then with two per cent. nitrate of silver solution, following this by washing the eyes frequently for twenty-four hours with two per cent. solution of salicylic acid. Encouraged by his success, but finding that the children of apparently healthy mothers occasionally took the disease, he treated all cases, and instead of washing the eyes with salicylic acid, he secured them for twenty-four hours with a bandage wetted with the solution. By these means he reduced his percentage of the occurrence from 13.6 to 0.5. The single case that went to make up this latter percentage was one where the treatment had been omitted. Olshausen, working at the same subject and at the same time, used a one per cent. solution of carbolic acid, which he pencilled over the eyes after birth, and thereby reduced his cases from 12.5 per cent. to 6 per cent. ; but latterly he has commenced treatment before the complete birth of the child, first pencilling the eyelids before they had been opened, and then washing the surface of the eye with a fresh piece of wadding, 1 per cent. carbolic solution being used for both purposes.　In this way he has brought his cases down to 3.6 per cent.　He also observes that the cases that have occurred have been much milder than were those before prophylaxis was practised, never going the length of ulceration of the cornea, and frequently only one eye being affected.　He suggests that a 2 per cent. solution might be more efficacious.　To guard against the infection of a sound from an affected eye, he recommends that the child should always be laid on the affected side, and that its hands should be tied.　The use of a bandage he disapproves of.　Haussmann, while agreeing with the others, recommends the use of antiseptic vaginal injections, especially in malpresentations and operative cases, as there is then a greater chance of the eyes being partially opened during birth.—*Edinburgh Med. Journal*, May, 1881.

Diabetic Cataract.

Dr. GALEZOWSKI contributes to the *Recueil d' Ophthalmologie*, August, 1880, an interesting paper on diabetic cataract, with the history of five cases of successful extraction.　He commences by remarking that diabetic cataracts are of two kinds, viz., those which depend on the presence of sugar in the blood, but more especially in the aqueous humour; and those which, occurring in diabetic subjects of a certain age, are simple coincidents, and do not stand in the relation of cause and effect.　Diabetic cataracts, according to the author, depend on the presence of saccharine matter in the aqueous humour rather than in the blood and tissues, and are more frequently to be met with in plethoric than in thin subjects.　As to the consistency of such cataracts, it will vary according as they are simply senile, or are dependent on the presence of glucose, and no hard and fast line can be laid down.　From his own researches, he is led to suppose that it is more especially at the posterior segment that diabetic cataracts commence; but they also occasionally arise simultaneously in one or more of the anterior and posterior layers, forming a sort of envelope around a transparent nucleus.　As to the prognosis of operation in such cases, it is by no means so desperate as some authors have taught.　A very careful opinion must, however, be given as to the amount of sight to be ultimately recovered, seeing that amblyopia, retinitis, atrophy of the papilla, paralysis of the sixth pair, and other complications, occur even more frequently than cataract in diabetic subjects.　Thus, in 108 diabetic patients suffering from disturbance of vision, only 37 had cataract.　As to the best method of extraction, the author holds that, while for soft cataracts the linear method may be allowed, for the hard, the only proper one is the peripheral flap operation with iridectomy.　The author sums up by saying that the existence of glycosuria should not be looked on as in any way a contraindication, so far as an operative interference is concerned; but that in all cases, both before and during the operation, extreme caution and a strictly antidiabetic regimen are necessary.—*London Med. Record*, April 15, 1881.

Treatment of Detachment of the Retina.

In an interesting paper on the treatment of detached retina, Dr. DIANOUX (*Archives d' Ophthalmologie*, Dec. 1880) insists on the therapeutic value of injections of pilocarpine.　He publishes a series of eight cases, in seven of which the improvement which followed this course of treatment was remarkable.　The first case occurred in a girl aged 21, very myopic, whose left eye was blind, while the right could do little more than distinguish light from darkness.　In the right the retina was almost wholly detached, except a small crescentic portion superiorly.

Within the first week of treatment the improvement was most marked, and continued to increase during nine months subsequently, until, with —10 D, vision was $= \frac{1}{10}$ for distance, and for near objects the finest type was legible. The second case occurred in a man aged 34, the sight of whose left eye had been previously lost by a detachment of the retina. The right eye was subsequently affected, and sight was reduced to counting of fingers at two metres. The inferior and external portion of the field alone remained. Six weeks after treatment vision had improved to $\frac{2}{3}$, and the detachment was limited to the inferior portion of the retina. Within a year vision had become normal; while, although the ophthalmoscope revealed no improvement in the condition of the other eye, vision had in a certain limited degree returned to it. The other cases are in the main similar to the above. In one, however, that of a woman aged 63, the treatment failed completely. In this case, the detachment had existed for three years, and was total, vision being limited to the perception of light. The author, in discussing these results, considers that a series of seven consecutive cases is sufficient to remove all suspicion of a merely fortunate coincidence. In a previous series of thirty detachments, treated by various methods, he had had but one case of cure. The drug acts as a derivative on the eye, probably by means of its action 'on the salivary, lachrymal, and other glands. Its action is rapid and prolonged, as, in all the cases in which it was beneficial, improvement took place before the tenth injection, and continued for months. The injections should be administered so as to keep the patient as long as possible under their influence. They should be used daily during ten or fifteen consecutive days, followed by a period of rest of ten days. This method should be persevered in, until it is evident that a stationary condition has been arrived at. The injections should be in sufficient doses to cause a copious salivation of at least au hour's duration. In most of his cases, the author commenced with six drops of a solution of twenty centigrammes of nitrate of pilocarpine to four grammes of distilled water (= 5 per cent. solution). The injection should be administered on an empty stomach to avoid vomiting.—*London Medical Record*, April 15, 1881.

Desquamative Syphilis of the Tongue.

M. PARROT has recently drawn attention (*Le Progrès Médical*, No. 11), in a clinical lecture with the above title, to an important and somewhat novel form in which hereditary syphilis sometimes manifests itself.

At the tip of the tongue, or along its edges, a small patch, from one to half a millimetre in diameter, shows itself; it is white, rounded in form, and on the surface of it the epithelium is somewhat thicker and whiter than normal. Very shortly, within twenty-four or twenty-six hours, in the place of this milk-like disk there appears a whitish ring circumscribing a red surface—the centre of the patch—where the epithelium is shed, and the papillæ are visible. From this time the affection spreads with remarkable rapidity, either towards the posterior parts of the tongue or towards its centre. The circles transform themselves into crescents or irregularly curved lines, the concavity of which is almost uniformly forward. This modification in the form of the disease is due sometimes to its attacking the borders of the tongue, where its eccentric course is arrested (for it rarely attacks the under surface), and sometimes to the coalescence of several crescents. In the latter case the surfaces which have most recently desquamated are limited by a kind of festoon. Each patch presents certain characteristics which deserve mention. At the periphery and along it there is to be seen a zone of a dead-white colour, which distinctly demarcates both by its colour and elevation between the portions of the tongue which have and those which have not been attacked. As regards the desquamated surface, this is found to vary in different parts; close to the epithelial zone, where the disease is most recent, the tongue is smooth and of a vivid red colour; while farther away this condition, though present in some degree, becomes less and less manifest until it shades off into the healthy appearance.

However rapid or active this affection may be, it is very rare for the entire tongue to be desquamated,by one of these patches; there nearly always remain, either behind or in the centre, some points which are not affected. Nevertheless, before one patch has completed its course, another one shows itself, and takes the same direction. In this way sometimes no less than three desquamating zones may be observed gradually spreading from the tip to the posterior region of the organ, not unlike the concentric successive undulations which may be seen on the surface of water after repeated shock of any kind.

The duration of the disease, considered in its *ensemble* or in any one of its stages, is very difficult to determine. The latter rarely lasts five or six days. The disease may remain dormant for several months, perhaps years, only to break out afresh during some period of activity, or under influences which up to the present time M. Parrot has not been able to formulate.

The diagnosis is simplified by this consideration—that the disease belongs essentially to childhood, though it is impossible to say that it may not also affect adults. The appearances are so peculiar and so typical, at whatever period observed, that it is impossible to mistake the affection after having once or twice attentively watched it. The scarlet fever tongue, in contradistinction, is despoiled of its epithelium very rapidly and over its whole surface. It is of such an intense red that one might think it would bleed if touched. Thrush also gives rise to desquamation, but very irregularly and not at all after the manner, in zones, just described. Besides, a microscopic examination, however rapidly made, would at once discover the spores and scolices of the parasite. Aphthæ cause not only simple desquamation, but also veritable ulcers sometimes, which, however, rarely extend beyond their first limits.

And as regards other affections of the tongue, such as pityriasis, lichen, psoriasis, or opaline syphilitic *plaques*, on which authors are at present far from agreed, and the signs of which are but badly defined, they may be left out of the question, as they are never found among young children. The pathological anatomy of the disease has yet to be determined. M. Renaut, of Lyons, on examining the scrapings of a tongue affected in this way, found a large quantity of epithelial cells, sporules, coagulated mucin, and embryonic cells in abundance. Such an examination, however, could not of course determine either the seat or the nature of the lesion. M. Martin, chief assistant in M. Parrot's laboratory, has examined microscopic sections of three tongues. From these it was found that the epithelium was tumefied and thickened. The cells of the corneous layer were increased in volume, as well as those of the Malpighian layer, which latter is further in a state of active cell-proliferation. There is also a large number of lymphoid corpuscles in the papillæ and adjacent portions of the derma, either scattered or in groups. M. Parrot thinks from these appearances that the derma is the principal and primitive seat of the affection, and that the superficial manifestations—the only ones visible during life—are secondary and consecutive.

As to the nature of the affection, M. Parrot thinks that it is certainly not parasitic, nor due simply to mal-assimilation, but that it is a manifestation of congenital syphilis: for of thirty-one cases, in no less than twenty-eight were the signs of this disease incontestable. Of these thirty-one cases, not less than twenty-two occurred in children of two years and under, while at from two years to six there were only nine. This is exactly the period when congenital syphilis is most active. The disease has manifest analogies with skin syphilis, which occurs in patches, with more or less concentric edges, which desquamates, and not infrequently occurs in successive crops, and which microscopically resembles closely the appearances above described in the tongue.

Why, of the whole buccal cavity, should the tongue alone be attacked? M. Parrot thinks because of its richness in nerves and bloodvessels, and of its great activity—conditions which favour diathetic manifestations. He thinks this affection is not contagions by contact, for there is neither erosion nor secretion, and the majority of the subjects attacked have passed the age when the disease is contagious.

The prognosis and treatment do not call for any special remarks, the indications being general rather than special.—*Med. Times and Gazette*, April 23, 1881.

—

Excision of the Tongue.

Mr. WILLIAM STOKES, of Dublin, at a recent meeting of the Clinical Society of London (*Lancet*, April 30, 1881), read a paper on this subject. He commenced by alluding to the change that surgical opinion has lately undergone in reference to the merits of excision of the tongue, and mentioned the views of Professor Gross and Mr. Collis on this subject. The particulars of six cases in which the writer had excised the tongue were then briefly stated, in which relief from suffering caused by enlargement of the tongue, difficulty of deglutition and articulation, discharge and pain, was obtained in all as an immediate result of the operation. In two of the cases a considerable time—twenty-two months and eighteen months—elapsed without any recurrence of the disease; in two others three months and four months elapsed; in one the patient was lost sight of immediately after the wound healed, and in only one of the cases was almost immediate return of the disease observable. Performing the operation at an early period of the development of the disease, if possible before glandular complications, was strongly advocated, and Sir J. Paget's views stated, as regards the small risk attending the operation.

The question of unilateral or bilateral ablation was then discussed, and the advantages of the latter pointed out. The question of what is the safest and best method of excision was then considered, as well as the two special dangers of the operation, hemorrhage and septic complications. The author observed that removal of the tongue by a cutting operation is not only more liable to be followed by hemorrhage, but also by septic infection, the outcome of which latter is in a large number of cases either pulmonary gangrene or septic pneumonia. These are not observable at all to the same extent in the cases operated on by the écraseur. In proof of this, the statistics of Dr. Scheffer and Mr. Collis were considered, in the former of which it was found that the percentage of mortality from septic causes in the cases operated on by incision reached the startling figures of 60, and in those of Mr. Collis 61. Mr. Barker's cases were also alluded to, but the number of cases (3) operated on by incision, in which there were no septic consequences, was not considered sufficiently large to materially affect the conclusions arrived at.

The disadvantages of certain of the écraseur operations were then pointed out, and the author concluded by describing the method of operating he preferred. He commences by transfixing the cheek at a point corresponding to the last molar of the lower jaw, and makes an incision downwards and forwards towards the angle of the mouth, terminating a few lines above it. All bleeding vessels being secured, and the parts retracted, a ligature is passed through the tip of the tongue to facilitate the drawing forwards of the organ by an assistant. This being done, a straight Liston's needle, armed with a double strand of carbolized silk, is passed through the base of the tongue at a point behind the foramen cæcum. In front of this the chain of an écraseur is passed round the tongue, and the organ gradually severed. This portion of the operation is done very slowly, taking from thirty-five to forty-five minutes. The author never witnessed in any of his cases any secondary hemorrhage, immediate or remote. The wound in the cheek is then brought together by a few points of interrupted suture. The free ends of the strand of silk passed through the base of the tongue are then fastened temporarily, by adhesive plaster, to the side of the cheek or forehead. This double thread, which, in the event of secondary hemorrhage or traction, would be of much assistance in enabling the surgeon to draw forwards the base of the tongue and secure the bleeding vessels, is removed usually on the third or fourth day after the operation. The author believed that, by the use of the écraseur employed in the manner he described, coupled with antiseptic measures during the healing of the wound, the operation is attended with little pain, with the minimum of risk as regards either primary or secondary hemorrhage, or those septic troubles which, after all cutting operations, are so fruitful a means of raising the mortality attending this important operation.

Mr. HEATH said that in this country the tongue was more freely operated upon than was assumed by the author. As to the question of growth after removal, in Mr. Barwell's case there was a considerable increase; and in his own case, where more than half was removed, the stump of the tongue nine years after appeared to have enlarged. The mode of operating was different in different cases. He had now entirely given up the galvanic écraseur, in favour of the chain écraseur, and had never found occasion either to pierce or incise the cheek; for, by bending the écraseur and pulling forwards the tongue, the instrument could be applied far back. Whether a unilateral or bilateral operation should be performed depended on the merits of the case; and he agreed with Mr. Baker that a unilateral operation should be done when necessary; it also enabled the surgeon to examine the two halves of the organ when split in the median line.

Mr. MORRANT BAKER advocated the unilateral method when the disease was sufficiently limited. The median incision avoided the severance of arteries and rendered the detachment of the organ more easy, and it allowed of removal of the other half if the disease were found to encroach near the median line. He thought division of the cheek might be more often done with advantage, especially when the disease extended far back. It allowed also of a better control of hemorrhage. He thought the tongue could not grow after incision, but that an apparent increase in size might result from the contraction of the cicatrix. And as to the retention of speech, it must be remembered that the tongue was not wholly removed when only the portion in front of the foramen cæcum was excised. When completely removed, the mouth has a very different appearance; there is a large hollow in the place of the root of the tongue, and the arches of the palate are approximated. Mr. Gant had recently exhibited a case of nearly entire removal, which had been effected much on the plan adopted by Collis. That patient could hardly articulate. Mr. Baker had not himself found tracheotomy necessary; but in a case where he assisted, tracheotomy had to be done on account of blood flowing into the trachea. A fresh hemorrhage occurred just before the removal of the tongue was completed, and the blood flowed more readily into the trachea than when there was no tube in it. Of course it might be said that the pharynx should have been plugged.

Mr. MacCORMAC pointed out that the trachea itself might have been plugged. He asked Mr. Stokes what measures had been taken to remove the diseased glands, which occurred in some of his cases. Permanent success depended upon this. Any modification of the operation, by splitting the cheek, etc., was justifiable if it facilitated the removal of the diseased tissues in the floor of the mouth. The difficulty of removal of infiltrated glands was considerable, and he should like to know whether the plan followed by Mr. Stokes enabled him to effect their removal. He was surprised to learn that an operation producing a crushed and bruised surface (as did the écraseur) is followed by less risk of septic processes than a simple cut wound. However, the fact remained. He had once or twice divided the tongue without any hemorrhage of moment occurring.

Mr. BARKER said that the list he had furnished to Mr. Stokes somewhat altered the relative rate of mortality after different methods of operation. At University College Hospital, from 1871 to 1879 inclusive, there had been 51 cases of lingual epithelioma, in 34 of which excision was performed. 11 of these cases died in consequence of the operation ; 5 from septic pneumonia, 2 from septic bronchitis, 2 from septicæmia, 1 from pyæmia, and 1 from œdema of the glottis. A large proportion thus died from septic causes. Of these cases 25 were operated on by the galvanic écraseur, with 9 deaths ; 7 by the wire écraseur, and 1 death (from pyæmia) ; 3 by the knife, no deaths ; and 1 by ligature, fatal (from septicæmia). These figures, although few, condemned the galvanic écraseur. Did Mr. Stokes include the galvanic écraseur in his statistics ? Mr. Barker agreed with Mr. MacCormac as to the preference to be given to the knife. The tongue should be split in the median line, and the base cut across, this measure allowing of the ready control of bleeding vessels and of their ligature in the ordinary way, and was far less open to danger of septic trouble than after crushing. Tracheotomy was sometimes called for in cases where much hemorrhage was to be anticipated, or the diseased tissues were of wide extent. The risk from hemorrhage could then be met by plugging the trachea, or by means of a sponge in the pharynx. In three cases he had no trouble in retaining a sponge there ; but if the trachea were to be plugged, Trendelenberg's tampon should be used, care being taken in its inflation, since, as Dr. Semon had shown, its over-inflation caused dyspnœa.

Dr. DOUGLAS POWELL asked Mr. Barker what was meant by " septic" bronchitis and " septic" pneumonia. Did he imply that in such cases there was general septic infection ; and were other organs affected, as in such septicæmia ? If there were only bronchitis or pneumonia, that might possibly be produced by the passage of irritant matter into the bronchi or lung, and would be met by measures preventing such gravitation. .

Mr. T. SMITH asked whether Mr. Stokes made any incision in the sublingual tissues. He believed that only a portion of the tongue could be pulled forward, and that the organ could not be wholly removed unless the subjacent tissues were divided. As he understood it, the septic pneumonia of these cases is produced by blood, etc. trickling down the air-passages. The discharges were more copious after the use of the galvanic écraseur, owing to the slough it produces.

Mr. MARSH, in two or three instances of unilateral excision, had been disappointed with the result, the longitudinal cicatrix holding the tongue down, and the muscles of the remaining half turning it over, a condition giving rise to discomfort. It was plain that opinion was adverse to the galvanic cautery. He was acquainted with cases of secondary hemorrhage following its use, and with one or two of fatal complications By first dividing the muscles attaching the tongue to the lower jaw the base of the epiglottis can be reached. The experience of St. Bartholomew's Hospital did not accord with the statistics given by Mr. Barker.

Dr. COUPLAND urged Mr. Barker to reply to Dr. Powell's question. In postmortem examination of cases of cancer of the tongue, foci of broncho-pneumonia were common, and to be attributed, not to septic infection in the ordinary sense, but to the inhalation of irritant and putrid materials.

Mr. BARKER said the question was an important one. No doubt sometimes there were pulmonary abscesses of truly pyæmic (embolic) kind; but the lungs might be also affected by blood trickling down the trachea during the operation, or fetid discharges similarly passing; also, he believed, by the simple inhalation of very acrid emanations from these wounds. In one instance the house-surgeon and nurse in attendance on the case became affected with sore throat. He did not think these different modes of lung complication should be confused.

Dr. POWELL said the point was one of great practical importance. He had asked if there was any evidence of general blood-poisoning to which the lung disease was secondary. If in all such cases the infection was local, then a remedy might be sought in antiseptic inhalations and in enforcing a prone position, so that the blood and discharges might not pass down the air-passages.

Mr. BARKER said that in one case there was distinctly a general pyæmia, developing long after the operation, with abscesses in the liver and in the vicinity of the kidney, as well as the lung. In the other cases there was no involvement of other organs.

Mr. STOKES in reply said, that he had not included Mr. Barker's statistics in his lists, but he had made a percentage mortality of about sixty in the cases of simple excision by the knife; and he admitted that it was remarkable that there should be apparently less danger from septicæmia in such cases than in those treated by the cautery. He was glad to find Mr. Marsh preferring the bilateral method, and could indorse what he had said as to the greater inconvenience both as regards deglutition and articulation resulting from one-half of the organ being excised than when both sides are removed. He knew of one case where the patient came to have the other half removed because of the difficulty in articulation and because it kept getting between his teeth. He was also pleased to hear Mr. Barker suggesting a preliminary division of the cheek, which greatly facilitates the operation. He had performed division of the sublingual tissues in such cases where the thickening and enlargement of the tongue called for it.

—

Extirpation of the Larynx for Malignant Disease.

Dr. WHIPHAM and Mr. PICK communicated to the Clinical Society of London (*Lancet*, April 2, 1881), a case of extirpation of the larynx for a growth originally affecting the left ventricular band and vocal cord, which subsequently involved the whole larynx.

The patient, a commercial traveller, aged thirty-nine, consulted Dr. Whipham on May 27, 1876, on account of huskiness and a constant desire to "clear the throat," which had come on suddenly and without apparent cause. He had been previously free from all throat affection, and there was no history of syphilis. The man was very nervous, and it was not till June 8 that a view of the larynx was obtained. It was then found that a warty-looking growth rather larger than a pea arose from the anterior part of the left ventricular band and vocal cord. After repeated examination and the passage of brushes into the larynx, with a view of preparing the patient for operation, his nervousness was so far under control on July 29 that two small portions were removed by evulsion, with great relief to the huskiness. The case was constantly under observation, but no further operative interference was required until March 3, 1877, when three pieces of the tumour (which microscopically presented for the most part the appearance of papilloma, but in which at one or two spots there appeared to be a tendency to the production of epithelial cells) were removed by the forceps. The whole of the warty portion was removed at this time, but the vocal cord was thickened generally ; the voice recovered tone to a great extent. Subsequently, however, it was found necessary to apply the forceps to a recurrence of the growth on several occasions—viz., June 16, 1877 ; January 5, 1878 ; March 23, 1878 ; April 19, 1878 ; December 31, 1878.

Early in 1879 the patient had a severe attack of catarrhal laryngitis, and on June 23 in that year he complained of having lately suffered from great dyspnœa, with tenderness over the thyroid cartilage and some external swelling in this situation. He was admitted into St. George's, and in the course of the following six weeks several pieces of the tumour were removed. Again in October, 1879, a large piece was taken from the larynx. By March, 1880, a great change had occurred in the state of the parts ; the growth involved the whole ventricular band and vocal cord ; the left ala of the thyroid cartilage was pushed outwards, and was tender ; dyspnœa being at times urgent. Towards the end of April, the dyspnœa threatened suffocation, and Mr. Pick, after examining the patient, performed tracheotomy, from which the recovery was perfect. During the next six months the disease progressed rapidly, the whole larynx being involved by the middle of October, when a large lobulated mass was felt in the position of the left ala of the thyroid cartilage. In the early part of November, 1880, some hemorrhage occurred through the tube, and at the end of the year he was readmitted into hospital with a view to the performance of some operation. Shortly after his readmission this hemorrhage recurred rather freely.

After consultation with his colleagues on the previous day, Mr. Pick proceeded to extirpate the larynx. Having introduced a tampon canula, Mr. Pick made an incision on January 16, 1881, two and a half inches in length in the median line of the neck, and a second incision at right angles to it across the middle of the thyroid cartilage. On reflecting the skin the growth was found to involve the left ala of the cartilage. The thyroid cartilage was then divided vertically in the median line, and the two halves separated, when the whole larynx was found occluded by the growth. The left ala was removed, and subsequently the right also. The cricoid, with the remains of the arytenoids, were then freed from their attachments, and removed, and finally the epiglottis, which was involved in the disease, was cut away. The wound was carefully explored, and all traces of the growth as far as possible were removed. No vessel required ligature. The operation occupied three-quarters of an hour, and the patient was not much exhausted at its close. The wound was plugged with sponges. Slight hemorrhage occurred after the operation, which was arrested by the introduction of an additional sponge. Nutrient enemata were ordered every four hours, and for the first two days the patient's progress was satisfactory. On the third day, however, his temperature rose to 103.2° F., and his skin became dry ; his pulse ran up to 142. On the fourth day he complained of severe pain about the ensiform cartilage ; his expression became anxious. Rapid exhaustion set in, and he died on the morning of the fifth day after the operation. At the autopsy, right pleurisy and pericarditis, presumably pyæmic, were the chief lesions found.

Among the many points of interest in the case, the following were brought before the notice of the Society : 1st. That for three years the microscopic appearances of the growth were for the most part those of papilloma. 2d. That the duration of the disease (four years) was rather in favour of its having been an innocent growth in the earlier stages, although microscopic examination showed that, even at the onset, there was, in one or two places, a tendency to epithelial proliferation. 3d. That the above facts, and the limitation of the growth to the larynx, were favourable to the success of the operation of extirpation. 4th. That if the operation had been undertaken as soon as the malignant aspect of the discase became manifest, success might have been the result. 5th. That the plan of dividing the thyroid cartilage and removing each half separately is preferable to the method adopted by Dr. Foulis of removing the larynx entire, and for these reasons: (1) that by separation of the alæ a good view of the extent of the disease is obtained at an early period of the operation; and (2) there appears to be less danger of wounding important structures.

Dr. SEMON was gratified that Mr. Pick had found his modification of Trendelenberg's tampon canula useful; and he drew attention to the liability to dyspnœa being caused by over-inflation of the tampon. This occurred in a case of thyrotomy he had recorded, and was attributed by him to pressure upon the tracheal branches of the vagus nerve. Similar attacks occurred in two cases by Dr. Bosworth, and also in one by an Italian surgeon, and another by an English surgeon. The dyspnœa at once ceased on allowing some of the air to escape from the tampon. In Mr. Pick's case there could be no doubt that the disease was epitheliomatous at the time of operation. Extirpation of the larynx was not necessary for papillomata, which could be removed by endo-laryngeal operation or by thyrotomy. He believed that for a simple growth to become malignant there must be a constitutional tendency to malignant degeneration, which would manifest itself whether the growth had been interfered with or not. To show what may be done by persistent endo-laryngeal operation, obviating recourse to the formidable operation of extirpation, he quoted a case recently published in the *Berlin. Klin. Wochenschrift*. It was a child eleven years old, in whom a papillomatous growth had been removed by thyrotomy, sub-thyroid laryngotomy, and thyrotomy again, with invariable recurrence; extirpation of the larynx was advised, but declined; and for six months Dr. Bucher persistently treated it by endo-laryngeal methods, so that he succeeded in completely removing the growth. Fifteen months later the child was free from the growth. In fact, papillomatous disease does not give any indication for extirpation of the larynx.

Mr Pick agreed that extirpation was not called for so long as the growth could be removed by the forceps. In this case it would have been better to remove the ala of the thyroid when the tracheotomy was done, for the growth had already perforated the cartilage.

——

First Endolaryngeal Operation during Anæsthesia.

By this operation, the successful removal of a papilloma laryngis from the larynx of a boy eight years old, under the influence of ether, Prof. SCHNITZLER has shown for the first time that an anæsthetic may in certain circumstances be used during endolaryngeal operations. Prof. Schnitzler describes (*Wiener Med. Presse*, 1880, Nos. 48, 49) the operation as follows: "An assistant seated opposite me took the boy on his knees and held him fast. Ether was then administered. So soon as the boy was narcotized, an assistant opened the mouth with a suitable dilator, drew forward the tongue with a forceps, and, taking hold of it with his left hand, held it so that I could not only pass the laryngoscopic mirror conveniently into the throat, but could also direct into the cavity of the mouth by means of a reflector on my forehead, the light of a gas flame situated on the patient's right. Holding the mirror with the left hand, I introduced the laryngeal polypus forceps with my right, and, notwithstanding the secretion collecting in the throat, I succeeded in rapidly seizing and extirpating the new growth." A slight recurrence was readily removed by the application of caustic.
—*London Med. Record*, April 15, 1881.

Extirpation of the Thyroid Gland.

Dr. RICHELOT (Annales des Malad. de l'Oreille, du Larynx, etc., Dec. 1880) reports a case in which he removed this gland for "colloid goître," associated with dyspnœa, in a woman aged 25. The first commencement of the tumour was at the age of 11 years, with great increase between the ages of 15 and 17. Six years before admission, M. Gosselin employed puncture, with the application of caustics and drainage. The tumour on examination was of the size of half a fist, the central lobe being especially large, hard, and non-fluctuating. There was habitual dyspnœa, with dysphagia and weakness of voice. Whilst the patient was in the hospital there was an attack of subacute thyroiditis, after cessation of which the operation was undertaken. The gland was removed through a curved incision with its convexity downwards, extending to the common carotid on each side, and passing immediately above the sternal notch in the median line. The trachea was found strongly curved to the right and slightly flattened from before backwards, but not softened or degenerated. It was intimately adherent to the gland, from which it was removed from below upwards. There was very little loss of blood during the operation. Silk ligatures, which were first employed, were mostly replaced by catgut ones, and the wound was united by wire sutures. There was severe dysphagia for several days, followed at the end of a week by an attack of bronchitis and tracheitis. The result was complete cicatrization of the wound in the fifth week, accompanied by complete and persistent aphonia.—London Medical Record, April 15, 1881.

Statistics of Mammary Cancer.

Not long ago we drew attention to some of the clinical aspects of cancer of the female breast, and especially as to its causes. We now propose to speak of it as seen in the post-mortem room, and of the metastatic deposits (verified after death) which occur in different organs, and which give to this disease one of its most terrible characteristics. Drs. TÖRÖK and WITTLESHÖFER have recently analyzed the statistics of the Viennese Pathological Institute from 1817 to 1879, including the post-mortem reports of no less than 72,000 bodies. The results of this exceedingly interesting study are given in Langenbeck's Archiv für Klinische Chirurgie, vol. xxv., page 873 et seq., and from it we extract the following as relating to mammary cancer. Of the 72,000 bodies of both sexes, 366 were reported to have died with cancer of the breast, i. e., about ½ per cent. ; of these, in eight cases only was there any doubt as to the diagnosis. Of course the figures can only have a relative value, for it is quite probable that breast-cancer is a more frequent cause of death than appears, seeing that cases, not adapted for operations would not be admitted, while many might be discharged after admission, as incurable cases. In 351 cases the affected side is given—161 cases right, 144 left, and 46 on both sides. Several authors seem to have noticed this fact, and associate it with the more frequent occurrence on the right side of diseases predisposing to cancer, such as puerperal mastitis. Of these cases (366) only three were males. As to the age at which death occurred, the results correspond very nearly with the clinical deductions of Dr. A. Winiwater. Between twenty-five to forty-five years, 29 per cent. ; forty-six to fifty-five years, 34 per cent. ; over fifty years, 37 per cent. From these percentages the authors framed the following rule for practice : The less the age seemed to render an operation advisable, either in consequence of special circumstances, or because of the shock of the operation, the greater the number of cancer deaths at that age. In estimating the value of an operation, attention was given to the occurrence of metastases (i. e., of metastatic deposits) in those who had undergone operation and in those who were not operated on ; for the operation can be considered advantageous then only, when it makes a radical cure of the disease possible. The following figures show how this stands :—

Operated	.	. 184	{ With metastatic deposits .	79	—
			{ Without " " .	—	105
Not operated .	.	182	{ With metastatic deposits .	141	—
			{ Without " " .	—	41
		366		220	146
				366	

It follows, therefore, that operation in 146 cases would have allowed of complete removal of the carcinoma. A further proof of the great value of early operation is afforded; for otherwise there is always a chance that metastases may have occurred.

Coming to the subject of the secondary growths, reference is just made in support of the common belief that in the generalization of cancer, before the outbreak actually takes place, a local proliferation in the immediate neighbourhood of the primary growth frequently occurs, either as a direct outgrowth, or in the form of new deposits. To this local dissemination is shortly added induration of the nearest lymph-glands, through which the cancer-cells first get into the lymph-stream, and thence into the various internal organs through the blood-current. Thus, in considering secondary deposits of cancer, it will be well to divide the subject into three stages—local infection, lymph-gland infection, and infection of internal organs. Local infection is where the cancer spreads by direct continuity. Among the 366 cases, there were 192 of local infection. Of these the skin of thorax 148 times, skin of abdomen 5, pectoral muscles 58, intercostals 22, ribs 29, sternum 20, clavicle 3, anterior mediastinum 4, pleura 25, pericardium 2, peritoneum 2, liver 2. Thus it will be seen that the skin and subcutaneous tissue were affected in about three-quarters of the whole cases ; while the pectoral muscles were much less frequently so. Thus the ribs and the pleura, and in about an equal number of cases, which must be regarded quite as exceptional and accidental, the pericardium and peritoneum. Of the 148 cases above given, in which the skin was affected, there was ulceration in 110 cases, and in 38 there were disseminated nodules near the original growth. If the entire number of cases (192) of local dissemination be considered in its relation to axillary glandular affection, and metastases in internal organs, a very similar percentage is found both in those with ulceration and those in which there was no ulceration : thus there were about 73 per cent. of cases of internal metastases in each group ; while the axillary glandular affection was present in 44 per cent. of the cases with ulceration, and in 59 per cent. of the group without ulceration. If the two groups, however, taken together, be compared with the cases in which there were no secondary local growths, then in only 45 per cent. of the cases were internal metastases present, and only 42.5 per cent. of axillary glandular implication. Thus it would seem that internal metastases are much more frequent in cases where local recurrence takes place, than in cases in which there is no such recurrence. And thus one is led to believe that the cells of a rapidly growing cancer more easily find their way into the blood and lymph currents, and so into internal organs, where they set up metastatic growths, than would the cells of a more purely local, and probably slower-growing, growth.

As regards the affection of the lymph-glands, it has generally been taught that this is the first stage of a general infection ; for, in accordance with our present views, the generalization of cancer takes place through the lymphatics ; hence the absence of glandular affection—other things being equal—is always thought to be a favourable omen. In this particular, however, the results of the present inquiry do not agree, for they show that in the 366 cases, axillary glandular affection was present in only 175 cases, with internal metastases in 57.7 per cent., while in the remaining 191 cases without axillary affection there were 62.3 per cent. of internal metastases. Of course, it is possible that these figures are not accurate ; for the glandular swelling may have been overlooked, or it may accidentally have escaped being recorded. The affection of other glands—cervical and supraclavicular,—as is well known, is very much below that of the axillary glands ; thus, in the cases now under consideration, it is only recorded in 6.3 per cent. of the total. The relative frequency with which internal organs are secondarily affected has been variously given ; but a consideration of the cases before us, when tabulated, points with great force to the lymphatic, respiratory, and digestive tracts as the "seats of election." All organs which are rich in blood and in lymphatics—such as the lungs and liver—are specially predisposed to metastatic disease. The bones, genital organs, and central nervous system are less liable to be infected with secondary deposits. The urinary apparatus is still less often infected ; while the skin and muscular system are much more generally affected by direct continuity of growth. The organs of sense sometimes suffer ; but these cases are extremely rare.

We have only been able to give a brief *résumé* of this interesting paper, to the original of which we would refer the reader who wishes for further details. On the whole, the result of this post-mortem research tends to confirm the conclusions which have gradually been arrived at from the many clinical studies on the subject that have been made ; and on this if on no other ground it is extremely interesting.—*Med. Times and Gazette*, March 26, 1881.

—

Final Results of Operations for the Radical Cure of Hernia.

BRAUN communicates (*Berl. Klin. Woch.* Nos. 4, 5) the results of nineteen such operations performed by Professor Czerny on sixteen patients. The indications for radical operations were : 1, strangulation ; 2, impossibility of keeping up the hernia with a truss ; 3, adhesion of the hernia, preventing its return ; and, 4, fecal fistula in the hernial sac. One case died from pyæmia ; another from convulsions independent of the operation. Ligature of the neck of the sac and suture of the hernial aperture was done in nine inguinal herniæ, and in two omental herniæ in the linea alba. Six inguinal herniæ in adults recurred, but remained small and could be kept up with a truss. One child had remained cured for three years. Partial constriction of the sac with suture of the hernial aperture was done in two children, and in both cases the hernia returned. The hernial aperture alone was closed in two adults and two children. In both adults the hernia recurred, and also another inguinal hernia appeared on the other side. The children remained cured nineteen and thirty-four months. The neck of the sac alone was ligatured in an adult, and a small local recurrence took place.— *London Med. Record*, May 15, 1881.

—

Treatment of Aneurism by the Elastic Bandage.

At a late meeting of the Surgical Society of Dublin, Mr. WHEELER communicated two cases of popliteal aneurism cured by the elastic bandage. The first case was that of a man aged thirty-seven years ; the tumour being as large as a small orange. In that case the blood was "locked" in the aneurismal sac, the limb being bandaged from the foot up to the inferior margin of the aneurism ; and a second bandage was applied, commencing at the superior margin of the tumour. The compression which was made with the elastic bandage was borne for sixty-five minutes; a tourniquet was then applied over the femoral artery, and the bandage gradually loosened. Pulsation returned in the sac, but not so forcibly as before, and the tumour felt more solid. In the evening, the bandage was reapplied in a similar manner, and in a little more than half an hour the compressing band was removed with the same precautions. The pulsation had then ceased; but compression, by means of a tourniquet, was exerted over the femoral artery for some hours after, to moderate the flow of blood. The second case was that of a young gentleman aged twenty-three years. The tumour was in the right popliteal space, and seemed about the size of a walnut. The only history as to its causation was over-exertion when playing cricket. He was of a nervous and excitable temperament. A somewhat similar mode of treatment was adopted in that case. The limb was elevated for a few minutes before applying the bandage, which was done continuously from the foot upwards, but very lightly over the aneurism. On removal of the bandage in forty-five minutes, all pulsation had ceased. The tumour was solid, and in five weeks after had almost completely absorbed.

Mr. TUFNELL said that he had had an opportunity of examining the first case mentioned by Mr. Wheeler, and that the result was most satisfactory. A question arose as to whether it would be safe to adopt that line of treatment in the country, where the surgeon might not have the patient under his immediate observation.

In reply, Mr. WHEELER said that he had been particular to state that, in both cases, he had applied compression to the femoral artery before removing the elastic band, which was, moreover, done very gradually. Lest the sudden return of the blood might damage the recently formed coagulum in the sac, he was of opinion that it would be advisable to compress the main artery, either by digital or instrumental means, before applying the bandage,' for the cure of aneurism in persons advanced in years, in order that the collateral circulation might be somewhat established.—*British Medical Journal*, April 16, 1881.

Iodoform as a Dressing in Tuberculosis of the Bones and Joints.

Dr. MIKULICZ (Vienna) at the recent Congress of German Surgeons read a paper on this subject. Mosetig had published a report of twenty cases, in which, no antiseptic precautions being used, wounds were treated by simply sprinkling iodoform on them, whereby their course was rendered quite aseptic, and the so-called local tuberculosis was healed. In consequence of this, the remedy had been used in Billroth's clinic since the beginning of the year, with a similar striking result. Wounds made in the extirpation of tumours, when sprinkled with iodoform, and covered with a dressing of cotton-wool, healed without secretion, just as wounds heal by granulation under a scab; ichorous sores, under the influence of this remedy, soon lost their putrid smell, and rapidly became clean; tubercular processes also, in the skin, as well as in the joints and bones, were definitely healed by this treatment. The remedy is especially to be recommended in wounds connected with cavities, which come into contact with readily decomposed fluids; as after extirpation of tumours of the pharynx and tongue. In cases of suspected tubercular disease of joints, the injection of an ethereal solution of iodoform appears to be sufficient. If, however, fistulæ be present, the primary focus must be exposed, scooped out, and filled with iodoform; and the fistulæ themselves must be treated with iodoform and gelatine bougies. For injection, an emulsion of iodoform with mucilage of acacia and water is recommended, or a solution of 1 part in 10 of ether, or of 1 in 5 of ether and 5 of oil. Iodoform does not excite any influence at a distance ; so that, while very severe local disorders may be healed, death may occur from tubercle of internal organs. Hence the constant contact of iodoform with the diseased granulating surfaces appears to be necessary. Lupous ulcers heal rapidly under iodoform, without previous scraping. According to the researches of Mikulicz, the antiseptic action of iodoform is small but constant ; this explains the necessity of its constant contact with the granulating surface. Iodoform does not prevent the formation of micrococci in blood and serum, nor of bacteria in Pasteur's fluid. Its active principle is iodine, which in the tissues is transformed into iodides of potassium and sodium. Toxic symptoms occur only in cases of large wounds, and are of short duration. Dr. Gussenbauer could confirm the excellent action of iodoform, which he placed before all other known antiseptics as a means of producing healthy granulations. In nineteen cases of tuberculous affections, he had hitherto met with seven rapid recoveries. In a case of extensive tuberculous ostitis of the tarsus, he had poured a large quantity of iodoform into a cavity in the os calcis, with the result of producing a high aseptic fever, which soon passed off. The case was still under treatment. A similar affection of the carpus was healed, with retention of free action in the joint.—*London Med. Record*, May 15, 1881.

Resections of Joints and Antiseptic Dressings.

In a recently published memoir (*Revue Mensuelle de Méd. et de Chir.*, No. 12, 1880) M. OLLIER points out in the first place that the value of the antiseptic method in resections of joints varies according to the nature of the indications for the operation. The category of what are called orthopædic resections, the sole object of which operations is the restoration of the form and function of an anchylosed joint, has profited the most from antiseptic practice. In recent times, and since the introduction of the antiseptic method, the indications for operation on deformed joints and distorted bones have multiplied to such an extent that this chapter of surgery, M. Ollier states, requires now to be wholly rewritten. With regard to the utility of antiseptic dressings, on the other hand, in cases of traumatic and pathological resections, it is necessary, in order to appreciate this, to distinguish whether such operations are performed for suppurative or for non-suppurative lesions. In the class of non-suppurative lesions, comprising recent articular fractures, plastic osteo-arthritis of rheumatic or traumatic origin, and neoplastic affections, the antiseptic method can be applied with almost as much advantage as in the category of orthopædic resections. In cases, however, of chronic inflammatory lesion with suppuration, the presence of numerous fistulæ, and the formation of fungoid tissue within the joint and along the fistulous tracks, the case is different, and the surgeon cannot obtain complete immediate reunion after resection, and has, during the after-treatment, to deal always with more or less abundant suppuration. Still, in such cases, this suppuration is considerably diminished by carbolized dressings, and in all kinds of traumatic and pathological resections, antiseptic methods, according to M. Ollier, are imperiously demanded.

The antiseptic method, whilst it has extended the range of operative surgery in one region of articular and osseous lesions, has contracted its application in another. As this method prevents suppuration after an orthopædic or a primary traumatic resection, so also will it act after an accidental wound into a joint with fracture of the articular extremities of the long bones, and thus prevent the complication which alone indicates resection in many of such cases. In many traumatic lesions of this kind, antiseptic cleansing of the wound, and the removal of detached splinters will, it is stated, suffice for the preservation of the limb ; and in others, a more or less extensive removal of fragments will replace a true resection. Thus the antiseptic treatment has reduced very much the number of primary traumatic resections, and especially those resections called by M. Ollier preventive, because they have been practised with the view of preventing the dangers to which formerly the subject of a contused wound of a large joint was always exposed.

During six months of the last year, M. Ollier, applying exclusively Lister's method of antiseptic dressing, performed seventeen resections of large joints, one resection of a pseudarthrosis, and two operations for osteotomy. In all these cases, the patients, so far as concerned the immediate result of the operative treatment, recovered without the occurrence of any infectious complications. M. Ollier, deprecating any desire to exaggerate the merits of Lister's antiseptic method, states that, in comparing this series of cases with those previously observed by him, he is compelled to recognize the fact that in the Hôtel-Dieu of Lyons he has never had a series so invariably satisfactory, with regard both to the simplicity of the processes of cicatrization and to the final result. Through comparison of a series of cases of any operation treated with Lister's dressing with analogous series of cases treated by other antiseptic methods, M. Ollier has been led to give the preference to the former. During the last four years he has performed resection of the elbow in thirty-two cases, in all of which the patients recovered. In nine only of these cases was Lister's dressing applied. In some the wound was uncovered; in some it was treated according to a plan of so-called immovable antiseptic occlusion, and in others by an imperfect dressing of carbolic acid. But though these different methods had all the same result with regard to the preservation of life, they varied with regard to complications. Whilst in the nine cases treated strictly according to Lister's method, no serious complication was observed, in many of the other cases the cicatrizing process was interrupted. In five of these last cases erysipelas occurred, and in two local gangrene. From his own experience of Lister's dressing in cases of resection, M. Ollier has made out that this prevents inflammation of wounds without arresting the physiological processes of repair. The cicatrization and repair of osseous structure progress equally with the reunion of skin, and are not affected by the antiseptic treatment. Indeed, the organization of bone, and the ossification of the periosteal sheath, are rather accelerated than retarded by this plan of dressing, since this protects the wound and the internal layer of granulation-tissue from danger of infection. In every case of resection treated according to Lister's method, whether the operation be practised for deformity, injury, or chronic disease, M. Ollier endeavours to establish free drainage by a multiplicity of tubes, and refrains from applying sutures along the whole extent of the wound. In cases of chronic joint-disease, where the synovial membrane is much thickened and vascular throughout, the superficial portion is excised or scraped away, and the deeper portions destroyed by the actual cautery or some chemical agent (chloride of zinc, nitrate of silver, perchloride of iron). Thorough ablation of this thickened granular layer is not practised by M. Ollier in every case. Though it may be right to attack with the curette all tuberculous fungosities, and whatever tissue resembles such structures, it should not be forgotten that the exuberant fungous growths about fistulous tracts either waste or become further organized, after, through the extraction of a sequestrum or some other dead material, the source of the suppuration has been removed. The thick granular layer of a diseased joint, when the result of simple inflammation, is useful, M. Ollier thinks, after it has been altered, in the repair of the bones and the articular structures, and, therefore, ought not to be wholly removed. A portion only should be cut or scraped away, or the surface should be touched by the actual cautery, which is regarded as an excellent agent for converting a fungous into a plastic process. The subsequent suppuration on this part of the wound will, it is stated, be of no consequence so long as the superficial structures and the edges of the wound do not become inflamed, and so long as fever and symptoms of septic absorption are absent. Lister's antiseptic method is of great value, M. Ollier holds, when applied in cases of subperitoneal resee-tion. By preventing inflammation, this method guards against destruction of the osteogenetic elements attached to the inner surface of the periosteum, and arrests any diffuse suppuration which, besides the accidents common to all resections, would prove a positive obstacle to the accomplishment of the processes of repair. In almost all cases of resection, Lister's method is valuable, not only in guarding the patient against dangerous septic affections, but also, as it accelerates the heal-ing of wounds, in its enabling the surgeon to arrest, after the operation, those changes in muscular and nervous tissue which are the result of prolonged suppu-ration, associated with prolonged immobility of the limb. The application of Lister's method, in cases of severe open wound of a bone or joint, should, in M. Ollier's opinion, lead to a difference in the treatment of such injuries. In case of a wounded joint with fracture, instead of resorting to a resection, that is to say, to an operation consisting in the removal of all free fragments, and in bringing together the ends of the remaining ·portions of the injured bones, the surgeon might rest content in freeing the wound of foreign bodies and loose fragments of bone, leaving in place the fragments that are still covered by periosteum, and even such as have been partially denuded. It is not the injury itself, M. Ollier points out, that causes the death of such fragments, but the inflammation and suppuration following such injury. Such fragments, as is well known, in cases of simple fracture usually unite with the rest of the injured bone.

A case of partial resection of the tibio-tarsal joint is reported, to show the good results of Listerism in operations for the partial removal only of one or both opposed surfaces of bone forming an articulation.

In conclusion, M. Ollier protests against an unnecessary and too widely ex-tended application of operative surgery with antiseptic precautions to deformities of the skeleton and its articulations, which have hitherto been regarded as ame-nable to ordinary orthopædic treatment.—*Lond. Med. Record*, April·15, 1881.

Midwifery and Gynæcology.

A Case of Extra-Uterine associated with Intra-Uterine´Fœtation, in which Abdominal Section was performed.

Dr. GALABIN related, at a recent meeting of the Obstetrical Society of London (*Med. Times and Gazette*, May 28, 1881), a case of extra-uterine associated with intra-uterine fœtation, in which abdominal section was performed. The patient, who was thirty-six years old, was married in the spring of 1878. In the summer of that year she had an abortion, and in April, 1879, was delivered, with the assistance of forceps, of a full-term child. She expected her second confinement in September, 1880, and engaged Mr. Thomas Duke, of Rugby, to attend her. During the fourth and fifth months of pregnancy she had considerable pain and tenderness in the right side of the abdomen. Two tumours were then discovered. That on the left side gave the usual evidences of fœtal life, and was clearly the pregnant uterus. Over the tumour on the right side nothing could be heard by auscultation; and Mr. Duke, as well as several other medical men who examined the patient, concluded that the case was probably one of an ovarian tumour complicating pregnancy. On June 16, symptoms of rupture suddenly occurred, followed by those of peritonitis, and the outline of the right-hand tumour was found to have disappeared. The patient's state having become very critical, the author was sent for, and reached Rugby on the evening of the 19th. He was inclined, from the history, to agree with the diagnosis of ruptured ovarian cyst, but the possibility of combined extra- and intra-uterine fœtation existing was entertained. He suggested an exploratory operation as the only chance for life, and performed this on the morning of the 20th. A large quantity of blood and clot was found in the peritoneal cavity, and an extra-uterine fœtus contained only in its thin membranes. The placenta, attached to the back of the pregnant uterus and the posterior surface of the right broad ligament, was left *in situ*, and a drainage-tube placed in the wound, entering the general peritoneal cavity. The operation was performed under carbolic spray. The patient appeared to be doing well for the first two days, and the temperature never rose above 99.8°. On the morning of the 22d, however, labour came on, and a child, which presented by the breech, was delivered stillborn. Though there was very little hemorrhage by the vagina, a great deal occurred through the drainage-tube. On the 23d the temperature was normal, but hemorrhage still went on through the drainage-tube, and she died, apparently from loss of blood, on the 24th. The author attributed the secondary hemorrhage to the shrinking of the uterus in the expulsion of the fœtus, and consequent further detachment of the extra-uterine placenta from its posterior wall. Both fœtuses appeared to be of about six and a half months' development, but the extra-uterine fœtus weighed only one pound and a half, the intra-uterine two pounds and three-quarters. A review was appended of similar recorded cases ; in all of which the extra-uterine pregnancy appeared to have been of the abdominal form, while in none of them was a complete diagnosis made while both fœtuses remained within the abdomen.

Dr. ROUTH congratulated the author on his skill and power of diagnosis. It appeared that death was due to the further detachment of the placenta in labour, and he suggested that it would have been expedient to reopen the abdomen, and arrest hemorrhage by the actual cautery. He had seen adhesions in ovariotomy, even adhesions to the liver, successfully treated by the actual cautery.

Dr. DUNCAN regarded uncontrollable hemorrhage as the great difficulty in surgical interference with extra-uterine pregnancy, and this even many months after the death of the fœtus. He did not look with much hope on the actual cautery as a means of arresting this or any other kind of hemorrhage, as he had used it, and seen it used, in vain.

Dr. GALABIN said that, on account of the distance of the patient, he had not had the opportunity of deciding on the expediency of reopening the abdomen. He thought that a styptic, such as perchloride of iron, would be more effectual than the actual cautery in arresting hemorrhage in such a case.

———

Phlegmasia Dolens with Lymphatic Varix.

Dr. MATTHEWS DUNCAN, at a late meeting of the Obstetrical Society of London (*Med. Times and Gaz.*, May 28, 1881), read a paper on a case of phlegmasia dolens with lymphatic varix. The author was disposed to support the view of Tilbury Fox and others, that phlegmasia dolens is due to venous and lymphatic inflammation and obstruction, and that of these two the lymphatic disease is the more important, especially as being probably present in every case, while the venous disease is occasionally absent. The case of white-leg occurred in the downward progress of a characteristic case of cancer of the womb. During its presence there appeared lymphangiectasis of a part of the skin of the thigh, and this disappeared as the phlegmasia disappeared.   The part visibly affected was at the upper and outer part of the anterior surface of the left thigh, and constituted an oval or triangular area, broader above than below, and of such extent as might be nearly covered by the hand.   There was no pain or tenderness.   The projecting vessels, covered by epidermis having a yellowish-white tint and pearly lustre, were seen and felt, and the prick of the small point of a knife allowed a large drop of limpid lymph to immediately exude.   A similar affection of lymphatics occurred during a slight attack of phlegmasia in the right limb, which began as the disease was slowly disappearing from the left.   The lymphangiectasis occurred in an area of skin mechanically weakened by being the seat of closely set spindle-shaped ribbon-like skin-cracks.   These cracks were obscured by the lymphatic distension, and did not subsequently become again visible as skin-cracks, except in small parts.   The lymphangiectasis was probably the result of general lymphatic tension in the whole limb, the special varicose lymphatics becoming so in consequence of being imperfectly supported by the weakened cracked skin.   Similar phenomena were observed in the abdominal skin-cracks of pregnancy, under circumstances not regarded as morbid.

Dr. PLAYFAIR said that many clinical facts proved that thrombosis of the veins was not of itself sufficient to account for the phenomena of the disease. Thus, there were cases of thrombosis of the veins of the lower extremities, occurring in gouty subjects, in connection with which nothing like phlegmasia dolens was observed.   Dr. Duncan's cases showed the probably intimate relation between a certain amount of septic absorption and phlegmasia, which was not uncommon in connection with cancer of the uterus.   He did not think that there was ground for assuming that lymphatic obstruction had more to do with phlegmasia than venous obstruction.   He had never seen any lymphangiectasis in puerperal cases, and in some instances thrombosis of pulmonary arteries preceded the phlegmasia.

Dr. GRAILY HEWITT thought that there was no doubt that in typical cases of this disease both lymphatics and veins were affected.   It was known that the venous obstruction originated in coagulation in the uterine sinuses extending to the iliac trunk, and it was probable that the lymphatic thrombosis occurred in a similar way.

Dr. DUNCAN would not attempt to estimate precisely the comparative influence in phlegmasia of venous and of lymphatic obstruction.   He would only say that while sometimes venous obstruction was certainly absent, we could not say the same of lymphatic obstruction.

Aphthous Vulvitis and Gangrene of the Vulva in Children.

Dr. PARROT contributes to the March number of the *Rev. de Méd.* an exhaustive treatise on aphthous vulvitis in infants, founded upon an experience derived from 56 cases.   Premising that the disease, even under this name, was known to Hippocrates, he proceeds to describe the result of his own observations. Whilst the vulva, especially the labia majora, and less often the labia minora and clitoris, are the constant seat of the disease, it is not necessarily limited to them, but often extends to neighbouring parts, such as the perineum, margin of the anus, the genito-crural folds, and groins, in different degrees of frequency, in the order enumerated.   The appearance of the disease varies at different stages.   At the onset, it consists of small rounded or semi-spheroidal elevations of the epidermis, pale, or grayish-white, often depressed in their centre, and with a diameter of 1 to 4 millimetres, and closely resembling buccal aphthous patches.   The surrounding integument is usually but slightly affected, though sometimes red, and slightly swollen.   They vary in number from six to fifteen, isolated or in groups, sometimes confluent. This condition lasts from thirty-six hours to three days, and is followed by the second stage, which is marked by ulcers with a gray or yellowish base, surrounded by a red zone, and accompanied by pruritus, which is often severe, and necessitates the employment of some means of restraint from scratching. When the ulceration extends, its edges are raised, and the neighbouring parts much swollen, and of a bright red, especially the labia minora and clitoris. This ulcerative stage constitutes the acme of the disease, whatever its subsequent course, and doubtless, Dr. Parrot observes, may be recovered from without treatment in healthy subjects ; though, since all his cases were subjected to systematic treatment, with the result of rapid improvement, he cannot assert this to be the case. Under unfavourable conditions, the ulceration gives place to gangrene, which is not to be regarded, properly speaking, as a complication of aphthous vulvitis, but rather a modification or one of the forms of the disease, which manifests itself under as yet little known conditions. The gangrene may spread to an enormous extent, involving the perineum, rectum, and integuments around the coccyx, large moist eschars sloughing away, leaving deep excavations. Even from such extensive destruction, recovery may take place with remarkable completeness of restoration, the reparative process seeming to vie with the destructive.

The extent to which the system is affected by the local affection, whilst in the aphthous and ulcerative stages, is but slight, and is involved in the general febrile state (measles, etc.) to which the disease is secondary. With the existence of gangrene, the usual severe constitutional symptoms set in, and may be fatal. In those cases which do not proceed to gangrene it is noticeable that the ulcers which spread over the perineum and the rectal mucous membrane extend more rapidly and last longer than those in other regions, probably because of their liability to disturbance and irritation by the excretions. Careful examination of these parts is, therefore, necessary before pronouncing that a cure is effected. It is a remarkable circumstance that enlargement of the lymphatic glands does not occur, or only to the slightest extent. The diagnosis of aphthous vulvitis is easy. The infecting chancre has its own characteristics, and affects the lymphatic glands. The vulvitis, which is often associated with variola and varicella, is indistinguishable from the aphthous form, but the eruption of these diseases reveals the nature of the case. Among the more interesting points in connection with the etiology of the disease are : 1. The age, the majority of the cases occurring from the second to the fourth year, the youngest of the 56 children being twenty months old, and the eldest $7\frac{1}{2}$ years. 2. The influence exercised by other maladies. Of the 56, there were associated with measles, 39 ; with whooping-cough, 4 ; with varicella, erysipelas, pneumonia, and diphtheria, 1 each ; and 9 independently of any other disease. The marked frequency of measles compels us to assume some intimate relation between these two states. What this is, the author confesses himself ignorant of ; but he points out that measles leads in many cases to an ulceration of the antero-external surfaces of the arytenoid cartilages, though not of an aphthous character. All the cases of gangrene were observed in children the subjects of measles, which may be explained by a tendency of the febrile blood to form thrombi in the pudendal vessels.

It is difficult to state the duration of the disease, but the most intractable ulcers yielded to treatment within eight days. Dr. Parrot does not hesitate to give a favourable prognosis in all cases, recovery from the local affection taking place even when the primary disease may be fatal. The treatment adopted by the author since 1873, whatever the stage of the disease, is to cover all the affected area with a uniform layer of iodoform, and over that a covering of lint. One application will often effect a cure, and rarely more than three are necessary, at intervals of twenty-four hours, preceded by careful washing of the parts. This treatment is sedative rather than painful, and since it has been pursued, cases of gangrene, which, under the old methods of poultices, charcoal powders, alcoholic applications, chlorate of potash, nitrate of silver, etc., were frequent, are now unknown.—*London Med. Record*, May 15, 1881.

Ovariotomy and Pregnancy.

The following three cases are related by Dr. J. PIPPINGSKÖLD in the *Finska Läkaresällsk. Handlingar*, Band xxii. :—

CASE I. A L. M., aged 41, menstruated first at the age of 15, and was married at 18. She had had ten labours, the last two and a half years since. A tumour was first observed in March, 1877; the menses had become irregular, and ceased in July, 1878. She was admitted to hospital at the end of January, 1879. Three days later, twelve and a half litres of ropy colloid material were removed by tapping. On the last day of February dyspnœa had increased, and pains resembling those of labour had set in; she was now again tapped, but only two and two-third litres of watery fluid escaped. As she had severe orthopnœa, and became worse during the next two days, ovariotomy was performed. As soon as a large portion of the contents of the cyst had been removed, she was found to be pregnant; the possibility of this had been borne in mind before the operation. The pedicle was cauterized, and secured by eleven ligatures. Immediately after the operation, the labour-pains, which had probably commenced during the previous night, became more powerful; seven hours later, the liquor amnii escaped, and a dead child was soon afterwards born. Dr. Pippingsköld attributes the death of the fœtus to extravasation into the placenta, and believes that it might have been born alive if the operation had been performed fourteen days earlier.

CASE II. L. S., aged 34, married six years, had two living children (the youngest three years old), had miscarried at the sixth month with twins two years before her admission to hospital in July, 1877. The catamenia, which had been normal, had disappeared three months previously. The abdomen had gradually enlarged after the miscarriage. The diagnosis of an ovarian cystic tumour on the left side was made. Ovariotomy was performed on July 27; on the eleventh day the patient left her bed, and returned home a few weeks afterwards. She was delivered of a fine girl on November 3.

CASE III. In the beginning of April, 1878, Mrs. A. was sent to Dr. Pippingsköld by another medical practitioner, who had diagnosed an ovarian cyst in combination with ascites. The patient was 24 years of age; she had been married three and a half years, and had had two children, the youngest being one and a half years old. After her last confinement, her abdomen began to enlarge, and was, when Dr. Pippingsköld first saw her, greatly distended; she had also prolapse of the uterus. A preliminary tapping was performed; after which an abdominal bandage was applied for twelve weeks, with a glycerine tampon, compress, and T-bandage to the uterus. On June 23, ovariotomy was performed; the cyst was found to be connected with the right ovary. On the left ovary were three small cysts with clear serous contents, which were opened and cauterized. The patient was kept in bed five weeks, during which a glycerine tampon was daily introduced into the vagina. She menstruated normally in July. After she had left her bed, the uterus was found to be in its normal position, and re-

mained so. On October 28, 1879, she was delivered of a child weighing more·
than ten and a half pounds, and made a good recovery.—*London Med. Record*,
May 15, 1881.

—

Removal of Uterine Appendages for the Arrest of Uterine Hemorrhages.

At a late meeting of the Royal Medical and Chirurgical Society (*Lancet*, May
28, 1881), Mr. LAWSON TAIT read a paper on this subject. He referred to the
use of the statistical method in testing the real value of operations, and especially
instanced ovariotomy as one which would not have obtained the complete acceptance it has received had not the careful statistical method of Mr. Spencer Wells
shown that its results could be favourably compared with those of every other
major operation in surgery. Mr. Lawson Tait wished to lay his experience
before the Society, in order to obtain its decision as a guide for the future for
himself and others. After protracted trials of drugs for the arrest of uterine hemorrhage, he had come to the conclusion that all were absolutely without effect,
save ergot and two salts of potash, the chlorate and the bromide, and these were
by no means uniformly successful in giving permanent relief. In all the cases
he had to relate these drugs had been fully tried before the question of operating
was discussed. He had entitled his paper "The Removal of the Uterine Appendages," because his experience seemed to show that the removal of the ovaries
was not a certain method of arresting menstruation, while removal of the tubes as
well seemed to be so.

The author then related thirty-one cases, of which four were fatal, twenty-seven
recovering from the operation. A summary table was appended to the paper,
which was a complete list of the operations and results.

The author summed up with the following conclusions, which he considered
might be legitimately drawn from them. 1. That, so far as its primary results
are concerned, removal of the uterine appendages for the arrest of intractable uterine
hemorrhage is an operation which is quite as easily justified as any of the major
operations of surgery. 2. That so far as its secondary results are yet know it is
an operation which yields abundant encouragement for its further trial; as conclusions which are indicated but not wholly proved, he thought he might formulate
a statement that removal of the ovaries alone is not sufficient to arrest menstruation,
but that removal of both tubes and ovaries does at once arrest it. So far as some
of these cases have gone the arrest would seem to be permanent. This conclusion is quite in harmony with what is known of removal of both ovaries for large
cystomata, for in such cases the tubes are almost uniformly included in the clamp
or ligature. Three at least of the cases, and probably two others, show that the
arrest of menstruation by this means leads or may lead to the atrophy of uterine
myoma. Finally, there is some close connection, here pointed out, he believed,
for the first time, and worthy of very close study, between uterine myoma and
its accompanying hemorrhages and cystic disease of the ovaries. In two of the
cases cystic disease seemed to be the cause of the hemorrhage without any
myoma intervening. One other conclusion, he thought, was justified, that the
whole subject is worthy of careful study, and should not be made the subject of
premature and hostile conclusions.

MEDICAL NEWS.

NOT A FAILURE OF VACCINATION AS A PROPHYLACTIC.

It can scarcely be doubted that the surest way to overcome the assailants of our great safeguard against variola is to determine with absolute accuracy the limits of its protective power, in order that we may not enthusiastically claim too much for Jenner's beneficent discovery. Hence a careful consideration of circumstances attending the recent complete destruction of a band of Esquimaux in France by smallpox is especially important at the present time, when vaccination is being so violently attacked by many ignorant or prejudiced enemies. From the official report of Dr. Leon Colin (Professor d'Epidémiologie du Val de Grâce), made after a thorough investigation of the whole subject, we learn that a party of eight Esquimaux brought from their native Labrador (probably to take part in some kind of exhibition or theatrical performance) disembarked at Hamburg the 26th of September, 1880, and visited in succession Berlin, Prague, and Frankfort, arriving at Darmstadt on the 13th of December, stopping at Crefeld, a small town of Rhenish Prussia, from the 18th to the 30th of that month, and reaching Paris, where they were taken to the Jardin d'Acclimation, on the last day of the year. On the 14th of September, just two weeks after leaving Prague, where an epidemic of variola was raging, a young girl of the troupe died of smallpox, the eruption being fairly apparent. At Crefeld, thirteen days afterward, the wife of one of the party died with the symptoms of hemorrhagic smallpox, but without any eruption being visible, and on the 31st of December, at the same place, another young girl died, exhibiting the characteristic eruption.

On the 1st of January, the day after their arrival, the remaining five Esquimaux were carefully vaccinated with animal vaccine virus, which had been preserved in tubes, and five days later the operation was repeated, in both instances, however, unfortunately without effect. This failure is attributed by Dr. Colin to the fact that, the systems of the Esquimaux being already infected with the variolous poison, they were all on both occasions in that stage of incubation of smallpox in which want of success in vaccination is (he states) the rule. It seems strange that, in view of the great previous mortality among the troupe, arm to arm vaccination was not daily practised, and varied, indeed, to different parts of the body, in order to give these unhappy exiles a chance of deliverance from the terrible disease which proved fatal to them all before the middle of January. And yet it is obvious that the time when the prophylactic should have been applied was when they first landed in Hamburg, or certainly at Prague, which was known to be the seat of an epidemic, or at any rate at Darmstadt, when

the death of a first victim, marked with the characteristic eruption, gave a
primary signal of the terrible danger to which the whole band was exposed.
But since the precaution was not thus resorted to *in time*, it is equally
manifest that there is no proof that the failure of vaccination to protect
these unfortunates from smallpox was due to aught but a neglect of the
proper method of its timely application, or in any sense owing to a deficiency in its prophylactic power.

The fact that all of the patients in this lamentable series of cases died
after a few days' illness, and two of them without showing any eruption,
suggested to some medical men in Paris that variola was here so modified
by racial peculiarities, or other causes, as to be less amenable to the influence of vaccination. But if we investigate the course of smallpox in
nations among whom it has not previously been prevalent, and where consequently there is, so to speak, a new field opened to its ravages, we will
find that it has often in the past history of mankind manifested the same
virulence and fatality. The circumstance also that no epidemic of variola
seems to have been originated by these Esquimaux, strongly indicates
that for their associates and caretakers, a certain amount of *inherited* in-
susceptibility (which probably exists in the inhabitants of countries, where
smallpox frequently occurs, and weeds out, as it were, the families which
are most easily affected by its poison) combined with the *acquired* protective influence of vaccinia to preserve them from its deadly power. All
the employés of the Garden of Acclimation were re-vaccinated with human
vaccine lymph taken from the arm of an infant on the eighth day, the
apartments occupied by the Esquimaux were disinfected with sulphurous
acid, and their effects either burned, or purified by prolonged exposure to
boiling or to dry heat of high degree. The Parisian Council of Health,
in seeking to profit by this remarkable example, urges upon the proper
authorities, the prompt vaccination immediately upon landing of all foreigners arriving at French ports, from countries such as Labrador, where
neither prevalent variola nor vaccine disease has tested their susceptibility
to smallpox. This wise precaution might well be adopted here in America
in regard to the arriving emigrants, annually crowding to our shores
from regions where systematic vaccination and re-vaccination are neglected,
especially as the health reports of our western States record numerous
local epidemics, the germs for which have been imported by Scandinavian
and other settlers. Furthermore, the Council earnestly advocates the
missionary work of introduction as rapidly as possible of the process of
vaccination among the various nations to whom it is comparatively unknown ; pointing out that the operation would not only preserve a few
individuals from the perils of variola attending a voyage to Europe, but
would protect whole populations from danger by the germs of smallpox,
imported by sailors or travellers, to which they are continually more or
less exposed without its aid.

INFECTED MEAT.

A short time since we called the attention of our readers to the danger of tuberculosis being transmitted by the ingestion of diseased meat, and the recent panic on the continent of Europe in regard to trichinosis in pork indicates that a knowledge of the exact extent of other dangers from infected animal food can scarcely be too often or too earnestly urged upon the community at large. Strenuous efforts, evidently inspired by the immense pecuniary interest involved, have been made to allay popular anxiety on this point, and a late account states that, among four hundred hogs examined at random in Chicago, no trace of Trichina was discovered. Investigations, which we may readily suppose were less partial, and, therefore, more searching, place the number of American hogs infected with trichina at four per cent., and when we consider that a large proportion of the cats and rats in cities contain trichina, and are occasionally eaten by swine, we comprehend at once why the wise old Hebrew lawgiver forbade pork to his followers. The obvious reason for our comparative immunity in this country from epidemics of trichinosis is found in our habit of *thoroughly cooking* all animal food, a culinary precaution which is infallible, and should never be omitted. Any one interested in this subject may consult with profit Dr. Noah Cressy's address on " Diseased Meat and its Consequences upon our Health and Happiness," published at Hartford, Conn., last year.

—

The American Laryngological Association.—The third annual congress of this Association convened in Philadelphia, on May 9, 1881, and continued until May 11th, holding morning and afternoon sessions. The meeting was held in the Hall of the College of Physicians, the use of which had been tendered by the College to the Association. A full attendance of the Fellows was present, and a number of candidates were elected. The meeting was presided over by Dr. J. Solis Cohen, and the papers presented were of great interest, and, as a rule, practical in their character; the discussions were spirited. Entertainments were tendered the Association by the President; and by the Philadelphia Laryngological Association. An excursion to Atlantic City on the afternoon of the last day concluded the exercises of the meeting, which was considered the most successful that has yet been held by the Association.

First Day's Proceedings.—The President, Dr. J. Solis Cohen, opened the session, at 10.30 A. M., on Monday, May 9th. Dr. Harrison Allen made a brief address of welcome, and the President then read his annual address.

The reading of papers being next in order, Dr. Frederick J. Knight, of Boston, read a clinical paper on Lupus Laryngis, followed by one on Lupus of the Pharynx and Larynx, by Dr. Morris J. Asch, of New York, which led to considerable discussion, in which a remarkable variety of opinions were upheld regarding the pathology of Lupus.

Dr. Andrew H. Smith, of New York, read a communication on Certain Neuroses of the Throat, in which laryngeal disorder was shown to exist in some cases as the result of reflex irritation, frequently uterine in its origin.

In the afternoon, papers were read by Dr. Beverley Robinson, of New York, on the Laryngeal Affections of Pulmonary Phthisis; by Dr. Wm. Porter, of St. Louis, on the Prognosis of Laryngeal Phthisis, and by Dr. F. H. Bosworth, of New York, on Tubercular Ulceration of the Mouth, with a report of Cases. In their essays, and in the discussion following them, a more hopeful view of the prognosis of laryngeal phthisis was given than is generally stated; the treatment being largely local by means of medicated sprays.

Second Day.—A business meeting was held from 10 to 11 o'clock, at which candidates were balloted for, and other private business transacted; reports of the Treasurer, of the Committee on Nomenclature, and of the Publication Committee were received and approved. The following were elected to active membership: Drs. D. Bryson Delavan, of New York; Urban G. Hitchcock, of New York; George W. Major, of Montreal; Ethelbert C. Morgan, of Washington; Herman Mynter, of Buffalo, and J. W. Robinson, of Detroit.

In regard to the following question, referred by the Council to the Association for their decision: Shall the inaugural theses of candidates for Fellowship be published as a part of the transactions of the Association in the Annual Volume? it was decided that it should be left to the discretion of the Council at each annual meeting.

Dr. Louis Elsberg, of New York, read a Contribution to the Histology of the Thyroid Cartilage, in which recent views on the structure of so-called hyaline cartilage structure were discussed, and the bio-plasmic character of the inter-cellular material maintained. He also exhibited an improved apparatus, by which the calcium light was made available for office use for laryngoscopic examinations, and, secondly, Trouvé's Galvanic Accumulator for illumination and cautery purposes. The President said that he had tried it as a means of illumination and for actual cautery, but it had not been satisfactory in his hands.

Dr. Wm. C. Glasgow, of St. Louis, read a paper On the Operation for Deviation of the Nasal Septum, in which Steele's method of cutting the cartilage by radiating incisions and restoring its position by pressure was advocated. The paper was freely discussed, this operation not being sanctioned by the Society generally.

An interesting essay, by Dr. Carl Seiler, upon the Effect of the Condition of the Nasal Cavities upon Articulate Speech, was listened to with marked attention, as it discussed the physical conditions of articulation and the functions of the upper air-passages in speech.

By permission, Dr. J. O. Roe, of Rochester, reported a curious case of Laryngeal Whistling; Dr. Glasgow also read a volunteer paper, containing the notes of a case of paralysis of the abductor muscles of the larynx.

Dr. Clinton Wagner read a paper On Sub-Hyoidean Pharyngotomy for the Removal of the Epiglottis, with an illustrative case; in which the advantages of the horizontal wound were discussed, and its enlargement by an antero-posterior incision recommended (a T incision) in difficult cases.

The question of Hemorrhage after Tonsillotomy was discussed by Dr. Geo. M. Lefferts, of New York, and the danger of serious bleeding pointed out, due, in the author's opinion, to section of the enlarged branches of the ascending pharyngeal arteries of the external carotid, rather than to the trunk of the internal carotid, as is usually stated by writers. In the free discussion which followed, the comparative advantages of the guillotine, the bistoury, the galvano-cautery, and the destruction by caustic applications, each found advocates.

A paper, by Dr. C. E. Sajous, on Paralysis of the Vocal Cords due to lead-poisoning, was read by title.

Third Day.—Dr. Wm. C. Jarvis read a paper on Chronic Irritative Hyperæmia of the Larynx, which was favourably discussed by Drs. Elsberg, Shurley,

A. H. Smith, Seiler, Cohen, and Bosworth. Dr. Jarvis also exhibited an ingenious instrument for removing hypertrophied tissue from the inferior turbinated bone.

Dr. J. O. Roe read a paper on the Comparative Value of Atomized Fluids in the Treatment of Diseases of the Larynx, which advocated this method of medication.

Dr. Delavan, of New York, by permission, also exhibited an instrument, which was an inverted Säss's tube for throwing an upward spray into the pharynx, and which was considered by several fellows as a decided improvement.

Dr. Wm. H. Daly concluded the public exercises by reading a communication upon the Relations of Hay Asthma and Nasal Catarrh, and the Congress went into executive session.

On motion of Dr. Knight, it was resolved that fellows who take no active interest, either by paper,or presence, in the sessions of the Congress for a period of three years, may, unless proper and satisfactory excuse to the Council be made, be dropped from the roll.

A communication was received from the editor of the *Archives of Laryngology*. On motion, the whole subject of publication of proceedings was referred to the Council with power.

The following fellows were elected Delegates to the Subsection on Laryngology of the International Medical Congress of 1881: Drs. Cohen, Lefferts, Lincoln, and Bosworth.

On recommendation of the Council, Dr. Morell Mackenzie, of London, was elected an honorary fellow, and Drs. M. Krishaber, Paris, L. Mandel, Paris, Karl Stoerck, Vienna, Leopold Schrötter, Vienna, Felix Semon, London, and R. Voltolini, Breslau, were elected corresponding fellows.

The following officers were duly elected for the succeeding year: *President,* Dr. F. J. Knight, of Boston. *Vice-Presidents,* Drs E. L. Shurley, of Detroit; Wm. Porter, of St. Louis. *Member of Council,* Dr. Harrison Allen, of Phila. . Next place of meeting, Niagara Falls, N. Y., during the month of June, the exact date to be decided by the Council, so that it shall not interfere with the meeting of the American Medical Association.

After the customary votes of thanks, the Association adjourned.

—

The Pennsylvania State Medical Society.—The thirty-second annual meeting of the State Medical Society was held at Lancaster, Penna., on May 11th, 12th, and 13th, 1881. It was the largest meeting of this Society that has ever been held, nearly three hundred members signing the register. The session was harmonious, and the proceedings were enlivened by many interesting papers and appreciative discussions.

The formal opening of the meeting by prayer was followed by an Address of Welcome from Dr. Henry Carpenter, of Lancaster.

Dr. Allis offered a resolution that the Philadelphia County Medical Society be made custodian of the publication of the Proceedings of the Pennsylvania State Medical Society and of the Transactions of such other State medical societies as shall exchange with it, until the Pennsylvania State Medical Society shall make other provisions for the same, and that the Publishing Committee shall be a Library Committee to report to next meeting of this Society. Adopted.

Dr. Sutton offered the following, which lies over under the rule :—

Section 2, Article III., of the Constitution shall be so amended as to read as follows :—

Every member of a county medical society in Pennsylvania shall, so long as he is in good standing, be a member of the State Medical Society and a delegate to its annual sessions.

In the afternoon, Dr. Albert H. Smith, of Philadelphia, offered a resolution in regard to giving the control of female insane patients in hospitals exclusively to women, and calling upon the Legislature to recognize this principle in making its appointments for the hospital at Warren, as had been done elsewhere in the State. After some discussion it was made the special order for the succeeding day.

Dr. S. M. Ross, of Blair Co., read the Address in Surgery, and several other papers were read, including one by Dr. S. D. Risley upon Diseases of the Lachrymal Passages, and one on the Pathology of Shock, by Dr. C. C. Seabrook, in which the phenomena are declared to be due to a paralyzing effect upon the vaso-motor centre in the medulla oblongata.

The President's Annual Address, by Dr. John T. Carpenter, of Schuylkill Co., was mainly devoted to the discussion of the management of the insane. He pointed out the defective system of treatment prevailing in many asylums in the United States, and urged the adoption of some comprehensive system of super-intendence of all the insane hospitals, with a view of securing an approach to uniformity in classification and administration.

A complimentary musical entertainment was given to the delegates, at the close of the President's Address, at Fulton Hall, which was well attended.

Second day.—After the appointment of the Nominating Committee, the resolution of Dr. Smith came up for action, and after considerable discussion the motion was lost. Several other amendments were adopted.

The amendment to the Constitution offered by Dr. Carpenter last year, allowing representation of the College of Physicians of Philadelphia, also failed to be adopted.

Dr. S. S. Schultz, of Danville, read a very interesting Report on Mental Disorders, in which the want of sufficient accommodation for the insane in our public institutions was pointed out, the number of the insane in our constantly growing population being steadily on the increase; he estimated the number of insane poor in this commonwealth at nearly 6000.

In a volunteer paper, Dr. John Curwen, of Dauphin Co., insisted upon the value of rest and careful attention to nutrition as restorative agents in nervous disease.

This was followed by an interesting communication from Dr. Traill Green, of Easton, entitled "The State Medical Society and the Preparatory Education of Medical Students," in which great stress was laid upon the necessity of proper preliminary studies for medical students.

Dr. O. H. Allis also read a paper upon the same question, "In what should Preliminary Examinations consist, and what step should be taken to make them uniform throughout the State?"

Dr. W. M. Findlay, of Blair Co., offered the following, which was adopted:—

Resolved, That a committee be appointed to prepare a schedule of subjects on which applicants for permission to study medicine shall be examined by the Board of Examiners of county societies.

The President appointed on this committee to report at the next meeting, Drs. O. H. Allis, Traill Green, W. R. Findlay, John B. Roberts, and W. B. Ulrich.

At the afternoon session, Dr. Wm. Goodell read a paper on "The Extirpation of the Ovaries for Insanity," in which some illustrative cases were reported, showing the value of this procedure in certain cases; the author noticing the strong hereditary tendency of mental disease, advocated the trial of this operation, which possessed the incidental advantage of preventing the propagation of insanity.

Dr. J. Aug. Uhler, Chairman of Committee on Nominations, made the following report: *President*, Jacob L. Ziegler, of Mount Joy. *Vice-Presidents*, 1. Jos. A. Reed, of Allegheny; 2. W. L. Roland, of York; 3. J. W. Houston, of Chester; 4. W. Murray Weidman, of Berks. *Place of Meeting*, Titusville, Crawford County, on second Wednesday of May, 1882. Adopted.

A Report on the State Board of Health was presented by the Permanent Secretary.

On motion John Norris, Esq., of the *Philadelphia Record* was allowed to address the association upon the progress of the bill to create a State Board of Health. A vote of thanks was subsequently tendered the *Record* for its services in aid of medical legislation and medical reform. Dr. R. L. Sibbett, of Carlisle, presented a report on Medical Legislation, which was adopted. A resolution was passed indorsing the bill then before the State Legislature for creating a State Board of Health, and regulating the practice of medicine.

Dr. Benjamin Lee, of Philadelphia, read the Annual Address on Hygiene, in which he discussed certain matters connected with the purity of the atmosphere, especially in large cities, calling especial attention to the dangers of inhaling street-dust, and of breathing sewer-gas in the houses; and recommending a mercury valve for water-closets.

Dr. R. G. Curtin, of Philadelphia, read a paper on Catarrhal Inflammation of the Pancreas, a heretofore undescribed Disease. The principal symptoms were diarrhœa, with fatty stools, followed by dyspepsia, and later symptoms of anæmia and starvation, to be treated in the early stages by the use of food containing little oily matter and inunction of oil by the skin.

Dr. O. H. Allis gave a short lecture on Why Deformity so frequently follows Fracture of the Lower End of the Humerus? and Why Fractures just above or below the Knee are so dangerous?—the latter being on account of the danger of hemorrhage, the former being due to rotation of the fragments, and vicious union. He recommended keeping the arm extended during the treatment of fracture of the condyles of the humerus, in order to prevent the sliding of the fragment.

Dr. Tyson read a short paper upon the Pathology of Albuminuria, which, with the preceding, was ordered to be published.

Third day.—Dr. Laurence Turnbull read a paper enlarging upon the dangers of Defective Hearing in Locomotive Engineers, and at his recommendation a resolution was adopted referring the consideration of the subject to a commission. He was then appointed Chairman of a committee to bring the subject before the railroad authorities, and to draft a memorial to present to the State Legislature.

The Address in Medicine by Dr. J. Solis Cohen, in which some new remedies were discussed and their dangers indicated, was well received, and led to an interesting discussion.

Dr. R. J. Levis explained his method of treating Hydrocele and Cystic Tumours by the Injection of Carbolic Acid (full strength from 20–60 minims may be used, half a drachm being usually sufficient).

Dr. Jacob Price read a practical paper on The Importance of Local Treatment in Congestion and Inflammation of the Cervix Uteri in Pregnancy, whose title indicates its scope. The local application used most frequently consisted of equal parts of iodine, phenol, and tannin, in four parts of glycerine.

The President appointed Dr. Chas. K. Mills to deliver the Address on Nervous Disorders at the next annual meeting.

The new incumbent, Dr. J. L. Ziegler, was escorted to the presidential chair, and the meeting was then adjourned.

The Sanitary Measures proposed by the National Board of Health for the control of New Orleans during the present Summer.—The National Board, in a letter to Dr. S. E. Chaillé, as Supervising Inspector, has set forth explicit instructions for his guidance. The Board desires to obtain the earliest possible information of the existence of yellow fever in New Orleans or its vicinity : to secure free commercial intercourse between New Orleans and other points, so long as such intercourse is unattended with danger; to so arrange matters when such intercourse must be restricted as to cause no more interference than is absolutely necessary; and in case of the appearance of yellow fever, to co-operate in every way to limit the spread of the disease and to stamp it out if possible. The Board of Health of Memphis, Tenn., of Shelby County, Tenn., and of Vicksburg, La., have communicated resolutions to the National Board, requesting early and efficient action on its part, anticipating the coming summer season as a critical one, and requiring clean bills of health, or inspection certificates, issued or countersigned by an inspecting officer of the National Board, from all water or land travel where it is deemed necessary, the Shelby County Board of Health also tendering the quarantine grounds and building on President's Island to the National Board for use as an inspection station.

The proper enforcement of these ordinances requires that the Supervising Inspector shall obtain suitable co-operation and information from the health authorities and physicians of New Orleans and the river parishes below New Orleans ; and, in furtherance of this object, the State Board of Health of Louisiana have tendered the use of a commodious room adjoining its own rooms to the inspector, and have requested his attendance at the meetings of the Board. The details of the instructions to the Supervising Inspector comprise regular daily reports from a National Board inspector at the Mississippi River Quarantine Station, who, in cases of difference between himself and the quarantine inspector, furnishes reports to both the Supervising Inspector and the President of the Louisiana Board of Health. All reports of deaths, in doubtful and suspicious cases, to be properly investigated, and information as to the presence of cases of yellow fever, or cases which are doubtful or suspicious to be furnished by request of health authorities of other States and municipalities, *with* the approval of the resident member of the Board and independent of the co-operation of the local board. Caution is enjoined in determining what constitutes dangerous infection to avoid, as far as possible, any undue restriction upon travel or traffic. The inspection of steamboats was to commence with the first of May, as conducted last year; two inspectors, and when necessary two sanitary policemen, being employed. No rigid railroad inspection further than the examination of freights is as yet recommended. The Supervising Inspector is advised to secure the co-operation of the Louisiana State Board of Health, so as to cause the passage by them of an ordinance similar to "resolution No. 6," as passed by the Sanitary Council of the Mississippi Valley, which, in effect, establishes a careful inspection of ships at Eadsport, the proper certificate from the inspector of the National Board at Ship Island Quarantine Station to be the only authority which would allow a vessel from infected ports to pass without inspection.

The Louisiana State Board of Health, at its meeting of May 19th, adopted the report of Dr. Formento, which was based upon these instructions to Dr. Chaillé, and which renders them nugatory in almost every particular, so far as the co-operation of the Board is concerned. Ship Island was not considered suitable for a quarantine station, and if it were, the State Board would not feel warranted in using it as such. The only station which the Board thought suitable was the State Mississippi River Quarantine Station, as the best equipped and organized outside of New York. The Board also took occasion to express its want of sympathy with the Mississippi Valley Sanitary Organization.

The National Board of Health, at its recent meeting, June 1st and 2d, has, it seems, taken no further action upon this condition of things.

—

Scarlet Fever in Charleston.—Dr. F. PEYRE PORCHER, of Charleston, writes us that "a severe epidemic of scarlet fever prevails in this city, many deaths have occurred in children—the throat being generally involved. As usual the cases vary; sometimes the eruption being not prominent. Deaths have occurred forty-eight hours after the invasion. Many recover. We are of the opinion that safety will be found in early treatment, by efforts to reduce the fever of the first few hours by fever mixtures, by repeated warm baths, cold sponging to the head and arms, and application to the throat externally and internally—Labarraque's solution of chlorinated soda and chlorate of potash being admirable in the composition of internal applications to the throat. Many have used a solution of sulphide of sodium as a prophylactic (ζj to water Oj—dessertspoonful t. i. d.), as recommended first, we believe, by Prof. Elliott, of Sewannee. We know of three instances where children had the disease, in a mild form, through taking this substance regularly.

"We prefer, and have used for this purpose, a combination of chlorate of potash, quinia, and hyposulphite of soda,[1] which we long since suggested and employed as the best prophylactic in diphtheria—to be taken by those exposed to these diseases. It is besides harmless and an excellent tonic. Some children of black persons have had the scarlet fever here, but there has been a most singular exemption in this race. The proportion of whites to blacks seized has, we believe, been as 100 to 1—perhaps much higher than this."

—

International Medical Congress, London, 1881.—The following general arrangements for the meeting of the Congress are announced.

An informal reception will take place at the Royal College of Physicians, Pallmall East, on Tuesday afternoon, August 2, from 3 P. M. to 6 P. M., at which the Executive and Reception Committees will meet the members of the Congress. The opening meeting of the Congress will be held in St. James's Great Hall on Wednesday, August 3, at 11 A. M. Entrances in Regent Street and Piccadilly. The other general meetings will be held in the Theatre of the University of London.

The Congress will be organized on Wednesday August 3. In the evening a conversazione at South Kensington Museum will be given by the English members of the Congress to the foreign members.

On Thursday Aug. 4, an address will be delivered by Prof. Maurice Reynaud, of Paris, on "Le Septicisme en Médecine, au temps passé et au temps présent." In the evening a banquet will be given at the Mansion House to certain members of the Congress by the Lord Mayor of London.

On Friday Aug. 5, Dr. J. S. Billings, of Washington, will deliver an address on "Our Medical Literature," and in the evening a conversazione will be given at the Royal College of Surgeons.

On Saturday Aug. 6, there will be no general meeting. The Sections will meet daily from 10 A. M. to 1 P. M. In the afternoon Sir J. D. Hooker will receive at the Kew Gardens, and Mr. and Mrs. Spencer Wells, at Golder's Hill, Hampstead.

[1] ℞.—Chlorate of potash, ζij; quinia, gr. xv; hyposulphite of soda, ζij; tr. chloride of iron ζij; water, ζvij.—Dessertspoonful t. i. d., used as a preventive.

On Sunday special services will be held at Westminster Abbey by Dean Stanley in the morning, and at St. Paul's Cathedral by Canon Liddon in the afternoon. Sir Trevor Lawrence, M.P., will entertain at luncheon a number of the members at his place at Boxhill, in Surrey.

On Monday Aug. 8, address by Prof. Volkmann, of Halle, and in the evening a dinner will be given to certain members of the Congress by the Society of Apothecaries in their Hall in Blackfriars, also a soirée in the Albert Hall.

On Tuesday Aug. 9, concluding general meeting. Address by Prof. Huxley "The Connection of the Biological Sciences with Medicine." After the conclusion of the meeting the members will be carried by special train to the Crystal Palace, and will be entertained at an informal dinner in the Concert Room. At dusk the fountains will play during a display of fireworks.

Arrangements have been made to enable the members to visit the prominent hospitals, the principal places of public interest, as well as a number of the private galleries in London. Attractive excursions have also been planned for Greenwich, Folkestone, Hampton Court, etc.

—

The Association of Medical Editors met at Richmond, on Monday evening, May 2. In the absence of Dr. J F. Shrady, President, Dr. Octerlony was called to the chair. Dr. D. S. Reynolds acted as Secretary.

Dr. Shrady's address was read and ordered to be printed.

The Committee on Nominations of Officers for the ensuing year reported as follows: President, Dr. Landon B. Edwards, Richmond, Va.; Vice-President, Dr. Ralph Walsh, of Washington; Secretary, Dr. D. S. Reynolds, of Louisville.

The Association adjourned to meet on Monday evening preceding the next Annual Meeting of the American Medical Association.

—

Health of New York.—The city's mortality has steadily diminished during the last month. The number of deaths for the weeks ending June 4 and 11 was, respectively, 660 and 633, while the numbers for the weeks ending May 1 and 15 were 814 and 822.

The number of new typhus fever cases developed during May was somewhat larger than in April. During the eighth week of the prevailing endemic (ending May 7), there were 28; in the ninth week 14; in the tenth week 34, and in the eleventh week (ending May 29), 13 cases were reported. Smallpox increased slightly in May, in spite of the energetic efforts of the Health Board to check its career.

The quarterly report of the Bureau of Vaccination, recently published, states that in the three months ending March 31, 3616 primary and 19,653 other vaccinations were performed by the Bureau. Several cases of smallpox have been discovered on incoming European steamships, and promptly quarantined. A number of new cases have also been reported in Brooklyn and Jersey City. On June 1 there were 129 cases of variola and 52 of typhus at the Riverside Hospital. Scarlatina has decreased during May, but diphtheria has slowly gained ground, and measles has rapidly increased. German measles has prevailed in almost epidemic form for some months. It has chiefly affected very young children. The heat was less intense in the latter part of May than in the second week of that month, but was sufficient to produce 20 cases of insolation on May 21, 2 of which were fatal.

A compromise street-cleaning bill was passed by the legislature, and received the Governor's signature. Although the time granted by the Governor to the proprietors of the factories on Hunter's Point and Newtown Creek for the abatement of the nuisances connected with their establishment has expired, the odours are as offensive as ever.

———

Indiana State Medical Society met at Indianapolis, May 18th, under the presidency of Thomas B. Harvey, M.D., of Indianapolis. The following officers were elected for the ensuing year: President, Dr. Marshall Sexton, of Rushville; Vice-President, Dr. F. J. Van Vorhis, of Indianapolis; Secretary, Dr. E. S. Elder, of Indianapolis.

———

Illinois State Medical Society held its thirty-first annual meeting at Chicago, May 17th, 18th, and 19th, Dr. George Wheeler Jones, of Danville, President, in the chair. A number of scientific papers were read, and the proceedings were of marked interest. The following officers were elected for the ensuing year: President, Dr. Robert Boal, of Peoria; Vice-Presidents, Drs. A. T. Darrah, of Tolono, and Ellen A. Ingersoll, of Canton; Assistant Secretary, Dr. Wm. A. Byrd, of Quincy. It was voted to hold the next meeting at Quincy.

———

Health of Chicago.—An epidemic of Rötheln or German measles is widely spread in Chicago. There were about one hundred cases of it in the Orphan Asylum. No case of death from the disease has been reported. A mild epidemic of diarrhœa, generally referred to the drinking water, also exists. Not long ago the Desplaines River overflowed its banks and a part of its stream entered the Chicago River, flooding the city in some places and carrying filth of the worst description into the lake as far as the Crib, whence Chicago gets its supply of drinking water.

Scarlet fever, diphtheria, and smallpox are still prevalent, and the mortality from each is high.

———

A New Home for Inebriates.—The laying of the corner stone of the " New York Christian Home for Intemperate Men," at the corner of Madison Avenue and 86th Street, took place on June 7. The Home will accommodate about seventy-five men. The cost of the site was $30,000, and the building expenses are estimated at about $60,000. The Home will be constructed of brick and brown stone. It will be four stories high, and its dimensions will be 60×100 feet. There will be private rooms for those patients requiring isolation, bath-rooms, sitting-rooms, a library and a chapel. The house will be ventilated, drained, and lighted by the most approved modern methods.

———

Registration of Plumbers.—The bill requiring New York and Brooklyn plumbers to be registered, and to subject all their work to the inspection of the City Health Board, has become a law.

———

The Sick Children's Mission.—A charitable institution under the direction of the Children's Aid Society, has begun its summer work of providing sick children of the lower classes, with gratuitous nourishment, medicines, and medical attendance. Druggists in different parts of the city will furnish medicines free of charge on the presentation of authenticated prescriptions from any of the twelve physicians whose services have been secured by the Mission. Substantial food and suitable delicacies will be furnished by the superintendent of the Mission, who will also provide trained female nurses for cases requiring their services.

Medical and Chirurgical Faculty of Maryland.—The 83d annual meeting of the Faculty was held in Baltimore, April 12 to 16, 1881, Dr. H. P. C. Wilson, of Baltimore, President, in the chair. The annual oration was delivered by Dr. William Goodell, of Philadelphia. A number of scientific papers were read in the sections. The following officers were elected for the ensuing year: President, Dr. Frank Donaldson; Vice-Presidents, Drs. A. H. Bayley and I. E. Atkinson; Secretary, Dr. W. G. Regester.

—

Instruction Preparatory to the Study of Medicine in the University of Penn-sylvania.—In the assignment of Prof. Joseph T. Rothrock to a Chair of Botany and Dr. Andrew J. Parker to a Chair of Biology in the Towne Scientific School, the Trustees of the University have not merely enlarged the curriculum of that school by the addition of two subjects of great importance, but they have also provided the means of rendering effective the *Sixth Course* as laid down in the general catalogue—*a course preparatory to the study of medicine.* The scheme of the course has not been fully elaborated, but, as now published, includes English Composition, History, Social Science, Latin, French, German, Physics, Chemistry, inorganic and organic, with laboratory practice, Botany, vertebrate and invertebrate Zoology, Mineralogy, and Geology. With the completion of the course, and the passing of appropriate examinations, the degree of Bachelor of Science is conferred.

It will be seen that this course includes a large number of subjects which not only lead to the higher culture so important to the physician, but directly pre-pare him for the special studies in human anatomy, physiology, medical chem-istry, etc., which should occupy him during the first year of his medical studies, as well as furnish the knowledge of physics and mathematics, now so essential to an intelligent study of certain branches of practical medicine, notably physical diagnosis, ophthalmology, laryngology, and otology.

Too high a value cannot be placed upon such a course. Since the establish-ment of scientific schools, both independently and in connection with colleges, courses have been adapted preparatory to the special studies of a large number of occupations, including now, with the establishment of the Wharton School of Finance and Economy at the University, the various branches of mercantile pur-suit. Not only has the mass of facts which the physician of to-day has to master increased a hundredfold, but he requires also rare mental qualities to be acquired only by training, in order that he may sift the true from the false, appropriately use the former and discard the latter. Much more, perhaps, to the study of medicine than to that of any other profession should be shaped the previous training and knowledge of the student.

So far as we know, the University of Pennsylvania is the first institution to adopt such a curriculum in its collegiate department, and we cannot but think that it will commend itself to students who desire to be thoroughly prepared to enter upon a medical course of study.

Still another advantage of such a course may be pointed out. It is constantly occurring that a young man looking forward to the study of medicine feels that he cannot, on account of his age or want of means or other sufficient cause, take a full collegiate course before beginning his professional studies, while he can still spend a year or more at college. To such a one the Sixth Course in the Towne Scientific School affords an admirable opportunity. For by a judicious selection he can avail himself of those branches a knowledge of which will be of the greatest use to him in his medical studies, and thus virtually prolong the period of those studies most advantageously.

With the better grade of material thus afforded, the Medical Department of the University hopes to be able also to make still more effective the measures of reform in medical education which it inaugurated four years ago.

—

Jefferson Medical College, Philadelphia.

The continued increase in the size of the Jefferson classes has rendered additional accommodations absolutely necessary ; hence, in the recess since the close of the winter term, the main building is being remodelled by an extension of the front, by adding a new story, and by constructing new Laboratory Rooms. By this extension of the front, the seating capacity of each lecture room will be materially increased. Thorough ventilation is secured to each lecture room by the introduction of the *Manchester system*. By the addition of another story a new and more commodious dissecting room will be constructed, and the present dissecting room will be converted into a laboratory for experimental therapeutics and pharmacy. A large, well-lighted room has been provided for practical obstetrics, and another with special reference to microscopic work, and for a laboratory of pathological histology and morbid anatomy.

The Faculty have made important changes in the curriculum. They have extended the winter term about one month, so that the Commencement exercises will take place at the end of March. Two very important objects to the student have been secured by this change ; the weekly number of lectures is reduced in some of the branches, which gives the student more time for practical and laboratory work, and affords him an opportunity to review and digest the lectures. The whole number of didactic lectures in each department will be about the same as before, the only difference being the distribution of the lectures over a longer period.

Courses of practical and laboratory instruction are to be given in connection with all the chairs, and are designed for, and obligatory upon, candidates for the degree—who are not already graduates of other schools—and are free of charge to them, except in the case of practical anatomy. Candidates for *partial examination* will be required to attend those branches on which they desire to be examined at the end of the session.

—

New York Academy of Medicine.—At a meeting of the New York Academy of Medicine, held May 19, Dr. E. G. Janeway, the retiring member of the Health Board, read a paper upon the present endemic of typhus fever in the city, tracing its course from its inception.

At the same meeting Dr. C. C. Lee offered a resolution congratulating Mr. Spencer Wells upon the completion of his one-thousandth case of ovariotomy, and upon his wonderful success in the operation—769 lives having been saved by his individual efforts. The resolution was unanimously adopted, and the president, Dr. Barker, appointed to personally present the same to Mr. Wells.

—

Louisiana State Medical Society.—The fourth annual meeting of this society was held at New Orleans, March 30th, Dr. C. W. Smith, President, in the chair. Dr. J. S. Herrick, Corresponding Secretary, reported that there are in the State 799 physicians, of which 642 are regular, 65 doubtful or unknown, and 92 irregular. The following officers were elected for the ensuing year: President, Dr. A. A. Lyon, of Caddo; Vice-Presidents, Drs. D. R. Fox, of Plaquemines, J. P. Davidson, of Orleans, A. B. Snell, of Iberville, R. H. Day, of Baton Rouge, W. W. Ashton, of Caddo, J. D. Hammond, of Morehouse; Secretary, Dr. L.

F. Solomon. The next annual meeting will be held in New Orleans on the last Wednesday in March, 1882.

———

New York Health Commission.—The Mayor has nominated Dr. Woolsey Johnson for the position of Health Commissioner in the place of Dr. E. G. Janeway, whose term of office has recently expired.

———

Iodine Fumigation of the Ear.—Dr. GUÉNEAU DE MUSSY speaks highly of the employment of iodine in affections of the cavity of the tympanum. A very firm little ball of iodized cotton surrounded by wadding is introduced into the meatus. The iodine gradually exhales, filling the tympanum with an iodized atmosphere. At the end of from twenty-four to thirty-six hours the cotton becomes decolourized and requires renewal.—*Med. Times and Gazette*, April 23, 1881, from *Journal de Thérapeutique*, March 25.

———

Prosecution of Unqualified Practitioners.—Still another unqualified medical practitioner is being prosecuted in New York for unlawfully practising in violation of Chapter 513 of the Laws of 1880. The prosecution was instituted by the Medical Society of the County of New York.

———

The Seaside Sanitarium, at Rockaway Beach, will soon be opened for the reception of destitute sick children. This institution was founded five years ago, and has received, during the summer months since its establishment, over 40,000 sick children from the tenement houses. 245 weekly inmates, besides 200 daily visitors, can be accommodated at the Sanitarium.

———

OBITUARY RECORD.—Died, in Philadelphia, on the 10th of June, aged 45 years, H. LENOX HODGE, M.D., Demonstrator of Anatomy in the University of Pennsylvania, and Surgeon to the Presbyterian Hospital and to the Children's Hospital.

Dr. Hodge was the son of the late Dr. Hugh L. Hodge, the eminent Professor of Obstetrics in the University of Pennsylvania. He was educated at the University, and graduated in the arts in 1855 and in medicine in 1858. He subsequently served a term as resident physician at the Pennsylvania Hospital. During the war he was attached to the Satterlee Hospital, at Philadelphia, and also served in the field with the Army of the Potomac. On the organization of the Presbyterian Hospital in 1872 he was appointed on the surgical staff. He was elected President of the Pathological Society in 187–. In 1870 he was appointed Demonstrator of Surgery in the University of Pennsylvania.

Dr. Hodge was distinguished for his integrity and uprightness. He was a conscientious student and pains-taking surgeon; and as a teacher he was always deeply interested in the welfare of his students, and, in turn, was greatly beloved by them. Charitable associations for the relief of the poor and afflicted found in him a ready co-worker, and at the time of his decease he was a director in the Pennsylvania Institution for the Deaf and Dumb, and President of the Society for the Organization of Charity. Of kindly nature and generous heart he was ever ready to give aid and counsel where it was needed, and deeply imbued with the true religious spirit, its practical lessons were beautifully exemplified in his daily life.

———

To Readers and Correspondents.—*The Editor will be happy to receive early intelligence of local events of general medical interest, or which it is desirable to bring to the notice of the profession. Local papers containing reports or news items should be marked.*

CONTENTS OF NUMBER 464.

AUGUST, 1881.

CLINICS.

MEDICAL NEWS.

THE

MEDICAL NEWS AND ABSTRACT.

VOL. XXXIX. No. 8.   AUGUST, 1881.   WHOLE No. 464.

· CLINICS.

Clinical Lectures.

THE TREATMENT OF THE NIGHT-SWEATING OF PHTHISIS.

A CLINICAL LECTURE DELIVERED AT THE PENNSYLVANIA HOSPITAL.

By J. M. DA COSTA, M.D.,

PROFESSOR OF PRACTICE OF MEDICINE AND OF CLINICAL MEDICINE AT THE JEFFERSON MEDICAL COLLEGE; PHYSICIAN TO THE PENNSYLVANIA HOSPITAL.

[Reported by Frank Woodbury, M.D.]

GENTLEMEN: The first case to which this morning I shall call your attention is that of Mary E., 26 years of age, unmarried. There is a bad family record; the mother is supposed to have died of pneumonia; more likely it was a tubercular affection, as she was ill for some time. The patient herself has never been in very robust health, and last August she had, it is said, an attack of intermittent fever, which lasted for four weeks. The menses were regular until April, since which time they have not appeared; and for the last three months she has had a troublesome cough, night-sweats, fever, and has lost forty pounds in weight. There has been no hæmoptysis. She has been obliged to work all the time, until she found herself absolutely unable on account of shortness of breath and debility. One point I want to make here clear to you—the thoracic symptoms came on suddenly, beginning in November, as a chest-cold following exposure.

Upon admission, she was found to have a cough and a troublesome hectic fever. Under the left clavicle the percussion-note was dull, and upon auscultation blowing respiration, and some moist râles indicated the advanced tubercular deposit. Her feet were œdematous, the urine was normal.

As regards treatment, she has been placed, since admission, upon pills of quinia, digitalis, and opium, and on these, with a liberal diet, she somewhat improved. But there was an element in the case which did not improve—her night-sweats—until, after being in the hospital for some time, the gentleman who had charge of her ordered her atropia (gr. $\frac{1}{80}$), to be given at night. The effect was most evident in putting a stop to one annoying symptom, the habit of getting up frequently at night to urinate.

Upon the sweating the influence of the drug was not so positive. It is, indeed, noted that even under one-sixtieth of a grain of atropia each night, with quinia, iron, and good food, the night-sweats continued, and the atropia was stopped. This note was made on the 13th of January, the atropia having been begun on the 8th.

I will not go on with the history of the case further than to say that a troublesome diarrhœa broke out about this time, and was met with bismuth and opium. The diarrhœa only for a time improved; she was then with better effect placed upon oxide of silver and opium. But what became of the sweats? They persisted. The atropia, as I have said, was discontinued after about ten days' trial, having produced some, but not a striking, effect; after the diarrhœa appeared it was not considered advisable to continue it. Upon the 28th of January, she was placed upon salicylic acid. It was noted at this time that the other symptoms were better; the diarrhœa no longer existed.

But what I wish to call your attention particularly to here, is the subsequent course of the fever and of the sweats, how influenced by salicylic acid, and what other remedies were made use of. The first effect of the salicylic acid given in doses of thirty-grains at night was an undoubted influence upon the sweats; they were less, they became localized more about the neck and face, and far less general. She slept well, her cough also was somewhat better, which cannot be attributed to the salicylic acid, but to the steady improvement in the nutrition, under good diet and the pills of quinia, opium, and digitalis, which kept the fever temperature in check. I exhibit to you the chart, which is the daily axillary thermometric record. You see it is sometimes as high as 103° or 104° in the evening and nearly normal the next morning; it seems almost like the record of remittent fever, so great is the difference between morning and evening. Her affection was therefore characterized by irregular fever, or rather by what is the regular fever of this type of pulmonary disease. The highest point reached was on the 4th of February (104.6° in the afternoon), while she was still taking salicylic acid.

I found that while the acid had some effect, it did not influence the sweats sufficiently, and a material change in the treatment was decided upon. I then put her upon a remedy to which I wish to call your attention—a remedy which I have been using in this hospital for the last three years—ergotine. The salicylic acid being suspended, she was ordered ergotine, two grains in pill, three times a day. The results were successful. I do not tell you that the salicylic acid had no effect, for it had, but the ergotine had a better effect. What is particularly observable is that the temperature has declined, the range is lower, and, indeed, it has been on several occasions lately a normal temperature. The highest point reached since taking the remedy is $101\frac{1}{2}°$, the lowest $98\frac{1}{2}°$.

Now having explained the case, and especially the treatment of the symptom for which I brought her before you, let us make an examination of her present state in order to compare it with her previous condition.

Her temperature this morning is $98\frac{1}{2}°$, normal; last night it was $100\frac{1}{2}°$. She says that she had a slight sweat last night about the face and neck; it was, however, of short duration, and nothing like as profuse as it has been. This was the first sweating for nearly a week. There has not even been any moisture.

As regards the physical signs, you observe dulness on percussion, still very marked at the left apex. Upon auscultation, I perceive harsh respiration, almost bronchial, with distinct prolonged expiration.   Harsh respiration extends all over the lung, with here and there moist crackling, but this is particularly noticed at the upper part of the lung, both anteriorly and posteriorly.   On the right side, the vesicular murmur is somewhat harsh, only there is no marked dulness, except immediately under the clavicle.   In other words, the signs of consolidation are here very light.

Her appetite is better, though the tongue is still somewhat coated.   She has, since Feb. 13, been taking the syrup of the iodide of iron in twenty-drop doses, the pills of quinia, digitalis, and opium having been stopped at that time.   The ergotine has been continued, and has been increased to four times a day.   [Let me add that sweating was never again marked. The patient died about a month afterwards from exhaustion.]

CASE II.—There was another case similar to this, occupying bed No. 1 which I shall bring before you.   I will give you very briefly her history. She has a tubercular deposit, especially in the right lung, of about one year's standing ; she lost a brother by tubercular consumption.   The history is that of a gradual disease with considerable wasting, purulent expectoration, and softening just beginning.   Her most troublesome symptom was night-sweating.   For this she was first ordered atropia, one-sixtieth of a grain at night on the 21st of December of last year, and the remedy was continued until Jan. 3, 1881, at first with good results, but finally losing its effect.   Oxide of zinc with hyoscyamus, aromatic sulphuric acid, strychnia, quinia, all answered partially for a time, but only partially, and salicylic acid, ten grains three times daily, was used for four or five days (the evening temperature being about 101°), with some, but not with very decided result.   On Feb. 6, ergotine, two grains four times daily, was ordered, while the same general tonic and nutrient treatment was continued.   After the second night she began to improve, and by the 13th the sweats had stopped, with the exception of the night of the 12th, when there was a little sweating on the face and breast.   From this time to the 28th, she took the medicine far less regularly, though she remained more or less under its influence.   For twenty days there was no night-sweating, only occasionally a little moisture about the face and breast ; with the stoppage of the exhausting discharge, her general health improved markedly. Unfortunately, by the 5th of March, the remedy began to lose its effect, and she soon afterwards left the hospital.   She returned in about one month for a few weeks, and the night-sweats, which, however, had never been so bad as prior to the ergotine treatment, were for a time again very favourably influenced by this agent.

I shall now call your attention to a couple of cases for some time under my observation in the men's medical, in which also profuse sweating was a very distressing symptom.

CASE III.—John McC., bed 37, a case of pneumonic phthisis of left lung, followed by tubercular complication of both.   There is beginning softening at left apex ; the cough is most troublesome, so are the night-sweats.   They have been going on for eight months, and gaining in intensity.   The patient is weak, but his disease was not actively progressing; the temperature was but little above the normal, and sometimes normal.   A treatment by pills of quinia, opium, and digitalis, and by the compound syrup of the phosphates improved his cough and general condition, but had no influence on the sweats.   A granule of one-sixtieth of a grain of atropia at night arrested them promptly, but though continned for a week had no permanent effect on them; oxide of zinc was temporarily of service; strychnia, one twenty-fourth of a grain three times a day, did better; and, being free from sweats for nearly two weeks, and under the effect of his general treatment, he improved decidedly. But the sweats returned, and he was placed, instead of on the strychnia, on ergotine, two grains three times daily. After the second night they were very much better, but they did not stop until the fourth. They were absent for a week, then he had a rather profuse sweat during a restless night. The ergotine was now given four times daily, and prevented further sweating. After about a week of this increased dose it was suspended, except occasionally, and though the disease was progressing, sweating was not again a prominent symptom.

CASE IV.—In this man of fifty years of age, a large cavity was found at the left apex, and, when he came under observation, decided night-sweats had existed for two months. The evening temperature did not exceed 102°. He passed six pints of urine daily of spec. gr. varying from 1007 to 1010, and free from albumen and sugar. Chlorodyne benefited his cough very much; the night-sweats were markedly and permanently controlled by ergotine in two-grain doses three times daily, which also strikingly lessened the quantity of urine passed.

But it is needless to multiply cases. I merely brought these forward because they were all marked instances of the symptom I wish to discuss with you—the night-sweating of phthisis; and they illustrate it in some of the various forms and different stages of the disease. Now sweating in phthisis is both an annoying and a serious symptom. It very often happens in the early morning hours, and the patient is languid all day from the drain. It may follow the decline of the paroxysm of the hectic fever, but also occurs in those who have but little if any fever, and certainly nothing like hectic paroxysms. To arrest it is not only to give the patient comfort, but to save his strength and thus to retard the progress of the disease. The remedies which influence the destructive malady and improve nutrition, restrain it; but they do so slowly, and we turn, therefore, naturally, to agents which, while they act much more quickly in so doing, assist at the same time the influence of the general treatment. A great many of these remedies are empirical: some take into account the supposed pathology of the sweats, and apply the fine experimental therapeutical research of the laboratory to the benefiting of a serious symptom. We might do this with even more accuracy if the pathology of the occurrence were better understood; if it were known how it is that the morbid conditions act on the sweat-centres which are so profoundly disturbed. Yet both physiology and pathology are in this matter of sweating, alike in health and in disease, still a good deal in the dark, notwithstanding such excellent observations as those of Luchsinger, Nawrocki, and Vulpian, and the increasing knowledge concerning the sweat-centres situated in the medulla and adjacent cord.

But I shall not wander away from my subject, the treatment of night-sweats in the light of actual experience. And here I shall select for discussion the action of such remedies as are valuable yet comparatively new, and not of such tried veterans as oxide of zinc, the mineral acids, tincture of iron, and decided doses of quinia.

Yet before I examine into the value of the medicinal substances I will allude to some subjects connected with clothing and with bathing which I know are constantly ignored and are yet of importance. The clothing is often much too heavy. Take a case just seen in the female ward. Her night-sweats were kept up by heavy clothing. We found her wrapped up in shawls; she said that she could not take them off because she felt chilly; she felt chilly, and next was sweating, then sweating and next chilly, and so she wanted still more clothes, and the sweating was kept up. I wish then to impress upon you that one of the first things to be taken care of in the management of night-sweats is to see that the patient's clothing is light, particularly that he be not weighted down with heavy bedclothing; and very often you may by paying attention to this simple means prevent or certainly very much lessen the exhaustive perspirations. In addition, direct your attention to the state of the skin; let the patient take a daily slightly astringent sponge-bath, having in the water alum, rock-salt, or even whiskey or alcohol, or let him be sponged with quinia dissolved in whiskey or alcohol, or with water to which a small amount of solution of ammonia has been added; and follow this by friction to give a healthy glow to the skin. You will find that in some persons very hot water checks the excessive sweating, but in the majority moderate friction, following astringent washes is better.

In reviewing the remedies with which the last few years have made us familiar, we find quite a number with which the experiments and the sagacious observations of Dr. William Murrell have acquainted us. In the *Practitioner* for 1879 and 1880 they are detailed in full, and a summary of the use of them might be thus made, which I think will be borne out by the experience of any one who will try them: *Muscarine* stops sweating on the second or third night without causing abnormal dryness of the skin. It is best given in three doses, at the interval of an hour, in quantity not less than five minims of a one per cent. solution of a liquid extract. *Picrotoxine* produces, generally, no effect the first night; may be given solely at bedtime, either in pill of one-sixtieth of a grain, or in solution with a little glacial acetic acid. *Nitrite* of *amyl*, a good, though not a very certain or pleasant agent. Dose from one to three minims.

Dover's powder, although it cannot be called a new remedy, since its use was advocated many years since by Stokes, has come again into prominence, and in doses of two to ten grains at bedtime undoubtedly shows power in controlling colliquative sweats. I wish I could give you a theory that accounts satisfactorily for its action. But I have none in my own mind to which I turn unfalteringly. There is the same difficulty in explaining its influence on pathological sweating that there is with all the agents, as, for instance, picrotoxine and jaborandi, which are excretors of perspiration. I suppose the solution will be found in their peculiar action on the sweat-centres; but we are still remote from it. Nor can I exactly tell you in what cases Dover's powder does better than the astringent class of remedies. I think, however, that it is in cases with decided rise of temperature. I am persuaded that it is to the ipecac in the composition that much of the good is due. For I have tried giving ipecac in small doses frequently repeated, about one drop of the wine every second hour, and have seen it have a most undoubted influence on the morbid discharge. In these small doses its action may be that of a tonic to the sweat-centres in the nervous system.

I have just referred to *jaborandi*. I shall presently explain to you how I have for some years used it, added in small doses to atropia, to correct some of the unpleasant effects of this. And it is while so using it that I began to be aware of its influence on night-sweating of phthisis. But I

only half knew the fact until I read the interesting observations of
Dr. John M. Keating,[1] who, prescribing it in small quantities of the
infusion, found it answer extremely well; he believes that it contracts
the capillaries, and thus explains its action.   Dr. William Murrell, whom
I have already quoted, has administered it or pilocarpine in thirty-three
cases, in all stages of the disease.   Of pilocarpine the dose employed was
generally $\frac{1}{20}$ of a grain, either at bedtime or three or four times daily.   It
acts somewhat slowly, but is said to be very efficacious, and even to lead to
permanent results.   I confess that I have not formed so high an estimate
of it.   Indeed, I cannot say that, given by itself, it ranks with me very
high.

Salicylic acid has attracted attention more for its supposed influence
on the febrile conditions of phthisis than as a remedy for the sweating.
Still it has been so employed.   Köhnhorn[2] has recommended dusting
with salicylic acid three parts, ten of starch, and eighty-seven of talc
earth, the entire surface of the body.   Internally salicylic acid has been
resorted to for night-sweats by my colleague, Dr. Hutchinson, and from
him I learnt its use for that purpose.   In some cases it seemed to have a
good influence, but the cases are not yet numerous enough to warrant a
definite conclusion as to its merits.

I was led to use *physostigma* for the same reasons which led me to investigate jaborandi, to try and counteract with it some of the disagreeable
effects of atropia, while preserving its useful ones.   But in doing so it
was first necessary to observe whether calabar bean had in itself any influence on night-sweats; and during the winter of 1879–1880, with the
active and zealous aid of Dr. Henry M. Wetherill, at that time the resident
physician in my wards, we tested the matter in this Hospital.   We found
that calabar bean had an influence.   To cite a few of the observations:
In a man with advanced tubercular consumption, attended with profuse
night-sweats, two minims of fluid extract of physostigma were given; he
was sweating at the time; his respirations were 30; the pulse, 120; the
temperature, 100°.   In an hour afterwards the skin was almost dry; respirations were 24; the pulse was 104; the temperature, 96.6°; it rose
in two hours after this to 97.8°.   There had been no unpleasant effects,
except great thirst.   In another case we first noticed the sweating carefully, while a placebo only was given.   It came on profusely at 12 P. M.,
and while profuse, the respirations were 32, pulse was 122, the temperature, 97°; the sweating lasted four hours; as it passed away, the respirations were 28, the pulse, 114, the temperature, 99.8°.   At the same
period of the next twenty-four hours, and when the sweating had fairly
begun, although the temperature then was 99.5°, a dose of two minims of
the fluid extract of calabar bean checked the sweating in an hour and a
half, the temperature rising to 100.6°.   In a third case of marked phthisis
with night-sweats, the temperature before the sweats at 3 P. M. was 100.5°;
in an hour afterwards, with a profuse sweat it had declined to 98.6°; four
minims of the fluid extract were then given, the sweat was completely
checked in an hour, the temperature rising to 99°; there was no decided
effect on the pupil, and no unpleasant symptom.   In a fourth case, the
profuse early morning perspirations were arrested in two hours by the
same dose, the pupils being slightly contracted, the pulse becoming less
strong, the temperature declining from 100° to 97.6°.   Now, both in
these and other cases the remedy was given in two minim doses, once or

---

[1] Phila. Med. Times, June, 1877.   [2] Berliner klin. Wochenschrift, No. 1, 1880.

twice in the evening, sometimes four minims at one dose (the preparation being of the strength of one of the bean to a minim of fluid), and the sweating was undoubtedly to a great extent prevented; but only in one instance was the effect at all permanent; and, on the whole, while the action of calabar bean is undoubted, it is decidedly inferior to atropia and to ergot.

I shall now pass to the two remedies which I think pre-eminent—atropia and ergotine. The use of *atropia* is now so widely known, and it has been so much resorted to, that, although having employed it systematically in this Hospital for night-sweats for years before it began to attract general attention,[1] we may claim for it the strong partiality of early knowledge, I shall only state that it is at present accepted as the most potent agent we possess to control inordinate sweating, particularly in consumption. Not one of the remedies which I have mentioned to you has, in my opinion, anything like its power. But atropia has a most serious drawback. Even the smallest dose, to be effective, $\frac{1}{80}$ of a grain, produces such a dry mouth and throat that it often keeps the patient awake, and, in not a few instances, increases his cough. Duboisia, so much like atropia, even in its influence on sweating, has the same unfortunate effect. Local remedies, such as sucking pieces of ice, chewing chamomile flowers or sassafras pith, sipping infusions of slippery elm, only afford partial relief, moreover they prevent sleep. And the inconvenience witnessed led me to a series of observations, that I have here carried on for the last four or five years, to find among the agents which possess a physiological antagonism to atropia one which, without materially, if at all, diminishing its action on the skin, might mitigate its influence on the salivary secretion. Not to detain you too long, I will speak particularly of strychnia, calabar bean, and jaborandi, added to belladonna or atropia. With reference to strychnia, it is in many respects not antagonistic to belladonna; one, indeed, may promote the activity of the other; and I was led to hope all the more from a combination being effective with a smaller dose of the belladonna or atropia, and was induced to persevere with my observations after reading Lauder Brunton's remarks on the unaided action of strychnia in the night-sweating of phthisis.[2] But this expectation has only been partially realized. The atropia preponderates, and even in decreased doses dries the throat.

From both calabar bean and jaborandi we get better results. I have already laid before you my observations with the former given alone, and you will recall the fact, which has been made very apparent by the experiments of Fraser, Bartholow, and other investigators, that in most respects it is a true antagonist to atropia. It leads to an increased flow of saliva, and is said to increase the perspiration. But it certainly does not do so in phthisis, whatever be the explanation; and if you add gr. $\frac{1}{8}$ to gr. $\frac{1}{4}$ of the solid extract, or two to three minims of the fluid, to $\frac{1}{80}$ or $\frac{1}{60}$ of atropia, you preserve or heighten the good effect of the latter, and lessen its evil ones. Still better I find is jaborandi. The drug, you are aware, illustrates in its action a complete antagonism to atropia and produces profuse secretion from the salivary glands. Yet, though in health it promotes the most active discharge from the skin, its powers in small doses to arrest morbid sweating have been abundantly proved, and added in small doses to atropia, say ten to fifteen drops of the ordinary

---

[1] Clinical Lecture, Phila. Med. Times, Feb. 15, 1871; and Ib., Oct. 1872.
[2] St. Bartholomew's Hospital Reports, 1879.

fluid extract to $\frac{1}{60}$ of a grain, or, as I have often done, a dose of this quantity given two hours in advance of the atropia, and repeated with it, the sweats will be as well influenced, while the discomfort arising from the dryness of the mouth will be greatly diminished. The effect of the combination is undoubted, and its power is not confined to the night-perspirations of phthisis. You will remember the man in bed 34 with chronic pleurisy and sweats, which here were increased by the doses of jaborandi he was taking to reduce the effusion. $\frac{1}{60}$ of atropia at night relieved the night-sweating completely, gave him in so doing comfortable nights, and enabled us to continue the other treatment. He had no inconvenience with his throat, until we suspended the jaborandi, placing him on iron, but continuing the atropia ; yet when this parched his throat, a single dose of jaborandi quickly relieved him.

Still we cannot, even by the combination of jaborandi with atropia, always remedy the annoyance. It is difficult to hit upon the exact dose, and the atropia will at times overpower the jaborandi. I have thus been led to look for an agent which should possess something of the certainty and permanence of action of atropia without its drawbacks, and I think I have found it in *ergotine*. My first observations, made some years ago, were with the fluid extract of ergot, but I have abandoned this for ergotine as better and more easily administered. The power ergot has of contracting the arterioles and of checking excessive discharges suggested its use, and the results have been very satisfactory. Ergotine was prescribed in the cases with which I introduced the subject to your attention this morning, and I could give you many more in illustration, showing its effects in the various forms of phthisis. The dose of ergotine I employ is usually two grains three or four times daily, and by the second night the influence begins to manifest itself. The remedy may then be continued and gradually abandoned ; it produces no annoyance or discomfort whatever, and its good effects persist after it is withdrawn. It will fail or lose its effect as every other remedy will fail or lose its effect in the treatment of such an unrelenting disease, but the proportion of failures is small compared with that of the successes.

You will ask for a comparative estimate between it and atropia. For immediate results ergotine is far inferior. If you see a patient in the morning in whom you wish to prevent a violent sweating in the evening, there is no remedy which for promptness can compare with atropia ; there is, moreover, no remedy which is so potent in cases where the skin pours forth quantities of fluid. But where such speedy and decisive action is not demanded, where you are obliged to keep up a remedy for some time, where to do so with atropia becomes very difficult or occasions first discomfort and then actual distress, you have then in ergotine an agent to which you can turn with confidence. Less prompt, perhaps less certain, it is better borne, and shares with atropia the valuable power of often making a durable impression. Nay, I have seen it do so when atropia has failed.

Gentlemen, I have now laid before you the results of a series of inquiries into a matter of deep and practical interest. In summing it up in your minds you will see that there are many articles, some of which do the work required of them well, others not so well. It is not easy to say which agent in a given case will succeed best, and you ought to be as accurately as possible acquainted with the action of many. Speaking generally there are remedies which act as astringents and as arresting the secretion; there are others which under normal circumstances promote per-spiration, and allay the morbid sweating, either because they substitute a normal discharge for an abnormal one, or, what is more likely, because given in small doses they tone up and gently stimulate to healthy action the sweat-centres and the respiratory centres. But whatever the explana-tion, the latter class of remedies, Dover's powder, jaborandi, picrotoxine, are, on the whole, greatly inferior to the former, and not so permanent. And it is permanency of action at which we must, as far as possible, aim. This gives time for the general treatment to take effect; it arrests a serious drain, and what I have endeavoured to show you in the case of several of the agents, if we once succeed in making for more than a very short period a decided impression, the annoying, dangerous symptom may be altogether relieved or at least for ever broken in intensity.

CLINICAL REMARKS ON TWO CASES OF TUMOUR OF THE BLADDER.

Delivered at the University College Hospital on January 17th.

By BERKELEY HILL, F.R.C.S.,
Professor of Clinical Surgery in University College, London.

GENTLEMEN : There have been recently in our wards some excellent examples of those rare affections, tumours of the bladder. I propose to-day to select for remark two of these cases, partly for their rarity, partly because we have the morbid growths themselves for your inspection.

In speaking of tumours, I mean true morbid growths; and exclude those swellings of the hypertrophied prostate met with in certain old men, which, by their deformity, produce a train of suffering sufficiently acute. During the year just past, we have had several such patients in our wards, affording examples of some or other of the consequences of hypertrophy of the prostate. But with such cases it is not my intention to occupy your time to-day.

The list of morbid growths comprises:—

1. *Fibrous polypi*, fibrous outgrowths from the surface of the bladder, an extremely rare affection, described by Civiale and one or two others. Of these growths, a few specimens are preserved in museums.

2. *Scirrhus and encephaloid* of the walls of the bladder, growths nearly always secondary to cancerous disease elsewhere, but occasionally occurring pri-marily in this situation.

3. *True epithelial cancer*, beginning in and slowly extending in the wall of the bladder.

4. *Villous tumour.*

These growths may all begin in the bladder itself; but affections of other organs may lead to projections into, and invasions of, the bladder, as, for example—

5. *Malignant disease of the prostate*, generally encephaloid in character.

6. *Tubercular disease* of the vesiculæ seminales, or of the vesiculæ seminales and prostate.

At this moment, there is an old man in Ward 10, seventy years of age, and in fair general health, who has, for the last eighteen months, been unable to void any urine by natural efforts. He draws it off through the catheter, by which the urethra is easily traversed until the prostate is reached, where, if not well curved or very supple, it stops short. There is no suprapubic dulness; but, when the prostate and floor of the bladder are examined *per rectum*, an irregular mass of stony hardness is felt; one firm nodule projects at the upper margin of the sphincter ani into the rectum. This condition of the base of the bladder not only obstructs the flow of urine, but is also the cause of the tenesmus to which he is frequently subject, though the rectum itself is at present free from the growth. The urine is normal, always clear, and free from blood or pus; but the increasing irritability of the bladder is the patient's constant torment. By night or day, he seldom passes an hour without being compelled to use his catheter; for, as soon as two or three ounces of urine collect, his bladder makes violent efforts to expel it. The wide extent of the induration of the prostate and floor of the bladder, and its irregular stony hardness, are the grounds on which we consider it to be a case, not of simple hypertrophied prostate, but of malignant, probably scirrhous, disease.

There is also at the present time, in Ward 9, a young man, whose life is tormented by cystitis and great irritability of the bladder, sometimes more, sometimes less acute, but of already more than twelve months' standing; and occasioned by a condition of the vesiculæ seminales which we believe to be tubercular. He has already undergone Syme's amputation at the ankle for strumous disease of that joint. On another occasion, I shall draw your attention to tubercular disease of this region, of which, from time to time, we get examples sent in as cases of stone. I will pass to the two cases of which the bladders are before you.

The first is the case of epithelial primary disease, whose history has been carefully recorded by Mr. A. J. Grant, the ward-clerk. The patient, No. 2448 in the hospital register, was sixty-three years old; and, until four months before his admission, had no sign of disorder of his urinary organs. The first symptom of his disease that attracted attention was hemorrhage. The urine became red, and the blood increased so much that in a week's time it came away from the bladder in clots. Soon, but after the appearance of clots, pain began to be felt; but only after the bladder was emptied. So long as the patient was still, and did not pass urine, he was free from pain. This character of the pains continued until after his admission to hospital; but, in a few days, there were added violent attacks of spasmodic effort to void urine, which, always painful, became excruciating towards the end of his life, growing more and more frequent, and at the end almost constant.

The frequency of micturition, at first not unusual for a man of his time of life —twice by night and about every four hours by day—steadily increased during the three months which elapsed after the first appearance of the blood, until the call to pass urine came every quarter of an hour. Up to this time, the urine, though bloody, was not offensive, and had no sticky deposit. At this stage of his malady, an irregular practitioner sounded the patient for stone. After this exploration of his bladder, which he described as being prolonged and very painful, his sufferings increased; micturition became necessary every quarter of an hour; and the urine, still loaded with blood, grew very offensive. Probably the exploration was the immediate cause of the cystitis, though this affection was almost certain to arrive sooner or later. Still, the danger of thus aggravating the patient's sufferings by instrumentation should always be kept carefully in view, when deliberating on the expediency of sounding a patient. On his admission, on December 7, 1880, he was found to be a fairly stout man, and in pretty good general condition; of this stoutness he lost little before death; but his state as to micturition was pretty much as already described; frequent (half-hourly) calls to pass urine.—its ejection being accomplished with much straining and pain, the latter referred to the end of the penis; and blood and ropy pus passed every time with the urine. The sound introduced into the bladder struck no stone, but caused great pain in passing over the neck ; indeed, the exploration could not be completely carried out, owing to the pain it excited. The prostate was not enlarged, nor could any unusual condition of the bladder be detected by rectal examination. There were no enlarged glands to be felt in the inguinal or the iliac regions.

Thereafter, various remedies were employed to allay the cystitis and consequent irritation of the bladder, but without avail. On one occasion, the patient was aræsthetized, the bladder carefully sounded, and its ammoniacal ropy contents washed out by Clover's bottle. As before, no stone was found ; but, in the purulent deposit from the fluid so exhausted, shreds of tissue were found on microscopical examination, by Mr. Stanley Boyd, our surgical registrar ; these consisted of patches of epithelial and nucleated cells, to some of which a shred of fibres was attached. In spite of anodynes, of attempts by tying in India-rubber catheters, or by washing out with quinine or astringent solutions, or simple warm water, to diminish the accumulation of fetid urine, the patient's sufferings increased ; the catheter could not be retained more than four or five hours; then the spasm it excited became unbearable. At this time constitutional disturbance began. His tongue became dry, and coated with brownish fur ; and his strength rapidly diminished. In these circumstances, I proposed to him that he should submit to operation—not with any expectation of cure, but, by establishing a free drain for the urine as fast as it reached the bladder, of relieving him of the constant pain and straining excited by its accumulation and putrefaction therein. With this object, on December 29th, I performed the usual lateral operation for the removal of stone from the bladder, making at first a small opening in the neck of the bladder, through which I introduced my finger, and recognized a soft mass projecting from the floor on the right side. By enlarging the incision in the neck of the bladder, I was able to bring away, in a lithotomy forceps, the mass I felt, which proved to be a pedunculated growth of cellular tissue, as large as a marble, but too much disorganized by sloughing for its structure to be minutely examined. By free injections of cold water, several such masses were washed out, along with much stinking pus and mucus. The hemorrhage during the operation was unimportant. The patient was but little relieved by the operation, though bleeding ceased and the urine drained away continuously through the wound. His spasms, though less frequent, continued with nearly the same severity until his death, on the third day after the operation.

 Post-mortem, the condition of the urinary organs was very interesting, and especially so when compared with that of the case of villous disease, whose examination we made on the same afternoon. The bladder was contracted, of about six ounces' capacity, and, when laid open along the mesial line from the neck by the anterior part to the apex and everted, it revealed this condition. There is a growth, which, commencing on the inner surface opposite the pubes, continues along the right side to the apex, and there crosses to the left. On the right, the growth is much the thickest ; while, on the left, its advancing margin is well defined, being raised near the apex a quarter of an inch above the general level of the mucous membrane. The surface of the growth is generally sloughy and very irregular ; long shreds hang down from the upper portion, and from the right side depends a finger-like process, one inch long and a quarter of an inch across. The mucous membrane of the bladder elsewhere is gray and pigmented, thus showing considerable chronic inflammation. The walls are rugose, from moderate hypertrophy of the muscular tissue. Here are some sections of the growth, showing the nests of nucleated epithelial cells, occupying the meshes of a fine connective network, freely supplied with capillaries. You should compare it with the specimen from the villous growth, showing the delicate branching processes hanging freely from the tumour. The ureters are but little, if at all, dilated, though, like the bladder, the mucous membrane and that of the pelvis, especially of the pelvis in the left kidney, are thickened, grayish, and marked with small hemorrhages. The kidneys themselves are congested and interstitially inflamed, the left particularly so. These changes in the kidney are of recent origin, set up by extension of the irritation from the bladder.

You will note that the condition of the body after death confirmed the indications of the symptoms during life, that the patient died of exhaustion consequent on the irritation of the bladder, and from the cachexia of the tumour. The general system was but to a small extent invaded. A few of the lumbar lymphatic glands were enlarged, and pale gray on section, but no consecutive multiplication of the growth beyond the bladder was found.

Next come the notes of the case of villous growth. J. M., 38 years old (No. 2615 in hospital register), a lamplighter, and, therefore, walking much daily, had been a healthy man, and noticed nothing unusual in his habit of passing urine until April, 1880, eight months before admission. Then suddenly his urine became red with blood after exercise, and flowed less freely than before. This red coloration was for some time only observed during and after exercise ; never on rising from bed in the morning. The intermixture of blood continued, without intermission, to be the main trouble until last Christmas, with the exception only of three or four days, during which his urine was of ordinary aspect. About Christmas new symptoms appeared, namely, constant desire to micturate and uncontrollable dribbling. On Christmas day, clots. of blood came away during the efforts to pass urine ; at the same time pain commenced to be felt in passing urine, and, for three or four minutes afterwards, at the end of the penis. When admitted on December 30th, he walked to the hospital from Kentish Town, and the urine passed on his arrival was dull crimson. The next day the patient was passing urine and blood every few minutes, with much painful straining to void the last few drops ; often black clots, without any urine, were then ejected. There were no renal or suprapubic tendencies ; no swelling of the testes or cords. The prostate was of normal size, but the trigone of the bladder, felt through the rectum, appeared to be thickened though yielding. The finger experienced the kind of resistance afforded by a moderately distended bladder. To clear up this doubt, a flexible *coudé* catheter was passed into the bladder, encountering no difficulty, and giving rise to no pain in its passage ; but, as only a few drops of blood escaped through it, some water was injected ; this returned almost untinged with blood, being forcibly driven out both through and along the sides of the catheter. The bladder being thus proved to be.empty, the catheter was withdrawn, and brought away in its eye a gray granulation. This was at once put under the microscope, when it was seen to be a compound papilla, covered by slender columnar epithelium. This discovery materially aided the diagnosis, otherwise difficult, of vascular tumour of the bladder. This diagnosis, suggested by the persistent painless hemorrhage, and by the fact that villous is the most frequent form of tumour of the bladder, was rendered certain by the structure of the papilla. This examination took place the day after the patient's admission, viz., December 31st. The treatment ordered was turpentine, in five-minim doses, every four hours, opiates to relieve spasm, rest in bed, and ice to the perineum. It was also determined that, if this did not check the hemorrhage in twenty-four hours, recourse should be had to subcutaneous injections of sclerotic acid, a form of the active principle of ergot. As the bleeding had not diminished by 11 A. M., on January 1st a subcutaneous injection was given, not of sclerotic acid, but of ergotine itself, specially prepared on a new method by Mr. Gerrard, the hospital pharmacist. The injection was repeated at 5 P. M., and again at 1 A. M. on the next morning (January 2d). On each occasion half a grain was injected, about half the dose usually employed. By 11 A. M. the hemorrhage had greatly diminished, though not wholly ceased, when suddenly syncope set in, and he died. *Post-mortem* examination twenty-seven hours after death. The body was somewhat blanched, and the viscera were all more or less drained of blood. The heart contained a small quantity of fluid blood, free from clot, and was firmly contracted in rigor mortis. The pulmonary arteries were clear of coagula. Owing to the obscurity surrounding the cause of death, all the viscera were carefully examined, and were all found to be free from disease, with the exception of the urinary organs. These, from the great size of the growth, formed an admirable example of a villous tumour in the bladder; such tumours usually are not larger than a marble or small strawberry; but this, you see, is as large as a hen's egg, measuring over two inches in length, by one and a half inches in breadth. The growth itself is formed of long delicate villi of deep red colour, and attached by a short pedicle, measuring less than half an inch across, to the margin of the orifice of the right ureter, around which it so grows that a probe passed down the ureter reaches the bladder only after traversing the growth. These growths are scarcely ever, if ever, found away from the trigone, and usually spring from one of the three orifices. In structure they are true papillomata, almost warts; and they prove fatal, not by any malignant character of their growth, but mainly by their mechanical action, wearing the patient out with pain and irritation, and partly by exhaustive loss of blood, for the structure of the tumour is loose and highly vascular, each of these delicate papillæ being provided with its capillary vessel, so that the frequent rupture of bloodvessels is an unfailing occurrence. We owe to our surgical registrar, Mr. Stanley Boyd, the preparation of the specimens for our inspection, and also these beautiful sections of the growths under the microscope now before you. You will at once recognize the fine branching papillæ, each one containing its capillary, and covered by slender columnar epithelium, of which the mass is almost entirely composed.

The bladder, ureters, and kidneys are excellent examples of the changes which take place as simple results of impediment to escape of urine from the bladder. The bladder itself is of ordinary capacity, its mucous membrane is healthy, not chronically inflamed as in the example of epithelial cancer. It is rugose and slightly sacculated from the great hypertrophy of the muscular coats, being half an inch thick in some places. The ureters are vastly dilated on both sides, that from the right kidney almost admitting the little finger, and having its coats much thickened, but, like the enormously dilated pelvis and calyces, presenting no trace of inflammation, either recent or old. The kidney itself shows an extreme result of distension, being little more than a bag of fluid. All signs of papillæ or pyramids are gone, their sites at the heads of the calyces being occupied by depressions. The cortex forms a thin layer, nowhere more than a quarter of an inch thick, and with the expanded pelvis and calyces constructs the bag which the kidney has become. The left kidney in all respects resembles the right, except that the dilatation of its several parts is considerably less. The cortex is of ordinary thickness, pale yellow, and of normal consistence; and a good deal of the pyramids still remains. It is obvious how these changes come about. The growth began at the outlet of the right ureter, consequently impediment to the escape of urine from the right kidney commenced very early, and was kept up, long before any difficulty occurred to the entry into the bladder of urine from the left ureter; thus expansion of the left ureter and kidney began only when the tumour had gained such a bulk that would enable it to overlie the

orifice of the left ureter, when it fell on the floor of the bladder, or was compressed against the trigone in the empty state of the viscus. So, again, the
hypertrophy of the muscular coat of the bladder was caused by the impediment
to the discharge of urine when the tumour blocked the neck. This position of
the tumour against the neck of the bladder probably excited the violent spasmodic
contractions which were so painful during the last days of the patient's life.

It is interesting to compare the absence of inflammation in this bladder with
the abundant evidence of cystitis, pyelitis, and nephritis in the case of epithelioma. There we have the slaty gray colour and punctiform hemorrhages in the
mucous membranes, the shiny muco-pus adhering to the walls of the bladder,
ureter, and pelvis, and the nephritis most decided in the left kidney, and not
quite absent in the right one. You will recollect, in the patient's account of his
state previous to his admission here, that his urine, though bloody, was neither
ropy nor offensive before the sounding by the quack ; in fact, probably it was
very similar to that which our patient with villous tumour passed—dark red,
though fairly clear, and with a sediment consisting almost wholly of blood-clots.
After the sounding the urine quickly changed, and showed evidence of cystitis.
Cystitis being set up, it was not difficult, in a bladder deformed by thickening of
its coats, for a shred of putrid muco-pus to slip into, or be driven into, the orifice
of an ureter during some expulsive effort of the bladder, and there excite inflammation, which would quickly travel along the irritated mucous surface to the
pelvis of the kidney. This is one mode, though probably not the only one, by
which pyelitis is set up in cystitis; but it is a mode that explains why, in cases
of cystitis and pyelitis set up by upwardly extending irritations, one ureter and
kidney shall be affected while the other escapes.

In both these patients the sign that enabled us to make a correct diagnosis
during life was the evidence obtained by putting under the microscope fragments
of the tumour itself, these fragments coming away in the fluid withdrawn from
the bladder in the one case, and being brought out in the eye of the catheter in
the other. But such good fortune is rare, and probably portions of the growth
are separated only when it has attained considerable development. Hence in
many cases the diagnosis (on which depends the treatment) has to be made on
symptoms. Now the three leading symptoms of tumour are—1. Irritable
bladder; 2. Hemorrhage; 3. Pain of a particular kind. But these symptoms
also often accompany several other affections, namely, stricture of the urethra,
stone, chronic retention from enlarged prostate, malignant and tubercular disease
of the prostate and vesiculæ seminales, and certain diseases of the kidney; even
piles or ulcer of the rectum are occasional reflex causes of irritable bladder. The
presence or absence of such possible causes as these must be ascertained by
physical examination of the parts. In these two cases the exclusion of all causes
of vesical irritative hemorrhage and pain, but stone, was easy during life. The condition of the urethra, and of the prostate and rectum, could be ascertained, while
the clinical symptoms, though not strongly indicative of stone, did not certainly
contradict that disorder.

Irritability of the Bladder.—In cases of stone, stricture, and prostatic retention, it usually happens that too frequent and somewhat painful desire to pass
urine is the first symptom for which relief is sought. When stone excites it,
irritability is an early sign, because the cause of irritation, the stone, most frequently lies on the neck, being continually thrown thither by the action of the
vesical muscles. Cases of tumour commonly differ from the rest, in that bleeding
is the first symptom to attract the attention. Irritability of the bladder is a late
symptom. It did not appear in our two patients for some time (four weeks in

one man, and several months in the other) after hemorrhage had become habitual. The early or late variation in the time of the appearance of frequent calls to pass urine in cases of tumour when bleeding has become a prominent feature of their malady, depends much on the position of the growth ; that is, in its proximity to the outlet from the bladder.   In our case of epithelioma, the morbid growth began at the right side of the bladder, and, spreading in all directions along the mucous membrane, soon reached the neck.   But in the case of villous tumour, the tumour was attached to the right ureter by a pedicle, and could affect the neck only when it had attained bulk sufficient to enable it to fall against that part.   In the former, irritation soon came; in the latter, only shortly before death.   Nevertheless, the character of the irritation they excited had features strongly unlike the irritability caused by calculus.

Hemorrhage.—The bleeding had characters differing from that customary with stone; it was the first symptom sufficiently urgent to attract attention ; it was from the beginning comparatively copious, and soon consisted in great part of clotted blood.   Again, the hemorrhage was persistent, and was almost throughout the leading symptom.   This is very characteristic of tumour, though intervals of cessation of hemorrhage do occur during the course of a tumour.   Even several weeks may at first intervene between the discharges of blood ; no other symptom is developed, and the urine may remain in the intervals quite free from blood or albumen.   But when once bleeding is set up, it becomes more and more copious, and the intervals between the bleedings grow more and more short, while the irritability is continuous, slight, or altogether absent.   When a stone causes hemorrhage, it is seldom copious at first, and never prolonged ; but it very rarely refrains from causing irritability.

Hemorrhage from calculus is caused by the stone eroding the mucous surface of the bladder where it lies, and opening a vessel whence blood escapes; but such vessels are commonly of small calibre, and are quickly closed by coagulation of the blood.   Hence, characteristic of such bleedings, is the small quantity lost, being often sufficient merely to furnish traces of albumen in the urine, or to appear as a few drops of blood *per urethram* distinct from the urine.   Copious intermittent hemorrhage may be caused by stone, but only in cases complicated by hypertrophied prostate, on which some dilated veins are coursing.   Such veins often bleed when grazed by a stone, just as they will bleed copiously for a short time, even when there is no foreign body in the bladder, if the organ become congested by exposure to cold, by venereal excitement, etc.   But, when the gorged vessels have drained themselves, and their orifices are plugged by coagula, the bleeding ceases until they are again over-distended, or again injured, and their coats give way anew.   There is no regular increasing frequency and gravity of the hemorrhages.   It is different with the bloodvessels of a rapidly enlarging tumour.   They are very numerous, have but thin walls, and are ill-supported in the soft cellular tissue, in which the fibrous element is but scanty.   In such new structures the vessels that first give way are plugged, and shrink, while new ones develop rapidly in their place, which are ruptured in a similar manner.   Thus a continual escape of blood from the surface of the tumour is maintained for some considerable time.

Pain.—I have spoken of the *irritable bladder* and of *hemorrhage* as symptoms of tumour, and how, in their niceties, they vary from the peculiarities of irritability and hemorrhage set up by stone.   The *pain* felt in these cases of vesical tumour closely resembles that due to stone, being felt at the end of the penis, sometimes elsewhere also ; but the pain of stone is most acute immediately *after* the bladder is emptied.   It is explained by supposing that the bladder's muscular contraction squeezes the stone against the ulcerated patch which it has worn for itself, and that the pain subsides when enough urine has trickled into the bladder to expand its sensitive surface away from the stone. This explanation is probably a true one in many cases, but not in all. The character of the pain in our case of tumour was not exactly of this kind. It was caused by micturition, it is true ; but during micturition it was most severe, and culminated in one or two agonizing spasms during the ejection of the last drops. It then began to subside, and soon disappeared, until the next act of micturition revived it. Hence the pain was one felt *during*, more than *after*, micturition. In the case of epithelioma there was ulceration of a great part of the surface of the bladder ; in the other patient there was no ulceration, but there was a foreign body, the villous growth, which was embraced by the extrusor muscles of the neck of the bladder, and prevented their natural contraction. Both conditions accounted for the agonizing spasms. These differences in the symptoms were not sufficient to warrant the exclusion of stone as the cause of the patient's sufferings. But they were so far different as to suggest tumour rather than stone. This exclusion of stone was rendered more probable in the case of epithelioma, by failure to detect it with the sound. Sounding is useful to gain information respecting the condition of the bladder, beyond the proof it affords of the absence of stone. The presence even of villous growths sometimes may be felt by the sound, while, when no such growth can be found, the sound forms an useful landmark for the finger in the rectum when searching all that portion of the bladder which can be reached by that means. Sounding should certainly have been performed in the second patient when the loss of blood had been somewhat checked, and the patient's condition improved by opiates and rest. As it was, instrumentation in both cases obtained positive evidence for us, though in that of villous growth the sound was represented by a soft, flexible catheter.

To sum up, then, gentlemen, the remarks which I have made. The symptoms of tumour of the bladder resemble very closely those of stone ; this, on reflection, we can see is only what we might expect on à *priori* grounds, for a tumour is, in all that concerns the functional activity of the bladder, as much a foreign body as a stone. The pain in tumour, though like that caused by stone, has its distinctions, which, though not very strong, are useful in diagnosis. It is due in some cases to ulceration ; in some, to the efforts at expulsion brought about by grasping of the tumour by the extrusor muscles. Hemorrhage is in tumours an early symptom, and, once established, is the most constantly present ; signs of irritation of the bladder are later on in their occurrence. With stone, the reverse holds good ; bladder-irritation is an early and almost constant symptom, and hemorrhage, as a rule, is not copious, and is always markedly intermittent ; in the cases where stone does produce copious bleeding, this proceeds from an enlarged prostate.

Exercise, perhaps, influences hemorrhage from stone more than bleeding from tumour ; though it has a marked influence over the latter. But exercise is most provocative of pain to the calculous patient ; witness the suffering caused by a ride in a jolting cart. On the other hand, exercise seldom causes pain to the patient with tumour. Sudden stoppage occurs with both classes of patients, though more frequently with the calculous ones. Owing to this want of broad distinction between the diseases, it will be proper in every case to sound the bladder, in order to gain all information possible respecting the state of the contents and of the neck and base of the bladder, and the structures in relation with it, by the sound and the finger.—*Brit. Med. Journal*, May 14, 1881.

Hospital Notes.

BELLEVUE HOSPITAL, NEW YORK.
(Service of Dr. AUSTIN FLINT, Sr.)
(Specially reported for the MEDICAL NEWS AND ABSTRACT.)

Diabetes Mellitus; Treatment with Codeia.

Peter S., æt. 35, Ireland, liquor dealer; admitted May 5th. In earlier life
the patient's occupations were of a laborious nature, and led to frequent exposures
and hardships. His later years have been spent in leisure. He has always
drank malt liquors, in moderation, but never was addicted to the use of spirits
until five or six months ago. Since then he has used them to excess, and often
upon an empty stomach. He had the initial lesion of syphilis twenty years ago,
which was promptly treated, and was not followed by secondary or tertiary
symptoms. He has not indulged in excessive venery. He has not had malarial
fever, gout, or rheumatism. The patient enjoyed perfect health until about six
months ago, when he became very dissipated. He spent almost every night, for
a number of consecutive months, in gaming and debauchery. He drank brandy
very often during the night, ate nothing, and, being absorbed with gaming,
habitually retained his urine longer than was natural. He suffered from gastritis,
with frequent vomiting. For four or five months he hardly took a substantial
nourishing meal. He cannot remember that he received any injury during this
time, to his head or abdomen. Three months since he began to be debilitated
and habitually constipated, having no fecal evacuations for eight or ten days at a
time. One day, after having induced free catharsis with a saline purgative, he
noticed that his urine became suddenly abnormally abundant. He believes that
he passed several gallons daily. He suffered from urgent thirst. A month later
his appetite became voracious. He was obstinately constipated. He suffered
from progressive asthenia, extinction of venereal desire, capricious appetite,
slight febrile movement, and progressive emaciation, but did not take to the bed
until his admission, on May 5th. He now complains of asthenia, but has no pain,
epistaxis, œdema, or emesis. He has great thirst and an enormous appetite. His
urine is pale, acid, sp. gr. 1036, and has no albumen nor casts. It contains thirteen
grains of sugar to the ounce.

Treatment.—His diet was restricted to meats, milk, fish, eggs, cabbage and
tomatoes, coffee, tea, and sherry wine. The only remedy employed in his case
consisted of codeia, gr. $\frac{1}{4}$, three times a day. On May 6th he passed 184 oz. of
urine; on the 7th, 170 oz.; on the 8th, 135 oz.; on the 9th, 130 oz.; and on the
12th, 140 oz. [He left the Hospital a few days later to go to Europe. The improvement was progressive, although not marked, up to the time of his departure.—REP.]

—

Acute Articular Rheumatism; Treatment with Salicin.

William N., æt. 26, Ireland, clerk; admitted April 30, 1881. The patient
states that he belongs to a healthy family, none of the members of which have
ever been afflicted with rheumatism. Five years ago, after exposure to inclem-
ent weather, he was attacked with acute pain in his left ankle, with marked redness and swelling of that joint. The inflammatory symptoms were subsequently
fully developed in the knees, hips, shoulders, elbows, and wrists. This attack
confined the patient to his bed for two entire months, at the end of which time
he resumed his occupations, but suffered from constant dyspnœa, vertigo, epistaxis, and cardiac palpitation. Two and a half years ago he had another attack
of acute articular rheumatism, which was milder, and incapacitated him for labour

only three weeks. The third attack occurred in March, 1881. He was admitted to Bellevue Hospital and treated during two weeks, with salicylate of soda. At the end of that time he was discharged quite cured, but returned on April 30th with acute inflammation in his knees and his left shoulder. His temperature was 101½°. His urine was normal. His heart was notably hypertrophied, the apex beat being in the 7th intercostal space. An organic systolic cardiac murmur was heard over the aortic orifice and was transmitted into the carotids. An endocardial systolic murmur was heard over the left ventricle, but was not transmitted.

Treatment.—Dr. Flint being of the opinion that endocarditis constitutes a contraindication to the employment of so powerful cardial depressants as salicylic acid or the salicylates, ordered salicin, grs. xx, to be administered every two hours, and sod. bicarb., grs. xxx, every three hours. On May 1st the urine had been rendered dististinctly alkaline. The temperature was 101°. The pain had not. been relieved. On May 2d the temperature was 100¾°, and the pain had almost disappeared. On May 4th not a vestige of inflammation could be detected in the affected joints, and there was absolutely no pain. The cardiac murmurs persisted. The patient was allowed to sit up, and on the next day to walk about.

May 12. There is still some slight stiffness in the joints, which were the seat of the inflammatory symptoms. Aside from this the patient is quite well. The heart murmurs are still audible, although the endocardial murmur is very faint.

Insolation; Treatment by Cold Shower-Bath; Recovery.

THEODORE TURNBULL, M.D., of Monticello, Florida, reports the following case :—

C. A., æt. seven years, female, rather delicate, while returning from school on the afternoon of May 15, 1881, became suddenly unconscious and fell headlong to the ground. Her companions thinking her playing, deserted their little schoolmate, but afterwards observed their mistake, and then alarmed the neighbourhood; she was removed to the nearest house, which was only a few yards. When I arrived a few hours later, I found her in a comatose state; pulse quick and feeble; temperature in axilla 106.5°; respiration stertorous and somewhat accelerated; relaxation of sphincter ani; sighing and moaning sounds on expiration; no tracheal râles or convulsions; pupil neither contracted nor dilated, but not responding to light.

The treatment consisted of the wet-sheet method advised by Dr. Flint. The girl was stripped and placed in a sheet, water being sprinkled over the whole surface at intervals of half a minute; whiskey was given at short intervals, and in small doses to prevent vomiting. She began to rouse up in about ten minutes, the shower-bath being kept up for at least half an hour, at which time her pulse was soft and slow; temperature in axilla 100°. After being removed from the wet sheet, she was wiped dry and put to bed, ordered whiskey and carbonate of ammonia every hour.

May 16. Feeling comfortable, dismissed.

Cases of sunstroke are exceedingly rare in this section of the country, yet persons who have never spent the summer in Florida generally suspect that the profession is often called on to treat such cases. The non-occurrence of insolation is due, perhaps, to our delightful summer nights, which counteract the heat of the day, as it were, which are very much unlike the oppressive nights experienced by the residents of large cities. The day was intensely warm, yet the sun was hidden by clouds the greater part of the time, and, as we afterwards observed, these few hours of intense heat were the forerunner of a heavy rain and wind.

MONTHLY ABSTRACT.

Anatomy and Physiology.

The Reflex Relations between Lungs, Heart, and Bloodvessels.

The influence which the respiratory movements exert upon the blood-stream in the lungs, heart, and bloodvessels is a subject which must always attract the attention of the physician and the physiologist. At first sight, it might appear that the problem was a simple mechanical one, explicable by physical laws; but here, as elsewhere within the body, it is necessary to take into account the nervous apparatus and the influence it exerts directly or in a reflex manner in modifying the action of the organs concerned. In considering the relation of the respiratory movements to the heart, lungs, and great vessels, it has recently been the practice to look, perhaps, too much to the subject as a physical problem, to the exclusion of the nervous apparatus and its effects thereon. We consider, therefore, that Dr. Julius Sommerbrodt of Breslau has done good service in directing the attention of physicians and physiologists to the "reflex relations between lungs, heart, and bloodvessels." Dr. Sommerbrodt shows that afferent nerve-impulses proceed from the lungs, and modify by reflex action the activities of the heart and bloodvessels in even a greater degree than is already known to be the case.

The recent histological investigations on the nervous apparatus of the lungs in the newt, frog, and other animals, by Egerow, W. Stirling, and Kandarazki, afford an anatomical basis in support of the physiological results. The results of these observers are conclusive that the lungs are supplied by a very large number of nerve-fibres—medullated and non-medullated—in the course of which many nerve-ganglia, as Remak showed, are intercalated. It is quite certain that all these nerve-fibres do not end in the non-striped muscle which exists in the bronchial wall and between the air-vesicles; but that many of them are afferent fibres, which convey impressions from the lungs to the respiratory and cardiac centres, so as to modify the activity of these centres by reflex agency. The present teaching on this question is that, during inspiration, the intrathoracic pressure is lowered, more blood flows from the veins into the right side of the heart, the blood-stream in the lungs is affected, so that more blood passes into the left side of the heart. Both these factors, as well as the increased number of heart-beats during inspiration, increase the arterial blood-pressure during inspiration. During expiration, the increased intrathoracic pressure causes a diminution of the supply of blood to the right and left heart; and the decrease in the number of heart-beats during expiration—through stimulation of the terminations of the vagus in the lungs—causes a fall in the arterial blood-pressure.

It has been attempted to show the influence of respiration on the circulation by sphygmographic investigations. In these investigations during normal breathing, the increase of the heart beats during inspiration, and the decrease during expiration, is scarcely perceptible, but occurs very markedly during forced respiration, or when the respiratory movements are interfered with (Marey). It would seem that all the phenomena of the influence of the respiration on the circulation are explicable on mechanical grounds, except the changes in the number of heart-beats, which are of a nervous nature. The first proof of a reflex relation between the lungs and the heart was given by Hering, who showed that moderate inflation

(30 to 35 millimetres of mercury) of the lungs in dogs caused an increase in the number of heart-beats. The first effect was always a fall of the blood-pressure; the second, an increase in the number of heart-beats, and that to the extent of double or treble the number of beats before the experiment. As soon as the inflation of the lungs was interrupted, the acceleration disappeared. Hering came to the conclusion that the afferent nerve-fibres of the lung bear the same relation to the inhibitory cardiac centre in the medulla that the depressor nerve bears to the vaso-motor centre. Both centres appear to be in a state of excitation, which is diminished by stimulation of certain afferent nerve-fibres.

There can be no doubt that one might expect to find a similar relation between the lungs and heart in man. Dr. Sommerbrodt has analyzed more than one thousand sphygmograms of the radial artery, especially during the performance of Valsalva's experiment, and during the inhalation of compressed air. During Valsalva's experiment, three marked changes occur in the sphygmographic curve: 1. When the expiration with closed glottis begins, the sphygmogram rises above the abscissa, then falls slightly, and rises again before the end of the experiment; 2. During the experiment, and for a few pulse-beats thereafter, the individual pulse beats become dicrotic; 3. The heart-beats are accelerated during the experiment, and for a few beats after free respiration. The rapidity of the rise in the sphygmographic curve depends on the rapidity, force, and duration of the expiration. The dicrotic or hyperdicrotic condition of the pulse-beats is always present, and is the most important sign of a diminished tension of the arterial wall and a fall of blood-pressure. The acceleration of the pulse-beat is always most marked in the latter half of the experiment, and the increase may reach 75 per cent. of the original number of beats.

With regard to inhalation of compressed air, its effects are twofold: first, purely mechanical; and, second, a reflex nervous action. The mechanical effects —apart from the ventilation of the lung and the gymnastics of the lung—are these. After a minimal increase, the blood-pressure in the aorta is much diminished, venous blood accumulates in the extrathoracic veins, the lesser circulation is thereby relieved, and the arteries become emptier. The reflex nervous effects are shown in the acceleration of the heart-beats, the diminution of the tension in the arterial wall, and the fall of the blood-pressure. Whilst the inspiration of compressed air is itself a hindrance to the circulation, its further effects exert a favourable influence on the circulation by accelerating the blood-stream. In cases of lesion of the valves of the heart, all of which hinder the circulation, inhalation of compressed air, as it favours the circulation, must be useful; and both Waldenburg and Sommerbrodt speak very strongly of its therapeutic effects in certain cases of valvular lesion of the heart.—*British Med. Journal*, June 25, 1881.

—

Nerve-plexuses of the Extremities.

Professors FERRIER and GERALD YEO have recently contributed a valuable monograph on this subject to the *Proceedings of the Royal Society*. They prove that a plexus has a great functional significance, and does not merely represent a convenient arrangement for the distribution of nerves to individual muscles. They rightly insist on the determination of the effects of excitation or destruction of the individual roots of a plexus, as being the only possible method by which we can discriminate between the sensory and motor constituents of the nerve-trunks, or indicate their functional relations and distribution. In order to throw light on these questions by physiological researches which may be regarded as almost directly applicable to man, these physiologists have made a series of experiments on the motor roots of the brachial and lumbo-sacral plexuses. Excepting in the absence of a branch to join the phrenic nerve, the brachial plexus is essentially the same in the higher quadrumana as in our own species. Reckoning the first lumbar as a thirteenth dorsal vertebra, and counting the last lumbar as a first sacral, then numbering the nerves in harmony with this arrangement, it is found that, in the old-world monkeys, the mode of distribution of the lumbar and sacral plexuses is the same as in man. In observing the effects of stimulation of exposed motor roots, after numerous precautions, attention was directed more especially to the resultant muscular combination, rather than to the mere number of muscles thrown into action; since the actions thus excited are all complex co-ordinated movements of great significance. It was found very difficult, when so many events are occurring simultaneously, to analyze each muscular combination into the individual factors at work; and, on that account, the muscles stated to be in action when any one particular root was stimulated, were only definitely registered as being thrown into action, under such a condition, after repeated observations, the suspected muscles being partially exposed when it was found difficult to be otherwise sure of their co-operation.

The movements resulting from stimulation of the individual roots of the brachial, lumbar, and sacral plexuses, appear to represent a highly co-ordinated functional synergy, and not mere contraction, more or less strong, of a given number of muscles, although many muscles are excited to contraction by more than one root, as previous observers have already discovered. The muscles thrown into action by irritation of each root being innervated, in most cases, by several nerve-trunks, it would appear that the plexuses which contiguous roots form with each other, serve to distribute the requisite motor fibres in different trunks to the various muscles engaged in each functional combination. Section of any motor root was found to paralyze, not the individual muscles involved, but their power of combination.

Irritation of the eighth cervical root, for example, caused firm closure of the fist, pronation and flexion of the wrist, extension of the forearm, and retraction of the upper arm; an action precisely imitated by pulling some object, hanging in front, downwards and towards the hip. Stimulation of the seventh cervical produced invariably a complex action, which brought the back of the hand against the nates. On irritation of the fifth lumber (the fourth, in man), the lower extremity was straightened directly backwards, in the position which immediately precedes the lifting of the foot to take another step forward in the act of walking. Although division of the roots above mentioned involved complete loss of voluntary exercise of the given combinations, it was found not to cause paralysis of the individual muscles contributing to each-combination. This is what was to be expected, since many of these muscles are innervated by more than one root, and hence, though weakened, they might still act in other combinations in so far as they were supplied by other roots. Panizza has gone so far as to believe, from experiment, that there is no absolute immobility of a limb until every root is cut.

In conclusion, these experiments tend to show that the cervical and lumbar enlargements of the spinal cord are centres of these highly co-ordinated muscular combinations. We understand that important work, to elucidate this question, is at present being carried on by the same physiologists—work that may bear fruit of great physiological and pathological value.—*British Med. Journal*, June 25, 1881.

Physiology and Pathology of the Excretion of Urea.

In a prize essay on the Physiology and Pathology of the Excretion of Urea, Dr. H. OPPENHEIM (Pflüger's *Archiv*, B. xxiii. p. 446) endeavours to ascertain the effects of food upon urea excretion. The observations detailed in this important paper were chiefly made upon the author himself, after the following manner. He was at pains to bring himself into such a condition that the quantity of urea excreted in the twenty-four hours remained nearly constant, and the urine and feces contained as much nitrogen as reached the body in the form of aliment. The urea-estimations were performed according to Liebig's method; and he believes that the results were free from the sources of error which, according to Pflüger, may occur in such analysis. During the first seven days, the quantity of urea excreted varied from 32 to 35 grammes in the twenty-four hours. The average hourly excretion of urea was 1.42 grammes. In the night (that is, in the hours after an albuminous meal) it stood at 0.13 gramme per hour over the average. The urea left the body in a solution which was never near saturation, but there was a distinct relation betwen the water and the urea excreted; so that, other things being equal, when the quantity of water passed was greater, the quantity of urea which it contained was also increased. The taking of coffee, while producing diuresis, caused a diminution in the quantity of urea, but along with this there was an increase in nitrogenous elimination by the bowel. Quinine caused an increase of the elimination of urea in the twenty-four hours to the extent of 4 grammes. This action began soon after taking the dose (2 grammes), and lasted for about twenty-four hours. The use of pilocarpin showed that the artificial production of great perspiration and salivation did not bring about any remarkable elimination of nitrogenous material from the body.—*London Med. Record*, June 15, 1881.

Materia Medica and Therapeutics.

Barium in Mineral Springs.

Dr. NEALE (*London Med. Record*), referring to the fact of the existence of barium in natural waters, says that we are not inclined to attach much importance to the presence of small quantities of barium in the Harrowgate waters, for several reasons; first, because their action (supposing it were to be considerable) must be greatly interfered with, when burdened with the presence of the large quantity of other salts. Next, the chloride of barium has been at times very extensively used, and in large doses; for instance, Hufeland used to give 4 to 5 grains of the crystallized chloride three or four times daily; and Lisfranc began with 6 and went on to 12 grains every hour, and at last gave 48 grains in one dose. Similar instances could be quoted, but we have said enough to show that probably the very small doses have not much operation. Further, chloride of barium and chloride of calcium had both fair trials, chiefly in glandular and scrofulous cases, but were both practically given up. Their effects were considered to be very similar, and some in those days thought that the calcium was more powerful than the barium. This, however, seems certainly not to be the case. Dr. Wimmer has called attention to the share which chloride of calcium may have in the operation of the Kreuznach and some other waters. We would venture to suggest that, as that salt is present in the Harrowgate waters in at least fifteen times the quantity of barium, it would be well worth Dr. Oliver's while to take up the consideration of the operation of a substance which occurs in so very tangible a quantity that its action must in all probability be stronger than that of the barium (*vide* Dr. G. Oliver's paper in the *Practitioner* for May, 1881, on "Barium in Medicinal Springs, with Special Reference to the Presence of it in some of the Harrowgate Waters").

Bromide of Ammonium in Whooping-cough.

As the result of five recently observed cases, KORMANN *(Jahr. für Kinder.,* Heft 1 and 2, 1880) asserts unhesitatingly that bromide of ammonium is more useful in whooping-cough than quinine. The bromide acts with greater certainty, and after a few doses (for young children, 5 centigrammes (¾ grain), for older children, from 25 centigrammes (4 grains), to 40 centigrammes (6 grains) every two hours) a marked improvement is observable. Should it be rejected by coughing, it must be repeated. There is only one contraindication to its use; and that is, when there is in addition chronic bronchial catarrh. The author was much struck by the wonderful efficacy of the bromide in whooping-cough, and is at a loss to understand the prejudice against it. In only a few cases was there marked drowsiness, and this was quickly overcome by suspending the remedy for a few hours. When the medicine is not retained, it should be abandoned, and tannic acid or quinine substituted, or an attempt might be made to give it in a syrup, or with liquorice. —*London Med. Record,* May 15, 1881.

The Action of Aconitine in Neuralgia.

M. DUMAS of Cette has been studying the action of aconitine in facial neuralgia, and comes to the following conclusions *(Journ. de Thérap.).* Crystallized aconitine is a powerful medicine. Very efficacious, especially in congestive facial neuralgia, and in some other forms of neuralgia *à frigore,* it is useful in the majority of catarrhal affections, in which it may replace the various preparations of aconitine. It deserves to be preferred over the other kinds of aconitine, which are ill-defined and unequal in their action. It is but slightly efficacious in tic-douloureux of the face, in which it only produces temporary sedative effects. As with the other alkaloids, it is tolerated when it is methodically administered. It may be long continued, without fear of the effects of an accumulation in the organism. It should be commenced in small doses and progressively increased. Unless in cases of tic-douloureux, the average dose should be restricted to two milligrammes daily. Carefully prepared granules containing a quarter of a milligramme (.0038 grain) of the alkaloid, or half a milligramme (.0077 grain) of the nitrate, deserve preference.—*London Med. Record,* June 5, 1881.

Aconite in Remittent Fever.

Dr. BOMFORD *(Practitioner,* March, 1881) records three cases of remittent fever treated with aconite. In its general course and uncertain duration, remittent fever somewhat resembles acute rheumatism, and especially on the West Coast of India is not uncommonly accompanied by slight inflammation of the joints. In the first of Dr. Bomford's cases, the patient, an officer, aged 20, had for four days been treated with large doses of quinine, but without effect. there being a daily exacerbation of fever at 3 P. M. On the fifth day the symptoms had increased in severity; the patient was sleepless, his tongue dry and glazed, skin dry, temperature in the axilla 103 deg., and pulse 88. The quinine was discontinued, and he was given one minim of tincture of aconite at 3 P. M., the dose being repeated every quarter of an hour until 4.30; it was given again at 5, and then every hour until 9. On the following day he was much better; he had slept well, his tongue was moist, the appetite was returning, the temperature was 100.4 deg., and the pulse 82. The tincture of aconite was again given in minim doses at 10.30 and 11 A. M., and then every hour until 7 P. M. At 3 P. M. there was free perspiration, temperature 99.5 deg., pulse 66. At 9 P. M., 97.5 deg., pulse 62. He had no relapse, and a week later returned to duty. The other cases are similar and equally striking. The author considers that the good effects of aconite in this class of fevers may be summed up as follows : 1. It reduces the temperature. 2. It reduces the rapidity of the pulse, and makes it full and strong. 3. It cleans the tongue, and restores the digestive functions. 4. It induces sleep. 5. It increases the quantity of the urine, and seems to have a direct effect in removing the symptomatic congestion of the kidneys. 6. It promotes perspiration. Dr. Bomford has often given aconite, sometimes for days together, to typhoid cases to clean the tongue and induce sleep. If pushed, it will reduce the temperature, but only slightly. The fall of temperature is not always accompanied by profuse sweating, and cannot be explained on the "heat-loss" theory as being merely the result of evaporation of the sweat. There can be no doubt that aconite acts best when given in frequent small doses.

Dr. William Murrell, of London, in commenting upon the above communication in the *London Medical Record*, makes the following practical remarks in regard to the administration of aconite in fever: "The author is quite right; aconite does act best in small doses, frequently repeated. Many practitioners get no good from aconite because they do not know how to use it. The dose of the tincture recommended in the *British Pharmacopœia*—from 5 to 15 minims— is absurdly large, and no one with any respect for his patient's safety or his own reputation would ever think of giving it. The best way is to put half a drachm of the tincture in a four-ounce bottle of water, and to tell the patient to take a teaspoonful of this every ten minutes for the first hour, and after this hourly for some hours. Even smaller doses may be given in the case of children. The great indication for the use of aconite is elevation of temperature; the clinical thermometer and aconite bottle should go hand-in-hand. If properly used, aconite is one of the most valuable and indispensable drugs in the *Pharmacopœia*."

—

The Arsenical Treatment of Chorea.

Arsenious acid is strongly recommended by Dr. SAWYER (*Brit. Med. Journ.*, Dec. 18, 1880) as being by far the best remedy for chronic chorea; and it is pointed out that the dose of liquor arsenicalis, as laid down in text-books, is too small. The quantity given should be cautiously increased. One exceptional case is mentioned, in which the dose was experimentally increased until as much as a drachm of Fowler's solution was given thrice daily, apparently with good effect on the chorea, until signs of gastro-intestinal irritation were produced.— *London Med. Record*, June 15, 1881.

—

Atropia in Vaseline.

Dr. KLEIN, of Vienna, recommends, in place of the ordinary solutions of atropin, to use an ointment prepared as follows : Sulphate of atropia, $\frac{3}{4}$ gr. ; vaseline, 160 gr. If the atropin salt be thoroughly triturated with the vaseline, it is unnecessary to use any solvent. The application of this ointment is much easier than the instillation of the solution. It is best applied by means of a camel's-hair brush to the inner surface of the lower eyelid pulled down.— *London Med. Record*, June 15, 1881.

—

Atropia as a more Effectual Remedy than Extract of Ergot in Menorrhagia and Hemoptysis.

TACKE (*Berl. Klin. Wochen.*, No. 6, 1881), having injected sulphate of atropia subcutaneously for eczema in a female patient ($\frac{1}{200}$ grain twice daily in dis-tilled water for two days), noticed that the menses, which had been very profuse, became moderate, and remained so. The same result he has seen follow five times in two other patients, and in a case of hemorrhage from the lungs the hemorrhage twice ceased immediately on the injection. He holds that as a remedy for visceral hemorrhage it is preferable to extract of ergot: 1st, on account of its certainty, and 2d, because, in the strength used by him (about ⅔ grain to an ounce of distilled water), it does not cause the inflammation which almost invariably follows the subcutaneous injection of extract of ergot.—*Lond. Med. Record*, April 15, 1881.

Administration of Cod-liver Oil.

Mr. FAIRTHORNE (*Pharmaceutical Journal*) suggests a new method of taking cod-liver oil, which consists of adding two drachms of tomato or walnut "catsup" (according to a new contemporary, the accurate and most appropriate orthography), to each ounce of the oil, the mixture being shaken before taken. He very pertinently remarks that taking an ordinary emulsion of cod-liver oil is like eating cod-fish or lobster with a dressing of sugar and gum. He has found the mixture of catsup and cod-liver oil to agree with many persons much better than in any other form in which cod-liver oil had been taken, and this he attributes to the association of substances generally employed as additions to food bringing into operation those digestive faculties of the stomach which might otherwise remain dormant when such incongruous substances as sugar, and one of the principal ingredients of fish, are introduced together into the stomach. Some years ago a paper was published in one of the scientific journals, showing that the condiments usually employed with particular kinds of food were the most appropriate ones, since they developed an electrical current, a phenomenon which did not appear to be indicated by the galvanometer when what would be considered by epicures to be incongruous articles of food were experimented with. Possibly the action of different adjuncts to food on the nervous system, and through it on the digestion, may deserve more attention than is generally devoted to that subject. Mr. Fairthorne also states that the following mixture is readily taken by the patient: Liebig's extract, ½ ounce; extract of celery seed, ½ fluidrachm; vinegar, 1 fluidounce; water, 2 fluidounces; cod-liver oil, 5 ounces. The extract of beef is dissolved in the water, the vinegar and oil are added, and the whole shaken with the extract of celery.—*British Med. Journal*, April 2, 1881.

Tetanus treated by Calabar Bean.

The case of a boy, aged 11, is related in the *Lancet*, Jan. 29, 1881. Tetanus followed a lacerated wound of the heel. Chloral and belladonna in full doses were first tried, but the patient became worse, and was presently unable to swallow his medicine, convulsive attacks being brought on by each attempt. Subcutaneous injections of morphia also caused convulsions and did no good. Gelatine lamels, containing one-sixtieth of a grain of extract of Calabar bean in each, were next obtained. One was given every four hours, being slipped between the teeth and allowed gradually to dissolve in the mouth. Improvement was noted two days later. The lamels were continued for seven days, by which time the boy was convalescing satisfactorily. He has since completely recovered. The case was an extremely unfavourable one at the time when the administration of Calabar bean was commenced. The boy's age, and his ability to take plenty of nourishment throughout his illness, were of course greatly in his favour, but the result affords a fair presumption that the drug had a beneficial effect. It, therefore, deserves a further trial (in the form of gelatine lamels) in similar cases.—*Lond. Med. Record*, June 15, 1881.

Resorcin in the Treatment of Cholera Infantum.

Andeer, of Würzburg, having asserted that resorcin ($C_6H_4(OH)_2$) has a marked antifermentative and antiputrefactive action, Dr. TOTENHÖFER, of Breslau, was induced to try it in an epidemic of cholera infantum during the summer of 1880 (*Breslauer ärztl. Zeitschr.*, 1880, No. 24). Of 91 children treated as out-patients in this way, there died 17. Of these last, three died from complications (pneumonia, croup, and meningitis); deducting these, the mortality was 15.4 per cent., against 34.4 and 30.7 per cent., the two previous years. The writer attributes the following actions to resorcin : 1. The vomiting ceases. 2. Symptoms of collapse are neither caused nor increased. 3. The number of stools is diminished. 4. Resorcin is not so irritant as carbolic acid, but quite as antimycotic. 5. It is readily taken without any corrigent, and is well borne. 6. It brings about rapid absorptive action in the stomach and intestine. Andeer gives adults internally a solution of 15 to 30 grains in $3\frac{1}{2}$ ounces of water; and in accordance with this the drug was administered to children during the first months of life, in a solution of $1\frac{1}{2}$ to 5 grains in 2 ounces of infusion of chamomile. Soltmann, in whose clinic the treatment was carried out, gives subcutaneous injections of ether when collapse is present, before commencing the resorcin treatment ; in cases of peritoneal irritation after removal of collapse, resorcin with one to three drops of tincture of opium.—*London Med. Record,* June 15, 1881.

—

Tannate of Quinia in Whooping-Cough.

In 1867 BINZ (*Berl. Klin. Woch.*, No. 9, 1881) was induced on theoretical grounds to employ quinine in the convulsive cough of children, other drugs having frequently failed in his hands to give relief. He found it most effectual in alleviating the violence and duration of the paroxysms of whooping-cough. The attacks became less frequent and less severe, and the vomiting ceased. When quinine was given quite at the commencement of the illness, the spasmodic element was suppressed, and the attack assumed the form of a severe, though manageable bronchitis. To obtain these good, results, it is necessary to give the remedy with no sparing hand. Twice a day the patient must take as many decigrammes as he is years old (a decigramme is a grain and a half), so that a child four years old would require 6 grains at a dose ; at ten years of age he would want 15 grains ; at fourteen, 21 grains, and so on.

The treatment must be steadily persevered in, for no immediate effect is observed. As a rule, there is no improvement until the patient has taken the full dose for three or four days, but then the progress is rapid. These results have been confirmed by one of Binz's pupils, JANSEN (*Klin. Beiträge zur Erkenntniss und Heilung des Keuchhustens*, 1868), and by HAGENBACH (*Correspondenz für Schweizer Aertz.*, 1881, and GERHARDT'S *Handbuch der Kinderkrankheiten*, 1877), who, as director of the Children's Hospital at Basel, has had many opportunities of investigating the subject. Hagenbach considers that, in the treatment of convulsive cough, quinine must be awarded the foremost place. The difficulties—at times insuperable—of inducing children to take such a bitter medicine as quinine, have been overcome by using the tasteless tannate of quinine. During a severe epidemic of whooping-cough in the neighbourhood of Rheindorf, Dr. Becker used this preparation with the greatest success. Hagenbach, in corroborating Becker's statements, says that it is best to give the tannate of quinine as early as possible, the dose being twice a day as many decigrammes as the child is years old. In his experience, the attacks have in a few days considerably abated, and the vomiting has ceased. He also used it with considerable success in the ordinary catarrhal affections of children. It is best given in a little sugar and water. In only one case did it induce constipation, whilst, in another, it arrested an attack of diarrhœa. Unfortunately, tannate of quinine is a very uncertain preparation, containing at one time 10 per cent., and at another 25 per cent., of the alkaloid. On this account it is a good plan to use the neutral tannate of quinine, made by precipitating the alkaloid with tannate of ammonia. The great objection to the employment of these salts is their expense, but there is good reason to suppose that they will soon be obtained by a new chemical method at a more reasonable rate.

It would appear that quinine produces its beneficial effects by a specific action on the organism which causes whooping-cough; salicylic acid and carbolic acid acting in the same way. Chloral-hydrate probably acts by lessening reflex action, and we know that its effects on the spinal cord are so marked that it is used as an antidote in cases of strychnia poisoning. The great objection to chloral in whooping-cough is, that it soon loses its effect unless the dose be increased. With quinine this is not the case; and, although it acts slowly, it is certain. It exerts no direct action on the nerves, but gradually destroys the poison itself. No hesitation need be felt in increasing the dose of tannate of quinine if necessary.—*London Med. Record*, May 15, 1881.

—

Use of Thymol in Burns.

Dr. FULLER, of Neukirchen, a mining district in which burns caused by explosions or fire damp or powder are frequent, has adopted a mode of treatment of burns by thymol, which he has found attended by most favourable results (*Hom. Rundschau* and *Therapeutic Gazette*). Each patient, as soon as admitted to the hospital, receives a warm bath. The burnt surface and its surroundings are then washed with an aqueous solution of thymol (1 to 1000), followed by the application of thymol spray for several minutes. The blisters are not disturbed, but are handled with extreme care. The raw surface is then painted with a one per cent. thymolized linseed oil. The patient is then laid on a waterproof mattress, the temperature of the room being kept comfortably warm. Particles of coal or other foreign matter, if not too minute, are, as a matter of course, at once removed. It is often very difficult to so lay the patient that the burned places are relieved of pressure, and it is frequently necessary to allow him to remain in a sitting posture, sometimes for several days, with support for the chin, or even *a la vache*, by suspending him by means of wide strips of muslin, passing under the chest or abdomen—the strips being fastened above. The application of thymol should at first be repeated every ten minutes; and as it relieves pain very remarkably, the patients themselves call for it. For this purpose large soft-haired paint-brushes are used. At first the oil is absorbed somewhat rapidly, and as soon as this has occurred a sensation of intense burning follows. The applications are gradually made less frequently; as an indication of their necessity, the appearance of the skin is sufficient. As soon as the oil is entirely absorbed, it should be replaced by a fresh portion, as it is important to prevent contact with the air. During the first few days the thymol spray is also applied as often as possible, which does much toward alleviating the pain.—*Lond. Med. Record*, June 15, 1881.

Medicine.

The Nature of the Infecting Agent in Diphtheria.

In an unusually interesting paper in the *British Medical Journal* for July 2, 1881, Dr. MICHAEL W. TAYLOR, of Penrith, discusses the Fungoid Òrigin of Diphtheria, especially as shown in an isolated outbreak in which dampness appeared to act as a favouring cause. In regard to the special agent he offers the following solution of the question:—

" The results of the investigations of scientific pathologists, during the last fifteen years, all tend to further the broad theory, that ' all contagia are probably particulate,' and that the infective particles enjoy endowments not known to exist otherwise than in association with life and organization ; and, moreover, microscopy and experimental inoculation have incontestably demonstrated the presence of distinct specific vegetative forms in the contagious liquids of at least four contagious diseases. These are smallpox, sheep-pox, splenic fever, and relapsing fever. It has been shown—first, that the minute organisms discovered infiltrating the tissues and blood in these diseases, which have been described, according to their form and structure, as the micrococcus, bacillus, spirilla, etc., are not congeneric with the animal body in which they are found, but are apparently of the lowest vegetable kind ; and, secondly, that they constitute the essence, or an inseparable part of the essence, of the contagia of these diseases.

" It has been proved, so late as the present year, by Toussaint, of Toulouse, that the very infectious disease amongst poultry, called the *cholera des poules*, consists of a minute bacterium, which is capable of cultivation out of the body, in chicken-broth ; and it has been long known that the epizöotic parasite which infests the silk-worm, and the house-fly, is a mould with fungal threads and mycelium, which is almost identical with oïdium, or peronospora, so well known in connection with the potato and vine plagues.

" Thus we see that the progress of modern research justifies the conclusion, that the vastly multiplied minute organisms and vegetable sporules, inducing and produced by the ordinary processes of fermentation and putrefaction going on in nature, may be absorbed into the blood of animals, or be engrafted on their tissues, so as to assume an intimate relationship with many of the diseases most fatal to human life. Hence there is really nothing startling nor singular in the proposition I enunciate, that the diphtheria in this particular instance had its origin in some of the fungoid sporules which infested this chamber.

" In the year 1858, Professor Laycock, of Edinburgh, put forth the theory, that diphtheritic exudation depended on ' oïdium albicans,' or potato fungus ;[1] the same conjecture was supported by Dr. Wilks and others ;[2] long before which— in 1844—Gruby, of Paris, and afterwards Ch. Robin, had shown, by the microscope, that in the pseudo-diphtherite, or muguet, and in thrush, the buccal pellicles displayed the tubular filaments and mycelium of a vegetable form analogous to the oïdium. This hypothesis, however, in regard to true diphtheria did not receive acceptation, in consequence of the general failure at that time of sufficient microscopic evidence, in the false membrane itself, of the presence of vegetable growths.[3] The more recent researches, however, of Nassiloff and

---

[1] Lancet, 1858. Laycock, Lecture on Diphtheria.

[2] Medical Times and Gazette, vol. xxxviii. On Diphtheria and its connection with a Parasitic Vegetable Fungus.

[3] Since I have been engaged with this paper, I find from a communication kindly · forwarded by the Rev. John E. Vize, M.A., Forden Vicarage, and published in 1880, that this able fungologist has strongly maintained the dependence of diphtheria on an oïdium.

Oertel in Germany, Leloir in France, Burdon Sanderson, and other workers in scientific pathology, show that pharyngeal diphtheria is a true mycosis, or infiltration of living tissue with micrococci, and that the development of these minute spheroids is intimately associated with the morbid process. It has been found that the pseudo-membrane consists of layers of stratified epithelium, more or less mingled with products of exudation from blood-plasma and some micrococci, but that, in the mucous and submucous tissues, the channels communicating with the lymphatics are filled with granular matter, which is mainly micrococci, or masses of vegetation; so that observation has tended to establish a certain analogy in the morbid processes of diphtheria with those in the respective diseases I have mentioned—splenic fever, or woolsorters' disease, for example, which we know to be produced by vegetable sporules existing outside of the body.

" As was well shown by Sir James Paget, in his masterly address at the Cambridge meeting of the Association, some of the obscure processes of human pathology are capable of receiving much elucidation from a comparative study of diseases in plants, and of the action of parasites on the vegetable kingdom. We have described to us, by the practical mycologist, an infinite multitude of distinct structural forms of fungi, each of which has its own habitat, and affects certain sites of decaying vegetable or animal matters, or preys on certain living species or natural orders of plants; each has its own feeding ground. We cannot advance far in this study without being struck with the marked parallelism which exists between the action of the parasitic spore in producing local and general morbid changes in the plant, and the action of a bacillus, or oïdium, affecting animal tissues. The resting-spore, let us say, of the peronospora infestans, capable of resisting the hardest winter frosts, and the greatest heats of summer, lies dormant underneath the ground, until the time of germination arrives; its habitat, or feeding-ground, is the potato; at the proper season it meets with a tuber; it attaches itself to the skin by its little lash-like appendage; it germinates there; it starts out its rootlets into the parenchyma of the tuber—this is its mycelium; it branches and penetrates in all directions; it poisons the tissues; the plant looks sickly; the stalk withers, and the leaves blacken; it has fulfilled its end, the reproduction of its kind. So, when the leaves of phanerogamous plants are attacked, the zöospores of the fungus gain entrance by the stomata, throw out their mycelium through the cellular tissue of the leaf; the thread-like filaments burrow underneath in search of food; whilst the epidermis is raised like a blister, and perishes and exfoliates, just as does the epithelial false membrane from a diphtheritic throat. No theory in regard to the essential cause of diphtheria explains so well many known facts in its history as that of its fungoid origin. For example, the persistence of vitality in the so-called resting-spores of fungi lying dormant in drains, or amid heaps of putrescible matter, for an indefinite time after an outbreak, affords a ready explanation why the disease so often inveterately clings to certain dwellings and localities."

Hay Fever.

M. DE BUDBERG, in a communication to the Société Vaudoise de Médecine, calls attention to the value of the method of treatment devised by Helmholtz, which is less widely known than it should be. The first case was observed by M. de Budberg in an Englishwoman, who had suffered from it for twenty years. The treatment employed consisted of nasal irrigations of solution of quinine, recommended by Helmholtz (1 part in 750 of water). This irrigation brought away masses of brownish mucus, in which were found small round yellow corpuscles, of smaller dimensions than the blood-corpuscles. It did not contain either vibrios or bacteria. After two or three douches, the patient was perfectly well. The attack was arrested from that time. A solution of chlorate of potash was employed, and no relapse occurred, although the patient frequently passed flowering meadows. Every time that she attempted to suspend the treatment, a relapse occurred, which, however, was promptly ameliorated by the use of the douche. M. de Budberg thinks that the yellow corpuscles found in the nasal mucus of this lady were pollen-corpuscles. The nasal douche freed the mucous membrane from them; hence its curative effect. In cases in which the mucus contained bacteria, Helmholtz's solution of quinine would probably be indispensable. In all cases, it is necessary that the douche should be made most carefully, so as to entirely wash out the whole of the nasal mucous membrane. Dr. Blackley, in his excellent monograph, relates that he induced hay fever in his own person by the introduction, on the nasal mucous membrane, of various kinds of pollen. He cites more than sixty different kinds of them—as a rule, graminaceous pollens.—*British Med. Journal*, July 2, 1881.

Treatment of Enteric Fever by Prolonged Lukewarm Baths.

For many years the reduction of the pyrexia of fevers by cold or lukewarm baths has been the subject of careful and extended inquiry both in this country and in Germany. Among those who have done much useful work in the investigation are Brand, Ziemssen, and Riess, while Dr. Wilson Fox's accurate and interesting observations on the reduction of the pyrexia of acute rheumatism have added much to our precise knowledge of the immediate and subsequent effect of such baths. The methods of the first three observers differ considerably. Brand uses largely, and more especially in severe cases, the general cold bath, cold affusions, and cold wet packings, the water being at a temperature of 50° F., and the affusions being continued for a quarter of an hour or thereabout. Ziemssen's method consists in placing the patient in a bath at 95°, which, in the course of half an hour or so, is gradually cooled down to 60°. He uses the cold wet packing as an adjuvant to the baths.

Riess's method (*Centralbl. für die Med. Wissen.*, July 24, 1880, p. 545) differs from both these in the duration of the bath, and also in the fact that the water is kept at a constant lukewarm temperature. His procedure is as follows: On the day succeeding the admission of a typhoid patient with high temperature, he is placed in a bath at 88° for twenty-four hours. The duration of the bath in the following days depends on the rectal temperature. So soon as the temperature reaches 101.5° the patient is placed in the bath, which is interrupted at 99.5°, until the temperature again rises to 101.5°. Riess claims for this treatment that it not only keeps the temperature in typhoid patients almost normal, but also that, under it, delirious and comatose patients return to full consciousness and gladly remain in the bath.

Notwithstanding the excellent results obtained by Riess, few test trials of this method have been published, and accordingly the detailed observations by AFANASSIEFF (*St. Petersb. Med. Woch.*, 1881, No. 7) of seven cases of enteric fever, treated by prolonged lukewarm baths, are possessed of some interest. In certain respects, Riess's method was not fully carried out. From circumstances of hospital convenience the bath lasted in general only three hours, being repeated twice daily if necessary, that is, if the rectal temperature rose above 101.5°. Sometimes, also, the baths were of a higher temperature than 88°, in one or two cases as high as 95°. As to the general course of the disease in these seven cases, two were specially severe, but in none was the "typhoid" condition developed. Consciousness was clear, headache slight or absent, and sleep good throughout the whole period of the use of the baths. The tongue was seldom coated, mostly clean and moist, and all the patients preserved a good appetite throughout the disease. Pain in the region of the cæcum and meteorism were generally present, but required no special treatment. Marked diarrhœa was not present in any of the cases, and the bowels were regularly and naturally opened. Two cases had bronchitis, passing over without treatment. The number of baths given was 114, of which 100 lasted three hours; 14 a longer or shorter time. As regards reduction of temperature: on two occasions the reduction was 5.8○; on seven, approximately, 5.5○; on twenty-one, 4.5○; on thirty-four, 3.5○; on twenty-four, 2.5○; on twenty-three, 1.5○; and on three, 1○. The last two classes were mostly those in which the baths lasted for only half an hour or an hour, the rectal temperature being only 101.5○. The temperature was taken in the rectum before and after the bath; and we must here note a practical point of which the observer seems to have been unaware. The temperature immediately after a bath by no means necessarily indicates the reduction of temperature accomplished by it; for Dr. Wilson Fox has shown, from his cases of acute rheumatism, that the temperature may continue to fall six or more degrees, forty or fifty minutes after the termination of the bath.

The conclusions arrived at by the observer are these: 1. The usual reduction is from 3○ to 4.5○. 2. In the later stages of enteric fever, the temperature yields more readily than at first. 3. The temperature sinks more readily in the evening than in the morning, the greatest reduction in the evening among his cases being 5.8○, while the greatest in the morning was 4.5○, both these meaning, however, a reduction to almost the normal temperature. The pulse and respirations also sank in number under the use of the bath. The fall in the pulse was in strict relation to the fall of temperature, the diminution being 20, 50, and in some cases even 70 and 90 per cent. The author considers the treatment well suited for hospital cases, and points out that the attitude of the patient in the bath ought to be as comfortable as possible, for which he recommends a waterproof mattress, covered with a sheet, and a movable pillow attached to the frame of the bath.—*London Med. Record*, May 15, 1881.

—

The Simulation of Typhoid Fever by Acute Tuberculosis.

Dr. SENATOR contributes to the *Berliner Klinische Wochenschrift*, No. 25, an article bearing on this subject, in which he relates a case of acute miliary tuberculosis that during life was supposed to be typhoid fever. The patient was a man aged forty-eight, who, three years before coming under observation, had gone through a severe attack of typhoid. During its third week a very stubborn and intractable hiccough came on, which lasted eight days. There had also been attacks of epistaxis, with hawking up of blood-stained mucus from the posterior nares; but he quite recovered. He subsequently broke his arm, and again recovered without further trouble. His last illness commenced, about five weeks before he came under Dr. Senator's care, with slight shiverings, malaise, depression, and dyspnœa, which obliged him to keep his bed for a few days. When taken into the hospital he was observed to be a fairly well-built man, well nourished, without cachexia, and with a good family history. There were no abnormalities in the circulatory or respiratory apparatus. After some days the spleen was felt to be enlarged, and several roseola spots showed themselves; then epistaxis came on, and some pulmonary catarrh also; and later, hiccough and slight deafness. About three weeks after admission some inflammation and suppuration occurred over and about the left parotid gland, sanious and fetid pus being discharged. The temperature varied from 100○ to 104○ Fahr. The patient then died. In view of the enlargement of spleen, the fever, and the roseola, a diagnosis of typhoid was made. The man, it is true, had once before passed through an attack of typhoid, but authentic cases are recorded where an individual may have the disease twice. Moreover, the occurrence of epistaxis and hiccough (which were marked symptoms during the first attack) occurred during his last illness. Finally, the occurrence of a suppurative parotitis seemed to favour the typhoid view. But at the autopsy, not only were there no appearances of typhoid—there were not even any traces of the previous attack. On the other hand, there was a general tuberculosis of both lungs, with enlargement of the bronchial glands. The spleen, the liver, and both kidneys were also tuberculous. —*Med. Times and Gazette*, July 2, 1881.

Massive Pneumonia.

GRANCHER was the first to point out the existence of a variety of pneumonia which showed most of the clinical symptoms of pleuritic effusion, and which deserved the special epithet of massive. Recently, two cases of this kind were observed at Professor Lasègue's clinic (*Arvhives Générales de Méd.*, Feb. 1881). The first was that of a labourer, aged 50, who developed an acute pneumonia. Examination revealed absolute dulness in front and behind on the right side. At the base and in the axillary region, resonance was still found; in the supraspinous and infraclavicular regions, absence of respiratory *bruit;* in the intraspinous region fine moist râles, but neither crepitant nor subcrepitant. Bronchial breathing was very marked at the inferior border of the scapula, extending from the axillary line to the vertebral column. Below this point there was a faint vesicular murmur, distant in sound and largely masked by sonorous *râles.* In front, similar conditions existed, but there was no respiratory murmur. On the left side there were apparently only the signs of bronchitis. There was little cough, and the expectorated matter was not characteristic of any special lesion. The febrile movement was not severe. The patient died soon after admission to the hospital. At the necropsy, the upper lobe of the right lung was found completely hepatized, having assumed a dirty yellowish colour. The other lobes and the left lung were not greatly altered; but the pathological condition which led to the clinical diagnosis of massive pneumonia was found to reside in the bronchial tubes distributed to the upper lobe. They were completely filled to their finest ramifications with a white, elastic, apparently fibrinous substance, which was not found elsewhere. Other cases are cited, and the writers, MM. Beurmann and Brissaud, finally conclude that, although massive pneumonia may at some time during its course closely resemble in its clinical aspects pleurisy with effusion, yet in certain cases bronchial breathing coexists with the dulness on percussion. This respiratory sound will be likely to exist at the beginning of the malady, when the fibrinous exudation has not yet advanced to the root of the lungs. In doubtful cases, an exploratory puncture would appear to be justified.—*London Med. Record,* June 15, 1881.

Progressive Painful Inflammation of Arteries.

Mr. J. H. MORGAN, in a paper read before the Clinical Society of London (*British Medical Journal*, April 23), describes the case of a middle-aged man, who during some years suffered at intervals from pain extending gradually from the trunk along the course of some of the main arteries, viz., both brachials, a carotid, a femoral, and extending from it to the arteries of the leg. The retinal vessels were very unusually small, indistinct, and exhibited a double contour. There was at no time any evidence of embolism. He contracted syphilis when eighteen years of age. The symptoms, according to the author, pointed evidently to disease of an artery, probably inflammation of the fibrous coat, since the pain passed from the centre to the periphery, was in the course of the various arteries, and was made intense by pressing upon the artery affected.—*London Med. Record*, June 5, 1881.

Cardiac Lesions in Locomotor Ataxy.

Dr. LETULLE publishes (*Gaz. Méd. de Paris*, 1881) two cases of locomotor ataxy, in which he met with cardiac lesions, already pointed out by M. Grasset of Montpellier. In the first of these cases, the patient, who died suddenly, had atheromatous lesions of the aorta and inefficiency of the aortic valves; in the other, there were also complex lesions of the aortic opening and mitral lesions.—*London Med. Record*, June 15, 1881.

Tuberculous Pericarditis.

Tubercular inflammation of the pericardium is a very rare lesion. Laennec only met with two instances of it, and Louis but one. Although cases have been from time to time recorded in medical literature, their total number is not large. Gray granulations in the pericardium have been met with in cases of general tuberculosis in children, unaccompanied by actual inflammation, but the condition of tuberculous pericarditis is most uncommon. An instance of the affection in a girl of nineteen has been lately recorded by Dr. VAILLARD in the *Journal de Médecine de Bordeaux*. The patient died from tubercular meningitis, with extensive enlargement and caseation of the lymphatic glands. The parietal and visceral layers of the pericardium were connected by soft adhesions, and each was covered by false membrane; the visceral layer was studded with granulations and small nodules of caseous tubercle. At a distance from these nodules the microscopical examination showed the proper tissue of the membrane to be somewhat thickened and continuous with a new membrane on the surface, which was almost perfectly organized. Sections through the yellow tubercles showed, even in the thickness of the visceral layer, a small oblong caseous mass, permeated by the remains of tracts of fibrous tissue in process of destruction. No giant-cells were seen in it. Around this caseous centre was a layer of embryonal cells, most marked in the deep layer of the serous membrane. Over the nodule extended the false membrane already described. The subjacent muscular fibres of the heart were fattily degenerated.

From the comparison of a considerable number of cases of tuberculous pericarditis, Vaillard concludes that it is much less common to meet with effusion than with the dry form, the latter having been met with twenty-seven times out of thirty-seven cases; in only ten was there effusion, of a citrine yellow or sanguinolent aspect. In all the cases of dry pericarditis, with one exception, there was complete adhesion of the two layers of the pericardium. Hence it would seem that adhesion is the habitual termination of this variety. The surfaces are covered by false membranes, in which the tubercles are scattered, as well as in the serous membrane proper. Tubercular granulations may, however, develop in the proper connective tissue of the myocardium, and Fauvel has even traced them through the whole thickness of the wall of the heart up to the endocardium. In the less frequent cases in which there is effusion, this is usually abundant, and may vary from 700 to 1600 grammes (Proust), and even 2800 grammes (Richard). This large effusion is so characteristic of the variety that, given a case of chronic pericarditis, the tubercular nature of the inflammation may be suspected from this characteristic. The layers of the pericardium present changes similar to those met with in the dry form, but the false membranes may undergo degeneration and ulceration, so that ulcers form similar in appearance to the specific ulcers of the intestine. The question has been discussed whether the formation of tubercles is primary and the inflammation secondary, or whether the opposite is the order of events. Cruveilhier, Empis, and Niemeyer have expressed doubts as to the occurrence of tubercles in uninflamed pericardium ; and, according to them, the formation only occurs in the depth of the newly-formed false membranes. The facts of the question have often been difficult to ascertain, in consequence of the close adhesion of the false membrane and serous layer, so that it is not always easy to say where one ends and the other begins. But many cases have been observed in which tubercles were seated in the thickness of the serous membrane without any trace of inflammation, as in a case in which, the patient having died from acute tuberculosis, miliary granulations were found on the parietal layer, and three similar nodules on the surface of the visceral layer. This renders it probable that, in some cases at least, the formation of tubercles is primary and the inflammation secondary. But it does not follow that this is the invariable order of events ; a simple pericarditis may be the occasion of the growth of tubercles in the inflammatory products.

The dry adhesive form of pericarditis is often overlooked during life. Its course is latent, and pericarditis not being expected in the course of phthisis, it is often discovered only at the autopsy. Any dyspnœa which it causes is obscured in the greater dyspnœa due to the condition of the lungs, and when adhesions form friction disappears. The occurrence of effusion renders the symptoms more obtrusive, so that this form is usually recognized during life. · If there are no lung symptoms it may be difficult even to suspect the nature of the pericarditis, but a correct diagnosis is, in these cases, of great importance, since the pericarditis is occasionally the first local manifestation of tuberculosis, as in cases which have been recorded by Virchow, Proust, and Richard.—*Lancet*, May 28, 1881.

———

The Phenomena of Neuro-muscular Superexcitability during Hypnotism.

MM. CHARCOT and RICHER, in a contribution to the study of Hypnotism in Hysterical Patients (*Le Progrès Médical*, Nos. 15, 16, 1881), draw attention to the phenomenon of exaggerated excitability of the nerves and muscles during certain forms of induced sleep. This phenomenon includes (1) great increase in the tendon-reflexes; percussion on a tendon giving rise to movements not only in the same limb but in the others, to sharper reflex contraction, to prolonged contraction, and to permanent contraction; the contraction may be brought about by kneading, friction, or simple pressure; (2) increased nervous excitability; pressure on nerve-trunks giving rise to spasm of the muscles to which their branches are distributed; (3) increased muscular excitability; pressure on a muscle causing it to contract; (4) a special increased excitability of the muscles of the face, which cannot be thrown into permanent spasm, but may be excited in any of the foregoing ways, and even by simply pressing each one with a small piece of wood, by which means they reproduced most of the experiments of Duchenne of Boulogne, on the partial action of the muscles of the face under the influence of localized faradisation.

The contraction resulting as above described is generally very intense, resisting the most forcible efforts to overcome it, but it may be made to yield, without force, by simply stimulating in the same manner the antagonist group of muscles. When the contraction is not destroyed during the hypnotic sleep, on awakening the patient, the contraction may disappear with the sleep; or it may persist after waking, if we render the patient cataleptic and awaken her during that state ; or it may in some cases persist whether the patient be awakened during either the lethargic or the cataleptic state. Such persistent contractions resemble those of hysteria; and for their reduction it is necessary to hypnotize the patient again, and then to excite the antagonist muscles.

The transference of artificial contraction by means of the magnet is well known, since the experiments at the Salpêtrière in 1878; but it was not known whether such transferred contraction affected exactly the same muscles as were involved in the primary contraction. One of the patients of MM. Charcot and Richer having been hypnotized, and her muscles completely relaxed, the ulnar group were stimulated by touching the right ulnar nerve at the elbow, and a magnet was then applied to the left arm, the muscles of which remained relaxed; at the end of two or three minutes the fingers of the contracted hand began slowly to open, while those of the opposite hand began to assume the position they were quitting, until the contraction was completely transferred. The same result followed when localized contraction was induced by exciting a tendon or the muscle itself.

Anæmia of a limb produced by Esmarch's bandage prevents the manifestation of contraction, so long as the anæmia persists; but as the blood returns to the limb the contraction shows itself. In the former stage, therefore, it may be considered to be latent. This latent contraction may also be transferred by the magnet; so that, while in the bloodless limb no contraction results from exciting the nerve, a magnet applied to the opposite arm develops in it the spasm of the ulnar group of muscles.—*London Med. Record,* June 15, 1881.

—

Glosso-labial Palsy.

Dr. ANDREW CLARK has recently had under his care a rapidly fatal case of glosso-labial palsy, which is reported in the *Med. Times and Gazette* for July 2, 1881. He says:—

"The chief features of this case are its rapid course (the patient being quite well three months ago), the transient attacks of loss of voice, the progressive emaciation, and the supervention of permanently dangerous and symptomatic phenomena only a fortnight before death—viz., inability to swallow, and loss of voice, and paralysis of the muscles of the pharynx—and the sudden death by syncope. The nerves involved in this disease are generally stated to be the seventh, the ninth, and the eleventh. In this case, the seventh was only very slightly involved, as evidenced by the slight drawing of the right side of the face. The ninth nerve, evidently, was chiefly implicated, as evidenced by paralysis of the azygos uvulæ and the palato-pharyngeus and palato-glossus of the left side, and the paralysis of the posterior portion of the pharynx. Some amount of loss of taste appears to point to impairment of its gustatory fibres also. The vagus had, no doubt, a share in producing the paralysis of the pharynx, and possibly in slowing the circulation by its inhibitory fibres, and causing the final attack of syncope. It is curious to note how partial is the paralysis in this disease very often. I have seen a case which had apparently become quite well under iodide of potassium, and in which the only lesion left was paralysis of the uvula. When we remember, however, how many individual fibres go to make up a nerve—*e. g.,* in the optic nerve probably some 100,000—the selection of these individual muscles becomes more intelligible. Glosso-labial palsy is somewhat rarer as an idiopathic disease than when occurring along with other well-marked nervous diseases. The causation is obscure, and in this case would appear to be from excessive heat and cold. These changes of heat and cold have a remarkable influence in inducing certain diseases of the nervous system—*e. g.,* progressive muscular atrophy, which Charcot has asserted to be very common amongst stokers. No doubt, had a post-mortem been made, a sclerosis in the medulla would have been found, involving the nerve-roots (or their cells) of the seventh, ninth, tenth, and twelfth. The disease is not always easy to recognize, but in a well-marked case the features are distinctive enough. The above case, however, had been treated for 'liver complaint' before being sent to the hospital.''

Paralysis from Apoplexy of the Medulla Oblongata.

Herr M. DE BON relates (*Nord. Med. Archiv*, Band xiii.) the case of an unmarried woman, aged 48, who had for two years had a constant dull pain in the neck, which was much increased when she bent the head forwards. In 1878, her sight began to fail. On April 2d, 1879, she had vomiting and giddiness. On May 2d, she had giddiness and nausea when she lay down. Afterwards, she had difficulty in speaking and swallowing; in the afternoon, she lost speech, and respiration became stertorous. The next day, there was complete paralysis of all limbs. The face was immovable; the right eyelid was paretic, and the right pupil dilated; the left eyelid was unaffected; respirations, 60 to 80; pulse, 150; consciousness appeared to be retained. She died on the same day. At the necropsy, the coats of the basilar artery were found to be much thickened, and its lumen reduced. The same condition, but in a less degree, was found in both vertebral arteries, for the space of about one centimetre. There were no dilatations nor depressions on the outer surface of the vessel. The basilar artery was empty; at the part next the vertebral arteries was a thrombus, half a centimetre (0.2 inch) long, which extended a centimetre into the right, and a centimetre and a half into the left vertebral artery. The pons Varolii was pale; the medulla oblongata was very pale and soft; and under the ependyma, corresponding to the eminentia teres, was a small hemorrhagic clot, which, on section, was found to be pale, soft, and homogeneous. Several small clots were found in the cerebellum. The occipital headache, for two years, might have been due to the anæmic condition of the posterior part of the brain and meninges, in consequence of the insufficient flow of blood from the obstructed basilar and vertebral arteries. The symptoms of affection of the medulla oblongata first appeared when thrombosis of the vertebral arteries, and consequent anæmia and softening of the medulla, took place. From this time, the symptoms became distinctly marked: on the second day, all the nervous functions were thrown into a state of inaction; and the patient died, unable to speak, swallow, or move herself, but apparently quite conscious. The thrombosis occurred, possibly, nearly at the same time in both vertebral arteries, since no unilateral paralysis was observed. No microscopic examination of the vessels was made.—*London Med. Record*, June 5, 1881.

Temporary Paralysis after Epilepsy.

Dr. HUGHLINGS JACKSON (*Brain*, Jan. 1881), by many and powerful arguments, supports, elaborates, and, we may say, establishes, the theory of Todd and Alexander Robertson, that temporary post-epileptiform paralysis depends on temporary central exhaustion, consequent on the excessive discharge during the paroxysm. Previous observation has shown that local temporary paralyses most usually occur after epileptiform seizures (the spasm commencing in the terminal part of a limb, or in the side of the face), as distinguished from epilepsy proper. Dr. Hughlings Jackson now shows that, in accordance with Todd and Robertson's theory, paralysis also occurs after true epilepsy; it is distributed over all parts of the body, and has hitherto been regarded as weakness, prostration, coma, etc. When the nervous discharge is partial in its distribution; when, for example, one limb only is affected thereby, that particular limb will suffer from the paralysis due to central nervous exhaustion in the paths or centres most intimately connected with it. If the nervous discharge be distributed along various paths to the whole of the body, then the whole body will be affected by the resulting central nervous exhaustion.—*London Med. Record*, June 15, 1881.

—

Softening of the Brain in Puerperal Pyæmia, as the Result of Infection with Micrococci.

In the *Breslauer Aerztl. Zeitschr.*, 1880 (S. 205), two cases are given by LAFFTER with autopsies. In the first, the woman was taken with pains in the abdomen eight days after delivery, these being followed by somnolence, and paralysis of the right side, extremities, and face. Death occurred three weeks after delivery. The following lesions were found at the necropsy: a pyæmic abscess of the lung, enlargement of the spleen, multiple abscesses in the kidneys, recent aortic endocarditis, and softened purulent thrombi in the plexus of veins around the vagina. In the left frontal lobe of the brain was a patch of red softening, almost as large as a hen's egg. On microscopic examination, numerous micrococcus-emboli were discovered in the vessels of the kidneys, and of the brain in the neighbourhood of the softened spot; the latter being in some cases tightly distended with colonies of micrococci, in others containing only scattered chains of micrococci arranged in a serpentine manner. In the second case, the signs of puerperal pyæmia and endocarditis were also found; and, in addition, a patch of red softening, about the size of a hazel-nut, in the right frontal lobe, and in connection with this a purulent meningitis over the convexity of the brain. The histological condition was identical with that of the first case. Clinically, somnolence only, and no local paralysis, was observed.—*London Med. Record*, June 15, 1881.

—

Determination of Albuminoid Degeneration.

Dr. C. ARNSTEIN, of Kasan (*Central. für die Med. Wiss.*, No. 13, 1881) says he has had the opportunity of examining certain growths from the eyelids sent him by Professor Adamuk, to investigate whether they were amyloid or not. He found that some were decidedly amyloid, but others, although the tissue was translucent, gave no amyloid reaction. In some of these latter there was no cell-proliferation; in others, the degenerated parts alternated with patches of cell-proliferation with numerous giant-cells. In one case he recognized the preliminary stage of hyaline degeneration, to which he gave the name of fibrinous degeneration. In the latter, he could distinguish, along the vessels, fibrous finely striated layers, which permeated the adventitia, and gradually became hyaline, in such a manner that the outer layers appeared already grass-like, while the inner were still finely striated. In the next stage, vessels could be seen, the wall of which appeared like thick clear glass rings or hollow tubes; the striation had completely disappeared, and the lumen of the vessel was reduced to a minimum, or quite obliterated. In the tissue itself, he could distinguish with high powers a finely fibrillated granular-looking reticulum, which, at neighbouring spots, was replaced by a bright hyaline stroma. In the narrow meshes of this stroma, nucleated cells and giant-cells were demonstrated by carmine. He has found cochineal-alum a valuable colouring agent for amyloid matter. The amyloid matter is coloured red, while, in the normal tissues, the nuclei are coloured violet, and the protoplasm and ground substance remain colourless.—*Lond. Med. Record*, June 15, 1881.

Formation of Hyaline Tube-Casts.

RIBBERT has already advanced the hypothesis that hyaline tube-casts are formed from altered albumen which has transuded into the glomeruli. This coagulation of albumen in the convoluted tubules he believes to be brought about by reason of the acid reaction of the urine. In order to prove this, he makes certain observations, proceeding upon the hypothesis that, if the acid reaction of the contents of the tubules so acted, then the artificial acidulation of the contents of the glomeruli by the injection of acids into the blood would cause a coagulation of the albumen in the Malpighian tufts. In each of two rabbits he clamped one renal artery, and, after an hour and a half, he injected 20 to 30 grains of a 2½ per cent. solution of acetic acid into the jugular vein. In the one animal, the kidney was extirpated thirty minutes after the operation; in the other, one hour. In both cases, hyaline masses of coagulated albumen were found in the glomeruli.—*London Med. Record*, June 15, 1881.

Quantitative Analysis of Chlorides in Urine.

For some time SALKOWSKI has employed Vothard's method for the estimation of chlorides in the urine by means of rhodan ammonium in the urine, which he carries out in the following manner. Ten cubic centimetres of urine are diluted to about 60 cubic centimetres, then acidulated with 2 cubic centimetres of pure nitric acid, and decomposed with 15 cubic centimetres of the silver solution usually employed for the estimation of chlorides (1 cubic centimetre = 0.01 NaCl). The mixture is then vigorously shaken until the fluid has become clear, diluted with distilled water to 100 cubic centimetres, and filtered through a dry filter-paper; 80 cubic centimetres of the filtrate are taken and to this are added 5 cubic centimetres of a cold saturated solution of rock salt; and then the quantity of silver estimated by means of a solution of rhodan ammonium. The latter solution is to be added to the silver until the red colour no longer disappears on shaking. The calculation is very simple.—*London Med. Record*, June 15, 1881.

Estimation of Urea.

In a paper in Pflüger's *Archiv*, Band xxi. p. 248, E. PFLÜGER gives in great detail his reasons for believing that Liebig's method is liable to error to the extent of 14 per cent., and indicates certain rules whereby such error may be corrected. Expressed shortly, the principal error in Liebig's work, according to Pflüger, is, that he assumes that if one have a solution of a substance A, and to it add the solutions of a second substance B, and of a third C, both of which have a chemical action upon A, the result is identically the same, whether B or C be the first to be added, which is not the case. Into the details of Pflüger's method (which he calls the static method) it is not possible here to enter. It depends in great measure upon accuracy of preparation, and upon the care with which the solutions required in the analysis are prepared. Very full directions are given in the original paper.—*London Med. Record*, June 15, 1881.

Surgery.

Arrow Wounds.

Dr. H. S. KILBOURNE, Captain and Assistant Surgeon, U. S. A., recently made some remarks upon arrow wounds before the Buffalo Medical Club, that form an interesting contribution to the literature of the subject.

As arrows were among the first offensive weapons used by man in ancient and barbaric times, so they are still the favourite weapon of many savage tribes. This antique weapon is, however, being rapidly displaced by rifles among those tribes whose enmities with the whites have taught them its superiority. An American Indian of the plains, who has seen a breech-loader and does not possess one, will part with all he has in the world to procure it. The bow and arrow is therefore disappearing, and with them the surgery of arrow wounds will become only a curious history.

The service bow of the Indian is quite a different thing from the dainty affair of the archery clubs. It is short, thick, and strong. It is made among the southwestern tribes of the bois d'arc or Osage range. The string is of raw hide, or buffalo sinew. The arrow is made of pecan or any suitable wood, not too heavy and having a straight, tough fibre. The arrow head, formerly of flint, is now usually made of soft iron, cut by a file into triangular shape. It is let into the split end of the shaft by a short shank and fastened by wrapping with strips of sinew, put on before it is dry.

In hunting and fighting, the warrior is mounted on a swift and active pony, and in using the bow he comes to close quarters. In action he rides at full speed, slipping over to the side of the horse and discharging the arrows from under the neck of the animal. The horse thus acts as a living shield for his body.

The rapidity, force, and precision of the shots are, in some instances, marvellous. As a rule, however, the accuracy is about that of a fair marksman with the pistol, as at a running mark.

There is in the Army Medical Museum, at Washington, a preparation of a portion of the left scapula of a buffalo, with an arrow head impacted in it. The barbed iron head of the arrow has entered the venter and the point protrudes from the dorsum, so that the missile must have passed through the thorax.

The specimen is from a buffalo killed at Fort Sedgwick, in 1860, by a Cheyenne Indian. There are also other specimens of bones, penetrated, perforated, and fissured in various ways, some of them resembling the appearance of glass, through which a pistol ball has been fired a few yards off.[1] The rapidity of the discharge of arrows rivals the fire of the first breech-loader I know of. The precision is sufficient to make it exceedingly uncomfortable for any one in the vicinity.

As the arrow head is secured to the shaft by strips of dried sinew, the wounds inflicted by it have this peculiarity: that in penetrating wounds, the fastening is softened by the fluids of the body, and, when not at once extracted, the head becomes loosened and is detached when extraction is attempted. In such cases it remains as a foreign body in the wound. If bone has been penetrated, the arrow head is impacted in it and held fast by the compact tissue, when extraction may become a difficult and hazardous operation.

The late Gen. Kearing suffered from a penetrating arrow wound of the superior maxillary bone, received in an affray with hostile Indians, about 1855 or 1856, until his death. The arrow head was so pinched and twisted by the hard bone, and attempts at removal were attended by such copious hemorrhage, that the iron was allowed to remain until a secondary operation was practicable. The missile was finally removed in St. Louis, after a severe operation, but the patient never entirely recovered from its effects. At short range, the arrow will perforate a flat bone, as a rib, making a clean cut, or a slight cracking or splitting. There is seldom any comminution or extensive fissuring like that produced by the impact of a conoidal rifle ball with bone.

---

[1] Dr. Otis, U. S. A., in Report in Surg. Cases in the Army.

In all the specimens showing penetration of the cranium, there is, according to Dr. Otis, little or no fissuring internally or externally. The inner and outer tables are both cleanly divided. This feature distinguishes arrow wounds of the calvaria from all others caused by weapons used in civilized warfare. Indeed, among all weapons I have seen, I know of none capable of making wounds so peculiar.

There are in the army museum specimens illustrating these features and also the impaction of arrow heads.

For the relief of these injuries, it is most natural to seize the arrow and draw it out of the wound. But that will never do. The head will part with the shaft and remain in the bottom of the wound. If not loosened by softening of the sinew, the head, if barbed, will catch in the soft parts and may, in certain regions, work irreparable injury.

Dr. Bill, of the army, has employed a device for these operations which is often of great service. He passes the loop of a wire snare down along the shaft and over the arrow head, and, when in place, secures it by traction on the outer end of the loop. The missile may then be carefully withdrawn entire. When the iron is impacted in the bone, he employs a loop of annealed wire, passed down along the shaft, which serves as a guide. The arrow head is snared by the loop; the ends of the wire are then passed through a long suture-twisters or double canula, which is passed down to the loop; the ends of the wire are then twisted or secured to the handle, and arrow and instrument are withdrawn together. In a case where a Navajo arrow had penetrated the lung to a depth of five inches, Dr. Bill removed it by means of the simple snare first described.

A prominent army officer, now retired from active service, when serving in Texas as a subaltern, was, while in an encounter with hostile Comanches, transfixed by an arrow. The weapon pierced the upper part of the right chest and passed nearly horizontally through the lung, the point protruding at the back, between the scapula and spine, on the same side. He informed me that, at his own request, a silk handkerchief was fastened to the shaft, which was then pushed on through the body, dragging the silk after it through the whole extent of this formidable wound. He recovered from the effects of the wound and from this novel surgical procedure, and served actively for many years after.

In the report of surgical cases in the army since the war, I find the following somewhat similar case, reported by Dr. Goddard, U. S. A. His employé at Fort Rice, D. T., was wounded in February, 1868, by an arrow, which entered his back three inches to the right of the fifth lumbar vertebra and emerged at a point two inches to the right of the ensiform cartilage. During the following evening the patient lost externally about eight ounces of blood, and a small (estimated) quantity internally. He was confined to his bed some two weeks, suffering from irritative fever and circumscribed peritonitis. In four weeks he was walking about, and on July 1st was actively employed. There are no further particulars or comments on this case.

The route of the missile is a mystery. It would seem impossible that it could have been direct between the two wounds, as the intestines, stomach, and liver lie in the way. Both the great cavities would also have been opened. Penetrating arrow wounds of the abdomen are usually mortal.

Of 9 cases reported in detail, 7 were fatal; and of the 2 which recovered, it is doubtful whether the peritoneal sac was penetrated. One of the fatal cases was mine, and, as it may be taken as a type of its class, I will give it here: A cavalry soldier was wounded while approaching an Indian camp at night, near the Canadian River, Texas, by an arrow which entered the abdomen in the left hypochondriac region, making a wound about three-fourths of an inch in length, through which about eighteen inches of the small intestine protruded. The gut was cut in four places. The wounds in the intestines were closed by sutures and the protruding portion returned through the wound, which was enlarged for the purpose. When found, the man had lain out all night, and was in a state of collapse. He was carried along with the column, in an ambulance, but died on the second day, never having rallied from the shock of the injury.

The great fatality of arrow wounds of the abdomen is so well known to the Indians that in action they usually aim at the umbilicus.[1]

Another case, which I personally observed, is so unique that I will briefly give its outlines. It is an example of a penetrating arrow wound of the lower part of the trunk. The operation for its relief was done at Fort Sill, I. T., by Dr. Forwood, of the army, who reports the case. I assisted him and saw the patient up to the date of his removal.

"Latimore, a chief of the Kiowas, aged 42 years, applied at Fort Sill for treatment, with symptoms of stone in the bladder. In 1862 he had led a band of his tribe against the Pawnees, and was wounded in a fight. Being mounted, and leaning over his horse, a Pawnee, on foot and within a few paces, drove an arrow deep into his right buttock. The shaft was withdrawn by his companions, but the point remained in his body. He passed bloody urine soon after the injury, but the wound soon healed, and in a few weeks he was able to ride without inconvenience. For more than six years he continued at the head of his band and travelled on horseback many hundreds of miles every summer. A long time after the injury he began to feel pain in urination, which increased, until he was forced to reveal the sacred secret, as it is regarded by the Indians, and to seek medical aid. The urine was loaded with blood, mucus, and pus; the introduction of a sound indicated a large, hard calculus in the bladder. Judging from the cicatrix and all the circumstances, it was apparent that the arrow had passed through the glutic muscles and the obturative (sciatic?) foramen into the bladder. On Aug. 23d I removed the stone by the lateral operation. The calculus was phosphatic, and weighed eight hundred and fifteen grains. On section of the stone, the arrow point was found imbedded near its centre. It was of iron, and had originally been about two and one-half inches long, by seven-eighths of an inch broad in its widest part. The urine began to pass by the natural channel on the third day, and on the seventh day it had nearly ceased to flow from the wound. But the restless spirit of the patient's band could no longer be restrained; open hostilities with the whites were expected to begin every moment, and they insisted on his removal. He needed purgatives on the eighth day, which they refused to allow him to take; on the following day they started with him to their camp, sixty miles away. Fourteen days after he is reported to have died. But his relatives have since assured me that the wound had healed, and that no trouble arose from it."

Notwithstanding a narrow pelvic outlet and the large size of the stone, there was every reason to expect a favourable result in this interesting case. These Indians possess remarkable powers of endurance and recuperation from wounds, due, doubtless, to their active life in the open air of the Western plains. But it is possible that the case may have been complicated by an induced disease of the kidneys.—*Buffalo Med. and Surg. Journal*, July, 1881.

—

Ununited Fracture of the Olecranon treated by Suture of the Bones.

At a late meeting of the Clinical Society of London (*Lancet*, June 4, 1881), Mr. MacCormac read notes of a case of Ununited Fracture of the Olecranon

---

[1] Dr. Bill, U. S. A.

Process, in which Bony Union was obtained by Sutures of the Bones. The patient (who was exhibited) was a piano-tuner, twenty-six years of age, who four months before coming to St. Thomas's Hospital had fallen upon the right elbow, and sustained a fracture of the olecranon. When admitted the limb was wasted, especially the triceps; there was no power of active extension; the line of fracture ran across the base of the olecranon, the detached portion being separated by two inches, and fixed to the back of the humerus, the condyles of which could be felt in the gap, no uniting medium being perceptible. On Jan. 6th Mr. MacCormac made a vertical incision three inches long, exposing the fractured bone and the articulation. There was no trace of uniting material, the fractured surfaces were covered with smooth fibrous tissue, and adhesions existed between the detached process and the condyles, and also between the end of the humerus and ulna. These adhesions were dissected out, and the periosteum being reflected, a thin layer of bone was cut off with a chisel, and by means of two wire sutures through holes drilled in the bone the surfaces were brought into close apposition. The wires were twisted and cut off so as to project at the centre of the wound, which was afterwards closed with catgut sutures. The operation was performed antiseptically, the joint being washed out with carbolic solution (1 in 30) before closing the wound. The first dressing was made on the fifth day, when the wound was found to be united, except where the bone-sutures emerged, and these were removed in twenty-one days. In forty days the patient left the hospital with very good active movement at the elbow-joint, and apparently firm bony union at the seat of fracture. From first to last he had no pain or inconvenience. The wound healed without a drop of pus; the temperature occasionally rose to 99°.8; it was otherwise normal throughout. He has now perfect power of active extension. The arm cannot be made absolutely straight, but he is able to follow his trade as well as before.

Mr. LISTER believed he was the first to perform an operation of a similar nature many years ago in Edinburgh. The patient was an engineer in the prime of life, who had sustained a fracture of the olecranon. Mr. Lister exposed the ends of the fragments by a longitudinal incision; and after paring away the surfaces, drilled the fragments and tied them together by strong silver wire, using a single suture, which was more convenient than a double suture, for it remained in the line of incision. The result was, as in Mr. MacCormac's case, there was no inflammatory or constitutional disturbance. The man left with bony union and resumed his occupation. Since then, at King's College Hospital, he had similarly treated another case with like result. In neither was the upper fragment fixed to the humerus, as in Mr. MacCormac's case; nor was the separation between the fragments so wide. It was refreshing to hear antiseptic dressings spoken of as a matter of course; but he supposed few members of the Society would perform such an operation as the free opening of a joint without such antiseptic precautions as we possess, which afforded such security against complications.

Antiseptic Osteotomy of the Tibia; Rapidly fatal Carbolic Intoxication.

Mr. PEARCE GOULD at a recent meeting of the Clinical Society of London (*Lancet*, May 21, 1881) read a paper on a Case of Antiseptic Osteotomy of the Tibia, in which rapidly fatal carbolic intoxication occurred. A lad, eight years of age, of robust appearance, was admitted, under his care, into Westminster Hospital in Oct. 1880, with rickety deformity of the legs, especially of the left tibia. Other treatment had been perseveringly tried at the National Orthopædic Hospital for some time without avail, and he was sent in for the purpose of having osteotomy performed. His general health was very good. On Oct.

30th chloroform was administered, and the left tibia divided with McEwen's chisel, with a careful observance of the details of Listerism. He quickly recovered from the effects of the chloroform, and slept well through the night; next morning (Oct. 31st) he took his breakfast and appeared quite well; temperature 98.4°. At 11 A. M. (twenty-one hours after the operation) he vomited; and vomited a watery fluid repeatedly up till 9.30 P. M. He also passed two orange-coloured loose stools. At 7 P. M. he was rigid, and at 8 P. M. very restless; at 9 P. M. he was almost unconscious, he was breathing hurriedly, pulse almost imperceptible at the wrist. At 10 P. M. Mr. Gould saw him; he was then conscious; lying quiet and quite flat, respiration 44 per minute, air entered lungs freely, pulse very small and rapid, pupils small. He died, asphyxiated, at 2.30 A. M., Nov. 1st, thirty-six hours and three-quarters after the operation. There was complete suppression of urine after 11 A. M. Temperature rose to 100.2°, and fell to 99.6° at 2 A. M. on Nov. 1st. The treatment consisted in the application of warmth and stimulants to the surface, and brandy internally. At the autopsy all the viscera were apparently healthy, with the exception of congestion of the tracheal and bronchial mucous membrane, and excess of mucus in these tubes, and slight congestion of the lungs. The left side of the heart was empty, the right side contained partly-clotted blood; blood in smaller veins all fluid, in the larger partly in soft clots, all of it black. No petechiæ; no staining of endo-cardium or intima; no sign of fat embolism. Bladder empty. A small blood-clot in the wound; no crushing of the medulla; no thrombosis of tibial vessels. Microscopic preparations of the organs were made for Mr. Gould by Dr. Heneage Gibbes, some of which were shown at the meeting. From these it was seen that there was thrombosis of the capillaries and smaller vessels of the lungs with minute spots of round-cell inflammatory exudation. Similar minute inflammatory foci were also found in the kidneys, while sections of the stomach showed intense inflammation of its mucous surface, only traces of its glands being visible, and at places the process was evidently advancing to suppuration. No sign of fat embolism.

In discussing the cause of death Mr. Gould pointed out that shock, chloroform, the acute specifics, erysipelas, septicæmia, pyæmia, and fat embolism might be excluded, as was also the ingestion of any irritant matter, but yet both the symptoms and pathological changes showed evidence of the circulation of some irritant in the blood. The symptoms were individually considered, and it was shown that the vomiting, diarrhœa with orange stools, collapse, rigidity, restlessness, loss of consciousness, very hurried respiration, slight rise of temperature, and death from asphyxia, were the symptoms observed in cases of undoubted carbolic intoxication. The urine passed before the onset of vomiting appeared to be normal, and was not preserved; the suppression of urine later on was a new fact in such cases. The softly coagulated and black blood had been noted before, but there was no record of any microscopical examination of the apparently healthy organs usually found. The quantity of acid absorbed was no doubt small, and the great susceptibility of the patient to its toxic effect must at present be spoken of as an idiosyncrasy; but from the absence of other cause, and of any facts to negative the supposition, as well as the agreement of the symptoms and post-mortem pathological changes in the main with those observed in cases of carbolic intoxication, he was forced to the conclusion that such poisoning was the cause of death.

Professor LISTER remarked upon the interest attaching to the suppression of urine, which he had not met with before. He had no doubt that Mr. Gould's view must be accepted, that this patient was one of those who had an unfortunate susceptibility to the toxic effects of carbolic acid. He had met with cases of such susceptibility, and one he called to mind was a lady whose breast he removed and dressed in his usual manner; intense symptoms of carbolic poisoning came on, and boracic lint was substituted for the gauze dressing, but the spray was used when the lint was changed, and this was sufficient to keep up the symptoms, which only abated when its use was discontinued. As an instance of the special local susceptibility of some patients, he mentioned a case of chronic synovitis of the knee-joint, which he opened and dressed antiseptically, and next day he found all the skin under the gauze intensely red and irritated. It had been stated that there was no antiseptic that could with safety replace carbolic acid, though several had been tried; but he was in a position to say that the oil of Eucalyptus globulus, if used properly, is a powerful and perfectly reliable antiseptic, and is also quite unirritating and without toxic effects. If the oil be made into an emulsion with spirit and water, and then used, it very quickly evaporates; but he had found that gum damar holds it exceedingly well, and the mixture remains soft and strongly odorous of the oil even at the end of several weeks. He had used a gauze prepared with a mixture of one part of the oil, three of damar, and three of paraffine, and he was able to assert that it might be thoroughly trusted as an antiseptic where carbolic acid was unadvisable.

Trepanation of the Ilium in a Case of Pelvic Abscess.

The patient, a tailor, aged 24, had disease of the lumbar vertebræ, a cold abscess starting from which had burrowed into the left hip-joint, and invaded the whole pelvis (*Deutsch. Zeitschr. für Chir.*, Band xii.). An opening above Poupart's ligament not affording sufficient drainage, Dr. G. FISCHER trephined the ilium at its upper and posterior part, and afterwards established a transverse drain across the pelvis. The patient died twenty-five days later from exhaustion, due to prolonged suppuration and progressive pulmonary tuberculosis. The necropsy showed that stagnation of pus had not taken place in any part of the pelvis; and hence Fisher considers that he has established the justifiability of trephining the ilium to obtain a counter-opening in cases of pelvic abscess.—*British Med. Journal*, May 7, 1881.

Resection of Large Trunk-Veins.

PILZER opposes strongly (*Deutsch. Zeitschr. für Chir.*, Band xiv. Heft 21) the prejudice against ligature of large veins, citing recently recorded cases to prove that the fear of pyæmia is groundless. He gives in detail six cases from the Heidelberg surgical clinic. In all six, malignant disease was present; and the internal jugular vein was resected in four cases, both internal jugulars in another, and the femoral vein in the sixth. All the cases recovered. Resection of the vein is much to be preferred to the dissection of it out of the tumour, with the great risk of recurrence of the tumour from fragments left on the vein.—*British Med. Journal*, May 7, 1881.

Treatment of Vascular Tumours by Electrolysis.

Dr. NIEDER, in the *Archives of Ophthalmology*, March, 1881, quotes some illustrative cases. In two of them, a tumour consisting of large veins exerted such a pressure on the upper eyelid that the eye could not be opened. In all instances, a complete cure was effected without any untoward symptoms. He employed from four to six cells (model of Spamer), with a key to connect or interrupt immediately. The needles may be of steel, although a platinum needle is preferable for the positive electrode, to prevent oxidation and permanent staining of the punctured spot. Both needles are introduced into the tumour, and left in place for the space of one to three minutes, whereupon the site of the negative pole is charged according to the size of the growth. The bubbles of hydrogen arising at the negative needle may disturb the tissues, but are harmless; moreover, they are readily dispelled by pressure. At each sitting a few punctures, not over five or six, are made, while the number of sittings varies according to the size and the location of the angioma. The immediate effect is hardening and shrinkage from coagulation of the blood. Some suppuration occurred in all instances but one, which resulted in loss of substance or formation of unexpected cicatrization. Antiseptic after-treatment was maintained.—*London Med. Record*, June 15, 1881.

Neuritis in Stumps.

In an original contribution to the first number of the *Revue de Chirurgie*, Dr. G. Nepveu, of Paris, after a short review of previously recorded cases of neuritis in stumps, relates a case, observed by himself, of ascending neuritis in the leg after amputation of the foot for gangrene from endarteritis. About four months and a half after the operation, the extremity of the stump ulcerated, and the patient, a man aged 44, suffered from severe shooting pains, which reached to the middle of the thigh, from painful contractions of the flexor muscles of the stump, and also from pain and convulsive movements of a similar character in the sound leg. Removal of the painful stump by amputation just below the seat of election was ultimately followed by complete relief, although the stump left at this second operation ulcerated and was very tender for about four months. On examination of the amputated stump, the posterior tibial nerve was found to be thickened and adherent at its lower extremity to the cicatrix; and the lower portions of the anterior tibial and internal saphenous nerves resembled fibrous cords. The microscopic appearances of these nerves even at their proximal extremities indicated a chronic interstitial and parenchymatous neuritis, that is to say, an inflammation affecting both the connective tissue and the nerve elements. This condition, M. Nepveu states, accounts for the convulsive movement of the stump, its ulceration, and the severe pain felt by the patient. Moreover, it enables us to understand why the sound limb had also been involved in the spasm, and why, after the second amputation, relief of the pain resulted very slowly and not immediately. Ascending neuritis in a stump affects, it is stated, two very different forms—the simple form and the complicated. Simple ascending neuritis may be accompanied by persistent neuralgia, or by trophic disturbances in the stump. The complicated ascending neuritis presents itself in one or other of two different aspects. Sometimes it attacks the other and sound limb on the side of the stump—ascending neuritis and unilateral myelitis. At other times the myelitis is called transverse, and then the surgeon has to deal with paralysis of the bladder, and paralysis, neuralgia, or contracture of the corresponding limb on the opposite side. The myelitis may be followed by rapid death. M. Nepveu regards his case as one of recovery. Attention is directed to M. Verneuil's practice of resecting nerve-trunks in the flaps during amputation. This resection, it is thought, would probably result in diminishing among those who have submitted to amputation the number of instances of neuritis, whether ascending or localized. In confirmed cases of neuritis of stumps, surgical intervention (reamputation, neurectomy) has been attended with varying success.—*London Med. Record*, May 15, 1881.

The Treatment of Neuromata by Enucleation.

Mr. E. DOWNES, in the *Lancet*, April, 1881, suggests that, in many cases of nerve-tumour, the morbid mass may be shelled out by a longitudinal incision, instead of excising the growth with a portion of the nerve itself, or amputating the limb, as in some cases has been done. Three cases are related in which this mode of treatment was successful, the nerve-fibres completely surrounding the tumours, which lay in the centre almost entirely unconnected with the nerve itself. In one case, in which a neuroma of the median nerve was treated by excising the mass with the included portion of the nerve, a large number of smaller neuromata spontaneously disappeared after the larger one was thus removed. [Prof. Kosinski narrated a somewhat similar case (*Medical Times and Gazette*, November, 1874, p. 558); here, after a neuroma of the small sciatic had been excised, a large number of similar tumours spontaneously disappeared.] —*London Med. Record*, June 15, 1881.

Removal of the Kidney for Nephrolithiasis.

At the Charing-Cross Hospital is a lad aged fifteen, from whom Mr. BARWELL removed a kidney on May 5th, and who is now convalescent. The boy had been under observation for about a year with pyelitis and retro-peritoneal abscess. An incision was made about ten months ago, with the effect of mitigating the symptoms. The wound had healed, leaving only a sinus. In April, by sounding through this passage, Mr. Barwell detected a stone. Yet although the lad was becoming very anæmic, with irregular hectic temperature, no consent for operation could be obtained until the above date, when lumbar nephrectomy was performed. Two peculiarities rendered the removal unusually difficult—viz., the dense thick cicatricial tissue and the proximity of the rib to the ileum. Mr. Barwell cut through the tissues, and came upon the kidney with the stone impacted. An endeavour to extract this latter caused copious bleeding, hence the operator rapidly enucleated the gland, and passed a ligature round the pedicle *en masse*. Since want of room forbade removing the kidney entire, it was divided and extracted in two parts. The operation was thus completed very quickly, and with scarcely any loss of blood. Since then the boy has been going on uninterruptedly well, his temperature becoming normal and regular, the wound being now nearly healed. This is, we believe, the second successful case of removal of the kidney for stone.—*Lancet*, June 4, 1881.

Rhinitis and Plugging of the Nose.

GOTTSTEIN, in the *Berl. Klin. Woch.* 1881, No. 4, defends his treatment of ozæna by means of a cotton-wool plug against the adverse criticisms of different writers. He holds to the following opinions: 1. Plugging is the best known means of preventing the formation of crusts in rhinitis having a tendency thereto. 2. Fetor arising from the so-called atrophic rhinitis is immediately removed by plugging, not so that arising from necrosis. 3. Plugging is effectual in atrophic rhinitis, only when the plug or tampon is in actual contact with the diseased mucous membrane. The tampon ought to be $1\frac{1}{2}$ to 2 inches long, and at the utmost a fifth of an inch thick, so that it may reach almost to the posterior nares. Both nasal cavities should never be plugged at the same time. The plug should remain, as a rule, two to three hours *in situ;* but sometimes it may remain as much as twelve hours, and some patients wear it during the night. Medical treatment is, he says, useless, but a vigorous nasal douche in the intervals is beneficial. In the hypertrophic form, the plug readily causes bleeding and pain. In defect of the septum with formation of crusts, plugging gives most excellent results.—*London Med. Record*, June 15, 1881.

Discovery of the Micrococcus of Syphilis.

Dr. AUFRECHT of Magdeburg (*Central für die Med. Wiss.*, No. 13, 1881) announces that he has discovered in syphilitic condylomota a micrococcus, which may be recognized by the following characters. The single cocci are of rather coarse grain; they are generally of the form of diplococci, or two joined together, and the number of these is greater than of the single cocci. They are very seldom in threes. They are stained deeply by fuchsin. He has found them in six cases; but in one, where the condyloma was ulcerated, and, in another, where it had been painted with corrosive sublimate, they were very scarce. He, therefore, excludes ulcerated condylomata, or those which have been treated specifically. To obtain the micrococci, the condyloma should be incised with a lancet, and the blood sponged away; then a drop of the serous fluid that follows should be collected on a cover-glass, which is put under a bell-jar for twenty-four hours to dry. At the end of that time, a drop of a half per mille solution of fuchsin is placed on an object-glass, and the cover-glass is laid on it. The excess of fuchsin is wiped away after two or three minutes, and the object examined with Hartnack's 9A immersion-lens. To preserve the object, he puts a little dammar varnish around the edge of the cover-glass.—*London Med. Record*, June 15, 1881.

—

Effects of Excision of the Syphilitic Chancre.

M. MAURIAC reports (*Gazette des Hôpitaux*, 1881, Nos. 7, 10, 14) seven carefully recorded cases in which he excised the initial lesion of syphilis. In six, excision was performed at periods varying from four to sixteen or eighteen days after the appearance of the sore. In the seventh case, the initial lesion was excised about fifty hours after it had been first noticed, and before there was the least trace of glandular enlargement; but in this, as well as in all the others, the operation was unsuccessful in preventing further development of the disease.—*London Med. Record*, June 15, 1881.

—

Pathological Anatomy and Pathogeny of Gonorrhœal and Urethral Epididymitis.

In a paper lately read before the Société de Chirurgie (*Bull. et Mém. de la Soc. de Chir.*, 1881, No. 2, pp. 119, 155), M. TERRILLON details his views on this subject, derived from a study of cases observed by himself and others, and of experiments made by himself on dogs, by injecting irrigating fluids into the vas deferens. 1. *Pathological Anatomy.*—There are four different degrees of inflammation of the vas deferens. (*a*) In the first, the mucous membrane is alone attacked, and presents all the characters of catarrhal inflammation. The epithelium loses its cilia, and the submucous tissue becomes swelled and infiltrated with lymph-corpuscles. The vas deferens is not altered perceptibly when examined externally, and, therefore, this degree of inflammation cannot be recognized clinically. (*b*) Much more frequently the inflammation extends to the fibro-muscular walls of the vas deferens, which becomes swollen to two or three times its normal size. The bloodvessels and lymphatics are also much dilated. (*c*) The inflammation may spread to the cellular tissue of the spermatic cord, when the whole becomes welded into a mass, of which the various constituents cannot be recognized. (*d*) The inflammatory process may reach the connective tissue and scrotum. During the course of the inflammation, the vas deferens contains a yellow fluid, with a large number of pus corpuscles, and a smaller number of large granular cells. Spermatozoa are at first present, but disappear if the inflammation be prolonged. The tail of the epididymis is the part chiefly attacked. On section, the colour is grayish-green; the tubes are mostly dilated, and little foci resembling abscesses are seen. The intertubular connective tissue is increased, hardened, and infiltrated with lymphatic cells and pigment-granules. In the body of the epididymis the changes are less marked, and still less so in the globus major. No appreciable alteration, except congestion, takes place in the testis proper. The tunica vaginalis is always affected in acute epididymitis, by the formation of false membranes and the effusion of serum. 2. *Results and Termination.*—The phenomena disappear in the inverse order of their appearance. In about a month, the globus minor and vas deferens only remain affected. The latter remains thickened for several months. The author does not agree with Gosselin, who is of opinion that the excretory duct becomes blocked. Terrillon thinks that obliteration is not necessary to explain the absence of spermatozoa; but that their absence is due in many cases to a modification of secretion—in short, to a persistent catarrh of the mucous membrane of the vas deferens and globus minor. In his experiments on dogs, the author found the spermatozoa absent, or nearly absent, from an early stage of the inflammation, and before obliteration had had time to take place. 3. *Development of Epididymitis.*—The sole theory which is admissible, and proved by pathological anatomy and experiment, is the propagation of the inflammation along the ejaculatory ducts and vas deferens. All clinical facts accord with this, viz., first, the appearance of epididymitis at the time when the inflammation has reached the prostatic region; second, the occurrence, in most cases, of swelling and pain in the course of the vas deferens before the epididymitis itself becomes affected. The theory of metastasis is untenable.—*London Med. Record*, June 15, 1881.

—

Colour-Blindness.

It has long been felt desirable that legislative measures should be taken to protect the public from the dangers to which they are exposed by the employment of the colour-blind in positions in which safety is dependent on colour-perception. Statistics have been industriously collected by our Continental and Transatlantic *confrères* as to the prevalence of colour-blindness, but it is obviously necessary that our legislative bodies should be supplied by trustworthy, accurate data as to the frequency of colour-blindness amongst our own population before they can be urged to frame laws for the public safety. The Ophthalmological Society has, therefore, done good service in instituting an inquiry into the prevalence of colour-blindness in the United Kingdom. The Report of the Committee appointed to inquire into defects of sight in relation to the public safety was read at a meeting of the Society held on the 7th inst. by Dr. BRAILEY, from whose lucid and able statement we gather the following particulars :—

The inquiry extended over five months, and the examinations were conducted by gentlemen of experience. The material was collected from various sources, consisting of public institutions, schools (public and private), the Metropolitan Police, and the Coldstream Guards. The number examined (18,088) was sufficiently large to justify deductions from the observations. The examinations were made by the matching of coloured wools, following, in the main, the method of Holmgren. Certain cases were also tested by coloured lights, as exhibited in the instrument of Donders, and also by means of a lamp designed by Mr. Nettleship, in which is employed the actual coloured glass used in railway signals.

Colour-blindness was taken as an inability to distinguish from each other two or more colours; but persons who had simply confused blue with violet, or green with blue, had not been ranked with the colour-blind. It was clearly distinguishable from a defective knowledge of the names of colours, and from defects of vision in other respects. Those were recorded as *slightly colour-blind* who had failed to distinguish from each other the pale shades only of different colours— mistaking, for example, gray or buff for green, and even mauve, yellow, or pink. Those who, besides failing as above, could not recognize the difference between red and green, matching either scarlet with green, or rose colour with green, gray, or violet, were considered *pronounced colour-blind*. Three cases only were discovered where there was a total failure of the recognition of *all* colours, these being only distinguished as shades. In the vast majority deficient recognition of two colours only was conspicuous. These associated colours were either red and green, or blue and yellow. Failure to recognize blue and yellow was rare, and from its little practical importance these cases were included as *slight* cases of colour-blindness. In every one of the *pronounced* cases of colour-blindness (617 in number) there was blindness to red and green.

All persons with pronounced blindness to red and green were found utterly incapable of naming with certainty a red or green light when exhibited singly. All failed, also, when the distance and intensity of illumination of the coloured light were unknown. The pronounced colour-blind were divided, as far as practicable, into two groups, in accordance with the definitions of Continental authorities. Those matching rose-coloured wools with dark-blues or violets, and scarlet with dark-greens or browns, were called *red-blind;* while those matching the rose with grays or greens, and scarlet with light-browns or greens, were called *green-blind.* Notwithstanding that many colour-blind stood, as regards the wools, in a position intermediate between the two groups, this division still appeared to the examiners to have a practical value, as the red-blind failed to appreciate at all, even as a light, except at a much shorter distance than normal, a light viewed through glass of the purest red obtainable; whereas the green-blind appreciate it at the full, or nearly the full, normal distance. Red-blindness appeared to be, in the United Kingdom, a little more common than green-blindness.

Coming now to the numerical results, we find that of the 18,088 persons examined, 16,431 were males and 1657 were females. Deducting from the males certain groups of cases specially selected in the expectation of finding peculiarities, there remained 14,846 with an average of colour-defects of 4.76; whilst among females, making similar deductions, there remained 489, with a percentage of only .4. Moreover, in addition to the striking difference in the prevalence of colour-defects in the two sexes, it should be mentioned that the forms encountered in females were nearly always slight.

In certain classes of persons exceptional prevalence of colour-blindness was found. Thus, among male Jews it was 4.9 per cent.; among male Friends, 5.9 per cent.; among the male deaf and dumb it reached the extraordinarily high rate of 13.7. Among females of each of these groups the percentage was less high. It appeared also, that the prevalence of colour-defects was lower among the more educated and socially higher classes. For example, at Eton the percentage was 2.46; among medical students and sons of medical men it was 2.5; in middle-class schools it was 3.5; and among the police, and schools of about the same class, 3.7. On the other hand, those with colour-defects were not intellectually inferior to those of the same class without these defects. Lunatics do not present the peculiarity more frequently than the sane. The prevalence was found to be about the same in adults and children, and in urban and rural districts. There appeared to be a higher percentage of colour-blindness in Ireland than in England, but this might be accounted for by the differences in the social classes examined.

With regard to the causation of colour-blindness, Dr. Brailey is inclined to regard it as due in most cases to a congenital physical defect, either in the eye or brain, occurring in the first instance as an accidental variation, and, when once existing, liable to be transmitted by descent. It was to the frequency of inter-marriage that the high percentage among the Jews and Friends was to be ascribed. The heredity of the defect was strikingly illustrated by some cases alluded to by Messrs. Frost and McHardy. The former referred to a colour-blind who had seven sons, six of whom were know to be colour-blind. None of the daughters had the defect, but one had a colour-blind son. Dr. Brailey is also of opinion that colour-blindness, especially the slighter forms, may arise from defective colour education in infancy, and hence it is that females, from the greater attrac-tion colours have for them at an early age, and the greater attention paid as a sex to colour-distinctions, are less frequently the subjects of the defect.—*Med. Times and Gaz.*, April 30, 1881.

Midwifery and Gynæcology.

The Earliest Recorded Case of Abdominal Section for Extra-Uterine Gestation.

At the March meeting of the Obstetrical Society of Edinburgh Dr. C. E. Un-derhill, in presenting a historical note of a remarkable case of abdominal sec-tion in the sixteenth century, said that "the triumphs achieved by abdominal sur-gery of late years lend a special interest to cases in which operations involving the opening of the abdomen were performed by the older surgeons. The case I am going to relate appears to be one of the first in which a surgeon ventured to make an incision into the abdomen for the purpose of removing the remains of an extra-uterine gestation; and it is the more striking as the operation was per-formed during the existence of a second and natural pregnancy, and the patient recovered without any interruption of the pregnancy, which terminated naturally in due course. I came across it in the voluminous collection of curious cases col-lected by John Schenck of Grafenberg, which was published in Latin in Frank-fort in 1609, under the title, *Observationum Medicarum, Rararum, Novarum, Admirabilium, et Montrosàrum Volumen.* The work is divided into seven books, and contains upwards of a thousand folio pages. The cases are collected from the writings of a large number of authors, of whose works a long list is given at the beginning of the volume. The case in question is quoted from the history of remarkable cases of Marcellus Donatus, and is to be found in Book IV. page 660, of Schenck's work. It was as follows: In the month of March of the year 1540, at Castrum Pomponii, commonly called Pomponischi, in the province of the Lords of Gonzaga, not far from the river Po, there lived a woman whose name was Lodovica; but, in consequence of her great size, she was commonly called La Cavalla. Now this woman had at one time been pregnant; the fœtus had died in utero, and the soft parts had become putrid and been discharged through the vulva, while the bony parts had been retained within her. When she had recovered her health, she again became pregnant. Her health soon be-came seriously impaired, and she passed into a condition of the greatest danger. At this time there chanced to come to these parts a certain surgeon, whose name was Christopher Bain, one of those who journey about, passing from town to town. As soon as he heard of this woman's condition, which was fully explained to him by some of the neighbours, he offered to try and restore her to health, on condition that they should put her unreservedly into his hands, including her body if she died (*ac mortuam*), and should agree to pay him ten golden pieces if she recovered. Her relatives, who were poor persons, accepted his offer, some of the wealthier people in the neighbourhood helping them and promising to pay the money. The man, who was ignorant of letters, but a bold fellow, had the woman tied up, and set about the operation. Having slowly dissected through the longitudinal muscles of the abdomen and the peritoneum, he at last opened the uterus itself, and extracted the skeleton of a male child. He washed out the uterus with warm wine mixed with certain aromatics, and united the lips of the wound by a suture, having burned with the actual cautery the part that was sewn in (*candentique ferro partem inconsutam inurit*). Wonderful to relate, the woman recovered, and in due time bore the other child, not only alive, but absolutely uninjured in any way. She subsequently conceived, not only once, but four times, carried her children to the full time, and was safely delivered. The case I have given is a remarkable one, but I am able to bring witnesses to its reality, namely, Dominus John Baptist Zorzonus, and Alexander Begher, Dominus Frederick de Felini, and Dominus Leonellus Zorzonus, and Antonius Maiochus or Mazzuchinus, and several others, who were present at the whole operation.—*Marcell. Donat. Hist. Med. Mirab.*, lib. 4, c. 22," from *Edin. Med. Journal*, July, 1881.

—

Another Successful Case of the Müller-Porro Operation.

Dr. A. BREISKY, of Prague, reports in the *Centralblatt f. Gynäk.* (p. 238) a successful case of Porro's operation. The operation was performed on a 28-year old woman, who had been in labour over two days. The pelvis was "asymetrical, generally contracted, flat, and rachitic," of the third degree of deformity, and with the conjugata vera measuring 2.7–2.9 inches. The child presented by the vertex in the first position. The patient was in good condition, and had no tenderness over the hypogastrium. Operation under thymol spray. Incision from a hand's breadth above the umbilicus. The unopened uterus was pulled forward through the wound, and two strong wire ligatures passed round the supra-vaginal portion. These could not be ligatured at first on account of the head bulging into the cervix. The uterus was opened, and the child with some difficulty removed. It was asphyxiated, but was soon brought round. The ligatures were, immediately on the birth of the child, drawn tight by means of a Cintrab's apparatus, and the uterus, with the placenta *in situ*, and ovaries cut off. No sponging of the peritoneum was necessary, as nothing had escaped into it. The stump was fixed by a long needle to the lower angle of the wound. The wound was closed with deep silver and superficial silk sutures. No drainage-tube was used. On the thirteenth day the needle was removed, on the fifteenth and sixteenth the ligatures, and on the twentieth the sloughing portion of the stump separated. The stump wound healed without leaving a fistula by the sixth week. The author states that the procedure he followed—Müller's modification of Porro's operation—is easily carried out, and is safer than any of the other methods, and that the intra-peritoneal method, by whichever way the stump is treated, is so unsafe as to be inadmissible.—*Edin. Med. Journal*, July, 1881.

—

Enucleation of Subperitoneal Fibromata through the Vagina.

CZERNY relates (*Wiener Med. Woch.*, April 30, 1881) two cases: the first done by Sutton, in which the vaginal roof was incised, and the tumour drawn out of the peritoneum through the vaginal incision. The tumour was attached by a broad pedicle to the posterior wall of the uterus. The pedicle was cut through, and the tumour delivered by an ordinary midwifery forceps. Some small intestine protruded, which was replaced with great difficulty. Death occurred after four days. Necropsy revealed perforation of the small intestine by the manipulations employed during the operation. The second case, by Derweer, was one of large retro-uterine fibroma, pressing on the ureters, and causing retention of urine. After incision of the posterior vaginal wall, the tumour was drawn outside the vulva by a small forceps, together with the uterus, and the left ligament and ovary. The capsule of the tumour was opened, and the tumour enucleated, without cutting into the peritoneum. Silk sutures were inserted into the wound. Recovery took place at the end of six weeks. The tumour weighed 324 grammes. The author thinks the operation was unsuitable in the first case, but indicated in the second.—*London Med. Record,* June 15, 1881.

Medical Jurisprudence and Toxicology.

A Case of Belladonna-poisoning treated with Pilocarpin.

A correspondent to the *Brit. Med. Journ.*, for April 16, 1881, Mr. NICHOLAS GRATTAN, reports the following case :—

Mrs. M., aged 42, drank by mistake a wineglassful of a liniment at 9 P. M., December 23d, 1880. Fortunately for her, she had had a hearty dinner about four hours before. She discovered her mistake, and took two teaspoonsful of mustard in water, with no effect; walked a short distance into town, purchased an emetic, which she drank, returned home, and felt dizzy, her sight going, and shadows before her eyes. She lost the power of speech, became greatly excited, had convulsions, and vomited slightly, and then lapsed into profound stupor. At 10.45 P M. I saw her for the first time. Her pupils were widely dilated, not acted on by light; her face was swollen, and of a bluish colour, more especially her lower lip, the mucous membrane of which appeared as if it had been blistered; the pulse was imperceptible in one wrist, almost so in the other; respirations 25. I introduced a stomach-tube, pumped in a mustard emetic, and washed out the stomach thoroughly. In half an hour she had vomited freely, and sensibility was slightly returning, but she soon lapsed again into complete stupor. From this time until 2 A. M. she was treated with cold affusion to the head, and flagellation with a wet towel over her heart. At 2 A. M. I heard from my friend Dr. Harvey (who had ordered the liniment for her) that she had taken two ounces and two drachms of belladonna liniment (*P.·B.*). There being no marked improvement in her condition I determined to try pilocarpin. This I procured at 3 A. M., and injected subcutaneously one-fifth of a grain every fifteen minutes. After the third dose, there was a decided improvement; consciousness was evidently returning, her countenance became more natural, her pulse could be distinctly felt, and she was able to raise her hands to her mouth and throat. At 3.45 A. M. I administered a fourth dose of one-fifth of a grain. This had an effect on both pupils, which began to contract under the influence of light. She was evidently fast recovering, had a drink of tea and milk, and was able to speak. At 4.30 A. M. she was so far recovered that I thought it safe to leave her, desiring her friends to send for me should she relapse into her former state. When I saw her again at 10 A. M., she had had a refreshing sleep, from which she awoke, saying that she did not remember anything that had occurred. She had had in all four-fifths of a grain of pilocarpin; it appears to act as a direct antidote to the belladonna; it did not cause the least perspiration. She continued to feel slight dizziness for two days, with dilated pupils; but was, in every other respect, quite well. I gave her half a drachm of tincture of opium each night. The third day she had perfectly recovered.

MEDICAL NEWS.

An Act "to provide for the Registration of all Practitioners of Medicine and Surgery," after passing the legislature, was signed by Governor Hoyt, June 8, 1881, and is effective at once. The object aimed at by the bill is to secure an authoritative list of practising physicians in each county of the State, which list shall be accessible by the public. It is based upon the registration law of New York. To insure against misapprehension the law requires the deposit of a duly attested copy of each physician's diploma to be deposited at the time of registration, and filed for future reference.

The bill has been carefully prepared, emanating, as it does, from the Committee on Medical Legislation of the State Medical Society; and it is chiefly due to the exertions of Dr. R. L. Sibbett, of Carlisle, the chairman of this committee, that it was finally passed. Its main features are as follows:—

Section I. requires the prothonotary of each county to keep a special book for the registration of physicians, in which also the subsequent death or removal from the county of a physician shall be duly inscribed.

Section II. declares that "every person who shall practise medicine or surgery or any of the branches of medicine or surgery for gain, or shall receive or accept for his or her services as a practitioner of medicine or surgery, any fee or reward, directly or indirectly, shall be a graduate of a legally chartered medical college or university having authority to confer the degree of doctor of medicine (except as provided for in section 5 of this Act), and such person shall present to the prothonotary of the county in which he or she resides or sojourns his or her medical diploma as well as a true copy of the same including any endorsements thereon, and shall make affidavit before him that the diploma and endorsements are genuine; thereupon the prothonotary shall enter the following in the register, to wit: The name in full of the practitioner, his or her place of nativity, his or her place of residence, the name of the college or university that has conferred the degree of doctor of medicine, the year when such degree was conferred, and in like manner any other degree or degrees that the practitioner may desire to place on record, to all of which the practitioner shall likewise make affidavit before the prothonotary; and the prothonotary shall place the copy of such diploma, including the endorsements, on file in his office for inspection by the public."

Sections III. and IV. provide that in case of the loss of a diploma a certified copy may be deposited, and in the case of a person commencing practice in this State after the passage of this act, who holds a foreign diploma, that the same shall be countersigned by the dean of one of the medical colleges of this Commonwealth, the faculty of said college, first "being satisfied as to the qualifications of the applicant and the genuineness of the diploma."

Section V. especially exempts those who have practised medicine without a diploma since 1871 from the penalties of the act, provided they make oath to this fact, and record it upon the register.

Section VI. establishes the registration fee at one dollar.

Registration in order to be efficient requires the active co-operation of physicians, and due provision should also be made for the publication in the daily papers once or twice a year, of an authoritative list of qualified practitioners with their place of graduation, if they have any, if not, let this fact likewise be stated.

It is to be regretted, that there was a misunderstanding among some of our principal physicians in regard to the bill for creating a State Board of Health, an important function of which would have consisted in carrying out the provisions of this law in regard to the practice of medicine. As the registration law is framed, it is left to some voluntary informer to prosecute non-registered physicians who are engaged in practice, as a reward he shall receive one half the fine ($100), and in the discretion of the court also half of the penalty (a year in prison), at least, so the law reads, owing to faulty construction of Section VII.

As all properly qualified physicians are interested in the success of measures tending to protect the public from ignorance, incompetence, and imposture, it devolves upon them to aid in making the law effective, by having a committee appointed in each county medical society, which will have the duty, and the courage to perform it, of prosecuting violators of the law. In the absence of a properly constituted State Board of Health this responsibility obviously rests upon the county societies. Should this duty not be performed, it is feared that the law will be a dead-letter. Physicians having urged the passage of this act, the community looks to them to take measures for its enforcement.

———

Annual Meeting of the American Surgical Association.—The American Surgical Association will hold its first regular meeting at the Oriental Hotel, Coney Island, September 13, 14, and 15. Papers are promised by several gentlemen.

———

Health of New York.—The advent of the heated term, always so prejudicial to infantile life, has caused a notable increase in the city's mortality during the last month. While the advent of the low temperature, which prevailed during the first weeks of June, was manifest in a reduced death-rate, viz., 660 for the week ending June 4, and 633 for that ending June 11; the figures for the following weeks are as follows: June 19, 637; June 26, 699; July 3, 906; and July 10 it reached 1144.

· The Board of Health has taken measures to avert this excessive great mortality from preventible disease, by appointing a corps of 50 tenement-house physicians, whose term of service will extend over five weeks. The corps, which commenced its duties on July 13, will visit every city tenement, at sufficiently frequent intervals, to examine into the health of the inmates and prescribe for the sick. The Board of Estimate and Apportionment has appropriated $30,000 for the salaries of special inspectors, physicians, and nurses, who will be appointed by the Board of Health to aid in combating contagious diseases.

It is noticed that typhus fever has perceptibly diminished during June. During the 12th week of the endemic (ending June 4) there were reported 32 new cases; in the 13th week, 37; in the 14th week, 16; and in the 15th week (ending June 25), 16. The total number of cases for May having been 125, and that for June 101, a reduction of 24 is seen to have taken place. Smallpox has, also, diminished. While 210 cases occurred in May, only 187 were reported in June. Of these 16 were discovered among newly-arrived English and Swedish emigrants. Several new cases developed in Brooklyn, and the disease also appeared in Newark, N. J.

Diphtheria is the only contagious disease which has not decreased during the last month. While there were 410 cases of this disease in May, 434 occurred in June. The number of scarlatina cases has fallen from 636, in May, to 435 in June; and rubeola from 587, in the former, to 430 in the latter month. German measles has diminished since the advent of the warmer weather. Eight cases of insolation were reported on June 29, 23 on July 7, 5 on July 8, and 6 on July 13.

—

The New York City Death-rate.—The reconstructed street-cleaning department is conducting its business with commendable thoroughness and dispatch, but the nuisances at Hunter's Point are still unabated. At a meeting of the Medical Society of the County of New York, held June 27, the chairman of the Committee on Hygiene stated that the death-rate of this city is the largest in the world, even exceeding that of London.

—

Honours to Professor Flint.—The degree of LL.D. was conferred upon Dr. Austin Flint, Sr., by Yale College, at its recent commencement. Dr. Flint is in Europe, whence he will return on September 1.

—

Chair of Gynæcology at the College of Physicians and Surgeons, N. Y.—Dr. T. G. Thomas has resigned the chair of Gynæcology at the College of Physicians and Surgeons, N. Y. City, and Dr. Paul F. Mundé has been appointed Clinical Lecturer on Gynæcology, for one year, at that institution.

—

Presentation to Dr. Shrady.—At a meeting of the New York Pathological Society, held on June 22, 1881, the members of the Society presented Dr. Geo. F. Shrady a massive silver pitcher and salver in token of their appreciation of his services as secretary. The presentation speech was made by Dr. A. Jacobi.

—

The New York Medical Mission.—The New York Medical Mission is the title of a religious and medical charity recently established in New York City. Its rooms at No. 5 East Broadway were formally opened on June 27. The opening exercises, which were conducted by Dr. C. A. Agnew, were largely attended by the poor people of the vicinity. A free dispensary, for the sick poor, will be attached to the institution, and a Gospel service will be held daily. The circulars of the mission state that " no recommendation will be required from patients other than that they are sick and poor." The circular also states that no fees will be exacted for medical treatment, although remuneration will be expected from such patients as are able to pay.

Patients whose complaints are so serious as to prevent them from attending the dispensary will be treated at their homes. The Board of Managers includes Mr. C. Vanderbilt, Dr. F. H. Markoe, and Dr. S. B. Bangs.

Practical Philanthropy.—A summer resort for young workingwomen has been recently opened at Atlanticville, near Long Branch, N. J. The establishment accommodates fifty guests at a time, is situated on the seashore, and has a private beach for surf-bathing. The terms are five dollars for one week, or ten dollars for two weeks, and the sojourn of each guest will be limited to the latter period, in order that the advantages of the institution may be extended to the largest possible number. Mrs. Fletcher Harper, Jr., is one of the leading managers.

Institution for the Care of Infants and Young Children in New York.—The New York Society for the Care of Infants and Young Children has established its temporary asylum at the corner of University Place and Ninth Street. The asylum has accommodations for one hundred and fifty children. The circular of the institution states that the plan of the society also embraces the establishment, at as early a period as practicable, of day nurseries in the most populous parts of the city, capable of receiving hundreds of poor children whose mothers are obliged to leave them, during the day, to gain a livelihood at a distance from their homes. The children admitted to the asylum are required to be under the age of three years, and of legitimate birth. A medical attendant resides at the institution, and daily visits are made by the members of the attending medical board.

Sanitarium for Children at Mott Haven, N. Y.—A free sanitarium for poor children has been opened in connection with the Old Men's Unsectarian Home at Mott Haven, N. Y.

The Working of the Registration Law in New York.—On July 2d two medical practitioners were charged, at the Jefferson Market Police Court, by Dr. A. E. M. Purdy, President of the New York County Medical Society, with practising without a license. In default of bail, these unqualified practitioners were held for trial.

Summer Home for Children at Bath, L. I.—The "Summer Home" of the Children's Aid Society, at Bath, L. I., was formally opened on July 8, 1881. The home has, however, been occupied since June 18. It was purchased, together with several smaller buildings, and presented to the Children's Aid Society by Mr. A. B. Stone. The institution will accommodate about two hundred inmates. The children, who come from various tenement districts, are taken to the home in companies of two hundred, and return to the city at the end of a week to make room for the same number of new-comers. Nearly one thousand children have already visited the home this season.

Commencement Long Island College Hospital.—The twenty-second commencement of the Long Island College Hospital was held in the Brooklyn Academy of Music on June 14 The graduating class contained fifty-one members. The alumni of the college held their first annual dinner at Coney Island on the preceding evening.

River and Seaside Trips for Poor Children.—The floating hospital of St. John's Guild, of New York, has been thoroughly repaired, and will make three regular weekly trips during the heated season. Tickets can be obtained for the sick children of the poor and their attendants at all the city dispensaries and of physicians. The most usual excursion routes of the floating hospital are up the Hudson, into Long Island Sound, or through the lower bay. Those children in need of treatment at a regular hospital will be transferred to the seaside nursery at Cedar Grove, Staten Island, which is under the direction of the St. John's Guild.

—

Adulteration of Food and Drugs.—At a special meeting of the New York State Board of Health held on June 23d, the duties imposed upon the board by recent legislation were considered. The act to prevent the adulteration of drugs and food was discussed, and it was decided to engage competent chemists to analyze suspicious samples.

—

The thirty-second annual session of the Medical Association of Georgia was held in Thomasville on April 20th and 21st, 1881. The following are the officers for the ensuing year; President, William F. Holt, Macon; First Vice-President, Eugene Foster, Augusta; Second Vice-President, T. M. McIntosh, Thomasville; Secretary, A. Sibley Campbell, Augusta; Treasurer, K. P. Moore, Forsyth. The next session will be held in Atlanta, on the third Wednesday in April (19th), 1882.

—

The New Hampshire Medical Society held its ninety-first annual meeting in Concord, on Tuesday and Wednesday, June 21 and 22. A large and enthusiastic meeting assembled, and the following officers were elected for the ensuing year: President, Dr. H. B. Fowler, Bristol; Vice-President, Dr. A. H. Crosby, Concord; Treasurer, Dr. D. S. Adams, Manchester; Secretary, Dr. G. P. Conn, Concord. Executive Committee, Drs. J. W. Parsons, Portsmouth; P. A. Stackpole, Dover; and M. W. Russell, Concord. Anniversary Chairman, C. A. Tufts, M.D., Dover; and a Council of twenty members. The next semi-annual meeting will occur in September, at the "Wentworth," a famous watering-place near Portsmouth; and the next annual meeting will be in Concord, on the third Tuesday in June, 1882.

—

Injection Brou.—The following is believed to be the formula of the much-vaunted gonorrhœal injection of this name, taken from the register in the French public office: ℞. Zinc. sulph. gr. viij; plumbi acet. gr. xv; tinct. catechu, ʒj; tinct. opii, aqua, āā ℥iij.

—

Change in the Manner of Publication of the Transactions of the Ohio State Medical Society.—By a resolution of the Ohio State Medical Society, its proceedings now appear in the new *Ohio Medical Journal*, of which Vol. I., No. 1, has just appeared. As the journal of the Ohio State Medical Society, it takes the place of the usual volume of *Transactions*, and will be issued monthly, being in reality the successor of the *Ohio Medical Recorder*, which no longer exists. The Editor-in-chief is the Secretary of the Society, Dr. J. F. Baldwin, of Columbus, who is assisted by four Associate Editors: Dr. J. H. Lowman, of Cleveland; Dr. T. C. Minor, of Cincinnati; Dr. Geo. A. Collamore, of Toledo; and Dr. W. J. Conklin, of Dayton. Ohio thus becomes the first State to take the new departure in issuing its proceedings, and, as one result, the papers presented get a circulation of three thousand copies, instead of less than five hundred, as under the old method.

———

The Kansas State Medical Society held its fifteenth annual session at Topeka, May 10, Dr. B. E. Fryer, of Ft. Leavenworth, President, in the chair. The following officers were elected for the ensuing year: President, Dr. J. H. Stuart of Lawrence; Vice-Presidents, Drs. G. W. Haldeman of Paoli, and F. M. Guibor of Beloit; Secretary, Dr. F. D. Morse of Lawrence. The next meeting will be held at Emporia, on the second Tuesday in May, 1882.

———

Ergot in the Treatment of Sea-sickness.—Dr. T. S. Hopkins of Thomasville, Ga., writes very enthusiastically in regard to the value of ergot for the relief of sea-sickness, from personal experience, in a passage from Savannah to Philadelphia. He considers the following formula as preventive as well as curative. R. Ext. ergot fld. (Squibb's) f$\tilde{3}$ss; potass. bromid. $\tilde{3}$ss; aquam ad $\tilde{3}$vj.—M. Dose, a tablespoonful two or three times a day.

———

Death from Chloroform(?)—Dr. O. B. Mayer, Jr., of Newbury, S. C., reports the following case of death during the administration of chloroform.

The chloroform was administered for the purpose of extracting a bullet from the hand, on June 13, 1881.

The patient, coloured, age 45 years, was an habitual drunkard, though rarely, if ever, sick, and appeared to be in good health. He had abstained from food and drink for twelve hours. When the chloroform was administered, the patient who had just arrived at the stage of excitement, was seized with an epileptiform convulsion, with marked opisthotonos. He was immediately turned on his side and artificial respiration commenced; stimulants were hypodermically administered, and the patient's head kept lowered. At no time was any evidence of returning life seen. The man died during the fit. He was not subject to epilepsy. A few weeks previously chloroform had been administered to a lady from the same phial successfully, though under its effects for thirty minutes. No autopsy was made.

———

Seaweed as a Substitute for Jam.—Among the few serious political papers published in Paris, we note that the *Temps* occasionally renders good service by describing, in popular language, frauds that gravely compromise public health. Thus on the subject of jellies we have some startling disclosures. We should remark that in France fruit preserves are generally sold as jellies, and not as jam, in which the seed, stones, and sometimes the outline or skin of the fruit itself can be discerned. Falsification is, therefore, more easy. For this purpose gelatine made from fish naturally suggested itself, but was found too expensive. Of late years, however, since the importation on such a large scale of Chinese and Japanese porcelain, etc., a new solution has been found to the problem. The objects imported are generally packed with a common maritime plant that is used instead of straw. This seaweed possesses, however, peculiar properties. When placed in a tumbler of water, it absorbs the water in a few minutes; then a number of shoots grow, and constitute a jelly nearly as transparent as the water from which it is made. This plant, the Arachnoïdiscus japonicus, only costs the trouble of bringing it over. The jelly it yields is easily sweetened with glucose, and cochineal or other colouring matter is added with equal facility to imitate the colour of the fruit. The perfume and the taste were the only real difficulties that remained to be overcome. After considerable study it was discovered that by mixing four parts of acetic ether and tartaric acid with four parts of glycerine and one part of aldehyde, formic ether, benzoic, butyric, butyric amyl, acetic, œnanthylic, methyl-salicylic, nitrous, reberythric, and succinic, a perfect imitation of the odour of raspberries was produced. By putting a little of this essence to the seaweed which has been allowed to develop itself in water, a substance is obtained which has the consistence of fruit jelly, though no fruit has been used, which is sweet, though no sugar has been employed, and which has the colour and fragrance of raspberries, though altogether destitute of that fruit. When this ceases to please, another very good fruit flavor is produced by treating castor oil with nitric acid ! Fortunately, though wonders are wrought with the Arachnoïdiscus japonicus, the result is not absolutely perfect. The jelly still retains a little of the fibrous nature of the plant, and has a tendency to split and fall to pieces, instead of forming adhesive lumps. Examined with the microscope, it has no resemblance to the jelly made from fruit. Then, as the jelly must be coloured, it is easy enough to discover the presence of an artificial dye. Without resorting to the laboratory, it suffices to dissolve a little of the suspected jelly in some tepid water, and dip a white silk ribbon in the solution. If it is a natural jelly, the ribbon will simply be a little soiled ; but if the jelly has been artificially coloured, the ribbon will also be coloured. By giving publicity to all these details, the frauds practised will be constantly discovered, and the perpetrators brought to justice. We fear also that the falsifications the French have contrived, the English will not be slow to imitate, unless it is generally known that the public are on the *qui vive*.— *Lancet*, Dec. 11, 1880.

—

The Rest.—A charitable institution, known as the "Rest," was founded, in January, 1881, at No. 4 Winthrop Place. Its object is the care of convalescent men who have been recently discharged from the city hospitals, but who are not sufficiently strong to undertake their usual occupations. The institution is under the management of the Sisters of the Stranger.

—

Removal of a Hypertrophied Spleen.—In even these days of "heroic" operations, it is very questionable whether the following operation reported in the *Gaz. Med. Lombardia* of April 9 can be justified : "Dr. Chiarleoni performed at the Casa di Salute, Milan, on March 26, splenectomy on a female patient suffering from paludal cachexia, in the presence of a large number of distinguished colleagues. The operation, executed with great method and freedom, was very laborious, owing to the extensive and strong adhesions of the spleen to the left edge of the liver and the diaphragm. It was impossible to tie all these adhesions before removing them, and a very considerable hemorrhage from the surface (*a nappo*) ensued, and this, conjoined with a certain amount of nervous exhaustion, caused the woman's death a few hours after the termination of the operation. As far as we are aware, so bold an operation has not been executed in Italy, except on one occasion by Drs. Zaccharelli and Fioravanti, at Naples, in 1549.—*Med Times and Gazette*, April 23, 1881.

—

Ultimate Effects of Tracheotomy.—In a note read at the Academy of Medicine (*Bulletin*, April 5), Dr. MONGEOT drew attention to the ultimately fatal results of tracheotomy. He had for a long time investigated the subject, and had come to the conclusion that children who had successfully undergone tracheotomy, and had worn a canula for a more or less prolonged period, did not live to attain their majority. He had long made inquiries among a great number of practitioners, and had only succeeded in discovering five or six adults who had undergone this operation in their infancy; while military surgeons, interrogated for more than twenty years past, all avowed that in examining conscripts they had never met with the scar characteristic of tracheotomy. He suggests further investigations on the subject by the military boards of Paris, seeing that the operation is performed about thirty-five times annually on hospital children. He also refers to Dr. Martin's proposal to cease the employment of metallic canulæ. —*Med. Times and Gazette*, April 23, 1881.

Statistics of Colour-Blindness.—The report of a Committee appointed by the Ophthalmological Society of the United Kingdom (*Lancet*, April 23, 1881) to collect statistics of cases of colour-blindness presents many features of special interest. The secretary of the Committee, Dr. Brailey, with the assistance of sixteen colleagues, has examined 18,088 persons of all classes, of whom 1657 were females. It is at once curious and suggestive to find that while the average percentage of colour defects among men is 4.76 and 3.5 for very pronounced defeets, it falls in women to the low figure of 0.4. This, if true, would seem to suggest a new sphere of labor for women. If women are comparatively free from colour-blindness, they are so far specially indicated for many of the less laborious occupations in which good colour-perception is desirable or absolutely indispensable.

Recent Health Legislation.—The New York Senate has passed a bill conferring upon the city health board the power of quarantining any building in New York City, which is used as a dwelling, when such a course seems necessary to prevent the dissemination of any contagious disease.

The New York Legislature has passed a bill for the prevention of the adulteration of food and drugs, which makes it a misdemeanor liable to punishment with a fine of $50, for the first and of $100 for the second offence, to sell any food or drugs adulterated within the meaning of the bill. The adulterations included within the meaning of the act are carefully classified, and the terms "drug" and "food" are stated to comprise every article used by man as food or drink as well as all medicines, whether for external or internal use.

Training-school for Nurses.—A new training-school for nurses in connection with Mount Sinai Hospital, has recently been opened at 852 Lexington Avenue, in convenient proximity to the hospital. One of the graduates of the Bellevue Hospital Training-school is the superintendent of the new school which numbers four trained head nurses and eight assistant nurses. The course of training covers two years' time.

Manufacture of Quinia.—A patent for the manufacture of quinia from coal tar has been applied for by a prominent drug house.

An Action for Malpraxis in Belgium.—The *Presse Médicale Belge* (April 24) refers to an action brought by the children of a person who had died after the injection of five milligrammes of morphia for the relief of severe pain. The experts called proved that the accusation (brought, it is said, at the instigation of a rival practitioner) was wholly groundless, the individual having in reality died from the natural results of organic disease. The tribunal not only acquitted the accused, but adjudged the persons who brought the accusation to pay 1000 fr.

damages to him.   If this latter action were followed up in other countries these unfounded accusations would soon diminish.—*Med. Times and Gazette*, May 7, 1881.

—

Professor Billroth's Fourth Case of Resection of the Stomach.—We learn from the *Wiener Medizinische Wochenschrift,* No. 22, that Prof. BILLROTH'S patient, on whom he performed excision of the pylorus for cancer on January 29, has just died in Vienna.   The case, surgically speaking, has become historical, for the operation was quite a new departure, and one which, but a short time ago, would have been considered impracticable.   The case is rendered more interesting by the fact that an autopsy was obtained, and that thus the condition of parts post mortem has been accurately studied.   Dr. Zemann— in the absence of Heschl, the Director of the Pathological Institute, whose death from the effects of a post-mortem wound has since occurred—conducted the examination.   He found that death had resulted from metastatic deposits of cancer throughout the entire peritoneum, the duodenum and jejunum being likewise coated with a similar deposit, so that it was impossible to separate them one from another.   As regards the stomach, it is stated that it retains its natural form, and that no one unacquainted with the operation to which it had been subjected would have observed anything remarkable about it, or guessed that fourteen centimetres had been removed from it."   The duodenum had been attached to its lesser curvature, so that a little pouching was observable along the greater curvature.   The woman had not suffered from any digestive troubles, but had taken and retained her food very well.   At the point of junction there was no stenosis, the thumb being easily passed through the orifice.   The union was perfect in all respects, so that hardly any scar could be perceived along the line of the suture.—*Med. Times and Gazette*, June 4, 1881.

—

Death of Professor Skoda.—The cable announces the death of Dr. JOSEF SKODA, the distinguished Vienna professor, on June 13, 1881.   He was born at Pilsen, Bohemia, December 10, 1805, graduated at the Vienna medical schools in 1831, distinguished himself in Bohemia during the cholera epidemic of 1832–33, became in the latter year second physician to the general hospital at Vienna, and became successively physician for the division of lung diseases (1840), chief physician of the hospital (1841), professor of clinical medicine (1846), and a member of the Vienna Academy of Sciences in 1848.   Professor Skoda was one of the first to popularize the use of the stethoscope of Laennec, was a great authority on pathological anatomy and on the new methods of auscultation and percussion.   His chief work was a "Treatise on Auscultation and Percussion" (1839, sixth edition, 1864).

—

Letter from Prof. Chaillé.

New Orleans, La., July 5th, 1881.

MR. EDITOR.

Dear Sir: Your Journals for July contain two statements in reference to my duties as the representative in New Orleans of the National Board of Health, which deserve correction.

I. The MEDICAL NEWS p. 442, states that "The Louisiana State Board of Health, at its meeting of May 19th, adopted the report of Dr. Formento, which was based upon these instructions [National Board of Health] to Dr. Chaillé, and which renders them *nugatory in almost every particular*, so far as the cooperation of the Board is concerned."   A more careful reading of the instructions on the one hand, and of the report on the other will show that, practically and in all essential particulars, the former were not rendered nugatory in any particular, *except in the single one* referring to the Ship Island Quarantine. A copy is inclosed of my reply to the report on this subject.[1]

II. The *American Journal of the Medical Sciences*, p. 240, referring to the unfortunate disagreement last year, respecting the diagnosis of certain alleged cases of yellow fever, states that "This unfortunate dispute has already been referred to in our columns, and we would therefore simply remark here, that the obvious lesson from its occurrence is in the future to secure so prompt and thorough an investigation, by representatives of all parties interested, of any 'suspicious cases,' that either there shall be no doubt as to their nature, or *the party in error shall be conclusively condemned by the whole country on the evidence of subsequent events.*" If the last clause, italicized, means anything, it must signify that in the writer's opinion, cases of veritable yellow fever must be followed by other cases of the same disease; for, no other subsequent event, except the presence or absence of subsequent cases could have any bearing on the issue. It is surprising to me, that any writer in a journal of such authority as the *American Journal of the Medical Sciences* should display so little knowledge of the history of sporadic cases of yellow fever in all of its noted habitats. In this city as elsewhere, one case alone, or several widely separated cases of *undoubted* yellow fever have repeatedly occurred, without being followed by any "subsequent events" whatever. Therefore, "the conclusive condemnation by the whole country" of a diagnosis of yellow fever, because followed by no subsequent events, would be an outrage upon medical and upon sanitary science. It is painful that your journal should be the instrument of teaching "the whole country" any such false and mischievous lesson, and it is hoped that you will have this error corrected.

Yours very truly, STANFORD E. CHAILLÉ, M.D.

[We gladly publish Dr. Chaillé's communication in deference to his wishes and to prevent any possible misunderstanding by others. It must be evident, however, to any one who has read the latter statement referred to, that it does not have the application that our correspondent has drawn from it, certainly no one would be so rash as to condemn the whole country on the negative evidence quoted in illustration; but where suspicious cases *are* followed by cases of veritable yellow fever the responsibility rests upon the physicians in charge of the early cases of not having made a correct diagnosis or of concealing it. In doubtful cases it is incumbent upon those in charge to take all the means required of securing full investigation and consultation in order that their true character may be brought out, and if the cases by some called "rice-fever," and others "bilious malarial" fever are found to be yellow fever, the proper authorities may then be promptly notified as in other epidemic diseases. If the sentence referred to by Dr. Chaillé means anything at all, it means this, in our opinion.

ED. MED. NEWS AND ABSTRACT.]

——

To Readers and Correspondents.—*The Editor will be happy to receive early intelligence of local events of general medical interest, or which it is desirable to bring to the notice of the profession. Local papers containing reports or news items should be marked.*

————————————

[1] Pamphlet inclosed entitled "Eadsport, Ship Island Quarantine and the National Board of Health." Reprint from the *New Orleans Democrat*, June 9, 1881. This is an open letter to the Louisiana State Board of Health, by Dr. S. E. Chaillé, in which he ably defends the legality, expediency, and efficiency of the Ship Island Quarantine. —ED. MED. NEWS AND ABSTRACT.

CONTENTS OF NUMBER 465.

SEPTEMBER, 1881.

CLINICS.

MEDICAL NEWS.

THE

MEDICAL NEWS AND ABSTRACT.

VOL. XXXIX. No. 9.   SEPTEMBER, 1881.   WHOLE No. 465.

CLINICS.

Clinical Lectures.

CLINICAL LECTURE ON CATALEPSY; TRICHINOSIS; AND THE TREATMENT OF PNEUMONIA BY BLOOD-LETTING, COLD SPONGING, AND THE WET SHEET.

DELIVERED AT BELLEVUE HOSPITAL, NEW YORK.

By AUSTIN FLINT, M.D.,
PHYSICIAN TO THE HOSPITAL.

GENTLEMEN : I shall introduce, to-day, several cases exemplifying different diseases, calling your attention, in connection with each case, to points of practical interest.

The first case is interesting as illustrative of a very rare form of disease, so rare that many of you will probably never meet with another example. The patient before you has catalepsy. As you see, she is a young woman, and appears to be tranquilly sleeping. Her eyes are closed. She is pallid, but the face is not cyanotic, and gives no appearance of distress. Her respirations are regular, in rhythm, and not accelerated. I now raise both arms so that they are perpendicular to the trunk. You will perceive that they will remain in this situation as long as the patient is in the amphitheatre. They are not kept in this situation by the volition of the patient. They will remain thus raised longer than would be comfortable, or perhaps practicable, by a sustained effort of the will. This is the symptom characteristic of catalepsy. Other parts of the body placed in positions not easily maintained by volition, continue immovable for a considerable period. There is, therefore, a tonic contraction of voluntary muscles, by which they adapt themselves to different positions of the body or of its parts, this tonic contraction persisting independent of volition. The contraction is easily overcome ; the positions of the body or of its parts may be readily changed, very little resistance being offered by rigidity of the muscles. As regards this point different cases differ. Aside from the symptom pertaining to the muscles which constitutes the pathognomonic feature of the cataleptic state, the morbid condition is that of hysterical coma. The coma is not complete. The patient can be aroused sufficiently to open the eyes and to protrude the tongue, but she takes no notice, and cannot be made to speak. She will not voluntarily take food or drink. It is necessary to nourish her by injecting food into the stomach. This is easily done by means of a tube introduced into the œsophagus through the nose, and Davidson's syringe. In order to illustrate the procedure, Dr. Anderton, the House Physician, will now inject into the stomach several ounces of milk. The patient, as you see, manifests some discomfort, but makes no resistance to the operation. This patient is a woman, but the affection is not confined to women. In the last case which came under my observation the patient was a boy, about 20 years of age, in this hospital.

I will now read the history of the case, as far as it has been ascertained, from the hospital records, as follows :—

" Minnie R., æt. 21, U. S., box-maker, admitted May 17, 1881. No history could be obtained from the patient, as she cannot be made to speak. She lies quietly, apparently paying no attention to events around her. Occasionally she moves her head on the pillow, but maintains her body in a state of perfect repose. The limbs remain in any position in which they may be placed, even though an uncomfortable one and difficult to maintain. When the limbs have been made to assume such positions they will support considerable weights for long periods. The limbs offer no resistance to passive motion, but remain fixed and immobile. Sensation is preserved and its existence betrayed by facial contortions, indicative of pain, when the cutaneous surface is pricked. The reflex movements are preserved. Slight irritation of the skin over the abdomen or thorax causes the patient to smile. When asked to protrude her tongue she does so, but quickly retracts it, as though she had committed an unintentional error in putting it out. The electrical excitability of the muscles and the tendon reflexes are well preserved. The temperature is normal, the pulse 78, and the respirations 20 per minute. The urine is reddish, acid, has a specific gravity of 1017, and contains no albumen.

" The patient refuses to eat, and is fed through a soft rubber catheter which is passed through the nose, and through which fluids are pumped into the œsophagus."

You may ask what is the pathology of this remarkable affection. I cannot give a satisfactory answer to this question. The condition of the patient is one which may be induced in some healthy persons who have a certain peculiar susceptibility of the nervous system. Thus induced, it was formerly included among the phenomena which were embraced under the names mesmerism and animal magnetism. The study of these phenomena within late years has been revived, and the term hypnotism is now applied to this voluntarily induced cataleptic state. The use of a new name is not an explanation, and I do not think that the phenomena can be better explained now than nearly half a century ago. The truth is, our present knowledge of the physiology of the nervous system is not sufficiently advanced to serve as the basis of an explanation of these and various other manifestations of perverted neurotic functions. We have no knowledge of the essential nature of the connection of nervous influences with muscular movements, either voluntary or involuntary, and of the tonic contraction of the muscles. We know not the nature of the agency which emanates from the brain, and is transmitted to the muscles in the exertion of the will. We are equally in the dark as regards the process which takes place within the brain whenever there is an act of volition.

Catalepsy is not an affection involving danger to life. This patient will recover. The first indication in the way of treatment relates to alimentation. Food must be introduced into the stomach until it is taken voluntarily. In order to arouse the mental faculties, "firing" may be resorted to. I shall prescribe this measure in this case. It may be employed by an instrument made for that purpose, but a common hammer dipped in boiling water suffices. It should be applied for an instant at different points over the spine and in other situations. The operation may be repeated two or three times daily. Electricity may also be employed with advantage.[1]

The next case is one of interest as a rare disease, and, also, for the reason that it has existed in the nosology for only a quarter of a century. Owing to its infrequency and the recent date of our knowledge respecting it, there is a liability to mistake it for other diseases; hence, the importance of its diagnostic features. The case is one of Trichinosis, Trichiniasis, or the Trichina disease. For a zoological history of the parasite which causes the disease, and a full account of its symptomatology, I refer you to text-books. I will just read the hospital record of the case, and afterward comment on some practical points.

"Peter Y., æt. 27; Germany; upholsterer; admitted April 15, 1881. The patient states that he ate pork, either raw or only partially cooked, several times during the week preceding March 21st, as also on that day and on the three succeeding days. On March 21st, up to which time he had been in perfect health, he was seized with a sense of oppression in the stomach, and with lancinating abdominal pains. He had also vomiting, which continued at irregular intervals for four days, and diarrhœa which persisted, in spite of domestic remedies, for two weeks. During this time he had occasional exacerbations of fever, most marked in the evening and at night. On April 1st his muscles began to be painful, particularly when they were made to contract, and they were tender on pressure. Deglutition became painful, and he suffered from asthenia and general *malaise*. On admission, April 15, 1881, he was found lying upon his left side with his arms and legs in the position of complete flexion. The thighs were strongly adducted. He moved his extremities without pain as long as they remained considerably flexed, but any attempt at extension occasioned great suffering. The abdomen was sensitive to pressure, as were the quadratus lumborum, the deltoid, and many of the muscles of the arm and neck. There was considerable œdema of the eyelids and of the lower limbs. The urine was normal, and no disease of any abdominal or thoracic viscus could be detected. The patient complained of great prostration. Temperature, $103\frac{1}{2}°$ F.; pulse, 118; respirations, 24 per minute. Three living trichinæ were found in a small piece of the deltoid muscle by microscopical examination, and many of the muscular fibres were seen to have undergone granular and fatty degeneration.

"*Treatment.*—Bicarbonate of soda, Ʒj, was administered every hour, until six doses had been given. Ol. ricini, flƷj, was then given, which produced very free catharsis. This treatment was repeated on the two following days. On April 17th the temperature was 101° in the forenoon and $103\frac{1}{2}°$ in the afternoon, and the muscular pain was so severe as to require the administration of morphia hypodermically. From April 18th

---

[1] Firing and electricity were employed, and, in addition to alimentation, constituted the treatment. The patient slowly improved, and in about two weeks was able to leave the hospital.

to April 21st the temperature ranged between 100° and 101$\frac{3}{4}$°.   On April 22d the temperature fell to 99$\frac{1}{4}$°, and on the 25th to 98$\frac{3}{4}$°.   During this time the muscular pains became less severe, the œdema disappeared, and the appetite returned."

This case was in the service of my colleague, Prof. Janeway, and the patient was convalescent when he came under my observation.   He is still confined to the bed, but the muscular pains have ceased, and he is able to bear considerable extension of the affected muscles.   He has no fever, and the digestive organs are beginning to resume the exercise of their normal functions.

You will connect the vomiting, diarrhœa, and colic pains with the development of the parasites within the alimentary canal, and their passage through the gastro-intestinal mucous membrane.   The fever and the general symptoms therewith associated are attributable to gastro-enteritis.   The muscular pains are caused by the presence of the parasites in the affected muscles.   The order of succession of these symptomatic events, and their occurrence shortly after pork, raw or imperfectly cooked, has been eaten, are diagnostic points ; but the diagnosis is made demonstrative by obtaining a small piece of an affected muscle, and subjecting it to microscopical examination.   In order to trace the disease demonstratively to its source, portions of the suspected article of diet should be microscopically examined.   This was not practicable in the present instance.

I call your attention to the treatment of this case under the direction of Prof. Janeway.   It consisted in the administration, for three consecutive days, of six drachms of the bicarbonate of soda, drachm doses being given hourly, followed by a cathartic of castor oil.   This treatment had for its objects the destruction of parasites, and their expulsion from the alimentary canal.   It is, of course, not proper to judge concerning the efficiency of treatment by the history of a single case, but it is noteworthy that, under this treatment, this case has progressed favourably, and the patient is now convalescent.[1]

The remainder of this lecture will be devoted to two cases of Pneumonic Fever or Acute Lobar Pneumonitis.   In one of these cases bloodletting was employed for a particular object, followed by sponging of the body as an antipyretic measure.   The other case was treated antipyretically by means of the wet sheet.   It is proper to state that the treatment in these cases was under the direction of Dr. W. B. Anderton, House Physician of the division of this hospital with which I am connected ; and that the treatment was directed by him without any instructions or suggestions from me.   I shall read the histories, with all the details respecting the temperature at different hours of each day, during the duration of the fever, in order to present as fully as possible the therapeutical indications, and the immediate effects of the treatment.   I hope you will not find these details tedious, when you consider the practical importance of the points which are involved.

The two patients are now before you.   I will take up first the case treated by means of the wet sheet.   The record is as follows :—

" Chas. L., æt. 32 ; Denmark ; labourer ; admitted May 16, 1881.   The patient has no regular occupation ; he has wandered about the streets, being exposed to all kinds of vicissitudes, and often remaining in wet clothes for hours.   Four days before his admission he was suddenly seized with a

---

[1] The patient was discharged well on May 30th.

severe chill, followed, very soon, by fever, pain in the right side, and cough. The next day he was on the street, as usual, though feeling very weak. From that time until his admission he spent the days in the Battery Park, and the nights in a poor lodging house. On his admission the face had a dusky flush and an anxious expression. He complained of cough, pain in the right side, anorexia, and weakness. The axillary temperature was 104°; the pulse was 90, and strong; respirations were 26 per minute. Over the lower and middle lobes of the right lung were dulness on percussion, increased vocal fremitus, pure bronchial respiration, and bronchophony. No râles.

" The expectoration was rusty and adhesive. The heart, liver, and spleen yielded no abnormal physical signs. The urine was normal.

" The wet sheet was applied, and the patient left, uncovered, beneath it whenever the temperature reached 103° F. The sheet was not removed until the temperature of the mouth had been reduced to 102° F.

" Sulphate of quinia, in five grain doses, was administered every four hours, and five grains of carbonate of ammonia every three hours.

" *May* 16*th.* 5 P. M., temp. 104°; the wet sheet was applied. 7 P. M., temp. 101°; the wet sheet was removed. 9 P. M., temp. 102$\frac{1}{4}$°. 11 P. M., temp. 102$\frac{1}{4}$°.

" 17*th.* 2 A. M., temp. 103$\frac{1}{4}$°; the wet sheet was applied. 4 A. M., temp. 102°; the wet sheet was removed. 8 A. M., temp. 101$\frac{3}{4}$°. 10 A. M., temp. 101$\frac{1}{2}$°; pulse 90; respiration 30. 12 noon, temp. 101$\frac{1}{2}$°. 2 P. M., temp. 102$\frac{1}{4}$°. 4 P. M., temp. 103°; the wet sheet was applied. 5 P. M., temp. 103$\frac{1}{4}$°; temp. taken by rectum, the sheet being still applied. 7 P. M., temp. 102$\frac{1}{4}$°. 8 P. M., temp. 101$\frac{1}{4}$°; the sheet was removed.

" 18*th.* 12 P. M., temp. 101$\frac{1}{2}$°. 6 A. M., temp. 100$\frac{3}{4}$°. 8 A. M., temp. 101$\frac{3}{4}$°. 10 A. M., temp. 101°; pulse 72; respiration 30.

" Over the middle lobe the bronchial has given place to broncho-vesicular respiration and bronchophony to increased vocal fremitus. Subcrepitant râles are heard. The pneumonia, however, has invaded the upper lobe, and dulness, bronchial breathing, and bronchophony extend upward nearly to its apex. Pleuritic friction sounds are heard over the entire anterior surface of the lung. Bronchial respiration, bronchophony, and crepitant râles are now heard over the whole lower and over the lower portion of the upper lobe.

" 18*th.* 12 M., temp. 102$\frac{1}{2}$°. 2 P. M., temp. 102$\frac{1}{2}$°. 4 P. M., temp. 101°. 8 P. M., temp. 101$\frac{3}{4}$°.

"19*th.* 12 P. M., temp. 102°. 4 A. M., temp. 101$\frac{1}{2}$°. 8 A. M., temp. 100$\frac{3}{4}$°; pulse 72; respirations 24. 10 A. M., temp. 100$\frac{1}{2}$°.

" The respiration is, now, broncho-vesicular at the right apex anteriorly. Behind the signs are the same as on yesterday.

" 12 M., temp. 101$\frac{3}{4}$°. 6 P. M., temp. 101$\frac{1}{2}$°.

" 20*th.* 8 A. M., temp. 101$\frac{1}{4}$°. 8 A. M., temp. 100°.

" 21*st.* A. M., temp. 98$\frac{1}{2}$°.

" 22*d.* Temperature, A. M., 98$\frac{1}{2}$°; P. M., 98$\frac{1}{2}$°. The bronchial respiration and bronchophony, over the lower lobe and over the lower portion of the upper lobe, are less marked. Friction sounds and crepitant râles are still heard over both lobes, anteriorly.

" 24*th.* Temperature normal. The respiratory murmur, over the affected lobes, is now broncho-vesicular in character, and bronchophony has been replaced by slightly increased vocal resonance. The patient sits up, and his appetite is excellent.

" *29th*. Resolution is complete, all the morbid physical signs due to consolidation having been replaced by the normal ones. Slight dulness still exists over the whole lower lobe, but this is referred to pleuritic thickening."[1]

The employment of the wet sheet as an antipyretic measure in the treatment of pneumonic fever is not a novelty in this hospital. In a lecture published in the number of *Gaillard's Medical Journal* for March, 1881, I reported three cases treated by this measure under the direction of Dr. Moeller, at that time House Physician of the division with which I am connected.[2] The treatment has been resorted to since the publication of that lecture in other hopital cases, and also in a few cases in private practice which have come under my observation. In all the instances thus far observed, the apparent effect of the treatment has been excellent. It remains to ascertain by clinical observation the circumstances, aside from the condition of hyperpyrexia, if there be any, which contra-indicate it. By the facts already observed I am justified in saying that in uncomplicated cases, a patient may remain in the wet sheet, with sprinkling of cold water at short intervals, without risk of harm, and with advantage, until the body-heat is reduced two, three, or more degrees, the period required for the reduction varying from a few to many hours, and that the measure may be safely repeated whenever the hyperpyrexia returns. In the case before us, it is fair to accord a certain amount of therapeutical influence to the quinia and the carbonate of ammonia which entered into the treatment.

Of the second of the two cases before you, the hospital record is as follows :—

" Sophia K., æt. 23 ; U. S.; domestic ; admitted May 9, 1881. On May 5th the patient had a well-marked chill, with vomiting, headache, fever, and pain under the left nipple. She grew weak, lost her appetite, and felt unable to exert herself; but, nevertheless, kept at work until May 9th, when she entered the hospital.

" On admission the cheeks presented a circumscribed flush ; the temperature was 102° ; the pulse 120, and the respirations 40 per minute. The patient complained of excessive weakness and of pain in the left mammary region, with cough and rusty expectoration. Over the lower lobe of the left side there was increased vocal fremitus, with dulness, bronchial breathing, and bronchophony. No râles. The thoracic and abdominal viscera, with the exception of the lungs, were normal, as was also the urine.

" *Treatment.*—Whiskey, fl℥ss every half hour ; ammon. carbonat. grs. v every two hours ; morph. sulphat. gr. ⅛, by mouth, every three hours ; infus. digitalis, fl℥ss, by mouth, every three hours.

" *May 9th.* 3.30 P. M. Œdema pulmonalis having been developed, Dr. Anderton performed venesection—removing twelve ounces of blood. This measure speedily relieved the symptoms due to the œdema. The latter became less marked, and the patient's general condition was considerably improved. 4.30 P. M., temp. 103½° ; ordered whiskey, ℥ss every hour. 6 P. M., temp. 104°. 7 P. M., temp. 104°. 12 P. M., temp. 103½°.

" *10th.* 10 A. M., temp. 103¼°. The patient suffered from intense dyspnœa, which was effectually combated by the inhalation of oxygen gas.

[1] The patient was discharged on June 3 completely recovered.
[2] For an account of these cases *vide* Medical News and Abstract for May, 1881.

At 12 M., temp. 104°, 2 P. M., temp. 104¼°, and 4 P. M., temp. 104¼°; considerable dyspnœa; gave oxygen. 6 P. M., temp. 103¼°. 8 P. M., temp. 103°. 12 P. M., temp. 103⅓°.

"11th. 9 A. M., temp. 103°. 12 M., temp. 104¼°. 2 P. M., temp. 104°; great dyspnœa; gave oxygen. Ordered the patient sponged with tepid water, only one extremity being exposed at a time. 4 P. M., temp. 104¾°. 5 P. M., temp. 103°. 7 P. M., temp. 104°. 8 P. M.. temp. 103°. 12 P. M., temp. 103°.

"12th. 5.30 A. M., temp. 103⅓°. 9 A. M., temp. 103¼°. 11 A. M., temp. 103¾°; sponge bath. 12 M., temp. 101¾°. 3 P. M., temp. 104°; sponge bath. 3.45 P. M., temp. 102¼°. 7 P. M., temp. 104°; sponge bath. 8 P. M., temp. 102°.

"13th. 1 A. M., temp. 102°. 7 A. M.. temp. 101¼°. 9.45 A. M., temp. 101°. 2 P. M., temp. 102°. 5 P. M., temp. 102°; normal alvine evacuation. 7 P. M., temp. 102°. 9 P. M., temp. 101½°.

"14th. 8.45 A. M., temp. 99¾°. 11 A. M., temp 99°. The patient's condition is materially improved. On percussion diminished dulness is found; on auscultation broncho-vesicular respiration, increased vocal resonance and *râles redux;* on palpation the vocal fremitus but slightly increased. The whiskey was reduced to fl℥ss every two hours. 6 P. M., temp. 99¾°; digitalis was discontinued.

"15th. 8 P. M., temp. 98¾°. 6 P. M., temp. 99¾°; stopped the carbonate of ammonia; ordered whiskey fl℥ss t. i. d.

"16th. A. M., temp. 98¾°. P. M., 99°. Physical examination now shows only slight dulness. The broncho-vesicular breathing has been replaced by natural vesicular respiration, and the vocal resonance is normal.

"18th. A. M., temp. 98¼°. P. M. 98½°. Ordered tr. ferri chloridi, gtt. xx t. i. d.

"19th. A. M., temp. 98¼°. The patient is now fully convalescent."[1]

An important event in this case was the occurrence of pulmonary œdema. Occurring in connection with pneumonia, and limited to the lobes not solidified by the pneumonic exudation, it is known as "collateral œdema." The diagnostic evidence of its occurrence is the more or less sudden development of rapid breathing and of cough with serous or serosanguinolent expectoration, these symptoms associated with subcrepitant râles over the lobes not affected by the pneumonia. The explanation implied in the term collateral is that the blood in consequence of the obstruction to the circulation in the solidified lobe or lobes, is determined in excess to the lobes not solidified. Were this the sole explanation, however, the so-called collateral œdema in cases of pneumonia and of pleurisy with effusion should be frequent. whereas it is of rare occurrence. Nor is it easy to understand why the œdema should occur suddenly, and when the obstruction has existed for some time as in the case under consideration. A better explanation is that the œdema is due to the same causes which induce it when pneumonia does not exist. The œdema implies pulmonary congestion, and the latter, in the second stage of pneumonia, cannot take place in a solidified lobe for an obvious mechanical reason; hence the congestion and œdema are limited to the lobes which are not solidified. As to the causes of pulmonary œdema I cannot go into their consideration now; but I would remark that my colleague, Dr. Wm. H. Welch, has demonstrated, experimentally, that the proximate cause is

---

[1] Recovery took place without any untoward symptoms.

weakness of the left ventricle of the heart, associated with either in.
creased or undiminished power of the right ventricle.

Pulmonary œdema existing in a degree to occasion notable embarrass.
ment of respiration is treated most efficiently by bloodletting.   Dr. An.
derton very judiciously adopted this measure in the case before us.   No.
table relief followed it, and the dyspnœa which remained was relieved by
the inhalation of oxygen gas.

In this case the febrile temperature indicated efficient antipyretic treat.
ment.   The wet sheet was not employed lest it might do harm in view of
pulmonary œdema having occurred.   The latter was perhaps not a contraindication, but if we must err in medical practice it is generally best to
err on the side of caution.   Sponging of parts of the body was, however,
resorted to, and with the effect of reducing the temperature.   Let me here
remark that sponging the surface of the body continuously for a long period,
will often accomplish all that is to be obtained by the wet sheet or the cold
bath.   This method of antipyretic treatment has the recommendation of
not appearing to be in such violent antagonism to popular traditional notions as the sheet or the bath.

CASE OF TREPHINING FOR ANOMALOUS CONVULSIVE ATTACKS, SUPERVENING SEVERAL MONTHS AFTER INJURY TO THE HEAD.

A Clinical Lecture.

By J. W. HULKE, F.R.C.S., F.R.S.,
Surgeon to, and Lecturer on Surgery at, the Middlesex Hospital.

GENTLEMEN: The subject of my last clinical lecture[1] was a little child who
had undergone secondary trephining for abscess following a punctured wound of
the vault of the skull, with lodgment of splinters of bone and hair in the brain.
The case to which I invite your attention to-day is that of a young man in Ben-
tinck ward who has recently been trephined for fits following an injury in the
right temple.

The following is the record abridged from my dresser's (Mr. Thane) notes :—

A ticket-clerk, aged twenty-one years, who as a youth was considered delicate
and to have phthisical tendencies, was admitted into the hospital on January 23,
1879.

Six months previously, at 5 A. M., he slipped off a railway-platform, which was
greasy with wet, and falling upon the line, about four feet lower than the platform, struck his right temple, it was supposed against the parapet of a dwarf wall.
He was stunned by the blow, which was severe, for although the distance through
which he fell was not great, he was running quickly at the moment which increased the impetus.   How long he continued unconscious is not known—probably
not longer than a few minutes.   On recovering consciousness he found himself
upon the ground.   He managed to rise, get upon the platform, and reach the
next station, about three-quarters of a mile distant, where he reported his accident to the station-master.   A bruise, and a bump of about the size of the last
joint of the thumb, were seen on his right temple by his father, a guard, and by
others.   His head ached greatly, and it felt very confused, but he managed to
perform his duty until mid-day, by which time the headache and confusion of mind

---

[1] See page 330, ante.

had become so great that he was compelled to leave work, and he then went to a friend's lodgings near the station, where he sat down in a chair.   About 4 P. M. his friend thought he had fallen asleep ; he had, however, become deeply unconscious, and could not be roused.   He was therefore put to bed, where he remained unconscious of what was happening during twenty-four hours, when he awoke, and was startled to find himself undressed, in his friend's bed, with two doctors examining him.

During about one month he continued deeply soporose, sleeping heavily during several hours, then waking and taking food.   He did not, however, feed himself, appearing to be unable to hold the cup or to manage a spoon.   He had complete control over his bladder, but it was necessary to place the vessel, for he seemed unable to arrange it or hold it himself.   He had also control of the bowels, and he always intimated his wants to those in attendance upon him.   Throughout this month he did not leave his bed ; he seemed to have become too weak to stand.

In the condition just described he was next taken to his parent's home in a seaport, seventy miles distant.   He did not appear to be much exhausted by the journey.   The quiet, the surroundings of home, and the fresh sea-breezes appeared to benefit him, and he slowly and gradually recovered, becoming able, at the end of a few weeks, to creep about in the garden.   At the end of two months (three months after the accident) he had improved so much that he made an attempt to resume work, but this aggravated the headache, which had never left him, and he could not bear even slight mental strain without becoming confused ; so that, after a fortnight, he was obliged to return into the country to his parent's with whom he remained until his admission into this hospital.   During all this time he was never free from headache, and latterly he occasionally had what were called slight seizures, twitchings, and very transient unconsciousness.

Five days before being brought to the hospital he was violently convulsed—in twenty-four hours he had fourteen very severe fits ; the convulsions were so strong that three men could not restrain him. ` During the fits and for some time after he seemed to be quite unconscious.   In the course of the next day and night he had ten similar fits, and on the third night he was convulsed with little intermission from 10 P. M. till 2 P. M. on the fourth day.   He did not bite his tongue nor foam.

When I saw him on the fifth day after his journey of 100 miles, he looked like a convalescent from a severe illness.   His face was pale, his pulse weak (100 per minute).   The surface of his body was mottled, and it felt cold to the hand.   The thermometer in the axilla, however, marked 99° Fahr.

His mind appeared to be unclouded ; his memory was good ; he gave a coherent account of the accident and his subsequent illness ; and when questioned, his answers were always pertinent.   His statements (corroborated by his father) were remarkably clear and consistent.

He complained of constant headache and dizziness, of a tightness as if a cord were tied round his forehead, and of a hammering in the back of the head.   His visual acuteness was unimpaired, but he said that on reading his sight soon failed. No indications of inflammatory or congestive disorder of optic nerves was discernible.   Just behind the right temporal ridge, about one inch above its origin, in the spot where the bump was noticed on the day the accident occurred, was a very limited area, pressure on which caused, he said, a darting sensation through his head.   This spot was marked with an ink-dot, and diverting his attention by questions referring to other matters, the smooth end of a pencil was repeatedly made to cross it in different directions, with the result that he always winced and exclaimed, "It darts through my head."   No scar was discernible here ; the soft coverings seemed to be quite natural, and no unevenness of the underlying bone could be felt.

At 7.20 P. M. he made a curious noise, so like a snarl or bark that the patients in the neighbouring beds thought a dog had got into the ward. His hands were then noticed to be clenched, and he became violently convulsed. The House-Surgeon, who saw him within a very few minutes of this attack, found him then quiet and apparently quite insensible; his eyes were strongly rolled upwards—the left appeared more elevated than the right. After about five minutes, the masseter muscles were observed to stand in tense relief, and the upper lip was raised, showing the teeth and gums. The teeth were tightly clenched. Then his fingers became flexed, and the arms rigidly stiff through violent contraction of their muscles. The muscles in the nape of the neck were soft, and not con-tracted. Seven such fits occurred at intervals of about five minutes, ushered in by the strange barking noise. There was then a calm interval of half an hour, followed by another fit, after which consciousness returned. He then asked for a chamber-pot, and micturated. At 11 P. M. he had two more fits. He passed the rest of the night quietly, appearing to sleep.

January 24. At 9 A. M., temperature 98.4°, pulse 84. Calm and sensible. Headache continued. At 3 P. M., two fits.

25th. 9 A. M., temperature 97.4°; pulse 86. Slept from eleven o'clock last night till seven this morning. Headache and dizziness unchanged. 9 P. M., temperature 98.4°. At 10 P. M., whilst apparently sleeping, began to mutter, then made a barking noise, and was convulsed six times in half an hour—after which he became conscious. In these fits there was extreme opisthotonus.

26th. 9 A. M., temperature 98°, pulse 78. More headache. At 7 P. M. a convulsion lasting five minutes; after which he continued unconscious during half an hour.

27th. In the course of the morning, five fits; and in the evening, four fits. Temperature 98.4°; pulse 84.

28th. During forenoon, three fits. Temperature 98.6°; pulse 96. Up to this time he had been taking large doses of potassium bromide. At mid-day he was placed under the influence of chloroform, and trephined at the spot in the right temple, where, as already mentioned, pressure always caused a darting pain through the head. In the soft coverings, and in the disk of bone removed, no trace of injury or structural change was discernible. The dura mater also appeared normal. An aspirator-needle was therefore pushed through this to the depth of rather more than an inch, upon which, as nothing escaped through it, the needle was withdrawn. For a few moments, cerebro-spinal fluid spurted in a slender stream through the prick in the dura mater to the distance of nearly a foot. The middle of the scalp-wound was purposely left open. Throughout the operation, and subsequently, strict antiseptic measures were observed.

During the next forty-eight hours no fits occurred. The temperature ranged between 98.4° and 99°, and the pulse averaged 80. He was cheerful but calm, and took fluid nourishment freely. His headache was, he said, much less. Move-ments of the lower jaw caused much pain, obviously referable to the division of the temporal muscle in the operation.

In the afternoon of the 30th he was allowed to see his father, which appeared to excite him. Later, at 5.30 o'clock, he seemed to become unconscious, and at 6.15 he was slightly convulsed.

February 1. At 1.15 A. M., a slight fit; at 11.45, a slight fit, preceded by unconsciousness of about twenty minutes' duration; and at 9.30 P. M., uncon-sciousness, which lasted twenty-five minutes, when he came-to without convulsion. Temperature ranged from 98° to 99°.

2d. One slight convulsion. Temperature 98.2°; pulse 84. Potassic iodide gr. x. t. d. now ordered.

3d. At 12.15 P. M., a strong fit.

4th. Had a calm day, followed at 8.40 P. M. by several violent fits.

5th. Between 7 and 9 A. M., six fits.

7th. Temperature 98°; pulse 56, in afternoon intermittent. The dose of iodide of potassium was diminished by half—to gr. v: t. d. 8.30 P. M.: Unconscious during five minutes, after which a severe fit of convulsions, lasting half an hour; followed by four more fits between 3.30 and 4 A. M.

On the 12th he began to take valerianate of zinc in doses of gr. iss, t d. On the 15th this was increased to gr. ij, 4ta quaque hora; then to gr. iij, gr. iv., and finally (on the 24th) to gr. vj, 4ta q. h.

After this date he had no fits until March 6, when he was unconscious during several hours, and was violently convulsed several times.

7th. Allowed to leave his bed and sit in an easy chair. The valerianate of zinc pills were now taken only four times in twenty-four hours. From this time he appeared to improve.

On the 15th he declared himself quite free from headache, and he had not had any fit for eight days.

On the 16th he returned home. At this time he could walk a little; had a good appetite, and was free from headache.

The early symptoms in this most remarkable case are those which are generally thought to indicate severe concussion of the brain. When death has occurred soon after an injury to the head, followed by such symptoms, not infrequently bruisings, slight lacerations, and small hemorrhages in the cortex of the brain have been demonstrated. The severity of the early symptoms, the tardy and imperfect recovery, warranted the belief that such surface-damage of brain had occurred here. The unconsciousness which supervened later on the day of the accident raised the suspicion that a coarse hemorrhage had happened; but the interval—twelve hours—between the accident and this unconsciousness was exceptionally great for it to have been due to pressure through hemorrhage, and the subsequent progress was also inconsistent with such a supposition.

What were the fits which came on six months after the time of the injury?

In those which occurred on the day he was taken into the hospital, the House-Surgeon noticed very marked *trismus;* the masseters became like rigid bars, and the lower jaw was tightly clenched.

In subsequent fits extreme *opisthotonus* occurred. The occiput and rump nearly touched.

Trismus and *opisthotonus* are, as you know, characteristic features in tetanus. Our patient, however, certainly had not tetanus, for during the cramp of the masseters the muscles of the nape were soft and uncontracted, those of the hands and forearms were as violently convulsed as those of the trunk, and in the intervals between these terrible fits none of the muscles were unnaturally rigid; whilst in tetanus, rigidity of the muscles of the nape is early associated with trismus, and it precedes the implication of the muscles of the trunk, the muscles of the hands and forearms usually escape, and between the convulsive paroxysms all the implicated muscles continue stiff through inordinate tonic contraction. It was evident, then, that these convulsive fits were not tetanic: were they epileptic?

The earliest seizures noticed at home, a few days before the first convulsions, were not unlike those of the least severe form of epilepsy—transient unconsciousness ("he seemed to lose himself for a moment") and slight twitchings. That epilepsy sometimes has a traumatic origin cannot be doubted. Its sequence upon injuries of the head affecting the brain has been observed too frequently to allow this to be regarded as a casual coincidence. We have had in the surgical wards within the last two years two instances of this. In the present case the increase of headache in the right temple, which often, he said, shortly preceded a fit, and the darting pain through the head on touching the site of the bruise at this part, favoured the supposition of a causal relation between the injury and the fits ; and this supposition was strengthened by the continuance of headache and dizziness during the intermediate time between the injury and the occurrence of the fits—symptoms suggestive of the existence of some chronic irritative process at the injured spot.

Against the idea that the fits were epileptic was the manner in which they often began : the patient, who a few moments previously had been talking rationally and coherently, appeared to lose the thread of the sentence ; he muttered disconnected words, repeating the same word again and again—mostly a word occurring in the last coherent sentence he had himself spoken, or in the last sentence addressed to him. He did not become unconscious instantly, but gradually, and a period varying from a few minutes to half an hour often preceded the convulsions. Occasionally the first convulsions had the aspect of purposive movement. He, on two occasions when I was myself present and saw it, distinctly made a snap at a dresser who happened to be at his bedside, and tried to seize him with his teeth. His tongue was never bitten.

As, however, the fits seemed to differ least from epilepsy, bromide of potassium, so useful in this disorder, was tried in large and frequent doses. It had not any controlling influence ; the fits continued with great violence. It was now that recourse was had to trephining. As you have already heard, nothing abnormal was discovered. The high intra-cranial pressure, sufficient to project a spurt of cerebro-spinal fluid to the distance of nearly one foot, is worth notice. The fluid continued to leak during several hours afterwards in quantity enough to wet the boric charpie with which the wound was covered, and the pressure will have been for some time lowered. Had this lessened tension any causal connection with the absence of fits during the next sixty hours or so ? On their return, iodide of potassium was next tried in doses of ten grains, diminished one-half when, after a few days, the pulse began to be very weak and to intermit. It was, however, soon apparent that this drug also was without influence over the malady. The similarity of the fits in respect of the occasional purposive character of the initial convulsions, and also in respect of the opisthotonus which sometimes occurs in violent hysterical convulsions, next led to a trial of valerianate of zinc, which was taken at first in doses of one grain and a half, and finally in six-grain doses at short intervals. Under this treatment the fits subsided, which favours the idea of their hysterical nature. In some recently published cases of violent hysterical convulsions in young women, it was related that pressure in the inguinal regions, directed so that it might be supposed to reach the ovaries, quickly arrested the convulsions. As an experiment, compression of the homologous organs, the testes, was tried here during some fits, but without any effect upon them.

Upon the whole the conclusion which has the largest support in the facts of this case is that the fits were hysterical, induced by the shock of the accident in a person whose nervous system was not particularly stable, and that they were not immediately dependent upon a local irritative process set up by the blow on the temple ; trephining, therefore, whilst it did not appear to have done any harm, was useless. In the case which I very recently brought before you, you will remember that the symptoms of cerebral disorder were one-sided : this gave them a very different signification to that of the convulsions in the present case, which were not restricted to one side, but implicated both sides equally.

Note.—After the patient's return home, he fell into what was called a "galloping consumption," and died on July 14 following. An examination of the head showed that the trephine-hole in the skull, which had measured eleven millimetres across, had been completely closed by new bone—a result probably referable to the small size of the trephine and the preservation of the pericranium, which was in a normal condition at the time of operation. No trace of the puncture with the aspirating-needle was discernible in the dura mater or brain.

. The brain weighed forty-eight ounces; it was well formed and symmetrical. The pia mater, especially that covering the posterior lobes, was congested. No trace of injury could be detected by most careful examination—no scar or depression or mark of former contusion or laceration; the surface of the brain appeared quite normal. The white and gray matter of the hemispheres were firm; the puncta vasculosa rather more conspicuous than usual. Each hemisphere was carefully sliced for traces of previous injury; none whatever were found. The only pathological conditions were four small yellowish nodules. One of these, about the size of a large pin's head, was in the gray matter of the anterior part of the corpus striatum, close to its upper surface; a second, slightly larger, was in the gray matter of one of the convolutions of the left frontal lobe; the two others were one in each cerebellar hemisphere—also in the gray matter, that in the right side being the larger, and about the size of a horse-bean.—*Med. Times and Gazette*, July 23, 1881.

Hospital Notes.

BELLEVUE HOSPITAL, NEW YORK.

(Service of Dr. AUSTIN FLINT, Sr.)

(Specially reported for the MEDICAL NEWS AND ABSTRACT.)

Transient Mellituria. Cardiac Disease.

Annie M., æt. 66, Ireland, domestic; admitted Dec. 6, 1880. The patient had malarial fever fifteen years ago. After that time she enjoyed good health until two years ago, when she had acute articular rheumatism involving the knees, ankles, and feet. The arthritic disease, having received no treatment, became chronic, and obliged the patient to seek admission to the hospital. On admission (Dec. 6, 1880), the patient had no pulmonary disease. The heart was hypertrophied, the apex being situated in the sixth intercostal space on the *linea mammillaris*, and the impulse being abnormally strong. A loud, musical, systolic murmur was heard at the apex, and was transmitted to the left, around the chest, being plainly perceptible behind, near the angle of the scapula. Another murmur was heard at the base, over the aortic valves, and was transmitted into the carotids. The patient had a good but not an unusually large appetite. She was not emaciated. She did not suffer from thirst. Her vision was not impaired. Her temperature was normal. She had no cutaneous eruptions or abscesses. Her tongue was moist, and her teeth perfectly sound. She micturated at natural intervals, and had no strangury or *ardor urinæ*. The vulva was not excoriated or tender. Her urine was pale, clear, acid in reaction, and its specific gravity was 1029. It contained an abundance of sugar, but neither albumen, casts, nor other abnormal ingredients. No medication was resorted to.

December 10. The urine has been carefully examined every day since the patient's admission and found to contain no sugar until to-day, when it was discovered to contain eight grains to the ounce. Some urine was withdrawn from the bladder by a catheter to prevent the possibility of deception, and was found to contain the same proportional quantity of sugar.

11*th*. The patient has passed only twenty-one ounces of urine during the last twenty-four hours. Its specific gravity is 1033, and it contains ten grains of sugar to the ounce.

12*th*. Amount of urine, twenty-four ounces; sugar in abundance.

13*th*. Amount of urine, twenty-two ounces; large amount of sugar.

21*st*. The amount of urine has averaged twenty-five ounces since the last note, and has contained about ten grains of sugar to the ounce. The patient's general condition is excellent, and all her bodily functions are naturally performed.

25*th*. No change in the urinary condition.

28*th*. To-day the sugar suddenly disappeared from the urine, and the amount passed was increased to four ounces.

January 19, 1881. Average daily amount of urine is now forty-five ounces, and it contains no sugar.

30*th*. A careful daily urinary analysis has failed to detect any sugar since last note. The average daily amount is now sixty ounces, and its specific gravity 1020.

February 18. The patient has no symptoms or signs of diabetes. Her urine is normal. She experiences no inconvenience from her cardiac disease, and has only slight stiffness in her rheumatic joints. She was to-day discharged.

Eliz. L., æt. 35, U. S., domestic; admitted Dec. 16, 1880. Six years ago the patient had her first attack of acute articular rheumatism which involved almost all her joints and was attended by præcordial pain and by dyspnœa. She has had several similar attacks since that time. Three years since she first noticed œdema of her lower extremities, which has persisted up to the present time. She has had abnormal frequency of micturition, but no diarrhœa, emesis, or headache. Has had a slight cough and scanty muco-sanguinolent expectoration. She has lost flesh, but has had no night-sweats. On admission she complained of dyspnœa, præcordial pain, and œdema of the legs and feet. The heart is hypertrophied, the apex-beat being situated in the fifth intercostal space, an inch to the left of the mammary line, and the impulse being unusually strong. A thrill is communicated to the palpating fingers. An organic mitral regurgitant and an aortic direct murmur are heard. A prediastolic murmur exists at the base. There is slight pleuritic effusion on the right side. The lower extremities are very œdematous. The temperature, pulse, and respiration are normal. There are neither excessive appetite, great thirst, nor other symptoms of diabetes. The urine, which is clear, alkaline, and has a sp. gr. of 1009, contains a trace of albumen and a considerable quantity of sugar. The quantity of urine passed in twenty-four hours is thirty-five ounces.

Treatment.—Infusion of digitalis, fl℥ss, every three hours, and a liberal diet of milk and eggs.

December 16. The patient has improved notably since her admission. The œdema and dyspnœa have diminished and the pleuritic effusion decreased. The average daily quantity of urine has been seventy ounces, and it has contained about six grains of sugar to the ounce.

17*th*. The sugar has disappeared. The digitalis was continued.

27*th*. The urine has been normal in quantity and chemical character since last note, and the patient is rapidly gaining strength.

January 10. The patient was discharged in good health, the pleuritic effusion, œdema, mellituria, and albuminuria having disappeared.

MONTHLY ABSTRACT.

Anatomy and Physiology.

Microscopic Structure of the Cortex Cerebri.

Professor BETZ (*Centralblatt für die Med. Wiss.*, 1881, Nos. 11, 12, and 13) has endeavoured, by his histological researches, to verify the statements of Hitzig and Ferrier respecting the localization of functions in the cortex cerebri. In 1874 he pointed out that the "motor zone" contained large cells, to which the name of giant-cells was given, though they have nothing to do with the giant-cells which play so large a part in the modern descriptions of new growths. He says, the cortex cerebri, as is well known, is composed of five layers, as follows : 1, a layer of neuroglia, containing small granular nuclei ; 2, in addition to the preceding, there are pyramidal cells of medium size, with the apices directed towards the periphery, and their bases towards the central parts ; 3, very large pyramidal cells, which are, however, fewer and scattered ; 4, small round or elliptical cells, constituting the "nuclear layer ;" 5, special fusiform cells.

This is the typical arrangement, but the various regions show differences. Thus, Meynert has shown that, in the neighbourhood of the calcarine fissure, the third layer is absent, and the structure in this region consists of two nuclear layers separated by a layer of nerve-fibres, on which lie by pairs large pyramidal cells. The hippocampus also is principally composed of the elements of the third layer. The claustrum consists of the elements of the fifth layer ; the ascending frontal, and the paracentral lobe, contain "giant-cells" grouped in nests.

He has examined 5000 preparations from brains of all ages, and has come to recognize, in addition to the above, certain other regional peculiarities.

The *ascending frontal convolution* in its upper two-thirds, presents the following characters. At first, just above the fifth layer, there are large cells, single or united by pairs, and at great intervals one from another ; higher up, these cells are grouped in threes and fours, and the intervals are less. Higher still, the groups are formed by a large number of cells, not less than four, often six or seven. In the third layer they present an uninterrupted series. In the second, they are scattered as in the fourth. Near the paracentral lobe, this series is again interrupted so as to form groups or nests. Nearer the lobe the cells become larger, until they pass into the condition of the true giant-cells of that region. These latter are never found in the ascending parietal.

The *convolution of the corpus callosum* is composed at its origin, beneath the anterior part of the lamina terminalis, almost exclusively of two layers, the superior and the fifth ; while the cells of the latter, instead of being parallel to the base of the convolution, are perpendicular, like the cells of the third layer elsewhere, and they are two or three times larger than the ordinary fusiform cells of the third layer. In the middle of this convolution, the "nuclear layer" (fourth), and the layer of pyramidal cells, reappear. In the posterior third, three new layers occur. The first, lowest, is composed of longitudinal fibres, forming an arch over the upper surface of the corpus callosum. The second layer, gray, is formed of small round cells ; the third, equally gray, contains pyramidal cells, and also large fusiform cells. These three layers become more and more important towards the extremity of this convolution, but never involve more than its inferior and internal portions. Where the convolution of the corpus callosum passes into the hippocampus, the layer of large cells suddenly increases, and goes to form the internal cellular layer of the hippocampus. The nuclear layer, above described, becomes the well-known nuclear layer of the hippocampus; and the layer of white fibres adjacent to the corpus callosum passes to form the reticular white matter of the hippocampus.

The *extremity of the hippocampus*, and the terminal part of the temporal lobe, present the peculiarity that the pyramidal cells of the third layer are found immediately beneath the first, and are arranged in groups like balls of thread, whence they have been named by Betz *cortical glomeruli*.

The *third frontal convolution* is separable into three parts, the most posterior extending from the ascending frontal convolution to the perpendicular branch of the fissure of Sylvius; the middle portion extends from this limit to the beginning of the orbital portion of the convolution; and the third, situated on the under surface of the brain, extends from the extremity of the convolution to the sland of Reil. The first portion contains in the third layer pyramidal cells of larger size than are found elsewhere in the frontal lobe; and in brains of persons of advanced age, there may be giant cells of small size, which pass into the extremity of the ascending frontal. The second portion contains, in the second and third layers, long, slender, pyramidal cells grouped together, and with their processes directed obliquely. The third portion contains chiefly cells on the type of the fifth layer, and of the size of those of the claustrum, arranged, generally, perpendicularly to the transverse section of the cortex; sometimes there are some cells of the third layer, but they are very small.

The *island of Reil* contains numerous small cells, like those of the fifth layer.

The *lingual lobe* possesses eight layers from without inwards : 1, the layer of neuroglia; 2, very small pyramidal cells; 3, nuclei; 4, horizontal fibres; 5, nuclei; 6, horizontal fibres; 7, triangular pyramidal cells; 8, fusiform cells.

The *fusiform lobule* has an analogous structure; but, as it approaches the occipital lobe, the seventh layer disappears, and at the end of the descending gyrus all the layers unite to form a homogeneous mass of nucleated cells, and a little row of fusiform cells.

The external portion of the *occipital lobe* has the second and third layers of pyramidal cells of the ordinary type, and here and there there are cells of large size.

The *angular gyrus* has an analogous structure, but the cells of the third layer are much larger than in the occipital lobe.

The *ascending parietal convolution*, and *superior parietal* and *inferior parietal lobules*, have the ordinary typical structure.

The three *temporal convolutions* are distinguished by the thickness of the fifth layer, and by the presence of small cells in the third.

The *parieto-temporal* and *transverse temporal* convolutions are of the ordinary type.

The *quadrate lobe* has near its upper border, in the third layer and above the fifth, two rows of pyramidal cells.

The *frontal convolutions*, excepting the lowest, already described, have a very thick third layer of large pyramidal cells, which almost obliterates the fourth layer.

The *straight gyrus* is very like the convolution of the corpus callosum.

In the *female*, the third layers in the frontal and parietal lobes are thinner, and the pyramidal cells fewer; while in the occipital lobes, the same layer presents larger and more numerous cells.

In the *embryo*, at seven months, the cortex is composed of only two layers, the first and fourth, and pyramidal cells may be seen only in the hippocampus.

In the *new-born child* the cortex is much the same, but the hippocampus has all its elements as visible as in the adult, and in the paracentral lobe there are some giant-cells, which may be distinguished by their pyramidal form and three prolongations. At the age of *six weeks*, the pyramidal cells of the third layer may be observed in several convolutions. ·

· In *children of eleven to twelve years* the giant-cells have still few prolongations, the apical prolongation is still short and pale, and no basal prolongation has been observed.

In the case of an *idiot* (Motté), the frontal lobe was composed of irregular, slender pyramidal cells, in which it was impossible to distinguish the five layers. The giant-cells of the ascending parietal and paracentral regions were narrow, oblique, and furnished with few prolongations, the basal prolongation being absent. The parietal and occipital lobes had the nuclear layer well developed, while the pyramidal layer was small, thin, and contained chiefly the small pyramidal cells of the second layer. The *hippocampus* had its white substance very well developed; its characteristic cellular layer was small, as was also the nuclear layer.

With respect to the origin of the olfactory nerve, the olfactory tubercle contains a first layer of small pyramidal cells, few in number; a thick layer of nuclei, and large cells in the fifth layer, like those in the convolution of the corpus callosum. There is, in the inferior portion of the tubercle, a bundle of white fibres, coming from the corpus callosum; and the same region contains a gray layer, consisting of oval ganglionic cells, of large size, and furnished with processes, recalling the cells of the cornua of the spinal cord. In the brain of Motté, this gray layer was much better developed than usual. This gray layer may be called the central ganglion of the olfactory tubercle.

These facts afford an anatomical confirmation to the researches of Ferrier. Convolutions are organs separated by sulci, or fissures, in which lie the blood-vessels supplying them. The larger the convolutions, the greater is the development of the particular organ; and the more numerous of the convolutions, the greater is the specialization of function.—*Lond. Med. Record*, July 15, 1881.

———

Anatomical Structure of the Mammary Gland.

In the *Verhandl. der Phys. Med. Gesellsch. in Würzburg* (Band xiv., Heft 3 and 4) Prof. KÖLLIKER gives a detailed descriptions of the minute anatomy of the male and female mamma at various ages. In the new-born infant, sex makes very little difference in the structure. At this period there are no terminal gland-vesicles, the ducts are lined with a single layer of cylinder epithelium or with a few layers of pavement cells, and end in club-like extremities. The ducts he finds in all cases irregularly dilated, the dilatations being filled with shed epithelial cells and a white granular material—forming the so-called "witch-milk," which he regards as normal. During the first year, the most noticeable point is the great dilatation of the ducts, giving the organ a cavernous appearance. The ducts are lined, according to the amount of dilatation, either with flattened epithelium or with several layers of round cells; and those which reach into the depth of the organ have now several club-like terminations. Strings of cells, afterwards developing into fat-cells, are also seen in the deeper parts of the gland. The above-mentioned dilatations gradually diminish during the latter half of the first year, till the lumen is normal, but in some cases swelling of the gland goes on, and a true mastitis results, from which, in all probability, follow those cases of imperfect development of the breast in otherwise well-developed women. From the age of one to ten little change takes place beyond the development of fat around the organ and the increase of the septa of connective tissue.

From ten to twenty, the male mamma changes but little, although the terminal gland-vesicles may develop here and there on one or both sides. From twenty to thirty, the male mamma reaches its highest development. The ducts divide dichotomously at their extremities, and send off cellular processes which develop into vesicles. The cutaneous papillæ, the smooth muscular fibre, and the sudoriparous glands, are also much developed. From thirty to fifty, regressive changes occur, gradual disappearance of the terminal vesicles from fatty degeneration of the epithelium with contraction of their lumen and a matting of the connective tissue. The ducts also become tortuous and varicose, and, in later life, there is a great enlargement of the sebaceous glands.

In the virgin mamma, there is no division into lobes. The great part of the gland lies underneath the areola and towards the lower segment of the organ. The cutaneous papillæ are not much developed, and the interstitial tissue is almost tendinous in structure. The gland-vesicles are few in number, even at the age of twenty. They are formed by cellular offshoots from the ducts, at first solid, but gradually acquiring a lumen. In pregnancy, this process goes on rapidly and in large extent. Circular and longitudinal smooth muscular fibres are present in considerable quantity; both classes of fibres being tolerably uniform on the nipple, while the circular fibres seem to preponderate in the areola. During menstruation, although the organ sometimes becomes harder and more sensitive, the author discovered no change. Probably the symptoms are caused by a temporary hyperæmia, producing more rapid growth. During pregnancy and lactation, the papillæ on the nipple are broad but not high, those on the areola are long and pointed. The rete Malpighii contains a thick layer of yellowish-brown pigment. From eighteen to twenty-two ducts converge to the depression of the nipple to open between the cutaneous papillæ, each of these ducts being made up of from four to fourteen branches. The connective tissue of the gland is loose and relatively less in quantity. The terminal vesicles are now well developed, forming a well-marked racemose gland. They are best developed in the deeper parts of the gland, the superficial part consisting mainly of excretory ducts and connective tissue. Between the papillæ of the areolar space are found the prominences of Montgomery's glands, especially developed sebaceous glands, about a dozen in number. Regressive changes follow pregnancy and lactation, general relaxation of the breast, the nipple and areola retaining their size, although the pigmentation slightly lessens in degree. The vesicles also lessen in size. The lobules become separated by more connective tissue. Later in life, the whole glandular tissue disappears except the excretory ducts; the fat also atrophies, and we have the pendent breasts of age.—*Lond. Med. Record,* July 15, 1881.

Materia Medica and Therapeutics.

Waldivin.

A short time since, M. Tanret separated a crystalline neutral principle from the fruit of *Simaruba Waldivia* (which should not be confounded with that of *S. Cedron*). Some physiological experiments carried out by M. Dujardin-Beaumetz (*Comptes Rendus,* tome xcii.) show that this principle, waldivin, is a powerful poison, but slow in its action, death in the case of dogs not occurring until from five to ten hours after injection, even when the dose is many times that necessary to produce death. In the human subject and in dogs it provokes vomiting when administered by the stomach, but rabbits fall into a profound stupor, which continues until death. In cases of snake-bite and hydrophobia it has failed to prevent a fatal termination, though, when administered to mad dogs in doses of one milligramme daily, it is said to cause an entire suppression of the exacerbations, the animals remaining insensible and dying without convulsions. Waldivin does not appear to exercise any influence in cases of intermittent fever. On the other hand, cedrin, the corresponding principle of *S. Cedron*, is less toxic, but possesses decided febrifuge properties, though the action is slower and less sure than that of quinine. Like waldivin, cedrin exercises no influence in cases of snake-bite; so that, if there be any foundation in the popular reputation in South America of the seeds of *Simaruba Cedron* as a specific against the bites of venomous serpents, it is not due to this principle. Neither substance produces toxic symptoms in frogs, even in large doses.—*London Med. Record*, June 15, 1881.

—

Xanthoxylum Naranjillo as a substitute for Jaborandi.

A rutaceous plant, growing wild in the Argentine Republic, where it is called "naranjillo," and which has recently been described as a new species by Griesbach, under the name of Xanthoxylum Naranjillo, has been examined by D. PARODI (*Revista Farmaceutica*, vol. xviii., and *Pharm. Jour.*). His attention was directed to it through its resemblance to pilocarpus jaborandi in its therapeutic properties, which are those of a sialogogue, sudorific, diuretic, and stimulant. He reports that he has separated a substance forming salts with acids, having a decided alkaline reaction, and giving all the reactions characteristic of an alkaloid, which he has named "xanthoxylina." The plant also yielded a hydrocarbon, "xanthoxylene" ($C_{10}H_{16}$), analogous to pilocarpin, a crystalline stearoptene, xanthoxylin, and finally an aromatic essential oil, having an odour between balm and lemon. From the great similarity of this plant to jaborandi, it appears worthy of further experiment in a therapeutic direction.—*London Med. Record*, June 15, 1881.

—

Oxidized Oil of Turpentine as a New Antiseptic.

Mr. C. T. KINGZETT, in the *Lancet*, June, 1881, p. 971, brings forward the oil of turpentine, through which air has been passed for a prolonged period, as a valuable antiseptic agent, being at the same time much cheaper than oil of eucalyptus and more intensely antiseptic than this drug, besides being free from all the objections that attend the use of this agent. Mr. Lister is making trial of the oxidized oil of turpentine, the result of which the profession will await with interest.—*Lond. Med. Record*, July 15, 1881.

—

Naphtha Oil in Affections of the Skin.

Prof. KAPOSI read a paper at the Vienna Medical Society (*Wien. Med. Zeit.*, May 10), in which he stated that he had employed this substance (the B naphtha oil, largely used by colour-makers) as an advantageous substitute for tar, being as useful, while not producing the same disagreeable effects as regards colour, smell, or spoiling linen. Hitherto he has used it only externally, but from its rapid absorption and excretion it may be used, probably with good effect, internally. How far this is the case, and to what diseases it is especially applicable, further trial must prove. At present, speaking from seventy-six cases, Kaposi has found it a useful remedy. Thus in scabies a 10 per cent. simple ointment followed by a compound ointment of 10 parts of naphtha oil, 50 of green soap, and 100 of lard, will effect a cure in two applications. In eczema, as with tar, the exact time of application is difficult to choose; but if this be well chosen, the itching is allayed, and a slow desquamation occurs. In psoriasis a 10 per cent. ointment produces the same effect as a chrysorabin ointment, without the discoloration caused by this. The ointment has also been used with good effect in ichthyosis, seborrhœa, and pityriasis versicolor; but it is of no avail in lupus vulgaris; while a case of lupus erythematosus was advantageously treated. The naphtha oil is easily soluble in alcohol and in oils or fats, but water requires equal parts of alcohol to be added to effect a solution.—*Med. Times and Gazette*, June 4, 1881.

Pepsine as a Solvent in Albuminous Obstruction of the Bladder.

Dr. Hollmann (*Nederl. Weekbl.*, 18, p. 272) reports the case of an old man, aged 80, suffering from retention of urine, in whom the introduction of a catheter failed to procure the desired result. It was found that the bladder contained coagulated albuminoid masses, mixed with blood. A few hours after the injection of about sixteen grains of pepsine dissolved in water, a large amount of a dark, viscid, fetid fluid readily escaped by the catheter.—*London Med. Record*, June 15, 1881.

Medicine.

Changes in the Salivary Glands in Lyssa.

Dr. A. Elsenberg (*Central. für die Med. Wiss.*, No. 13, 1881) has examined the salivary glands of twelve mad dogs and of two human subjects dying of lyssa. The principal changes in the dog were in the submaxillary and sublingual glands. The former, on section, were smooth, showed their acinous structure clearly, and were of a grayish-red colour. Under the microscope, the interstitial tissue was distinctly infiltrated with small cells with one or more nuclei, like colourless blood-cells. This infiltration was most marked around the medium-sized veins in the hilus of the acinus, diminished at the periphery, and was scarcely present at the hilus of the gland; in some places, the infiltration was of sufficient intensity to form a microscopic abscess. The fixed cells were slightly swollen, but showed no trace of division. The bloodvessels were filled with blood, containing many leucocytes, partly lying by the walls of the vessels, partly irregularly mixed with the coloured corpuscles. The alveolar epithelium, as well as the half-moon cells, were not unchanged. The contents of the secreting cells became, from a transparent mucous mass, at first slightly granular; then the granular mass gradually enlarged, while, at the same time, the circumference of the cell diminished by a third. The nucleus, from being flat, became round, enlarged, and, instead of lying peripherally, passed more to the centre. Such cells coloured readily with picrocarmin or hæmatoxylin; sometimes two nuclei were seen. The half-moon cells swelled up so as to fill two-thirds of the alveoli; at the same time their nuclei proliferated, so that each cell contained three or more times as many nuclei as a normal cell. Besides, there were sometimes in the alveoli round cells like white blood-cells, which had penetrated from the neighbouring interstitial tissue. The same appearances were found in the middle-sized ducts; the small cells, penetrating the walls, pushed up the epithelium, loosened the connection of the cells to one another, and forced them into the lumen of the duct. Around the nervous ganglia were similar infiltrations, which sometimes penetrated the ganglia. In the sublingual gland, the changes were similar in kind but less in degree. The orbital gland in dogs, which belongs to the salivary glands, was usually very little altered. The parotid showed badly marked changes in four dogs only ; the interstitial infiltration was usually mode-rate ; the gland-cells were a little enlarged, granular, and contained two or three nuclei, and similar changes were found in the epithelium of the ducts of middling calibre. In the human subjects he found scarcely any changes in the parotid, very little in the submaxillary, which was limited to small-celled infiltration of the tissue surrounding the ducts and veins of middling calibre ; the most marked changes were in the sublingual. These were less intense, but similar to those found in dogs. He concludes that these appearances are characteristic of an in-flammatory process, caused by an infectious material circulating in the blood and excreted by the saliva. As the changes are most marked in the submaxillary and sublingual glands, it is probable that the saliva of these glands principally, or perhaps exclusively, secretes the specific poison. These changes are suffi-ciently characteristic to permit the diagnosis of lyssa in dogs, but they are too feebly marked and too like what occur in other infectious diseases, or as the result of drugs, to be of the same value in man.—*London Med. Record*, June 15, 1881.

—

Turpentine in Diphtheria.

Dr. BOSSE (*Berlin Klin. Wochenschrift*, 1881, No. 9) illustrates this method by several cases. Of the pure oil of turpentine, an adult requires one large spoonful a day ; children from six to twelve years, two-thirds of the same ; children from one to two years, half of a large spoonful. The tolerance of this medicine is greater than might be expected. Out of eleven cases, only four vomited ; if rejected, the dose must be repeated after some hours. Generally, alvine evacuations follow, which possess a penetrating odour of turpentine. After these, the general symptoms, such as fever and headache, cease. There is a rapid recovery ; patients, who on the previous day took a spoonful of oil, already recovering the day after, or two days at the most, at least as regards the clearing of the throat, and the disappearance of the exudation. They would die only when assistance was rendered too late—*i. e.*, on the sixth or eighth day. Dr. Bosse attributes this effect of the oil of turpentine to its containing ozone. He denies that it has a caustic effect in swallowing, and mentions Naunyn's example, who (1868), in order to try the physiological effect of this remedy, took in company with his three assistant-surgeons 300 grammes of turpentine at one dose, 100 grammes thus coming to the share of each ; no pain, except a slight headache, was experienced by these experimenters ; neither albuminuria nor strangury followed.—*London Med. Record*, July 15, 1881.

—

Diphtheria in Russia.

In *Wratsch* (Nos. 49 and 51, 1880), BERG makes some remarks on 192 cases treated, in part in the ambulance, in part within the Children's Hospital at Charkow. A small number of observations are of especial value from this source, since little work has been published concerning the epidemics of diph-theria in Southern Russia, and because the cases were treated in hospital, and hence could be more carefully watched. The epidemic broke out towards the end of 1878, and continued throughout 1879. The interesting observation was made, that the number of cases always increased after a great change of tem-perature. Infection was usually the result of direct contact, but in one case in-fection was conveyed by a third person, who himself remained well. Of the patients treated in the hospital, 41 per cent. died, this large mortality depending on the fact that a great number of them were in a hopeless condition when first seen. The majority of the children were between two and eight years of age, the percentage mortality decreasing as the age rose. Berg divides the cases clinically into two classes—1. *Slight form*. Recovery took place after four to six days, the temperature never rising above 102.7. The membrane spread equally in all directions, healing progressing from periphery to centre. The membrane was yellowish-white in colour, easily detached, and odourless. The submaxillary glands were always swollen. 2. *Severe form*. The temperature rose to 103.2°. The membrane was usually distributed bilaterally, of a dirty tint, stinking, and rapidly invading the larynx. In the majority of the cases, death occurred in five to seven days from paralysis of the heart. The invasion of the larynx often resulted from the swollen and elongated uvula coming into contact with the root of the tongue and epiglottis, and so spreading the process. In two cases hemorrhages took place beneath the skin, and in one case there was subcutaneous emphysema in the neck. The treatment chiefly consisted in painting with a 10 to 15 per cent. solution of chloride of iron in glycerine, and the use of a 5 per cent. gargle of chlorinated potass. Other drugs were tried (in three cases benzoate of soda) without good results. Pilocarpin was not tried.— *London Med. Record*, July 15, 1881.

—

Vidal's Lotion for Diphtheria.

The following formula is given in *La Presse Méd.*, May, 1881. Take 10 grammes of tartaric acid; 25 grammes of hydrolate of peppermint; 15 grammes of pure glycerine; allow them to dissolve. With a brush steeped in this lotion, the diphtheritic patches are touched every three hours. They become reduced to a diffluent pulpy mass, which is afterwards easily removed. In the interval of the application of the tartaric acid, the false membranes are touched with lemon juice. An internal stimulating treatment is prescribed, with substantial and nourishing food.—*London Med. Record*, July 15, 1881.

—

Neuralgic Character of Certain Forms of Angina, and their Treatment by Sulphate of Quinine.

Dr. R. SAINT-PHILIPPE, surgeon to the Bordeaux hospitals, points out a certain number of cases of angina observed by him, and characterized by intermittent symptoms, so that the patient scarcely suffers at all in the morning, and is the victim of intolerable pain in the evening (*Jour. de Méd. de Bordeaux*, 20 Mars, 1881, p. 371). These forms of angina, which Dr. Saint-Philippe is inclined to refer to neuralgia of the median branch of the trigeminus, are amenable to treatment by sulphate of quinine. He prescribes from 40 to 50 centigrammes (6 to 7½ grains) two hours before the attack, and obtains cure. M. Marotte published analogous cases, in 1874, in the *Bulletin de Thérapeutique.*—*London Med. Record*, July 15, 1881.

—

Doliarin as a Remedy for Ankylostomum Dubini.

Doliarin is a crystalline substance extracted from a plant native to Brazil, the *Urostigma doliarium* or *Ficus doliaria*. The juice of this plant is used there as a remedy against a disease which seems to result, like the severe anæmia of the Gothard tunnel workers, from the ankylostomum Dubini. In any case, Dr. ROZZOLO has found it the most useful remedy against this parasite, although he does not deny that extract of male fern has been very successful in other hands than his.—*London Med. Record*, July 15, 1881.

Varix of the Œsophagus.

Among the extremely rare positions in which varicose veins may be found is the mucous lining of the œsophagus. An example was exhibited at the Pathological Society by Dr. Bristowe in 1856, in which "the veins of the mucous membrane were found to be enlarged and tortuous, especially in the lower part, having all the characters of varicose veins of the lower extremities." Death was caused by hemorrhage from the perforation of one of these dilated veins. C. J. EBERTH records a closely similar case in *Deutsches Archiv f. Klin. Med.* A man forty years of age had suffered for four years from hæmatemesis and bloody or tarry stools, and this had been repeated eight times within a year of his death. As there was pain over the region of the stomach, the symptoms were thought to depend upon an ulcer of the stomach. At last a fatal hemorrhage occurred, and it was then found that the veins of the mucous membrane were varicose over the lower half of the œsophagus, and that, reaching the size of pencils, they projected as soft cords from the surface. The hemorrhage was traced to an opening in one of these veins, about two centimetres above the cardiac orifice. Several minute white cicatrices were also found along the greater curvature of the stomach.—*Lancet,* June 4, 1881.

Typhoid Fever with Low Temperature.

FRANTZEL (*Zeit. für Klin. Med.,* Band ii. s. 217) describes severe cases of typhoid fever which attack exhausted individuals, and which run their course with low temperature or without fever, but in which occur general collapse, serious cerebral symptoms, and tendency to gangrene of the extremities, which run a strikingly acute course. Such cases indicate that high temperature is not the only cause of death in typhoid fever, but that cerebral symptoms are of great importance, and that patients even with low temperature must be carefully watched, to preserve them from the many evil consequences of even quiet delirium.—*London Med. Record,* July 15, 1881.

Desquamation and Infection following Scarlatina.

In the *Lancet,* June, 1881, p. 938, Mr. W. K. RIX, of the Fever Hospital, Bradford, states that in cases of fever, attended with intensely bright scarlet rash and high temperature, the desquamation may be completed in thirty days; that the great majority of cases, however, require from sixty to seventy-two days before they are fit to be discharged. In many cases, after nine weeks' quarantine, it is extremely doubtful whether the old thick skin from the heels has quite fallen off. That the dead skin from scarlatinal patients does carry infection, there appears to be little doubt; but that other factors are at work also appears certain, for frequently patients have been discharged, after all evidence of desquamation had long disappeared, the hair had been cut short, the clothes all changed, and every precaution possible taken to avoid infection, yet fresh cases have occurred within a week of the patient mixing with his brothers and sisters.—*London Med. Record,* July 15, 1881.

Theory of Mitral Insufficiency.

In most handbooks of medicine, in the chapter devoted to heart-affections, we find the theory of "compensation in valvular disease" based upon the law of retrodilatation and consecutive hypertrophy of the section of the heart situated above the lesion. According to this, mitral insufficiency should be followed by dilatation and hypertrophy of the left auricle, and shortly of the right ventricle

The fact that eccentric hypertrophy of the left ventricle is found in cases of simple mitral insufficiency has been frequently observed, but, nevertheless, scarcely rightly estimated.

Weil (*Berl. Klin. Woch.*, No. 7) agrees with Waldenburg in thinking eccentric hypertrophy of the left ventricle a necessary condition for efficient compensation for insufficiency of the mitral valve, dilatation and hypertrophy of the left auricle and right ventricle being of themselves insufficient to compensate for the lesion. Weil's argument is clear and simple. Mitral insufficiency is only compensated for, when, in spite of regurgitation of a portion of the contents of the ventricle into the auricle, the same quantity of blood enters the general circulation with each systole, as is the case with competent valves. Hence the ventricle must be capable of containing as much more blood as is regurgitated at each systole ; as a consequence it must be dilated, and, since the work is increased, it usually becomes hypertrophied. The clinical diagnosis of eccentric hypertrophy depends on the force of the impulse and on percussion. Exaggeration of the sounds over the aortic valves may be absent, since that is, merely indicative of increased tension in the aortic system. A further postulate of compensation is dilatation and hypertrophy of the left auricle, and, *hypertrophy of the right ventricle;* the latter may, however, be developed without accompanying dilatation. In proof of this, Weil has continually found eccentric hypertrophy of the left auricle, while he very commonly failed to discover any enlargement of the right heart. Exaggeration of the sounds over the pulmonary valves always existed, a sign of increased tension in the pulmonary circulation. The systolic murmur at the apex alone proves little. The existence of eccentric hypertrophy of the left ventricle with a normal pulse, allows the presumption of insufficiency of the mitral valve even before auscultation.

If with mitral insufficiency stenosis be associated, the hypertrophy may retrograde and altogether disappear, for the stenosis diminishes the amount of blood entering during diastole. The knowledge of this circumstance is the more important for the diagnosis of the combination of stenosis and insufficiency, since, in spite of serious stenoses, no presystolic murmur may exist.

If, however, on the *post-mortem* table eccentric hypertrophy of the left ventricle be seen associated with serious stenosis, it may in these cases be assumed that the hypertrophy is of older date ; in fact, dates from the time when the insufficiency of the valves prevailed.—*Lond. Med. Record*, July 15, 1881.

—

The Treatment of Phthisis by Residence at High Altitudes.

Dr. C. Theodore Williams, in a paper presented at the last International Medical Congress, first alludes to the effects of great altitudes (12,000 to 20,000 feet) on the human frame, as shown by the observations taken in the Alps, Rocky Mountains, Andes, and Himalayas by De Saussure, Lombard, Lortet, Marcet, Dennison, Zapatu, Jourdanet, and Henderson, and contrasts them with those of more moderate altitudes (from 4,000 to 10,000 feet), as given by Hermann, Weber, Clifford, Allbutt, Ormieux Coindet, Kellet, and others at Davos (Alps), Barèges (Pyrenees), Mexico, Blœmfontein (South Africa), and Landour (Himalayas), deducing that all advantages of mountain climates, without their disadvantages, can be obtained at moderate elevations.

Statistics are then given of cases of phthisis treated by residence at Davos, and in the South African uplands, and instances to illustrate the chief climatic effects on the various organs of the body.

Skin.—The influence on the skin is seen in the tanning of the complexion even during winter, which is due to the diathermancy of the air, and in the bracing effect on the sudoriferous glands causing cessation of night sweats.

Appetite and Weight.—Appetite is greatly increased, except in advanced cases of phthisis, and a gain of flesh (from 7 to 25 lbs.) is the result.

Muscular and Nervous Systems.—Daily exercise and frequent mountain ascents develop the muscular systems largely. The nervous system is stimulated and not unfrequently becomes over excited, and want of sleep follows, but as a rule less sleep seems necessary at high altitudes.

Temperature.—In healthy persons or ordinary chronic cases of phthisis there is little change. Where there is a tendency to pyrexia the exciting influence of the climate develops it, and if pyrexia already exists, it may increase. Mountain climates are generally contraindicated in pyrexial phthisis.

Circulation.—The first effect on consumptives is quickening of the pulse, followed later by a return to the normal rate, with a fuller vascular system, and a more powerful cardiac impulse. The pulse-rate of natives does not differ materially from that of lowlanders (Weber).

Respiration.—At the commencement of residence the respirations are more frequent than in the plains, their depth, as shown by Lortet's tracings being less; after a time they gain in depth and diminish in frequency, returning to the normal standard, as a gradual expansion of the thorax and lungs occurs. There is nothing remarkable about the respiration-rate of natives.

Changes in the Thorax.—Widening of the chest has been noted by Jourdanet and Walshe in cases of phthisis in Mexico and the Andes, by Rellet in consumptive soldiers at Himalayan stations, and by the author in cases returning from the South African mountains, by H. Weber, McCall Anderson, and the author, in patients treated at Davos.

This expansion was noticed by Dr. Ruedi in 95 out of 105 consumptives who passed the winter of 1880–81 at Davos, all stages and conditions of phthisis being here included, even some bedridden cases, and some who were losing weight. It may be concluded therefore that the enlargement of the thorax is not due to accumulation of fat and muscle, but to direct expansion of its walls from external pressure.

The amount of increase in circumference varies from 1 to 3 inches. Measurements taken at various levels, and cyrtometric tracings made by the author to determine the parts of the thorax involved in the expansion and their relation to the diseased lung, have led him to the following conclusions :—:

(1) That as a rule the portions of the chest wall overlying the *healthy* lung most frequently undergo dilatation.

(2) That this may be either in an antero-posterior, or lateral direction or sometimes in both directions.

(3) It is more common in the upper regions of the thorax than the lower.

(4) That if the disease be limited to the apex of the lung, the lower portion of chest on that side may become expanded, this leading to very remarkable deformities of the thorax. Observations on the length of residence required to produce this expansion of the thorax show that this varies, but often some months are necessary for the purpose, it being dependent on the respiration rate and on the yielding or non-yielding nature of the thoracic wall.

The length of time this expansion continues after a return to low levels also varies. In one case a considerable dilatation only lasted three months after return to England, in another about six months. In the majority of cases, however, it is of long duration and probably permanent.

Changes in the Lungs.—The changes in the thorax are accompanied, or preceded by marked increase of resonance over the whole chest, diminution of dulness over the affected areas, the substitution of dry sounds for moist, and the appearance of (emphysematous) crackle around the old lesions often masking other sounds. The tendency of cavities to contract does not seem greater than in patients treated at low levels. Over the healthy parts of the lungs the breath sound becomes harsh and puerile, the inspiration very long and the expiration short and feeble. Bronchophony and bronchial breathing become less distinct. The appearance of the thorax is striking, the intercostal spaces are hardly seen, the chest is full and well developed, but differs from the barrel-shaped form of large lunged emphysema.

The above phenomena indicate:—

(1) The development of vesicular emphysema around the affected portion of the lungs, thus localizing the disease and preventing its extension to healthy portions by infection from a caseous centre or from a secreting cavity.

(2) Absorption of some of the consolidations.

(3) The hypertrophy, or at any rate more perfect development of the healthy lung and of certain portions of the diseased one. These extensive changes in the lung-tissue necessarily lead to the dilatation of the thorax, the total result being due partly to the rarefaction of the air, and the consequent necessity at first of more frequent respirations, and later on of deeper ones, and partly to the species of lung gymnastics which the constant exercise, and especially the mountain ascents, induce.

The author is of opinion that the above constitute the principal elements in the curative process of mountain climates, but he does not undervalue the effect on the constitution generally of the dryness and purity of the air, and its freedom from septic materials.

Pneumothorax and Empyema.

H. SENATOR (Zeit. für Klin. Med., Band ii. s. 231) brings forward four cases to disprove the current opinion that fluid effused in the course of a pneumothorax must be purulent. He insists on the frequency of bilateral pleurisy in unilateral pneumothorax, and the occurrence of late pericarditis in cases of pneumothorax. When exudation takes place in pneumothorax due to internal injury of the lung, the fluid seldom putrefies in spite of the free access of air. He urges the point, overlooked in the text-books, that pleuritic effusion in children is generally purulent. With regard to the treatment of pneumothorax he lays down these rules. 1. If only air be present, no good can be done by operative interference. 2. If fluid be also present, the fluid should be tapped, not the air. 3. If the fluid be putrid, an incision must be made. Aspiration is indicated with serous or purulent exudations in phthisical patients. He recommends that the pus should be diluted by the injecting of an indifferent fluid, so that it will run better through a fine trocar, and what is left behind will be more easily absorbed. He avoids disinfecting the pleural cavity or emptying it completely.—London Med. Record, July 15, 1881.

Stertorous Breathing in Apoplexy.

In the Brit. Med. Journ., May, 1881, p. 845, Dr. ROBERT BOWLES again draws attention to the great value of position in relieving one of the most distressing and dangerous conditions of the apoplectic state, namely, stertor. [Previous papers may be consulted, Med. Times and Gaz., Jan. 1860, p. 126; Lancet, June, 1870, p. 875, Dec. 1880, pp. 971, 1018.] If a patient with an attack of apoplexy be laid on the side paralyzed, immediately the stertor ceases, from the fact that the tongue falls on one side, allowing free ingress of air to the lung on the sound side, which is better able to carry on its functions. The cerebral circulation on the diseased side is also, by this plan, relieved from all hypostatic congestion, and this may have a material effect in relieving the urgent symptoms. Dr. Bowles distinguishes several kinds of stertor: palatine, pharyngeal, mucous, nasal, laryngeal, and buccal stertor. Nasal stertor is readily removed by mechanically dilating the paralyzed nares. It is the pharyngeal form of stertor that so seriously aggravates the symptoms, adding suffocation to the apoplectic phenomena; and on removal of this symptom, by the simple act of change of position, the change from certain death to life is frequently obtained.—*London Med. Record*, July 15, 1881.

Pathological Changes in the Retina associated with Progressive Pernicious Anæmia.

In *Klin. Monats. für Augenheilkunde* (Dec. 1880), UHTHOFF describes the changes revealed by the microscope in the retinæ of six eyes removed after death from four cases of fatal penicious anæmia. They were, 1, hemorrhages, limited chiefly to the nerve-fibre and intergranular layers, and situated for the most part near the posterior pole, especially around the disk; 2 varicose hypertrophy of the nerve-fibres, affecting chiefly those of the most internal layers, so as to cause them to intrude upon the vitreous body, and consisting chiefly of the often-described shining, or finely granular masses of spherical, or spindle-shaped or retort-like form; 3, homogeneous colloid, or finely granular masses in the intergranular layer, present in one case only. It seems from these observations that progressive pernicious anæmia must be added to the list of morbid conditions which give rise to a peculiar varicose hypertrophy of nerve-fibres.—*London Med. Record*, June 15, 1881.

Cerebral Amblyopia and Hemiopia.

In this paper (*Brain*, part xii.), Dr. FERRIER furnishes material aid in explaining away the differences which have been hitherto apparent between the facts of clinical medicine and pathology, and those of physiological experiment, with regard to the relations of the eyes to the cerebral hemispheres. From numerous facts and arguments, the author arrives at the conclusion "that there is a twofold relation between the eyes and the cortical visual centres; the one mainly cross—the central portion of the retina probably bilaterally represented—by the angular gyrus; the other bilateral—the corresponding side of both retinæ being represented—by the occipital lobe, not alone, however, but in conjunction with the angular gyrus." From the nature of the impairment of vision existing in cerebral hemianæsthesia of organic origin, and which is due to lesion of the posterior segment of the internal capsule, external to the optic thalamus, the author concludes that the fibres which pass through the segment are specially in relation with the angular gyrus, and represent the opposite eye as regards those functions which are affected in hemianæsthesia. In cases of hemiopia, where central vision is retained for some degrees on all sides of the point of fixation, Dr. Ferrier considers that the cause is cerebral, not peripheral. In relation to this subject, numerous cases are discussed, and three unpublished ones are related.—*London Med. Record*, June 15, 1881.

Treatment of Epilepsy.

Dr. LASKIEWICZ (*Przeglad lekarsk.*, Nos. 4 and 6, 1881, *Centralblatt für Nervenheilkunde*, 1881, No. 6) commences the treatment of epileptic patients with bromide of potassium, of which a solution of one gramme is best given in the evening. As often as the attacks are repeated, the dose is increased one gramme daily, until 20, 25, and even 30 grammes are reached. The author mentions a case in which as much as 60 grammes' per day was given for some time. This remedy is very differently tolerated. The largest dose which has had an effect is to be continued for months and years, and then diminished with great care. Probably the patient will then be free from future attacks. If the remedy be not tolerated, atropine must take its place. This it is best to give as an alcoholic solution: 8 centigrammes of sulphate of atropine in 20 grammes of alcohol; this to be kept well closed in a glass. The dose is increased from one to ten drops, the largest dose for adults being twelve drops per day. It will be best to give it in milk or soup, about one hour before or after breakfast. The alkaloids of coffee, cocoa, or tea diminish the effect of atropine.—*London Med. Record*, July 15, 1881.

Compression of Carotid in Trigeminal Neuralgia.

Dr. SEIFERT (*Berlin. Klin. Wochensch.*, 1881, No. 11) publishes three cases of trigeminal neuralgia, in which he successfully employed compression of the carotid, as recommended by Gerhardt. The compression was made to last from fifteen seconds to one and a half minutes, and repeated as often as the pain was interrupted, while arsenic and quinine were likewise administered. Gradually, the intervals were lengthened.—*London Med. Record*, July 15, 1881.

Schiller on a Case of Catalepsy with Speech-reflexes.

SCHILLER (*Bres. Aertzl. Zeit.*, 1780, No. 21, and *Central. für die Med. Wiss.*, 1881, No. 17) reports the case of a previously healthy girl, aged 10 years, who became suddenly unconscious; the night before she had complained of stomach-ache, which had disappeared in the morning. The limbs could be moulded into any positions, and, in spite of their inconvenience, retained these for some time, and then gradually sank down again. Stroking from below upwards in the umbilical region made the child give a peculiar cry, which was not caused by deeper and sharper pressure on the same place. Also touching a place close to the manubrium sterni caused a peculiar cry. Strong electrical stimulation (the electric brush) and a vinegar enema, cured her after the lapse of one hour and a half. On other days, there were symptoms of commencing chorea in the facial muscles and fingers, which afterwards disappeared. The child has remained quite well for more than six months since the attack, of which she retains no recollection.—*London Med. Record*, July 15, 1881.

Formation of Trichinæ Cysts.

The mode of formation of the cysts of trichina has been studied by M. CHATIN and described in a communication to the Académie des Sciences. It was formerly said to be formed partly from the contractile tissue, and partly by a secretion from the nematoid, but this opinion was based only on some apparent differences in the thickness or aspect of the cyst wall, and not on any careful study of its formation, which necessitates the examination of animals dying or killed in different stages of the affection. When it arrives in the muscles the worm forms adhesions with the interfascicular tissue in which rapid changes occur. The elements increase in size, and during the growth of the protoplasm it assumes the appearance of an amorphous mass, in which, however, nuclei and vacuoles can be seen, which seem to indicate that the mass consists really of aggregated cells. By the growth of this the primitive fibres are compressed. In the new protoplasm fine proteoid granulations are first observed, and then other granulations which present all the reactions of glycogen. Then follow important changes in the periphery of the granular mass containing the trichina now curled up in the interior; the outer surface becomes distinctly thickened and indurated, and may then become lamellated or present granulations or folds. The sarcolemma takes no part in the formation of the cysts except occasionally furnishing it with a purely adventitious layer. Moreover, when the nematoid contracts its first adhesions to the sarcolemma, and not to the interfascicular tissue, it rapidly dies without determining a new formation.—*Lancet*, July 30, 1881.

The Need of Revaccination.

Dr. RENNER, in a communication to the *British Medical Journal* of June 4, 1881, shows in a very conclusive manner the very highly unprotected state of the adult population against smallpox, owing to the neglect of revaccination. In eighty-one cases in which persons had not been revaccinated since the first vaccination in infancy, ninety per cent. of the revaccination with calf-lymph proved successful; showing that, in ninety per cent. of those persons, the protection afforded during early life had worn out, and the necessary protection to be obtained by revaccination after the age of fifteen had been neglected, until the present alarm, owing to the epidemic prevalence of smallpox, had reminded them of the extreme danger of such neglect. As a matter of fact, it is essential, as a protection of the population from smallpox, that each individual should be successfully revaccinated after the age of fifteen. The rule is very simple, and the evidence overwhelming. Our soldiers, sailors, postmen, smallpox nurses, all of whom are revaccinated, enjoy an almost absolute immunity from smallpox, even during epidemic periods, and when surrounded with disease. The like immunity may be obtained by every rational member of the community who chooses to submit himself after the age of fifteen to revaccination. The present epidemic of smallpox is a lamentable monument of the human folly and neglect, which leave out of view a harmless and necessary precaution against so fatal and loathsome a disease. The responsibility of the misguided persons who seek to deter from obtaining this protection is great indeed; and it is difficult to use words of moderation in viewing all the fanatical ignorance and obstinate perversion of the truth of the facts with which they stimulate and maintain their reckless and mischievous crusade.

Ainhum.

Dr. FRANCIS GUYOT (*Le Prog. Méd.*, 1881, No. 19) gives a description of this peculiar tropical disease, and adds four cases observed by himself. It is met with in North Africa, in Southern India, Central America, and some of the Pacific islands. It affects generally the fifth toe, but sometimes the fourth, and more rarely many or all the fingers and toes. The chief symptom is an annular groove round the affected member, deeper on the palmar or plantar surface, growing deeper as it advances until amputation results. The surface of the fissure is normal; sometimes it is bathed in serous fluid, sometimes the segment above the fissure becomes swollen. In some cases the tissues of the stump are normal, more often atrophied or undergoing fatty degeneration, but preserve a healthy nucleus. There is neither inflammation, constitutional reaction, nor pain. It lasts often many years. It has no ultimate bad effects on the general health. The negroes attribute it to a parasite, but there is no evidence in favour of this view. Females do not escape. Consanguinity probably plays some part. No treatment is of use, though Da Silva Lima cured one case by an incision at right angles to the groove.—*London Med. Record*, July 15, 1881.

Antiseptic Inhalations in Pulmonary Affections.

Dr. J. G. SINCLAIR COGHILL, in the *Brit. Med. Journ.*, May, 1881, p. 841, has an interesting paper upon the value of antiseptic inhalations in all lung affections characterized by purulent expectoration. By this means we are enabled to dispense with cough-mixtures by arresting the secretion of the sputa; for, if sputa exist, cough must necessarily follow, and it is dangerous to arrest the cough under such circumstances. Dr. Coghill finds the following formula good: ℞ Tincturæ iodi etherealis, acid carbolici, āā ʒij; creasoti vel thymoli, ʒj; spiritûs vini rect., ad ʒj; M. If the cough be urgent, or breathing embarrassed, chloroform or sulphuric ether may be added at discretion. The mode of inhaling is most important. The patient should be carefully instructed to inspire through the mouth alone, and expire through the nose, as, by this means, the medicated air is forced into the remoter air-cells.—*London Med. Record*, July 15, 1881.

Surgery.

Removal of the Entire Tongue through the Mouth by Scissors..

In the Section on Surgery of the International Medical Congress, Dr. WALTER WHITEHEAD read a paper upon the removal of the tongue through the mouth with scissors, and gives the details of the operation. He says, "On November 3d, 1877, I removed the whole of the tongue through the mouth with scissors. (Vide *British Medical Journal*, 1877, Dec. 8, p. 303.)

"This case, to the best of my knowledge, was the first instance of the entire tongue having been removed for disease through the mouth by simple excision.

"More than thirty tongues have since been removed by the same plan.

"The operation is conducted in six stages after the following simple manner: 1. The mouth is opened to the full extent with a suitable gag; and the duty of attending to this is entrusted to one of the two assistants required. 2. The tongue is drawn out of the mouth by a double ligature passed through its substance an inch from the tip. 3. The operator commences by dividing all the attachments of the tongue to the jaw and to the pillars of the fauces. 4. The muscles attached to the base of the tongue are then cut across by a series of successive short snips of the scissors until the entire tongue is separated on the plane of the inferior border of the lower jaw, and as far back as the safety of the epiglottis will permit. 5. The lingual or any other arteries requiring torsion are twisted as divided. 6. A single loop of silk is passed by a long needle through the remains of the glosso-epiglottidean fold of mucous membrane, as a means of drawing forwards the floor of the mouth should secondary hemorrhage take place.

"The patient is fed for the first three days by nutritive enemata; satisfying thirst by occasionally washing out the mouth with a weak iced solution of permanganate of potash. The difficulties and dangers of the operation are few. Hemorrhage is easily controllable. I have twice removed the entire tongue without having to secure a single vessel, and more than once have only had to twist one lingual artery.

"A table of twenty-eight cases, with one death the immediate result of the operation (an old man æt. 62), accompanies the paper. Two other deaths occurred in consequence of the operation, but from remote causes.

"Taking the most unfavourable estimate, the deaths in the twenty-eight cases do not amount to 11 per cent., and, when contrasted with the 30 to 60 per cent. of deaths resulting from removal of the tongue by any other operation, I venture to affirm that substantial evidence has been submitted in favour of the removal of the tongue with scissors."—*Official Abstract of Proceedings International Medical Congress.*

Suprapubic Lithotomy.

In a recent contribution on "Lithotomy and Antisepticism" (*Archiv für Klin. Chir.*, Band xxvi., Heft 1, 1881), Dr. CARL LANGENBUCH of Berlin advocates the high (suprapubic) operation. In perineal lithotomy, the antiseptic method cannot be rigorously carried out, in consequence of the proximity of the anus, whilst in the high operation this method is applicable under very favourable circumstances. The risk of wounding the peritoneum in this latter operation is not so great as is generally supposed, since out of 478 cases of suprapubic lithotomy collected by Dr. Dulles, in thirteen only had this membrane been wounded, and of these three cases were fatal. It was shown also by the same author that any stone weighing more than two ounces could be removed with less risk by the high than by the perineal operation. This latter proceeding, however, in Germany, as in other countries, has long been almost exclusively favoured, high lithotomy having been resorted to in some few cases of very large and very hard stone.

The author considers whether this preference of perineal to suprapubic lithotomy can be supported by anatomical and physiological data and by clinical experience. Urinary infiltration of connective tissue, it is pointed out, is a danger common to both operations, which, however, in the suprapubic proceeding can be prevented. The danger of this infiltration, when it has occurred, is much less after the high than after the perineal operation, since the epi-cystic is more accessible and less confined than the peri-prostatic and circum-rectal connective tissue, can be more readily incised and disinfected, and, as it is not connected with any large venous plexus, is less likely through its decomposition to set up general septic infection. In the high operation, the incisions can be made carefully and precisely, and through structures that are freely exposed to view, and there is no necessity for forcible laceration and contusion of connective tissue and other soft parts. It may be said, the author suggests, that it is as difficult to set up urinary infiltration after the high operation, as it is to prevent such infiltration after lithotomy by the perineum.

In the high operation, when successfully performed, the only structures that are incised are integument, cellular tissue, and the wall of the bladder; all which structures are capable, after healing, of performing their physiological functions. In perineal lithotomy, on the other hand, many vascular and glandular structures must necessarily be wounded, and some of these are liable to be permanently injured. The latter operation may, it is true, be very often considered as successful; the stone has been removed, and the patient recovers; but it cannot be denied that it is often followed by one or more of such results as urethral stricture, incontinence, impotence, urinary fistula, recto-vesical fistula. With regard to the danger of wounding the peritoneum in the high operation, it is stated by the author that the topographical conditions of the para-cystic peritoneal fold in adults are not so unfavourable as is commonly supposed. Petersen of Kiel has shown by recent experiments on the dead body that, though the bladder is inaccessible when empty, yet, by the injection of water into this viscus and also into the rectum, the peritoneal reflexion can be elevated to an average distance of one inch and a third above the upper margin of the symphysis pubis. In a smaller series of experiments, Langenbuch has been able, by extreme distension of the bladder by injected fluid (800 to 1000 cubic centimetres), to raise above the symphysis from two inches to three inches and a third of uncovered vesical wall. In some of these experiments, it is stated that the bladder was filled almost to the point of bursting. With this question two factors, one negative, the other positive, come into play. In cases of calculous impaction at the neck of the bladder, especially when the stone is large, it will often be found impossible to introduce any quantity of fluid into this viscus. On the other hand, there is no necessity for free incision into the bladder, since the vesical wall, unless much thickened, is very elastic, and a small orifice can be readily dilated by traction in different directions. Langenbuch concludes that in ordinary cases sufficient room can be obtained above the symphysis for the performance of the high operation, by injecting the bladder, or, if this cannot be effected, by distending the rectum.

The risk of wounding the peritoneum in the high operation is no reason, Langenbueh holds, for preferring perineal lithotomy in these days of antiseptic surgery, when many laparotomies are performed yearly with little mortality. Much depends on whether the peritoneum be wounded before or after incision of the wall of the bladder. In the former, no danger is likely to result if the operation be performed under antiseptic conditions, and if the opening of the bladder be postponed for a time, and until after the cicatrization of the superficial wound. If the peritoneum be accidentally wounded after the vesical wall has been incised, then there is great risk of decomposed urine passing into the abdominal cavity and setting up fatal peritonitis.

For the removal of a large stone—one with a maximum diameter of about two inches—the safest proceeding, Langenbuch thinks, is the high operation performed in two stages, and under strict antiseptic conditions. To meet the case of a monster stone, measuring from four to seven inches in diameter, the extraction of which in the second stage of the high operation would probably cause much laceration of the recently healed superficial parts, and also of the peritoneal fluid, he proposes a complicated proceeding. A description is given of a high operation in two stages. In the first stage, the anterior surface of the bladder is freed to some extent of its layer of peritoneum, and a plastic operation is performed on this membrane. In the second stage—that of extraction performed after an interval of from five to eight days—elaborate precautions are taken to disinfect the bladder.

Dr. Langenbuch does not undertake in this paper to discuss how far the indications for lithotrity might be modified by a general acceptance of his proposed antiseptic high operation performed in two stages, but points out that, in the first place, the invention and development of lithotrity are due to the dangers of lithotomy, and that, in the second place, the former proceeding, as is well known, is not free from danger, nor capable in every case of effecting complete cure.— *London Med. Record*, June 15, 1881.

—

Treatment of Blood-Cysts of the Thyroid Gland by Electrolysis.

M. BERGER, in the name of M. Onimus and himself, read a communication on this subject at the last meeting of the Paris Société de Chirurgie (*Bull. Gén. de Thér.*, May 15, 1881). A lady had suffered for a year and a half with a tumour on the left side of the thyroid gland, and, latterly, it had rapidly increased in size. The first puncture was almost immediately followed by a relapse. The tumour rapidly became as large as an apple; it was movable, colourless, fluctuating, and already gave rise to disturbances in the action of the air-passages. M. Onimus proposed to treat it by electrolysis. On the 30th of January, MM. Berger and Onimus made a puncture, which gave issue to about 150 grammes of a chocolate-coloured liquid. A carbolated injection was then made by the channel; then an injection of a solution of iodide of potassium of ten degrees of strength. There was then introduced into the cystic cavity, filled with this solution, a metallic stem placed in communication with the positive and negative poles of the electric pile, of from 24 to 36 elements, whilst the other pole was applied on the periphery. There was a little hemorrhage. In a short time the cavity refilled itself, and the tumour was as large as ever. The day after the operation there was an attack of intermittent fever, which was only one of those diathetic reminders pointed out by M. Verneuil. M. Berger gave up the patient five months ago, being persuaded that it was a bad case. Four weeks ago he discovered that from the size of an apple the tumour had become reduced to that of a nut, and since that time it had decreased in considerable proportion. M. Boinet also related several cases in which he obtained excellent results after puncture, followed by the iodized injection. It was a mistake to believe that the iodized injection was also followed by acute inflammation, for in the cases to which he alluded there was neither inflammation nor suppuration. M. Delens remarked that he could not quite understand the curative action of electrolysis in M. Berger's case. The treatment was complex ; there had only been one application. Generally the action of electrolysis was much more slow, and it was necessary to repeat it frequently. M. Desprès pointed out that there were serous cysts with thin walls, which were cured with one simple puncture, and there were others with anfractuous walls, with syrupy and sticky contents, on which treatment was excessively difficult. In fact, in these cases the iodized injection did not succeed better than anything else. M. Le Dentu agreed with the last speaker as to the fact that there were mild cysts, and there were others in which the treatment was very difficult. It was not always easy to ascertain which variety was present. A puncture was made, blood flowed, and sometimes there was great difficulty in arresting the hemorrhage. The therapeutic treatment should therefore be varied according to the cases in serous cysts. The iodized injection left excellent results in sanguinous cysts. There was often a gangrenous inflammation, which might go on to elimination of the sac. The effect of electrolysis had yet to be determined. M. Berger concluded by owning that he was opposed to iodized injection, but he believed that in certain sanguineous cysts electrolysis brought on coagulation.—*London Med. Record*, July 15, 1881.

Symptomatology of Mediastinal Tumours.

A. SCHREIBER (*Deutsches Archiv für Klin. Med.*, Band. xxviii. s. 52, *Central für die Med. Wiss.*, No. 17, 1881) bases his remarks on four cases observed in Ziemssen's clinic. 1. A girl, aged 21, complained for some months of palpitation and breathlessness. There were physical signs of left-sided pleuritic effusion ; later on, a peculiar dulness developed, which began at the right costal cartilages and ran across the sternum to the left anterior axillary line, then downwards and backwards, and finally, horizontally, to the spine. The pleura was punctured many times with temporary benefit. There were then some difficulty in swallowing, and slight right-sided pleuritic effusion. There was a fibro-sarcomatous tumour as large as a man's head. 2. A baker, aged 17, complained for eight days of cough, pain in the chest, and loss of appetite. The expression of his face was anxious, the skin was yellowish, the veins of the neck were distended. He had a barking cough. There were paralysis of the right vocal chords, and multiple swollen lymphatic glands. He had slight fever. Later on there was increased glandular swelling, especially along the lower border of the pectoralis major. He had increasing breathlessness. There was dulness above the heart, reaching up to the clavicle and to the axillary line. Section showed a round-celled sarcoma of the anterior mediastinum, with numerous metastases which pressed on the vena cava and recurrent nerve. 3. This case was that of a woman, aged 35, with diffuse fibro-sarcoma of the mediastinum, which led to metastases in the lungs, and to closure of the vena cava and subclavian vein. 4. A peasant, aged 31, had been ill eight and a half years. He was breathless and had swollen veins on the thorax. There was a resistant tumour in the left supraclavicular region. He had œdema of the face. There was protrusion of sternum and superior thoracic region. There was absolutely empty note over the whole sternum and along the right sternal border. The dulness was limited to the left by a line drawn from the attachment of the third rib, outwards and downwards to a centimetre outside the nipple.—*London Med. Record*, July 15, 1881.

—

Causes of Death from Burns.

LESSER (Virchow's *Archiv*, Band lxxix.) first of all combats the deductions drawn by Sonnenburg from his experiments (*Deutche Zeitsch. fur Chir.*, Band. ix.), and, supported by his own experiments, conclude that irritation of the terminations of the cutaneous nerves is of no special importance in death rapidly following burns. He then passes on to demonstrate the changes which take place in the blood circulating in the skin in burns of the surface of the body ; and further, the changes induced in the body by these alterations. He has come to the conclusion that (apparently without essential destruction of the red corpuscles) the red colouring matter of the blood becomes diffused in the plasma. He proves this by transfusing defibrinated blood heated to above 70 deg. Cent. (158 deg. Fahr.), as well as that of previously burned animals. The diffused colouring matter is chiefly excreted by the kidneys in the urine, as is evident from examination of the urine and kidneys. The excretion begins about an hour after the burning, and may continue as long as two days. On *post-mortem* examination, extravasations of blood were discovered in various organs, and in the kidneys large collections of blood-colouring matter especially within the convoluted tubes, pigment-granules between the epithelium, hyaline cylinders, etc. On the ground of previous, as well as some more recent, experiments, Lesser discusses the possible causes of death ; and, after eliminating numerous possibilities, advances the theory that a relatively too large number of red disks (through separation of the blood-colouring matter and consecutive damage) become fully developed, so that a sufficient quantity of blood for the completion of the respiratory processes necessary for the prolongation of life is no longer furnished, and, as a consequence, paralysis of the respiratory and circulatory centres ensues.

Lesser thinks that the injurious effects of burns on the general system depend neither on the thickness and capacity for resistance of the skin, the extent of the burned region, nor on the intensity or length of the operation ; but that for seriousness of the burns it is necessary that the circulation should be kept up in the burned parts, and that new masses of blood should constantly stream through the heated skin and muscles ; the longer this is continued, so much the greater being the number of the red corpuscles robbed of their vitality. At a later period, death may result from septicæmia.

Lesser speaks strongly in favour of the method of treatment already recommended by Ponfick for severe burns ; viz., transfusion, in addition to local antiseptic treatment, and is of opinion than transfusion may still be useful at a later period, if the patient do not recover his strength.—*Lond. Med. Record*, July 15, 1881.

Rupture of the Bladder.

In a paper read at the German Medical Society of St. Petersburg (*St. Petersburg Med. Woch.*, June 11), Dr. ASSMUTH stated that he had brought forward two cases of rupture of the bladder from muscular exertion in consequence of the rarity of the accident; for, although these two cases were admitted into the Obuchow Hospital in two successive years (1879 and 1880), yet Bartels, in his monograph on the subject, states that among 10,867 surgical cases, treated at the Bethanieu in Berlin (1869–76), only three cases of rupture of the bladder occurred, and in 16,711 surgical cases at St. Bartholomew's only two cases occurred. Of the 169 cases collected by Bartels, not one arose from mere muscular exertion.

The subject of the *first* case was a man, thirty-two years old, who, while removing a heavy sack of flour from a railway platform to a cart, was seized with a violent pain in the hypogastrium. Trying some time after to make water, he only passed a few drops of blood. He came to the hospital on foot two days afterwards. His pulse was then 88, and his temperature 37.7° C. There was great tenderness in the hypogastrium, and a catheter only withdrew a few drops of blood. His general condition, and the apparent absence of any cause for it, prevented the diagnosis of a ruptured bladder, which the local symptoms would have justified. He soon, however, became much worse, and died on the sixth day after the accident, without having passed a drop of urine. The autopsy exhibited recent general peritonitis, and a rupture, two centimetres and one-third in length, at the upper part of the posterior wall of the bladder, a little to the right of its apex. The *second* case occurred in the person of a man forty years of age, who, two days prior to admission, had been seized with a violent pain in the hypogastrium while endeavouring to raise a very heavy burthen. He died on the sixth day after the accident. Peritonitis with purulent exudation was found, together with a rupture, three centimetres in length, at the right side of the posterior wall of the bladder, about two centimetres from the apex. The mucous membrane of the bladder was quite normal in appearance, and no trace of coagulum was found within the organ or in its vicinity. Of the urine, which during life had in both cases collected in the right hypogastrium, there was but little found after death, it having evidently become diffused by the intestinal movements. The local tenderness in that region became less concentrated in that spot; and after death a diffused peritonitis was found to be present.

In both these cases the muscular exertion required to raise a heavy burthen was obviously the cause of the rupture, and although hitherto no example of such an occurrence has been published, yet an analogous action in the production of fractures and dislocation is not rare. Although both patients denied that the urine had been long held in the bladder, there can be little doubt that considerable distension must have existed. In practice we frequently meet with very erroneous statements as to the fulness of the bladder, and that not only from defective self-observation, but also from impaired elasticity of the walls of the bladder, preventing a right judgment being formed as to its distension. In both cases the localization of the rupture of the bladder was the same; and Dr. Assmuth deduces from Hyrtl's description of the anatomy of the bladder that this was at the feeblest part of the organ.—*Med. Times and Gazette*, July 23, 1881.

Cancer of the Breast and Meninges.

The following case is related by Dr. OTTO LUND, in the *Norsk Magazin for Lägevidensk* for 1880. A woman, aged 59, was operated on, in October, 1869, for a cancer of the right breast; and in November, 1876, for a cancerous infiltration of the glands in the right axilla. In the interval, three years after the first operation, the patient—who was said to have suffered several times while young from convulsions and attacks of giddiness, and afterwards also from migraine— was again seized with giddiness, which came on, or was made worse, when she turned her head to the right, while lying in bed. The attack of giddiness passed off gradually; but, after some years, she had sciatic pains in the left lower limb, and periodical pains in the right half of the forehead, and in the right temple, with tenderness on pressure. There was no disturbance of intelligence; weakness of memory was first observed in 1880. In February she had an epileptiform attack, with loss of consciousness and tonic convulsions, during which the head and eyes were turned to the right side; after the attack, there was found to be paralysis of the upper and lower limbs. The intellect also became disturbed; and she died on March 29th, fourteen days after a similar attack to that above described. On *post-mortem* examination, a cancerous nodule, of the size of a nut, was found in the left breast (this had been observed during life); there were two disk-shaped cancerous growths, respectively 5 and 3 centimetres (2 inches, and 1.2 inches) in diameter, and about half a centimetre thick, in the arachnoid in the right parietal region, and a smaller similar tumour on each side of the crista galli. There was fatty degeneration of the heart.—*London Med. Record,* June 15, 1881.

Of Syphilis Fungus.

Dr. BERMANN of Baltimore describes (*Archives of Med.*, Dec. 1880, p. 263) certain microscopic growths which he found in syphilitic primary sores, and which he believes to be peculiar to that disease. The author begins by quoting Klebs's experiments on the subject, and states that, before the publication of that observer's views, he had already discovered certain fungoid growths in a freshly excised prepuce obtained from Zeissl. What first attracted Dr. Bermann's attention was a singular collection of micrococci and fungoid growths, firmly adhering to and partly filling up the lumen of most of the lymphatic vessels. Some of the arteries also contained these growths, intermixed with blood-corpuscles. The growths were found in all the hundreds of sections made by the author. The micrococci are small, strongly refracting spherical bodies, and resemble those illustrated by Klebs; but the bacteria, described by the same observer, Dr. Bermann found only in a few instances, and then only in the arteries. The principal changes take place in the lymphatics, and chiefly in those at some distance from the initial sclerosis, which explains, according to the author, why others have been unsuccessful in discovering these organisms.—*London Med. Record,* June 15, 1881.

Case of Hepatotomy for Hydatids.

Mr. LAWSON TAIT, in a communication to the *British Medical Journal* for July 16, 1881, says: "The following notes briefly give the details of the sixth case of this operation which I have performed; and, like the others, it has been remarkable for the speedy and complete recovery of the patient from the operation, and the thorough cure of the disease from which she was suffering.

" A. M. S., aged 7, was admitted to the Women's Hospital early in May last, suffering from severe symptoms due to a tumour which existed on the right side and above the level of the umbilicus, which was clearly cystic, and in all probability connected with the liver. It gave the patient great pain; and I diagnosed it to be a hydatid tumour of the liver. She had been under the care of my friend

Dr. Welch at the Children's Hospital, who has kindly favoured me with the following notes.

"The child never was strong; on the contrary, she had always been regarded as delicate. A year ago, her mother noticed that her motions were rather white-coloured. A swelling was noticed in the abdomen about November last, and she complained of pain across the back and shoulders. When she was admitted to the Children's Hospital, in December, 1880, there was a firm tumour just below the ensiform cartilage, the dulness extending round the side. It was noticed in February that there were some nodules on the surface of the liver, also that the tumour was more freely movable.

"When she was admitted to the Women's Hospital, under my care, she had a tumour about the size of a fœtal head, which was extremely tender to the touch. The child was very sick and ill, and altogether her appearance warranted interference. I therefore opened the abdomen on May 20th, making an incision about three inches long, an inch and a half to the left of the umbilicus, the lower end corresponding to the umbilical level. When the cavity was opened, it was perfectly clear that the tumour was situated in the liver, and was a hydatid cyst. I removed from it, by means of an aspirator, about twenty-six ounces of clear fluid containing a large number of scolices. I then enlarged the aperture in the liver to about an inch and a half, and secured its edges to the edges of the parietal wound by means of a continuous suture, and fastened in a wide soft India-rubber drainage-tube about six inches long. She went on perfectly well; her severe symptoms were immediately relieved, and on May 26th the mother-cyst came away entire. The drainage-tube was removed on May 30th; and on June 2d she left the hospital with the wound quite healed, having gained greatly in weight, and having acquired a perfectly healthy appearance.

"No attempt was made to conduct the case upon Listerian principles, the only dressings used to the wound being lead lotion and absorbent wool."

—

Treatment of Intra-Thoracic Suppurating Hydatid.

At the April meeting of the Medical Society of Victoria, Dr. S. D. BIRD reported two cases in which intra-thoracic hydatid cysts, which had advanced to the stage of death and decomposition, were got rid of by incision between the ribs. Such treatment is, of course, a more complete and radical cure than any system of tapping, injection of parasiticide fluids, or electricity can be, as the latter always leave with the cyst the possibility of its refilling if its vitality is not completely destroyed, of which we cannot be absolutely sure. On the other hand, extraction is a much more serious operation, and one that requires considerable time and patience for its successful accomplishment, as well as the existence of certain conditions without which such a procedure would be hardly allowable.

To my mind the conditions that justify incision between the ribs, with the view of extracting hydatid cysts, are—*First*, any case of hydatid in the pleural sac, in which situation the cyst always enlarges with great rapidity, and even when emptied of its contents, or dealt with in any way short of removal, remains a permanent source of irritation to the serous surface, with consequent pleuritic pains, febrile irritation, and even inflammatory effusion. The question now naturally arises as to the possibility of the differential diagnosis of pleural hydatid from one in the lower lobe of the lung, or in the convex surface of the liver, especially on the right side. In most cases it will be very difficult to decide before operation, the only special physical sign of pleural hydatid being that the usual rounded area of dulness is to some degree alterable by change of position, which is not the case if the cyst is embedded in the lung substance. In my cases the pleural cyst has always been loose, and has not contracted adhesions to the serous surface.

The *second* set of cases demanding incision and extraction are those of large old suppurating cysts of the lung which have generally found their way into a bronchus, and fragments of cyst and fetid pus are being constantly expectorated with great labour and distress to the patient.   Such cases are generally in the lobe, and if of long standing, adhesions will almost certainly be found to have taken place, so that the operation will be comparatively safe and easy. I have seen over a dozen of such cases, and in no one has the result been other than completely successful. I shall now proceed to read notes, hitherto unpublished, of two cases, one of pleural and the other pulmonary hydatid, treated in this way.

Mrs. G., æt. 26, married lady with two children, native of a neighbouring colony, consulted me for a condition which had been diagnosed variously as pleurisy with effusion, enlargement of the liver, and abscess. On examination, the right side measured one and a half inches larger than the left, intercostal spaces not bulged. There was no febrile pleuritic history, but she described stitchy pains all over the side of a distinctly pleuritic character, and also pains in the point of the shoulder that were suggestively hepatic. On percussion and auscultation the question of pleuritic effusion was set at rest, as the rounded area of dulness characteristic of hydatid presented itself in the lower part of the right chest, while the breath sounds and percussion note at the apex were normal, even when the hips were raised above the level of the thorax. The rounded dull area shifted a little with gravitation in this position, but hardly enough to convince either the late Dr. Martin (who consulted with me) or myself, of the diagnosis of pleural hydatid absolutely, for of course a large cyst in the convex surface of the liver would shift and alter the relations of the diaphragm to its parallel ribs by the weight of that heavy bulky viscus in the inversed position of the body. In any case, it was determined to introduce a trocar, which was done in the seventh intercostal space, when three pints of semi-purulent fluid escaped, showing plenty of hooklets on microscopic examination. Not much relief followed, and there was ill-defined dulness about the base of the right lung, with pleuritic stitches, and persistent high pulse and temperature, evidencing a local source of irritation in the pleura. Feeling convinced now that the case was one of pleural hydatid, I determined, with the concurrence of Dr. Martin, to remove it, as the only method of accomplishing a cure.   On the tenth day after the first tapping, I made a free incision between the seventh and eighth ribs at the same position, and accordingly removed, without any difficulty, a large semi-decomposed hydatid cyst, broken into several fragments. The site was now beyond doubt, for I passed my little finger through the wound, and felt the round surface of the liver through the thin interval of the pleura and diaphragm. A few ounces of pus and broken-down fragments of hydatid followed the main cyst, and then rather a free discharge of venous blood, which, however, soon ceased. I left a piece of drainage tube in the pleura as a precaution.   The patient experienced the greatest relief from the operation ; the febrile symptoms and pain all left her, and the physical signs gave no evidence of any further foreign body in the cavity of the thorax ; in fact, for several days everything promised a speedy recovery. I had the advantage of Mr. Fitzgerald's opinion on the case, and he concurred in the diagnosis and treatment.   However, about a fortnight after the removal of the cyst, the patient began to complain again of dyspnœa and oppression of the chest, and on exploring the cavity of the pleura with an elastic catheter, to my great disgust I burst into another cyst, from which ran about ten ounces of perfectly clear hydatid fluid, swarming with echinococci in full vigour and vitality. I succeeded in removing this cyst also, and irrigated the pleura frequently with weak solutions of iodine, with a view of destroying any lurking ova. Again great relief followed, but the poor patient was doomed to be the victim of the parasite, for soon heart distress commenced, exactly similar to that experienced by another case of pleural hydatid recorded by me in my pamphlet on this subject.

Sudden and alarming attacks of dyspnœa, generally ending in syncope, with cardiac murmurs terribly jumbled and confused. These symptoms increased in intensity till in one of them the poor lady died suddenly, the pleura and lung being apparently quite restored to their normal condition. Unfortunately there could be no post-mortem, but I have no doubt that the cause of death was hydatid of the pericardium, similar to that in my other patient, a preparation of whose heart is in the University Museum. It seems almost as if, when hydatids attack one serous sac, similar cavities are more attractive to them than the solid viscera. A very remarkable feature in these two cases was the extraordinary rapidity with which the new cysts developed in the pleura and pericardium, a few days only being sufficient to cause urgent symptoms in one case and death in the other.

The other case being one of hydatid of the lung substance had a more happy result. A girl nine years old was brought to me by her parents from a township in the northeastern district, about seventy miles from Melbourne. She was excessively emaciated with intense hectic and rapid pulse. Cough constant and violent, with expectoration of pus and fragments of cyst of horrible fetor. She was only able to breathe in one position, lying over and partially prone on the affected side. Any change from this caused alarming symptoms of suffocation, and as the poor child had been in the same state for over two months bedsores on the side were very distressing. A large trocar introduced between the fifth and sixth ribs gave exit to many ounces of fetid pus and fragments of cyst, giving great relief. After two days I enlarged the opening, and succeeding in removing the parent cyst, and left a piece of drainage tube in the nidus of the parasite which was frequently washed out with weak solution of Condy's fluid. In less than a month from her arrival the child returned to her home in perfect health, the wound having healed up from the bottom. I rather pushed on the treatment in this case as the symptoms were so urgent, but I am convinced that in the majority of cases one of the great factors of the constant success that attends them is to take time over the different steps of the operative procedure, so as to allow the lung time to expand, especially in adults.—*Australian Medical Journal*, April 15, 1831.

Early Resection in Tuberculous Disease of the Joints.

Dr. König, of Göttingen, in a paper read before the recent congress of German surgeons, ascribed only a limited value to early resection in tuberculous disease of joints. In a case of white swelling of the knee, with fistulæ and abscesses, he had obtained a cure by expectant treatment; and, in a case of coxitis, with large abscesses reaching to the middle of the femur, he had laid the parts freely open, and scraped the bone, without any disturbance of motor power. He had also acted in the same way, producing only slight impairment of motion, in a case of contraction of the adductor muscles, with a slight shortening of the limb. It was only when the patient's general condition was seriously implicated by the local disease, or when there was danger of the occurrence of this, that resection should be done without delay. In a large number of cases, resection might be done to a very limited extent, especially when the neighbouring joint was not implicated in the disease of the bone. Up to 1879 he had successfully treated in this way five cases of this kind, but afterwards he had twenty-one cases. Of these, the elbow-joint was affected in eleven cases; the hip in four;

the tarsus in six ; and the knee in five. Ten recovered with useful limbs ; in twelve, small fistulæ still remained ; one died of erysipelas ; and the result in one case was not known. Such diseases of bone usually revealed themselves by abscesses affecting the epiphysis, and by little pits on the surface of the bone, which denoted the commencement of fistulous tracks. An accidental opening of the joint in operating was harmless, under antiseptic protection. Cases might occur, though rarely, in which the morbid deposit in the bone could only be reached through the joint.—*London Med. Record*, June 15, 1881.

Ozæna ʼfrom Retained Secretion.

Dr. KENDAL FRANKS, in a paper read before the Dublin Biological Club, and published in the *Dublin Journal of Medical Sciences* for June, 1881, reports several cases of this not rare form of ozæna. He makes the following remarks upon this important subject :—

In treating of the subject of ozæna in general we must distinguish between two classes of morbid conditions in which fetid nasal breath is a prominent symptom. I exclude at once all cases in which the fetor is due to diseases in the deeper structures of the nasal cavity, as ulceration, caries of the bones, and abnormal growths, or when foreign bodies are the immediate cause.

But, independently of these, we find two distinct classes—one in which the ozæna is due to some lesion of the mucous membrane, most frequently the result of a dyscrasia ; the second class comprising those cases in which there is no such lesion to which to attribute the disease, or in which an altered state of the mucous membrane is the result of the ozæna, and not its cause. This form has till the last few years been apparently quite overlooked, and it at present forms the subject of an interesting and animated controversy with our Continental brethren. It is to this latter form that I desire to call your special attention.

In all the standard works in which the subject of ozæna is discussed we find no allusion to this form of the disease. In Ziemssen's Cyclopædia, ozæna, the "Stinknase" of the Germans, the "punaisie" of the French, from its fancied resemblance to the smell of crushed bugs, is classed under the same heading as chronic rhinitis, and it has origin accordingly in a dyscrasia. "Acute rhinitis," Fraenkel tells us, "may pass into the subacute or chronic forms, and yet in the vast majority of cases this *only takes place in persons suffering under a dyscrasia.* Scrofula and syphilis are particularly liable to induce this transition. . . . We can distinguish two forms of chronic catarrh in the nose—the hyperplastic and the atrophic forms. They often coexist, but in most cases the atrophic form seems to be the result of the hyperplastic ; at least it is most commonly found in old cases, and after the prolonged continuance of the hyperplastic." This is the order of events which we find in the pharynx : The three stages of chronic follicular pharyngitis are repeated in the nasal cavities, beginning as a chronic catarrhal pharyngitis, going on to hypertrophy of the follicles and mucous membrane, and finally, as the follicles wear out, the retrograde process taking place, and atrophic pharyngitis or pharyngitis sicca being the result. In the nose we have the same sequence—a chronic rhinitis is established. This is the result of an acute attack occurring in persons presenting other symptoms of dyscrasia ; or "in persons having no dyscrasia, an acute rhinitis under bad care, continuance of the irritant, and under injurious influences, may relapse and finally terminate in the chronic form." This chronic form is at first of the hypertrophic kind, the mucous membrane being thickened and red, the secretion being of a muco-purulent character, and abundant in quantity. Morgagni relates a case in which it amounted to an ounce per hour. Should the mucous membrane be sufficiently tumefied to cause obstruction of the nose, the secretions are retained and by degrees decompose, their composition giving rise to the fetor of ozæna. This, however, is not a very frequent occurrence during this stage of the disease. It is in the later stage, when the hyperplasia gives place to atrophy, that this symptom declares itself with all its unpleasant consequences. To this latter stage Gottstein applies the term, "chronic atrophic rhinitis." Robinson, in his recent work on "Nasal Catarrh," calls it "the dry form of chronic coryza." It seems to be brought about in the following way: During the hypertrophic stage there is deposited in the deep layer of the mucous membrane new formations of connective tissue and hyperplasia of the normal elements found there. This new tissue so presses upon the glands and follicles that their function is almost, if not entirely destroyed, and they consequently atrophy, or as the inflammatory products become organized and contract, they so constrict the glands that atrophy is the result. In proportion to the activity or intensity of these processes is the rapidity with which these changes occur; and hence, though we generally find the atrophic stage coming on at a late period after the hypertrophic stage has existed for years, still we need not be surprised if we find them coming on at a comparatively early epoch, so that the early stage of enlargement of the glands, thickening of the mucous membrane, and abundant secretion, may almost be overlooked. The appearance of the nasal passages and of the naso-pharyngeal space is very characteristic. The first thing we observe is an abnormal dryness of the mucous membrane in these regions. It has a glazed, parchment-like appearance, and is covered with inspissated mucus. This is very thick, and has a tendency to form crusts: "These," says Fraenkel,[1] " become firmly attached to the subjacent surface, perhaps owing to the large amount of albumen they contain, and by reason of their wealth in morphological elements (numerous epithelial cells) and their dearth of fluid constituents, are easily dried by the air passing over them." The tenacity with which these crusts cling to the mucous membrane beneath is exhibited when trying to remove them—sometimes they resist even a stream of water directed against them; and this tenacity is characteristic also, though in a less degree, of the dry pellicle of mucus which has not gone so far as to form crusts. The amount of secretion is very great, and is poured out as thick viscid mucus. It, however, rapidly dries, and if retained, as it will be unless proper means be used to get rid of it, it decomposes and gives rise to the characteristic stench. Fraenkel attributes the retention and drying of the secretion to the abundance of cells, the paucity of water, and its stickiness, but considers that defective cleaning of the nose aids in accomplishing the result: "This may be owing to habitual failure to blow one's nose, to feebleness of the expiratory current of air at the point affected (stenosis), or to diminished reflex irritability and an absence of a disposition to sneeze." Cohen, in his lecture on Naso-pharyngeal Catarrh,[2] takes a more histological view of the case when he attributes these conditions to a destruction of the epithelium. I need scarcely remind you that the epithelium lining the respiratory tract, with a few exceptions, is of the ciliated variety, and that the cilia have a continuous waving motion towards the exterior. In the nasal passages these cilia are continually brushing away excess of mucus. The diseased condition of the mucous membrane in chronic rhinitis causes destruction of numbers of the ciliated epithelia, and these are not reproduced. Hence this *potent* cause, according to Cohen, is absent, and retention is the result.

On removing the dried mucus and crusts from the surface, the mucous membrane has a remarkable appearance—it is reddened, the result of the cleansing

---

[1] Ziemssen's Cyclopædia, vol. iv. p. 138.
[2] Medical News and Library, October, 1879.

process, and looks dry and raw. Looking up into the naso-pharynx, by means of the rhinoscope, the same condition is seen, and tumefied masses of glands and follicles are visible on the vault and sides. The posterior portions of the turbinated bones present the same dry crusts and pledgets of mucus, and sometimes an entire turbinated bone is covered over as if with a false membrane. Anteriorly the same appearance is seen. The turbinated bones are distinct and normal in size, the mucous membrane covering them thin and atrophied, the secretion dry and encrusted. The symptoms which this condition give rise to are similar to those observed in the next class of ozænæ, to which I will now call your attention.

In this class of ozænæ no lesion is found, no disease of the mucous membrane, to which this disagreeable condition can be assigned; cases in which there is no previous history of a catarrh, or of a period at which there was an abundant odourless discharge. To account for such cases, to determine the true cause for a most pungent symptom, where to all appearance no disease exists, has been the endeavour of several astute observers in Germany. Several, among whom I may mention Gottstein, have attempted to class these cases under the third or atrophic form of chronic catarrh; but this is eminently unsatisfactory, as there has never been a second or third stage—and for other reasons to which I shall have occasion to refer again, I pass by this opinion as untenable. There still remain two views, which have been put prominentlyforward by their exponents. The first we shall consider is that propounded by Michel.[1] Recognizing the fact that the mucous membrane of the nose and pharynx is more or less healthy, and that its condition is quite insufficient to account for the ozæna, he lays emphasis on the exceeding abundance of the discharges. The mucous membrane of the nasal passages he considers is incapable of secreting so abundantly; for, if altered, it is on the side of atrophy. Whence then does the discharge come? Evidently not from the nose, but from the accessory cavities. The only cavities which could be the cause of it are the sphenoidal and ethmoidal sinuses, since anatomical considerations preclude the other sinuses from being the chief factors. Thus the opening of the antrum into the middle meatus of the nose is situated in the upper part of the internal wall, so that any flow of mucus from it could only be by overflow, and there are no evidences that the antrum is full of fluid. The frontal sinuses could not discharge fluid on to the upper surface of the middle turbinated bone, where it is seen to exist, as their openings into the nose are situated below the anterior extremity of this bone. Hence he concludes that a chronic catarrh exists in the sphenoidal and ethmoidal sinuses, which by retaining the secretions allows them to decompose, and by then discharging them over every portion of the nasal cavity gives rise to ozæna.

Now this theory, which is very plausible, is not sustained by facts. In the first instance, the grounds on which it is based are hypothetical, for the author has failed to demonstrate that any catarrh of these sinuses does actually exist; whilst, on the other hand, in a well-marked case of the disease, Hartmann, who made a *post-mortem* examination, could detect no abnormal condition of these cavities.

The second view enunciated is by Zaufal,[2] and the cases which I shall lay before you seem to me to support this view. He states the case thus: This class of ozæna, in which no lesion is found, affects children, and especially girls arriving at the age of puberty. The parents usually state that the fetor began to show itself within the last few months. The child finds great difficulty in blowing its

---

[1] Maladies du Nez et du Pharynx Nasal. Berlin, 1876. Traduction Franç. Par A. Capart. Paris, 1879.

[2] Aerztliches Correspondenzblatt aus Böhmen, No. 23, 1874.

nose, and the particles emitted are composed of horribly fetid, greenish crusts. The young patient is pale and dispirited, complaining sometimes of cephalalgia. The scrofulous diathesis is not specially marked ; the nose is flattened, the septum is deflected to one side; so as to compress the lachrymal canal and cause epiphora. The alæ nasi are enlarged, but the nasal fossæ specially have a remarkable aspect to those who are well acquainted with their usual appearance. Instead of the normal narrowness of the passages between the septum nasi and the middle and inferior turbinated bones, a true cavern is seen to exist, due to the almost complete absence of these two turbinated bones, especially of the inferior, which are reduced to mere ridges, thus exposing to view the trumpet-shaped opening of the Eustachian tube, all the movements of which during phonation and deglutition are clearly seen. The whole septum and back of the pharynx are well exposed. Abundant semi-inspissated or dried crusts cover over the various parts, and if they be removed by irrigation the mucous membrane beneath is found to be reddened, but without any trace of ulceration. At the same time it seems to be atrophied. Over the inferior turbinated bone the erectile structure has disappeared, and a probe comes into immediate contact with the turbinated bone. This characteristic conformation may exist only on one side, or it may be hereditary, the mother who brings the child having a nose formed absolutely in the same way.[1]

Michel, who has seen this condition and recognized it, in holding to his own view, does not consider the malformation sufficient explanation of the disease ; whilst Gottstein considers that the small size of the bones is part of the general atrophic process which goes on during the third stage of the catarrh. But then Michel's theory does not explain why the ozæna should be hereditary, why it appears always at puberty, or why it may sometimes be unilateral ; and Gottstein does not state why in some cases of atrophic catarrh the turbinated bones do not share in the process.

On the other hand, Zaufal maintains that this excessive arrest of development explains these points, as well as accounting for the occurrence of ozæna. The ozæna is simply the result of the size of the nasal fossæ. The mucous secretions are no longer driven forwards little by little, as takes place in the normal condition when the expired air plays on the turbinated bones. The air goes out more slowly ; the mucus, no longer drawn with it, retains its position and decomposes. Moreover he points out that there is not an abnormal increase in the secretion, as stated by Michel, but that it is only apparent, and results from the fact that the patient cannot blow his nose. The disease does not make itself apparent in early life. The child is born with rudimentary turbinated bones.. During the first few years, the nose being very small, the disease does not declare itself ; but, as the child grows, the bones of the face gradually develop, the turbinated bones remain stationary, and at or about puberty ozæna appears.

The retention, drying, and decomposition of the secretion on the surface of the mucous membrane reacts in an injurious way on this membrane, with whose function it interferes, and thus causes it to undergo a process of atrophy more or less pronounced, so that this atrophy, instead of being the cause is in reality the consequence of the ozæna.

—

Blindness after Glaucoma.

KUBLI reports the following case of total blindness from glaucoma simplex, in which vision was restored. The patient, a man, aged 21, stated (*Klin. Monats. für Augen.*, Oct. 1880) that his sight had been steadily failing for twelve months,

---

[1] Hayem. Revue des Sciences Médicales, April 15, 1880.

with occasional appearance of a coloured ring around the light, and that two months ago he had suddenly become totally blind. No other symptoms were complained of. On admission, both eyes presented T + 2, glaucomatous cupping of the disks, total absence of perception of light, oval dilatation of the pupils. The pupils gave no reaction to light, but contracted with movements of convergence, and were contracted strongly by eserine. Iridectomy upwards was performed on each eye. Perception of light returned the following day. Vision ultimately reached 3-100; whether in both eyes, or in one only, is not stated. [The strong contraction of the pupils by eserine is worthy of note in connection with the exceptionally good result. There is no reason to believe that such contraction in a glaucomatous eye indicates that the angle of the anterior chamber, though compressed, has not reached the stage of solid adhesion.—*Rep.*] —*London Med. Record*, June 15, 1881.

Operation for Trichiasis.

FÆSCHE recommends (*Klin. Monats. für Augen.*, xix. Jahrg., January) the following modification of Arlt's operation for trichiasis. In the first act, the upper lid is split into an anterior and a posterior part, as in Arlt's operation. In the second act, the anterior part is pushed up on the posterior about 1-12th to 1-10th of an inch, and fixed with three sutures on the tarsal cartilage. The middle of the three sutures is applied transversely, and includes about 1-8th of an inch, the other two sutures are vertical. The raw surface thus left, in place of being allowed to heal by granulation, as in Arlt's method, is covered with a thin strip of epidermis taken from the upper arm with a razor. With proper care, this transplanted strip heals in its place in twenty-four hours. Immediately on the eye the author lays a protective disinfected with salicylic and boracic acid, then a fold of lint similarly disinfected, over this salicylic cotton-wool, and over all, carbolized gauze. The first dressing may remain on for forty-eight hours. The author has used this method in twelve cases, and is thoroughly satisfied with it.—*London Med. Record*, June 15, 1881.

Midwifery and Gynæcology.

The Broad Ligament and Pelvic Cellulitis.

The anatomical and pathological relations of the broad ligament to the cellular tissue of the pelvis have recently been occupying the attention of several distinguished French authorities. The internal female organs lie very conspicuously in the pelvic cavity, and are so characteristic in outline as to be fairly familiar to every student. Much has been written on the nature of pelvic cellulitis and pelvic peritonitis by the greatest authorities on the diseases of women, and it is easy to beg the question, and to accept the doctrine, not as yet entirely discarded, that injuries and diseases of the vagina and uterus may set up forms of inflammation in the cellular tissue of the broad ligament, ending in the formation of an abscess within that structure. The layers of this ligament, closely applied to each other between the Fallopian tube and the ovary, diverge widely below the ovary ; and the anterior continues forwards, to form the serous investment of the bladder, the posterior passing backwards as the peritoneum forming Douglas's pouch. It is a common idea that the pelvic cellular tissue fills up the lower part of the broad ligament, where the peritoneal layers are diverging towards the bladder and rectum, and, passing upwards, forms a thin but distinct stratum of cellular tissue between the folds of the ligament as far as to its very uppermost limit below, or rather around, the Fallopian tube.   If this were really the case, the formation of abscess between the folds of the broad ligament would be of very frequent occurrence in pelvic cellulitis.

The presence of a distinct layer of cellular tissue in the interior of the ligament is, indeed, taught by the authors of one of the best and most widely studied French text-books ; for in Cruveilhier and Sée's *Traité d'Anatomie*, it is written : " The broad ligaments are formed by two peritoneal folds and by an intermediate layer of cellular tissue, through which pass the numerous vessels and nerves supplying the uterus and ovary, as well as a quantity of muscular fibres derived from the uterus." Whatever may have been the views of past authorities on the anatomy of the ligament, they almost universally admitted the frequency of abscess within it.   Dr. Matthews Duncan has shown, in his work *On Perimetritis and Parametritis*, that such a condition is " very far from being common." The error, he believes, arose from the frequency of the presence of pus within the veins and lymphatics of the ligament, in fatal cases of puerperal fever.   At necropsies, these purulent collections were taken for circumscribed abscesses.

MM. A. GUÉRIN and LEBEC have recently made the broad ligament an object of special study, and the fruits of their researches will be found in the *Gazette Hebdomadaire de Médecine et de Chirurgie*, April 15th.   They insist on the selection of perfectly normal adult bodies for the dissection of these parts, subjects not easy to obtain ; for slight attacks of adhesive inflammation in the parts around the internal organs are very common.   In detaching the peritoneum from the bony walls of the true pelvis, a layer of cellular tissue is pulled up with it ; this layer, almost as aponeurotic as the pelvic fascia itself, they call the fascia propria.   This layer seals up hermetically the outer extremity of the broad ligament, which lies entirely below the fimbriæ of the Fallopian tube and the ovary. Another layer of dense cellular tissue is given off horizontally from the fascia propria, and forms a complete floor to the broad ligament.   Hence the interior of this ligament is bounded by the uterus internally, by the tube above, and by the fascia propria below and antero-externally.   The amount of cellular tissue between the layers of the ligament is very small, and cannot be said to constitute a " layer."   By carefully scratching a hole in the anterior layer of the ligament, a few grammes of coloured fluid or tallow may be injected between the layers, care being taken to stop the injection the moment that slight resistance is felt, otherwise the material will force itself under the peritoneum to an indefinite extent.   When properly injected, the real cavity of the broad ligament, thus produced, measures a little over an inch vertically, somewhat less laterally, and not quite half an inch antero-posteriorly.   Its boundaries will be those given above as bounding the broad ligament, except that it does not extend so high as the tube ; and it will be found to be cut off from the walls and the lower part of the pelvic cavity by the fascia propria.   Now, a parametric phlegmon, long held to be entirely situated between the layers of the ligament, forms a mass far bulkier than the cubic capacity of the cavity of the ligament.

It might, however, according to older theories, be believed that abscess could actually begin between the layers of the broad ligament, and readily extend lower and lower into the pelvic cellular tissue below.   Guérin and Lebec deny that this extension of suppuration can occur, as the horizontal layer of their fascia propria seals up the lower limits of the ligament.   The development and extension of inflammatory deposit in the pelvic cellular tissue must be traced to their sources ; in short, to the lymphatic vessels.

The lymphatics of the vagina empty into larger vessels, which join each other at the level of the superior *cul-de-sac*—the level, in fact, of the body and the cervix of the uterus.   Under the cervical mucous membrane is a very dense lymphatic plexus, which communicates with the large vessels of the upper part of the vagina. From these united vessels, one or two large trunks pass outwards towards the pelvic walls, running along the base of the broad ligament, but entirely below it, and therefore separated from its cavity by the impermeable flooring of fascia propria. The trunk-lymphatics ultimately empty themselves either into one single gland, or else, more commonly, into a series of glands situated on the inner aspect of the ischium, close to the obturator foramen. From thence, lymphatic vessels ascend behind the pubes, and directly communicate, at the level of Poupart's ligament, with vessels from the thigh. They then ascend, in front of the peritoneum and behind the rectus and its sheath, and follow the epigastric vessels upwards. The lymphatics of the body of the uterus, on the other hand, actually pass between the layers of the broad ligament on their way to the lumbar glands, but they pass in its very uppermost part, quite above its cavity.

The course of the lymphatic vessels from the vagina and cervix explains certain symptoms frequent in pelvic inflammation, symptoms which cannot be logically referred to abscess in the broad ligament, but which represent what M. Guérin terms *adéno-phlegmon juxta-pubien*. Postpubic lymphangitis will sound a trifle less objectionable to British ears ; but rather let us banish such terms, and say that, according to M. Guérin, pelvic cellulitis (evidently the same thing) begins as lymphangitis, produced by any severe irritation to the vagina or cervix ; then the large lymphatic trunks below the broad ligament become involved ; the gland or glands close to the obturator foramen enlarge, and may be detected on digital examination by the vagina ; and the inflammation may extend to behind Poupart's ligament, or even form a hard mass palpable through the rectus, and following, from the groin upwards, the course of the epigastric arteries, as in a case described by M. Rigal. When the morbid process extends, the tissue round the lymphatics may become indefinitely involved, and abscess form at any point along the track above described. This condition represents the "parametritis anterior" of some authors. Hence the ill-defined extensive hardenings and the scattered collections of pus frequent in pelvic cellulitis. In short, says M. Lebec, the anatomy of the lymphatics of this part thoroughly explains the clinical symptoms of pelvic cellulitis. The structure of the broad ligament proves how rarely this affection can start from that appendage of the uterus ; so that we may say, with M. A. Guérin, that the clinical symptoms of abscess situated actually and primarily between the layers of the broad ligament have yet to be discovered. —*Brit. Med. Journ.*, June 4, 1881.

—

Obstetrical Auscultation.

In a clinical lecture (reported in the *Revue Médicale*, No. 7) Prof. DEPAUL, after adverting to the history and progress of obstetrical auscultation, to which no one has contributed more than himself, proceeded to explain to his class how best to perform it. The woman should be laid on a bed on her back—for although she can be auscultated while standing, this is very inconvenient, and may give rise to serious mistakes. The abdomen should be exposed free from all garments, especially among common women, whose coarse clothing might give rise to difficulty in the perception of sounds. In private practice it may be possible to make an examination over a chemise of fine linen. The physician must place himself on her left and right side alternately, so as to make the examination of both sides, the most complete silence being observed. The auscultation must be made by means of the stethoscope ; and after having tried the various forms of this instrument, Prof. Depaul has finally adopted one of medium length, having its auricular surface slightly excavated and the edges of the opposite aperture sufficiently thick to prevent disagreeable or painful sensations being caused. The wall of the abdomen and that of the uterus must be somewhat depressed, but only moderately so, as any strong pressure would modify the sounds to be perceived, and especially the *souffle*. Some women refuse to allow of auscultation, but a little persuasion and explanation of the objects in view usually overcome their objections. There are others, again, who have the abdominal surface in a state of hyperæsthesia, the slightest touch, according to their account, causing pain. Moreover, in morbid conditions of the respiratory organs, the various pathological sounds produced may render the uterine auscultation difficult.

It is towards the third month and a half, or the fourth month, that auscultation is of service; and the sounds produced are of two kinds, those proceeding from the pregnancy itself, and those which are independent of it. Of the first, there are the uterine *bruit de souffle* and the double sound resulting from the contractions of the fœtal heart, the fœtal *souffle* dependent upon the circulation of the fœtus, and the uterine *souffle* dependent upon the maternal circulation. Finally, there are sounds due to the active movements of the fœtus, as the *bruits de choc*, which may be both perceived by the hand and heard by the ear. We may also perceive by palpation, as well as by the ear, a friction sound (*bruit de frottement*). As to the sounds independent of pregnancy which are heard in women with child, it is of importance not to confound them. They may arise from the constriction of the muscles of the abdomen, or from the vesicular expansion of the lungs, which in some women extend from above downwards. So also the sounds produced by the beating of the heart of the mother may be transmitted to the cavity of the abdomen, and these are to be distinguished from those of the fœtus by their isochronism with the pulse. Finally, there are the pulsations of the aorta, and the sounds due to the presence of gas in the digestive canal, especially in nervous and impressionable women.

The maternal *souffle* has been designated by various names, but Prof. Depaul prefers that of "uterine *souffle*," given it by Paul Dubois; and although it is not the most important of the sounds inherent to pregnancy, it is very desirable that it should be known. It is a *souffle* without pulsations isochronous with the maternal pulse. It is more or less strong and intermittent in the great majority of cases, having a certain interval between two successive *souffles*. It is sometimes musical or sibilant, analogous to the sound produced by a large bass-string —at least, these are the typical sounds, of which, however, numerous shades exist, and which may be modified at intervals of a few instants in the same subject. There is no part of the uterus at which this may not be heard, but still there are generally three points of predilection—at the right and the left (sometimes both sides in the same woman), and at the fundus. This uterine maternal *souffle* may sometimes be absent on the first examination, for it is capricious, and not being constant, like the beatings of the heart, it may disappear and reappear occasionally. It is heard from the fourth or fifth month until the end of pregnancy. Nearly everybody is agreed in admitting that this sound is produced within the interior of the walls of the uterus, and that its mobility is due to the movements of the child, which compress this or that artery according to the position it occupies at the moment.—*Med. Times and Gazette*, July 23, 1881.

—

Pilocarpin in the Treatment of Puerperal Convulsions.

In the *British Medical Journal* for April 2, 1881, Dr. A. HAMILTON reports the following interesting case.

M. J. E., aged 22, domestic servant, a primipara, and previously healthy, was suddenly seized with convulsions. When seen by me, she was in a violent general convulsion, which had continued for two hours. On examination, I found her to be in the sixth or seventh month of pregnancy, the os rigid and undilata-ble, and the urine loaded with albumen. The convulsions continuing, and it being impossible to give anything by the mouth, I injected hypodermically, six hours from her seizure, fifteen minims of a two-per-cent solution of pilocarpin. This was followed in about two minutes by very profuse salivation and perspiration; the convulsions ceased, and strong uterine contractions soon became evident. After an interval of an hour, she had seven fits in quick succession. Mr. Taylor then saw the patient with me; and, with his concurrence, I gave, two hours after the first, a second injection of pilocarpin. The salivation following this was so copious as to threaten suffocation, and, although the convulsions became weaker and less frequent, the breathing was so much embarrassed as to make the patient's recovery almost hopeless. Pains, however, became stronger and more frequent; the fœtus being expelled ten hours after the last injection. The woman remained unconscious for two days, and then recovered rapidly.

In puerperal convulsions, I have found the best treatment to be dilatation of the os uteri, with or without chloroform, and speedy delivery; but in the fore-going case, one of the worst I have ever seen, the convulsions seemed to be so much controlled by the pilocarpin, that I shall certainly use it again in such cases. I may also say that I have used jaborandi with very good results in cases of Bright's disease and spasmodic asthma.

Medical Jurisprudence and Toxicology.

Cadaveric Alkaloids.

The very serious question, from the medico-legal point of view, of the sponta-neons development of cadaveric alkaloids and their toxic power, was first raised by M. Selmi of Bologna. After many vicissitudes of alternate favour and dis-credit, this subject has been revived in France by the researches of MM. Brou-ardel and Boutmy, in Germany by those of M. Husemann, and in Italy by the *résumé* of all the information on the subject recently published by the original discoverer, M. Selmi. These researches are succinctly summarized in the *Gazette Hebdomadaire*, and their results given in a concise form as follows: Last year, at the Congress of Rheims, M. Boutmy read, in his own and M. Brouardel's name, a paper which excited much attention, and in which the joint authors, after having shown that the existence of cadaveric alkalies has been erroneously contested, insisted on the toxic properties of ptomaïnes, pointing out that the activity of some of these substances is in no degree inferior to that of the strongest poisons. They demonstrated that there are many distinct ptomaïnes, each showing special chemical and physiological characteristics; and noted the following fact, of which the im-portance is clear: that one of these ptomaïnes, extracted from a corpse which had been eighteen months in the Seine, had all the properties of veratrine. Since the time they read this paper, its authors have followed up their researches by devoting themselves to the determination of the differences, either chemical or toxicological, which might prevent the confusion between the poisons formed by putrefaction and the venomous substances absorbed during life.

One of the first results of their labours is a paper presented to the Académie de Médecine on May 10th, in which they point out the property of the ptomaïnes to bring back the ferricyanide of potassium to the condition of ferrocyanide, which is capable of forming Prussian blue with, for instance, the chlorides of iron. The same reagents, however, in presence of pure alkaloids or extracts from a corpse after poisoning, do not undergo any change. These researches are being continued, and doubtless new facts will corroborate the facts already obtained. MM. Bergeron and l'Hôte, who have been studying the toxic effects of amylic alcohol, point out that, this alcohol being employed in the extraction of ptomaïnes, it becomes a question whether the toxic action of these alkaloids may not be partly due to amylic alcohol, frequently mixed with butylic alcohol, used to extract them. MM. Brouardel and Boutmy, however, state that they have not fallen into the probable cause of error here pointed out. Husemann (*Les Ptomaïnes et leur Signification en Chimie Légale et en Toxicologie*) has taken up the study of ptomaïnes from another point of view. He has felt doubtful whether these substances may not account for the poisonings by alimentary substances and putrid infections. The researches of Hoppe-Seyler, Schmidt, Schmideberg, and Panum have shown, in alimentary substances in a state of putrefaction, the presence of alkaloids analogous to ptomaïnes (Schmidt's and Schmiedeberg's sepsine and Panum's putrid poison). Husemann concludes that, as a matter of fact, the majority of the accidents observed in persons who had partaken of food in a state of commencing putrefaction are to be imputed to these alkaloids, which are of similar constitution to ptomaïnes (Schmidt's *Jahrbücher*, 1880). M. Selmi, in his recent work on the subject (*Les Ptomaïnes, les Alcaloïdes Cadaveriques, et les Produits Analogues des certaines Maladies dans leurs Rapports avec la Médecine Légale*), has collected his former researches on ptomaïnes and the method of distinguishing them from the true alkaloids, and has added a paper on the technical method of extracting ptomaïnes, and on the chemical differences which differentiate them from colouring and resinous matters. An interesting paper relating to the toxic effects produced by the extractive substances obtained from the urine of certain patients will also be found in this volume.—*British Med. Journal*, July 30, 1881.

—

The Influence of Ammonia in Chloroform-Poisoning.

Dr. SIDNEY RINGER, in a paper published in the *Practitioner*, June, 1881, p. 437, shows, by experiments, the rapid influence ammonia exerted in a frog's heart, whose action had been arrested by an overdose of chloroform. The chloroform evidently paralyzes the heart's muscular substance, affecting the ganglionless and nerveless portion of the ventricle exactly in the same way as any other part of it. [In the *Medical Times and Gazette*, May, 1871, p. 616, Dr. Neild reports a case of apparent death from chloroform inhalation, which recovered from the alarming state of syncope after four half-drachm injections of liquor ammoniæ into the median cephalic vein.—*Rep.*]—*London Med. Record*, July 15, 1881.

—

Poisoning by Potassium Bichromate.

Dr. WM. A. M'LACHLAN reports the following case of this rare form of poisoning:—

James W., aged 60, of spare build and nervous temperament, followed the occupation of a goods clerk. He had been complaining for some time with a dull pain in the hypochondriac regions, and had been doctoring himself with a variety of medicines. One of his fellow-workmen suggested to him a trial of bichromate of potash and rhubarb. Acting on his advice he procured these at a registered druggist's. While returning home with his medicines, he met in with a friend, and adjourned to his neighbour's house. Here he unfolded the packet of bichromate of potash, and after explaining its supposed utility, took fully three drachms of it. He dissolved it in cold water, then drank the solution. This was shortly after 3 P. M., on 9th March, 1880. He had not taken it more than one-quarter of an hour, when the symptoms of an irritant poison began to manifest themselves in the form of excessive vomiting and purging, accompanied with violent abdominal cramps. At this time, the woman of the house he had entered gave him an emetic of common salt and plenty of water to drink. At 5 P. M., when I was called, I found him reclining on a chair moaning and complaining of cramps in the abdomen and lower limbs. The surface of his body was cold. His hands and fingers were shrivelled, wrinkled, and dusky, much like those of a person in the advanced stage of cholera. His face and lips were very dusky. His beard was coloured chrome yellow. The mucous membrane of his mouth and throat was dark coloured. His breath was cold and his voice very feeble and tremulous. He was vomiting occasionally tough mucus mixed with blood. The mucus was very tenacious, and was with considerable difficulty removed from the mouth. His thirst was excessive. Pulse very weak and barely perceptible at the wrist. Respiration hurried. Urine suppressed. Mental faculties unimpaired.

Treatment.—He was covered up in bed, with hot blankets and hot jars placed in close proximity to him. Had olei ricini ℥ss at once. Then a dessertspoonful of brandy in hot water every quarter of an hour; also, water slightly acidulated with citric acid *ad lib.*, and milk gruel occasionally.

10 P. M. Much better. Slight perspiration on surface of body, trunk much warmer. Extremities still cold and cramped. Pulse 120 per minute, feeble, regular. Vomiting much less. Mucus much less tenacious. Thirst less; pain in abdomen less. Urine suppressed. Respiration still accelerated. Continue same diluents and give the brandy hourly.

March 10, 9 A. M. Has passed a restless night, slept very little. Vomiting almost gone. Cramps in the extremities still continue, the interval between them is much longer than last night, and the spasms themselves are not so prolonged, nor is the pain of them so severe. Thirst is not so excessive though still considerable. The heat of the body is much better. Pulse 120, better in volume, regular, though still feeble. Respiration more equable, though occasionally there is slight irregularity in the movements of the chest. Urine suppressed. Diminish the brandy to one teaspoonful every hour. Also to have liq. bismuth. ʒj every hour. Continue same diluents.

8 P. M. Patient is still better. Pulse 120 per minute, of better volume, regular. Respiration better. Cramps of extremities gone. There is still pain over the epigastric and umbilical regions. Vomiting almost gone. Urine suppressed. Continue treatment.

11*th*. 9 A. M. Patient still improving. Slept moderately well during the night. Vomiting entirely gone. Abdominal tenderness much less. Pulse 120 per minute, much stronger. Conjunctiva coloured a deep yellow. About one and a half ounces of urine have been passed since last visit—it is coloured chrome yellow. To have milk diet only. Also the following medicine: ℞. Pot. cit. gr. xxx; spt. æth. nitrosi, ʒij. Sig.—To be taken every three hours.

12*th* Still better. Urine abundant—still coloured deeply yellow. Bowels normal. Can take liquid food, but finds his digestion very weak. Pulse 76 per minute, still feeble. Respiration normal.

It would thus seem that the specific remote effects of this salt not only manifest themselves by producing yellow discoloration of the conjunctiva, but also by causing enervation of the kidney, with suppression of urine, which in this case was well marked.—*Glasgow Med. Journ.*, July, 1881.

MEDICAL NEWS.

THE INTERNATIONAL MEDICAL CONGRESS.

The recent meeting of the International Medical Congress in London, the seventh of the kind, from the reports which have reached us, appears to have been an unqualified success; the weather was favourable, the arrangements carefully made, the attendance very large (between three and four thousand), the addresses excellent, and the proceedings in the Sections distinguished by papers of unusual interest and importance. Upon another page will be found a brief but graphic account, from the pen of the Editor of this Journal, of the proceedings, and of the entertainments given to its members, from which it appears that the occasion was diligently and enjoyably improved. By a judicious arrangement, the committee obtained in advance abstracts of papers to be read; and these, in English, in French, and in German, were published in a portly volume of over 700 pages, and distributed on the first day of the session. It not only formed a valuable guide to the discussions, but also affords a very fair *résumé* of the intended proceedings. The meetings commenced on Aug. 2d, and continued with daily sessions until Aug. 9th, in accordance with the following programme :—

Tuesday, Aug. 2. 10 A. M. to 6 P. M. : Registration of Members. 3 to 6 P. M.: Informal reception at the College of Physicians. 9.30 P. M.: Conversazione given by President of Odontological Society to the members of Odontological Section.

Wednesday, Aug. 3. 11 A. M.: General Meeting at St. James's Hall; Chairman Sir William Jenner. The Prince of Wales will declare the Congress open. Inaugural Address by Sir James Paget. 3 P. M.: Meeting of the Sections. 4 to 7 P. M.: Musical Promenade in Royal Botanic Society's Gardens. 4.30 P. M.: General Meeting. Address by Professor Virchow. 9.30 P. M.: Conversazione at South Kensington Museum.

Thursday, Aug. 4. 10 A. M. to 1 P. M. : Meetings of Sections. 1.30 P. M.: Visits to Hospitals. Demonstration of Natural History Collection at South Kensington by Professor Owen. 2 P. M.: Meetings of Sections. 4 P. M.: General Meeting. Reading of the late Professor Raynaud's Address by his friend Dr. Féréol. 6.30 P. M. : Banquet given by the Lord Mayor at the Mansion House.

Friday, Aug 5. 10 A. M. to 1 P. M. : Meeting of Sections. 12.45 P. M. : Visit to Mr. Penn's Works at Greenwich. 1.30 P. M. : Visits to Hospitals. Demonstration of Natural History Collection at South Kensington by Professor Owen. 2 P. M.: Meetings of Sections. 4 P. M. : General Meeting. Address by Dr. Billings. 8 P. M. : Conversazione at the Guildhall. Soirée at the Royal College of Surgeons, free to members of the Congress.

Saturday, Aug. 6. 10 A. M. to 1 P. M. : Meetings of Sections. 12.15 P. M. : Excursion to Croydon Sewage Farm. 1.45 P. M. : Excursion to Folkestone— Unveiling of Harvey Memorial Statue. 2 P. M. : Excursion to Hampton Court, and Garden Party at Normansfield, given by Dr. Langdon Down. 4 to 7 P. M. : Reception at Kew Gardens by Sir J. D. Hooker. Garden Party at Hampstead, given by Mr. and Mrs. Spencer Wells. Garden Party at Wimbledon, given by Mr. and Mrs. Saunders. 6.30 P. M. : Dinner at Richmond, given by the United Hospitals Club. Reception by the Foreign Secretary to the Foreign Members of the Congress.

Sunday, Aug. 7. 10 A. M. : Full Choral Service and Sermon in Westminster Abbey. 3.15 P. M. : Full Choral Service, and Sermon by Canon Liddon, in St. Paul's Cathedral. 1.30 P. M. : Excursion to Boxhill. The Gardens of the Royal Botanic Society, Zoological Society, and at Kew and Hampton Court, will be open to Members of the Congress.

Monday, Aug. 8. 10 A. M. to 1 P. M. : Meetings of the Sections. 11 A. M. : Visit to the Docks. 2 P. M. : Meetings of Sections. 4 P. M. : General Meeting. Address by Prof. Volkmann ; Garden Party by Lady Burdett-Coutts Bartlett. 6.30 P. M. : Dinner given by the Masters and Wardens of the Society of Apothecaries. 9.30 P. M. : Conversazione given by the Royal College of Surgeons.

Tuesday, Aug. 9. 10 A. M. to 1 P. M. : Meetings of Sections. 2 P. M. : General Meeting. Address by Professor Huxley. 4 P. M. : Visit to the Crystal Palace ; Informal Dinner, and Display of Fountains and Fireworks, etc.

In this connection, and as an instance of medical journalistic enterprise, we note that the *Boston Medical and Surgical Journal* for August 18th, but issued two days in advance of date, contains in full the opening address by the President, Mr. James Paget, the Introductory Remarks delivered upon the opening of the Section in Pathology by Samuel Wilks ; on Surgery by John Eric Erichsen ; in Obstetrics by Alfred McClintock ; and in Anatomy by Prof. W. H. Flower ; and an interesting letter from London on the subject of the meeting ; altogether forming a most interesting, timely, and valuable issue of this representative Journal.

—

THE SANITARY CONDITION OF SUMMER RESORTS.

The Isle of Wight, sometime known as the Garden of England, but according to the *Practitioner* now deserving of a much less complimentary and euphemistic title, as a summer resort is under a cloud. It appears that the Local Government Board, having had its attention directed to the matter, resolved to subject the sanitary administration of the island to investigation, and delegated the task of inquiry to an energetic health officer, Dr. Ballard. From the official report of this observer, just made public, it appears that this particular garden-spot is one to be carefully shunned by all summer tourists who have the slightest regard for their health. The *Practitioner*, in a very forcible editorial upon this subject, based upon Dr. Ballard's report, says that it appears that "the sanitary affairs of the island are in the utmost state of confusion, and that the authorities, who should be responsible for keeping the island free from those accidental sources of impurity which necessarily accompany houses and communities, have done nothing of the sort, or done so only in the incompletest fashion ; and that the island has become defaced by conditions detrimental in the highest degree to its own inhabitants and peculiarly detrimental to the health and well-being of visitors."

One of the earliest and most important results of such neglect of proper sanitary regulation, of which Wight is by no means an isolated example, is the pollution of the water supply, and this is the very subject which must be kept constantly and prominently before the authorities of small out-of-the-way communities periodically subjected to overcrowding by summer visitors. The bill of indictment against Wight is clear, and carries conviction with it; the report of Dr. Ballard not only should be read by sanitarians and physicians, but it has its lesson as well for every summer tourist. That the Isle of Wight is peculiar among summer resorts in England or the Continent in its defective sanitation, no one will assert; they may " do these things better in France," but we have serious doubts whether there are many popular places of resort where in the details of scavengering, practice will at all approach theory, even in the native home of sanitary science. The earnest recommendation made only a short time ago, by the editor of the *British Medical Journal*, to tourists to carry their water supply with them, or at least to drink nothing while travelling on the continent except Apollinaris, is still fresh in our minds, and emphasizes the point that we wish to insist upon.

If we inquire further and ask the sanitary status of similar places upon the American continent, we find that the mushroom growth of many of our summer resorts has, almost without exception, effectually militated against anything like intelligent hygienic administration. The summer visitors take the ordinary hygienic conditions for granted on account of the great natural advantages principally in the way of ventilation, which usually are found at localities selected for summer habitation; if they are taken sick the water disagrees with them, and they go away, blaming their weakness rather than the water; but others come to fill their places probably to go through a like experience. In an excellent report on the Drainage of Summer Hotels and Boarding Houses,[1] Mr. Ernest W. Bowditch, an engineer of Boston, gives the results of investigations into the sanitary condition of one hundred and fifty of these "health resorts" (*lucus a non lucendo*), which were found to be almost-without exception unsatisfactory and liable to become at any time breeding places for epidemics of typhoid fever, diphtheria, and other infections diseases. These New England hotels and boarding houses are the prototypes of others all over the country; no doubt in many places the conditions are even worse, for these examples, it should not be forgotten, are taken from a section of the country noted for its thrift and cleanness. At Newport some years ago, matters became so serious that the inhabitants were forced to adopt prompt measures for self-protection, which fortunately resulted in the establishment of a very efficient system of sanitary inspection and control

---

[1] First Annual Report of the State Board of Health, Lunacy, and Charity of Massachusetts, 1879. Supplement containing report and papers on Public Health, Boston, 1880.

which now serves as a model for other places of resort.[1] Some portions
of Long Island are notoriously unhealthy. New Jersey has a large
number of watering places upon its coast, which are visited by enormous
numbers of people every year. Atlantic City and Cape May in particular are poorly drained, and still retain the primitive method of water supply, by rain water collected from the roof, left as regards cleanliness to
individual enterprise without any attempt at the much-needed systematic
filtration. There are also some surface-wells which are occasionally
resorted to by the poorer classes. At the former place during the past
summer some activity has been manifested, and a system of sanitary inspection and scavengering projected, which we hope will be freely matured
and actively in operation before next season. Fair Point, Chautauqua,
was recently in such bad sanitary condition as to attract public attention,
on account of the presence of a large number of persons dwelling in tents
and temporary structures. Under the efficient direction of the very intelligent administration, acting under the suggestion and advice of Prof. Lat-
timore, we believe this has been largely corrected, but there is yet much
to be done to make it what its natural advantages entitle it to be. We
need not pursue this subject further by multiplying illustrations, but would
direct professional and public attention to the drainage, sewage, and water
supply of our places of summer resort as a subject worthy of earnest and
careful consideration. In 1875, Dr. Henry Hartshorne read before the
American Public Health Association a brief paper entitled a " Preliminary Report on the Sanitary Conditions of American Watering Places,"[2]
and urged that " the same principles of sanitary science and practice,
essentially, are capable of illustration in camps and in places of summer
resort " owing to the great periodical increase in the population at places
where everything is temporary, as it were, and migratory, not permanent.
We mention this matter particularly at the present time, in order that the
intelligent and enterprising proprietors of places of summer resort may
see the necessity of satisfying popular opinion in this matter of sanitary
reform, and in putting their houses in order for next season they may adopt
the latest methods of scavengering and the greatest precautions to insure
uncontaminated water supply. We hope that they will not forget to
invite a thorough examination by competent authorities of their premises,
and in next season's circular, we shall be glad to see due prominence
given to the announcement of the satisfactory sanitary condition of the
house, with the examiner's certificate appended.

[1] See an article by Horatio R. Storer, M.D., on "The New Principles of Protective
(Private) Sanitation in its Relations to Public Hygiene;" Transactions American
Medical Association, vol. xxx., 1879, p. 357. Also one on "Sanitary Protection in
Newport;" Public Health Papers and Reports, vol. vi., Boston, 1881.

[2] Public Health Reports and Papers, vol. i., presented at the meeting of the American
Public Health Association in the year 1874–5, N. Y., 1876.

INTERNATIONAL MEDICAL CONGRESS, LONDON, AUGUST 2–9, 1881.

(SPECIAL CORRESPONDENCE OF THE MEDICAL NEWS AND ABSTRACT.)

The seventh meeting of the International Medical Congress was formally opened in St. James's Hall, London, on Wednesday morning, August 3d, by his Royal Highness, the Prince of Wales, in the presence of about 2500 members. The Prince of Wales, on his arrival at the Hall, was received by Sir William Jenner, Sir William Gull, Sir James Paget, Mr. Mac Cormack, and the other members of the committee, and conducted to the platform ; a little later the Crown Prince of Russia entered and took a seat on the left of the chairman. The large hall was crowded to its utmost capacity with eminent members of the profession, gathered together from every part of the world. Among the many distinguished persons present we recognized Virchow, Langenbeck, Charcot, Esmarch, Flint, Cardinal Manning, the Archbishop of York, the Bishop of London, Volkmann, Lister, Pasteur, Brown-Séquard, Fordyce Barker, Ranke, J. S. Billings, Kister, Snellen, Warren Bey, Sir William Gull, Spencer Wells, J. C. Hutchinson, Sapolini, and many others of equal prominence.

Sir William Jenner, K.C.B., President of the Royal College of Physicians, as chairman *ex-officio* of the general committee, called the Congress to order in a short address, in which he offered the acknowledgments of the profession to the Prince of Wales for the support which his Royal Highness had accorded to the Congress, and then referred to some of the objects which were to be attained by such an international gathering as was then assembled. He concluded by referring to the incessant and arduous labours which had devolved upon Mr. William Mac Cormac, the Hon. Secretary-General, in the devising and executing the preliminary arrangements for this Congress, and said that every member owed to Mr. Mac Cormac a deep debt of gratitude, which ought to be most heartily acknowledged.

Mr. William Mac Cormac, the Hon. Secretary-General, read the report of the Executive Committee, which contained a sketch of the origin of the meeting and of the steps that had been taken to insure to it a truly international character.

Sir J. Risdon Bennett, Chairman of the Executive Committee, then offered a resolution accepting the official list of officers nominated, and appointing Sir James Paget, Bart., President of the Congress, a number of honorary vice-presidents, including as American representatives Drs. Billings of Washington, Barker of New York, Bigelow of Boston, and Flint of New York, with Mr. William Mac Cormac, Hon. Secretary-General. Prof. Donders, as President of the preceding Congress, held at Amsterdam in 1879, seconded the motion in a short speech, in which he paid a just tribute of praise to the admirable arrangements which had been made for the meeting of the Congress. The resolution was carried by acclamation.

Sir William Jenner then presented to the Prince of Wales a medal struck in commemoration of the meeting of the Congress, and resigned the chair to Sir James Paget, the President-elect.

The Prince of Wales cordially greeted the President, and in a short and admirable address expressed his interest in the meeting, and the confident anticipation he felt in the great international benefits which must accrue from the conferences of men of science from all countries, and he formally declared the Congress open.

Sir James Paget then delivered his inaugural address, which was a thoughtful, philosophic, and eloquent statement of the true aims and objects of an international gathering such as this Congress was, and he concluded with the following peroration, which, for nobility of thought and beauty of expression, fully justifies Sir James's high reputation as an orator :—

"And then, let us always remind ourselves of the nobility of our calling. I dare to claim for it, that among all the sciences, ours, in the pursuit and use of truth, offers the most complete and constant union of those three qualities which have the greatest charm for pure and active minds—novelty, utility, and charity. These three, which are sometimes in so lamentable disunion, as in the attractions of novelty without either utility or charity, are in our researches so combined that, unless by force or wilful wrong, they hardly can be put asunder. And each of them is admirable in its kind. For in every search for truth we can not only exercise curiosity, and have the delight—the really elemental happiness—of watching the unveiling of a mystery, but, on the way to truth, if we look well round us, we shall see that we are passing among wonders more than the eye or mind can fully apprehend. And as one of the perfections of nature is, that, in all her works, wonder is harmonized with utility, so is it with our science. In every truth attained there is utility either at hand or among the certainties of the future. And this utility is not selfish : it is not in any degree correlative with money-making; it may generally be estimated in the welfare of others better than in our own. Some of us may, indeed, make money and grow rich ; but many of those that minister even to the follies and vices of mankind can make much more money than we. In all things costly and vainglorious they would far surpass us if we would compete with them. We had better not compete where wealth is the highest evidence of success; we can compete with the world in the nobler ambition of being counted among the learned and the good who strive to make the future better and happier than the past. And to this we shall attain if we will remind ourselves that, as in every pursuit of knowledge there is the charm of novelty, and in every attainment of truth utility, so in every use of it there may be charity. I do not mean only the charity which is in hospitals or in the service of the poor, great as is the privilege of our calling in that we may be its chief ministers; but that wider charity which is practised in a constant sympathy and gentleness, in patience and self-devotion. And it is surely fair to hold that, as in every search for knowledge we may strengthen our intellectual power, so in every practical employment of it we may, if we will, improve our moral nature; we may obey the whole law of Christian love, we may illustrate the highest induction of scientific philanthropy.

"Let us, then, resolve to devote ourselves to the promotion of the whole science, art, and charity of medicine. Let this resolve be to us a vow of brotherhood ; and may God help us in our work."

The first general meeting then adjourned.

In the afternoon the Sections organized as follows : Section I. Anatomy, President, Prof. Flower. Section II. Physiology, President, Dr. Michael Foster, of Cambridge. Section III. Pathology and Morbid Anatomy, President, Dr. Samuel Wilks. Section IV. Medicine, President, Sir William Gull. Sub-section. Diseases of the Throat, Chairman, Dr. George Johnson. Section V. Surgery, President, Mr. John Eric Erichsen. Section VI. Obstetric Medicine and Surgery, President, Dr. McClintock, of Dublin. Section VII. Diseases of Children, President, Dr. Charles West. Section VIII. Mental Diseases, President, Dr. Lockhart Robinson. Section IX. Ophthalmology, President, Mr. Wm. Bowman. Section X. Diseases of the Ear, President, William B. Dalby, Esq. Section XI. Diseases of the Skin, President, Mr. Erasmus Wilson. Section XII. Diseases of the Teeth, President, Mr. Edwin Saunders. Section XIII. State Medicine, President, Mr. John Simon. Section XIV. Military Surgery and Medicine, President, Surgeon-General Professor Thomas Longmore. Section

XV. Materia Medica and Pharmacology, President, Prof. T. R. Fraser, of Edinburgh. In many of the Sections, the President delivered introductory addresses.

Subsequently, the Congress again met in general session to listen to an address on the Value of Pathological Experiment, by Professor Virchow.

In the evening a conversazione was given by the English members to the foreign members and ladies, at the South Kensington Museum, which was graced by the presence of their Royal Highness the Prince of Wales, the Crown Prince of Russia, and his eldest son Prince Henry. The beautiful courts and picture galleries of the Museum with their exquisite art treasures, combined with the brilliant illumination and the presence of the ladies, constituted a scene of rare beauty which will long be remembered by all who participated in it.

On Thursday, August 4th, the Congress met in Sections in the morning, and in the afternoon in general session, to listen to an address which was written for the occasion, and finished just before his untimely death, by the late Prof. Maurice Raynaud, of Paris, on "Le Scepticisme en Médecine, au temps passé et au temps présent," which was read by his friend Dr. Féréol. In the evening a banquet was given to a certain number of the members of the Congress by the Lord Mayor of London, at the Mansion House, at which were present the following representatives of the United States: Drs. Fordyce Baker, H. J. Bigelow, J. S. Billings, V. T. Bowditch, J. Solis Cohen, R. B. Cole, Austin Flint, Wm. Goodell, S. W. Gross, I. Minis Hays, A. Jacobi, M. A. Pallen, L. A. Sayre, and Wm. Thomson.

On Friday, August 5th, the sections again met in the morning, and in the afternoon the Congress met in general session to listen to an address on "Our Medical Literature," by Dr. J. S. Billings, of Washington, U. S. Dr. Billings considered his theme in reference to the growth of medical literature all over the world, and gave interesting statistics in regard to subjects written upon and the nationalities of authors. He then ably discussed the character and value of our literature and presented some valuable reflections on the making of it and on its utilization. Dr. Billings's address was often witty, and was very enthusiastically received, and the thanks of the Congress were tendered to him for it, by Sir James Paget, in most complimentary terms. In the evening a conversazione at the Guildhall was given to the members of the Congress and their ladies, by the Lord Mayor and corporation of the city of London.

On Saturday, August 6th, the Sections met in the morning, and in the afternoon garden parties were given by Sir Joseph Hooker, at Kew, by Mr. and Mrs. Spencer Wells at Golder's Hill, Hampstead, and by Mr. and Mrs. Saunders, at Fairlawn, Wimbledon. Excursions were also made to Folkestone, to witness the unveiling of the Harvey memorial statue; after which ceremony the Mayor and corporation of Folkestone entertained the visitors at a banquet in the Town Hall. At the invitation of Dr. Langdon Down, a number of the members visited Hampton Court and then proceeded by river to Hampton Wick, where they were entertained by Dr. Down at a garden party at his residence, Normansfield. Excursions were also made to the Croydon Sewage Farm, and to Hanwell Lunatic Asylum. In the evening a party of the members were entertained at dinner by the "United Hospitals Club," at the "Star and Garter," Richmond Hill, Mr. Thomas Bryant, of Guy's Hospital, in the chair. A reception at his residence, Carlton House, was tendered to the foreign members of the Congress, by His Excellency Earl Granville, K. G., Her Majesty's Minister for Foreign Affairs.

On Sunday, August 7th, a full choral service was held in Westminster Abbey, and the sermon was preached before the Congress by the Rev. Canon Barry; and in the afternoon at St. Paul's, with the sermon by the Rev. Canon Liddon.

Visits were also made by special parties to Bethlehem Convalescent Hospital, Witley, Surrey, to the Margate Hospital, where the new wing of the Royal Sea-bathing Infirmary for Scrofulous Disease was inspected, and afterwards the party were entertained at lunch by Mr. Erasmus Wilson. In the afternoon Sir Trevor Lawrence, Bart., M. P., entertained at luncheon a party at Burford Lodge, his residence in Surrey; and Mr. Lennox Browne entertained a number of the members of the Section of Diseases of the Throat at a very handsome dinner, at the "Star and Garter," Richmond Hill.

On Monday, August 8th, the morning was devoted to sectional meetings, and in the afternoon a general meeting was held, at which Prof. Volkmann, of Halle, delivered an address, entitled "Ueber Moderne Chirurgie," and Professor Pasteur communicated the results of his most recent investigations in vaccination in relation to the prevention of chicken cholera and splenic fever.

For the entertainment of the members a visit was made to the Docks under the guidance and hospitality of Sir George Chambers; Baroness Burdett-Coutts gave a beautiful garden party at her residence, Holly Lodge, Highgate; the Society of Apothecaries, a dinner at their hall in Blackfriars; and the Royal College of Surgeons, a conversazione; and at the same time an opportunity was afforded the members to view the Hunterian Museum.

On Tuesday, August 9th, the Sections met in the morning, and at 2 o'clock the sixth and concluding general meeting was held, at which Prof. Huxley delivered an address on "The Connection of the Biological Sciences with Medicine."

Mr. William Mac Cormac, the Hon. Secretary-General, then presented his report, in which he stated that 3210 persons had registered as members of the Congress; that 119 meetings of Sections had taken place, which had sat in the aggregate for 293 hours, or 12 days and nights. The attendance at the sectional meetings had been very large, and 464 written and 360 spoken communications had been made, and in their discussion great interest had been shown. Many additional hours had been spent in visiting hospitals and museums, where there had been demonstrations of various diseases. Some hours had also been spent in listening to the addresses in the general meetings and at the museum of the Congress, which had been crowded with visitors.

The President, Sir James Paget, announced that resolutions had been received from the Sections of Physiology and Ophthalmology, and that they had been very carefully considered in their respective Sections, and it was now judged best that there should now be no discussion on them; that they would be submitted to the meeting, which would adopt them or not, and if any member dissented from the action of the Congress he could have his vote recorded.

The resolution from the section of physiology was, "That this Congress records its conviction that experiments on living animals have proved of the utmost value to medicine in the past, and are indispensable for its future progress. That, accordingly, whilst strongly deprecating the infliction of unnecessary pain, it is our opinion that, alike in the interests of animals and of men, it is not desirable to restrict competent persons in their experiments." The resolution was received with great applause, and was carried without a single dissentient voice.

The president then explained that the Ophthalmological Section had prepared a series of tests which it recommended for persons working signals on land and sea, and that its views were about to be drawn up in due form by a committee. In the mean while the Section recommended that its action should be adopted as the action of the Congress in order that the recommendations might be forwarded by the Secretary-General to the President of the Board of Trade, the First Lord of the Admiralty, and the Secretary of State for Foreign Affairs, with an expression of the desire of the Congress that they should be favourably entertained, and, if approved, be recommended for adoption by foreign governments. The resolution was unanimously adopted.

On motion of Mr. Bowman, seconded by Mr. Lister, medals of honour were presented to the President of the preceding Congress, Prof. Donders, of Utrecht, and to the Secretary-General, Dr. George, of Amsterdam, to Madame Raynaud, as a souvenir of her husband, whose untimely death rendered necessary the reading of his address by his friend Dr. Féréol, and to the readers of the general addresses, Drs. Féréol, of Paris; Billings, of Washington; Pasteur, of Paris, Volkmann, of Halle ; and to Prof. Huxley, of London.

Prof. Von Langenbeck moved that the executive committee should convey the thanks of the Congress to those non-members whose hospitality the Congress had received. Adopted.

The President moved that the decision as to the next place of meeting be left to the Executive Committee. Adopted.

Dr. Billings, of Washington, moved that the best thanks of the Congress be tendered to Mr. Mac Cormac, the Hon. Secretary-General, for the able and painstaking manner in which he had successfully discharged the multifarious duties of his laborious office. Adopted.

Prof. Charcot, of Paris, moved a vote of thanks to Sir James Paget, the President, for his services as presiding officer, which was carried with great enthusiasm, the whole meeting rising and cheering.

Sir James Paget said he had now the privilege of returning his thanks for the second time ; at first for selecting him as as their president, and now for saying that he had done the work fairly well. If he had worked hard with them all, every day of work had been a day of pleasure, for he had been associated with so many whom he much desired to meet, and had laid the foundation of friendships to make old age happy. (Cheers.) In so vast a work there must have been some lapses. (Cries of " No, no.") If there had, he begged to apologize. The meeting had been one of a rare amount of work, and the time occupied by the sittings of the Sections had been more than that spent in the meetings of the whole thirteen considerable London Medical Societies in a year. It was now time to say good-bye. It was not possible that all the work which they had done should be without good fruit, that all the mental force they had put forth should be lost. He would then say good-bye, not from himself to them, or from them to him, but to all good-bye, in its full meaning, namely, good be with them all in the future, especially that good which comes from doing good. (Cheers.)

The Congress then adjourned *sine die*. After the adjournment a large number of the members went to the Crystal Palace where they informally dined together. Afterward the fountains played, and there was a beautiful display of fireworks. The closing piece consisted of three colossal portraits of Charcot, Paget, and Langenbeck, which, as they became recognizable, were received with the utmost enthusiasm.　　　　　　　　　　　　　　　　　　　　　　　I. M. H.

Scarlatina in Charleston, South Carolina.

Dr. F. Peyre Porcher, under date of July 20th, writes : " In our last communication we stated, with regard to scarlet fever (which has very much abated), that at the commencement of the epidemic there had been an extraordinary exemption of the coloured race. This was true. The ward physicians and others note that subsequently the disease began to show itself more frequently in negroes, and some deaths have been reported among them.

" It seems to us that, having passed through any epidemic, a physician should have more precise opinions regarding the disease, and his practice should be more fixed and precise with the fresh recollection of his recent experience.

Without pretending to a very extensive one, we have come to these conclusions : Scarlet, like yellow, fever should be treated early ; efforts to control the fever should be made *from the beginning*, and the temperature, if possible, not be allowed to remain over 103° for any length of time. As in yellow fever continned high temperature and rapid combustion lead to black vomit and to uræmic poisoning, so in scarlet fever they intensify the tendency to and the grade of the throat affection as well as the congestion of the kidneys. To reduce the temperature and maintain it at a safe standard, the best means are naturally, after a mild laxative, the *early* use of alkaline fever-mixtures containing potash, spiritus mindereri, etc., the frequent application of ice-water to the head and hands, two or three warm baths daily, and greasing the entire surface of the body. Local applications to the throat internally of Labarraque's solution, chlorate of potash, tincture of myrrh, etc., should also be used. This, however, is not the place to go into detail on such matters, but the above we believe to be *essential* for success in the treatment of the disease. We would decidedly favour the trial of prophylactics in all children exposed to this disease and to diphtheria."

—

Health of New York.—The city's mortality has been somewhat smaller during the past month than in the preceding one. There were, however, 4378 deaths in July, against 3487 in July, 1880. Intense heat prevailed on August 5th, 6th, and 7th, the thermometer registering about 90° in the shade. On these three days 60 cases of insolation were reported. On July 11, 14, 22, and 26 there were 5, 4, 6, and 5 cases of sunstroke, respectively. Two cases of yellow fever have reached the port from Havana during the month. These are the only cases of yellow fever which have been received at quarantine this year. Last year patients sick with that disease arrived at quarantine almost daily from June till October. The special medical corps of the Health Board still continue their work in the tenement districts. Their visits cover the whole of Manhattan Island, this year, for the first time. On August 2d the Board of Health ordered the lodging-house at 61 Thompson St. closed for the reason that 22 undoubted cases of typhus fever were removed from that house between April 8th and July 21st, and that it would probably have become a focus for the disease with the advent of cold weather and the invading army of tramps.

Typhus fever has steadily abated during July. In the sixteenth week of its prevalence (ending July 2d) there were 11 new cases ; in the seventeenth week, 10 ; in the eighteenth week, 24 ; in the nineteenth week, 19 ; in the twentieth week (ending July 30), 10 cases. There were, thus, 74 cases in July, against 101 in June and 124 in May. Variola has also diminished to an encouraging extent. While 187 new cases of this disease were reported in June, and 210 in May, only 99 were discovered in July. Measles has also notably diminished, only 231 cases being reported for July, against 430 in June, and 587 in May. Scarlatina has increased from 435 in June, to 575 in July ; and diphtheria from 434 in June, to 521 in July.

Dr. Nagle, Registrar of Vital Statistics, has recently published New York's mortality report for the six months ending June 30th. From his report it appears that the deaths from zymotic diseases have increased 40 per cent. during that time. The death-rate from diphtheria is twice as great, and that from scarlet fever five times as great as in the preceding period of six months. The mortality for this year is further shown to be 20 per cent. greater than for a corresponding period in 1880, the actual excess in deaths being more than 3000. The death-rate during the last six months has been about 30 per 1000, while it varied between 24 and 26 per 1000 for the corresponding six months of 1880.

Appointment at the New York University.—Dr. F. R. S. Drake has been appointed Clinical Professor of Practical Medicine in the University Medical College of New York.

———

New York Physicians at the International Medical Congress.—New York was well represented at the International Medical Congress recently held at London, by many of her eminent physicians, among whom may be mentioned Drs. Barker, Flint, Sayre, Mundé, Sands, Arnold, Bosworth, Purdy, Satterthwaite, Schaffer, and Taylor.

———

Regulation that does not Regulate.—The Censors of the New York County Medical Society complain that their efforts for the suppression of unqualified and irregular medical practitioners have not been properly seconded by the grand jury, which body recently dismissed a case in which the law regulating the practice of medicine had been manifestly violated.

———

Meeting of American Ophthalmological Society.—The American Ophthalmological Society held its annual meeting at Newport, R. I., on July 27th and 28th, 1881. The following officers were selected for the ensuing year: President, Dr. H. D. Noyes, of New York; Vice-President, Dr. W. F. Norris, of Philadelphia; Secretary and Treasurer, Dr. R. H. Derby, of New York; Committee on Publication, Drs. D. B. St. John Roosa, R. H. Derby, and E. G. Loring; Corresponding Secretary, Dr. J. S. Prout, of Brooklyn.

———

Organization of the Barren County Medical Society, Kentucky.—The Barren County Medical Society, at Temple Hill, Kentucky, was organized June 20, 1881. Officers as follows: R. H. Grinstead, President, Glasgow; J. J. Jepson, Vice-President, Glasgow; Geo. S. Leach, Secretary, Glasgow; C. T. Grinstead, Corresponding Secretary, Temple Hill; S. T. Batts, Treasurer, Dry Fork.

———

Meeting of the American Otological Society.—The American Otological Society held its fourteenth annual meeting at Newport, R. I., July 26th, 1881, after the transaction of the ordinary business, and listening to papers by Dr. Theobald, of Baltimore; Roosa, of New York; Orne Green, of Boston; Burnett, of Phila.; Kipp, of Newark; Blake, of Boston; Buck, of New York, and others, the Society adjourned to meet next year at Lake George, on the day previous to the meeting of the Ophthalmological Society.

———

Ice for the Sick Poor in New York.—The Earle Guild has inaugurated a novel charity, the object of which is the supplying of the sick poor with ice during the heated term. The circumstances and condition of each applicant for ice will be investigated before relief is extended, unless such applicant be provided with a voucher from a reputable physician. The Guild will issue tickets to families in distress for a two, three, or four weeks' supply of ice, which will be delivered daily anywhere in the city. On Saturday a double quantity will be delivered. Books containing ten orders, each one of which is good for a two weeks' supply, will be sold to the sick, who are able to pay a small sum for relief, at the rate of $5.00.

———

New Summer Cottage Charity.—The Sisters of St. John Baptist, of No. 233 E. 17th Street, New York, propose to erect a house, at some convenient place on Long Island, which will be known as St. Anna's Cottage. The house will be designed to give the benefit of fresh air and recreation to mothers of families, with their children, whose means are too limited to admit of their procuring these essentials to health during the hot weather elsewhere. It is proposed that the sojourn of the women and children shall extend from three days to a week, so that large numbers can be successively entertained. This charity is intended for the special benefit of the Germans living on the east side, between the East River and Avenue A.

Seaside Sanitaria.—The Seaside Sanitarium, at Rockaway Beach, which was mentioned in the July number of the "Medical News and Abstract," has been in successful operation for nearly two months, and has already afforded entertainment to several thousand sick children from the tenement districts. The managers have this year set apart a portion of one building for the use of respectable working girls and women who cannot pay the price demanded at ordinary seaside resorts. The price of a week's board is $3.50, including the fare to and from the Sanitarium.

The Seaside Nursery of St. John's Guild, N. Y., situated at Cedar Grove, Staten Island, and referred to in the May number of the "Medical News and Abstract," was formally opened on July 28th. It is located on Prince's Bay, below the Narrows, and commands a fine view of the lower Bay. Is is a two story, wooden structure, with piazzas along the entire front of both stories. The house is very well ventilated. The main building is 25 by 60 feet, and there are to be two wings, each 25 by 95 feet. Only one of these is now completed. Fifty children and their mothers can now be accommodated, but three times as many will find room when the second wing is completed.

The grounds of the Guild comprise ten acres, including a cedar grove. The bay frontage is 600 feet. Sick children, whose complaints are too serious to be relieved by an excursion on the Floating Hospital of the Guild, are transferred to the Seaside Nursery. The Floating Hospital takes on an average over a thousand mothers and children on an excursion thrice weekly.

Working of the Sick Children's Mission, New York.—The number of applicants for medical aid for sick children at the office of the Sick Children's Mission of New York has been unusually large this season. This institution has been in operation for twelve years, and has been the means of considerably diminishing infantile mortality in the city. Twelve visiting physicians are employed by the Mission; and six druggists, in convenient localities, furnish medicines upon these physicians' orders. The physicians are also authorized to give orders on the Mission for any kind of nourishment needed by the sick children, if the parents are too poor to provide it.

Country Week for Sick Children.—The Rev. Willard Parsons has arranged with the farmers in various towns in the Naugatuck Valley, Conn., to board a certain number of poor children from New York city, for a period of two weeks free of charge. The object of this arrangement is the removal of the children from the city during the season of most intense summer heat. Forty children were sent to Woodbury, Conn., in pursuance of this plan, on July 23d, and other detachments were sent to adjoining towns. The two weeks' sojourn in pure country air has, in past years, exerted a uniformly beneficial effect upon the city children.

To Readers and Correspondents.—*The Editor will be happy to receive early intelligence of local events of general medical interest, or which it is desirable to bring to the notice of the profession. Local papers containing reports or news items should be marked.*

CONTENTS OF NUMBER 466.

OCTOBER, 1881.

CLINICS.

CLINICAL LECTURE.

ADDRESSES.

MONTHLY ABSTRACT.

ANATOMY AND PHYSIOLOGY.

MATERIA MEDICA AND THERAPEUTICS.

MEDICINE.

VOL. XXXIX.—37

MEDICAL NEWS.

THE

MEDICAL NEWS AND ABSTRACT.

·VOL. XXXIX.   No. 10.   OCTOBER, 1881.   WHOLE No. 466.

CLINICS.

Clinical Lectures.

THE RELATION OF CLEANLINESS TO THE PREVENTION OF PUERPERAL SEPTICÆMIA.

A CLINICAL LECTURE.

BY ALBERT H. SMITH, M.D.,
LECTURER ON PRACTICAL OBSTETRICS TO THE PHILADELPHIA LYING-IN CHARITY.

ONE of the greatest steps in the progress of modern obstetrics is the full recognition, which has at last been brought about, of the causal relations of septic absorption to the great train of inflammatory and febrile troubles, attendant upon the puerperal condition, and upon the after stage of abortion, embracing those fearfully fatal maladies which have, since obstetrics could be considered to be an art, been the opprobrium of that department of medicine. When we bear in mind that the process of parturition is simply a physiological one; that it is to a human being what the ripening and falling off of the fruit is to the tree; that it is really but a natural function of the reproductive organs, and ought not to be attended with any more danger than the functional operation of any other organs, provided the mother be placed in circumstances favourable for the free course of nature's laws;—we find it a lamentable thing, surely, and a source of the deepest humiliation, that there can arise in the newly delivered woman, a disease, whose source we cannot trace, whose outburst we cannot anticipate, whose course we cannot control; further and more deplorable, that the disease may attack the healthiest, the most robust, the most buoyant, the woman of best previous condition for health, the woman surrounded by the most favourable relations for resisting pestilence, the woman with everything to live for and everything to make her live; that it converts the simple physiological process, which nature ought to guarantee and protect against danger, into a cause of agonizing death, and into the house where the highest joys of life have just been realized, brings, as it were in an instant, the deepest grief and desolation.

We cannot wonder, then, that for ages the teachers and practitioners of the obstetric art should have felt this reproach and bestirred themselves earnestly to remove it. And, we find upon this one subject continuous discussion and the arising from time to time of opposing schools as to the causations and the treatment of this fearful scourge, each school making an honest and conscientious effort to get at the true cause from its own stand-point of observation, and each founding its treatment upon reasonable deductions from its views of the pathological conditions. We have had in turn the earnest partisans of the doctrine of acute inflammation, of specific fever, of contagion, of epidemic influence, of typhus, and of thrombosis; and the appropriate treatment insisted upon for each. But the true causation of the puerperal diseases was first suggested by Semmelweiss, as being the absorption from open surfaces of decayed animal matter, resulting in a true blood-poisoning, operating either by the production of an erysipelatous inflammation at the point of absorption and gradually travelling to adjacent tissues, and secondarily through the lymphatics and by blood-infection producing a blood-phlogosis and death; or, when the poison was exceedingly virulent being carried by absorption directly into the blood without the previous, or even intercurrent, development of any local phlegmasia, going on to rapid blood-disorganization and death. In other words, he announced the theory that all puerperal fevers, peritonitis, arthritis, cellulitis, and the whole range of those serious lesions appearing a few days after labour, attended by high temperature, increased pulse rate, and various local inflammations, are merely different forms and manifestations of one and the same pathological condition, and that that was septicæmia. The profession, especially the English and the American teachers, were slow in adopting this view, but it has now become so thoroughly proven by clinical observation, and comparative symptomatology, that but little opposition is made to its recognition. It is agreed then at present that these diseases are precisely analogous in their causation, their pathology, their course of development, their urgent need of prophylaxis, and their treatment, to septic inflammation and fever found in surgical practice, their differences dependent only upon the peculiarity of the tissues involved in parturition, upon their exceeding capacity for absorption and transfer of poison, and upon the many points likely to be presented where such absorption may take place.

Another consideration in connection with these diseases, is the vastly greater number of cases needing care than in any other class of practice; also the greater number of sources from whence the poison may be accidentally conveyed to the absorbing surfaces; also, lastly, the greater caution to be used in watching against accidental or thoughtless conveyance from such sources. It is upon this last point which I wish mainly to dwell in this lecture, that is, upon what is called the antiseptic management of labour and the puerperium, the prophylaxis of septicæmia, which, as in all other antiseptic treatment, means simply the maintenance of cleanliness, as far as possible absolutely, in opened surfaces, until they have either united or granulated.

How to keep the genital canal clean during and after parturition is then the great question in the prevention of this horrible malady. The study of this question involves the consideration of the points where absorption may take place, the sources from whence poison may be conveyed, and the precautions to be used against such conveyance.

First, then, as to the points liable to absorb poison. We know that any surface upon which there is loss of integrity of the external investment (whether epidermis upon the integument, or epithelium upon the mucous membrane) is capable of absorption; and we know well how a very slight opening into the integument upon the hands, a scratch, of which one was not even conscious before, will smart when introduced into any acrid liquid, or may absorb the fatal poison from the cadaver when it was not even suspected. How much more then might we expect, upon theoretical grounds, that the highly vascular tissues of the genital canal, as we find them in their increased vitality in pregnancy and even more especially during parturition, would be quick to take up any noxious material which comes in contact with fissures or abrasions upon their surfaces; and unfortunately our practical experience gives sad confirmation of the theory. We know how, even in the unimpregnated uterus, the gentlest use of a mechanical dilator may lacerate the mucous surface of the cervix, producing, perhaps, tears that the naked eye could scarcely detect; and we know so well, if any broken-down or decaying tissue from a malignant growth or from the scraping of vegetations, so often recklessly done, should come into contact with this point of opening, how a fire is lighted up, and we are startled by the outbreak of a series of symptoms, the meaning of which we know so well: the high temperature, and the rapid pulse, and the quickened respiration, and then the pain and the tenderness—pelvic and abdominal—and the chill, and the other evidences of the septic metritis, and cellulitis and parametric phlegmon, and, perhaps, peritonitis and death. And yet in the process of labour, we have not only the little fissure to absorb, but also, especially in the primipara, large open surfaces, superadded often one upon another, from the cervical canal to the integument of the perineum. Now these are altogether unavoidable to a large extent; in a greater or less degree we may consider that they are present in every case of labour. There is probably not one case in a thousand in which there is not before the process is completed some solution of continuity. This may occur very superficially without any bleeding, but when there is blood there must necessarily be a surface to bleed, and how very rare is it to go through the management of a case where there is no stain of blood before the head is expelled. The "show," that is, the plug of tinged mucus, which sometimes and often amounts to a free discharge of blood, is recognized by the monthly nurse as the diagnostic sign that labour has begun, so uniformly is this present.

This, then, is the beginning of the lacerations, and the first appearance of blood in normal labour, or when there is no premature placental detachment, or mis-implantation of that organ. This discharge arises, undoubtedly, from the rupture of some minute fibres of the uterine lower segment, probably in the expansion of the internal os, as the contractions of this body drive the membranous pouch or the presenting part of the child into it, at the same time loosening up the plug of cervical mucus, which comes away stained with the momentary discharge from the lacerated surface. How far this continues to tear, we cannot say, but I have no doubt that fissures in the canal are much more frequent than we have any positive means of proving, for we often have free, and even profuse, bleedings from the cervix after the expulsion of the placenta, when no fissure in the rim of the os can be detected, yet the firm contraction of the uterine body and the bright red colour of the flow, and sometimes even the arterial jet, show that it cannot come from patulous venous sinuses opening upon the placental site. There is no blood from these tears while the head is passing, because the compression of the surface then prevents it. As the distension goes on, just before the os is fully open, a violent expulsive effort will often drive the presenting part of the child so forcibly, that the most prominent projection upon the circumference of the head-globe, making a sudden strain upon the rim, where it impinges, will tear

through, either in the line of a fissure already made, or, starting an entirely new laceration, until a gap is produced involving the whole distance
from the rim to the vaginal reflection. And then, after the head has
cleared the os uteri, and meets the resistance of an undilatable canal, and
especially in the posterior occipital position, when the forced flexion drives
the occiput at each recurring pain violently against the posterior vaginal
wall, how often does the finger detect the opening of a little fissure upon
the mucous surface, as the head recedes after the subsidence of the pain;
and with each successive pain finds the fissure deepening into a furrow,
which causes the observer great anxiety for the safety of the perineal
body, lest it should involve the deep tissue of the recto-vaginal septum,
and unless prevented by judicious labial incisions, even cut through the
perineum and the sphincter into the rectum. Then as the head passes
the vulvar outlet, there may be minor separations of tissues, even if the
perineum proper be saved; and sometimes when no laceration can be
found upon the mucous surface, the perineal integument in the line of the
raphé may yield superficially before the great tension.

Thus we see how many ways there are in which the surfaces of the parturient canal may be opened for absorption of poison, and we have in addition to all these the large placental site, covering one-fourth of the whole
superficies of the uterine cavity. It will be easily recognized, why in the
primipara, with her rigid tissues never before subjected to dilatation and
strain, the probabilities will be vastly greater of vaginal and vulvar, and
somewhat greater of cervical, laceration, than in the pluripara, with her
previous distension.

Having now considered briefly the causes and the character of the various
absorbing surfaces in the lying-in woman, let us call to mind the sources
from whence poison may come. The septic diseases of childbed have been
divided into *autogenetic* and *heterogenetic*, more for the ease of mind of
the accoucheur than from any real distinction in the nature of the poison
or of the results that attend its absorption. The autogenetic infections
are those which originate from the absorption of poison generated in the
body of the mother; the heterogenetic, those in which the septic matter
is conveyed to the maternal tissues from extraneous sources through the
neglect or ignorance of the accoucheur or the nurse.

From her own fluids the mother may be infected during her labour, when
she has been the subject of any disease of her uterine or vaginal canal,
attended by a discharge or casting-off of broken-down or sloughing tissue;
a scirrhus or epithelioma which has undergone softening within the cervix, upon its external surface, or anywhere in the vaginal canal, or upon
the vulva, where the discharge may come in contact with any open surface or point; a polypus or other non-malignant growth, from whose surface there may be a discharge, or which may be caused to slough from
pressure in labour; and, more commonly, any ulcerated surface or erosion
upon the cervix or vagina, discharging pus or a muco-purulent discharge,
which, if allowed to remain in the vagina for any length of time, becomes
virulently poisonous.

There is another autogenetic source of infection during the process of
parturition, to which, as far as I know, attention has never been called,
and yet, which I doubt not, is one of the most fertile causes of septic fever
in cases of prolonged labour. This is the accumulation and continued exposure to atmospheric influence in contact with the warm tissues of the
mother, of the *natural and healthy discharge* of mucus with its admix-

ture of blood from the cervix and vagina, while the tissues are gradually relaxing for the passage of the child. This discharge, perfectly healthy and clean, as it exudes from the vaginal canal, bathes the vulva and perineum, and the thighs and pubic region ; it agglutinates the tissues, matting up in thick adhesive masses upon the labial surfaces, as can be seen when the patient is cleansed after her labour, if it has not been scrupulously cleansed before, requiring vigorous efforts with soap and water to remove it. It remains exposed to the warm air of the chamber upon the warm surface of the body. Decay, with its resulting sepsis, must soon, under these circumstances, begin its work, and the poisoned moisture outside will readily impart its virulence to the fluids of the lower vagina, and as the head passes through the vaginal canal making its attacks upon the natural barriers provided against infection, and opening one or many doors for the enemy to enter, it is there in full force prepared to insinuate itself into tissues well prepared by their unusual vitality and turgescence to receive it.

Of the autogenetic causes acting after parturition is over, the main source of infection will be the decomposition of the lochial discharge or of clots of blood or pieces of membrane retained in the uterus from deficient cleaning after labour, or from defective involution. This source will, probably, rarely be a fruitful one upon the cervical or vaginal lacerations, for these will begin to suppurate and granulate in their effort at repair in from twenty-four to thirty-six hours (unless made to unite by sutures), and up to that time the lochial discharge rarely becomes foul or likely to infect. After granulation begins there is no absorption, so that it could only be by a re-opening through some disturbance of the granulating surface, such as might occur from the passage of a large clot through the now contracted vagina, or even the presence of large, hard, fecal masses in the lower rectum. But we may easily have, as we can often recognize, septic fever developed by the absorption of poisoned lochia, or of decomposing clots pent up within the uterine cavity, through the imperfectly closed orifices of vessels opening upon the placental site of the too slowly involuted womb. The poisoning from the amniotic fluid from around a dead fœtus is so questionable as to its occurrence that it is scarcely worth while to mention it.

The *heterogenetic* sources of infection will be found in poisonous matter conveyed by the hand or the clothing upon the arm (either an enveloping towel or sleeve) either of the doctor or nurse, or upon the surface of the instruments used either during or after labour. Upon the hands of the accoucheur may be carried any septic matter with which they have come in contact, even for several days, unless care be taken with such methods of cleansing as will be suggested hereafter. The worst and most rapidly violent poisons are those from the autopsies or manipulations of tissues of persons dead with blood-diseases ; but any autopsies, or handling of pathological specimens or decaying or broken-down tissues from the body living or dead ought to be avoided as death-carriers by the accoucheur, and, unless under some peculiar circumstances which might rarely render such handling necessary, ought to be conscientiously avoided. But there are equally noxious matters with which the hand of the obstetrician may be unavoidably polluted in the necessary exercise of professional duty, after contact with which the only thing is thoroughly to cleanse. Vaginal examination in cases of malignant disease, especially in operative work, when the hands are long in the vagina ; examinations also of any tumours in a

sloughing condition; of a uterus dilated by tents; of any diseased conditions, even of an inflammatory character, with discharge; of simple
leucorrhœa; any of these might be the source of such contagion.   And
especially would I caution earnestly against careless use of the hands after
contact with the disorganized clots in a case of hemorrhagic abortion, the
foul odour from which is as penetrating and as persistent upon the hands,
and the poison as virulent, in my opinion, as that of a sloughing cancer.
All discharges from wounds of the body in surgical practice should also be
sedulously removed.   In short, organic matter of any sort should be removed promptly and thoroughly from the hands of the obstetric practitioner, lest he should be caught with a case unexpectedly, when active
detergents and disinfectants could not be obtained as quickly as an examination might be needed.

But infection may take place from the finger of the obstetrician, after
the most scrupulous cleansing from any previous infection, by carelessly
carrying back to the patient's person her own discharge, in the frequent
examinations of a long labour.   This is a point upon which I do not think
any one has made suggestions, but it is easily seen that if the woman may
poison herself by the retention upon her external tissues of decomposing
discharges, ever so healthy at first, so may the doctor by carelessly retaining upon the hand these same fluids perfectly harmless previously, return
them after they have decomposed under the nails and upon the fingers to
the abraded vagina, to poison the woman whom he has been selected to
protect.   How often have I seen a doctor after an examination simply
wipe his hands upon a towel, and make a subsequent examination without
any washing in the interval.

So, also, the doctor cannot be too cautious about any sores upon the
hands, or upon any part of his person with which the hands may come in
contact; granular ophthalmia, otorrhœa, and what may be so easily overlooked, the discharge from a purulent coryza, or more especially from a
foul ozæna.   There is an historical case, to which I had better call attention
in this lecture, of a physician in the early middle part of this century, who,
practising in this city, was followed about from case to case almost in scores
by the fearful scourge of puerperal fever, as it was then called, a man
truly a " colporteur of pestilence," as Professor Schroeder would aptly
have termed him; who used every means that could be thought of to
cleanse his person, and to purify and regularly change his clothing, but to
no effect; his touch was poison, and yet no one ever dared to suggest to
him, and perhaps no one ever thought of it until too late, that the reason
why his work everywhere was accompanied by the fearful disease, when
other men were free from it, might be that he had a foul chronic ozæna,
the thoughtless contact of his finger with which could carry poison to the
tissues of his patient.

From the clothing both of the physician and nurse pestilence can be
conveyed, and I would suggest that in all cases the sleeve of the doctor
should be drawn up a short distance at least from the wrist and the latter
closely enveloped in a napkin tightly held between the fingers and the
palmar surface of the hand, and not pinned permanently.   For upon the
sleeve may accumulate little by little discharges from various examinations and operations, unconsciously to the physician, which when brought
to lie against the mother's tissues, warm and moist, would be a fruitful source
of infection.   If the arm is covered with a napkin, to avoid a disagreeable
impression, the sleeve may be rolled up to the elbow.   But my suggestion

about the napkin not being kept permanently upon the arm during many successive examinations follows naturally upon what I had said before about the neglect to wash the hands during the intervals between the same. A towel saturated around the wrist with vaginal discharge would itself be a fertile source of infection if again brought into close proximity to the genitalia at a subsequent touch. Where at all possible, a towel even used in a lying-in chamber by the physician should be carefully put out of reach until the labour is over, or if it must be used again, thoroughly washed and disinfected in the interval. How often this is neglected by a nurse, or others in the room, a towel already soiled ever so little with blood and discharges, being handed to the accoucheur again to wipe his hands before making an examination.

Monthly nurses cannot be too scrupulous in regard to personal cleanliness in going from one case to another, and especially in going directly from the dressing of suppurating wounds or cases attended with foul discharges. In attendance upon such cases they should always wear wash dresses, and put them through the boiling process before again wearing them.

In enumerating the sources of puerperal septicæmia, I do not mean to ignore certain meteorological or atmospheric influences, present during *epidemics* of puerperal fever, so called, which predispose the patient to respond more readily to the poisonous impression of septic absorption, nor do I question the predisposing influence of malaria, and some of the eruptive fevers, to magnify such a septicæmia as in a majority of cases used to be developed upon the third day, and erroneously called *milk fever*, but which nature could often throw off unaided,—to magnify, I say, such a condition into a malignant case of septic fever, perhaps ending fatally. But I am thoroughly convinced that whatever be the predisposing condition, the immediate exciting cause of the fearful malady in all its various phases, is the absorption by open surfaces of disorganized animal matter.

It is easy to see why primiparæ are more likely to be victims to this disease than pluriparæ, when we consider the greater likelihood of injury to the mucous surface of the genital canal, the longer period of exposure of the vulvar orifice to atmospheric influence before the external surface is cleansed, and the necessity for more repeated and prolonged manipulation especially upon the perineum, in the neighbourhood of which the tissues are so very apt to be more or less impaired in their integrity.

We arrive then finally at the purpose of this lecture, to see how we can most effectually carry out that indication which must be the clear one to any mind, the PREVENTION of such poisoning; and the essential means of such prevention is *cleanliness*, the keeping clean of the tissues before and after the production of lesions of their surface, and of everything that comes in contact with them ; the purifying and removal of all morbific materials, and the prevention by suitable means of their reproduction. The antiseptic treatment in surgical cases is really only a systematic method of cleanlinesss.

First, in regard to the care of the physician's person. After laying down the rule that the hands should be carefully washed and cleansed with disinfectants after handling any animal matter, I would still further say that the person of the patient should not be approached without a most thorough and complete repetition of such process, between which cleansing and the examination of the patient, nothing should be touched except what is known to be perfectly clean. No driving should be done, no gloves worn, nothing should come in contact with the hands of a doubtful character. This cleansing should be done by soaking the hands and arms first in warm water, then with a *stiff* nail-brush with soap, scrubbing most carefully under the nails, where the poison is retained most persistently; and then the whole hands and wrists; a clean water is then to be used with the nail-brush, and the hands allowed to soak in it, medicated in the proportion of two and one-half per cent. of carbolic acid, or six to eight per cent. of good recently-made Labarraque's solution; that is about seven fluidrachms of a ninety-five per cent. solution of crystals of the former, and about a fluidounce of the latter to the pint of water. I always order as part of the preparation for labour, a bottle of each of these antiseptics to use under different conditions as may be required; and usually prepare for myself in each case, some washed lard carbolized to about five to ten per cent. The hands should be washed as directed always before the first examination, and after each examination and again before the subsequent they should be thoroughly washed with the nail-brush in one solution or the other. My preference is rather for the chlorinated water, as it is a more thorough disinfectant, and in such proportion as is necessary for the purpose, does not burn the skin nor obtund the tactile sense, as does a carbolized solution. Any instruments which can possibly be required in the labour, forceps, vectis, or catheter, should be treated in the same way with brush, soap, and disinfectant solution always both before and after use. Neither hands nor instruments should ever be wiped upon a towel previously used or soiled; it is better to let both go unwiped, where not a matter of importance, than to risk wiping them upon a doubtful towel.

During the labour systematic cleanliness with the patient should be rigidly observed. If practicable at the onset of parturition, she should take a general bath at about 95 to 100° F., which is useful not only for detergent purposes but also as a promoter of the action of the skin, and as relaxing the muscular fibre, and the tissues generally. After a rectal enema a vaginal enema either of the carbolized or chlorinated solutions above suggested may be given, if the membranes are not ruptured; if they are, or if there be any doubt about it, we should not risk the throwing in of these solutions into the uterine cavity in contact with the foetus. But the external genitalia should be frequently bathed with one of these solutions, and a soft cloth moistened with the same passed up inside the vaginal cavity from time to time, as far as the finger of the physician or nurse can carry it. The use of the *spray* during the whole process of labour, seems to me to be not only unnecessary, but very annoying to the patient, if done thoroughly enough to be of any service. It involves the necessity of keeping it under the constant observation of an assistant and the genitalia constantly exposed to view; the bed clothing and the patient's person kept all the time wet with it. If a carbolized spray be used the patient's tissues would be irritated and benumbed, and to keep a patient in the agonies of labour in a fixed position in order for this, which is an annoyance to her at any rate, would be a tax upon her forbearance which would be unreasonable. Then again, if it be only during the manipulation of the accoucheur, a carbolized spray would be just as annoying to him as it would be to the patient; saturating the clothing and benumbing the hand and arm. Instead I find perfect satisfaction in keeping at the side of the bed, during the whole time of my manipulations, a dilute Labarraque solution, double the strength of that mentioned; I put into a half-pint toilet cup an ounce of the solution, and fill the cup nearly full of water; in this I keep a small soft cloth of old muslin or linen ; whenever I make the touch I dip the finger into the cup, and from time to time bathe the genitalia with the cloth wrung out in the liquid removing all mucus and blood accumulated, and as the head is descending through the vaginal canal I frequently pass the cloth freshly wrung out in the cup up into the cavity as far as to reach the head.   As the head is passing the vulva, distending the perineum, I often keep the cloth in continuous contact with the tissues.   Thus there is no possibility of infection taking place either autogenetically or heterogenetically.   If any decomposing mass were in the pelvic cavity, a scirrhus or epithelioma, the cleansing would have to be even more vigilant and repeated.

After the delivery of the placenta, I wash out the uterus at once with a syringe with hot water at 115° to 120°, either chlorinated, or acidulated with vinegar, about twenty-five per cent.   I formerly used carbolic solution for this, but in two cases in the last year, I saw symptoms which confirmed Fritsch's statements as to the absorption of carbolic solution by the uterus, in the appearance of carbolic poisoning immediately.

For four days after the labour I have the nurse wash out the vagina with carbolized or chlorinated water about 110° F. every four to six hours, If any offensive lochia appear with the least symptom of septic poisoning, I wash out the uterus with the strong ten to fifteen per cent. Labarraque with a double canulated uterine tube, using a siphon generally in preference to a forcing syringe, to avoid the passage of the fluid into the peritoneal cavity.

ADDRESS ON OUR MEDICAL LITERATURE.

Delivered at the International Medical Congress.

By JOHN S. BILLINGS, M.D.,
Surgeon, U. S. Army.

When I was surprised by the honour of an invitation to address this Congress, my first thought was that it must be declined ; for the simple but sufficient reason that I had nothing to say that would be worth occupying the time of such an assemblage as it was evident this would be.   But while thinking over the matter, and looking absent-mindedly at a shelf of catalogues and a pile of new books and journals awaiting examination, it occurred to me that perhaps some facts connected with our medical literature, past and present, from the point of view of the reader, librarian, and bibliographer, rather than from that of the writer or practitioner, might be of sufficient interest to you to warrant an attempt to present them ; and, the wish being probably father to the thought, I decided to make the trial.   •

When I say '' Our Medical Literature,'' it is not with reference to that of any particular country or nation, but to that which is the common property of the educated physicians of the world as represented here to-day—the literature which forms the intra- and inter-national bond of the medical profession of all civilized countries ; and by virtue of which we, who have come hither from the far West and the farther East, do not now meet for the first time as strangers, but as friends, having common interests, and though of many nations, a common language, and whose thoughts are perhaps better known to each other than to some of our nearest members.

It is usual to estimate that about one-thirtieth part of the whole mass of the world's literature belongs to medicine and its allied sciences. This corresponds very well to the results obtained from an examination of bibliographies and catalogues of the principal medical libraries. It appears from this that our medical literature now forms a little over 120,000 volumes properly so called, and about twice that number of·pamphlets, and that this accumulation is now increasing at the rate of about 1500 volumes and 2500 pamphlets yearly.

Let us consider the character of this annual growth somewhat in detail, first giving some figures as to the number of those who are producing it.

There are at the present time scattered over the earth about 180,000 medical men, who, by a liberal construction of the phrase, may be said to be educated—that is, who have some kind of a diploma, and for whose edification this current medical literature is produced. Of this number about 11,600 are producers of, or contributors to, this literature, being divided as follows: United States, 2800; France and her Colonies, 2600; the German Empire and Austro-Hungary, 2300; Great Britain and her Colonies, 2000; Italy, 600; Spain, 300; all others, 1000. These figures should be considered in connection with the number of physicians in each country; but this I can only give approximately, as follows: United States, 65,000; Great Britain and her Colonies, 35,000; Germany and Austro-Hungary, 32,000; France and her Colonies, 26,000; Italy, 10,000; Spain, 5000; all others, 17,000.

It will be seen from these figures that the number of physicians who are writers is proportionately greatest in France and least in the United States. As regards France, this is largely due to the requirement of a printed thesis for graduation, which of itself adds between six and seven hundred annually to the number of writers.

Excluding popular medicine, pathics, pharmacy, and dentistry, all of which were included in the figures for the annual product just given, we find that the contributions to medicine, properly so called, form a little over 1000 volumes and 1600 pamphlets yearly.

For 1879 Rupprecht's Bibliotheca gives as the total number of new medical books, excluding pamphlets, periodicals, and transactions, 419; divided as follows—viz.; France, 187; Germany, 110; England, 43; Italy, 32; United States, 21; all others, 26. These figures are, however, too small, and especially so as regards Great Britain and the United States. The Index Medicus for the same year shows by analysis that the total number of medical books and pamphlets, excluding periodicals and transactions, was 1643; divided as follows: France, 541; Germany, 364; United States, 310; Great Britain, 182; all others, 246. This does not include the inaugural theses, of which 693 were published in France alone.

The special characteristics of the literature of the present day are largely due to journals and transactions, and this is particularly true in medicine. Our periodicals contain the most recent observations, the most original matter, and are the truest representations of the living thought of the day, and of the tastes and wants of the great mass of the medical profession, a large part of whom, in fact, read very little else. They form about one-half of the current medical literature, and in the year 1879 amounted to 655 volumes, of which the United States produced 156, Germany, 129, France, 122, Great Britain, 54, Italy, 65, and Spain, 24. This is exclusive of journals of pharmacy, dentistry, etc., and of journals devoted to medical sects and isms. In a table I have drawn out it appears that the total number of volumes of medical journals and transactions of all kinds was, for the year 1879, 850, and for the year 1880, 864. The figures for 1880 are too small, but the real increase is slight. During the year 1879, the total number of original articles in medical journals and transactions which were though worth noting for the Index Medicus was a little over 20,000. Of these there appeared in American periodicals 4781, in French 4608, in German 4027, in English 3592, in Italian 1210, in Spanish 703, in all others 1248. The figures for 1880 are about the same. It will be seen that at present more of this class of literature appears in the English language than in any other, and that the number of journal contributions is greatest in the United States. The actual bulk of periodical literature is, however, greatest in Germany, owing to the greater average length of the articles. With regard to the mode of publication, I will only say that in all countries except Spain the greater number of medical periodicals are monthly, while in Spain they are semi-monthly. It is this periodical literature which, more than anything else, makes medicine cosmopolitan, and although as regards new discoveries or methods of treatment it is still somewhat farther from London or Berlin or Paris to New York than it is from New York to either of these places, the discrepancy is gradually becoming less.

Many of the medical journals are very short lived, but the total number is increasing. In 1879, 23 such journals ceased, but 60 new ones appeared, and in 1880 there were 24 deaths and 78 births in this department of literature. Over one-third of this fluctuation occurs in the United States alone, France being next in the scale, Spain third, and Italy fourth, while Great Britain is the most stable of all.

This merely quantitative classification gives of course no idea as to the character, and very little as to the value of the product. Let us now consider it by subjects. During 1879 there were published 167 books and pamphlets and 1543 articles relating to anatomy, physiology, and pathology—that is, to the biological or scientific side of medicine. Dividing this again by nations, we find that Germany produced a majority of the whole, France being second. The proportionate production by nations of this class of literature is perhaps better shown by an analysis of the bibliography of physiological literature for the year 1879, as published by the *Journal of Physiology*. This shows 59 treatises and 500 articles in German, 17 treatises and 227 articles in French, 5 treatises and 77 articles from Great Britain, 8 treatises and 41 articles from Italy, and 2 treatises and 24 articles from the United States. The number of authors for this product was— German, 393; French, 119; English, 59; Italian, 39; United States, 19; all others, 41. For the year 1880 the same journal reports 62 treatises and 452 articles from Germany, 23 treatises and 216 articles from France, 12 treatises and 76 articles from Great Britain, 4 treatises and 51 articles from Italy, 6 treatises and 25 articles from the United States, and 10 treatises and 31 articles from all other countries.[1]

When we turn to the literature of the art, or practical side of the profession, the figures are decidedly different. We find over 1200 treatises and 18,000 journal articles which come under this head, and the order of precedence of countries as to quantity is France, United States, Germany, Great Britain, Italy, and Spain. The tables I have constructed give still further subdivisions, showing by nations the number of works and journal articles upon the practice of medicine, surgery, obstetrics, hygiene, etc., for the years 1879 and 1880, and some of the figures will be found interesting. A marked increase has occurred in the litera-. ture of hygiene during the last two years, and this especially in England, France,

---

[1] The difference between these figures and those of the Index Medicus is due, on the one hand, to the fact that the Journal of Physiology includes articles which are placed under other headings in the Index Medicus, and, on the other hand, to the fact that the Journal has a different standard of excellence from that of the Index, rejecting many articles which the latter must accept as original.

Germany, and the United States. The literature of diseases of the nervous system, of ophthalmology, otology, dermatology, and gynæcology is also increasing more rapidly than that of the more general branches.

It would, of course, be extremely unscientific to use these figures as if they represented positively ascertained and compared facts, the accuracy of which, as well as of the classification, could be verified. They represent merely the opinions of an individual—first, as to whether each treatise or pamphlet included in these statistics was worth noting, and second, as to how it should be classed. Had everything been indexed, the figures, for journal articles at least, might have been nearly doubled; while if the selection had been made by a more severe critic they might have been reduced one-half.

If I had to do the work again I should not obtain the same results. The prevailing error is that as regards journal articles the figures are too large, for some of those included are of so little value or interest that they are, I fear, never read by more than two persons.

Be that as it may, I think we can take them as indicating certain differences in the direction of work of the medical authors of the great civilized nations of the earth; but they must be considered as approximations only; and the statistical axiom must be remembered that the results obtained from a large number of facts are applicable to an aggregate of similar facts, but not to single cases. There will be a certain number of medical books and papers printed next year just as there will be a certain number of children born—and as we can within certain limits predict the number of these births and the proportion of the sexes, or even of monsters—so we can within certain limits predict the amount and character of the literature that is yet to come, the ideas that are yet unborn. The differences are due to race, political organization, and density of population. As Dr. Chadwick has pointed out in speaking of the statistics of obstetric literature, one of the chief causes of the multiplication of medical societies is geographical. "In England it is possible for those who are specially interested in gynæcology and obstetrics to attend the meetings of the Obstetrical Society of London, whereas in America the distances are so great that this is impossible." Speaking broadly we may say that at present Germany leads in scientific medicine both in quantity and quality of product, and that the rising generation of physicians are learning German physiology. But the seed has gone abroad, and scientific work is receiving more and more appreciation everywhere.

Seven years ago Professor Huxley declared that if a student in his own branch showed power and originality he dared not advise him to adopt a scientific career, for he could not give him the assurance that any amount of proficiency in the biological sciences would be convertible into the most modest bread and cheese. To-day I think he might be bolder, for such a fear would hardly be justifiable—at all events in America, where such a man as is referred to could almost certainly find a place, bearing in mind the professor's remark that it is no impediment to an original investigator to have to devote a moderate portion of his time to giving instruction either in the laboratory or in the lecture room.

Within the last ten years the literature of France, Germany, Great Britain, and the United States has contained much with regard to medical education and the means for its improvement. In all these countries there is more or less dissatisfaction with the existing condition of things, although there is no general agreement as to the remedy. Solomon's question, "Wherefore is there a price in the hands of a fool to get wisdom, seeing he hath no heart to it?" is now easily answered, for even a fool knows that he must have the semblance of wisdom, and a diploma to imply it, if he is to succeed in the practice of medicine, but to insure the value of a diploma as a proof of education is the difficulty.

This evidence of discontent and tendency to change is a good sign. In these matters stillness means sleep or death—and the fact that a stream is continually changing its bed shows that its course lies through fertile alluvium and not through sterile lava or granite.

I have said that as regards scientific medicine we are at present going to school to Germany. This, however, is not the case with regard to therapeutics either external or internal—in regard to which I presume that the physicians of each nation are satisfied as to their own pre-eminence. At all events it is true that for the treatment of the common diseases a physician can obtain his most valuable instruction in his own country, among those whom he is to treat. Just as each individual is in some respects peculiar and unique, so that even the arrangement of the minute ridges and furrows at the end of his forefinger differs from that of all other forefingers, and is sufficient to identify him; and as the members of certain families require special care to guard against hemorrhage, or insanity, or phthisis; so it is with nations and races. The experienced military surgeon knows this well, and in the United States, which is now the great mixing ground, illustrations of race peculiarities are familiar to every practitioner.

Neither the tendency nor the true value of this current medical literature can be properly estimated by attending to it alone. It is a part of the thought of the age—of that wonderful kaleidoscopic pattern which is unrolling before us, and must be judged in connection with it. From several sources of high authority there have come of late years warnings and laments that science is becoming too utilitarian. For example, Prof. Du Bois-Reymond, in his address upon civilization and science, says that that side of science which is connected with the useful arts is steadily becoming more prominent, each generation being more and more bent on material interests. " Amid the unrest which possesses the civilized world, men's minds live as it were from hand to mouth. . . . And if industry receives its impulse from science, it also has a tendency to destroy science. In short, idealism is succumbing in the struggle with realism, and the kingdom of material interests is coming." Having laid down this rather pessimistic platform, he goes on to state that this is especially the case in America, which is the principal home of utilitarianism, and that it has become the custom to characterize as " Americanization" the dreaded permeation of European civilization by realism. If this characterization is correct, it would seem that Europe is pretty thoroughly Americanized as regards attention to material interests and appreciation of practical results. But the truth of the picture seems to me doubtful. Science is becoming popular, even fashionable, and some of its would-be votaries rival the devotees of modern æstheticism in their dislike and fear of the sunlight of comprehensibility and common sense. The languid scientific swell who thinks it bad style to be practical, who takes no interest in anything but pure science, and makes it a point to refrain from any investigations which might lead to useful results lest he might be confounded with mere " practical men," or inventors, exists and has his admirers. We have such in medicine, and their number will increase.

The separation of biological study from practical medicine, which has of late years become quite marked in the literature of the subject, has its advantages and disadvantages. Thus far the former have far outweighed the latter, and both the science and the art of medicine have been promoted thereby. But are not the physiologists, or, as I believe they prefer to be called, the biologists, separating themselves too completely from medicine for the best interests of their own science, in that they are neglecting human pathology? In our hospital wards, and among our patients, nature is continually performing experiments which the most dextrous operator cannot copy in the laboratory; she is, as Pro-

fessor Foster says, "a relentless and untrammelled vivisector, and there is no
secret of the living frame which she has not, or will not, at some time or place,
lay bare in misery and pain."

Now, while it is true that Professor Foster, in his address before the British
Medical Association last year (which address is the clearest exposition of the
aims of the physiology of the present day that I have seen), insists upon the fact·
that all distinctions between physiology and pathology are fictitious, and declares
that attempts to divide them are like attempts to divide meteorology into a science
of good and a science of bad weather, his conclusion that the pathologist should
be trained in methods of physiological investigation seems to me to be only a part
of the truth.   The tacit assumption is that all, or at least the most important,
phenomena of human disease may be reproduced in the physiological laboratory.·
If this were only true what a tremendous stride would have been taken towards
making medicine a science.   Unfortunately, it is not so.   Many of the most interesting of these phenomena, the most interesting because as yet the most unex-
plainable, can only be observed in the sick man himself.   Nor have the physiologists as yet made much use of that field which ought to be specially inviting to
them—namely, comparative pathology, although the literature of the present
time already indicates that a change has begun in this respect.

While it is true that to the graduate of thirty years ago much of the physiological literature of the present day is an unknown tongue, it is also true that the
physiologist of the present, who confines himself to laboratory work, will find
himself distanced by the man who keeps his clinical and pathological studies and
his experimental work well abreast.   .

The increase in both the amount and value of the literature of the several
specialties in medicine is readily seen by a comparison of recent catalogues and
bibliographies with those of twenty or thirty years ago, and this increase still continues at a greater rate than prevails in the more general branches.   There are
great differences of opinion as to the relative value of this increase and as to its
future effect upon the profession, but there can be no doubt as to the fact.   There
must be specialties and specialists in medicine, and the results will be both good
and evil; but the evils fall largely upon those specialists who have an insufficient
general education, who attempt to construct the pyramid of their knowledge with
the small end as a foundation.   It has been said by Dr. Hodgen that "in medicine a specialist should be a skilled physician, and something more ; but that he
is often something else—and something less."   There is truth in this ; truth which
the young man would do well to consider with care before he begins to specialize
his studies; but, on the other hand, it is also true that the great majority of men
must limit their field of work very much and very clearly if they hope to achieve
success.   The tool must have an edge if it is to cut.   It is by the labour of specialists that many of the new channels for thought and research have been opened,
and if the flood has sometimes seemed to spread too far, and to lose itself in shallow and sandy places, it has nevertheless tended to fertilize them in the end.

The specialists are not only making the principal advances in science, but they
are furnishing both strong incentives and valuable assistance towards the collection and preservation of medical literature and the formation of large public
libraries.

Burton declares that a great library cannot be improvised, not even if one had
the national debt to do it with—thinks that 20,000 volumes is about the limit of
what a miscellaneous collection can bring together, and refers especially to the
difficulty in creating large public libraries in America.   My experience would
show that these statements do not apply to medical books.   Of these the folios
and quartos of three and four hundred years ago seem to have had great capacity

for resistance to ordinary destructive forces.   Perhaps much of this is due to the fact that they are not usually injured by too much handling or perusal.   True, they are gradually becoming rarer, but at the same time by means of properly organized libraries they are becoming more accessible to all who wish to really use them, and not merely to collect and hide them away.   They drift about like the seaweed, but the survivors are gradually finding secure and permanent resting places in the score of great collections of such literature which the world now possesses.   At present the currents of trade are carrying them in relatively large numbers to the United States, where medical collectors and specialists are among the best customers of the antiquarian booksellers of Europe.   I could name a dozen American physicians who have given to European agents almost unlimited orders for books relating to their several specialties, and upon their shelves may be found books of the 15th and 16th centuries, which may be properly marked as "rarissime."

Not that the rarest books are by any means the oldest.   The collector who seeks to ornament his shelves with the Rose of John of Gaddesden, or the Lily of Bernerd de Gordon, the first folios of Avicenna or Celsus, or almost any of the eight hundred medical incunabula described by Hain, will probably succeed in his quest quite as soon as the one who has set his heart on the first editions of Harvey or Jenner, the American tracts on inoculation for smallpox, or complete sets of many of the journals and transactions of the present century.

Whatever may be the chosen line of the book collector, he is the special helper of the public library, and this whether he intend it or not.   In most cases his treasures pass through the auction room, and sooner or later the librarian, who can afford to wait, will secure them from further travel.   Thanks to the labours of such collectors, I think it is safe to say—what certainly would not have been true twenty years ago—that if the entire medical literature of the world, with the exception of that which is collected in the United States, were to be now destroyed, nearly all of it that is valuable could be reproduced without difficulty.

What is to be the result of this steadily increasing production of books?   What will the libraries and catalogues and bibliographies of a thousand, or even of a hundred years hence be like if we are thus to go on in the ratio of geometric progression, which has governed the press for the last few decades?   The mathematical formula which would express this, based on the data of the past century, gives an absurd and impossible conclusion, for it shows that if we go on as we have been going there is coming a time when our libraries will become large cities, and when it will require the services of every one in the world, not engaged in writing, to catalogue and care for the annual product.   The truth is, however, that the ratio has changed, and that the rate of increase is becoming smaller.   In Western Europe, which is now the great centre of literary production, it does not seem probable that the number of writers or readers will materially increase in the future, and it is in America, Russia, and Southern Asia that the greatest difference will be found between the present amount of annual literary product and that of a century hence.

The analogies between the mental and physical development of an individual, and of a nation or society, have been often set forth and commented on, but there is one point where the analogy fails as regards the products of mental activity— and that is that as yet we have devised no process for getting rid of the exuviæ. Growth and development in the physical world imply the changes of death as well as of life—that with the increase of the living tissues there shall also be the excretion and destruction of dead, outgrown, and useless matters which have had their day and served their purpose.   But *litera scripta manent*.   There is a vast amount of this effete and worthless material in the literature of medicine, and it is increasing rapidly. Our literature is, in fact, something like the inheritance of the golden dustman, but with this important difference—viz., that when the children raked a few shells or bits of bone from the dustman's heap, and, after stringing them together and playing with them a little while, threw them back, they did not thereby add to the bulk of the pile; whereas our preparers of compilations and compendiums, big and little, acknowledged or not, are continually increasing the collection, and for the most part with material which has been characterized as "superlatively middling, the quintessential extract of mediocrity." A large medical library is in itself discouraging to many inquirers, and I have become quite familiar with the peculiar expression of mingled surprise, awe, and despair which is apt to steal over the face of one not accustomed to such work when he first finds himself fairly in the presence of the mass of material which he wishes to examine for the purpose of completing his ideal bibliography of—let us say epilepsy, or excisions, or the functions of the liver.

Let such inquirers, as well as those who regret that they have no access to large libraries, and must therefore rely on the common text-books and current periodicals for bibliography, console themselves with the reflection that much the larger part of all of our literature which has any practical value belongs to the present century, and, indeed, will be found in the publications of the last twenty years.

There are a few books written prior to 1800 which every well-educated medical man should—I will not say read but—dip into, such as some of the works of Hippocrates and Galen, of Harvey and Hunter, of Morgagni and Sydenham; but this is to be done to learn their methods and style rather than their facts or theories, and by the great majority of physicians it can be done with much more profit in modern translations than in the originals. The really valuable part of the observations of these old masters has long ago become a part of the common stock, and the results are to be found in every text-book.

If, perchance, among the dusty folios there are stray golden grains yet ungleaned, remember that just in front are whole fields waiting the reaper. There is not, and has not been, any lack of men who have the taste and time to search the records of the past, and the man who has opportunities to make experiments or observations for himself wastes his time, to a certain extent, if he tries to do bibliographical work so long as he can get it done for him. He wishes to know whether this problem has been attacked before, and with what result—whether there are accounts of any other cases like the one he has in hand. In ninety-nine instances out of a hundred if the answers to these questions are not given in the current text-books or monographs it is not worth prolonged search by the original investigator. Yet he should know how to make this search, if only to enable him to direct others, and it is for this reason that a little acquaintance with bibliographical methods of work ought to be obtained by the student.

When a physician has observed (or thinks he has observed) a fact, or has evolved from his inner consciousness a theory which he wishes to examine by the light of medical literature, he is often very much at a loss to know how to begin, even when he has a large library accessible for the purpose.

The information he desires may be in the volume next his hand, but how is he to know that? And even when the usual subject-catalogue is placed before him he finds it very difficult to use it, especially when, as is often the case, he has by no means a well-defined idea as to what it is he wishes to look for. Upon the title-page of the Washington City Directory is printed the following aphorism, "To find a name you must know how to spell it." This has a very extensive application in medical bibliography. To find accounts of cases similar to your own rare case you must know what your own case is.

To return to the subject-catalogue. If it is a classed catalogue—a catalogue raisonnée—it will often seem to be a very blind guide to one who is not familiar with the classification and nomenclature adopted by the compiler. And certainly some of these classifications are very curious—reminding one of Heine's division of ideas into reasonable ideas, unreasonable ideas, and ideas covered with green leather. But if the inquirer has mastered the arrangement of the catalogue, it is two to one that it will not help him. It is a catalogue of the titles of books, but very often the title of a book gives very little information as to its contents, if, indeed, it is not actually misleading. Now, suppose the particular case he has in hand is one of a new-born infant having one leg much larger and longer than the other. He will find no book title relating to this. There may be a book in the library on diseases of the lymphatics which contains just what he wants, but unless he knows that his case is one affecting the lymphatics, he will hardly get the clue. There may also be in the library twenty papers, in as many different volumes of journals and transactions, the titles of which show that they probably relate to similar cases, but the titles of such papers do not appear in the catalogue.

It should also be observed that subject-catalogues may easily be put to improper uses, or thought to give more information than they really do. They are not bibliographies, but mechanical aids in bibliographical work.

You will perhaps pardon me for taking as an illustration the Index-Catalogue of the Library of the Surgeon-General's Office, in Washington, as being one with which I am familiar, and which I can venture to comment on without risk of its being thought that I wish to depreciate its value. Taking any given subject in medicine, it is possible for a fairly educated physician to obtain from this catalogue a large proportion of all the references which have any special value, and by so doing to save a vast amount of time and labour. On the other hand, he will find, when he comes to examine the books and articles referred to, that at least one-half of them are of no value so long as the other half are accessible, seeing that they are dilutions and dilatations, rehashes and summaries of the really original papers. If the seeker is in the library itself this does not cause a great waste of time, as he can rapidly examine and lay aside those that do not serve his purpose. But if he is using this catalogue in another library—say here in London, the case is different. It is highly improbable that he will find in any other collection all the books referred to, and then comes the annoyance of the doubt as to whether he may not be missing some very valuable paper. How is he to know whether or not Smith in his pamphlet on the functions of the pneumogastric has antici-pated his own theory of its relations to enlarged tonsils? And in all such cases *omne ignotum est pro magnifico*. In a bibliography of the subject, prepared from the same material as the catalogue, he would either find no mention of Smith's paper, or, better still, a note that his paper is merely an abstract or compilation. The fact that he does not find Smith's book in the London library, nor any allu-sion to it in the best works on the subject, ought to induce him to ignore it alto-gether.

In proportion to the energy of the young writer, and his determination to not only note everything that has been written about his subject, but to carry out the golden rule of verifying all his references, he is apt to be led off from his direct research into the many attractive by-paths of quaint and curious speculation which he will find branching off on every side, and this danger must be guarded against, or he will find that he is wasting his time and energy in turning over chaff which has long ago been pretty thoroughly threshed and winnowed.

It is, however, no part of my present purpose to set forth the methods and principles of bibliography, it is sufficient to point out their importance, and to call attention to the point that a knowledge of how and where to find the record of a fact is often of more practical use than a knowledge of the fact itself, just as we value an encyclopædia for occasional reference, and not for the purpose of reading through from cover to cover.

Instruction in the history and literature of medicine forms no part of the course of medical education in English and American schools, nor should I be disposed to recommend its introduction into the curriculum if it were to be based on French and German models, but it does seem possible to take a step in this direction which would be of great value ; not only as a means of general culture, as teaching students how to think, but from a purely practical point of view, in teaching them how to use the implements of their profession to the best advantage—for books are properly compared to tools of which the index is the handle. Such instruction should be given in a library, just as chemistry should be taught in a laboratory. The way to learn history and bibliography is to make them—the best work of the instructor is to show his students how to make them.

In the absence of some instruction of this kind the student is liable to waste much time in bibliographical research. There has been much more done in this direction than many writers seem to suppose, and there are not many subjects in medicine which have not been treated from this point of view. Of course, all is not bibliography which pretends to be such, very many of the exhaustive and exhausting lists of references which are now so common in medical journal articles have been taken largely at secondhand, and thereby originate or perpetuate errors. It is well to avoid false pride in this matter. To overlook a reference is by no means discreditable—but a wrong reference, or an unwitting reference to the same thing twice gives a strong presumption of carelessness and secondhand work. Journal articles, however, and especially reports of cases, undergo strange transmogrifications sometimes, and I have watched this with interest in the case of a French or German paper, translated and condensed in the *London Record*, then appearing in abstract under the name of the translator in a leading journal, then translated again, with a few new circumstances, in a continental periodical, and finally perhaps reversed and appearing as an original contribution in the pages of the *Little Peddlington Medical Universe.*

In this connection it is well to remember that a mere accumulation of observations, no matter how great the number, does not constitute science, especially if these observations have been recorded under the influence of the same theories and in essentially similar conditions.

Science seeks the law which governs or explains the phenomena, and when this is found the records of isolated instances of its action usually become of small importance so far as that law is concerned. We care little now for the records of the chemical experiments of a century ago, and the many detailed accounts of the earlier cases of the use of ether or chloroform are of so little interest at the present time that it is not worth while to refer to them in a bibliography of the subject. And although much has been done towards classifying and indexing our medical records (more, in fact, than most physicians suppose), still, as Helmholtz points out, such knowledge as this hardly deserves the name of science, since it neither enables us to see the complete connection nor to predict the result under new conditions yet untried.

Do I seem to depreciate the value of the thoughts which our masters have left us, and which have furnished the foundations on which we build ?—or to undervalue the importance of the great medical libraries in which are stored these thoughts ?—or to speak slightly of the utility of the catalogues, and indexes, and bibliographies, without which such libraries are trackless and howling wildernesses ? If so, I have said what I did not mean to say. The subject has been considered from the point of view of what used to be called the division of labour, but which now I suppose should be called evolution and differentiation; and this has been done because "life is short and the art is long," with fair prospect of becoming longer. It is surely unnecessary for me to enter upon any panegyric of books or libraries. As Dr. Holmes says, "It is not necessary to maintain the direct practical utility of all kinds of learning. Our shelves contain many books which only a certain class of medical scholars will be likely to consult. There is a dead medical literature, and there is a live one. The dead is not all ancient; the live is not all modern. There is none, modern or ancient, which, if it has no living value for the student, will not teach him something by its autopsy. But it is with the live literature of his profession that the medical practitioner is first of all concerned."

In medicine, as in social science, we must depend for many facts upon the observation of conditions which occur very rarely, and which cannot be repeated at pleasure. I have already alluded to the importance of Nature's vivisections to the physiologist, and a record of a case written a century ago may be just the link that is needed to correlate the results of his experiments of yesterday with existing theories. The case which at first seems unique and inexplicable both receives and furnishes light when compared with ancient records.

A science of medicine, like other sciences, must depend upon the classification of facts, upon the comparison of cases alike in many respects, but differing somewhat either in their phenomena or in the environment. The great obstacle to the development of a science of medicine is the difficulty in ascertaining what cases are sufficiently similar to be comparable, which difficulty is in its turn largely due to insufficient and erroneous records of the phenomena observed. This defect in the records is largely due, first, to ignorance on the part of observers; second, to the want of proper means for precisely recording the phenomena; and, third, to the confused and faulty condition of our nomenclature and nosological classifications.

Let us consider each of these points briefly. Very, very few are the men who can by and for themselves see and describe the things that are before them. Just as it took thousands of years to produce a man who could see what now any one can see when shown him, that the star Alpha in Capricorn is really two separate stars, so we had to wait long before the man came who could see the difference between measles and scarlatina, and still longer for the one who could distinguish between typhus and typhoid. Said Plato, "He shall be as a god to me who can rightly divide and define." Men who have this faculty—the "Blick" of the Germans—we cannot produce directly by any system of education; they come, we know not when or why, "forming a small band, a mere understanding of whose thoughts and works is a test of our highest powers. A single English dramatist and a single English mathematician have probably equalled in scope and excellence of original work in their several fields all the like labours of their countrymen put together."[1]

But cannot we do something to increase the number of observers by telling them what to observe? It is probable that much may be accomplished in this direction provided that care be taken to limit the field. Manuals of "what to observe at the bedside and in the post-mortem room" are very well in their way, but can never be made to reach the great majority of the profession, nor would they be of much use if they did. If a few, a very few, distinct specific questions are brought to the attention of the general practitioner, he will often be on the alert for their answer. And it should be remembered that chance may present to the most obscure practitioner an opportunity for observation which the greatest master may never meet.

---

[1] Iles, Mathematics in Evolution. Pop. Sci. Monthly, 1876, ix. p. 207.

The great difficulty is to get such questions prepared. They must relate to matters that are just in the nebulous region between the known and unknown— to points not yet clear, but of which we know enough to make it probable that by observing in a definite direction they can be made clear; and to prepare them requires not only knowledge, but a certain reaching out beyond knowledge. It usually happens that the man who has this faculty strives to answer his questions himself, and no doubt he can usually do it better than another. But much can be done towards defining and marking out what we do not know, and this has been a powerful aid to the progress of physiology in recent years. I have had occasion to refer to this in speaking of Prof. Foster's work on physiology, in each section of which an attempt is made to separate that which may be considered as proved from that which is merely probable; and thus almost every page becomes suggestive of work to be done.

Another example of what I mean will be found in a paper on the collection of data at autopsies by Professor H. P. Bowditch, of Boston (Trans. Mass. Med.-Legal Soc. 1, 1880, p. 139). Taking the results of an investigation into the absolute and relative size of organs at different periods of life, and in connection with different morbid tendencies, recently published by Professor Beneke, of Warburg, Dr. Bowditch urges the securing as large a number as possible of such data, and selects certain of Professor Beneke's results for special inquiry; as, for instance, that "the cancerous diathesis is associated with a large and powerful heart, capacious arteries, but a relatively small pulmonary artery, small lungs, well developed bones and muscles, and tolerably abundant adipose tissue." It can hardly be doubted that those who read the papers of Professors Bowditch and Beneke will be induced to examine things which before would have had for them no interest, and, therefore, to make and record observations in pathological anatomy which otherwise would have been lost.

The second difficulty referred to—viz., the want of means for making accurate records—is one that is yearly growing less. It behooves us to be modest in our predictions as to what may be accomplished in the future towards the solution of our Sphinx's riddle. We see as through a glass darkly, and except through the glass in no wise; but, at least, we have made such progress that what we do see we can, to a great extent, so record that our successors yet unborn can also see, and it is owing to this fact that a part of the medical literature of the last quarter of the nineteenth century will be more valuable than all that has preceded it.

The word-pictures of disease traced by Hippocrates and Sydenham, or even those of Graves and Trousseau, interesting and valuable as they are, are not comparable with the records upon which the skilled clinical teacher of the present day relies. Yet how imperfect in many cases are even the best of these records as compared with what might be given with the resources which we have at our command. The temperature chart has done away with the errors which necessarily follow attempts to compare the memory of sensations perceived last week with the sensations of to-day—and the balance and the burette enable us to estimate with some approach to precision the tissue changes of our patients by the records of change in the excretions which they furnish; but we must still trust to our memory, or to the imperfect descriptions of what others remember, when we attempt to compare the results obtained on successive days by auscultation or percussion, although the phonograph and microphone strongly hint to us the possibility of either accurately reproducing the sounds of yesterday, or of translating them into visible signs, perhaps something like the dot and dash record of the telegraph code, which could then be given to the press, and so compared with each other by readers at the antipodes.

We are beginning to count the blood corpuscles, and to use photomicrography, but we do not yet apply the latter process to the former so as to enable every reader to count for himself.

The connections of medicine with the physical sciences are yearly becoming closer, and the methods by which these sciences have been brought to their present condition are those by which progress has been, and is to be, made in therapeutics as well as in diagnosis or in physiological research. These methods turn mainly upon increasing the delicacy and accuracy of measurements; of expressing manifestations of force in terms of another force, or of dimension in space or time. The balance and the galvanometer, the microscope and the pendulum, the camera, the sphygmograph and the thermometer are some of the means by which investigators, at the bedside and in the laboratory, are seeking to obtain records which shall be independent of their own sensations or personal equations; which shall be taken and used as expressing not opinions, but facts; and with every addition to or improvement in these means of measurement and record, the field of observation widens, and new and more reliable materials are furnished for the application of logical and mathematical methods.

Upon the third difficulty which has been referred to, viz., our confused and defective terminology, I need not dwell. "Science," said Condillac, "is a language well made," and though this is far from being the whole truth, it is an important part of it. In examining medical reports and statistics, it is necessary to bear constantly in mind that to understand many terms you must know what the individual writer means by them. When, for example, we find in such statistics a certain number of deaths attributed to gastro-enteritis, or croup, or scrofula, we have to take into account the country, the period, and the individual author, in order to get even a fair presumption as to what is meant.

The three difficulties which have been referred to, although the most important, are by no means the only causes of the confusion and imperfection of our records.

Prominent among the minor troubles of the investigator are defective or misleading titles, and in behalf of the readers and bibliographers of the future I would appeal to authors, and more especially to editors, to pay more attention than many of them do to the matter of titles and indexes. The men to whom your papers are most important, and who will make the best use of them provided they know of their existence, are for the most part hard workers, busy men who have a right to demand that their literary table shall be provided with properly prepared materials and not with shapeless lumps.

The editors of Transactions of Societies, whether these are sent to journals or published in separate form, often commit numerous sins of omission in the matter of titles. The rule should be that every article which is worth printing is worth a distinct title, which should be as concise as a telegram, and be printed in a special type. If the author does not furnish such a title, it is the editor's business to make it; and he should not be satisfied with such headings as "Clinical Cases," "Difficult Labour," "A Remarkable Tumour," "Case of Wound, with Remarks." The four rules for the preparation of an article for a journal will then be: 1. Have something to say. 2. Say it. 3. Stop as soon as you have said it. 4. Give the paper a proper title.

Some societies and editors do not seem to appreciate fully their responsibility for the articles which they accept for publication; a responsibility which cannot be altogether avoided by any formal declaration disclaiming it. This is due to the fact that while the merits of a paper can usually be determined by examination, this is by no means always the case. In every country there are writers and speakers whose statements are received with very great distrust by those best acquainted with them. Supposing these statements to be true, the papers would be of much interest and importance; but the editor should remember that a certain number of readers, and especially those in foreign countries, have no clue to the character of the author beyond the fact that they find his works in good company. In medical literature, as in other departments, we find books and papers from men who are either constitutionally incapable of telling the simple, literal truth as to their observations and experiments, although they may not write with fixed intentions to deceive, or from men who seek to advertise themselves by deliberate falsehoods as to the results of their practice. Such men are usually appreciated at their true value in their immediate neighbourhood, and find it necessary to send their communications to distant journals and societies in order to secure publication.

I presume that you are all familiar with the peculiar feeling of distrust which is roused by too complete an explanation. The report of a case in which every symptom observed, and the effect of every remedy given is fully accounted for, and in which no residual unexplained phenomena appear, is usually suspicious, for it implies either superficial observation or suppression, or distortion of some of the facts. A diagrammatic representation is usually much plainer than a good photograph, but also of much less value as a basis for further work.

No fact is more familiar to this audience than the vast extent of the field of the science of to-day—so vast that few may hope to master more than a small part of it, and yet so closely connected that even the small part cannot be fully grasped without some acquaintance with a much wider field.

But little over a hundred years ago, Haller, in Göttingen, was professor of anatomy, botany, physiology, surgery, and obstetrics, and lecturer on medical jurisprudence At the same time he was writing one review a week, and summing up existing medical science in his "Bibliotheca." To-day any one of these branches requires all the time of the most energetic and learned of our contemporaries; but, on the other hand, the well-educated medical graduate of to-day could give Haller valuable instruction in each of the branches of which he was professor. It is also true, as I have pointed out, that our actual progress is by no means in proportion to the work done, nor as great as these merely quantitative statements would seem to make it.

Science has been termed "the topography of ignorance." From a few elevated points we triangulate vast spaces, inclosing infinite unknown details. We cast the lead, and draw up a little sand from abysses we shall never reach with our dredges.

If it is true that we understand ourselves but imperfectly in health, it is more signally manifest in disease, where natural actions imperfectly understood, disturbed in an obscure way by half-seen causes, are creeping and winding along in the dark towards their destined issue, sometimes using our remedies as safe stepping-stones, occasionally, it may be, stumbling over them as obstacles.[1]

In days of old, when the profession of medicine, or of a single medical specialty, was an inheritance in certain families, a large part of their knowledge and the efficiency of their remedies was thought to depend upon these being kept a profound mystery. Among the precepts of magic there was no more significant one than that which declared that the communication of the formula destroyed its power, and that hence attempts to reveal the secret must always fail.

We have changed all that. Every physician hastens to publish his discoveries and special knowledge, and a good many do the same by that which is not special, or which is not knowledge. For the individual, in a degree—for the nation or the race in a much greater degree—the literature produced is the most endur-

---

[1] Border Lines of Knowledge, etc., by O. W. Holmes, Boston, 1862, pp. 7, 8.

ing memorial. The whole result of civilization has been cynically defined as being roughly, "Three hundred million Chinese, two hundred million natives of India, two hundred million Europeans and North Americans, and a miscellaneous hundred million or two of Central Asians, Malays, South Sea Islanders, etc., and over and above all the rest the Library of the British Museum. This is the net result of an indefinitely long struggle between the forces of men and the weights of various kinds in the attempt to move which these forces display themselves."[1]

And thus in our great medical libraries each of the folios or quaint little black-letter pamphlets which mark the first two centuries of printing, or of the cheap and dirty volumes of more modern days, with their scrofulous paper and abominable typography, represents to a great extent the life of one of our profession and the fruit of his labours, and it is by the fruit that we know him.

After stating that modern physicists have concluded that the sun is going out, that the earth is falling into the sun, and therefore that it and all things in it will be either fried or frozen, Professor Clifford concludes that "our interest lies so much with the past as may serve to guide our actions in the present, and with so much of the future as we may hope will be affected by our actions now. Beyond that we do not know and ought not to care. Does this seem to say, Let us eat and drink, for to-morrow we die? Not so, but rather, Let us take hands and help, for this day we are alive together." To this I join a verse from the Talmud, which will remind you of the first aphorism of Hippocrates, and is none the worse for that: "The day is short, and work is great—the reward is also great, and the master presses. It is not incumbent on thee to complete the work, but thou must not therefore cease from it."—*Lancet*, Aug. 13, 1881.

TRANSLATION OF AN ADDRESS ON THE GERM THEORY.

Delivered at the International Medical Congress, London, August, 1881.

BY PROFESSOR PASTEUR.

GENTLEMEN: I had no intention of addressing this admirable Congress, which brings together the most eminent medical men in the world, and the great success of which does so much credit to its principal organizer, Mr. Mac Cormac. The good-will of your esteemed President has decided otherwise. How could one, in fact, resist the sympathetic words of that eminent man whose goodness of heart is associated in no small degree with great oratorical ability? Two motives have brought me to London. The first was to gain instruction, to profit by your learned discussions; and the second was to ascertain the place now occupied in medicine and surgery by the germ theory. Certainly I shall return to Paris well satisfied. During the past week I have learned much. I carry away with me the conviction that the English people are a great people, and as for the influence of the new doctrine, I have been not only struck by the progress it has made, but by its triumph. I should be guilty of ingratitude and of false modesty if I did not accept the welcome I have received among you and in English society as a mark of homage paid to my labours during the past five-and-twenty years upon the nature of ferments—their life and their nutrition, their preparation in a pure state by the introduction of organisms (*ensemencement*) under natural and artificial conditions — labours which have established the principles and the methods of microbie (microbism), if the expression is allowable. Your cordial

---

[1] Liberty, Equality, and Fraternity, by James Fitz James Stephen, N. Y. 1873, p. 178.

welcome has revived within me the lively feeling of satisfaction I experienced when your great surgeon Lister declared that my publication in 1857 on milk fermentation had inspired him with his first ideas on his valuable surgical method. You have reawakened the pleasure I felt when our eminent physician Dr. Davaine declared that his labours upon charbon (splenic fever or malignant pustule) had been suggested by my studies on butyric fermentation and the vibrion which is characteristic of it. Gentlemen, I am happy to be able to thank you by bringing to your notice a new advance in the study of microbie as applied to the prevention of transmissible diseases—diseases which for the most part are fraught with terrible consequences, both for man and domestic animals. The subject of my communication is vaccination in relation to chicken cholera and splenic fever, and a statement of the method by which we have arrived at these results—a method the fruitfulness of which inspires me with boundless anticipations. Before discussing the question of splenic fever vaccine, which is the most important, permit me to recall the results of my investigations of chicken cholera. It is through this inquiry that new and highly important principles have been introduced into science concerning the virus or contagious quality of transmissible diseases. More than once in what I am about to say I shall employ the expression virus-culture, as formerly, in my investigations on fermentation, I used the expressions, the culture of milk ferment, the culture of the butyric vibrion, etc.

Let us take, then, a fowl which is about to die of chicken cholera, and let us dip the end of a delicate glass rod in the blood of the fowl with the usual precautions, upon which I need not here dwell. Let us then touch with this charged point some *bouillon de poule*, very clear, but first of all rendered sterile under a temperature of about 115° Centigrade, and under conditions in which neither the outer air nor the vases employed can introduce exterior germs—those germs which are in the air, or on the surface of all objects. In a short time, if the little culture vase is placed in a temperature of 25° to 35°, you will see the liquid become turbid, and full of tiny microbes, shaped like the figure 8, but often so small that under a high magnifying power they appear like points. Take from this vase a drop as small as you please, no more than can be carried on the point of a glass rod as sharp as a needle, and touch with this point a fresh quantity of sterilized *bouillon de poule* placed in a second vase, and the same phenomenon is produced. You deal in the same way with a third culture vase, with a fourth, and so on to a hundred, or even a thousand, and invariably within a few hours the culture liquid becomes turbid and filled with the same minute organisms. At the end of two or three days' exposure to a temperature of about 30° C. the thickness of the liquid disappears, and a sediment is formed at the bottom of the vase. This signifies that the development of the minute organism has ceased—in other words, all the little points which caused the turbid appearance of the liquid have fallen to the bottom of the vase, and things will remain in this condition for a longer or shorter time, for months even, without either the liquid or the deposit undergoing any visible modification, inasmuch as we have taken care to exclude the germs of the atmosphere. A little stopper of cotton sifts the air which enters or issues from the vase through changes of temperature. Let us take one of our series of culture preparations—the hundredth or the thousandth, for instance—and compare it in respect to its virulence with the blood of a fowl which has died of cholera; in other words, let us inoculate under the skin ten fowls, for instance, each separately with a tiny drop of infectious blood, and ten others with a similar quantity of the liquid in which the deposit has first been shaken up. Strange to say, the latter ten fowls will die as quickly and with the same symptoms as the former ten; the blood of all will be found to contain after death the same minute infectious organisms. This equality, so to speak, in the virulence both of the culture preparation and of the blood is due to an apparently futile circumstance. I have made a hundred culture preparations—at least, I have understood that this was done—without leaving any considerable interval between the impregnations. Well, here we have the cause of the equality in the virulence. Let us now repeat exactly our successive cultures with this single difference, that we pass from one culture to that which follows it—from the hundredth to, say, the hundred and first, at intervals of a fortnight, a month, two months, three months, or ten months. If, now, we compare the virulence of the successive cultures, a great change will be observed. It will be readily seen from an inoculation of a series of ten fowls that the virulence of one culture differs from that of the blood and from that of a preceding culture when a sufficiently long interval elapses between the impregnation of one culture with the microbe of the preceding. More than that, we may recognize by this mode of observation that it is possible to prepare cultures of varying degrees of virulence. One preparation will kill eight fowls out of ten, another five out of ten, another one out of ten, another none at all, although the microbe may still be cultivated. In fact, what is no less strange, if you take each of these cultures of attenuated virulence as a point of departure in the preparation of successive cultures and without appreciable interval in the impregnation, the whole series of these cultures will reproduce the attenuated virulence of that which has served as the starting point. Similarly, where the virulence is null it produces no effect. How, then, it may be asked, are the effects of these attenuating virulences revealed in the fowls? They are revealed by a local disorder, by a morbid modification more or less profound in a muscle, if it is a muscle which has been inoculated with the virus. The muscle is filled with microbes which are easily recognized because the attenuated microbes have almost the bulk, the form, and the appearance of the most virulent microbes. But why is not the local disorder followed by death? For the moment let us answer by a statement of facts. They are these: the local disorder ceases of itself more or less speedily, the microbe is absorbed and digested, if one may say so, and little by little the muscle regains its normal condition. Then the disease has disappeared. When we inoculate with the microbe the virulence of which is null there is not even local disorder, the *naturæ medicatrix* carries it off at once, and here, indeed, we see the influence of the resistance of life, since this microbe, the virulence of which is null, multiplies itself. A little further, and we touch the principle of vaccination. When the fowls have been rendered sufficiently ill by the attenuated virus which the vital resistance has arrested in its development, they will, when inoculated with virulent virus, suffer no evil effects, or only effects of a passing character. In fact, they no longer die from the mortal virus, and for a time sufficiently long, which in some cases may exceed a year, chicken cholera cannot touch them, especially under the ordinary conditions of contagion which exist in fowl-houses. At this critical point of our manipulation—that is to say, in this interval of time which we have placed between two cultures, and which causes the attenuation—what occurs? I shall show you that in this interval the agent which intervenes is the oxygen of the air. Nothing more easily admits of proof. Let us produce a culture in a tube containing very little air, and close this tube with an enameller's lamp. The microbe in developing itself will speedily take all the oxygen of the tube and of the liquid, after which it will be quite free from contact with oxygen. In this case it does not appear that the microbe becomes appreciably attenuated, even after a great lapse of time. The oxygen of the air, then, would seem to be a possible modifying agent of the virulence of the microbe of chicken cholera— that is to say, it may modify more or less the facility of its development in the body of animals. May we not be here in presence of a general law applicable to all kinds of virus? What benefits may not be the result? We may hope to discover in this way the vaccine of all virulent diseases; and what is more natural than to begin our investigation of the vaccine of what we in French call charbon, what you in England call splenic fever, and what in Russia is known as the Siberian pest, and in Germany as the Milzbrand. In this new investigation I have had the assistance of two devoted young *savants*—MM. Chamberland and Roux. At the outset we were met by a difficulty. Among the inferior organisms, all do not resolve themselves into those corpuscle germs which I was the first to point out as one of the forms of their possible development. Many infectious microbes do not resolve themselves in their cultures into corpuscle germs. Such is equally the case with beer yeast, which we do not see develop itself usually in breweries, for instance, except by a sort of scissiparity. One cell makes two or more, which form themselves in wreaths; the cells become detached, and the process recommences. In these cells real germs are not usually seen. The microbe of chicken cholera and many others behave in this way, so much so that the cultures of this microbe, although they may last for months without losing their power of fresh cultivation, perish finally like beer yeast which has exhausted all its aliments. The anthracoid microbe in artificial cultures behaves very differently. In the blood of animals, as in cultures, it is found in translucid filaments more or less segmented. This blood or these cultures freely exposed to air, instead of continuing according to the first mode of generation, show at the end of forty-eight hours corpuscle germs distributed in series more or less regular along the filaments. All around those corpuscles matter is absorbed, as I have represented it formerly in one of the plates of my work on the disease of silkworms. Little by little all connection between them disappears, and presently they are reduced to nothing more than germ dust. If you make these corpuscles germinate, the new culture reproduces the virulence peculiar to the thready form which has produced these corpuscles, and this result is seen even after a long exposure of these germs to contact with air. Recently we discovered them in pits in which animals dead of splenic fever had been buried for twelve years, and their culture was as virulent as that from the blood of an animal recently dead. Here I regret extremely to be obliged to shorten my remarks. I should have had much pleasure in demonstrating that the anthracoid germs in the earth of pits in which animals have been buried are brought to the surface by earthworms, and that in this fact we may find the whole etiology of disease, inasmuch as the animals swallow these germs with their food. A great difficulty presents itself when we attempt to apply our method of attenuation by the oxygen of the air to the anthracoid microbes. The virulence establishing itself very quickly, often after four-and-twenty hours in an anthracoid germ which escapes the action of the air, it was impossible to think of discovering the vaccine of splenic fever in the conditions which had yielded that of chicken cholera. But was there, after all, reason to be discouraged? Certainly not; in fact, if you observe closely, you will find that there is no real difference between the mode of the generation of the anthracoid germ by scission and that of chicken cholera. We had therefore reason to hope that we might overcome the difficulty which stopped us by endeavouring to prevent the anthracoid microbe from producing corpuscle germs and to keep it in this condition in contact with oxygen for days, and weeks, and months. The experiment fortunately succeeded. In the ineffective (*neutre*) *bouillon de poule* the anthracoid microbe is no longer cultivable at 45° C. Its culture, however, is easy at 42° or 43°, but in these conditions the microbe yields no spores. Consequently it is possible to maintain in contact with the pure air at 42° or 43° a *mycélienne* culture of bacteria entirely free of germs. Then appear the very remarkable results which follow. In a month or six weeks the culture dies—that is to say, if one impregnates with it fresh *bouillon*, the latter is completely sterile. Up till that time life exists in the vase exposed to air and heat.   If we examine the virulence of the culture at the end of two days, four days, six days, eight days, etc., it will be found that long before the death of the culture the microbe has lost all virulence, although still cultivable.   Before this period it is found that the culture presents a series of attenuated virulences.   Everything is similar to what happens in respect to the microbe in chicken cholera.   Besides, each of these conditions of attenuated virulence may be reproduced by culture ; in fact, since the charbon does not operate a second time (*ne récidive pas*), each of our attenuated anthracoid microbes constitutes for the superior microbe a vaccine— that is to say, a virus capable of producing a milder disease.   Here, then, we have a method of preparing the vaccine of splenic fever.   You will see presently the practical importance of this result, but what interests us more particularly is to observe that we have here a proof that we are in possession of a general method of preparing virus vaccine based upon the action of the oxygen and the air—that is to say, of a cosmic force existing everywhere on the surface of the globe.   I regret to be unable from want of time to show you that all these attenuated forms of virus may very easily, by a physiological artifice, be made to recover their original maximum virulence.   The method I have just explained of obtaining the vaccine of splenic fever was no sooner made known than it was very exten- sively employed to prevent the splenic affection.   In France we lose every year by splenic fever animals of the value of 20,000,000f.   I was asked to give a public demonstration of the results already mentioned.   This experiment I may relate in a few words.   Fifty sheep were placed at my disposition, of which twenty-five were vaccinated.   A fortnight afterwards the fifty sheep were inoculated with the most virulent anthracoid microbe.   The twenty-five vaccinated sheep resisted the infection ; the twenty-five unvaccinated died of splenic fever within fifty hours.   Since that time my energies have been taxed to meet the demands of farmers for supplies of this vaccine.   In the space of fifteen days we have vacci- nated in the departments surrounding Paris more than 20,000 sheep and a large number of cattle and horses.   If I were not pressed for time I should bring to your notice two other kinds of virus attenuated by similar means.   These experiments will be communicated by and by to the public.   I cannot conclude, gentlemen, without expressing the great pleasure I feel at the thought that it is as a member of an international medical congress assembled in England that I make known the most recent results of vaccination upon a disease more terrible, perhaps, for domestic animals than smallpox is for man.   I have given to vaccination an ex- tension which science, I hope, will accept as homage paid to the merit and to the immense services tendered by one of the greatest men of England, Jenner. What a pleasure for me to do honour to this immortal name in this noble and hospitable city of London!—*Lancet*, Aug. 13, 1881.

ADDRESS ON THE CHANGES WHICH SURGERY HAS UNDERGONE DURING THE LAST TEN YEARS.

Delivered at the Meeting of the International Medical Congress, London, 1881.

BY PROFESSOR VOLKMANN.

GENTLEMEN : It is with hesitation and only in accordance with the wish of my London friends that I have undertaken to speak before such a distinguished assembly, and to make an attempt to sketch a hasty picture of the changes which surgery has experienced in the last fifteen or even ten years. And I trust that in this attempt I may rely on your special indulgence; for great and unparalleled in the history of medical science have been those changes. Problems thousands of years old have been solved, or are at any rate approaching a sure solution; the desires of our fathers have been fulfilled beyond their hope or expectation. But all our practice and theories have been also fundamentally altered. The position of our science, the position that we ourselves occupy towards invalids, have become entirely different. And this revolution, in the midst of which we still stand, although the first wave has exhausted itself, has been called forth by the one incontestable fact, that all those countless and disastrous disturbances by which the wounds and hence also the life of those operated on or injured are threatened are only the consequences of particular processes of decomposition of the animal fluids, brought about by the intrusion of lower organisms.

For with the recognition of the manner of their origin, and with the knowledge of their nature, we have also gained the power of preventing these disturbances. Conscious of our aim, we are able so to act as to prevent the evil influences of these micro-organisms. The fate of countless invalids is from henceforth placed in our hands. In the place of blind chance, in the place of fortune or misfortune, which formerly played so great a part in the work of the practical surgeon, there now appear, in quite a different degree, knowledge and ignorance, capability and inability, care and carelessness. But a short time ago the surgeon, when he had, according to the rules of his art, made a wound, was like the husbandman who, when he has sown his field, patiently awaits the harvest, and accepts it as it may turn out, powerlessly exposed to the elements which may bring him rain and sunshine, storm and hail. Now he is the manufacturer from whom we expect good wares. By rescuing from the domain of chance the results of our labours, as far as they depend on operations and the treatment of wounds—and this will always remain the chief and especial work of surgery— the antiseptic method has elevated surgery to the rank of the latest experimental science.

Never has a discovery been made in surgery which has even approached this in its benefits to humanity in general. Many thousands of human beings have in the short space of time that has elapsed since then preserved life and limbs, and been spared pain and a long confinement to a sick-bed; and millions will yet share in these benefits, for the principles of the antiseptic treatment of wounds will *never* again be abandoned as long as the whole of our knowledge is not lost, no matter how our art or the points of attack may change. Perhaps we may some day succeed in treating injured limbs simply in heated or filtered air, or may learn to strengthen the living power of resistance of the tissues and organs so that they can of themselves resist the action of those invisible enemies. The protection afforded by vaccination makes it appear possible that in this direction also new paths are opening out to us.

England may be proud that it was one of her sons whose name is inseparably connected with this the greatest advance that surgery has ever made. Without envy other nations may yield her the crown. For the long and silent labour which made the ripening of the seed possible, which we now reap so quickly and fully, was quite international, and especially France and Germany took part in it in an equal degree. Nor did any one more fully recognize the importance of those who worked before him than Mr. Joseph Lister.

Moreover, it has happened with the discovery of the antiseptic method as with so many great discoveries; years, sometimes centuries, prepare them, they are in the air as it were, until one day, to the surprise of mankind, they suddenly seem to fall down from heaven. Nothing is more instructive than to reflect the light of our present knowledge on the endeavours of past times, and to see how since the beginning of this century the most heterogeneous opinions have been held concerning the treatment of wounds; how methods apparently the most opposite have been employed, in all of which we may, however, now recognize a certain value—how wounds were treated with ice, with the cautery iron, with alcohol; how they were ventilated or hermetically closed; how the subcutaneous mode of operation was resorted to without deciding the question why the air coming into contact with the injured tissues of the body in one series of cases causes such deleterious results, in others appears perfectly harmless; how, seeking without any firm leading principle, experimenting and often abandoning one's self to the rudest empiricism, yet the goal was approached nearer and nearer— so near, that we might suppose it was almost possible even then to grasp the truth, and that every one ought to have recognized it, and then, when daylight is approaching, and even when the chief problem has been solved, that then the complete failure of our art was shown by the adoption of the open treatment of wounds.

I consider the directions given by Stromeyer and Pirogoff, especially for gun-shot wounds, and in their time perfectly justified, never to probe a fresh wound, is here carried out to actual nihilism, and, to our shame, proofs are given that with passive looking on and the renunciation of quick healing by first intention, with good cicatrizing, the results were on an average better than in all active methods of treatment practised up to that time. Gentlemen, I wish not to be misunderstood. I do not mean that open treatment of wounds which is at this day employed in the most efficacious manner in combination with strictly antiseptic measures where the locality or serious disturbances already caused in the wound do not permit of the usual appliances, or where after an operation performed with all the means of protection which modern surgery affords us, we may so safely count upon a healing by first intention that further measures seem unnecessary. I will also point out that the German surgeon who first employed the open treatment of wounds and gave it its name, and achieved excellent results with it— Burow—introduced in connexion with it a remedy which we now know as one of the strongest antiseptics—i. e., the argilla acetica. But I speak of that open treatment of wounds which, rejecting all the attainments of modern surgery, was so emphatically lauded as a special method to be preferred to all other modes of treatment.

Gentlemen, in speaking of the open treatment of wounds, I have touched on the opposition which the new doctrine at first met with on so many sides. You all know well how violent this was. Even in science great changes cannot be brought about without injury to numerous personal interests. But I insist that nowadays no serious opposition exists, that there is no surgeon who would dare at the operating-table or in the treatment of the wounded quite to renounce antiseptic methods; who calmly and with a good conscience would tread the paths in which fifteen years ago we all followed like cattle. Even the most obstinate have had to give way to the great principles of the new era, and often in a much higher degree than they acknowledged to themselves or others; the necessity not only of the disinfection of hands, sponges, instruments, and bandages, but also the necessity of a primary disinfection of fresh wounds, is, I believe, universally acknowledged.

In this respect, then, the time that we have lived through stands alone. In a period of a few years a new revolutionizing doctrine and a new difficult method of treatment which increases to the utmost the responsibility of the surgeon treating the case has celebrated its triumph through the whole of the educated world.

I hope you will think it natural if I, in the attempt to sketch the most essential points by which modern surgery differs from that of past times, place in the first ranks the immense diminution of mortality after serious operations and severe injuries. It seems natural to prove the advances made in this respect by comparing the mortality under the old surgery with that of the present day. But in spite of all trouble and labour, the only result of such attempts is the conviction that our present results are incomparably better. How great used to be the average losses caused by important operations and serious injuries we shall never learn. One thing is certain, that they were much greater even than most of the available calculations made them appear. But this second fact is just as certain ; that the calculation of averages had at that time scarcely any value, because the mortality was subject at different times, in different hospitals, and under different surgeons, to the most enormous variations, as a glance into the celebrated work of Malgaigne will show. Average numbers can only be of value when the variations take place within certain fixed limits. The high tables of mortality of old surgery have been obtained by the addition of series of cases which differed from one another fivefold or tenfold ; and as soon as they were applied by the sick-bed or in the judgment of the results of treatment, they let any result appear satisfactory, and, if fatal, excused it.

We may therefore say without exaggeration that the old statistics of surgery were of no use, but only did harm, and we may oppose to their sad, unsatisfactory figures the simple demand that *no* person should die of an injury unless its severity directly threatens his life, and that no person injured or operated on should perish through a secondary inflammatory disturbance developed from the wound. Every loss of this kind may be traced to some mistake on our part.

But we, who have ourselves groaned beneath the weight of the old surgery, and have now made the new our own, possess comparative statistics that are infinitely more valuable to us than all those that our opponents have held up against us, statistics which we have fought for in the last few years. The time is long enough to have excluded all the old theories of chance. During ten years it is not possible to be always lucky, always to have good cards, as even Pirogoff still ventured to assert of certain privileged surgeons.

And if we compare our former with our present results we find a difference like that between day and night, the feeling of a great victory after long and severe defeat ; and never do I feel more solemnly and gratefully inclined to Providence, who has permitted me to live to see this blessed change, than when I make this comparison.

Professor Nussbaum has drawn this comparison between then and now in his clinic in clear traits and with manly candour ; he has shown that for forty years, under his own direction as well as under that of his predecessors, among whom was Stromeyer, fatal wound diseases raged, that nearly all patients with compound fractures died of them, and that even those with the slightest injuries often succumbed to them ; that erysipelas and abscess were matters of daily occurrence, that during the latter years hospital gangrene also appeared and attacked the dreadful number of eighty per cent. of all wounds and sores, that he stood helpless and powerless before all these conditions, and that at one step, after the general introduction of the antiseptic method, all this ceased, and instead, even after great operations, healing by first intention was introduced as an entirely new result.

I have also tried already at the third German Congress of Surgeons to draw a similar comparison ; it is not essentially different from Nussbaum's. Since then many years have elapsed ; and in all countries, but perhaps most of all in Germany, a great mass of experience has been collected, and it might perhaps be now possible by a comparison of large numbers to discover with some amount of certainty what is really the chief question; how far we have got in the control of accidental wound diseases; what dependence is to be placed on our present technical aids; where and how often they leave us in the lurch, and where the limits to our present power are placed. Time and place do not permit me to make this attempt, and perhaps it would be beyond my power. But, with your permission, I will lay before you some data bearing on these questions, and if I take these chiefly from my own experience, you may be convinced that this is only because these are most accessible to me, and because I can myself vouch for their accuracy. For the satisfaction of personal vanity I should probably have chosen another subject than this which shows what can be achieved by a method in the invention of which I had no share, and should have brought forward other results than those which were only achieved by submitting entirely during the first years to the prescriptions of Joseph Lister, and resisting every temptation to do better and more simply than he. Most of the unfavourable judgments passed on this method are due to the fact that surgeons who had not yet learnt to experiment *with it* already made *it* the subject of their experiments.

Two examples will suffice, compound fractures and major amputations. The mortality after compound fracture had, during the long labours of my predecessor as well as during my own, reached the sad height of forty per cent. When I adopted the antiseptic treatment of wounds my last twelve patients, with compound fracture of the leg, had all died of pyæmia or septicæmia. From that time up to the present day I have treated one after another 135 compound fractures, and not a single patient has succumbed to either of these accidental wound diseases; 133 were cured, two died, one of fat-embolism of the lungs, during the first few hours, and one, a drunkard, of delirium tremens.

For amputations one assertion will almost suffice, which I beg you to regard seriously; I now cure every year more cases of amputation of the thigh than during all the rest of my labours before the introduction of the antiseptic method. The number of the amputations of the larger limbs which I have undertaken during the last few years amounts to more than 400. If I subtract those cases where death did certainly not result in consequence of the operation, but independently of this from some other serious complication, there results a mortality of four to five per cent., and the same number, as far as I can discover from the communications before me, was obtained in the other German hospitals in which antiseptic surgery is practised in full strength.

My friend Dr. Schede has made a calculation which will, I believe, interest you. He has studied the reports of a great number of amputation cases of the old period, so that he was able to distinguish those in which death resulted from pyæmia or septicæmia—those therefore which we now save—and the mortality of the remaining cases also amounted to about five per cent. In these four to five per cents., besides those fatal cases caused by mistakes in treatment, those are also included which in amputations after serious injuries must be laid to the door of the shock caused by the previous serious loss of blood. We may therefore declare that amputation of the larger limbs has been almost absolutely free from danger—at any rate, much less dangerous than many small operations were formerly, whose mortality was never discussed. After extirpation of sebaceous cysts in the head, occasionally one or other of those operated on perished; and a by no means small part came off only with their lives. It is true, I must not disguise the fact, that my numbers have been slighted. It has been said that I kept back the unfavourable cases, and thus improve my figures of mortality. Quite lately a French colleague of mine declared that in France it would not be possible to agree to my sort of statistics!

But, gentlemen, what do we want? Do we want to count the amputated limbs like fallen apples, which are picked up from under the trees? Or do we want to gain figures that answer questions which have a practical importance? If we want to know how dangerous *per se* is amputation at the upper part of the thigh, we cannot learn this from the patients who already suffer from severe septicæmia, or who, besides, suffer from severe brain injuries; and if we want to know how dangerous it is to remove *one* thigh, we cannot make use of cases where both have been amputated. But I will not complicate these statistics in order, as my opponents say, to contrast the most favourable with the most conceivably unfavourable cases. During the time of which I speak 57 large limbs were amputated—lost according to common parlance—because of acute progressive septic processes, chiefly patients with severe open fractures, wounds of the joints, and laceration of the soft parts, who were brought to us too late from the country, cases of embolic mortification and large putrid abscesses. All patients in whom signs of mortification had shown themselves, were not counted. Of these 57 amputated cases, in which, in almost half the cases, the operation concerned the thigh, fully 70 per cent. were cured. A mortality of 30 per cent. is lower than I formerly attained to in cases of primary amputation. It shows best how erroneous are the views of those who contend that antiseptic surgery can only attain results in prophylaxis. Far more rapidly than by means of figures and a survey of successes, we can attain to a comprehension of the enormous advance achieved by modern surgery when we see what is actually done in the domain of operations—what is held permissible, and what is done and risked daily without danger to the patient. For this it is not needful to be a surgeon, not even a doctor, in order to testify to the changes that have come about. Operations are now conducted which fifteen years ago would have been regarded as madness, or as crimes. And often it is the younger doctors who have not had much experience of independent practice who have this advantage over their more venerable colleagues—that they have faith in the infallibility of the antiseptic principle, and have a courage that has not yet been daunted by ill-success; and it is they who venture upon operations of which formerly the most daring surgeons did not think, and attain results concerning which these shake their heads.

But do you think, gentlemen, that one of us older ones could so easily take up the idea of Ogston's operation? For this one must be young, and have grown up in the new thoughts and surroundings, and only know the sad experiences of older surgery as a legend. It is far from me to wish to discuss the value of the operation for the cure of genu valgum. I only wish to show from what one does not shrink. It will always remain of historical interest that, a few years after a great war, in which we were obliged to let the greater number of our wounded die in whom a ball had pierced the knee-joint capsule without hurting the bones; we dared to saw off in the dark within the joint a condyle, leaving blood and saw-dust behind. Further, it would be easy to produce numbers of as apparently venturesome operations of which no one doubts the necessity or that they should be permitted.

For a large enchondroma in the costal pleura that occupied the left wall of the thorax, Professor Fischer removed a large piece of the chest-wall and ribs, so that the heart and lungs were exposed and an opening as large as a child's head was made, and yet the patient was able to be discharged from the hospital after four weeks.

In the case of a large echinococcus of the liver, which in front and at the side was covered with thick layers of liver tissue, and which projected into the thoracic cavity after resection of the seventh rib, I opened the healthy pleural cavity, which was free from adhesions. The thorax was freely open, the thin diaphragm cut into, the echinococcus sac opened, the animal bladder extracted *in toto*, and

the patient recovered without complication. A similar operation, with like results, was conducted by Mr. Israel of Berlin. Mr. Hahn, also of Berlin, in two
cases of wandering kidney, where the mobility and the discomfort induced thereby had attained an unusually high degree, drew out the organ in question through
a large wound in the loin, and sewed it into the same. Both patients recovered
and lost their pain. The opening of the joints seems a most innocent performance. Hips and knees are cut open in order, in a case of luxation, to search for
the obstacle which opposes itself to reduction, in order to suture the ruptured
tissues, and in obscure symptoms to clear up the diagnosis *in vivo* by means of
autopsy. More than two hundred times I alone, without in one instance bad
results following, have incised, drained, and washed out diseased knee-joints
without exciting suppuration.

Bone and marrow tissue will submit to every kind of treatment without putre-
fying and without suppuration. Orthopædics celebrated their greatest triumphs
in the saving and straightening of limbs. We read that Mr. McEwen alone has
performed 835 osteotomies, of which 827 were healed without suppuration, and
he lost no patient from the operation itself or from its consequences. To facilitate
the healing of empyemic cavities, Mr. Schneider resected from six to nine ribs,
and even also the clavicle. In very painful cases of syphilitic hyperostosis I myself have repeatedly exposed the tibia in its whole length, and knocked off with
a chisel a whole handful of bone shavings. The cure was rapid ; the pains disappeared. The old opinion that in cases of strumous suppuration wounds heal
less well has been set aside—the largest scrofulous abscesses, even if they come
from the spinal column, can be opened not only without danger, but often healed
in a brief time through a special kind of first intention. The feat of excision of
part of the stomach has excited the whole world, perhaps to excess, since the
same operation has been already effected upon the intestines with the happiest
results. Weak, paralyzed persons, who usually are anxiously shielded from every
injury, have had their main nervous system exposed, to subject it to thorough
manipulation.

And now leave the writings and let us realize the teachings of the greatest
masters of the first half of this century, of those who were equally great as doctors and as men ; for instance, Sir Astley Cooper, whom we may regard as the
representative of the highest development of the older surgeons, and you will be
convinced that their firm and leading principle, the moral standpoint on which
they stood was this, that every operation is dangerous, and should if possible be
avoided. There is not one of us who, led by B. von Langenbeck, did not stand
on the same ground during the great wars of 1866 and 1870, in his treatment of
the wounded. Only since 1870 the new views have forcibly made their way.

Cast a glance at the surgical clinics of hospitals, where these are conducted by
men who have willingly given up the hardly won results of their own work, and
have entirely adopted the knowledge and power of our new art, and here too
you will see the greatest changes ; cases of operations and wounds without fever
and pain, a happy result being regarded as certain; no traces of blood and wound
secretions on the bandages, let alone on the body and bed linen ; disappearance
of that incessant activity of untrustworthy and senseless assistants, the continuous
putting on and taking off of compresses and cataplasms, the regular change of
bandages repeated every morning and evening. It would thus appear that in
association with anæsthetics and the bloodless method, antiseptic surgery has
deprived all important operations of their terrors. Certainly the preparations
for an operation are often tedious, the first cleansing and preparation of a fresh
wound circumstantial and lengthy, but with the first dressing an immense amount
of work has been obviated, which formerly extended over the following weeks

and months. The later course, the fate of the wounds of the patient, is as a rule determined and assured by this first dressing ; we can often heal an amputation wound with one or two dressings.

Our views on the nature of contagia in the surgical department of hospitals, on their origin and breeding places, have entirely changed.   There is no hospital that is so bad that it can excuse failure in the treatment of wounded and operated patients.   If we had no other task in the treatment of our sick but to guard against the purely relative interruptions of the normal process of wound healing, we could be content with the old close and over-filled houses, and the splendid piles we now erect would be superfluous.   We well know plague-stricken hospitals, where, from wound to wound, from sponge to sponge, from compress to compress, fungous formations in countless generations have grown to the highest degree of adaptation to the fluids and wound secretions of the human body.   But it lies in our power to disinfect them.   By no ventilation in the world can septicæmia, pyæmia, and erysipelas be blown out of the hospitals ; not even by the most assiduous care in ordinary life can they be avoided, but only by the conscientiousness and prudence of the surgeon.   If ever the excellent Simpson was right in his assertion that far more operated patients die in hospitals than in private practice, modern surgery may rather declare the contrary.   If there is any danger of a mistake in the treatment of a wound, it is more likely to happen in a private house where it is more difficult to satisfy the accurate demands of modern surgery than in the hospitals.

Gentlemen, weighty circumstances and daily occurences have always made surgeons as well as laymen recognize the importance of those problems which are solved by the discovery of the mycotic nature of wound diseases.   The contrast between open and subcutaneous wounds must have been known as long as men have worked hard and have fought each other with weapons.   And not only was this known, that simple fractures are not dangerous and heal without suppuration, but also the experience had been gained that there will be no suppuration, no matter if the individual concerned is young or old, robust or decrepid, scrofulous or syphilitic—whether he has this or that constitutional condition, this or that individual disposition.   And this also has long been known, that the danger in a compound fracture is very great ; if only on the lower thigh the skin, very poorly supplied by nerves and vessels and scarcely for an inch in area be sharply perforated by one of the fractured ends.   But the consequences of these facts were not seen.   They were too much opposed to the prevailing doctrine which regarded not only the suppuration, but also the serious disturbances resulting from it, as only *quantitative* increase of the process of reaction following on the injury.   The whole of antiphlogistic therapeutics was based on this supposition.   And yet the history of fractures might long ago have afforded the most conclusive proofs that it could not be the intensity and extent of the injuries of the tissue which determine the severity of the inflammation and the suppuration, that these latter had in reality nothing to do with the traumatic reaction, but must be some other thing essentially different.   For even a good number of simple fractures are by no means such simple things as was formerly imagined, since they often do not occur without serious crushing of the marrow, tearing off of the periosteum, laceration of muscles, fissures, and splinters ; certain forms of fracture, especially those of the cervix femoris, and of the spine, are good examples of destruction and crushing of the tissues.   And yet even in these cases, suppuration of the greatest intensity does not occur.   To attain the conviction that mechanical obnoxious influences, however severe, cannot of themselves produce suppuration, no myologic examination would have been required.   The importance of this fact was only revealed to me in its full bearings in examining the wounded on the

Bohemian battle-fields.   Among the great number of gunshot fractures which I had to treat there, there was a not inconsiderable number of cases where cure resulted after the usual course, as after a subcutaneous fracture without suppuration and without discharge of splinters; and I considered it obvious that here only that explanation was admissible which Stromeyer had given to these cases —namely, that the ball, passing at a tangent, had broken the bone flat, as in the simplest subcutaneous fracture.   But of those so successfully cured, two of those who had been injured in the upper part of the thigh died from the results of other wounds inflicted at the same time; and when I examined these supposed bone-fractures, I found to my surprise that just here the most extensive destruction had taken place.   In the one case twelve splinters, in the other about twenty, of a size varying from several inches to that of a pea, were caked together by fresh callus without any suppuration or necrosis, and in another similar case there lay firmly inclosed in the callus a little piece of cloth from the uniform.

Then, in the year 1870 Professor Klebs discovered that even in the internal organs, which are considered so vulnerable—as brain, lungs, and spleen,—no inflammatory reaction occurs, if the path of the bullet is so long and narrow that it prevents the admission of air; and that even weeks afterwards, macroscopically, no changes can be traced in the tissues shot through, while microscopically the process of healing can only be recognized by a minimum of cellular activity.

And now antiseptic experiments which exclusively belong to Mr. Joseph Lister, to whom I therefore here offer a small part of the gratitude that German surgery owes him, show us that, after an amputation, on the fourth or sixth day the ends hang down in just as limp and unchanged a manner as immediately after the operation, just as if it had been performed on a dead body and not on a living being; that after a great plastic operation, in spite of countless sutures, no trace of œdema or reddening, and no pain, occur.   India-rubber tubes passed through dropsical joints may remain lying there for weeks without causing suppuration, and they may, slipped unnoticed into the cavity, heal so firmly into the armpit that a year after they may be mistaken for well-defined cancer tubercles, and be extirpated.   Into the open peritoneal cavity a piece of gauze larger than a table napkin, and pressed together like a handkerchief, can be put, and remain for several days, without fever or clinical appearances of fever resulting.   And I should like to mention one more experiment, which, it is true, will not always succeed.   Suppose we have a case of limited fistulous caries of the foot before us; five or six times we introduce the glowing Paquelin cautery iron to the depth of an inch and a half, and carbonize the dissected tissues.   Then we cut the skin in a circle round the former fistula at a breadth of two lines, and let the blood, mixed with a disinfecting fluid, flow into the deep spherical cavity, fill it out, and coagulate.   In a fortnight or three weeks the upper layer of the coagulum scales off and the burn is cicatrized without any reaction, suppuration, or falling off of the scab.   So that in man also Professor Hueter's five experiments on animals are confirmed.

After such facts there can be no further doubt that we have hitherto studied traumatic reaction of open wounds on tissues infected at the same time that the four cardinal symptoms of inflammation—robor, calor, tumor, dolor, even in the severest open wounds—are not developed when disturbing agencies have no access, or do not find soil fitted for their development.

Seriously, we have now to consider the question whether mechanical irritations, such as the surgeon's knife and saw cause, and the injuries of the social life, are at all capable of alone bringing about those processes which have at all times been designated as inflammatory.

I do not consider this latter question as yet fit for decision, although the extreme radicals already advance weighty reasons to refuse even to thermic and chemical irritants the power of causing inflammation ; so long as in the erythema of burns and the dermatitis from iodine painting associated with abundant exu_ dation of leucocytes the influence of organic germs is not proved, and so long as the same proof is wanting for carbolic erythema, I believe that we ought at any rate to wait for the results of further investigations.

Gentlemen, I have touched on traumatic reaction of the tissues to show how distinctly modern times have influenced even the oldest dogmas of our science ; how we are obliged to abandon almost everything that our schools have taught us in order to gain for our scientific opinion a newer, firmer foundation.

I am coming to an end. I have already occupied your attention for a longer time than may appear fitting to some of you. I have spoken of the advances in surgery. There is one I have not yet mentioned. It has never hitherto been so deeply and universally realized that the interests of our practice must coincide entirely with those of our patients ; never before was the feeling of responsibility for our actions so great as at the present day. The breach which divides us from the older surgeons is immense here. We do not refuse to let our capability be entirely measured by our successes. For even if the surgeon of former times willingly submitted to this measure, when it was only a subcutaneous fracture without essential displacement or the straightening of a club-foot that was to be dealt with, yet, as soon as it was a matter of preserving life after an operation, or even of preventing serious disturbances, he might decidedly reject this standard. No surgeon, however learned and skilful he might be, would have been willing then to promise or guarantee, or in case of ill-success to reproach himself; he is almost certain in this important point to have, like every other surgeon, the sad privilege of not being responsible for uncontrollable circumstances.

To-day we may say with the deepest conviction that the surgeon is responsible for every disturbance that occurs in a wound ; that it is his fault if even the slighest reaction or redness is developed in it, or if an amputation is not healed by first intention. He must reproach himself severely if after an operation bag- ging of pus occurs, and especially if death occurs from pyæmia. He who cannot attain to this degree of perfection may be converted from his former method of treatment to antiseptic methods like one who, having hitherto always prescribed senega for catarrh, now uses ipecacuanha. Of the storm that has swept over the fields of surgery during the past ten years he has not experienced a breath.

Justice requires us to recognize that the higher moral aspect of this question has come to us from England. It was the English ovariotomists, with Mr. Spencer Wells at their head, who first showed us how to approach an operation at that time looked on as fatal, how to take on one's self the whole responsibility of success or failure, and to keep no other goal in view than this one, to save the patient, and, by a constantly improving and perfecting of our art and carefully keeping everything injurious at a distance, gradually to become more and more master of one's actions. At that time we began to recognize that at the ope- rating-table there are other matters of importance than to shine by quickness, elegance, and security in the use of the knife.

Yes, gentlemen, our labours have become more blessed and more joyful. We know that a great responsibility rests upon us, but we also know that with honest will, knowledge of our subject, and use of all our powers, we are able to satisfy its demands. And because we believe that this feeling of responsibility is living and constantly increasing in the younger generation, we trust that surgery will overcome the dangers that doubtless lie in the rapid changes it has experienced, and is being led towards a further development.—*Lancet*, Aug. 13, 1881.

MONTHLY ABSTRACT.

Anatomy and Physiology.

An Experimental Inquiry into Human Milk, and the Effects of Drugs during Lactation on either Nurse or Nursling.

Mr. THOMAS M. DOLAN and Mr. W. H. WOOD commence, at p. 85 of the *Practitioner*, for 1881, a series of interesting papers on this subject, undertaken by Mr. Dolan in order to answer the frequent question, " Will my medicine have any effect upon the child?" That medicines and foods do affect the milk, and consequently the child, is certain. Frequently, a wet-nurse, on her first arrival, causes the child to thrive; but soon all becomes changed, because, from a laborious out-door life, with few luxuries, the woman is surrounded with good living, and has very little exercise, and consequently her milk ceases to nourish the child. Cause her to resume, as near as possible, her former mode of life and food, then her nursling quickly recovers. A clear description of the best method to analyze human milk is then given, which is, however, too long for insertion, and cannot be condensed. The practical outcome of these elaborate papers is summed up at page 337. 1. All therapeutical agents intended to act on the mammary gland must first enter the blood. 2. All drugs derived from the natural orders Liliaceæ, Cruciferæ, Solanaceæ, Umbelliferæ, etc., enter the blood and impregnate the milk, hence caution is needed in giving such drugs to nursing women. 3. The only approach to a true galactagogue is jaborandi. 4. Belladonna is an antigalactagogue. 5. In inaction of the mammæ, the milk may be increased and influenced by medicines. 6. The milk of the mother may be increased in heat-forming elements by the administration of fats. 7. The salts of milk may be improved by the administration of medicines. 8. Various physiological actions—purgative, alterative, diuretic, etc., may be produced in the child by administering drugs to the mother. 9. If we are to expect any improvement in milk-secreting power, both as to quantity and to quality, we must look to diet for the attainment of that object.—*London Med. Record*, July 15, 1881.

Materia Medica and Therapeutics.

Pilocarpin.

Dr. WILLIAM SQUIRE read a paper at the London Congress on the physiological action and therapeutic use of pilocarpin, which is the alkaloid obtained from the leaves of jaborandi, on which the efficacy of that drug, long known in Brazil, in producing sweating and salivation, depends. Another alkaloid, of different, and even antagonistic properties, named jaborin by Harnack and Meyer, coexists with it, and renders the infusion or tincture of jaborandi less certain, and perhaps, less safe than that of the pure alkaloid. It is possible that pilocarpin itself has not always been obtained quite free from admixture with its associated but antagonistic jaborin. Muriate of pilocarpin, in simple solution, is the best form to use —1 grain to 15 minims of water for hypodermic injection—1 grain to 4 ozs. of water for internal use are convenient proportions; $\frac{1}{8}$d grain is the largest, $\frac{1}{15}$th of a grain the smallest dose needed. Mr. S.'s plan is to give a full dose at once; others give small doses every hour with some warm drink or alcoholic stimulant, till perspiration and salivation are freely established. A drachm of the tincture, made with 30 grains of leaf, is equivalent to $\frac{1}{4}$d of a grain of pilocarpin; $\frac{1}{4}$th of a grain of the muriate, injected hypodermically, will in a few minutes produce suffusion of the face, quickened pulse, some throbbing in the neck, and a general feeling of warmth, followed by free perspiration; this is soon streaming profusely from all parts of the surface, and continues long after the skin has become pale, or even cool; the pulse subsides, while the force of the heart's impulse is rather increased; there is a tendency to sleep, and generally a fall of temperature; the perspiration goes on for three or four hours; there is an increased flow of saliva, and some increase of pharyngeal, and sometimes of bronchial mucus, that may give rise to trouble during sleep, and require attention; such a quantity of saliva may be swallowed as to excite vomiting. No headache, sickness, or depression has been noticed by me as a direct result of this medicine. All the secretions of the body, except the intestinal, are increased by it; the quantity of urine, hardly lessened during perspiration, is increased afterwards. Dr. S. has not met with dysuria. Swelling and tenderness of the submaxillary salivary glands has remained for a day or two after profuse ptyalism. The action of the drug is on the peripheral secreting apparatus, and not on the nerve centres, except so far as the first action on the vaso-motors may dilate the vessels, and allow the agent freer access to the glands.

Atropia is directly antagonistic to it in this respect. Aconite dilates the vessels, but weakens the heart, while pilocarpin, having no such effect, may even allow of small hemorrhages occurring. It is not anæsthetic. The perspiration induced by it does not relieve dysmenorrhœa, sciatica, or colic. Pilocarpin does not moderate specific fevers; but given near the time for the separation of the false membranes in diphtheria, it aids the fall of temperature, and favours sleep. Where there is already a tendency to collapse, of course it can do no good. It is useful in the febrile relapse of scarlatinal nephritis. Dr. S. has met with no confirmation of the observation that small doses ($\frac{1}{20}$th of a grain) will check perspiration; a similarly homœopathic view, that particular diseases must have particular remedies, has led to the statement that pilocarpin is unsuited to renal disease. The use of it has been chiefly in the different kinds of Bright's disease; it may be unsuited to that particular form where dilated vessels and diminished blood-pressure are associated with a large quantity of albumen; yet, in these very cases, it is serviceable to the intercurrent exacerbations and conditions of accidental congestion, not infrequent in their course, and it is preferable to the hot pack, or vapour bath. In the early stages of interstitial nephritis of gouty origin it is of great benefit; in the chronic course which these cases generally follow, it is often useful; it may be resorted to in some of the extreme effects of renal dropsy, and the relief obtained is not accompanied by great depression. In the chronic results of parenchymatous nephritis, as after scarlet fever, it has been found useful; and that it need not be withheld in some cases of scarlet fever itself is proved by the remarkable results obtained from it by Guttman in the treatment of the allied disease diphtheria.

—

Physiological and Therapeutic Action of some new Active Principles
(Pelletierine, Valdivine, and Cedrine).

Dr. DUJARDIN BEAUMETZ was the author of a paper with the above title, read at the London Congress, of which the following is an abstract:—

Pelletierine is the alkaloid obtained from pomegranate-bark. It was discovered by Tanret, on the 26th of August, 1878. Its name commemorates the services of the French chemist, Pelletier, the discoverer of a large number of alkaloids and, in particular, of quinine. Pomegranate root contains a series of alkaloids: Pelletierine ($C_{16}H_{15}NO_2$), Isopelletierine ($C_{16}H_{15}NO_2$), Pseudopelletierine ($C_{18}H_{15}NO_2$), and Methyl-pelletierine ($C_{18}H_{17}NO_2$). The author has investigated the action of all the above alkaloids, more especially of the sulphates of pelletierine and isopelletierine.

To the lower animals these alkaloids are speedily fatal. Rabbits are killed by a dose of 0.15 to 0.20 centigramme; frogs, by the hypodermic injection of one or two drops of a solution of one in ten. These effects are due to a paralyzing action upon the motor nerves, on muscular contractility, and on sensibility. The alkaloids are " curarizing poisons;" there is no difference between a curarized frog and one poisoned by the salts of pelletierine.

In the human subject, the sulphate of pelletierine, or of isopelletierine, administered hypodermically in a dose of from 30 to 40 centigrammes, gives rise to motor paresis with vertigo; the latter being due to well-marked congestion of the fundus oculi, and of the whole encephalon.

Pelletierine has been chiefly used as a remedy for tape-worm. The author and M. Bérenger-Férand have shown that, of the four alkaloids, pelletierine and isopelletierine alone are endowed with tænicide properties. The author prescribes the sulphate of pelletierine in combination with tannin. A mixture of 30 centigrammes of the sulphate, in a solution containing 90 centigrammes of tannin, is given on an empty stomach; this dose is followed by one of 30 grammes of compound tincture of jalap. This treatment is followed by the expulsion of the tapeworm, with its head, in a majority of cases (9 out of 10). The above dose is only suited for adults. Children about thirteen years of age should not take more than 0.15 centigramme of the sulphate of pelletierine, and infants not more than 0.10 centigramme.

The author has prescribed pelletierine with success in Menière's vertigo; he recommends it in all those cases in which curare is indicated (tetanus, rabies) and in those ocular affections in which it may be necessary to excite rather active congestion of the fundus.

Valdivine and cedrine have been extracted by Tanret from cedron seeds. Of these seeds there are two distinct kinds, which have hitherto been confounded with each other. One of them is derived from the simaba cedron (Simarubaceæ), the other from the valdivia, also a simarubaceous plant, but which belongs, according to Planchon, to the genus picrolemma (picrolemma valdivia). Both of these species grow in Columbia.

Valdivine ($C_{16}H_{24}O_{20}, 5HO$) crystallizes in hexagonal prisms. It is not, strictly speaking, an alkaloid, but a glucoside, not entering into combination with acids. It requires 30 parts of boiling water for its solution. Its bitterness is intense.

The author has investigated the action of this substance together with M. Restripo. It is extremely poisonous, a dose of 0.002 milligramme being sufficient to cause the death of a rabbit in ten hours. Increase of dose does not much increase its toxic activity, which appears to be greater in proportion to the place of the animal in the scale of organization. Thus, frogs are not susceptible of the poisonous effects of valdivine.

In the human subject, a dose of 4 milligrammes, given subcutaneously, excites vomiting in from one to two hours.

The administration of valdivine in cases of intermittent fever, snake-bite, and rabies, yielded negative results in all save the last-named affection. Experiments made at the veterinary school of Alfort showed that a dose of 4 milligrammes of valdivine administered to rabid dogs abolished the paroxysms, without, however, preventing the fatal issue of the disease.

Cedrine has been extracted from cedron seeds. It was first described by Lewy, who seems, however, to have confounded it with valdivine. Cedrine has not been crystallized. It is much less poisonous than valdivine, 10 milligrammes being required to kill a rabbit in forty-eight hours.

Cedrine does not cause vomiting. Subcutaneously injected, in doses of from 3 to 5 milligrammes per diem, it exerts a real influence on intermittent fever. But its activity is inferior to that of sulphate of quinine.

Against rabies and snake-bite cedrine is absolutely devoid of efficacy.

Medicine.

Connection of Chorea with Rheumatism.

Prof. STEFFEN, of Stettin, made some interesting remarks at the London Congress, on this subject, of which the following is an abstract :—

A definite interdependence between chorea and rheumatism is not as yet proved. That both of these morbid states are often joined with endocarditis cannot be used as evidence of such a connection.

The relation between chorea and endocarditis cannot be fixed anatomically or pathologically. Probably the chorea is always the primary morbid phenomenon.

The chief symptoms of acute endocarditis are active fever, dilatation of the heart, with enlargement of the area of dulness, a systolic blowing murmur, and an accentuation of the second sound in the area of the pulmonary artery. The dilatation precedes the murmur, if the endocarditis has originally or exclusively attacked the heart walls. In primary inflammation of the valves the opposite takes place.

When an endocarditis which exclusively involves the heart-walls recedes, the dilatation of the heart disappears first, and then, gradually, the blowing murmur. If the valves are also attacked, the systolic murmur remains after the dilatation has disappeared. Dilatation and hypertrophy may afterwards develop afresh as a secondary process.

Acute dilatation of the heart is observed without endocarditis in grave and acute obstruction of the pulmonary circulation, and in septic processes.

Cardiac murmurs occur in chorea without endocarditis. These depend on impaired function of the heart, not only through nervous influence, but also through the obstruction to the circulation of the blood, which occurs as a result of the spasmodic movements of the body.

—

The Modifications of Syphilis in the Tuberculous, Gouty, and other Constitutions.

At the London Congress M. VERNEUIL, of Paris, read a valuable paper on this subject, of which the following is an abstract:—

Syphilis may coexist with any other constitutional taint. There is often simple coexistence of the two conditions, but not unfrequently one has an important influence on the other.

Though referred to by Hunter, Ricord, Revillet, and others, there is, at present, no complete work on syphilitic hybrid disease.

The author's observations have been principally directed to hybrids between syphilis and scrofula and syphilis and cancer.

Scrofula usually precedes syphilis, and exerts an influence upon it ; but, occasionally, syphilis in a youth or young adult, brings out struma which has been latent from infancy. Scrofula attracts syphilis to the organs it most commonly itself affects, skin, glands, periosteum, etc., and is apt to set up suppuration in these, a result not common in simple syphilis. Scrofula modifies secondary and tertiary syphilitic ulcerations, so as to make the diagnosis often difficult. It does not aggravate syphilis, but perhaps renders its local manifestations more permanent, while, as a rule, it removes the element of pain.

Tuberculosis, on the other hand, if it does not actually favour the occurrence of severe and intractable syphilitic lesions, certainly makes some tertiary manifestations persist indefinitely. Stricture of the rectum, for example, is commonly complicated with pulmonary tuberculosis.

In treating such conditions, it is well to combine antiscrofulous with antisyphilitic remedies, but, on the whole, the indications are similar in the two diseases.

When cancer is combined with syphilis, it is the former which is modified by the latter. The cases are rare. There are hardly any which prove the existence of the opposite condition. The author has seen cancer attack a testicle in which a gumma had existed which had been cured two years previously, no doubt a *locus minoris resistentiœ.*

The diagnosis of such hybrid cases is difficult. Enlargement of the lymphatic glands favours the idea of the existence of a new growth. The almost complete indolence which is so frequently noticed, and the comparative benignity of these cases, are due to the syphilis; but the constant advance, the infection of the system, and the fatal termination depend upon the new growth, the latter always asserting itself at last. In doubtful cases, antisyphilitic remedies should always be tried. They sometimes produce remarkable improvement, and raise the hope of a cure. This temporary arrest of the growth may well surprise when it is remembered how useless, if it be not actually harmful, is the administration of mercury and iodide of potassium in ordinary cases of epithelioma or cancer.

———

On the Rôle of Syphilis as a Cause of Locomotor Ataxy.

Prof. W. Erb, of Leipzig, in a paper read at the recent International Medical Congress, said: "My own recently published statistics on 100 new cases of typical tabes in male adults (*Medicin. Centralblatt,* 1881, Nos. 11 and 12), showed:—

	Per cent.
Cases *without* previous infection	12
Cases *with* previous infection	88
(Amongst them, *with secondary syphilis*	59
And *with chancre, without secondary syphilis*	29)

(Up to to-day—June the 1st, 1881—I have observed 13 further cases; amongst them there is *but one without* previous infection; of the remaining 12 eight have had secondary syphilis, four only a chancre; the proportion in these cases is, therefore, still somewhat more unfavourable.)

With regard to the *time of appearance of the first symptoms of tabes after infection,* my cases show, that by far the most occur from the 5th–15th year after infection; a considerable fraction, however, occurs 3–5 years after infection.

In order to control these statistics, I have made a *counter proof* extending over all male adults over twenty-five years old, of my clientèle, who do *not* suffer from tabes, and not directly from syphilis. I have carefully examined up to to-day nearly 500 persons with regard to this question, and I find præter propter:

77 per cent. were *never infected.*

12 per cent. who had formerly *secondary syphilis;* and

11 per cent. who had only a *chancre.*

The simple confrontation of these facts is forcible enough, and convincing for every one who does not shut his eyes purposely. The only possible logical conclusion from these facts is *that there must be a certain etiological connection between syphilis and tabes.*

The remark which has been made repeatedly before this, viz., that it is just the milder and apparently harmless syphilitic infections, which are followed later on by severe syphilis of the nerves, intrudes itself also with regard to tabes, according to my observations.

The author's experiences push him more and more towards the unitarian view of syphilis. At any rate, the *absence* of most, or even of *all*, the so-called secondary manifestations of syphilis, is by no means a proof for the *non-syphilitic* nature of the previous chancre.

Only after the decision of the question in the unitarian sense, would we be entitled to state *that tabes in* 90 per cent. *of all cases is occasioned by syphilis as one of the etiological factors.*

The Analytical Study of Auscultation and Percussion, with reference to the Distinctive Characters of Pulmonary Signs.

In the Medical Section of the London Congress, Dr. AUSTIN FLINT, of New York, read a paper, the object of which was to indicate the pulmonary signs which are determinable by the analytical method of study, and the characters by which they may be readily distinguished. The auscultatory signs referable to respiration, the loud voice, and the whispered voice, were considered ; and, afterward, the signs produced by percussion. The characters of the normal respiratory or vesicular murmur were brought into comparison with those of the sign known as the bronchial or tubular respiration. Under the head of bronchial respiration, a new term—broncho-vesicular respiration—was proposed to mark the different grades of solidification below the amount requisite for bronchial respiration. Cavernous respiration was shown to have characters clearly distinguishing it from bronchial respiration. Modifications of cavernous respiration, determinable by means of analysis and comparison, were distinguished as broncho-cavernous and vesiculo-cavernous respiration. A prolonged expiratory sound was stated in the paper to denote either solidification of the lung, or absence of solidification, by characters relating to pitch and quality. The existence or the absence of solidification could thus be ascertained by characters pertaining exclusively to expiration, when an inspiratory sound was wanting. The foregoing respiratory signs, referable to the loud voice, were next taken up. The distinction between simply increased vocal resonance and bronchophony was the object of analytical study. Ægophony was shown to be a modification of bronchophony, differing from the latter in an apparent distance of the resonance and an interrupted or tremulous character. Pectoriloquy, the transmission of speech or articulated words, denoted either a cavity or solidification of lung. The sounds caused by the whispered voice were considered of sufficient practical importance to form a distinct group of physical signs. The abnormal modifications of the normal bronchial whisper were as follows : (1) increased bronchial whisper ; (2) whispering bronchophony ; (3) cavernous whisper ; (4) whispering pectoriloquy. Whispering pectoriloquy might signify either solidification of lung or a cavity. The characters associated with the pectoriloquy enabled the auscultator to decide which one of these two anatomical conditions, in individual cases, was represented by the sign. The paper concluded with the results of the analytical study of the physical signs obtained by percussion. The number of morbid signs furnished by percussion need not exceed six, namely : (1) absence of resonance, or flatness ; (2) diminished resonance, or dulness ; (3) increased or vesiculo-tympanitic resonance ; (4) tympanitic resonance ; (5) amphoric resonance ; and (6) cracked-metal resonance. These were discussed in succession.

Dr. DOUGLAS POWELL (London) said it was a pity Dr. Flint did not lay down general laws, rather than refer to particular cases. Many of the sounds of prolonged expiration heard in bronchitis and emphysema were really *râles* produced by an interruption of the current of air passing down the tubes; and often there was no such sound if it was not interrupted. With regard to bronchial and cavernous breathing, all had seen the fixed character of the chest in pneumonia, and in lungs which had caverns in them; it was impossible to explain the sounds heard over such lungs by the to-and-fro passage of air: but these sounds might occur by conduction from the glottis.

Dr D'ESPINE (Geneva) thought that Dr. Flint's paper pointed to the uncertainty of always knowing whether we are listening to a bronchial or a vesicular sound. He had been taught in Germany that, when the sound came from the lung, the consonant v could be used with the sound produced; but, if from the bronchial tubes, the aspirate H could be produced with the sound. The binaural stethoscope was a great aid to diagnosis, as, by its means, the superficial sounds of the chest were best detected; but to the ear alone, or an ordinary single tube, the deeper sounds were given off.

Sir WILLIAM GULL (President) asked if it were possible to diagnose a cavity in the lung by any means whatever; or to distinguish always the sounds over a cavern from those over some bronchial tubes.

Dr. MAHOMED (London) said that students had great difficulty in distinguishing chest-sounds. What was wanted was a correct definition of the terms in general use; and, if the Congress were to appoint a committee to determine the meaning of these terms, it would be a good step in the right direction. For instance, "rhonchus" and *râles* were in many text-books used synonymously; also the terms "bronchial and cavernous respiration." Again, "pectoriloquy" was limited by some to the transmission of whispered sounds, as compared to that caused by the resonance of the larynx. Numerous other examples showed that the confusion of terms was extreme.

Dr. THEODORE WILLIAMS (London) said that, before arriving at the conclusions which Dr. Mahomed desired, it would be necessary to unite in using and speaking of one code of instruments. All the first works on auscultation were written when one instrument, the simple tube, was in existence; but now there was in very general use a binaural stethoscope, manufactured of totally different material, which conveyed to the ears sounds totally different from those of the single one; and, further, the description of sounds detected by these instruments did not correspond.

Dr. FLINT, in reply, said that, as regards bronchial and cavernous respiration, Skoda said they were the same in character; but he (Dr. Flint) thought the one was distinct from the other. Bronchial respiration was high-pitched, tubular; and the expiratory sound was also high-pitched. Cavernous respiration was low in pitch, non-tubular; and the expiratory sound was still lower in pitch, and also non-tubular. He agreed with Dr. Mahomed's suggestion. Bronchophony and pectoriloquy were often confounded; and a committee would do good, if they settled the value of the terms. As regarded the stethoscope, the binaural had a great advantage over the single one; as, although the area of sounds was limited with the former, still it distinguished chest-sounds to a remarkable degree. Dr. Flint had used it for a quarter of a century, and advised its use. Although the instrument did give off a sound of its own, still the mind soon became accustomed to the sound, and finally disregarded it.

Sir W. GULL proposed, "That Professor Ewald (Berlin), Professor D'Espine (Geneva), Dr. Douglas Powell (London), Professor Austin Flint (New York), and Dr. Mahomed (London), do constitute a committee to consider, and, if possible, to fix on, some definite terms to be used in auscultation of the chest, so as to form a uniform nomenclature; and to report the result of their labours to the next Congress, wherever that may be held." This was carried unanimously.—
British Med. Journal, Aug. 27, 1881.

Surgery.

The Healing of Wounds.

The treatment of wounds always occupies so large a share of the attention of every surgeon, that it was only meet that the several important questions in connection with it should have been freely raised at the recent Congress. The Surgical Section devoted a whole morning to the consideration of the means best calculated to secure primary union of wounds, and although there were some differences of opinion, in the main the old classical principles were reasserted. As in so many other cases, it is well to approach this subject through the study of the simplest cases. In the treatment of a simple cut of the finger, or after the operation for hare-lip, the essential principles to observe are to adjust as perfectly as possible the clean-cut surfaces, hold them in exact apposition, and keep the part at rest and free from all disturbance until union has occurred. A simple observance of these particulars is all that is necessary to obtain union by first intention, and every one of these is essential. If the surfaces are not placed in apposition, if they are not retained in contact, or are not at rest, union by first intention does not occur. Now in all this we have not had occasion to say anything about germs, or sprays, or antiseptics. We suppose no one regards the one as dangerous or the other essential in treating such simple incisions; and Professor LISTER has himself brought forward evidence to show that healthy blood-serum and blood-clot are not favourable nidus for the development of bacteria. We may advance further to large incised wounds, such as of the abdominal wall in ovariotomy, where observance of the same principles is sufficient to secure primary union. But if we go beyond this we reach cases of larger or irregular wounds, such as in an amputation, where the conditions are seriously modified. If we attempt to carry out the treatment on the same lines, we are at once confronted with the circumstance that the *exact apposition* of the wound surfaces is impossible; the edges of flaps may be brought together and carefully united, but no suturing, be it ever so skilful, is able to place every portion of wound surface in close contact with some other portion of wound surface and retain it so. One of the necessary conditions for primary union being wanting, failure results. As a consequence of this want of exact apposition, fluid accumulates in the spaces and interstices, and may so distend them as to irritate the nerves of the part and thus lead to inflammation, or may decompose and then excite inflammation by its directly irritating properties, or, being absorbed, may lead to general blood-poisoning. In either case the wound fails to unite throughout by first intention. The difficulty thus raised has presented itself in various ways to many minds, and hence has arisen the divergence in practice. Some surgeons, such as Messrs. Savory and Gamgee, make it their aim to carry out the three cardinal principles of wound treatment as far as possible in these complicated cases, and then by simple means prevent the ills to which they are exposed. They urge that such wounds should be treated in a great degree like simple wounds; that the parts—not the edges alone—should be adjusted with the greatest care, and retained in that position, and perfect rest secured, while the fluid exuded into the unavoidable spaces should be drained off and received into some kind of dressing in which its decomposition is prevented. The special means used are pressure, drainage-tubes, and an absorbent antiseptic dressing. Another school of surgeons, while not professing to neglect the principles named, are yet so impressed with the evils attending the decomposition of retained fluids, and rightly tracing such decomposition to the influence of minute organisms introduced from without, that they concentrate their attention—in some cases their sole attention—upon the prevention of the access of these "germs" to wounds. Here, at once, two new elements are introduced. First, some agent has to be used which acts destructively upon the "germs," and, as these germs are organic, they share to some extent the properties of all organized structures, and the strongest antiseptics are injurious in their action on the human body also. A very careful adjustment of means to ends is thus required, the imperfection of which has made us familiar with constitutional disturbance, amounting even to death, from the effects of the agent employed to ward off decomposition. The second element introduced arises from the fact that the effused fluids are organizable, and if preserved from contamination, even in large quantity, can organize and so cicatrize a wound. In one particular the divergence in practice has recently became greater, for while the one school of surgeons look upon primary union of a wound as the surest safeguard against septic mischief, the other school, confident in its own power of preventing septic mischief, will forego the primary union of a wound in attaining this end. The difference between the two parties may, indeed, be roughly expressed thus: that while the one, confronted by complex conditions, proceeds as far as possible along the lines observed in the simpler, the other attacks them by entirely novel, methods. We say "roughly" advisedly, because, as was well pointed out in one of the recent debates, where primary union is achieved, sepsis is prevented by that very condition. Which of these two lines of practice will ultimately prove the more successful it would be foolish and useless to attempt to predict. At present the general statistics of the one bear comparison with those of the other, and it may be that each will have to accept a part of the other, or seek its aid in certain classes of cases.

We have, of course, been referring to so-called "Listerism," but we have purposely avoided using that name, and one reason for so doing is that it is unjust to so great a man to use his name in connection merely with a special means of dressing wounds. We consider Mr. Lister's work as far too great to be narrowed down to be a mere matter of spray and gauze. It is not a mode of dressing wounds that he has introduced, but a surgical revolution that he has accomplished. There is not a hospital in the whole civilized world that has not been affected by his teaching and labours, even if a spray, or gauze, or even carbolic acid, have never been found in its wards. He has gone far towards abolishing suppuration, and taught us all to consider it a preventable accident in the healing of an operation wound. And it is to him above all others that we owe it that septic diseases are now generally held to be avoidable, and their occurrence a serious reproach. His work, in fact, has been far greater than the perfecting the form of dressing that bears his name, and he can fairly count among his disciples many whose outward ritual differs *in toto* from his own.

It is interesting to notice the development which the antiseptic method of dressing wounds is undergoing. Carbolic acid has evidently had its day; the cause of immense good, its use has yet been attended with such inconveniences, and in some cases peril, that it has been, or shortly will be, replaced by other and safer means. The spray, which by some has been considered one of the pillars of the system, has been abandoned by many of Mr. Lister's most ardent followers, and he himself has spoken of it as likely to become unnecessary. The gauze, too, is being replaced in some hospitals by more absorbent, softer, and more elastic materials; so that Esmarch—an antiseptic surgeon whose brilliant statistics would be incredible from any less trustworthy source—dresses his cases far more after the fashion of Mr. Gamgee than that of Mr. Lister, and has shown that the transition from one to the other is neither difficult nor illogical. We cannot doubt that, amid all this development and change, surgery is advancing, and truth is being preserved; and Mr. Lister is far too wise a man to think that finality has been attained in the so-called "Listerian" dressing. Side by side, however, with this development, another fact is prominent. Our hospitals, previously dirty, have become clean; surgeons, before too careless, are now scrupulous in their attention to cleanliness in all its details. And, as Mr. Lister himself says, it is "bits of dirt" that do the harm. Is it that his crusade has to a very large extent—would we could say entirely!—prevented these "bits of dirt" from being deposited on or in wounds, and that so previously necessary antiseptic precautions are now dispensed with in safety ? Or did his earlier teachings err in considering the invisible floating particles in the air as more dangerous than they really are ? Whatever may be the truth in the matter, it seems plain that the great lesson of antiseptic surgery has been widely learnt, and bids fair soon to be universally mastered. We now want to assign it its proper place in the management of wounds, as one of the elements—not the sole—to be considered by the surgeon; and it will not be surprising should the next few years witness a great simplification of its details as a juster conception of its influence and worth is attained. The danger has been that the "system" should blind some of its followers to the fact that Nature works along certain lines or according to certain principles, all of which must be understood by the successful surgeon; and surely when primary union of a wound is dispensed with in order that the "system" may be carried out, this danger has become real indeed !—*Lancet*, Sept. 3, 1881.

—

Treatment of Detachment of the Retina by Injections of Pilocarpine.

Dr. DIANOUX, of Nantes, stated at the London Congress that he had treated sixteen cases of detachment of the retina by methodical injection of nitrate of pilocarpine only, of which there were cured 6, improved 8, and unsuccessful 2. In his opinion treatment by methodical injections of pilocarpine should be employed from the beginning in all cases of detachment not symptomatic of hopeless disease. It is greatly superior to other modes of treatment. It is harmless, and in some cases no other plan is applicable. The dose should be strong at first, then moderate (salivation of at least two hours' duration). There should be a series of fifteen consecutive injections; and then a rest of eight days, etc. .

Treatment should be kept up at least three months. When the result is favourable at first, the treatment should be continued till a decidedly stationary condition is reached.

The case should be kept under care and the injections resumed if there be the least evidence of a relapse.

—

The Relation between Ophthalmoscopic Conditions and Intra-Cranial Disease.

Dr. BOUCHUT, of Paris, in some remarks before the London Congress, held that all the important diseases of the brain and cord, as well as the serious diathetic diseases, may be recognized by ophthalmoscopic examination, and he applies the term cerebroscopy to this use of the method.

Thus, congestion and swelling of the optic nerve indicate congestion of brain, meningitis, compression of brain, or commencing spinal disease. Œdema of disk and neighbouring retina shows œdema of meninges and obstruction to circulation in the sinuses and meningeal veins, in tubercular meningitis, in acute and chronic hydrocephalus, in cerebral hemorrhage, in certain cerebral tumours accompanied by encephalitis, etc. Complete anæmia of the nerve and retina shows arrest of cardiac and cerebral circulation. Death is thus easily diagnosticated by the ophthalmoscope. Retinal varices and thromboses indicate thrombosis of the sinuses and meningeal veins. Miliary aneurisms of the retinal arteries show miliary aneurisms of the brain.

In fevers and diseases of the nervous system retinal hemorrhages indicate either compression of the brain by a copious effusion, the hemorrhagic diathesis, cardiac obstruction to the cerebral circulation, or changes in the cerebral and retinal vessels caused by chronic albuminuria, glycosuria, syphilis, and leucæmia. Miliary tubercles of the retina and choroid show tuberculosis of the brain or meninges. Lastly, in nervous diseases, atrophy of the disk or sclerosis of the optic nerve always indicates a disseminated sclerosis of the brain or of the anterior columns of the cord.

———

On the Relations between Adenoma, Sarcoma, and Carcinoma of the Mammary Gland in the Female ; their Diagnosis in the Earlier Stages of Disease, and the Results of their Treatment by Operations.

Dr. SAMUEL W. GROSS, of Philadelphia, in a paper read at the London Congress, presented the results which he has obtained from an elaborate study of this subject, and offered the following propositions :—

1. That from a genetic stand-point there is a distant connection between adenoma and carcinoma, since they both originate from the glandular constituents of the mamma. In the former neoplasm, however, there is a numerical increase of the lacteal glands ; in the latter, there is merely a multiplication of the epithelial cells, the descendants of which extend into the lymphatic vessels and the perivascular sheaths of the bloodvessels. From a clinical standpoint, adenoma is a benign tumour, and carcinoma is a malignant growth.

2. That sarcoma has neither a genetic nor a structural affinity with adenoma or carcinoma, but that it resembles the latter in its malignant attributes.

3. That, in view of the recurring tendency of adenoma after simple enucleation, the entire breast should be extirpated with it.

4. That surgical intervention in sarcoma and carcinoma not only retards the progress of the disease by preventing local dissemination and the development of visceral tumours, but it also not infrequently results in permanent recovery.

5. That local reproductions in sarcoma and carcinoma do not militate against a final cure, provided they are freely excised as soon as they appear.

6. That lymphatic evolvement does not forbid operations in carcinoma, since infected glands were removed in nearly one-third of the examples of permanent cure.

7. That the subjects of sarcoma and carcinoma are, almost without exception, safe from local and general reproduction if three years have elapsed since the last operation.

8. That all sarcomata and carcinomata of the mammary gland, if there are no evidences of metastatic tumours, and if thorough removal is practicable, should be dealt with as early as possible by amputating the entire breast and its integuments, and dissecting off the subjacent fascia. In carcinoma, moreover, the axilla should be opened with a view to its exploration and the removal of any glands which were not palpable prior to interference.

———

Etiology of Aural Exostoses and their Removal by a New Operation.

Dr. JAMES PATTERSON CASSELLS, of Glasgow, read a paper on this subject at the London Congress, of which the following are the conclusions :—

The osseous tumours of the external meatus are of two kinds, the one, named hyperostosis, being a hyperplasm ; the other, exostosis, being a new growth. These differ from each other in origin, site, shape, structure, and number.

Hyperostosis is never seen till the osseous meatus is completely ossified ; exostosis appears before the complete ossification of the meatus. Exostosis is found arising from a point near the junction of the osseous canal with its cartilaginous portion; hyperostosis is seen only in the inner, or osseous end of the external auditory canal. Hyperostosis is always conical in shape, never pedunculated; in exostosis, on the other hand, there is always a pedicle, and its shape varies. Hyperostosis is of ivory hardness; exostosis before complete ossification has taken place in the tumour, can be pierced to a varying depth. Hyperostosis is not movable on pressure; exostosis is slightly movable, even when complete ossification has taken place. Hyperostosis is often seen without any other disease of the ear, and if an ear disease exists, there is no causative relation between them; they exist altogether independently, and apart from each other. Exostosis is nearly always complicated with another affection of the ear, past or present. Hyperostosis, therefore, may exist in the meatus with normal hearing. Exostosis, on the other hand, is almost always attended by a defect in the hearing. The deafness which accompanies hyperostosis, in the absence of any other disease of the ear, is due to the size of the growth, and is mostly mechanical, or it is due to the presence of *débris* between or behind the tumours. In exostosis the defect in the hearing may also be mechanical; this defect, however, is generally due to ear disease, either past or present.

The operation for the removal of hyperostosis is only justifiable, when its mechanical presence has been ascertained to be the sole cause of the deafness, or when a coincident ear discharge exists, the escape of which may be hindered, or altogether arrested by the presence of the tumour. The commonest cause of deafness in hyperostosis is the presence of *débris* around the tumours, either cerumen, epidermic masses, or other matters, or to mechanical irritation and inflammation of the tissues that cover them. The hearing is mostly restored on the removal of the *débris* or inflammation. The operation for the removal of hyperostosis is best effected by a mechanical drill, such as dentists use; this is the safest method of removal.

For the operation of the removal of an exostosis a gouge is the best instrument, because the tumour can be removed at one operation, whereas a hyperostosis usually demands several operations, as well as separate sittings, for its complete removal, when this is possible. There may be several hyperostoses in an ear, but hardly ever more than one exostosis. Both classes of tumours may exist together in the same ear.

———

Laparotomy and Cystorrhaphy in Cases of Perforating Wound of the Bladder.

Dr. E. VINCENT, of Lyons, presented at the London Congress the results of a new series of experiments performed upon rabbits, and the following conclusions which he deduced therefrom :—

I.—1. The contact of urine with the peritoneum is not such a fatal accident as is usually supposed.

2. Suture of the bladder by interrupted metallic stitches, the serous surfaces being brought into contact, and the stitches left in the abdomen, may be practised with almost a certainty of success.

3. Whatever the cause of rupture, the animal can almost invariably be saved if the vesical suture be practised immediately or within a very short time, even if grave complications be present.

4. The animal may be saved even if a considerable time be allowed to elapse after the injury

5. When the operation was delayed longer than sixteen hours, some animals died from urinary intoxication without true peritonitis; others survived owing to a spontaneous closure of the opening in the bladder.

6. The spontaneous closure is exceptional, and, therefore, laparotomy and cystorrhaphy should be at once practised.

II.—Taking into consideration these and previous experiments, and the result of a case in which a large piece of the bladder was excised accidentally during an ovariotomy, the author would formulate the following propositions as applicable to the human subject:—

7. Considering the almost invariable mortality which follows wounds of the bladder, however produced, laparotomy and crystorrhaphy should be resorted to immediately. The chance of success diminishes in proportion to the length of time that has elapsed since the accident.

8. As the employment of antiseptic means has removed the danger of operations involving the peritoneum, ought we not to prefer suprapubic lithotomy to any of the perineal methods, retaining only two operations for stone; lithority, if it be friable and small; suprapubic lithotomy, if it be very large or hard?

Pathology and Treatment of Genu Valgum.

Mr. BERNARD E. BRODHURST was the author of a paper on this subject read at the London Congress, of which the following is a full abstract:—

Genu valgum is regarded as a constitutional rather than as a local defect; and it is shown to be accompanied for the most part by a relaxed condition of the ligamentous system in general, and to be preceded by flat-foot. Especially the ligaments on the inner side of the ankle, and those in the sole of the foot, having yielded, the arch of the foot becomes flattened, and the foot itself everted; the inner malleolus projects inwards and is lowered towards the ground, and the shaft of the tibia is inclined outwards.

Thus the weight of the body is thrown unduly to the inner side of the limb, and is borne rather on the inner margin of the foot than on the entire breadth of the sole of the foot.

Secondly, the long axis of the femur becomes inclined inwards, the inner condyle protrudes, and the internal lateral ligament yields to the superincumbent weight, and the weight of the body being no longer borne in a vertical line and transmitted through the long axis of the femur and the tibia to the arch of the foot, is thrown to the inner side of the knee and of the foot. These, then, being the relative positions of the femur and the tibia, the former inclined inwards and the latter outwards, the condyles of the femur necessarily assume an oblique position from without inwards.

In the normal condition of the bone, there is usually some difference in the length of the condyles: in a rickety bone the inner may be one inch longer than the outer condyle; in the rickety bone the inner condyle is nipple-shaped, and the outer is undeveloped, or almost absent; so that the superincumbent weight could never have been borne on the foot, but it was probably borne on the knee. The length of the inner condyle varies according to the healthy development of the bone. The difference in length may be less than 1-10th of an inch, or it may be in an ordinarily healthy bone as much as half an inch.

In its commencement genu valgum is only apparent in the erect position, and it ceases in the horizontal position, just as is observed in scoliosis and in flat-foot; in an early stage of development these disappear in the horizontal position.

After some time, knock-knee becomes permanent. Even now, however, splints firmly supporting the knee, together with the horizontal position, are sufficient to remove this deformity.

As deformity increases, the biceps femoris becomes tense, and the ilio-tibial band and the external lateral ligament are rendered rigid. Then the right line of the limb being destroyed, the question arises how is it to be restored, so that it shall pass through the long axis of the femur and of the tibia, and impinge on the arch of the foot?

Various operations have been proposed to restore the straight line of the limb, such as forcible straightening, osteotomy, and tenotomy.

Tenotomy, however, or that operation known as Guérin's, is sufficient; without either force or osteotomy, to remove the most severe forms of genu valgum.

Perforating Ulcer of the Foot as connected with Progressive Locomotor Ataxy.

Prof. BENJ. BALL, of the Paris Faculty, and Dr. THIBIERGE, presented the following conclusions in a joint paper on this subject read before the London International Medical Congress :—

1. Perforating ulcer of the foot is, in such cases, the consequence of the spinal disease, as in the "joint disease," which has been brought before the medical public by Charcot and myself.

2. The local disease is more especially connected with certain symptoms of locomotor ataxy, such as shooting pains, absence of tendon reflex, and other trophical lesions.

3. The perforating ulcer may be cured while the symptoms of locomotor ataxy follow their progressive course.

Midwifery and Gynæcology.

Parallel between Embryotomy and the Cæsarean Section.

Dr. G. EUSTACHE, of Lille, in a paper read at the London Congress, presented the following conclusions, which he believed should be the future rules of practice :—

Considering, on the one hand (1), the recent results of ovariotomy, and of all other abdominal sections; (2), the improvement in the prognosis of all surgical inquiries under antiseptic treatment; (3), the success of Porro's operation; (4), the immensely favourable results both to mother and child after the Cæsarean section, which have been published during recent years.

And considering, on the other hand, that embryotomy, while it always sacrifices the child, exposes the mother to as grave dangers as the Cæsarean section; that it is inapplicable in many cases of deformed pelvis, *e.g.*, when the conjugate is 5 centimetres and under.

I conclude :—

1. When the child is living at the beginning of labour, and when the pelvic strait is under 78 mm.—the extreme limit for the application of the forceps—the Cæsarean operation should be performed early, that is to say, as soon as labour has really set in, and with antiseptic precautions.

2. If the child is dead, and the superior strait measure 5 centimetres, recourse should be had to embryotomy. Below 5 centimetres the Cæsarean section becomes an operation of necessity.

To sum up, the Cæsarean section should be the method of election, embryotomy that of exception.

The Curability of Uterine Displacements.

Dr. PAUL F. MUNDÉ, of New York, finding that the text-books either entirely omit all mention of the possibility of permanently curing displacements of the uterus by any of the methods in use, or give but vague statements on the subject, and impressed with the importance of having some positive conclusions on this matter, both for the sake of the patient and the satisfaction of the physician, in a paper presented to the London Congress has analyzed the numerous cases of displacements which have come under his care (895), and arrives at the following conclusions : —

1. Displacements of the uterus are permanently curable in the large majority of cases only when recent, or when a complete tissue metamorphosis, as occurs during pregnancy and after parturition, takes place.

2. Chronic cases (of more than a year's standing) are but rarely curable permanently, except occasionally under the last-named circumstances. Apparent cures reported by some authors and witnessed by many physicians, soon show themselves to have been but temporary.

3. Pessaries form unquestionably the most practical, rational, and (temporarily) the most efficient means of treating uterine displacements. Cures are but rarely accomplished by them.

4. Medicated, chiefly astringent, tampons, intelligently applied every day by the physician, give the best chances for permanent cure. This is particularly true of prolapsus, but holds good for all forms.

5. Electricity locally applied deserves more extended application.

6. All methods should be persevered in for months and years before success is to be expected.

—

Removal of both Ovaries for the Cure of Insanity.

Dr. T. B. WILKERSON, of Youngs Cross-roads, Granville, N. C., reports in the *North Carolina Medical Journal*, June, 1881, the case of a young woman 19 years of age, in which he successfully extirpated both ovaries for insanity with strong erotic tendencies of two years' duration. At the end of three weeks she recovered from the operation, and there was a gradual improvement in the mental condition, and three months after the operation sanity was perfectly restored. Nine months after the operation she is reported as being "gay, lively, cheeks ruddy, and in the full enjoyment of a vigorous mental and physical health."

———

Hygiene.

Influence of Milk in Spreading Zymotic Disease.

At the London Congress Mr. ERNEST HART, the talented editor of the *British Medical Journal*, submitted an abstract, giving in a tabular form particulars of 71 recent epidemics due to infected milk, that have been recognized and made the subject of detailed observations in Great Britain, 67 of them since the Marylebone milk typhoid epidemic, traced and reported by Dr. Murchison and the author, in 1873. The particulars of the epidemics are given in the abstract under the following headings : —

1. Date of outbreak ; 2. Locality ; 3. Reporter ; 4. Total number of cases ; 5. Deaths ; 6. Number of cases amongst drinkers of infected milk ; 7. Percentage to total cases (col. 6 to col. 4) ; 8. Number of families supplied by milkmen ; 9. Number of such families invaded ; 10. Percentage (col. 9 to col. 8) ; 11. Sanitary circumstances of farm or dairy from which milk was derived ; 12. Exciting cause of outbreak ; 13. Circumstances implicating milk ; 14. Facts showing special incidents of the disease ; 15. References to sources of information.

The three diseases which have as yet been recognized as capable of being spread by milk are typhoid fever, scarlatina, and diphtheria. There is nothing in the analogy of epidemics to limit the list permanently to these ; and already there are indications of other cognate diseases being spread by the same agency. The number of epidemics of typhoid fever recorded in the abstract as due to milk is fifty, of scarlatina fourteen, and of diphtheria seven. The total number of cases traced to the drinking of infected milk occurring during the epidemics may be reckoned in round numbers as 3500 of typhoid fever, 800 of scarlatina, and 500 of diphtheria. As regards typhoid fever, the most common way in which the poison has been observed in these epidemics to reach the milk is by the soak-age of the specific matter of typhoid excrements into the well-water used for washing the milk cans and for other dairy purposes, and often, it is to be feared, for the dilution of the milk itself—for which, in official reports, "washing the milk cans" has become a convenient euphemism, advisedly employed to avoid raising unpleasant questions.

In twenty-two of the fifty epidemics of typhoid fever recorded this is dis-tinctly stated by the reporters to be the case, and in other cases it was more or less probable.

When a dairy is unwholesomely or carelessly kept, there is obviously a great variety of ways in which the poison may reach the milk. (Numerous instances of this kind are given.) ·

Scarlatina being almost invariably spread by contagion and by the inhalation of the bran-like dust which is thrown off from the body during the disease, we should expect in epidemics of milk-scarlatina to receive evidence of this dust having access to the milk ; and in the majority of recorded epidemics it was found that persons employed about the dairy operations were in attendance at the same time on persons sick of scarlatina.

In none of the seven recognized outbreaks of *diphtheria* due to milk, has it yet been possible to trace the exciting cause of the outbreak, though as to the dis-ease being spread by milk there could be no doubt whatever. It has indeed been suggested whether a disease of the udder of the cow, called " garget," may not so affect the secretion of milk as to give rise to diphtheria in the human sub-ject. So far, this notion is a mere conjecture unsupported by fact.

The great majority of the cases give statistical as well as experimental support to the conclusion that the responsibility of the epidemic lay with the milk.

It is upon the largest drinkers of the milk (those, namely, who, consuming the greatest quantities, have a correspondingly greater chance of imbibing disease germs), that the incidence of the disease chiefly falls.

Thus young children (ordinarily little liable to attacks of typhoid) who are accustomed to drink milk largely in the raw state, domestic servants, who, after children, drink the most raw milk, and large milk drinkers of every rank and station, furnish by far the largest quota of cases in each epidemic.

People, too, who drink exceptionally of the implicated milk are attacked, although the milk taken at their own houses is derived from other sources.

The houses invaded during the epidemics are found to be commonly of the better class and in healthy situations. The poor, who take very little milk, and that only in tea or coffee, commonly escape the disease.

The striking fashion in which the disease " picks out" the streets supplied by the implicated dairy, and the houses in those streets receiving the milk, is note-worthy. People in adjacent houses, and who drink milk supplied by different retailers, escape ; and when supplies from two sources enter the same house, the disease only attacks those drinking that from the infected source. The contem-poraneous invasion of so many households at once can only be explained on the hypothesis of a common cause acting on a particular set of persons, and on no others

MEDICAL NEWS.

The Case of President Garfield.

The publication in the current number of the *American Journal of the Medical Sciences* of the official report of the autopsy upon the body of President Garfield will, we trust, while satisfying the legitimate curiosity of the profession and of the laity, at the same time effectually and permanently quiet the unfriendly criticism of the surgical treatment of the case, in which part of the daily press has so freely indulged, and from which, we regret to observe, some medical journals without full knowledge of the case have not thought proper to abstain. The discoveries of the autopsy, taken in conjunction with what is known of the clinical history, will at once make apparent to the profession the good common sense, admirable conservatism, and sound surgical judgment which have characterized the management of the case from first to last, and, although the non-medical mind may be slower to comprehend the questions at issue, it will not be long before the same conviction forces itself upon the people at large.

We know now beyond the possibility of doubt that no human skill could have averted the fatal result, but we find moreover that, even in the searching light of the careful and thorough post-mortem examination, it is difficult, if not impossible, to suggest any modification of the treatment even in minor points, which would have made it better adapted to the exigencies of the case.

Directly after the shooting, the symptoms of impending collapse, so severe as to threaten immediate dissolution, and possibly, in the absence of hemorrhage, depending largely upon spinal concussion and mental shock, received, as was proper, the greatest attention.

Later in the day, after reaction had been established, a cautious examination with a probe and with the finger disclosed the fact that the eleventh rib had been struck and broken, and that the ball had passed onward into the abdominal cavity. In accordance with one of the best-established rules of surgery, further exploration was desisted from, and two days later, at the time of the first consultation, the same praiseworthy conservatism was observed in spite of the senseless clamour for the extraction of the ball which was already being raised, and which, to their shame, be it said, was aided and encouraged by a few prominent members of the profession who had possessed neither the details nor a personal knowledge of the case. Although, at that time, the surgeons were governed by general principles, and were necessarily ignorant of the course and situation of the

ball, the wisdom of their inactivity has been made clear by the disclosures
of the autopsy, and we can all recognize now that an operation for extraction would have been not only fruitless, but almost certainly fatal,
while, on the other hand, it is shown that the ball itself, after effecting its
lodgment, had ceased to be a factor in the production of disease. We
know also, that, as it had passed through the fibres of the psoas muscle,
which, running longitudinally by the side of the spine, had closed over it,
persistent probing would only have been productive of increased laceration of the parts with no possibility of the discovery of the track of the
ball.

It seems not improper to say in this connection that weeks ago, when
the daily press was filled with fictitious accounts of the exact situation
of the ball, and of certain imaginary movements which it had made, Dr.
Agnew, who, doubtless, in this, as in other matters, represented accurately the sentiment of the surgical staff, assured us that he did not know
the position of the ball, and knew of no safe means of determining it.

The vomiting immediately after the accident, and the temporary retention of urine were common symptoms of shock, and received all the attention they required; so, too, the pains in the feet and ankles and the
scrotal hyperæsthesia—both possible results of nerve-injury or of concussion of the spine—called for no special treatment, and subsided, together
with the abdominal tympany, in from one to two weeks. At no time was
there any loss of muscular power. The rigors which occurred about the
end of July were immediately associated, in the first instance, with the
formation of a small abscess under the erector spinæ muscles, possibly
caused by the irritation of fragments of the broken rib, and next, with the
obstruction of the outlet from this pus-cavity by one of these fragments.
A free incision in the one case, and removal of the spicula of bone in the
second, caused an immediate cessation of the chills, followed by subsidence
of the temperature. It seems probable that about this time the blood
received its first septic impression; but this is not to be wondered at when
we recall the fact that suppuration occurring in this region is rarely circumscribed, the pus, owing to the scanty amount of connective tissue and
to the presence of loose masses of fat, finding its way freely through the
surrounding parts, and thus affording the best possible condition for decomposition and for the absorption of poisonous matters. When, too, we
remember the laceration of the cancellated structure of the first lumbar
vertebra, it seems rather remarkable that these symptoms did not make
their appearance earlier, and the injustice of attributing them to improper
or insufficient treatment becomes evident.

The discovery of a point of induration in the right iliac fossa, and the fact
that a small flexible catheter could be carried downward from the wound in
that direction for several inches, led very naturally to the harmless belief
that this was probably the original track of the ball; but, while the au-

topsy shows that this was not the case, it also develops the fact that the wound proper was thoroughly drained through this channel, and that the operation of August 8th, which, by an opening below the twelfth rib and directly through the quadratus lumborum muscle, effectually drained the space between that muscle and the peritoneum, and, indeed, the whole iliac and lumbar regions, also aided in carrying away the products of suppuration from the neighbourhood of the wounded vertebra.

The drainage of the long, narrow passage into the iliac fossa by a counter-opening at its lower extremity, which it has been asserted was an indication not met by the surgeons, would have necessitated an abdominal section, displacement of the viscera, and division of the posterior layer of the peritoneum, and would have resulted in absolutely no benefit, as in the recumbent position the pus would have continued to gravitate toward the opening in the lumbar region, as it did throughout the entire case.

The fact that drainage was thorough and complete, and that no portion of the unfavourable symptoms was due to neglect in this respect, is finally and fully established by the circumstance that no accumulations of pus were found at the autopsy, either along the track of the ball or in the passage caused by the burrowing of the pus. There was no time previous to the first operation at which the accumulated pus did not pass out of the original wound, but its exit was favoured by gravitation after the two operations which brought the external openings on a lower level, and enabled them not only to drain completely the iliac and lumbar regions, but also to carry away any discharge that may have come from the fractured vertebra.

Throughout the whole treatment antisepsis was employed to the fullest possible extent, although a more unfavourable case in which to obtain its peculiar benefits could hardly be imagined.

The irritable stomach, a relic of old dyspeptic troubles, the parotitis, a not uncommon accompaniment of exhausting fevers, the bronchitis and broncho-pneumonia, partly the results of recumbency and partly of the septic state of the blood, were the subsequent complications through which the President was being so skilfully, and we may say, successfully carried, when the ulceration of the splenic artery, a slowly developing result of inflammation extending from the contiguous track of the ball, terminated the case; the rigors preceding death being doubtless due to the successive hemorrhages which are indicated by the lamination of the blood-clot found in the peritoneal cavity. The edges of the ulceration in the splenic artery were adherent to the posterior surface of the peritoneum. It will be seen that no metastatic abscesses were discovered, the only accumulations of pus which were found being a cavity on the under surface of the liver which may have been a result of contusion by the broken rib at the time of the injury, and at any rate did not communicate with the wound, and another, one-third of an inch in diameter, just beneath the capsule of the left kidney. With the exception of the moderate broncho-pneumonia the viscera were free from all acute pathological changes.

From this general consideration of the history of the case, viewed in the light thrown upon it by the details of the autopsy, we may safely conclude :—

1st. That the treatment at the time of the reception of the injury, and immediately subsequent to it, was that rendered proper by the condition of collapse which then existed.

2d. That on reaction taking place, a sufficiently thorough and careful examination was made with the finger and the probe.

3d. That when the consulting surgeons were called in, and found that this had been done, they very properly, and in accordance with well-established and universally recognized rules of surgery, refrained from repeating that examination.

4th. That even if these rules had been disregarded, and such examination had been made, it would have determined nothing of practical importance as regards the subsequent treatment.

5th. That wherever pus accumulations had taken place, they were properly opened by free incisions made at the most dependent portions.

6th. That these incisions drained not only the course of the abscess, but communicated freely with that portion of the spine which had been penetrated, and, therefore, with the track of the ball, and the completeness of the drainage is shown by the absence of pus accumulations either in the locality traversed by the ball or in the iliac or lumbar regions.

7th. That the damage done to the cancellated tissue of the lumbar vertebra was sufficient in itself to explain the septic state of the system, which in time, and independent of the ball, which proves to have become harmless, would have destroyed the life of the patient.

If it be thought that these conclusions need to be substantiated by a more detailed acquaintance with the surgical history of the case, it may be said that such a history giving minutely all the particulars of symptoms and treatment is now in process of rapid preparation, and in our opinion will serve to confirm and strengthen the above assertions.

Of the sympathy of the nation and of the civilized world with the distinguished victim, of the universal respect and affection called forth by his quiet, patient endurance of his sufferings, of the admiration excited by the persistent, almost heroic, struggle which he sustained against overwhelming odds, of his watchful and tender nursing, of the thoughtfulness which anticipated every want and of the ingenuity which devised new appliances for his comfort or his transportation, enough has been written in well-deserved commendation.

But for the men who took the crushing responsibility of his case, who spared neither time nor labour nor health in its conduct, who remained prudent and far-seeing and self-reliant under an electric light of criticism such as has been directed upon no other physicians in the history of the world, and who have in our opinion reflected credit upon the profession and upheld the reputation of American surgery, there has been written scarcely a word of praise, but oftentimes columns of unmerited censure.

—

INTERNATIONAL MEDICAL CONGRESS, LONDON, 1881.

The International Medical Congress which has just adjourned at London, was the most notable medical gathering which has ever assembled in any part of the world. The Congress was honoured by being held under the patronage of Her Majesty the Queen, and of His Royal Highness the Prince of Wales. Its membership was alike international, and representative in character; and in the magnitude of the Congress, in the amount of work it accomplished, and in the attractions which it offered to those who attended it, it surpassed all its predecessors. Official representatives were sent by the governments of the United States, France, Germany, Russia, Italy, Denmark, Norway, Sweden, and by Roumania. The Prince of Wales, and the Crown Prince of Russia showed their interest in the Congress by being present at the opening meeting, and by subsequently on the same day taking luncheon with Sir James Paget, dining with Sir William Gull, and by being present at the conversazione at the South Kensington Museum in order to meet the chief notabilities of the profession who had assembled from all parts of the world to attend the Congress. The Empress of Germany graciously expressed her personal interest in the meeting by deputing Prof. Küster, Principal Surgeon of the Augusta Hospital, to attend as her special representative.

Of the scientific work done in the Sections we can only here say that the large number of papers read were, as a rule, markedly valuable contributions to our science, and the summaries of the more important will be found in our *Monthly Abstract,* and in the current number of the *American Journal of the Medical Sciences.* Some conception of the number and extent of these communications may be formed from the fact that the official volume of abstracts printed in English, French, and German, covers over 700 closely printed royal octavo pages, and contains 325 communications, extending over the entire range of medicine and surgery. The devotion of the members to the serious work for which they had assembled was most marked, and the general sessions and sectional meetings were always largely attended, and the discussions were as full and as interesting as time would permit.

Of the addresses that were made in the general sessions that of Dr. Billings, of Washington, was received with marked favour, and the sallies of wit with which it sparkled elicited cordial applause from the large audience whose attention was closely held during its entire delivery. This

able address we have laid before our readers in full, as well as that of
Prof. Volkmann, who is one of the most prominent advocates of antiseptic surgery in Germany, and that of Prof. Pasteur, of Paris, which, from
a scientific standpoint, is the most valuable of all, dealing, as it does, with
new and original investigations, the importance of which can be scarcely
over-estimated.

The social entertainments given to the Congress as a whole, or to select
parties of its members, were so numerous and brilliant as to constitute a
marked feature of the meeting.   Indeed such a spontaneous outburst of
generous hospitality as was daily met with, we believe is without parallel
in the history of any scientific or popular Congress.   The magnificent
hospitality of the corporation of the City of London was shown in the
sumptuous conversazione at the Guildhall; and the Lord Mayor of London officially entertained at dinner at the Mansion House as many members of the Congress as the Egyptian Hall would hold.   Among the many
notable private entertainments it is impossible not to refer to the brilliant
dinner at Willis's Rooms, given by Sir William Gull, to a select number of guests invited to meet the Prince of Wales.   Among the distinguished company who were not members of the profession, besides the
Prince of Wales, were observed the Crown Prince of Germany, Prince
Henry of Germany, Cardinal Manning, the Archbishop of York, the
Bishop of London, and the President of the Royal Society.   Of the members of the Congress from America there were present Drs. Billings, Solis
Cohen, Austin Flint, Minis Hays, T. M. Lefferts, and D. W. Yandell.

Sir James Paget fulfilled the duties of the Presidency of the Congress
with a dignity, zeal, discretion, and grace which won for him universal
praise.   To the unswerving energy, and quiet courtesy of the Hon. Secretary-General, Mr. William Mac Cormac, much of the superb success of
the Congress is unquestionably due, and we are happy to learn that in
recognition of the value of his services in promoting the Congress the
Queen has signified her intention of conferring upon him the honour of
knighthood. ·

At a meeting of the members of the Congress from the United States,
held at the close of the Congress, the following resolution was passed :—

Resolved, That we highly appreciate the privilege we have enjoyed of
attending this Congress, which has been, in every sense, a great success.
That we offer our thanks to the officers of the Congress for the manner in
which they have organized and conducted its meetings, and also to the
corporations, societies, and individuals of whose unbounded hospitalities
we have had such ample experience ; and that we shall always preserve
the most pleasant and grateful memories of the uniform courtesy and kindness which we have received, and which will strengthen the ties of friend-
ship which exist between the United States and the mother country.

American Dermatological Association.

The fifth annual meeting of this Association was held at the Ocean House, Newport, R. I., Aug. 30th, 31st, and Sept. 1st. The proceedings opened with an able and scholarly address by the president, Dr. James Nevins Hyde, of Chicago, on *the Relations of Dermatology to Periodical Medical Literature.* A comparison of the articles published during the last few years with those of an earlier date showed a very marked improvement. Allusion was made to the importance of correct diagnosis, and some of the diseases were referred to where mistakes are frequently made. Some of the popular errors in etiology and pathology were also considered, and the injudicious use of well-known and powerful remedies, as mercury, arsenic, and iodide of potassium, strongly denounced. "He who would specially devote himself to the investigation of the diseases of the skin requires fully as much as his fellows the amplest preparation in a finished medical education and experience, and when at last ready for his work he will discover, if he has not done so before, that he needs to be a physician in the highest sense of the term. There is no organ of the body, in health or in disease, which it may not become his duty to explore and investigate." Appended to the address, the reading of which was listened to by the members of the association with the deepest interest, was a general alphabetical index, by authors and subjects, of all original communications which have appeared in the several dermatological journals.

The first paper read was one by Dr. Charles Heitzmann, of New York, on *The Minute Anatomy of the Hair*, the ground being taken that the anatomy of this structure had heretofore been incorrectly stated by authors. Dr. James C. White, of Boston, next read a paper on the *Limitations of Internal Therapy in Skin Diseases*, referring to the differences of opinion regarding the value of internal remedies among dermatologists of equal experience, and stating that in his opinion but few diseases of the skin were under the direct control of internal medication and in any uniform or marked degree. We would encourage experimental studies, empirical or philosophical, but thought that a frank confession of our present inabilities was an essential step towards real advance. This article was followed by one by Dr. Arthur Van Harlingen, of Philadelphia, describing an interesting case of *Lymphangioma cutis Multiplex.*

The next paper was one by Dr. Louis A. Duhring, of Philadelphia, on *The Small Pustular Scrofuloderm*, the disease being undescribed and rare, and characterized by small, disseminate, chronic, pustules with a hard base of a cold violaceous tint, the eruption resembling the small pustular syphiloderm.

The second day's morning session was devoted to an interesting series of articles on leprosy, and to the valuable report of the Committee on Statistics presented by the Chairman, Dr. James C. White. The first paper was on a *Case of Tubercular Leprosy*, occurring in a native of Maryland, who had never been beyond the limits of the State, and who was of healthy parentage, by Dr. I. Edmondson Atkinson, of Baltimore. Dr. Hyde, of Chicago, presented a case of acute *Tubercular Leprosy*, and read a paper by Dr. H. D. Schmidt, of New Orleans, *On the Pathology of Leprosy.* The day's proceedings were concluded by a paper by Dr. Edward Wigglesworth, of Boston, on *Buccal Ulcerations of Constitutional Origin*, the difficulties of diagnosis between lupous, tubercular, syphilitic, and cancerous disease being dwelt upon.

On the third day Dr. Heitzmann, of New York, contributed papers on *Clinical Experience in the Use of the Solution of Oxysulphuret of Calcium*, and on the use of a *Kido-Galvano-Cautery for Depilation*, his results justifying the highest claims made for the operation.

The committee on the microscopic examination of a specimen of ainhum, presented at a former meeting, reported through its chairman, Dr. Heitzmann, that the appearances presented no pathological changes to account for the result, which can only be explained by the supposition that a system of self-mutilation is practised by the negroes.

The officers elected for the ensuing year were as follows:—

President, Dr. James Nevins Hyde, of Chicago; Vice-Presidents, Drs. George H. Fox, of New York, and W. A. Hardaway, of St. Louis; Secretary, Dr. Arthur Van Harlingen, of Philadelphia; Treasurer, Dr. I. E. Atkinson, of Baltimore.

—

Tribute to the Memory of the late Dr. Otis at the London Congress.—During a discussion in the Section of Military Surgery and Medicine, on the transport of sick and wounded in the field, Dr. Gori (of Amsterdam) made reference to the death of Dr. Otis, which drew forth the following remarks from the President, Surgeon-General Longmore:—

"This seems to be a very fitting occasion, representatives as we are of the science and practice of military surgery in all countries, for us to express our profound regret at Surgeon Otis having been taken away from among us before he was able to complete the greatest of all his many valuable professional works, as he had hoped to do; and it seems also to be a fitting opportunity to convey to Surgeon-General Barnes, and, through him, to all the medical officers of the United States Army, our heartfelt sympathy with them on the great loss their medical service in particular, and at the same time military surgical science in all parts of the world, has sustained in the death of their great colleague. I say these few words in the presence of an eminent friend and fellow-labourer of Dr. Otis—Dr. Billings, who occupies an important part in the Surgeon-General's Office at Washington—and I beg to propose to the meeting that Dr. Billings be asked kindly to allow himself to be made the medium of communicating this, I may truly say, international expression of feeling—for I see plainly you all share with me in sentiments I have tried to express—to the distinguished chief at the head of the Department, and to his colleagues, on his return to Washington."

Dr. Billings, in reply, said: "In behalf of the Medical Department of the United States Army, of the Surgeon-General, and of the colleagues and friends of Dr. Otis, I desire to return thanks for, and to express the highest appreciation of, the eloquent tribute which Surgeon-General Longmore has paid to the memory of Dr. Otis. I shall not attempt to add to the eulogy which Surgeon-General Longmore has pronounced upon my friend and colleague; I can only say that I find I want words to express the emotion with which I have listened to it, and that I shall convey the message with which he has charged me, to the best of my ability. You will all, I am sure, be glad to know that before his death Dr. Otis had completed so much of the Surgical History of the War, upon which he was engaged, as relates to wounds of the extremities. There remains yet to be completed the account of the complications of wounds, such as gangrene, tetanus, septicæmia, etc. Another surgeon of the Army will be assigned to complete this history, and you can hardly conceive how difficult he will find it to prepare a report which will be the continuation of, and be constantly compared with, the work of Dr. Otis."—*Med. Times and Gaz.*, Aug. 13, 1881.

—

Health of New York.—The average mortality for August has been considerably smaller than that for July. During the latter month 4378 deaths occurred, while only about 3000 were reported for August. In the week ending Aug. 6, there were 839 deaths, and in that closing Aug. 13, 849. For the weeks ending

Aug. 20th and 27th, the numbers were respectively 682 and 679. This decrease in the death-rate may in part be attributed to the low average temperature which prevailed during the month, whereby the infant mortality was materially reduced, and to the indefatigable efforts of the tenement-house medical corps appointed by the Health Board. The special physicians of the corps completed their labours at the middle of the month, after a service of five weeks' duration.

The progressive abatement of typhus fever manifested throughout the month was the source of great rejoicing among all classes of society. In the 21st week of the fever's prevalence (ending Aug. 6), there were only 2 new cases; in the 22d week, 12; in the 23d week, 4 cases; in the 24th and last week (ending Aug. 27), only 1 case. 19 new cases were, therefore, reported against 124 in May, 101 in June, and 74 in July. In the last four numbers of the MEDICAL NEWS AND ABSTRACT, the reader will find a numerical history of the endemic, and will see that the entire number of cases reported during its course was 527. During the weeks ending Sept. 3d and 10th no cases were discovered, and the disease is, therefore, regarded as arrested. The last case of typhus was discharged from the Riverside Hospital ten days since. All the contagious diseases have decreased during August. 75 cases of smallpox were reported against 99 in July, and, on Sept. 7, only 12 cases of that disease remained at the Riverside Hospital. The number of scarlatina cases fell from 575 in July to 320 in August; diphtheria from 521 to 355; and rubeola from 231 to 96. The most intense heat of the season prevailed on Sept. 6, 7, 8, and 9. On the 6th inst., the thermometer reached $97\frac{1}{2}°$; on the 7th inst., 100°; and on the 8th, 103°, in the shade. The total number of insolations reported for these days amounted to about 75. On Sept. 9, 26 additional cases occurred. Nearly one-third of all the cases were fatal. Such excessive heat as that just recorded has not been experienced in New York since 1871.

—

New York State Health Board held a meeting at Niagara Falls on Aug. 11th, at which Dr. Harris, the secretary, read a paper proposing a plan of State vaccination for the purpose of eradicating variola. A resolution recommending the establishment of a State vaccine farm was carried. A resolution to the effect that the State Board co-operate with the National and local boards for the prevention of the introduction of variola into the United States, by emigration, was adopted. The Board has commenced to investigate the subject of adulteration of food in accordance with the provisions of a law recently enacted by the Legislature. The Board has appointed special officers to obtain and analyze samples of pharmaceutical preparations, and of the most commonly adulterated varieties of food. Among those claiming special attention are cheese, milk, butter, sugar, quinia, beer, honey, molasses, syrups, fish, baking-powders, soda-water, ice cream, teas, cocoa, canned fruits and extracts, wines and spirits.

—

Regulation of Medical Practice in New York.—On August 8th Dr. A. M. Purdy, President of the New York County Medical Society, appeared in behalf of the Society in the Police Court as complainant against three unlicensed medical practitioners. The offenders were each placed under $500 bail to await examination. The censors of the society in question are determined to deal summarily with prescribing druggists and unqualified practitioners.

—

Honours to the Secretary-General of the London Congress.—It is gratifying to find that the valuable services of Mr. Mac Cormac in organizing the London Congress are being recognized outside of his own country, and the profession will learn with pleasure that, in addition to the honour of knighthood which Queen Victoria has intimated that it is her pleasure to confer on Mr. Mac Cormac, he has also received from France the Cross of the Legion of Honour.

—

Transactions of the International Medical Congress.—We learn that the Transactions of the London Congress will probably fill three bulky volumes, and that the first volume, containing the Addresses, will be put to press immediately.

—

Abatement of Noxious Odours.—The Committee on Hygiene of the New York County Medical Society is at present interesting itself with the abatement of noxious odours emanating from city stables, and with the prevention of smoke from kindling-wood and box factories.

—

The New York City Health Board is rigidly enforcing the act pertaining to the registration of plumbers and to the submission of their plans, for new plumbing work, to the Board for approval. The result of this commendable legislation has been to materially improve the drainage and ventilation of all recently constructed houses.

—

Prize Essay of the American Medical Association.—The committee of selection appointed by the chairman of the section on Practical Medicine, Materia Medica, and Physiology, at the June meeting of the American Medical Association, have selected, and announce, as the subject for the prize to be awarded in 1883, the following question:—

" What are the special modes of action or therapeutic effects upon the human system, of water, quinia, and salicylic acid, when used as antipyretics in the treatment of disease ?"

The essays must be founded on original experimental and clinical observations, and must be presented to the chairman of the committee of *award* on or before the first day of January, 1883.

—

OBITUARY RECORD.—At Breslau, on August 10th, of kidney disease, in the fifty-second year of his age, Dr. OTTO SPIEGELBERG, Professor of Midwifery and Director of the Obstetric Clinic in the University of Breslau.

Dr. Spiegelberg graduated at Göttingen in 1853, and in 1858 published his first work, a *Compendium of Midwifery.* In 1861, he was appointed Professor of Obstetrics and Gynæcology in the University of Freiburg. In 1864, he accepted a similar professorship at Königsberg ; and in 1865 accepted the professorship at Breslau. Since that time, he has been distinguished for literary activity. In conjunction with Dr. Credé, of Leipsic, he established the *Archiv für Gynäcologie,* of which seventeen volumes have appeared, and which contain numerous contributions by himself and his assistants. About five years ago, he published a *Text-book of Midwifery,* the second edition of which he had almost completed at the time of his death. He distinguished himself by his readiness to adopt all new improvements in the obstetric art. The first ovariotomy in Breslau was performed by him, and he operated in all in considerably more than one hundred cases. By his death, the obstetric branch of medicine has, in Germany, suffered a severe loss.—*British Med Journal,* Aug. 20, 1881.

—

To Readers and Correspondents.—The Editor will be happy to receive early intelligence of local events of general medical interest, or which it is desirable to bring to the notice of the profession. Local papers containing reports or news items should be marked.

CONTENTS OF NUMBER 467.

NOVEMBER, 1881.

MEDICAL NEWS.

THE

MEDICAL NEWS AND ABSTRACT.

VOL. XXXIX. No. 11.   NOVEMBER, 1881.   WHOLE No. 467.

CLINICS.

Clinical Lectures.

ON INJURIES OF THE SPINE.

A CLINICAL LECTURE.

By WILLIAM HUNT, M.D.
SENIOR SURGEON TO THE PENNSYLVANIA HOSPITAL.

GENTLEMEN: The years circling about 1850 were troublesome times in Philadelphia. Political differences, race prejudices, an inefficient police, and, more than all, a volunteer fire department were causes of disorder and riot which at times raged rampant. The typical firemen of that day represented a race which is now extinct. Jakey, Mose, and Sykesey have disappeared. The only impress they have left is one upon the language of political slang. To "run with the machine," in those days meant what it said; now it means absolute fealty to party and obedience to the "boss."

What characters they were!

The rough of to-day only replaces them in his roughness. In no other respect does he resemble them. One of the most noble motives that can incite men to great deeds was the cause of their existence, that of saving life and property from destruction by fire. But the same enthusiasm that led them to do this, with a bravery and a risk to life and limb that were both reckless and astonishing, also excited such rivalry among the different organizations, that bitterness, enmity, and hatred, leading to frequent riots and bloodshed, were the result.

Jakey was a picture, with a high cocked hat surmounting his soap-locks, generally close shaved, except before parade days, when the big fellows let their beards grow, so as to appear as ferocious pioneers with their fire axes, prognathous, a defiant leer on his lip, between his teeth a segar held so tightly that its free end took an upward pitch, neck long, sinewy and open, a red cravat loosely tied with a large bow under a low-down collar, except when there was a red shirt, lithe and long of limb, arms akimbo and swinging free from the shoulder, a rough coat, long boots, with trowsers turned up at the bottom, here we have Jakey, brave to a fault and ready at any time for a fire or a fight.

Now what, I hear you say, has all this to do with a clinical lecture? It has this to do with it, that these same brave, rough and ready fellows, always had a respectable quota of their number, whether from fire or battle, in the wards of this hospital. After a riot they fairly filled it. Let me give you an idea of the times we went through. I lived here day and night, in the latter part of 1849 and through the years 1850 and 1851. This was the only accident hospital at that time of any account in the city, and as a matter of course, nearly all of the wounded were brought to it. The firemen were generally good and grateful patients. Many a Moya, Fairmount, Goodwill, or Perseverance Hose fellow would have willingly risked his life for me. I nearly laid down my life for them. Two young resident doctors succumbed and died, greatly owing to their over-work and exposure in the house. I had an attack of typhoid fever, which became historic, and was a theme for the medical lecturers, in their clinics, for many years. I had, according to the opinions of most distinguished attendants (Drs. G. B. Wood, W. W. Gerhard, and the elder William Pepper), every symptom of having perforation of the bowels. The accident was made out completely, but I treated science so disrespectfully as to get well, and so gave no opportunity to confirm the diagnosis.

After one riot (which, by the way, I believe was more a riot of the mob against the firemen than the firemen with each other), there were admitted no less than ten seriously wounded men. The slightly wounded were dressed and sent home. Gunshot wounds of the skull, trunk, and extremities were among them. Three alone of this lot died. So vivid is the impression of these times, that I remember the cases perfectly, their respective beds in the wards, and even the names of some of them. There was McShane, with his brains oozing from a depressed gunshot fracture of the skull; Westerhood, with his leg shattered by a bullet; Shearer, with his bad wound of the thigh, and the genial Jim Beesley of savory memory.

It is no exaggeration to say that in this hospital we saw more cases of gunshot wounds, through those disturbed periods, than were seen by most medical officers of the army and navy in the times before the war. But sad to say, it was not always the participant in the battles who were struck. Women and children on the outskirts of the crowds were sometimes the victims. In this way little Johnny Farley, aged eleven, was fatally wounded. He was brought into my ward, and I at once saw that he had a compound comminuted fracture of the head of the left humerus, which would probably require operative interference. He was in profound shock, and before sending a note calling the visiting surgeon on duty, I resorted to the usual means to bring about reaction.

This was the case that thus early in my surgical life strongly impressed me with the phenomena that occur in serious injuries to the spinal column and cord or to either of them. In those phenomena, I have ever since taken a deep, though melancholy scientific interest, melancholy, because of the utter hopelessness of recovery for most of the victims; scientific, because these and brain cases are those which give us more knowledge of the physiology of the nervous system than anything else.

They are cruel, accident vivisections, vivisections performed on the highest of God's creatures. I dislike vivisection, although I have done something at it in my day; but I have frequently thought when standing helpless at the bedside of one of these terrible cases of spinal injury, that if a dog could be wounded and give me any light for the relief of the man, it ought to be done. I think of him who said "ye are of more value than many sparrows," and I say ye are of more value than a few dogs.

Now note what happened. After Johnny had warmed up a little in bed, I turned down the covers to apply artificial heat to his feet. He complained of pains in his legs, and I noticed something that then surprised me. Gradually his penis began to swell, and in a few moments complete priapism was established. I then felt his feet, and tickled them on the soles; there was response and complaint, but soon no notice was taken of what I was doing. I brought my hands up the limbs and found that both sensation and the power of voluntary motion were gradually going; soon they were entirely gone. The pains disappeared; nothing was complained of or felt on either side below a line a little above the umbilicus. The case was clear. The ball had not only broken the humerus, but it had passed along the posterior aspect of the thorax, and had wounded the spinal column and cord, and I caught a view of the phenomena that were thus produced, *right in the act*, as clearly as if I had performed a vivisection in the same region. In this case the cord, as was shown *post mortem*, was not entirely compressed or lacerated, otherwise complete paralysis would have come on at once. Its gradual approach was explained by partial wounding and pressure, which latter was made complete through effusion of blood, as reaction came on, and the force of the heart was restored.

The fracture was of one of the dorsal vertebra, at or below the third, for there were no nerve symptoms involving the upper extremities. The brachial plexus and the intercosto-humeral nerves were not affected. It was a matter of indifference where the ball was. It had either passed on, or it was lodged in the column where in fact it was afterwards found. Johnny lived seventeen days. His may be taken as the type of an acute case of severe wound of the spine and cord. He passed through all of the phenomena incident to such cases, and had one (which I shall discuss fully further on) to an extreme degree. The priapism continued unabated for fourteen days. What else? There was complete paralysis both of sensation and motion on both sides downwards, from a line just above the umbilicus. The functions of organic life went on. The patient breathed, ate, and slept, and his food was digested, voluntary power over the bladder was lost, and the urine had to be drawn off with the catheter; the urine itself became ropy with mucus, ammoniacal and fetid. The bowels, at first torpid, relaxed, and there were involuntary stools. The pulse was always rapid. We did not take definite temperature in those days, but there were alternations of heat and cold. I was stricken with the sickness to which I have alluded, a few days before the death of the patient. My friend Doctor, now Professor, Penrose took charge of the case. The *post-mortem* examination completely confirmed the diagnosis. The line of injury was through the shoulder-joint into the chest and along its posterior face. The 4th or 5th dorsal vertebra was broken in fragments, the cord was lacerated, and the ball was found projecting into the spinal canal, where it was held and supported by spiculæ of bone. I looked over the University Museum yesterday for the specimen, where I thought it was; it was in the possession of Dr. Edward Peace, the chief surgeon for many years. I fear it has been lost.

I will now take up a case at the other end of my experience to this time, and then sum up what I have seen in a general way between the two periods. It also is typical, in that it illustrates a class which unfortunately are too common in accident hospitals. The victims truly "languish, and, languishing, they die."

Peter Green, adult, was admitted August 26, 1880. He died July 19, 1881—that is, 327 days after the injuries which killed him were received. He was in a stooping position, when a partition wall fell upon and crushed him.

The last dorsal and first lumbar vertebra were fractured, and a loose piece of one of them could be felt. There was immediate paralysis from the hips downward. In this case there was no priapism. The urine at first had to be drawn off with a catheter. The bowels were sluggish also, but soon became uncontrollable. Tympanites was a prominent feature. There was at times burning pain in the rectum. There was rapid emaciation, particularly noticeable in the limbs. At times there were attacks of local peritonitis. The pulse range for 42 days was from 108 to 72; temperature during the same period, $101\frac{1}{2}°$ to $98\frac{1}{2}°$; and respiration averaged 22.43. After this, as the case became chronic, and was almost one thing from day to day, the records were not regularly kept. Bed-sores formed, the urine dribbled, the feces oozed out. But the brain was perfect, the heart was sound, as also were the lungs; the stomach performed its digestive duties.

If no fortunate accident intervenes, as hemorrhage, for example, there is nothing for such patients but to be worn out. Food and care prolong their lives to an indefinite extent. It is nothing but a question of endurance. Barring accident or intercurrent disease, death takes place at last through exhaustion, and sometimes suddenly, from heart embolism, a stoppage of the circulation occurring at once, and thus mercifully ending a life which might still further be prolonged. Peter died from exhaustion. There was no autopsy granted, nor was it necessary. The case was too well known to require it.

Now during the time between these two cases, I do not know how many of the kind I have seen and have had under my care.

I have had them injured in every region of the column, from the atlas to the sacrum, cervical, dorsal, and lumbar, and in various parts of these regions. Understand, they do not all die, but the slightly injured, and even seriously injured, provided the cord is not too much involved, may get entirely well, or make partial recoveries. Sometimes the paralysis remains through a full length of days, and the patient is otherwise in reasonably good health. Again, the paralysis may be partial, or one side may recover to a much greater extent than the other. It is much easier to understand these cases in an anatomical, physiological, and pathological sense, than it is to cure them. Those who get entirely well are, I think, mostly cases of shock to the cord, through injury to the column, without lesion of its contents. In a letter I have written about President Garfield's case,[1] I have described such a case as this which came under my care last summer, and which fully proved that such shocks occur, for I had my fingers directly on the broken vertebral bones in the operation for removing the ball. Symptoms of shock to the column were present at first, but they rapidly disappeared. The President's case was also one of the kind, but the wound was in an inaccessible place. The spinal symptoms having gone so soon, is it any wonder that the true diagnosis was missed?

How easy such a diagnosis is when the symptoms remain and are more or less permanent, as in those I have described. As the letter is published

[1] See page 700.

in this number of the *Medical News* it is unnecessary to allude to it further. To give you an idea of the number of cases that are sometimes under notice, I remember on one occasion that Dr. Weir Mitchell asked me to let him know when I had any of them in my wards, as he wished to study certain points about them. I was able at that very time to show him five—three on one side, and two on the other, of the long ward alone. I have not given you nearly all the points, but only the striking ones. This is a clinical lecture, and the subject is one for a volume. Volumes have been written on it. I have not referred to them, but only give you a hasty sketch of my own experience. I will now relate another case, to show what inflammation of the membranes and softening of the cord do, where there is no injury to the bone, and thus you will understand how the bones, provided they are not displaced, are not at all necessary factors in producing the dreadful symptoms I have described, and also how, through the application of anatomy and physiology, we are sometimes able to locate the trouble precisely.

In the summer of 1859, a gentleman, 52 years of age, began to complain of pain posteriorly, over a limited space, at the root of the neck, which at first was slight, but it was continuous and annoying. There were also sensations of a peculiar kind down both extremities, more of uneasiness and want of confidence than of pain. The fingers became numb, and things did not feel right in them; this was more noted in the right hand than the left, but only owing to the fact that the use of the right was wanted more than the left, and consequently its defects were noted. At this time there was no tottering in gait. Travel was tried for a few weeks, but the patient returned somewhat worse than when he went away. The symptoms were more pronounced. The pain was greater, the gait somewhat uncertain, a pen could not be held rightly. There was no trembling nor spasmodic jerking. The functions of the body were properly performed; the intellect was clear; there was some mental depression and anxiety. Business, however, was attended to. The patient was president of a corporation. Counter-irritants and other remedies were of no avail to check the progress of the disease.

The pains became more severe and sometimes were very bad; they did not spread, but were distinctly localized, and kept to the same region. The difficulties about the extremities grew worse. Finally the patient stayed at home, and soon took to his bed. His sufferings increased, and then he lost the use of all his limbs—of the legs first, and then of the arms. There was no priapism. The diagnosis was, that there was, first, a local spinal meningitis, and a subsequent inflammation and softening of the cord. The pain became intense; as a measure of the suffering I shall never forget what he said when the actual cautery was applied to the back. Dr. Joseph Pancoast, who attended the case with me, did the operation. The patient would not take ether, and as the white hot iron was seething through his skin and flesh, clear down to the bone, he said, "Oh, that is better than the pain!"

But all efforts to check the disease were in vain. Paralysis of the animal life of all parts below the root of the neck came on. Voluntary motion and sensation here were gone. We knew the part of the cord affected was below the origin of the phrenic nerve, for the diaphragm acted perfectly. It was by this muscle and through physical laws that the patient breathed. We knew the lesion was just below this nerve, for the parts supplied by the brachial plexus were paralyzed.

The intercostal muscles did not act. The abdomen became enormously distended, by reason of flatus accumulating in the bowels, the abdominal muscles having no power to control or repress it. In this case I did what I have never done since, although I have tried it. I have seen it denied in a French journal that it can be done. Regularly every morning, with a large stomach tube, which I passed as much as eighteen inches up the bowel, I drew off the flatus and relieved the pressure, as an engineer would relieve the pressure of steam on his boiler. The abdominal walls fell flaccid, but incapable of resisting, they arose again from the same cause in the following twenty-four hours. The urine, which early in the case had to be drawn away, now dribbled, and a flexible catheter was kept in the bladder. Peripheral nutrition was interfered with; there were huge sloughs of the skin, particularly of the back, in spite of all that wealth could purchase, in the way of peculiarly constructed beds and cushions, and all that the best nurses could do. The fault was within, and not without. The patient was vegetating below the root of the neck; all there was of animal life in him was above it. The heart, supplied from its cardiac plexus, most of which comes from above the origin of the brachial nerves, continued to act; the stomach did its digestion; the sympathetic nerve, which was not involved, regulated the secretions and the supply of blood to it, which in its turn it furnished with new material. But day by day there was loss, and death took place in the beginning of the following year, six months having been required with all these terrible things to destroy life. Now what was the cause of all this? The post-mortem examination, made by Dr. James Darrach and myself, showed it to be an inflammation of the membranes of the cord and a softening and destruction of the cord itself, for a space of about two and a half inches. The lesion was below the phrenic nerve, and where the cord gives off its branches to form the brachial plexus. *Everything else was normal.*

I will now detail a case of severe spinal *shock*. On the 6th of May, 1881, a man aged 21 was brought to the Hospital, paralyzed in both lower extremities. He fell from a height (about twenty feet) and landed directly on his feet. It was at first thought there was fracture of the lumbar vertebra, but nothing of this kind could be found on examination. Both calcanea were found to be fractured. The escape of the spinal column from severer injury was thus explained by the feet receiving the greater force of the blow, as much of it must have been expended in breaking such well-protected and thick bones. Enough of the shock however was transmitted to the spinal cord to produce most serious results. The paralysis of the left leg was not so great as that of the right one. There was dribbling of urine from loss of control of the bladder and overdistension. The catheter had to be used for a few days. There was no priapism. The bowels were torpid, and there was tympanites. There was much pain in the legs. Sensation was not affected at any time to the same degree as motion, although it was impaired. Nutrition went on uninterruptedly. The bones of the feet united as rapidly and as firmly as though nothing else was the matter. There was no particular trouble with bedsores. To aid in preventing them the patient was at first put on a waterbed.

In a short time he became very tired of the unsteadiness of this, and asked for an ordinary bed. His request was granted without any bad result. Whilst his bones were mending, the spinal trouble was slowly and surely disappearing. Sensation improved quite rapidly. On the 31st of the month the patient was able to lift the left leg. Through the following two months he gained power over the right one, and in the mean time perfect control was gained as to the other functions.

The injuries of the feet and cord together required the use of crutches after the patient left his bed. He soon learned to walk, and was discharged on the 31st of August.

Contrast this case with the one of gunshot fracture of the spine and that of myelitis or inflammation of the cord which I have given you, and there will be no difficulty in noticing the distinctions. Sometimes after such falls the feet take all of the force of the blow. I once saw a man who fell in the same way as the one I have just described, but from a much greater height. The bones of both legs were driven out at the ankle-joints, and the limbs had to be amputated. There were no spinal symptoms whatever in this case. Some cases of spinal shock are so severe as to go on to death through disorganization of part of the cord. Then the progress is like one of progressive myelitis.

The way in which the spinal cord is suspended in the canal without nearly filling it, as the brain fills the cavity of the cranium, is the reason that some surgeons deny the occurrence of spinal shock ; what they mean is that some lesion takes place at the same time, for instance a local stasis of blood, or may be ruptures of small vessels. The same thing is more than likely true of many concussions of the brain, which all admit occur frequently. Concussions of the spine are of all grades from the unpleasant temporary jar that one gets when he is ignorant of or does not see a step in his way, and suddenly leaves a level, to the severe ones, such as that which has been described.

Railroad presidents and officials, and their lawyers, are the greatest skeptics about spinal concussion. The reason is, that it is the injury above all others that is simulated by dishonest claimants for damages after railroad accidents, so much so indeed that the name of "railroad spine" has absurdly been given to the cases. Spinal shock from other causes does not differ in its symptoms and progress from that which is produced on railroads. It is the degree of all of them that determines their gravity.

The possible results of a severe spinal shock can hardly be exaggerated. At the same time its symptoms and progress have been studied and imitated with a most astonishing minuteness. Judges, lawyers, and doctors have all been deceived, for after a supposed most pitiable victim of injury has recovered damages, he has also recovered health.

You should study these cases well, otherwise one of these doubting lawyers will twist you on the witness stand worse than the claimant's spine has been wrenched. I believe in spinal shock whatever its pathology may be, but I also know that it is a most difficult matter to distinguish the real from the spurious cases, especially where there is an insufficient or vague account of the accident which is supposed to have caused it.

I said I would discuss the symptom of priapism, which so often takes place after injuries to the spine, and which, if it does occur, is such a sure index of that injury. I have seen it follow, after accidents to all parts of the column, from the axis, of which I remember one particular case where it was present, down to the fifth lumbar vertebra. It is by no means a constant symptom. It may be but momentary, and, as we have seen, it may continue for days.

Also, as shown in the case I have last described, it is not apt to come on in disease of the membranes and cord, not the result of injury.

It may show itself rather late in such a case by extension outwards, but I have never met with it.

All these facts are puzzling, and I have never found a satisfactory explanation of them until now it dawns upon me. I suppose the same thing is in some book or lecture, but I have never seen it, and can not look for it now. I know this: that I have asked men most learned in nerve matters about it, and they have given me no satisfaction, and have acknowledged the puzzle. The fact is, we do not want the cerebro-spinal axis at all to explain it. Hilton, I think, goes to the brain for a reason for it, but we do not want the brain. We want the brain and axis to explain normal erection where there is sensation accompanying it, for in the form I am considering there is no sensation.

Now call to mind the sympathetic system of nerves. It is composed of a chain of ganglia and peculiar nerves lying along the spinal column, on the outside of the vertebral bodies, near the junctions of the ribs with the vertebra, and the intervertebral foramina, in the dorsal region; further forward on the bodies, in the lumbar region; and latterly with very long ganglia, in the cervical region.

Again, you all remember the rabbit that is brought out, in the lectures on inflammation, to show how the bloodvessels of the ear become engorged when the sympathetic nerve is divided in the neck. Whatever else this nerve may do, it is acknowledged to be the great vaso-motor regulator of the bloodvessel system; it is, as Draper says, the "fly-wheel" of the economy. The fibres of this nerve are abundantly distributed along the spermatic cord, which is mainly composed of the bloodvessels of the genital organs and the spermatic duct. In a normal erection the inhibitory power of the sympathetic is overcome by the fierce intensity of sexual emotion transmitted through the brain and cord. Local irritation through reflex also conquers the inhibition. This inhibitory power is also overcome when the trunk or ganglia of the sympathetic is abnormally irritated, lacerated, or divided. When this is the case, the blood rushes into and engorges the highly vascular tissue of the penis, and erection takes place, exactly as it rushes to the ear of the rabbit when the nerve is cut in the neck. If the ear was composed of what is called erectile tissue, which is highly vascular and elastic tissue, with fine muscular fibres, it would swell enormously from the same cause.

Thus it is not necessary to trouble one's self about a special nerve centre ruling over the function we are considering. Thus also this symptom in accidents to the column and cord is explained; also why some have it and others do not, why it is evanescent in some and in others almost constant, why it may appear in injuries occurring anywhere along the spine, why there is no sensation when it occurs as an accompaniment of laceration or pressure on the cord, for communication with the brain is cut off, and why also it is rare to find it in disease of the membranes or cord.

When the wounding missile or crushing force breaks the spine and involves the cord, and there is accompanying priapism, then the neighbouring ganglia or nerves of the sympathetic are bruised or wounded at the same time, from being caught in the line of the crush or wounding missile. When this symptom does not occur, the sympathetic has escaped. I have no doubt that when it occurs in hanging, the superior cervical ganglia of the nerve are caught in the squeeze. In most cases of disease the lesion is within the canal, and the sympathetic fibres or ganglia are not involved.

I shall say but little of the treatment of these cases. They are those to which as much as any other class the popular solecism is applied, that "the doctor can do nothing for them," meaning that he cannot cure them. Do nothing for them? Why everything has to be done for them. The bad ones are themselves helpless.

How hospital nurses dislike to see them come into the wards! How hospital governors and managers deplore the expense of maintaining them! How residents and chiefs get tired of seeing them, day after day, slowly but surely losing ground! What a relief it is to make a morning visit and find the long occupied bed empty! There is respite for a while only, for soon another will come in. Individuals perish, the race survives, and so it is with accident and disease. We have their victims always with us. Where we cannot aid to bring about recovery, we can alleviate and prolong life, although, if we were the judges, we would often say it was not desirable to do so. The details, for instance, of what was done for Peter Green, during the 327 days he was in the hospital, would fill pages, and I have not time to give to them now.

ADDRESS ON PUBLIC MEDICINE.

Delivered at the Opening of Section XIII. State Medicine, of the International Medical Congress.

By JOHN SIMON, C.B., F.R.C.S., D.C.L., LL.D.

GENTLEMEN: In preventive, just as in curative, medicine, it occasionally happens that consequences more or less valuable result from some mere chance-hit of discovery; but, except so far as this may sometimes (and but very rarely) happen, disease can only be prevented by those who have knowledge of its causes—knowledge which does not deserve to be called knowledge, unless in proportion as it is conclusive and exact; and thoroughly to investigate the causes and their mode of operation is the quite indispensable first step towards any scientific study of prevention. Essentially, we know how to prevent by having first learnt exactly how to cause. Therefore it is that preventive medicine has had almost no development until within these later times. The germinal thought of it may be traced in even the first days of our profession. The spirit in regard of which Hippocrates has been aptly called the Father of Medicine—the scientific spirit of observation and experiment, as distinguished from the spirit of priestcraft, was one which his medical writings equally showed in their preventive as in their curative relations; and when he, some twenty-three centuries ago, expounded to his contemporaries that pathology is a branch of the science of nature—that causes of disease are to be found in physical accidents of air and earth and water, and in quantities and qualities of food, and in personal habits of life, he (not without risk of being denounced for impiety) virtually proclaimed for all time the first principle of preventive medicine, and indicated to his followers a new line of departure for those who would most largely benefit mankind. His followers, however, have had their work to do. True knowledge of morbific causes could only come by very slow degrees, and as part of the development with which the physical and biological sciences have, little by little, with the labour of ages, been building themselves up; and so no wonder that, despite the lapse of time, even the most advanced of nations are hitherto but beginning to take true measure of the help which preventive medicine can render them.

Now what is the nature of that study of causes through which we may gradnally arrive at counter-causing or prevention?

Addressing a skilled audience I shall utter what to them is the merest commonplace when I say that, in the physical and biological sciences, we acknowledge no other study of causes than that which consists in *experiment*. And the study of morbific causes is no exception to that rule; it is solely by means of experiment than we can hope so to learn the causes of disease as to become possessed of resources for preventing disease.

· The experiments which give us our teaching with regard to the causes of disease are of two sorts—on the one hand we have the carefully prearranged and comparatively few experiments which are done by us in our pathological laboratories, and for the most part on other animals than man; on the other hand we have the experiments which accident does for us, and, above all, the incalculably large amount of crude experiment which is popularly done by man on man under our present ordinary conditions of social life, and which gives us its results for our interpretation.

When I say that experiments of those two sorts are the sources from which we learn to know the causes of disease, I, of course, do not mean that the mental process by which an experiment becomes instructive to us is the same in regard of the two sorts of experiment. On the contrary, the etiological problem (so long as it is a problem) is approached in the two cases from two opposite points of view; and the dynamical continuity of relation, which we call cause and effect, is traced, in the one case from the one pole, and in the other case from the other pole of the relation. In the one case, starting with knowledge of our own deliberately-prepared *cause*, our question is, What will be its effect? In the other case, starting from a certain *effect* presented to us, our question is, What has been its cause? But in the second case, just as in the first, when the question is answered, when the problem is solved, when the relation of cause and effect has been made clear, we recognize that the conjuring power which has brought us our new knowledge is the power of a performed experiment.

Let me illustrate my argument by showing you the two processes at work in identical provinces of subject-matter. What are the classical experiments to which we habitually refer when we think of guarding against the dangers of Asiatic cholera? On the one side there are the well-known *scientific* infection experiments of Professor Thiersch, and others following him, performed on a certain number of mice. On the other hand, there are the equally well-known *popular* experiments which, during our two cholera epidemics of 1848-9 and 1853-4 were performed on half a million of human beings, dwelling in the southern districts of London, by certain commercial companies, which supplied those districts with water. Both the professor and the companies gave us valuable experimental teaching as to the manner in which cholera is spread. I need not state at length the facts of those experiments, probably known to all here, but may rather justify my parallel by referring to an etiological question which will presently be discussed in our Section. It concerns the *causation of tubercle*—the most fatal by far of all the diseases to which the population of this country is subject. On that subject for the last sixteen years we have had a new era of knowledge. It was the great merit of a Frenchman, M. Villemin, that he, in 1865, first made us fully aware that tubercle is an infectious disease. He did this by certain laboratory experiments performed on other animals than man. He found that general and fatal tubercular infection of the animal was produced when he inoculated it subcutaneously with a little crude tubercular matter from the human subject. That first laboratory investigation of the subject has been followed most extensively by others; and the further experiments, while entirely confirming M. Villemin's discovery, have shown that subcutaneous inoculation is not the only mode by which the tubercular infection can be propagated. Dr. Tappeiner and others have shown that the same effect is produced on the animal if tubercular matter (such as the sputa of phthisical patients) be diffused in spray in the air which the animal breathes; and Professor Gerlach, of Hanover, showed twelve years ago with regard to the bovine variety of tubercular disease (the Persucht of the Germans) that its infection can be freely introduced through the stomach if bits of tubercular organs be given in the food, or if the healthy animal be fed with milk from the animal which has tubercle. That the communicability of tubercle from animal to animal is also being tested to an immense extent by popular experiments on the human subject is what a moment's reflection will tell; and from that wide field of experiment I select one instance for illustration. I have every reason to believe that Professor Gerlach's experiments on the communicability of tubercle by means of milk are very extensively parodied by commercial experiments on the human subject. I learn, on what I believe to be the highest authority in this country, that tubercle (in different degrees) is a malady which abounds among our cows; and that so long as the cow continues to give milk, no particular scruple seems to prevent a distribution of that milk for popular use. To the persons who consume that milk an important question as to the causability of tubercle is put in an experimental form. Whether they will become infected with tubercle is a question which the individual consumers do not stand forward to answer for themselves, like the animals of the laboratory experiments; but Dr. Creighton's lately published book, entitled "Bovine Tuberculosis in Man," and a paper in which I am glad to say he brings under notice of our Section the very remarkable series of facts on which he grounds that startling title, seem to suggest a first instalment of answer in accordance with Professor Gerlach's experimental finding.

The two sorts of experiment—the scientific and the popular—differ, as I have noted, in this particular: that the popular experiment is almost always done on man; the scientific almost always on some other animal. It is true that many memorable cases are on record, where members of our profession have deliberately given up their own persons to be experimented on by themselves or others for the better settlement of some question as to a process of disease; have deliberately tried, for instance, whether, in this way or in that, they could infect themselves with the poison of plague or of cholera; and as regards one such case which is in my mind, I think it not unlikely that the illustrious life of John Hunter was shortened by the experiments which he did on himself with the ignoble poison of syphilis. There have been cases, too, where criminals have been allowed to purchase exemption from capital or other punishment at the cost of allowing some painful or dangerous experiment to be performed on themselves. And cases are not absolutely unknown where unconsenting human beings have been subjected to that sort of experiment. But waiving such exceptions, the rule is, as I have said, that scientific experiments relating to causes of disease are performed on some animal which common opinion estimates as of lower importance than man. Now, as between man and brute, I would not wish to draw any distinction which persons outside this room might find invidious; but, assuming for the moment that man and brute are of exactly equal value, I would submit that, when the life of either man or brute is to be made merely instrumental to the establishment of a scientific truth, the use of the life should be economical. Let me, in that point of view, invite you to compare, or rather to contrast with one another, those two sorts of experiment from which we have to get our knowledge of the causes of disease. The commercial experiments which illustrated the dangerousness of sewage-polluted water-supplies cost many thousands of human lives; the scientific experiments which with infinitely more exactitude justified a presumption of dangerousness, cost the lives of a few dozen mice. So, again, with experiments as to the causation of tubercle; judging from the information which I quoted to you, I should suppose that the human beings whose milk-supply on any given day includes milk from tubercular cows might be counted, in this country, in tens of thousands; but the scientific experiments which justify us in declaring such milk-supply to be highly dangerous to those who receive it were conclusive when they amounted to half a dozen. So far, then, as regards the mere getting of experimental knowledge, we must not, with a view to economy of life, be referred to popular, rather than scientific, experiment. And, in the same point of view, it perhaps also deserves consideration that the popular experiments, though done on so large a scale, very often have in them sources of ambiguity which lessen their usefulness for teaching.

Let me now briefly refer to the fact that, during the last quarter of a century, all practical medicine (curative as well as preventive) has been undergoing a process of transfiguration under the influence of laboratory experiments on living things. The progress which has been made from conditions of vagueness to conditions of exactitude has, in many respects, been greater in these twenty-five years than in the twenty-five centuries which preceded them; and with this increase of insight, due almost entirely to scientific experiment, the practical resources of our art, for present and future good to the world, have had, or will have, commensurate increase. Especially in those parts of pathology which make the foundation of preventive medicine, scientific experiment in these years has been opening larger and larger vistas of hope; and more and more clearly, as year succeeds year, we see that the time in which we are is fuller of practical promise than any of the ages which have preceded it. Of course, I cannot illustrate this at length, but some little attempt at illustration I would fain make.

First let us glance at our map. When we generalize very broadly the various causes of death (so far as hitherto intelligible to us), we see them as under two great heads, respectively autopathic and exopathic. On the one hand there is the original and inherited condition-under which to every man born there is normally assigned eventual old age and death, so that sooner or later he "runs down" like the wound-up watch with its ended chain; and, as morbidities under this type, there are those various original peculiarities of constitution which make certain individual tenures of life shorter than the average, and kill by way of premature old age of the entire body, or (more generally) by quasi-senile failure of particular organs. On the other hand, as a second great mass of death-causing influence, we see the various interferences which come from outside; acts of mechanical violence for instance, and all the many varieties of external morbific influence which can prevent the individual life from completing its normal course.

As regards cases of the first class—cases where the original conditions of life and development are such as to involve premature death (which in any such case will commonly show itself as a fault in particular lines of hereditary succession)— the problem for preventive medicine to solve is, by what cross-breeding or other treatment we may convert a short-lived and morbid into a long-lived and healthy stock; and this, at least as regards the human race, has, I regret to say, hardly yet become a practical question. But as regards cases of the second class, evidently the various extrinsic interferences which shorten life have to be avoided or resisted, each according to its kind; and here it is that the scientific experimenters of late years have been giving us almost daily increments of knowledge.

Two early instances, vastly important in themselves, though of a comparatively crude kind, I have already mentioned; and I now wish to glance at some illustrations of the immense scope and marvellous exactitude of the newer work.

The invaluable studies of M. Pasteur, beginning in the facts of fermentation and.putrefaction, and thence extending to the facts of infectious disease in the animal body, where M. Chauveau's demonstration of the particulate nature of certain contagia came to assist them—they, I say, partly in themselves, and partly in respect of kindred labours which they have excited others to undertake, have introduced us to a new world of strange knowledge. We have learnt, as regards those diseases of the animal body which are due to various kinds of external cause, that probably all the most largely fatal of them (impossible yet to say how many) represent but one single kind of cause, and respectively depend on invasions of the animal body by some rapidly self-multiplying form of alien life. This doctrine, which scientific experiment initiated, has for the last dozen years been extending and confirming itself by further experiment. As soon as the doctrine began to seem probable, science saw that, should it prove true, it must have been the most important corollaries. If the cause of an infecting human disease is a self-multiplying germ from the outside world, the habits of that living enemy of ours can be studied in its outside relations. It becomes an object of common natural history; it has biological affinities and analogies. We can cultivate it in test-tubes in our laboratories, as the gardener would cultivate a rose or an apple, and we can see what agrees and what disagrees with its life. And then, as the next and immeasurably most important stage, where nothing but experiment on the living body will help us, we can try whether perhaps any of our modifications of its life have made it of weaker power in relation to the living bodies which it invades, or whether, through our more intimate knowledge of its vital affinities, we can artificially give to bodies which it would invade a partial or complete protection against it. Such, at first blush, were the obvious possibilities of research which the new doctrine of infectious disease suggested to the mind of the pathologist; and never since the profession of medicine has existed had a field of such promise been before it. The promise has not been belied. A host of diseases has been worked at in such lines as I just now indicated, and with many of them important progress has been made.

It would be impossible for me even to name a twentieth part of the investigations which have been more or less successful. As regards some which have most struck me, I pass with but a word—Dr. Klein's investigation of the pneumo-enteritis of swine; Professor Cohn's and Dr. Koch's and Dr. Buchner's respective contributions to the natural history of the anthrax bacillus; Dr. Böllinger's recognition of the microphytic origin of an important cancroid disease of horned cattle; with Dr. Johne's illustration of the inoculability of this disease; the research of Drs. Klebs and Tommasi-Crudeli into the intimate cause of marsh-malaria; and, not least, the demonstration (as it appears to be) which Dr. Grawitz has recently published, that some of the commonest and most innocent of our domestic microphytes can be changed by artificial culture into agents of deadly infectiveness. I pass these and others in order that I may more particularly speak of some which have already shown themselves practically useful; for in respect of some of them the time has already come when abstract scientific knowledge is passing into preventive and curative act.

First, and not in a spirit of national partiality, I will mention the application which M. Pasteur's doctrine has received at the hands of Mr. Lister, with regard to the antiseptic treatment of wounds, an application which, enforced and illustrated at every turn by Mr. Lister's own eminent skill as an experimentalist, has been confirmation as well as application of the parent doctrine, and the beneficent uses of which, in giving comparative safety to the most formidable surgical operations, and in immensely facilitating recovery from the most dangerous forms of local injury, are recognized—I think I may say by the grateful common consent of our profession in all countries—to be among the highest triumphs of preventive medicine.

Secondly, out of the experimental studies of anthrax—chiefly out of those of Dr. Sanderson and Mr. Duguid in this country, and those of Dr. Buchner in Germany, and M. Toussaint in France—has grown a knowledge of various ways in which the contagion of that dreadful disease can be so mitigated that an animal inoculated with it, instead of incurring almost certain death, shall have no serious illness; and the further knowledge has been gained that the animal submitted to that artificial procedure is thereby more or less secured against subsequent liability to the disease. In other words, with regard to that disease, an infliction which sometimes spreads to man from his domestic animals, and one which in some parts of Europe is of serious consequence to agricultural interests, as well as to animal life, the later experimenters—of whom I may particularly name M. Toussaint, and our countryman, Professor Greenfield—seem to be giving to the animal kingdom, and to the farmers, the same sort of boon as that which Jenner gave to mankind when he taught men the use of vaccination. Quite recently our great leader, M. Pasteur, seems to have made, by new experiments, still further progress in the mitigation of anthrax. ·

Thirdly, a similar discovery has been made by M. Pasteur, with reference to the contagium of a very fatal poultry disease, known by the name of fowl's cholera; he has learnt to mitigate that contagium to a degree in which, if fowls be inoculated with it, they will suffer no serious ailment, and he has found that fowls so inoculated—or, as he, in honour of Jenner, would say, "fowls so vaccinated"—are proof against future attacks of the disease.

Fourthly, Professor Semmer, of Dorpat, through experiments done under his direction by Dr. Krajewski, has made a similar discovery in regard to the infection of septicæmia—has found, namely, that, by treatment like that with which M. Toussaint mitigates the contagium of splenic fever, he can bring the most virulent septic contagium into a state in which it shall be mild enough to serve for harmless inoculations, which inoculations, when performed, shall be protective against future infections.

Finally, in a different direction of experimental work, let me name the recent most admirable research which Dr. Schüller, of Greifswald, has made, nominally in respect to certain surgical affections of joints, but in reality extending to the inmost pathology and therapeutics of all tubercular and scrofulous affections. A knowledge of the fatal infectiveness of crude tubercular matter has been given (as I before said) by Villemin and those who followed him, and Professor Klebs, four years ago, declared the infective quality to be due to the presence of a microphyte (micrococcus), which he had succeeded in separating from the rest of the matter by successive acts of cultivation in fluids of inorganic origin. Dr. Schüller solidly settles, and widely extends, that teaching. According to his, apparently quite unquestionable, observations and experiments, the micrococcus which characterizes tubercle characterizes also certain affections popularly called "scrofulous"—namely, "scrofulous" synovial membrane, "scrofulous" lymph-glands, and lupus; so that these diseases may be defined as essentially tubercular, and that inoculation with matter from any of them, or with a cultivation-fluid in which the micrococcus from any of them has been cultivated, will infect with general tuberculosis. The rapid multiplication of the tubercle-micrococcus in the blood and tissues of any inoculated animal can be verified both by microscopical observation and by inoculative experiment; and an extremely interesting part of the research in explanation of certain of our human joint-diseases is the demonstration that if in the inoculated animal a joint is experimentally injured, that joint at once becomes a place of preferential resort to the micrococcus which is multiplying in the blood, and becomes consequently a special or exclusive seat of characteristic tubercular changes. Even thus far the practical interest of Dr. Schüller's book is such as it would not be easy to overstate, but still greater interest attaches to the last chapter of the book, in which, confidently resting on the pathological facts which I have quoted, he makes proposals for the treatment of tubercle on the basis of its microphytic origin, and shows the successful result of such treatment as he has hitherto tried from that basis on animals artificially infected by him.

I venture to say that in the records of human industry it would be impossible to point to work of more promise to the world than these various contributions to the knowledge of disease, and of its cure and prevention; and they are contributions which from the nature of the case have come, and could only have come, from the performance of experiments on living animals.—*Lancet*, Aug. 20, 1881.

Hospital Notes.

BELLEVUE HOSPITAL, NEW YORK.

(Service of Dr. AUSTIN FLINT, Sr.)

(Specially reported for the MEDICAL NEWS AND ABSTRACT.)

Chronic Nephritis. Uræmic Convulsions (Unilateral). Phthisis Pulmonalis.

Jennie C., æt. 40, Irish, domestic; admitted Sept. 20, 1881. About sixteen months since the patient had the initial lesion of syphilis, which was followed by secondary manifestations of the same disease. She was subjected to a course of treatment with mercurials, under the use of which the syphilitic symptoms disappeared in Aug. 1880. From that time until May, 1881, she enjoyed good health, having no prodromata of any disease whatever. At that time she suddenly became unconscious, and, falling to the ground, had several convulsions. Recovering from these, she pursued her ordinary avocations without applying for medical aid. Since then, however, she has had a convulsion almost every week, and sometimes twice a week. She has often bitten her tongue and foamed at the mouth during the convulsions, which have, however, been of brief duration, continuing only a few moments at any one attack. On Sept. 19, 1881, she had an unusually severe and protracted convulsion.

On admission (*September* 20, 1881), she was somewhat stupid, but conscious, and complained of loss of power in her left side. Suddenly, while undergoing examination, she became convulsed, the left side of the face and the extremities of the same side being most affected. The eyes were fixed, and blood-stained froth came from the mouth. Paroxysms similar to that just described recurred at short intervals during the night and on the following morning.

Physical examination revealed the second stage of phthisis pulmonalis at the left apex. The urine was acid and clear, had a specific gravity of 1021, and contained ten per cent. of albumen by volume, together with large and small hyaline and granular casts. The quantity of urine in twenty-four hours was ten fluidounces. Two drops of Ol. tiglii were administered, inasmuch as another uræmic convulsion was apprehended, and produced a small fecal evacuation.

September 21. The patient is still stupid, and has slight *subsultus tendinum.* One-tenth of a grain of elaterium was now exhibited every three hours until three doses had been administered. The result of this medication was to produce several watery movements and to relieve the ataxic symptoms.

22d. The amount of urine for the past twenty-four hours has been only eight fluidounces. The patient had one attack of eclampsia in the morning, followed by profuse diaphoresis. She was placed upon the use of infusion of digitalis, one-half ounce, and bitartrate of potassium, one drachm, every three hours.

23d. Patient had two violent convulsions during the night, but soon completely recovered from them. Urine in twenty-four hours, sixteen fluidounces.

24th. One convulsion occurred during the night. Urine passed, thirty-six ounces. The same treatment is continued.

25th. Amount of urine, forty-seven ounces. No convulsion occurred.

26th. No eclampsia. Amount of urine, forty-two ounces. Appetite has returned.

28th. Amount of urine, thirty-seven ounces. It is clear, has a specific gravity of 1025, and contains albumen, 5 per cent., by volume, with a few granular and hyaline casts. The digitalis was discontinued.

October 8. No convulsions have occurred since last note. Patient's general condition has improved. Urine, forty ounces, and contains no casts, although some albumen still remains.

12th. The patient is so well as to desire her discharge.

—

Recurrent Fibroid Mammary Tumour.

An interesting case of this kind recently came before Mr. GAY, at the Great Northern Hospital. He had removed the mammary gland a twelve-month previously. There was no axillary complication, and the wound healed well in about three to four weeks. The patient was a lean person, aged fifty-four years. When she presented herself again, two painful growths had recurred on the axillary side of the site of the former operation, and had ulcerated on their surfaces. The bases were of almost a scirrhous hardness, but unadherent to the subjacent structures. The ulcerated surfaces were flattened, and had the appearance of being made up of eversion, from central gaps of the skin and, might be, allied structures.

Mr. Gay said he deemed the case one of considerable interest, as illustrating a by no means uncommon instance of fibro-recurrent or recurrent adenoid growth, such as he had described repeatedly in the Pathological Transactions, and which has a history, both clinical and pathological, of its own. Mr. Gay had no difficulty in distinguishing the case from absolute cancer, although it appears to stand close on the immediate confines of that disease. Originally a growth from the mammary fibrous structures, its recurrence is never prevented by the ablation of the gland. It is but slightly infective, so that the axillary glands do not show any marked disposition to enlargement, either by contamination or sympathy; and in the event of their becoming enlarged, the swellings usually either subside, or ulcerate after the fashion of the parent growths. It is at certain stages spindle-cell shaped in its histological characteristics. The tendency of these tumours to grow, as well as to ulcerative degeneration, is in the direction of the skin. They admit of removal in any stages of their career, and certainly with much temporary advantage to the patient, as the disease seems to have a specifically local character, and does not usually invade vital organs. On the other hand, with removal, the patient is very prone to improve in constitution, and to get healthy and fat. Such cases must have come under the observation of other surgeons; but, as far as Mr. Gay was informed, have not met with much attention.—*Lancet*, October 8, 1881.

MONTHLY ABSTRACT.

Anatomy and Physiology.

The Origin of the Liquor Amnii.

Dr. WIENER, of Breslau, has experimentally investigated upon dogs and rabbits the above subject, with special reference to the part played by the fœtal kidneys in the production of the amniotic fluid. His results are communicated to the *Archiv für Gynäcologie*. The amnion is of course a fœtal membrane, and therefore it might be supposed that, at least in the early months of pregnancy, the fluid within it was in some way furnished by the fœtus. From the fact that the liquor amnii contains urea, some have supposed that the fœtus passed urine into it. But some experiments which have been made by Kuntz, and confirmed by the author, show that when a solution of an indigo salt is injected into the maternal blood, the liquor amnii becomes coloured by the pigment, although none of it enters the fœtal circulation or stains the fœtal tissues. And according to Fehling and Ahlfeld, the secretion of urine by the fœtus during intra-uterine life is very scanty and slow. If these facts be correct, it would seem that the liquor amnii in the later months of pregnancy is mainly furnished by the mother, and that fœtal urine does not, as a rule, form a part of it. To determine both whether the kidneys act, and whether their secretion does add to the amount of the liquor amnii, Dr. Wiener injected the indigo solution, with a hypodermic syringe, directly into the fœtus. This, he says, is not difficult to do. He found that when introduced thus into the fœtal circulation, it was excreted by the kidneys, and tinged the liquor amnii. He concludes, therefore, that the kidneys do actively act in intra-uterine life; that the urine is passed into the amniotic sac ; and that the liquor amnii largely consists of fœtal urine. His experiments give a little additional support to what might have been inferred from the facts, that, as mentioned, the liquor amnii commonly contains urea, and that in cases of malformation and occlusion of the fœtal urethra, the bladder and kidneys are found distended with urine.—*Med. Times and Gazette*, Oct. 8, 1881.

Heat Dyspnœa.

Several physiologists have lately turned their attention to the interesting phenomenon known as "heat" or thermal dyspnœa, and a *résumé* of the results obtained is given in the last number of the *Revue Scientifique*. It is well known that when the temperature of the blood increases, the respiratory rhythm becomes more frequent, dyspnœa supervenes, and those phenomena are observed which are properly attributable to exaltation of temperature. The interesting question arises, Where are the points of attack for the increased temperature? Does it act on the cerebral convolutions primarily, and through these on the respiratory centres, or does it act on the skin first, or on the pulmonary endings of the vagus first, or, finally, does it act directly on the nerve-centres which govern the respiratory movements? Goldstein believes he has proved that increased temperature does not act by way of the skin, because in a heated animal cold affusions do not at once destroy its effects; that it does not act through the cerebrum, or is owing to any feeling of uneasiness on the part of the animal, because it is not

prevented by morphia injected into the veins; that it does not act by the pulmonary expansion of the vagi, because it is not prevented by their section; but
he endeavoured to show that it is occasioned by the direct action of heated blood
on the respiratory nerve-centres by employing a method of increasing the temperature of the blood without exciting the sensory nerves at their periphery.
This method consisted in exposing the carotid of a rabbit, and without otherwise
disturbing the circulation through it, surrounding it with hot water, which of
course heated the blood passing to the brain and medulla oblongata.   Goldstein
came to the conclusion that as heat dyspnœa then set in, it was clearly due to the
action of the warm blood upon the respiratory nerve-centres.   M. Gad and M.
Mertchinsky have made a series of experiments on rabbits in this mode, and on
registering by means of a pneumograph it was found that about thirty seconds
after the heating of the carotidean blood the respiratory rhythm became four or
five times more frequent, and ten seconds later heat dyspnœa was fully established.   The same result was obtained by another experimenter, and in an article
in M. Foster's *Journal of Physiology*, contributed by M. Sihler, that observer
considered that it was attributable partly to pain and partly to an increase in the
amount of carbonic acid contained in the blood, and to the augmented molecular
changes naturally consequent on an elevated temperature.   But this conclusion
is disputed by the most recent experimenters, Mertchinsky and Gad, on the
ground that the type of thermic dyspnœa differs from that of asphyctic dyspnœa.
In heat dyspnœa respiration is short and shallow, whilst in asphyctic dyspnœa
it is deep.   According to Mertchinsky moderate doses of chloral do not modify
thermic dyspnœa, whilst toxic doses almost entirely prevent it from supervening,
or at least cause it to appear at a much later period and in a much less marked
form.   The section of the two pneumogastrics was without effect.   Section of
the fifth pair did not prevent it from occurring, but it was much less distinctly
marked.   Hence he concludes that it is not a reflex action consecutive to excitation of the sensory nerves of the face by heat.   Moreover, the respiratory excite-
.ment is observed in as distinct a form after ablation of the encephalon as before.
Hence Mertchinsky maintains that the type and rhythm of the respiratory acts
depend on the temperature of the inspiratory nerve-centres situated in the medulla oblongata.—*Lancet*, Oct. 8, 1881.

Materia Medica and Therapeutics.

Absorption of Mercury.

After the inunction of the ointment of mercury in rabbits and men, FURBREN-
GER failed to discover any trace of mercury in the rete Malpighii of the skin, but
globules were visible in the hair-follicles and in the sweat-ducts. If, however,
the epidermis was first removed, the metal was then found in the corium, but
only a few isolated globules could be seen in the deeper layers of the skin and in
the subcutaneous tissue.   After exposure to mercurial vapour no mercury could
be found in the hair-follicles or sweat-ducts, although the surface of the skin was
covered with a gray deposit. Twenty-four hours after an injection of a mercurial
emulsion into the jugular vein the presence of dissolved mercury in the blood
could be demonstrated in five out of eleven experiments, and the liver always
contained mercury in a state of solution.   Hence it seems certain that metallic
mercury becomes dissolved in the blood.   The metallic mercury in the hair-follicles was considerably diminished in quantity in eight days, and those globules
which remained were oxidized on the surface, angular, and dirty-black in colour.

It is probable that the fatty acids of the skin assist in the solution. Oberländer has found that silver could be detected in the urine 190 days after the cessation of a course of inunction. The excretion was not, however, uniform, but presented remissions and exacerbations, the former occasionally of ten days' duration. A course of treatment by sulphur waters seemed to make no difference to the excretion, and no influence could be ascribed to salt baths, soda baths, or vapour baths. He concluded from his experiments that mercury is probably excreted largely by the liver and intestine. Although the action of mercury has been much studied, little attention has been given to the lesions which are found when death results from its action. Mering has produced in cats all the symptoms of chronic mercurial poisoning by injecting daily a solution of oxide of mercury in glycocoll—stomatitis, salivation, anorexia, diarrhœa, anæmia, prostration, albuminuria. After acute poisoning the autopsy uniformly revealed intense hyperæmia of the gastro-intestinal mucous membrane, and often actual erosions. The lesions were most intense in the lower part of the small intestine. Occasionally hemorrhages were found in the cardiac muscle, and ecchymoses in the bladder. The liver and kidneys were intensely congested. After chronic poisoning there was found a similar inflammation of the gastro-intestinal mucous membranes, ulceration in the small intestine, and a still more severe affection of the large intestine. Ulceration in the mouth and necrosis of the maxillary bones were also common. These effects are regarded less as due to a general cachexia than to the localized action of mercury on the different organs.—*Lancet*, Sept. 24, 1881.

—— ·

Carbolic Acid as an Antipyretic.

At a recent meeting of the Soeiété de Biologie, M. Raymond gave an account of the markedly antipyretic qualities possessed by carbolic acid, which he has administered in cases of typhoid fever. The acid is given simultaneously by mouth and rectum, to the amount of one gramme per diem, fifty centigrammes being divided into three pills, and a like quantity used in enemata. He declares that its administration on this plan is very soon followed by a great reduction in temperature—viz., to the extent of 3° or 4° C., and within half an hour most profuse diaphoresis is established. To ascertain whether this hypothermic effect was produced by the direct action of the carbolic acid, or indirectly through the diaphoresis, M. Raymond suppressed the latter by the injection of duboisin, and found the lowering of temperature to be unaffected. He found also that the antipyretic action was increased the longer the administration was continued. By employing larger doses—viz., two grammes, toxic effects were produced, the temperature fell to 34°, convulsive tremors occurred, and carboluria appeared. At the suggestion of M. Vulpian, carbolate of soda was given in doses of one gramme and a half, instead of the free acid, and the patient kept under the influence of the drug. The toxic effects did not appear, but the antipyretic action was still marked. The remedy does not, according to M. Raymond, limit the duration of the stages of typhoid fever; it controls the pyrexia of idiopathic erysipelas in a similar way, but has no influence on that of tuberculosis. It was pointed out that the antiseptic could not, of course, pass through the alimentary canal unchanged, so as to reach the ulcerated small intestine, and it would seem simply that it acted through the spinal cord and the vascular system.

M. Hallopeau thought the acid might have a topical effect on the typhoid ulcers. M. Dumontpallier pointed out that it was not so good a regulator of the fever as refrigeration. M. Hanot made some curious observations, which he detailed more at length at the next sitting of the society. He said that in two cases of adults suffering from typhoid fever, whom he had treated by carbolate of soda given internally, defervescence was determined on the fourteenth day in one case, and on the sixteenth in the other, the temperature falling 3° to 4° C. on the second or third day of treatment. In each case a peculiar rash appeared at the same time as the fall in temperature, the rash becoming pustular and vari-oliform in a short time. The pustules, on microscopical examination, were found to be formed almost wholly of bacteria mingled with a small amount of pus. The urine also contained bacteria. M. PAUL BERT, in commenting upon this, went so far as to say that carbolic acid renders the organism unfit for the development of the bacteria, and causes the particular material in which they thrive to be eliminated by the skin and kidneys, and the bacteria following its elimination are found in these parts. Upon what slender facts are marvellous and weighty theo-ries sometimes raised!—*Lancet*, Aug. 20, 1881.

Merits of Hospital Kwass.

This, an old popular Russian drink, is included in the obligatory diet of the military hospitals in that country, being given out (in full diet) in allowances nearly one litre. Iljinsky, at the request of his senior medical officer, undertook the task of overlooking the preparation of the beverage, and daily analyzing it as to its contents of acids, alcohol, and extractive matter. For the preparation of 5496.161 litres (80 eimers), the following ingredients are made use of: Bar-ley malt, 104.950 litres (4 tschetwerik); rye malt, 1638.4 to 4095.10 grammes (4 to 10 Russian pounds); rye meal, 24,570.60 grammes (60 Russian pounds); yeast, nearly ¾ of a litre (¾ of a "krug"); peppermint, 2047.55 grammes (5 Rus-sian pounds); wheat meal, 819.2 grammes (2 Russian pounds). When brewed under observation, the specific gravity was 1012 to 1021, although formerly it was 1004 to 1006, and Dr. Georgievski gives 1006 to 1007 as the average specific gravity of kwass. Hence it appears that in general 70 per cent. of the officially determined quantities of ingredients are, for economical reasons, not used. The analysis showed it to contain a series of valuable nutritive constituents, thus: lactic acid (according to Preyer a nerve-sedative), acetic acid (a thirst quencher), and, further, alcohol and carbonic acid, both of which hinder tissue change, and thus, to a certain extent, lower the temperature. The day's hospital ration of kwass contains: albuminates, 5.5 grammes; carbon hydrates, 33.0 grammes. The merits of the drink may be thus summed up: it excites appetite, acts both on the nervous system and on tissue-change, and is to a certain extent nourishing. When it is rapidly cooled after boiling, as is done with beer, a beverage resem-bling stout, but of more nutritive value, is obtained.—*London Med. Record*, July 15, 1881.

Fernet's Method of Introducing Food and Medicine by the Nostrils.

M. FERNET (*Revue de Thérap.*) wishes to popularize the method of intro-ducing liquid or semi-solid elements, and certain drugs, by the nostrils. The author has seen it employed successfully in newly-born infants, too weak to take the breast or milk from a spoon. He proceeds as follows: The patient being laid on his back, a little raised, the end of a spoon or, better, the spout of a close vessel, is brought near to one nostril, and its contents are poured in gently at in-tervals. The liquid slides over the floor of the nasal fossæ and the roof of the palate, and reaches the pharynx, where it induces movements of regular degluti-tion. If the operation be well done, the liquid never returns by the other nostril. This method may be applied in certain cases of apoplectic coma, when the patient cannot drink for three or four days successively, in the tuberculous meningitis of children, etc.—*London Med. Record*, July 15, 1881.

—

Preparations of Digitalis.

Dr. FRANKEL (*Charité-Annal.*, Band vi.) says, that the leaves of digitalis have an effect upon the circulation, which differs greatly according to their source, and possibly also to their freshness. The German Pharmacopœia prescribes a watery extract prepared from the pressed leaves; an alcoholic and an ethereal extract; and, finally, one obtained with the help of vinegar. The tinc-ture is made by treating crushed portions of the fresh plant with six parts of alcohol; while the acetum is obtained by maceration of the dry leaves with a mixture of one part of alcohol and nine parts of vinegar. About ten grammes of the tincture are considered equal to one part by weight of the leaves of digitalis. Digitalis, when given in small doses, has a very different effect from that obtained by large quantities. The latter are chiefly administered in cases of acute inflammation, attended with fever, while the former are employed to remove the troubles observed in heart-disease, in the so-called stage of compensatory disturbance. While the effect of smaller doses (0.5 to 0.75 gramme daily) is retardation of the contractions of the heart with increased arterial tension, larger doses (1.0 to 1.5 gramme daily) are followed by diminished arterial expansion and reduced frequency of the pulse, not unfrequently accompanied by collapse and vomiting. These latter doses were therefore administered as an antiphlogistic and antifebrile in pneumonia, pleurisy, pericarditis, and acute rheumatism, especially when the disease was naturally inclining towards a crisis and recovery. Traube explained this influence of digitalis in reducing temperature by its action upon the vaso-motor nervous system, and the vascular expansion of the skin especially. Traube's experiments have shown that the smaller doses in heart-diseases, by exciting the vagus nerve, retard the beating of the heart, and, by increasing the pressure of the aorta, regulate the adduction of a sufficient quantity of arterial blood to the myocardium, so that this organ recovers from its previous state of exhaustion, and is once more enabled to contract energetically. Only when the poisonous effect increases, paralysis of the cardiac nervous system and sinking of the blood-pressure set in. Böhm has since proved, by experiments on the exposed hearts of frogs, that digitalin has a specific effect upon the cardiac muscle itself, and upon the terminal branches of the vagus nerve connected with it, whereby the remarkable phenomena in the action of the heart are chiefly called forth. In order to test the activity of the different preparations of digitalis used in practice, dogs of middle sizes were curarized and injected subcutaneously with the infusion, the tincture and the acetum (the alcohol and vinegar having been removed), and the beginning of the retardation of the pulse and the enlargement of the single beats were considered as the commencement of the action. The following were the results. 1. The tincture, and also the acetum and the infusion of digitalis, are capable of exercising an exciting influence upon the inhibitory nerves of the heart, and upon the vaso-motor centre; but there are unmistakable grades of distinction in the action of the three preparations. 2. The tincture is the least reliable. 3. The action of digitalis—retarding of the pulse and increased blood-pressure setting in, after divers large doses of both the infusion and the acetum—sets in according to the individuality of the animals, and other accessory circumstances. 4. The acetum digitalis is the most powerful.—*London Med. Record*, Aug. 15, 1881.

Dangers of Peritoneal Transfusion.

Professor MOSLER (*Deutsch. Archiv für Klin. Med.*, vol. xxviii.) refers to the successful cases of Ponfick with injection of defibrinated blood into the abdomen (already recorded in the *London Medical Record*, vol. viii. p. 12), and to the observations which we have also recorded of Golgi and Bizzozero (*Ibid.*), indicating the excellent effect of such injections in increasing the richness of the blood, as tested by observations on the increase of blood-corpuscles and hæmoglobin. Mosler assumes as an indication for transfusion the leukæmic quality of the blood ; and the observations of himself and others on the effect of transfusion in leukæmia indicate that it should be done repeatedly in similar cases. It could not as yet be repeated often enough, on account of the dangers and difficulties of transfusion into the vessels. It being reported by Ponfick and Bizzozero that peritoneal transfusion presented greater advantages, the author resolved to try it on his patients, and especially to study the influence of repeated transfusion in the same patient. The first patient who appeared adapted for peritoneal transfusion was a man, aged 27, who had had sixteen parenchymatous injections of Fowler's solution of arsenic into a chronic tumour of the spleen without any symptoms of irritation of the peritoneum. Peritoneal transfusion appeared to be indicated by the anæmia, which had set in in a very high degree ; besides, it was of especial interest to be able to state whether the splenic tumour, which had considerably diminished after the injection of Fowler's solution, would show a yet greater diminution. After repeated peritoneal transfusion, microscopic examination of the blood showed, besides a diminution of the red corpuscles, a large number of microcytes. The origin of the tumour was referred to intermittent fever and syphilis. On December 8, 1880, 40 centigrammes of defibrinated blood were slowly injected, by means of a well disinfected injecting apparatus, through a puncture made in the left side of the abdominal wall. On the place of puncture a carbolized compress was laid, fastened with a gauze bandage ; and above this a bag of ice was placed. In the morning and evening the patient received a dose of 15 milligrammes (nearly a fourth of a grain) of pure opium. He complained of pains in the place of puncture, both during the operation and for some time afterwards. The temperature in the evening was 38.4 deg. Cent. (101 deg. Fahr.) ; the following morning 37.2 deg. Cent. (99 deg. Fahr.) ; no alteration could be noticed in the urine and blood. On December 21, the peritoneal transfusion was repeated with the same apparatus. The place of puncture was the linea alba, about 7 centimetres below the navel. The transfusion, of 130 cubic centimetres of blood, was done gradually. The patient complained while the puncture was made, and also afterwards, of pains in the place of puncture, and upwards. Hourly measurements, after the transfusion, showed a moderate elevation of temperature. The pulse was 110 per minute. In the night the pains increased. On December 21, in the morning, the temperature was 39.6 deg. Cent. (103.3 deg. Fahr.), pulse 128 ; there were symptoms of peritoneal irritation. The abdomen was distended ; he had considerable difficulty in breathing ; the heart's action became irregular ; and death occurred on the following night. The *post-mortem* examination showed diffuse peritonitis, a tumour of the spleen, and a high degree of syphilis of the liver. In this case, observation shows that peritoneal transfusion cannot be recommended in all conditions of the vascular system. The author suspects that the repetition of the transfusion was the cause of the peritonitis ; since neither were the instruments dirty, nor was there any injury to the intestine, nor abnormality of the injected blood. In this case an interval of twelve days occurred between the two operations, in which the patient showed no signs of peritonitis. He is inclined to think that the immediate cause of peritonitis here was an increased vulnerability of the peritoneum, due, probably, to the previous transfusion, as well as to the disease from which the patient suffered. He points out that peritoneal transfusion at short intervals must not be regarded as a harmless operation; and that it is probably contra-indicated in inflammatory and other diseases of the abdominal organs attended with a tendency to peritonitis.—*London Med. Record,* Aug. 15, 1881.

New Method of Producing Anæsthesia of the Larynx.

Prof. ROSSBACH, in the *Ann. des Maladies de l'Oreille, du Larynx, et des Organes Connexes,* Sept. 1881, describes his method, which consists in an attempt to suspend the conductibility of the trunk of the sensory nerve of the larynx so as to produce complete anæsthesia of that organ. The trunk of the sensory branch of the superior laryngeal nerve reaches the interior of the larynx by penetrating the thyro-hyoid membrane, below the extremity of the greater horn of the hyoid bone. At this point the nerve trunk is very superficial, and it is very easy, by means of ordinary agents, to destroy its conductivity. The author uses subcutaneous injections of morphia, 0.005 grm. at this point on both sides of the neck. Success was complete. He also found, by experiments made on healthy subjects, that the conductivity of this nerve could be suspended by cold. He used for this purpose a Richardson's atomizer, with two jets so arranged that the spray is thrown on both nerves at the same time. A spray of ether served in less than two minutes to render the interior of the larynx entirely insensible of contact with a foreign body. The author thinks that this method might be of use in cases of reflex spasm, where the point of departure is in the interior of the larynx, as well as in painful affection of this organ.

Medicine.

Presence of Bacilli in Typhoid Fever.

As a conclusion of his earlier communications on this subject, EBERTH reports the results of the examination of seventeen cases of typhoid fever. For the sake of comparison, he contrasts these cases with eleven examples of different forms of infection, in which, with the exceptional occurrence of micrococci in the lymphatic glands, no bacilli were found, and with thirteen cases of tuberculosis and phthisis, in which, in spite of the extensive ulceration of the intestinal canal, no allied forms of organism were found in the spleen or lymphatic glands. The ulceration of the intestine did not here, as in typhoid fever, favour the introduction of organic forms. Among the cases of typhoid fever, bacilli were found in six instances, especially in the infiltrated lymphatic glands, more seldom in the enlarged spleen, and in eleven cases they were absent. In the cases in which these organisms were found, as in his earlier observations, the duration of the disease was, as a rule, larger; the number of bacilli, however, with the exception of one case of fourteen days' standing, in which they were found in great abundance, was less. The bacilli agreed in their general characteristics with those previously described by the author and by Klebs; in addition, however, to the usual forms, longer and broader threads were noted, which were perhaps only other developmental forms.—*Centralblatt f. d. Med. Wissenschaft,* Sept. 10, 1881.

Treatment of Typhoid Fever by Salicylate of Soda.

M. CAUSSIDOU made a communication to the meeting of the French Association for the Advancement of Science at the Congress of Algiers, which was based
on thirty-two cases of typhoid fever treated by salicylate of soda, and in which
the rise of the temperature and the influence of this drug on the febrile process
had been registered with the greatest care, as attested by numerous tracings shown
by the writer. M. Caussidou arrived at the conclusion, in opposition to the facts
observed in several wards of the Paris hospitals, that salicylated medication gives
larger, more certain, and more permanent effects than refrigeration. M. Caussidou has even been in doubt if, by administering salicylate of soda from the outset of typhoid fever, it would not be possible to limit the duration of the disease
to the first week (?), and if, at least, it would not be possible to obtain a number
of cases belonging to the abortive form. Nevertheless, M. Caussidou does not
conceal the dangers of salicylate medication. Like other observers, he has
noted dyspnœa, precordial trouble, and exhaustion in patients where the salicylate of soda brought on a too sudden apyrexia. To avoid these objectionable
results, he proposes to administer salicylate of soda in fractional doses of one
gramme given every two hours, and to stop as soon as the temperature falls below
38° Cent. (100.4° Fahr.) In a complicated case of erysipelas, the salicylic medication was powerless to produce a febrile recrudescence brought on by this complication. M. Hérard declared that he had nothing but commendation for the
use of antiseptics, such as carbolic and salicylic acids, in the treatment of febrile
diseases.—*London Med. Record*, July 15, 1881.

—

Period of Latent Muscular Excitation in Different Nervous Diseases.

This paper (*Archives de Physiologie*, No. 2, 1880) is a continuation of MEN-
DELSSOHN'S previous communication (*Travaux du Laboratoire de M. Marey*,
1880), in which he had given the results obtained by him in the physiological
laboratory from experiments on frogs and healthy human subjects. The main
conclusion which he had reached in the latter was, that the time of latent excitation is not constant, but varies even in the same subject, with variable conditions
of nutrition, rest, amplitude of muscular curve, strength of exciting current, etc.
In the frog it averages .008 second; in man, .007. Generally speaking, the
duration of latent stimulation bears an inverse ratio to the muscular excitability
and contractility. Experiments in diseased conditions bear out these physiological data. There is a diminution of the lost time in hemiplegic late rigidity, an
increase in hemiplegic muscular atrophy, and so on in the whole list of diseases
with tendency either to contracture or to atrophy. The author found considerable variations prevail in hysteria, but noted that shortly before an attack the lost
time was shorter. In artificial catalepsy, it sunk to .001 second. [Waller
(*Brain*, No. 10, 1880), in a recent paper, assumes the time of latent contraction
of healthy human muscle to be .02 second, and gives tracings in support of his
view. It will be remembered that Helmholtz (1852) had estimated the same
period (in frogs) at .01 second, and that his determination has since been generally accepted and reproduced in text-books.—*Rep.*]—*London Med. Record*,
June 15, 1881.

—

Spinal Myosis and Reflex Pupillary Rigidity.

Prof. W. ERB (*Centralb. für die Med. Wiss.*, No 17, 1881) has found that,
out of 84 cases of tabes dorsalis, 59 had absolute reflex pupillary rigidity, 12
showed very feeble and low reaction to light, and in 13 the reaction was normal.

In 5 cases the symptom was unilateral, in 7 there was more or less advanced atrophy of the optic nerve. Out of the 71 cases in which more or less rigidity was present, 37 had distinct myosis, 34 had normally wide pupils, sometimes unequal. Myosis was absent in quite half the cases. Of the 71 cases, 43 were in the initial stage; in the remaining 28 the ataxy was already manifest. These symptoms may therefore appear quite early in the disease, or, on the other hand, be absent after it has existed for years; a closer connection between syphilis and pupillary rigidity appears not to exist in tabes. Out of 16 cases of progressive cerebral paralysis, he found the pupils only twice normal; in 10 they were unequal, but of these only 3 showed rigidity; in 4 cases there was myosis combined with rigidity. All this holds good also of the earlier stages of the disease. Very much more often were pupillary differences observed, 10 times in 16 cases; the reflex rigidity, on the other hand, only 7 times (once unilaterally). This symptom was also noticed several times in other diseases (anæmia, syphilis, tumours); in myosis after disease of the cervical sympathetic, the reaction to light is generally preserved, as well as in lesions of the cervical part of the spinal cord. Myosis and rigidity do not appear to occur together in healthy persons; in uncomplicated senile myosis, the reaction to light is unaffected. They must, therefore, be regarded separately. Respecting the former, it is most probable that the pupil-dilating centre, or its tract in the spinal cord or in the cervical sympathetic, is paralyzed; the rigidity, on the other hand, seems to be due to some change in the reflex arc, which lies between the centres of the optic nerve and the third nerve. Further observations, by irritation of the peripheral cutaneous nerves, showed that not only was there paralysis of the reflex contraction of the pupil, but also of the reflex dilatation, so that the expression "reflex rigidity" is doubly correct.—*London Med. Record*, July 15, 1881.

—

Magnet, Statical Electricity, and the Tuning-Fork, in Pseudo-Syphilitic Paralysis.

Drs. CH. MAURIAC and R. VIGOUROUX (*Le Progrès Méd.*, 1881, No. 19, 21, and 22) have published two examples of what they describe as a rare form of nervous disorder occurring during the course of syphilis, but of which it is difficult to determine exactly what part syphilis plays in their determination. The first case was that of a man, a haircutter, aged 22, who had chancres, followed by roseola, crusts on the scalp, sore mouth, with headache, fever, and night-sweats. After treatment for two months he was discharged cured, but soon returned with a painful tumour over the inner aspect of the arm, along the inner border of the triceps; under large doses of iodide of potassium this rapidly disappeared, but the limb became anæsthetic, with loss of motor power, and preservation of normal electrical reactions. This did not improve under iodide; but the application of a magnet caused headache, and complete transfer of the anæsthesia and paralysis to the sound arm; repeated applications cured these for a time, but he relapsed after a few days. Statical electricity, repeated three times, produced no effect but slight numbness of the fingers and dorsum of the hand. By introducing the sound hand into the resounding box of a large tuning-fork (ut 3), transfer of the affection was effected, and at the same time there was produced hemianæsthesia of the sound side, with loss of taste, smell, hearing, diminution of the field of vision and visual acuity, and complete colour-blindness; in every respect this resembled hysterical hemianæsthesia. By the following day the phenomena had changed sides, even the artificially induced hemianæsthesia having become transferred. By repeated applications, a cure was effected: the patient went home, relapsed again, was put on iodide of potassium, and after taking it for some time, got well suddenly, and has remained well. The second case was that of a man, aged 40, who denied all venereal antecedents, and the diagnosis of constitutional syphilis rested on the presence of a fissured and atrophied tongue. He had been epileptic when young, and his mother suffered from the same disorder. After suffering from diffuse superficial headache, worse at night, he became hemianæs-thetic, the anæsthesia affecting the special senses, with some loss of power in the lower extremity. The magnet and tuning-fork caused malaise and insomnia, but had no influence on the neurosis. Statical electricity caused transfer, and cured him after twenty sittings of forty to forty-five minutes each. The authors admit that the evidence of syphilis was not clear, but the lesion of the tongue was regarded as syphilitic, both at the Hôtel-Dieu and at St. Louis. The phenomena were not those of ordinary syphilitic paralysis, yet a localized lesion in the poste-rior part of the internal capsule would be capable of giving rise to these symp-toms. The early epileptiform attacks in the first case, and the existence of hys-tero-epilepsy in the mother of the second, indicate that in both there was a predisposition to nervous affections. The inefficacy of ordinary antisyphilitic remedies is opposed to the notion that these symptoms depended directly on syphilitic lesions ; but syphilis probably played the part of an exciting cause.— *London Med. Record*, July 15, 1881.

The Cephalic Souffle in the Adult.

In 1838, Dr. Fisher, of Boston, published in the *American Journal of the Medical Sciences*, a paper in which he described the *bruit de souffle* in the head, and stated that he had met with this sound in auscultation of the cranium in cases of chronic hydrocephalus, cerebral congestion, either simple or coincident with dentition or whooping-cough, in acute encephalitis or meningitis, in suppu-ration of the brain, induration of that organ, etc. Other authors recognized the same sound later, and reported it with other affections ; among others, M. Henri Roger, who found it only exceptionally after the closure of the fontanelles, and expressed the opinion that cranial auscultation is not really applicable to persons past the first two or three years of life. Subsequent writers to M. Roger have, as a rule, agreed with him in this opinion, though it has, perhaps, not been al-together denied that the cerebral *souffle* might occur in the adult also.

M. RAYMOND TRIPIER, in a memoir published in the *Revue de Médecine* (the continuation of the *Revue Mensuelle*), Nos. 2 and 3 of this year, takes up the subject anew and reports six cases of the occurrence of this intracranial *souffle* in the adult, with a very thorough discussion of the conditions of its occurrence and its significance. The following are the conclusions of his memoir :—

1. The cephalic *souffle* occurs in the adult as Fisher and Whitney have stated, and, contrary to the opinion of M. Henri Roger, now generally accepted.

2. I have met with it in one case of anæmia from neuralgia, in several cases of chlorosis, in one patient suffering from cachectic anæmia, in one case of intra-cranial tumour, and in a case of hydrocephalus.

3. It is a profound systolic *souffle* that can be heard over the whole cranium, but principally over the lateral portion at the horizon of the temples ; its maxi-mum intensity is in the right temporal region, and it does not appear to be modi-fied by changes of position of the head and trunk.

4. The patients in whom it occurs have no intermittent sound synchronous with the *souffle* heard on auscultation, and, consequently, with the cardiac sys-tole, the intensity of which is in direct relation with that of the cephalic *souffle*.

5. Both this subjective sound and the *souffle* may be modified or suppressed momentarily by the compression of the carotid on the side auscultated, or even that of the opposite side. Simultaneously we observe in the anæmic patients the

production of a general *malaise*, with numbness of the hand of the side opposite the compressed carotid. These phenomena are most marked, or are only produced by compression of the right carotid.

6. The cephalic *souffle* may be diminished or disappear with a cure or an aggravation of the disorder which it accompanies.

7. The cephalic *souffle*, being perfectly synchronous with the carotid systole, ought to have its origin in the arterial system. It is not due to a transmission of the systolic *souffle* of the heart that we observe in anæmic or chlorotic patients, nor to that of a *souffle* occurring in the arteries or veins in the neck. By exclusion, we locate it in the terminal portion of the internal carotid, at the point where it enters the cranial cavity. Not only are there many reasons militating in favour of this location, but in one case there was found a small tumour, situated alongside the artery at this horizon, which gave rise to a sound altogether similar to that found in the other cases. The *souffle* may be produced on both sides, or only on one side, and that, preferably, the right.

8. In anæmias due to hemorrhages or to cachexia, as well as in chlorosis, the cephalic *souffle* is met with when the symptoms of anæmia are especially intense and of long duration, notably when there is a very pronounced discoloration of the integuments, palpitations and breathlessness with the slightest exertion, digestive disturbances, and especially vomiting, together with great weakness.

9. In these cases there exists a cardiac systolic *souffle*, which is lacking in cases connected with an intracranial lesion.

10. A cephalic *souffle* without any corresponding sound at the base of the heart, and especially without coexisting anæmia, ought to suggest the possibility of compressions of the internal carotid in its terminal portion, when there is no disease of the orbit.

11. The cephalic *souffle* can be distinguished by the above condition from the continuous *souffle* with reinforcements, which may appear intermittent, produced by communication of the carotid with the cavernous sinus, as well as from the intermittent *souffle* due to aneurisms of the carotid and the ophthalmic arteries, since in both these cases there are characteristic symptoms on the part of the orbit.

12. We have not met with the cephalic *souffle* in the cerebral affections mentioned by Fisher and Whitney, with the exception of hydrocephalus.

13. We have also not found it in the healthy adult.

14. Is there a continuous cephalic *souffle?* We have not met with it in the adult. But the patients may hear sounds that are probably venous *bruits*, either continuous or intermittent, but which must not be confounded with those accompanying the cephalic *souffle*.

15. The cephalic *souffle* may afford important indications for the diagnosis, prognosis, and the treatment of the disease in which it occurs.

Parotitis as a Complication of Ovariotomy.

Dr. MÖRICKE, in a communication to the *Zeitschrift für Geburtshülfe und Gynäkologie*, narrates five cases in which inflammation of the parotid gland followed ovariotomy, and in four of them went on to suppuration. He refers to the well-known connection between inflammation of the testis and of the parotid gland, and quotes cases from other authors in which affections of the female genitals—swelling of the labia, vulvo-vaginal catarrh, swelling and pain in the breasts, swelling and pain of the ovary—came on in the course of mumps. He thinks these instances point to a connection between the parotid gland and the ovary, similar to that which exists between the parotid gland and the testicle. In support of this view he further states that he has never seen parotitis follow any other operation on the female genitals, although the operations of this kind which he has done far exceed in number his ovariotomies. In one of his cases there was the possible source of fallacy, that some children suffering from mumps were in the hospital at the time, and a nurse caught the disease. But the ovariotomy case was kept separate from the other patients, had her special nurse, and no other patients in the hospital caught the disease The criticism, that parotitis is not uncommon in the course of the acute infectious diseases (typhus, scarlatina, etc.), and in pyæmia, he anticipates by saying that his patients were not suffering from any of these diseases ; nor was the inflammation so acute or so dangerous as in the pyæmic form. In time of occurrence and in frequency it closely resembled the orchitis which complicates mumps. The parotitis came on five times out of 200 cases of ovariotomy, and began from the third to the seventh day after the operation. Orchitis in mumps is said to occur once in sixty cases, and to come on, as a rule, about the sixth day.—*Med. Times and Gazette*, Sept. 3, 1881.

—

Peripheral Temperatures in Lung Diseases.

ANREP has made a series of observations on fifty cases of lung disease, with a specially constructed thermometer, which may be described as an ordinary clinical thermometer in which the bulb has been flattened out horizontally, and is protected from draughts by a glass bell springing from the sides of the tube below the index. With two such instruments accurately compared beforehand, he observed (*Verhandl. der Physik. Med. Gesellsch. in Würszburg*, Band. xiv. Heft 1, 2) the temperature on opposite sides of the thorax of healthy individuals. He found the average to be about 96.3 deg. Fahr. ; but the temperatures were very rarely the same, the difference varying from 0.2 deg. Fahr. to 0.5 deg. Fahr., sometimes on the one side, sometimes on the other. The cases of lung disease observed were pleurisy, croupous pneumonia, and chronic catarrhal pneumonia. In pleurisy the cutaneous temperature of the affected side (thermometer in an intercostal space) is higher than the axillary temperature of the opposite side, and the highest temperature corresponds to the time of most rapid effusion. The cutaneous temperature of the opposite side is also slightly raised. In pleurisy without effusion, the rise of cutaneous temperature is neither so great nor so long continued. In cases of croupous pneumonia, the difference between the two sides amounted to as much as 2.7 deg. Fahr. ; and from the tables given by Dr. Anrep it can be seen that those parts of the lung in the first stage of inflammation, before crepitation has appeared, give a higher temperature than those completely solidified. In chronic catarrhal pneumonia, the cutaneous temperatures closely agree with the local progress of the disease ; and in one case fully recorded the rapid rise of temperature over the apex, followed by a fall as the symptoms of a large cavern developed themselves, is very striking, more especially as the temperature over the cavern continued lower than all the rest of the chest. The author believes that the observation of cutaneous temperatures is, even at the present, of practical value ; and when the clinical thermometers now in use are replaced by thermomultipliers, we shall be able to derive from it most valuable information.—*London Med. Record*, July 15, 1881.

—

Typhoid Pleurisy.

In certain very rare cases, acute pleurisy may take on a typhoid form which is extremely serious, and almost always ends fatally. Dr. A. GOUMY, who has studied this disease very carefully, thus summarizes in his inaugural thesis the indications for treatment (*Revue de Thérap.*, p. 331). To keep up the general condition of the patient by hygienic measures, tonics, in large doses, given at an early stage, are the most urgent indication. Subsequently, the pleural liquid must. be evacuated as early as possible. One puncture is made, then a second, and if the general condition do not improve, pleurotomy is resorted to. Professor Bouchard is greatly in favour of this treatment; two out of three cases, under his care, recovered under this treatment. The incision of the thoracic wall disengages the lung, and favours its gradual and progressive expansion. Antiseptic washings-out prevent any danger of putrid infection ; for this purpose carbolic acid, sulphate of zinc, a three per cent. solution of salicylic acid which has been employed by Potain, and a five per thousand of chloral which has been employed by Villemin, are all recommended. According to the recent statistics compiled by Robert, pleurotomy has yielded 78 cures out of 114 cases. These figures are satisfactory, especially if the frequency of symptomatic pleurisy be taken into account.—*London Med. Record*, Aug. 15, 1881.

—

Favourable Influence of Hydro-Pneumothorax upon the Progress of Pulmonary Tuberculization.

This paper (read at the meeting of the French Association for the Advancement of Science at Algiers by Dr. HÉRARD, Physician of the Hôtel-Dieu) was intended to show that, whereas ordinarily the occurrence of hydro-pneumothorax in the course of phthisis forms a serious and often fatal complication, in a certain number of cases, more frequently than is supposed, it exercises a favourable influence on the progress of the malady, may arrest its progress, and become an unhoped for means of safety to the patient. Dr. Hérard had collected a certain number of observations, which established in the clearest and most positive manner this salutary influence of hydro-pneumothorax. An illustrative case was that of a youth, a mechanic, aged 17, who was admitted into the Hôtel-Dieu on July 15, 1880. His mother died of chest-disease, and his father from tuberculosis. He had been delicate from childhood, and had suppuration of the right ear since three or four years of age. Since a sudden chill in May he had had a constant cough, with expectoration, which became muco-purulent. Loss of strength and appetite, sweating, and profuse diarrhœa followed. These symptoms, together with great emaciation and hectic fever, were present on his admission.

Auscultation showed the existence of blowing respiration and subcrepitant *râles* at the right apex. Over the left apex there were cavernous breath-sound and gurgling, especially marked behind. There was dulness on percussion over the left apex, and some loss of resonance over the right. The vesicular murmur over the rest of both lungs was nearly normal. On August 10, on making a hasty movement, he was suddenly seized with an acute pain in the left side, and with intense dyspnœa ; his face was pale and anxious. Tympanitic resonance was found all over the left side, except for about four or five finger-breadths at the base, where there was marked dulness. Amphoric voice and breath-sounds with metallic tinkling were heard on auscultation, the thoracic vibrations were abolished, and succussion could be easily felt, even by the patient himself.

For some days the patient was alarmingly worse ; the lower limbs became œdematous, and the evacuations were involuntary ; he was thought to be on the point of death ; but, after a struggle of several weeks, about the end of September, a favourable change took place, and from that moment he continued to mend daily. The dyspnœa diminished ; strength, appetite, and sleep returned. The cough diminished ; and the expectoration, before so abundant, almost completely disappeared. The physical signs at that time were dulness, and resistance to the finger at the left base behind, exaggerated resonance in the other parts of the chest; the amphoric breath-sound and the metallic tinkling had disappeared, but succussion was still perceptible; the cavernous blowing and the subcrepitant *râles* had notably diminished. The heart remained displaced to the right. At the end of November he was able to return to his home in the country. Had he been able to pass the winter in a favourable climate, Dr. Hérard believes he might have been completely restored to health. Such cases as these are not rare or isolated ones; twenty such are collected in the thesis of Dr. Toussaint, from different authors.

How shall we explain the favourable influence of hydro-pneumothorax in these instances, and what is the mechanism by which a cure is effected? Is it possible to foresee in what cases such an issue may be hoped for, and in what cases a fatal event may be anticipated? Bearing in mind the anatomico-pathological conditions under which hydro-pneumothorax may occur, we may arrange the cases under three categories, founded on the state of the tuberculous lung.

In the first category, the lesions of the lung are in their earliest stage. The lung presents scattered granulations or small caseous nodules, in the midst of a tissue more or less hyperæmic, but in a condition in which any sudden compression might reduce it to a small volume. The occurrence of hydrothorax in such cases is not rare. All that is necessary in order to establish a communication between the bronchi and the serous cavity, is the softening of one of these small tuberculous masses on the surface of the lung. The first effect of such an accident is the compression and flattening of the lung by the escaped air and the liquid effusion which rapidly follows. Later on, false membranes envelop the organ in a sort of thick resistent shell, and maintain it reduced often to quite an insignificant volume against the vertebral column and groove. The lung, under these circumstances, is dense and carnified, and its functional activity is greatly diminished or completely suppressed; we can readily understand how, in such a case, the tuberculous evolution is checked, or sometimes altogether arrested.

In the second category the pulmonary lesions are much more advanced, and the phthisis has reached the second or third stage only, and this is the important point; these changes are limited to the upper lobe, the other lobes presenting merely granulations or small caseous masses, surrounded by more or less congested lung-tissue. As in the first category, the effect of hydro-pneumothorax, by compressing the lung, is to arrest its functions, and in diminishing the afflux of blood, to prevent the nutrition of the morbid products, and to stop, in short, the tuberculous process. At the same time another remarkable phenomenon takes place in the upper lobe; the walls of the cavities, yielding to compression, come together, become agglutinated, and sometimes even cicatrize; the pulmonary suppurations and excessive bronchial secretion diminish, and, as in the case cited, the expectoration is completely suppresed. This suppurative process being arrested, the consequent hectic fever, sweating, diarrhœa, etc., disappear also, and the patient passes from the most alarming state into one of sensible amelioration, and even of real cure. But to insure so favourable a result, it is necessary that the opposite lung should be and remain free from disease.

One of the cases cited by Dr. Toussaint gives anatomical demonstration of the cicatrization of cavities under such conditions. A young soldier presented all the signs of pulmonary tuberculosis in the third stage, gurgling, loud cavernous blowing, metallic bruits at the left apex, and a few subcrepitant *râles* at the right apex; abundant purulent expectoration, great emaciation, profuse sweatings, hectic fever, intractable dyspepsia. A few days after admission into hospital, a sudden access of suffocation, with pain in the left side, drew attention to the occurrence of hydro-pneumothorax. For some days the patient seemed on the point of death, when slowly and unexpectedly he began to revive; the dyspnœa abated, the fever disappeared, and the appetite became good. The sweatings ceased, and the expectorations changed completely in character, and became scanty and glairy. This amelioration was maintained and augmented until some months afterwards, when an exudation into the right pleural cavity gradually increased, in spite of all that could be done, and the patient died. The necropsy showed the existence of double pleural effusion. The left lung was flattened and compressed upwards and backwards, and strongly bound down, so that it did not reach below the fourth rib; at its apex there were traces of a large cavity, the walls of which were in contact and had become agglutinated and cicatrized; it was represented by a gray, irregular band, about the size of the little finger. Two smaller bands indicated the existence of two other smaller cavities. These were surrounded by masses of hard cretaceous tubercle. The right lung presented at its apex a few small masses of hard tubercle. These observations show the important part which the compressibility of the pulmonary tissue takes in the cure of such cases.

In the third category we find the whole of the lung invaded by tuberculous lesions (granulations and broncho-pneumonia); the organ is hard, compact, resistant, irreducible by compression; in such cases, hydro-pneumothorax can only increase the peril which already exists.

It is incorrect, then, to regard the occurrence of hydro-pneumothorax in the course of phthisis as always fatal; on the contrary, in certain well characterized cases, it may be of favourable import.—*London Med. Record*, Aug. 15, 1881.

Heart Symptoms of Chorea.

Dr. OCTAVIUS STURGES, Physician to the Westminster Hospital, London, publishes in *Brain*, July, 1881, an interesting paper, in which he shows that in chorea the heart is apt to sympathize with the voluntary muscles at all ages up to the adult period, this sympathy being shown as well by dynamic murmur as by accelerated action, unevenness of rhythm, and, not seldom, the excited impulse common in hysteria, the particular manner of response being dependent upon the age of the patient. The hypothesis is that these several modes of heart affection correspond with as many modifications of chorea, which are exhibited not in the heart only, but in the voluntary muscles as well; these several regions sharing jointly, each in its own degree and after its own manner, in a disorder the area of whose influence is coextensive with that of ordinary emotional disturbance; and particularly that in all such variations the motor element of the affection is represented mainly by irregularity and unevenness of cardiac rhythm, the emotion element by acceleration, and the paresis element by dynamic murmur.

Treatment of Cardiac Diseases.

According to Prof. RENZI, bromide of potassium diminishes the anxiety of patients with heart disease, and renders their respiration easier. Under its influence sleep is more tranquil, easier, and lasts longer. The number of cardiac pulsations and respiratory movements diminishes; the cough, however, seems to be aggravated by this remedy. Iodide of potassium succeeds better, particularly in ameliorating the respiratory symptoms and in overcoming dyspnœa. Hydrate of chloral serves to overcome the insomnia in cases of heart disease, but in general it does not diminish dyspnœa of cardiac origin. It tends, moreover, to increase cerebral torpor and somnolence, and when combined with iodide of potassium it tends to produce a serious and persistent somnolence.—*Journ. de Méd. de Paris*, Sept. 10, 1881.

A Case of Prolonged Intestinal Obstruction.

Dr. F. W. DRAPER, of Boston, reports the following case. The patient was a man, aged thirty-three, of sedentary habits. For six years, dating from an attack of "inflammation of the bowels," he had been subject to recurrent attacks of obstinate constipation, in one instance lasting ten days, and accumulation of flatus. On June 28, 1880, after indulgence in iced water, he was attacked with slight vomiting, distension of the abdomen, and moderate pain. The matter vomited was of a bilious character. The abdomen was uniformly distended and tympanitic, without tenderness, and careful palpation and percussion detected no region presenting exceptional signs. After the second day vomiting ceased spontaneously; there was obstinate constipation, which lasted for twenty-one days, in spite of the employment of laxatives, turpentine stupes to the abdomen, and stimulating enemata. Sulphate of magnesia was once employed, but increased the patient's misery; belladonna was employed until its physiological effects gave warning to desist. The intestines were four times aspirated, and large quantities of gas removed; large enemata of warm water were also employed without effect. On the twenty-first day flatus escaped from the anus, followed by scybalous fæces, and on the next morning a normal stool was voided; and for nine days, though weak, the patient appeared to be in good health and spirits. On the ninth his symptoms returned, but with increased severity, and death occurred seventy-two hours after the onset of the attack.

An autopsy was made thirty-two hours after death : The abdominal walls were distended to the utmost; when the usual longitudinal section was made, the intestines escaped through the incision in huge convolutions. The entire length of the small intestine and the ascending and transverse portions of the colon were fully loaded with mingled liquid and gaseous contents. The peritoneum was everywhere injected, and the vessels of the omentum were especially engorged. In the dependent portions of the abdomen there was an effusion of dark-red, thin fluid, amounting, by estimate, to eight fluidounces. The colour of the small intestine was a dark purple; its diameter was that of a large orange; its contents consisted of dark-brown, fetid liquid feces. The distended large intestine was of a pale colour; its diameter was six inches and its contents semi-solid fæces. Search was made for the points of puncture by the aspirator needle, but no remnant of that operation was found. There was no agglutination of the intestinal folds or other indication of peritonitis, beyond the intense general hyperæmia and the fluid exudation.

At the junction of the transverse and descending portions of the colon (splenic flexure) there was a cicatricial constriction. In the concavity of this flexure the three coats of the intestine were drawn into a firm, dense mass of tissue, the puckered folds of which contraction had reduced the calibre of the gut so as scarcely to admit the tip of the little finger. Above this stenosis the intestine was dilated into a great bag or reservoir filled with semi-solid fæces; below it the gut was contracted to its normal dimensions. Seen from within the intestine showed nothing remarkable at the constriction beyond the puckering of the mucous lining; on the outside (peritoneal surface), however, the stenosis was marked by a roughened, elevated ulceration of the size of a silver quarter-dollar. A fold of the jejunum was attached by loose adhesion of its free border to this ulcer, and its peritoneal coat presented a corresponding, though more superficial, loss of tissue. The situation and relations of the constriction were such that it could easily be plugged by a fæcal mass of slight consistency.

Upon the surface of the large intestine, just above the ulceration, was a minute perforation which hardly admitted the head of a probe, and through this small opening enough fæcal matter had probably escaped to develop the peritonitis which destroyed the patient.—*Boston Med. and Surg. Journ.*, Sept. 22, 1881.

Amyloid Degeneration of the Kidney.

In the twenty-eighth volume of the *Deutsches Archives für Klinische Medicin*, WAGNER publishes an interesting paper upon amyloid degeneration of the kidney. In regard to etiology, out of 265 cases, Wagner found that 136 accompanied phthisis; 56 occurred along with disease of bone (non-syphilitic); 36 accompanied syphilis; 30 were found in connection with certain rarer diseases; and with regard to 7 no probable mode of origin was apparent. The more interesting portion of this paper is that in which the author deals with the symptomatology of waxy kidney. In comparatively few of these cases were the symptoms observed during life so closely as to be of service; only twenty-four appear to have been available, and of these the majority were only under observation for very limited periods; the longest apparently only during a few months. Studying these cases in detail, Wagner separates them into four groups: 1. Slight amyloid degeneration of the cortical or the medullary substance, or of both, without alteration of the epithelium or of the stroma; this variety was hardly observed clinically; 2. Greater or less waxy degeneration of the cortical or medullary portion, with a varying amount of fatty degeneration of the epithelium, without changes in the stroma; 3. The same waxy degeneration, along with fresh interstitial changes; 4. Waxy-contracted kidney. In regard to this last-named condition, Wagner adopts the view held by Cohnheim, Bartels, Rokitansky, etc., viz., that the waxy change occurs in the kidney after it has become cirrhotic. With regard to the condition of the urine in these cases, Wagner found that it was almost invariably diminished in quantity, and this without diarrhœa, perspiration, or increasing œdema being present. In a few cases the urine was of normal quantity, and only in two does it appear to have exceeded that amount. The quantity of albumen was in thirteen cases of the fifteen belonging to the first two groups, in medium or in great amount ($\frac{1}{4}$, $\frac{1}{2}$, $\frac{1}{3}$, or even ^{1} volume); but in two cases it was at the commencement small in quantity, afterwards increasing. The tube-casts varied much in number from one day to another. They were for the most part of medium diameter, and usually hyaline, sometimes fatty. Wagner believes that œdema is more rarely met with in such cases than is generally supposed. In conclusion he observes that, while waxy kidney may often be diagnosed with care, there are many cases in which such a diagnosis cannot be arrived at with any certainty.—*Lond. Med. Record*, July 15, 1881.

The Pathogenesis of Albuminuria.

The physiological experiments of Gull and Stokvis, of raising the arterial pressure in the kidneys by ligaturing arteries or compressing the abdominal aorta, showed that high pressure alone would not determine albuminuria. This may seem at variance with the clinical fact of the presence of albuminuria in interstitial nephritis with hypertrophied heart; but M. CHARCOT, in a recent lecture (*Le Progrès Médical*, 1881, No. 19), explains this by the fact that some of the glomeruli are more or less profoundly altered, in consequence of which both the pressure and the rapidity of the blood-current are diminished. [It is obvious that, if the changes in the glomeruli are to be called in question at all, M. Charcot is departing from the mechanical theory he has propounded.—*Rep.*] On the other hand, Overbeck's experiment of reducing the blood-pressure by introducing a sound into the right ventricle, carrying a small bladder which can be inflated at will, is always followed by albuminuria. Here the condition of things is diminution of pressure and rapidity. Such a condition is met with clinically in valvular disease of the heart, chronic disease of the myocardium, and some pulmonary diseases. In cases of mitral insufficiency, Rosenstein observed that the albumen disappeared as the urine increased, and returned as it fell in quantity. The cardiac kidney is not the cause of the albuminuria of heart disease, but the consequence of the state of things which causes the albuminuria. The albuminuria of Asiatic cholera and other acute diseases is also explained by this theory. The anatomical theory which refers albuminuria to a lesion of the renal epithelium, supported of late by Lécorché, is opposed by the experiments which show that albumen is excreted by the glomeruli, and that its presence in the convoluted tubules is a pathological occurrence, and by the fact that the epithelium may be profoundly altered or destroyed, as in granular kidney or in phosphorus poisoning, without albuminuria.—*Lond. Med. Record*, July 15, 1881.

Simultaneous Existence of Albumen and Sugar in the Urine.

In a paper read before the Berlin Medical Society, and published in the *Deutsche Med. Woch.*, No. 24, 1881, Professor FRERICHS says that the coexistence of albumen and sugar in the urine occurs under various conditions, which must be carefully discriminated. Three forms of this anomalous process of secretion must be distinguished : one occurring in glycosuria, another in diabetes mellitus, and a third in chyluria. In glycosuria—by which Frerichs denotes cases in which small quantities of sugar are discharged within a longer or shorter time without having any obvious influence on nutrition—albuminuria is frequently met with. Of thirty cases observed and collated by Frerichs, albumen was found in fourteen, that is, in nearly one-half. They were partly acute, partly chronic, diseases of the brain. Three times albumen and sugar were observed in the urine of patients affected with cerebral aneurism, which had burst into the ventricles ; four times in extensive apoplexies ; twice in purulent cerebral meningitis ; and once in chronic tuberculous basilar meningitis. In all these cases the ventricle was found to contain blood, with the exception of one case, in which the apoplectic focus extended to part of the cerebellum and to the cerebral peduncle. The chronic form of the disease lasted for years, and there was no opportunity of making a *post-mortem* examination. In these cases Frerichs three times observed albuminuria, and also, in the further progress of the disease, simultaneous paresis of the facial nerve. The sugar in these cases amounted to from $1\frac{1}{2}$ to 2 per cent., while the quantity of albumen varied. Sometimes the sugar disappeared, and then the albumen, until in some cases there was a retrogression of the renal secretion. At the same time polyuria existed ; in other cases it was absent.

In all these cases of glycosuria, Frerichs thinks the secretion of albumen and sugar to have the same source, namely, a lesion of the fourth ventricle, since, when the injury is situated higher, there is secretion, not only of sugar, but of albumen also. In such cases, the prognosis must depend upon the nature of the cerebral lesion. Severe apoplexy, with lesion of the lateral ventricle, usually proves fatal in a few days ; so also does cerebral aneurism. The course is more favourable in meningitis, in which recovery occurs in some circumstances. Frerichs reports two cases, in which the secretion of albumen and sugar ceased, and all symptoms disappeared.

In the chronic form, the prognosis must be cautiously made, for this mostly affects persons whose health is impaired by mental excitement or overwork, who complain of headache and indisposition, and are unable to attend to their daily avocations. Apoplectic injuries are associated with remarkable frequency with glycosuria, a circumstance that points to an effusion of blood into the fourth ventricle.

In the same manner may be explained the coexistence of albumen and sugar in cases of poisoning, especially by carbonic oxide gas. In 12 out of 17 cases there was sugar; in three there were albumen and sugar; and in one only albumen, together with cylinders.

In diabetes mellitus, the condition is altogether different. It is assumed by many that diabetes mellitus will lead to nephritis. Griesinger, in 64 *post-mortem* examinations of cases of diabetes, found 32, that is, one-half, complicated with nephritis. Seegen found nephritis in 20 of 30 cases in the Vienna *post-mortem* house; while Dickinson found 25 of 27 cases in the St. George's Hospital to have nephritis. With that, however, Frerichs's experience does not agree. In true diabetes, albuminuria is not frequent, nephritis rare, and occurs only in certain conditions. Out of 316 cases of diabetes mellitus, which Frerichs partly observed for ten, twelve, and even fifteen and sixteen years, there were only 16 cases of nephritis (5 per cent.). Cases in which small quantities of albumen were occasionally found in the urine were never pure and simple cases, since it could be proved, at least in most of them, that other processes were involved, which of themselves could produce nephritis. Of 16 cases, 6 were complicated with arterial sclerosis; in 3 others there was pulmonary phthisis; in 2 cystitis; and in 2 arthritis with renal calculi. Therefore, only three cases remain in which no co-operating cause could be suggested. Thus it becomes evident that the general belief that the increased action of the kidneys in diabetes mellitus leads by fluxion to albuminuria and nephritis is erroneous, notwithstanding that it has numerous followers. According to Frerichs's *post-mortem* examinations, which comprise more than 50 cases, true nephritis is hardly ever met with in diabetes; and where it did occur, it was of a parenchymatous nature, moderate hyperæmia of the renal substance, or there was shrivelling of the kidney. It has been believed that the changes of the epithelium of the gland, now and then occurring in diabetes, and lately described by Ebstein, might contribute towards the production of albuminuria. These changes in the epithelium have been searched for in the clinic, and have been found where there was no albumen in the urine; so that Frerichs feels rather disinclined to go as far as Ebstein does in drawing conclusions. All cases which were complicated by pulmonary phthisis proved fatal, while in all cases in which albuminuria was produced by additional cystitis, nephritis, or arthritis, there was a favourable course. An old gentleman, aged 79, who was attacked with pneumonia while in Carlsbad, and was afterwards lying ill in Nice, suffered from albuminuria, on which cystitis supervened. Gradually the sugar disappeared, and albuminuria, with cylinders, set in. Then the albumen disappeared, and at present he may be regarded as cured.

There is yet another condition in which sugar, albumen, and fat occur together—chyluria. It remains, however, an open question how the sugar is transmitted into the urine along with the albuminates. Whether, as some believe, there is a damming back into the lymphatic vessels or a transition into the urine, consecutive upon chylosis, has not yet been determined by anatomical observation. One thing only has been established by Brieger—that fat disappears from the urine, if it be withdrawn from the patient's food, and that it reappears in the urine as soon as it again becomes part of the food. It is much to be regretted that the experiment was not made with regard to sugar.—*London Med. Record,* August 15, 1881.

Urinary Analysis.

A new method for the quantitative analysis of the extractive matters of urine has been worked out by MM. CHAVANÈ and RICHET, who claim for it the advantage of much greater simplicity than that of the methods at present in use. A solution of biniodide of mercury and iodide of potassium, to which potash has been added, is blackened by urine, and oxide of mercury is precipitated. The reaction takes place even in the cold, but is facilitated by heat. Neither the urea, chlorides, phosphates, nor sulphates are precipitated, but uric acid causes a white deposit from which heat causes oxide of mercury to separate. Alkaloids, formiates, and acetates have no influence. If the reaction of the mixture is acid the precipitate does not form, a soluble salt of mercury being produced, but the alkalinity of the test solution is usually sufficient to insure the reaction. Salts of ammonia, moreover, mask the reaction by dissolving the oxide of mercury. Chloral, aldehyde, sugar, and all readily oxidizable substances also precipitate the oxide of mercury. Normal urine contains substances which have the same action, viz., nitrogenous substances soluble in ether and in alcohol. Hence this method gives a simple means of ascertaining the amount of colouring matter, extractive matter, and nitrogenous substances other than urea. The exact mode of proceeding is as follows: The composition of the solution is 10 grammes of binoxide of mercury, 20 of iodide of potassium, 50 of caustic potash, and 930 of distilled water. One burette is filled with the solution, another with urine. Fifteen drops of each are allowed to fall into a porcelain capsule, and it is heated and urine added until the mercury is proved to be precipitated by the absence of the reaction given by an alkaline solution of tin, with a small quantity taken up by a capillary tube. A litre of normal urine precipitates about five grammes of mercury.—*Lancet*, Sept. 24, 1881.

Surgery.

Antiseptic Treatment of Abscess.

Dr. LUCAS-CHAMPIONNIÈRE recommends the following procedure: Before opening an abscess, in whatever region it may be placed, we should carefully wash the skin, especially if it has been covered by a poultice, with a strong carbolic acid solution (crystals 50 parts, glycerine 50 to 75 parts, and water 1000 parts). The bistoury should also be dipped in the solution. The contents of the abscess are to be discharged, and some of the above solution injected, care being taken that the injected liquid has a free issue. The end of a caoutchouc tube is introduced into the wound, having a thread attached to it to facilitate its removal, and it is then covered by a thick layer of charpie, impregnated with a solution of carbolic acid 25 parts, glycerine 25 parts, and water 1000 parts. Finally, over all is laid a layer of gummed silk. At the end of twenty-four hours the tube is removed in order that it may be cleansed and shortened, when it is again covered with the charpie moistened with the weaker solution. Under this treatment the amount of suppuration is diminished, the redness of the wound becomes insignificant, and the cicatrices which result are much less apparent. Dr. Lucas recommends this procedure especially in abscess of the breast. — *Med. Times and Gazette*, October 8, 1881, from *Union Médicale*, September 15.

Treatment of Malignant Lymphosarcoma with Arsenic.

Dr. F. THOLEN (*Arch für Klin. Chir.*, Band xvii.) reports four cases of lymphosarcoma, in three of which the course of the disease was greatly influenced by arsenic, while in the fourth case the disease had already advanced too far towards a fatal result. The first case was that of a man, aged 47, who suffered from an infiltrated epithelioma in the right angle of his lower jaw, of three months' duration. It could not be operated upon, because of the extent and infiltration of the neighbouring lymphatic glands, and was therefore treated with arsenic. From May 26 until the end of December, 1872, the patient took Fowler's solution; partly internally, from five drops a day to fifteen drops twice a day, and partly in the form of parenchymatous injections into the tumour, ten drops each time, amounting altogether to 748 drops internally and 76 injections. This treatment resulted in the complete disappearance of the tumour. The patient was discharged on January 15, 1873, and on returning in April, 1873, and in February, 1874, he showed no sign of recurrence. Examination of a small particle taken from the margin of the ulcerating tumour indicated a lamellar epithelioma, yet the appearance of the disease, as well as the favourable action of the arsenic, rather suggested an infiltrated malignant lymphosarcoma. The author, therefore, thinks it probable that epidermic cells from the adjacent healthy epidermis might have been present when the examination was made. From these cases, although few in number, Tholen is led to ascribe to arsenic a positive salutary action against cancerous ulcers, especially lymphosarcomata, which, in fact, are nearest to inflammatory neoplasms, and are quickly dispersed by other agents as well. A mischievous result has been several times observed by Billroth to follow this rapid breaking up, when iodide of potassium was energetically administered. —*London Med. Record*, August 15, 1881.

Treatment of Burns by Bicarbonate of Soda.

J. TROIZKI adds his testimony to that already published as to the value of solution of bicarbonate of soda as a dressing for burns (*Wratsch.*, 1881, No. 4; and *St. Petersburg Med. Woch.*, 1881, No. 19). He says that during the previous year he noticed twenty-five cases of burns, mostly of a severe nature. Sixteen of them were received in a fire in a village, during a strong wind, when the inhabitants, in order to save their property, were obliged to work in the flames. In all these twenty-five cases bicarbonate of soda was exclusively applied. The result of this treatment was so favourable, that the author considers himself justified in pronouncing this remedy the best and most efficient in burns of all kinds and degrees. Even in extensive burns of the second and third degrees, the pain was soon alleviated by the application of compresses soaked in a solution of bicarbonate of soda; and the wounds soon healed, leaving but few scars, and no impairment of the functions of the affected parts. No evil results from this extensive application of bicarbonate of soda, which might suggest the reception of carbonic acid into the blood, were noticed. Of the ten cases of which a detailed account is given by the author, one rather serious case may be related, in which the burns had spread over half the body. The whole face was stripped of epidermis, the hair was singed off, and the front of the neck, chest, and abdomen, and the dorsum of the foot, presented burns of the second degree; burns of the third degree were also found on the right mammary gland and on the right forearm, all the muscles of which were exposed as if prepared by dissection. A solution of the bicarbonate of soda was applied to these burns with a most conspicuous success: the patient felt relieved, and a cure was effected in four weeks; but the healing of the burns on the right breast and on the forearm lasted two months. The scars which were left were insignificant, and the mobility of the fingers was nearly normal. As regards the application of bicarbonate of soda in burns, the author distinguishes three methods. 1. Powdered bicarbonate of soda is strewn over the burned parts. 2. Linen rags, sprinkled with a solution of bicarbonate of soda (1 in 50) are laid on; as soon as these rags become dry, they are replaced by others or are moistened again in the solution. 3. Linen rags are applied in the same manner, but are kept constantly upon the burns, and moistened by pouring the solution on them. The first method suffices only for burns of the first degree. Change of the moistened rags is chiefly adapted for burns of the third degree, attended with much suppuration. In exchanging the dry rags, the pus which has accumulated underneath them must be carefully washed off, that it may not be received into the blood; and then a fresh rag soaked with the solution must be placed upon the clean granulating surface. The third method is applied solely in burns of the second degree. Changing the compresses would in these cases only irritate the exposed surface, and, by causing a more copious suppuration, delay the healing process. The beneficent effect upon burns of the solution of bicarbonate of soda the author considers to be due to the anæsthetic, antiseptic, and disinfecting property, which the bicarbonate owes to the ready disengagement of carbonic acid from it. Herr Troizki has also made experiments with other antiseptic and disinfectant agents, but has come to the conclusion that these are inferior to the bicarbonate of soda in their effect upon burns. Besides, the application of some of these, as for instance of carbolic acid upon large surfaces, would be dangerous; on small surfaces they very thoroughly disinfect the secretions of wounds; but these disperse more slowly than by the use of soda, and the anæsthesia, so desirable for the patient, is not so complete as when soda is applied.—*London Med. Record*, Aug. 15, 1881.

—

Case of Coin in Air-passages treated by Inversion of the Patient.

Mr. JOSEPH BELL, Surgeon to the Royal Infirmary, Edinburgh, reports (*Edinburgh Med. Journ.*, June, 1881) the case of a waiter who amused himself by throwing into the air a sixpenny-piece just received from a traveller. He intended to catch it in his mouth, but the coin disappeared. Fancying it had passed into his œsophagus, he came to the Infirmary, where he was seen by the house-surgeon, Mr. Ross, who failed to find any evidence of its presence in either œsophagus or stomach, for the examination of the throat caused vomiting, and the coin was not found. No laryngeal or pulmonary symptoms were present, though patient pointed to his left chest as being painful. A laryngoscopic examination, however, satisfied Mr. Ross and Dr. Maxwell that the coin was lying edgeways in the left bronchus, just at the bifurcation. There being no symptoms, he was left quiet, all preparations being made for tracheotomy if necessary, and Mr. Ross slept in the side-room of the ward.

Next day Mr. Bell carefully examined chest and air-passages, with negative results; immediately after this, however, when he was in the act of operating on a sarcoma in the theatre, the patient was reported to be choking. Mr. Ross found him in a paroxysm of coughing, and when it passed off he described a feeling of fluttering or flapping in his windpipe. Dr. Wyllie and Mr. Bell then made a most careful laryngoscopic examination, and though they saw the tracheal rings most clearly, no foreign body could be made out.

The history and the symptoms of the one attack were to Mr. Bell's mind so convincing that the coin was in the air-passages, that, with the approval of his colleague, Mr. Duncan, he at once prepared to perform tracheotomy in the event of the failure of inversion. So, having obtained the patient's leave, and all things being ready, he was held by the heels by two dressers standing on the operating-table, and a smart blow was struck on his back opposite the left bronchus, while he was instructed to keep his mouth open and to breathe freely. The sixpence at once fell into his mouth; a pretty smart cough coincided with its passing the glottis.

Cases of this kind are comparatively rare, and this one is an encouragement to attempt the inversion method. The surgeon must, however, be prepared to perform tracheotomy at once if the coin sticks in larynx and excites spasm, or lodges flatwise in upper part of trachea, and thus prevents ingress of air.

Gastrotomy in Stricture of the Œsophagus.

A paper by Dr. T. F. PREWITT on gastrostomy in stricture of the œsophagus will be found in the *St. Louis Cour. of Med.* It is accompanied by a table of fifty-nine cases. Dr. Prewitt considers the great difference in mortality from the operation in cases of this class, when compared with the same operation for the removal of foreign bodies, to be due to the exhausted condition of the subject. It is his belief that it can be greatly lessened if the operation be performed early. In a large percentage of fatal cases, even though union had taken place, no peritonitis existed, and death was due to exhaustion. Gastric fistula is not incompatible with long life. Of the forty-nine cases tabulated, forty were malignant, twelve cicatricial, three syphilitic, and in four the nature of the stricture was not given, but was almost certainly malignant. Of these cases, operated upon for malignant disease, the patients lived from fourteen days to six months, and one patient is still living comfortably. In the cicatricial variety six recovered, as also one where the stricture was of syphilitic origin. In but seven of the whole number is peritonitis stated to have existed. Exhaustion alone is assigned as the cause of death in the large proportion of cases.—*London Med. Record,* July 15, 1881.

Perineal Calculi.

Dr. C. MAZZONI, Professor of Clinical Surgery at Rome, read a paper on this subject at the London Congress which contained the following conclusions:—

1. Perineal calculi may originate in the bladder.

2. They may be formed in perineal fistulæ communicating either with the bladder or ureter.

3. They may be contained in a cyst formed by the walls of the ureter.

4. They may be found in the scrotum, and have no connection at all with the ureter.

Treatment.—In such conditions as are included under headings 1, 2, and 4, extraction of the stone results in a cure of the fistula. For those of class 3 it is imperative to make a permanent perineal opening into the urethra.

Midwifery and Gynæcology.

Time of Ligation of the Umbilical Cord.

Dr. J. G. SINCLAIR COGHILL, in his address in Obstetric Medicine, before the British Medical Association, called attention to an extremely interesting and valuable communication with reference to the time and mode of separating the fœtus and umbilical cord which has been made by Ribemont, in a recent number of *Les Archives de Tocologie,* and which shows satisfactorily the great influence of the "thoracic aspiration" of the fœtus on the umbilical circulation before its ligature. This was first pointed out by Budin; but is denied, among others, by Schücking. Determined by the manometer, it was found that—1. Tardy ligature of the cord benefits the child by increasing the quantity of blood which is required for the establishment of the third circulation, that is, the fœtal pulmonary. 2. The immediate ligature of the cord deprives the infant of a quantity of blood, larger or smaller in proportion to the time of ligature; and it especially deprives it of necessary blood if the ligature has been applied before the child has breathed. 3. The early ligature of the cord thus compels the abstraction of the blood necessary to establish the pulmonary circulation from the general circulation. The result is a diminution of the arterial tension equal to one-third of the initial tension. 4. The cause of the penetration of the blood into the pulmonary circulatory system of the child is the "thoracic aspiration." This is proved by the constant superiority of the pressure of the blood in the umbilical arteries to that in the umbilical vein. Again, the thoracic respiration is observed to produce considerable oscillations in the tension of the arterial and venous blood. The uterine contractions are utterly insufficient to force any blood along the umbilical vein when the arterial pulsations of the cord have ceased. 5. Thoracic aspiration causes the *sufficient* and *necessary* amount of blood to enter the pulmonary vessels; *sufficient* because, under these circumstances, the tension in the arterial system does not fall; necessary because the arterial tension in the umbilical cord of a newly-born child is never seen to rise after tardy ligature of the cord. Professor W. T. Lusk, of New York, in corroborating Ribemont's views, says that, in children born pale and anæmic, and suffering from syncope, late ligation of the cord furnishes an invaluable means of restoring the equilibrium of the fœtal circulation.—*British Medical Journal*, Aug. 20, 1881.

Membranous Dysmenorrhœa in relation to Normal Menstruation.

In a paper read at the Académie de Médecine, Dr. SINÉTY stated that it resulted from the observations which he had made on a great number of women, that, in the physiological condition, the uterine mucous membrane is not, as is generally taught, eliminated in menstruation; but, under certain pathological conditions, the mucous membrane of the body of the uterus exfoliates, and is expelled at the catamenial period. This phenomenon, designated as "membranous dysmenorrhœa," is usually accompanied by severe pain and loss of blood. It does not constitute a special disease or morbid entity, and is observed under very variable conditions, with or without metritis. The exfoliation is the result of an exaggeration of the normal menstrual process, inducing a too great infiltration of the deeper layers of the mucous membrane and compression of the vessels of this region, and leading to elimination of the tissues situated above this layer. It will be thus understood that anything which prevents the blood issuing, as in the normal state, by the superficial vascular network of the mucous membrane, may be a cause of membranous dysmenorrhœa.—*Med. Times and Gaz.*, Sept. 24, 1881.

Local Treatment of Chronic Metritis.

Prof. AMANN, of Munich, read a paper on this subject, at the London Congress, of which the following is an abstract:—

Most cases of chronic metritis require local treatment for their cure. If the disease be limited to the mucous membrane of the cervical canal the treatment is comparatively simple, and cure can be affected by various harmless means. Greater difficulty is met with when chronic inflammation of the body or of the body and neck of the uterus calls for local treatment. For many years I have carefully tested the various means recommended during the last twenty years in the treatment of the affection in question, in hospital and private practice, in more than 3000 cases, and have come to the conviction that only one method acts with certainty without being troublesome and *dangerous*.   This is new only in the manner of its execution, and consists in the systematic cauterization of the cavity of the body, and eventually of the cervix of the uterus by means of an instrument like a sound, into a hollow in the upper end of which is fused lapis mitigatus.   This can be employed as is self-evident, according to the behaviour of the endometrium, and the resisting power of the uterus in individual cases, at one time more frequently and thoroughly, at another more rarely and cautiously, and will have, according to the peculiarities of the special case, by itself alone, or in conjunction with other means (topical blood-letting, scraping off of growths of the endometrium), almost sure results.   Only in a few cases of large tumours or severe bleeding granulations of the endometrium is the employment of the galvano-cautery or thermo-cautery necessary.   The intra-uterine application of *lapis mitigatus* is, with the necessary caution, absolutely free from danger, and in a small number of cases only does it cause pain, which, however, is usually of short duration ; sometimes also it gives rise to considerable but transient bleeding. Once only have I noticed, after a severe cauterization of the whole of the uterine cavity, dangerous metritis or peri-metritis, which, however, ended in a few weeks in complete recovery.   Even slighter degrees of acute endometritis and acute metritis occur according to my experience in barely 2 per cent. of all the cases.

One of the chief advantages of the proceeding in question is, that it can be carried out without assistance in at least 95 per cent. of cases, and usually in five, exceptionally in ten minutes.   Within this time, moreover, the cleansing of the uterine canal from mucus, a necessary preparation for cauterization, as well as the dilatation of the narrow canal by means of metallic dilators, can be accomplished. Further this procedure is applicable, when the condition is complicated by severe flexions and versions, either after straightening the organ immediately before cauterization, or if the canal be of normal width by cauterizing with the sound-like instrument forthwith.   This is done without a speculum just as the sound is introduced.   By reason of the rapidity of the cauterization, which is finished in three to five seconds, and because, by the revolving of the caustic holder, contact of the caustic with the individual parts of the endometrium is extraordinarily short, coating of the caustic with coagulated albumen is prevented.   Immediately after cauterizing a large tampon of wadding soaked in a solution of tannin should be introduced into the vagina in order to prevent the caustic dissolved in the uterine cavity from escaping into and through the vagina.

—

Total Extirpation of the Uterus for Cancer.

This operation may be said at present to be on its trial ; for surgeons are not yet agreed as to whether the prospect of benefit outweighs the risk.   The statistical accounts that have as yet been published are incomplete, and therefore not quite in agreement.   We want figures to show us, first, in what number of cases the operation itself proves fatal, and then, in how many of those who recover from the operation the disease returns.   The statistics are not in agreement ; first, because improvements are being made in the *technique* of the operation, and in estimating the probable future mortality of an operation, we must reject cases in which the operation was not done in the way which better knowledge has shown to be the safest, and also because some cases, published as cures, have afterwards relapsed. Bearing in mind these errors, the following statistics will be interesting : MIKU-LICZ (*Wiener Medizinische Wochenschrift*, 1880, No. 47) quotes from Ahlfeld a table of 66 cases, out of which 49 proved fatal, in 4 the operation could not be completed, and of the 13 who recovered, in 6 relapses occurred ; of the remain-

ing 7, in some the period since the operation, at the time the figures were compiled, was too short to allow the occurrence of relapse to be considered improbable. Some later statistics are more favourable. KLEINWACHTER, writing at
the beginning of the present year, collected 94 cases of operation, with 24 recoveries; but KALTENBACH, writing about the same time, out of 88 cases enumerates 30 as successes. These figures evidently want sifting. They all relate to
cases in which the uterus has been extirpated by abdominal section. OLSHAUSEN
has collected (*Berliner Klinische Wochenschrift*, No. 35, 1881) 41 cases in which
the uterus was removed by the vaginal method; of these 29 recovered and 12
died. To these he adds 6 performed by himself, all of which, so far as the operation was concerned, were successful.—*Med. Times and Gaz.*, Sept. 24, 1881.

———

The Ovary in Incipient Cystic Disease.

Dr. VINCENT D. HARRIS, Demonstrator of Physiology at St. Bartholomew's
Hospital, and Mr. ALBERT DORAN, Surgeon to Out-Patients, Samaritan Free
Hospital, having enjoyed exceptional opportunities for studying incipient cystic
disease of the ovary, have, in a joint paper, contributed the results of their observations to the *Journal of Anatomy and Physiology*, July, 1881. In over one-
eighth of the cases operated upon at the Samaritan Hospital Dr. Bantock and
Mr. Knowsley Thornton find that, after the removal of a large ovarian cyst, the
opposite ovary presents such distinct symptoms of early cystic disease, that they
remove it, knowing that otherwise a second operation will almost assuredly be
necessary at no very distant date. A large number of such ovaries have been
collected, and their appearances, when fresh, carefully described; the history of
the patients, and notes as to the absence or regularity of the menstrual functions,
together with records of abortion, parturition, or sterility, have also been preserved. The ovaries, within a few hours after removal, were placed within a
half per cent. solution of chromic acid mixed with equal parts of methylated
spirit. When sufficiently hardened, sections were prepared from them by means
of Williams's freezing microtome. These sections were stained in logwood solution, and then mounted. Lastly, all have been since examined minutely by Dr.
Harris and Mr. Doran, and separate notes carefully compared.

The results of their researches are summarized as follows:—

1. There is strong evidence that multilocular cystic disease of the ovary may
arise from two totally different ovarian elements.

2. Cysts may arise from partial dilatation and partial obstruction of enlarged
and thickened bloodvessels, as Noeggerath maintains,[1] and we think, as he does,
that many errors have arisen from imperfect knowledge of the appearance of
bloodvessels in the ovarian stroma.

3. Cysts more frequently appear to originate in changes in those Graafian follicles that undergo involution without having ever ruptured; this includes a large
majority of the follicles, when we remember the vast number found in the ovary
at birth, and bear in mind that involution of many follicles takes place between
birth and puberty.

4. The morbid changes which replace normal involution of the follicle are an
active ingrowth from the stroma, and a long persistence of the cloudy tube-like
bodies that represent the remains of the membrana propria of the follicle. These
two processes sometimes proceed at an equal rate, sometimes irregularly.

5. When the relics of the membrana propria are slow to disappear, and the
stroma slowly sends ingrowths amongst these relics, we find the cystic bodies

_____

[1] "The Diseases of Bloodvessels of the Ovary in Relation to the Genesis of Ovarian
Cysts." Amer. Journ. of Obstetrics, etc., vol. xiii., 1880.

described as seen in the fourth case, containing myxoma-cells partly, at least, connected with the outgrowths. Such delicate tissue, made up of these cells, must soon break down as the cyst becomes larger.

6. When the process of ingrowth of stroma into the follicle, during involution, is particularly active, the ingrowths interlace and rapidly form cystic spaces, including portions of the cloudy relics of the membrana propria, giving the appearances seen in the third case.

7. On the other hand, the stroma may show little or no tendency to develop ingrowths, but the relics of the membrana propria may break down very slowly, and end, not in simple effacement and incorporation with the stroma, but in slowly breaking down, as in the second case. This must necessarily end in the formation of a cyst full of a colloid or semi-fluid material, the completely broken down granulosa, etc.; previous theories on colloid degeneration of the stroma itself may be based on the overlooking of the intra-follicular origin of the colloid collections. In all cases of myxomatous or colloid changes, or simple rarefaction of tissue, we found full evidence that those changes were in degenerate follicles and never free in the stroma.

8. All these changes in the degenerating membrana propria and the tissue surrounding the follicle, begin as exaggerations of the normal process of involution, which is never a mere disintegration and degeneration of the follicle. Slavjansky, in the work we have quoted, gives accurate drawings of the normal process. Patenko traces these abnormal changes to sclerosis of the follicle-wall, under different conditions.[1]

9. These changes in the follicle do not appear due to inflammation; indeed, in old inflamed ovaries the atrophy of the follicles appears to be quicker and more complete than in healthy ovaries, so that no trace of them is left, excepting certain granular masses.

10. The manner in which the young cyst first becomes invested with its characteristic epithelium is obscure. We found that the "germinal epithelium" of the tunica albuginea and the cells of the granulosa of normal follicles never invaded the ovarian stroma, and the epithelial relics of the Wolffian tubes, that are usually found loose about the stroma, were never in close relation to any of the bodies we have described. In the case of the dilated vessels, the endothelium must be the most natural starting point of the epithelial lining of cysts derived from such vessels. Remembering the changes in the mucous membrane of a prolapsed vagina, the endothelium may, we can conceive, alter its character when the nature of the free space on which it borders has become completely altered. Should the theory of Cripps[2] be even partly correct, that nuclei in lymphoid or connective tissue may gather protoplasm around them till they form real epithelioid bodies lining spaces deeply situated in solid structures, we could readily account for the origin of the epithelial lining of any cyst. We do not profess to accept as positive that observer's theory, that the nuclei in the submucous tissue of the rectum are normally the parents of the columnar epithelium of the mucous membrane, although microscopical evidence tends to support it; his other opinion, expressed above, that such nuclei may become epithelioid, is far more probable. An area in any tissue, with such nuclei, breaks down—the nuclei bordering on the broken-down region must be placed at once in different circumstances to their normal state, deep in tissue and away from any free surface. We do not find such nuclei on free surfaces; we do find epithelium. In other words, we

---

[1] In Virchow's Archiv, May, 1881, he demonstrates the manner in which this process ends in the formation, not of cysts, but of "corpora fibrosa."

[2] Cancer of the Rectum. See particularly Pl. III. fig. 1, in that work.

see no difficulty in supposing that the epithelial lining of ovarian cysts is probably developed from nuclear elements in the bodies above described. It seems, on mere reasoning, less far-fetched to assert that this epithelial lining is derived from pre-existing epithelium. To this we reply that, on actual observation, detecting incipient cystic cavities and also healthy epithelium on the tunica albuginea, in the follicles, and, as embryonic relics in the stroma, often in one single section, we find no connection between the cavities and any of these three normal epithelial elements. We must not conclude that when the mucoid contents of the imperfectly involved follicles have broken down to their utmost, the cellular elements immediately adjacent to the resulting semi-fluid material, simply assume the epithelial type. Only as long as the source whence normal epithelium is renewed remains obscure, so long must this question remain unsettled.

Remarks on Antiseptic Ovariotomy.

Mr. KNOWSLEY THORNTON made the following remarks to a number of the members of the International Medical Congress who assembled at the Samaritan Hospital, on Aug. 3d:—

This being, he said, the last of our regular operation days before the hospital is closed for its autumn cleaning, I think it is a good opportunity to make a statement as to the work done in my wards since the 1st of January in this year. I have performed ovariotomy twenty-eight times, and I have only lost one patient, a child of fifteen, from whom I removed a solid carcinoma of 7 lbs. weight, involving both ovaries, the cæcum, and sigmoid flexure, so that I had to carve the intestines out of the solid growth. She died of exhaustion in forty-eight hours. Every one of these operations was performed with the $2\frac{1}{2}$ per cent. spray, and solutions of absolute phenol (pure carbolic acid), and in no case was drainage employed. All the wounds healed by first intention, and the dressings were changed for the first time as a rule from the ninth to the twelfth day, when all the sutures were removed. Nineteen of the patients recovered without fever (i.e., the temperature never rose even during reaction beyond 101° F.); five had temperatures from 101.6° to 103.4° during a few hours, but required no special treatment; four had temperatures from 102.8° to 104.6°, and required the use of the ice-water cap during periods of from thirty-nine hours to sixty-eight hours. These nine cases were all of more than usual gravity, with large tumours, extensive adhesions, long exposure, and much sponging. Only two of the patients remained in the hospital twenty-eight days after operation: one a patient from whom I removed an extensively adherent tumour weighing 80 lbs.; and the other one of the cases requiring the ice-water cap; a case of ruptured colloid, which I kept in bed longer than usual. The average stay in hospital after operation of the other patients was twenty days and a half, the shortest seventeen days. There were no adhesions in fourteen cases, slight adhesions in one case, and extensive adhesions with other complications in thirteen cases. In nineteen of the cases only one ovary was removed; in the others both were diseased and removed. To these twenty-eight cases of my own, I may add four cases operated upon in my wards by my colleague, Mr. MEREDITH, in which strict Listerism without drainage was also employed; all recovered. So that we have thirty-two Listerian ovariotomies without drainage with only one death, and that a case of cancer. I have also performed eight other abdominal sections: A removal of uterine fibrocyst, weighing 23 lbs., together with both ovaries; a removal of several sessile and pediculate fibroids; an enucleation of a uterine fibro-cyst weighing 10 lbs.; a complete hysterectomy, with removal of both ovaries; and three coöphorectomies, undertaken for various conditions. All the patients recovered with the exception of the hysterectomy, and she died of septicæmia. I had to open a much enlarged uterine cavity, which contained putrid material, and I failed to correct the putrefaction. This was the only case in which it was impossible to perform a strictly aseptic operation, and it was the only one terminating fatally. The total result is forty abdominal sections, with two deaths—a mortality of only 5 per cent. I may add that in no case were there symptoms of carbolism, though the 2½ per cent. solutions were used with all necessary freedom, and some of the patients had albuminuria before the operation.—*Lancet,* Aug. 20, 1881.

Medical Jurisprudence and Toxicology.

Notes of a Case in which Chrysophanic Acid was Administered Internally by Accident.

Mr. JOHN GLAISTER reports in the *Glasgow Med. Journ.* for October, 1881, a case in which the patient was given a powder containing, by accident, a three-grain dose of chrysophanic acid, having been in fairly good health before. Within two hours after she was seized with the symptoms of irritating poison—burning pain in stomach, vomiting, pain in bowels, diarrhœa, hæmaturia, and pain over bladder, with tenesmus. It would, therefore, seem clear that the symptoms followed the medicine—*post hoc propter hoc.* It was also very evident from the symptoms that considerable irritation was produced in the gastro-intestinal and urinary tracts, occurring in that order. Hence, Mr. Glaister infers that a dose of three grains acts as a strong irritant. The colour of the matter first vomited, and the urine, point to the chrysophanic acid, because it is well known to produce coloured stains on linen coming in contact with it when used in an ointment.

But what are we to say about the bladder condition ? The prolonged retention of urine pointed to one of two things—paralysis of the bladder through inflammation or disinclination to initiate the act of micturition owing to the great pain felt during that time. That there was inflammation of the bladder there can be no doubt, the persistent pain over that region indicating as much ; and that this inflammation had ended in ulceration Mr. Glaister is inclined to believe, although some may gainsay it. He feared that the catheterism had had something to do with its production, but it was after the lengthened use of the catheter, when the parts had become accustomed to it, that the blood made its appearance, consequently he inclines rather to the previous explanation.

Previous to this case Mr. Glaister was not acquainted with the internal use of chrysophanic acid, and it was only in looking into the literature of this drug that he fell upon the recorded observations of Dr. Ashburton Thompson in the *British Medical Journal* for 19th May, 1877, pp. 607–8, where he calls chrysarobin—the powder in which chrysophanic acid exists to the extent of 80 per cent.—"a new emetic purge." The action of the powder in doses of six grains to children of twelve, according to this experimenter, produced the following effects :—"Vomiting is always the first sign of action. This is not attended by any depression at all comparable with that caused by tartar emetic or ipecacuanha. In the doses presently to be named, it has not caused any distressing retching ; and in children, as well as in adults, the acts of vomiting varied between nine in three out of the number, and six in two out of the whole number. They were usually two or three ; very often only one. The action on the bowels was much more variable—from none in a few cases to nine or ten in equally few cases ; most often the range was between three and seven. There is no griping pain, but the nausea continues more or less markedly until the bowels recover. . . . If the dose be taken into a full stomach, that delays its action and determines it to the bowels." Dr. Thompson concludes "that chrysarobin is, in a dose of twenty-five grains for adults, or of six or more grains for children, an emetic purge of which the action is unattended by any inconvenient symptoms." Then as to the action of chrysophanic acid, pure. The same observer says that its action "is similar to the action of chrysarobin, with this difference, that while in a suitable dose each will cause vomiting and purging, if the dose be too small, chrysarobin is most likely to purge only, while chrysophanic acid is most likely to cause vomiting only." . . . A dose of "from fifteen to twenty grains will always both vomit and purge the patient very freely, at the same time that it causes an inconvenient amount of either of those effects very rarely indeed. Farther, there is but little danger of inconvenience from too large a dose."

The dose of the drug, as recommended by Dr. Thompson, is from six grains upwards.

Wood, in his *Treatise on Therapeutics*, p. 437, speaking of the action of this acid, says that "according to Schlossberger, Bucheim, Meykow, and Auer, it is not purgative; but Schroff has found it to be so."

In Professor Charteris' cases, recorded in the *Lancet* lately, where comparatively large quantities of strong chrysophanic acid ointment were used externally, symptoms of gastro-intestinal irritation always asserted themselves in the early part of the treatment, but afterwards disappeared. It is therefore quite clear that this acid acts as a gastro-intestinal irritant; the question which then naturally suggests itself is, Can it be given internally in doses which would produce therapeutic action, and fall short of producing severe symptoms such as experienced by my patient? In answer to this, Dr. Thompson, after an extended series of observations in the use of the drug, says that such a dose can be given without producing severe results. This case of Mr. Glaister, however, shows that even such a small dose as three grains will produce effects which *are* unpleasant and very severe; and it also points to the fact that its effects are not always to be referred to the gastro-intestinal tract simply, but to the urinary tract also. The question has now arisen in the minds of some of those who are accustomed to the use of this drug externally in skin diseases, whether the same beneficial effect now obtained by such use could not be more speedily and comfortably got by its internal administration. This has arisen from the fact that, in some cases, where the acid ointment has been applied only to one side of the body, the other, perhaps equally as much affected, has been nearly as quickly cured; and this would point to the absorption of the drug into the body. Every one knows that it cures skin affections by the irritant action it produces where it is applied—by its altering the character of the inflammatory condition producing the chronic disease, and giving it, as it were, a more acute tone. But how does it act internally? It certainly acts as an irritant, but whether directly as the metallic irritant poisons, or indirectly as apomorphia, is a question not yet settled. The presence of food in the stomach prevents its early action, thereby pointing in the direction of the behaviour of an ordinary metallic irritant. Its mode of exhibition, too, influences the rapidity of its action; when given with an alkaline solution, it acts more quickly, things being equal, than it does undissolved, as in water or an acid medium. So that, given in a powder, as in the case of my patient, and into an empty stomach, it will, by reason of its being undissolved in the water used as a vehicle for taking it, and also because it would remain undissolved in the acid contents of the stomach, probably act as a direct irritant; when, however, it has been exhibited dissolved, as in an alkaline solution, or where it has passed from the stomach with food and only been dissolved by contact with the alkaline juice of the pancreas, and then absorbed, it will probably act as an indirect irritant.

In the light of the foregoing case, Mr. Glaister confesses, even in the face of the recorded observations of Dr. Thompson, that he would be very chary as to the dose he would administer internally. Probably an unpleasant introduction to the use of a drug regulates one's feelings as to its general behaviour, and possibly that may be so in my case: in any case, I would prefer to begin its administration internally in much smaller doses than are recommended by Dr. Thompson.

Possibly, again, the element of idiosyncrasy had something to do with its severe behaviour in the person of Mr. Glaister's patient; that much might be argued; but he doubts if any one would question the severity of the effects, which were carefully noted as they appeared, more with the view of being recorded as the eccentric behaviour of the euonymin, no suspicion having arisen in my mind at the time as to an error in the dispensing of the powder.

A Case of Nicotine Poisoning.

A case of poisoning, with sudden death, is reported by L. L. DORR, occurring in a cigar-maker 49 years of age, and apparently due to excessive smoking and prolonged presence in a room filled with tobacco smoke. At the autopsy, the description agreed with von Borek's description of the morbid state (*vide Ziemssen's Cyclopædia*), viz., "The heart is generally empty, and the blood in the vessels is of a dark-red colour. The liver, spleen, and kidneys are generally hyperæmic. Vascular engorgements of the brain and its membranes, and serous fluid in the ventricles of the brain, are mentioned in almost all published reports."—*New Remedies*, March, 1881.

Iron as a Poison.

ORFILA demonstrated that large doses of sulphate of iron will cause death with symptoms of collapse and insensibility, and, post mortem, congestion and ecchymoses in the gastro-intestinal mucous membrane, and remarkable black discoloration of the blood. Frank arrived at similar results, employing the citrate or bromhydrate. Recently MEYER and WILLIAMS have found similar effects from the subcutaneous injection of the potassio-tartrate of iron, slightly alkalized. About seventy-five thousandths of a grain constitutes a poisonous dose for the frog, and about six-tenths of a grain for a rabbit. In the frog, after absorption, there are paralysis of movement and disappearance of muscular irritability, without affection of the heart. In rabbits a great acceleration of the respiratory movements is first produced, and at the end of a little time diarrhœa comes on, with muscular weakness, while paralysis of movement, dyspnœa, and convulsions precede death. The lungs and heart are found healthy, the duodenum is swollen and hyperæmic, the mesenteric glands are engorged, and the liver, kidneys, and spleen are congested. Similar effects are produced in the cat by four or five tenths of a grain, and in the dog by rather more per pound of body weight. The toxic symptoms are accompanied by a remarkable diminution of blood-pressure, explicable by vascular paralysis. There is also observed the black tint of the blood signalized by Orfila, which is not, as might be imagined, due to the accumulation of carbonic acid in the blood, since analysis proves that this is really diminished.—*Lancet*, Sept. 24, 1881.

Hygiene.

Prevention of Scarlet Fever.

Dr. DAVID PAGE, at the London Congress, made some interesting remarks on this subject, in which he said, at the outset, that those precautions which, in respect of scarlet fever, prove successful for the protection of a neighbourhood or a household, must also be the real defences for the community which is immediately concerned, and therefore for other and more distant communities. All national or international preventive measures against the diffusion of such a disease as scarlet fever must, in their essence, be measures for effectual individual control. These measures ought to give practical effect to the questions :—

1. What ought to be done with the infected individual or patient ?

2. How long may the patient continue to be a possible source of infection ?

3. What is the latest period, after exposure to infection, at which the disorder will show itself in a person who has received the infection into his system ?

4. How soon may a person who has been exposed to risks of infection be pronounced safe against attack ?

Two main clinical facts are involved in these questions :—

1. The duration of the incubation period of scarlet fever.

2. The modes of exit from the system of the fever poison.

A knowledge of the incubation period essential in disposing for the time of a person, who, having been exposed to chances of infection, may have contracted the disorder. In this case an appreciation of the maximum period of latency required. Literature of subject vague and untrustworthy.

The author's observations coincide with those of the late Dr. Murchison, and may be summed up :—

1. The common duration of the incubation period in scarlet fever is from twenty-four to forty-eight hours.

2. The period is occasionally longer, lasting from three to five days.

3. In rare instances practically absent, the symptoms following quickly upon exposure to infection.

Based upon these conclusions, the author requires that a person who has been exposed to infection should, before being pronounced safe from its probable consequences, be kept under surveillance for a week, and only then, after change of clothes, and baths, be set at liberty.

Of even greater importance than this is the action which ought to be taken in regard to the fever patient himself. This action is rendered difficult by reason of diversity and inconstancy of what are commonly looked for as the diagnostic features of scarlet fever.

An estimate of the real value of desquamation of the cuticle as a trustworthy guide in preventive measures must be based upon knowledge of irregularity of process in relation to time, quantity of eruption, or intensity of attack. Error of regarding infective process at an end before cessation of desquamation and *for some considerable interval afterwards*. Importance of pathology of scarlet fever as regards the nature of the eruption and the tendency to albuminuria, as a guide to preventive action and treatment.

The author's experience points to the necessity for isolation of the scarlatinal patient for a period of not less than eight weeks, and he would state the rule of Nature to be isolation for this period as a minimum, and, in cases of protracted desquamation or of relapse, until entire cessation of the process *and for a fortnight afterwards*.

For the rest, official action should include :—

1. Due provision for the separation of the sick from the healthy in the way of hospitals and convalescent homes.

2. Notification of the occurrence of cases of infectious disease.

3. Continuous supervision of all scarlatinal convalescents.

4. Control of school attendance of children belonging to infected families.

5. Disinfection and purification of infected houses and things.

MEDICAL NEWS.

Defective Plumbing and Drainage.

Our publication in the present number of the excellent plan of plumbing and drainage, approved by the New York City Board of Health, will we trust direct attention to a subject which requires the most careful consideration, not only in this community, but also in every town and even in every village throughout our country. The people of America stood aghast, as they well might, before the devastation caused a few years since by yellow fever, in New Orleans and Memphis; and yet it is probable that twice as great a proportionate annual mortality occurs, in every closely built city, from typhoid fever, diphtheria, and allied diseases, resulting from sanitary faults in plumbing and drainage.

That these dangers to our health and our lives are real and imminent, is shown by a moment's glance at the record of facts brought to light by Dr. H. R. Storer in his valuable report of the workings of the Sanitary Protective Association of Newport, R. I., in which he relates that the inspecting engineer of the society had found soil pipes both of iron and clay cracked, that joints were discovered having no cement or solder whatever, while frequently they were merely plastered over, leaving spaces whence sewage escaped; other joints being found so imperfectly closed, that rootlets of trees had entered, and by their growth entirely plugged up the pipe, with the result of backward flow and leakage of sewage. Soil pipes were likewise met with where old fractures had been plugged with wood, which in time, of course, had rotted away, and allowed sewer-gas to escape. Direct communications were unearthed moreover, between house and cess-pool, with no intervening trap, detection being made through inspection alone, there being no perceptible odour, although such must have been the state of things for more than a year, in some instances.

Last but not least in the long list of faults actually revealed by inspection, in the houses of subscribers to the Newport Association, it is to be noticed, that cess-pools were constantly discovered in close proximity to wells, thus suggesting an examination of the well water, which was rarely found good in any portion of the city.

Among medical men of the present generation, there exists, it is to be hoped, little need of dwelling upon this unsavory subject, but we desire to urge on every physician whose eyes these remarks meet, the vital importance of impressing upon his circle of friends and patients, how dangerous to health are these constantly occurring blunders of defective plumbing. Thousands of valued lives have been sacrificed by typhoid fever, through the ignorance of architects and builders in regard to the first principles of sanitary drainage; and tens of thousands of beloved children have died from diphtheria and other filth diseases, in consequence of culpable carelessness or deceit on the part of plumbers.

The philanthropic efforts of sanitarians would probably be much aided, if the public could be persuaded to understand, that the risk of contaminating the human organism with the poison of typhoid fever (and perhaps of other diseases) is twofold; that is to say, the typhoid germ may enter our bodies by way of drinking-water (into which it finds its way in consequence of faulty construction and arrangement of drain pipes, etc.); or it may gain access to our systems through the lungs, by our breathing-air (if that air becomes mingled with sewer- or cess-pool gas), as a result of leaky and defective pipes, traps, or reservoirs for sewage. Moreover, it must always be remembered that no plumber's work, however complete it may be at first, can be relied upon to remain perfect; and that therefore the only sewage and drain-pipe arrangement, which is worthy of any confidence, is one in which nothing is concealed, but all parts may be easily inspected and repaired, whenever and wherever the slightest defect is found to exist.

In his efforts to secure due attention in the community to this all-important subject of proper plumbing and drainage, the sanitarian is baffled by an incredulity as to the impending danger, based upon the circumstance that individuals were known to have drunk water contaminated with the soakage of a cess-pool, or breathed air rendered foul by the emanations of a leaky trap or drain pipe, *for years* without apparent injury. Hence it is furthermore very important to disseminate in the community a knowledge of the fact that air or water rendered impure by admixture with simple ordinary filth, may be taken into the economy for a long time without obvious ill effects, but if this filth becomes infected with the specific poison or *germ* of typhoid or diphtheria (as may happen at any time, by the passage into it of the excretions from a person affected with either of these maladies), it is changed at once into the virulent carrier of disease. No better illustration of this great truth could well be given than the remarkable instance recorded by Prof. Flint, in which a young man travelling by stage coach in Vermont, fell ill with typhoid, was left at the hotel of a wayside hamlet, and within a week infected with his malady (through his intestinal discharges) all the families on the tavern side of a creek, which divided the village, *except one* whose head had quarrelled with the landlord, and drank none of the water from his well. Doubtless in this case the tavern-keeper's well-water had been contaminated with sewage from the hotel for years, and it would seem without serious injury to those using it, yet directly after the simple filth it previously contained was impregnated, *in addition*, with the self-propagating germ of typhoid fever, this hitherto comparatively innocent water was altered into a powerful and deadly poison, for those who drank it. So strong is this single item of evidence, in regard to the dangers arising from impure water, that could it alone, without any other testimony, be heard by every one, we might soon expect a vast diminution in the evils from defective plumbing and drainage throughout the civilized world.

———

Rules for Drainage and Plumbing.—A system of rules to govern the plumbing and drainage of all buildings hereafter erected in New York has been adopted by the Health Board, in accordance with the power conferred upon it by the statute enacted by the State Legislature June 4, 1881. These rules were distributed to plumbers on October 11, and are as follows :—

1. All materials must be of good quality and free from defects; the work must be executed in a thorough and workmanlike manner.

2. The arrangement of soil- and waste-pipes must be as direct as possible.

The drain-, soil-, and waste-pipes, and the traps, should, if practicable, be exposed to view for ready inspection at all times, and for convenience in repairing. When placed within walls or partitions, they should be covered with woodwork, fastened with screws, so as to be readily removed. In no case should they be absolutely inaccessible.

It is recommended to place the soil and other vertical pipes in a special shaft, between or adjacent to the water-closet and the bath-room, and serving as a ventilating shaft for them. This shaft should be at least two and a half feet square. It should extend from the cellar through the roof, and should be covered by a louvered skylight. It should be accessible at every story, and should have a very open but strong grating at each floor to stand upon.

3. Every house or building must be separately and independently connected with the street-sewer by an iron pipe caulked with lead.

4. The house-drain must be of iron, with a fall of at least one-half an inch to the foot, if possible.

It should run along the cellar-wall, unless this is impracticable, in which case it should be laid in a trench, cut at a uniform grade, walled up on the sides, and provided with movable covers, with a hydraulic concrete base of four inches in thickness on which the pipe is to rest.

It should be laid in a straight line, if possible. All changes in direction must be made with curved pipes, and all connections with Y-branch-pipes and one-eighth bends.

It must be provided with a running trap placed at an accessible point near the front of the house. The trap must be furnished with a hand-hole for convenience in cleaning, the cover of which must be properly fitted and the joints made tight with some proper cement.

There should be an inlet for fresh air entering the drain just inside the trap of at least 4 inches in diameter, leading to the outer air and opening at any convenient place not too near a window.

No brick, sheet-metal, or earthenware flue shall be used as a sewer-ventilator, nor shall any chimney-flue be used for this purpose.

5. Every soil-pipe and waste-pipe must be of iron, and must extend at least two feet above the highest part of the roof or coping, of undiminished size, with a return bend or cowl. It must not open near a window nor an air-shaft ventilating living rooms.

Horizontal soil- and waste-pipes are prohibited.

There should be no traps on vertical soil-pipes or vertical waste-pipes.

6. All iron pipes must be sound, free from holes, and of a uniform thickness of not less than one-eighth of an inch for a diameter of two, three, or four inches, or five thirty-seconds of an inch for a diameter of five or six inches; and for large buildings the use of what is known as extra heavy soil-pipe is recommended, which weighs as follows:—

2 inches,	$5\frac{1}{2}$ pounds per lineal foot.			
3 "	$9\frac{1}{2}$ "	"	"	
4 "	13 "	"	• "	
5 "	17 "	"	"	
6 "	20 "	"	"	
7 "	27 "	"	"	
8 "	$33\frac{1}{2}$ "	"	"	"
10 "	45 "	"	"	
12 "	54 "	"	"	"

Before they are connected they must be thoroughly coated inside and outside with coal-tar pitch, applied hot, or some other equivalent substance.

Iron pipes, before being connected with fixtures, should have openings stopped, and be filled with water and allowed to stand twenty-four hours for inspection.

7. All joints in the drain-pipes, soil-pipes, and waste-pipes must be so caulked with oakum and lead, or with cement made of iron filings and sal ammoniac, as to make them impermeable to gases.

All connections of lead with iron pipes should be made with a brass sleeve or ferrule, of the same size as the lead pipe, put in the hub of the branch of the iron pipe and caulked in with lead. The lead pipe should be attached to the ferrule by a wiped joint.

All connections of lead pipe should be by wiped joints.

8. Every sink, basin, wash-tray, bath, safe, and every tub or set of tubs, must be separately and effectively trapped. The traps must be placed as near the fixtures as practicable. All exit-pipes should be provided with strong metallic strainers.

9. Traps should be protected from siphonage by a special metallic air-pipe not less than one and one-half inch in diameter; if it supply air to a water-closet trap, not less than two inches in diameter, the size to increase with the number of water-closets.

These pipes should extend two feet above the highest part of the roof or coping, and, if independent of the upper end of the soil-pipe, this extension should not be less than four inches in diameter to avoid obstruction from frost. If, however, they are branched into a soil-pipe, it must be above the inlet from the highest fixture. They may be combined by branching together those which serve several traps. These air-pipes must always have a continuous slope, to avoid collecting water by condensation.

10. Every safe under a wash-basin, bath, urinal, water-closet, or other fixture must be drained by a special pipe not directly connected with any soil-pipe, waste-pipe, drain, or sewer, but discharging into an open sink, upon the cellar-floor, or outside the house.

11. No waste-pipe from a refrigerator shall be directly connected with the soil- or waste-pipe, or with the drain or sewer, or discharge into the soil, but it should discharge into an open sink. Such waste-pipes should be so arranged as to admit of frequent flushing, and should be as short as possible, and disconnected from the refrigerator.

12. All water-closets inside the house must be supplied with water from a special tank or cistern, the water of which is not used for any other purpose. The closets must never be supplied directly from the Croton supply pipes. A group of closets may be supplied from one tank, if on the same floor and contiguous.

The overflow-pipes from tanks should discharge into an open sink or into the bowl of the closet itself, not into the soil- or waste-pipe, nor into the drain or sewer. When the pressure of the Croton is not sufficient to supply these tanks, a pump must be provided.

13. Cisterns for drinking-water are objectionable; if indispensable, they must never be lined with lead, galvanized iron, or zinc. They should be constructed of iron or of wood, lined with tinned and planished copper. The overflow should be trapped, and should discharge into an open sink, never into any soil- or waste-pipe or water-closet trap, nor into the drain or sewer.

14. Rain-water leaders must never be used as soil-, waste-, or vent-pipes; nor shall any soil-, waste-, or vent-pipe be used as a leader.

When connected with the house-drain, the leaders should be trapped beneath the ground, with a deep- seal, to avoid evaporation, and, if placed within the house, must be made of cast-iron, with leaden joints.

15. No steam-exhaust will be allowed to connect with any soil- or waste-pipe.

16. Cellar- and foundation-walls should be rendered impervious to dampness, by the use of asphaltum or coal-tar pitch in addition to hydraulic cement.

Subsoil drains should be provided whenever necessary.

17. Yards and areas should always be properly graded, cemented, flagged, or well paved, and drained by pipes discharging into the house-drain. These pipes should be effectively trapped.

18. No privy-vault, or cesspool for sewage, will be permitted in any part of the city when a sewer is accessible.

—

Raid on Poor Milk.—The New York Health Board is at present engaged in very energetic efforts to prevent the sale of inferior milk. The milk inspectors make careful examinations of the milk when it reaches the city, and pour into the street all that does not conform to the standards and tests established by the Board. 5000 quarts of poor milk were thus spilled during the last week in September. A large number of milk dealers have also been arraigned and fined for the sale of adulterated and inferior milk.

—

The International Pharmacopœia.—A project of no small importance—viz., construction of an International Pharmacopœia, which should include a common mode of preparing and prescribing the more important drugs—has been considerably advanced during the last month, as the result of the conference of the International Pharmaceutical Congress held in London. The following resolutions were unanimously passed at this Congress; and will, we believe, be practically acted upon:—

" 1. The fifth International Pharmaceutical Congress, held in London, confirms the resolution passed at the previous Congresses, as to the utility of a Universal Pharmacopœia, but is of opinion that it is necessary at once to appoint a Commission, consisting of two delegates from each of the countries represented at this Congress, which should prepare within the shortest possible time a compilation in which the strength of all potent drugs and their preparation is equalized. 2. The Executive Committee of this Congress is requested to take the necessary steps that the resolution be speedily carried out. 3. The work, when ready, should be handed over by the delegates to their respective Governments or their pharmaceutical committees. 4. It is desirable that the Committee suggest an uniform systematic Latin nomenclature for the Pharmacopœias of all countries. 5. It is desirable that the Committee take measures that an official Latin translation be made of the Pharmacopœias of different countries which are not now published in that language. 6. It is desirable that the Committee be put in possession of all the manuscripts, including the documents relating to the Universal Pharmacopœia, compiled by the labours of the Society of Pharmacists of Paris, presented at the fourth meeting of the International Congress of St. Petersburg by the Society of Pharmacists of Paris. 7. That the pharmaceutical societies of the respective countries be requested to nominate those members of the Commission not appointed by this Congress, and to fill up any vacancies which may arise from time to time."—*British Med. Journal*, Aug. 20, 1881.

The representatives of the United States on this Committee are Mr. J. M. Maisch, of Philadelphia, and another to be chosen.

—

Health of New York.—The city's mortality for September somewhat exceeded that of August. For the week ending Sept. 3, there were 864 deaths. For the weeks ending Sept. 10, 17, and 24, there were respectively 866, 688, and 705 deaths. The total number for September thus amounted to upwards of 3100, while that for August was about 3000. The increased mortality may in a measure be accounted for by the fact that unseasonable, and, at times, excessive heat prevailed during almost the entire month, and gave rise to many fatal cases of infantile gastro-enteritis. The records of the Bureau of Vital Statistics show that 28,567 deaths have occurred during the past nine months. This number exceeds that for the corresponding period of 1880 by 4715. The total number for 1880 was 31,866, while the present indications are that this year's mortality will reach nearly 38,000. This death record, if actually reached, would be the highest known since the establishment of the Bureau, the next highest being that of 1872, which was 32,647.

The Board of Health cherish strong hopes that their strict suspension of all new plumbing work, and their active crusade against bad milk, will notably improve the city's sanitary condition in future by diminishing the cases of zymotic disease.

One case of typhus fever was discovered in the city during the week ending Sept. 24, but the premises upon which it was detected were so thoroughly fumigated and cleansed that no extension of the disease is apprehended. All the infectious diseases have diminished to a very encouraging extent during September. Only 46 cases of smallpox were reported as contrasted with 75 in August. Diphtheria diminished from 355 in August to 276 in September, while scarlatina and rubeola fell from 320 and 96 in August to 259 and 36 respectively in September. So excessive was the September heat that a number of sunstrokes occurred during the month.

—

The American Gynecological Society held its sixth annual meeting in New York, at the hall of the Academy of Medicine, on Sept. 21, 22, and 23. Owing to the absence of the President, Dr. Byford, of Chicago, the duties of presiding officer were discharged by the First Vice-President, Dr. Thaddeus A. Reamy, of Cincinnati. The address of welcome to the delegates was delivered by Dr. Fordyce Barker, President of the New York Academy of Medicine. Receptions were held during the session of the Society by Drs. Isaac E. Taylor and T. A. Emmet. Lunch parties were given by Drs. Sims, Thomas, Barker, Byrne, and Skene. Papers were read by Drs. Thomas; A. H. Smith, of Philadelphia; Campbell, of Augusta, Ga.; Taylor, of N. Y.; Goodell, of Philadelphia; Lyman, of Boston;

Garrigues, of N. Y.; and others. The officers elected for the ensuing year are as follows: President, Dr. T. A. Emmet, of New York; Vice-Presidents, Dr. George H. Lyman, of Boston, and Dr. E. Noeggerath, of New York. Council, Drs. Geo H. Bixby, of Boston; Jas. D. Trask, of Astoria, N. Y.; H. J. Garrigues, of New York; and G. J. Englemann, of St. Louis.

Epidemic of Typhoid Fever.—An endemic of typhoid fever which recently occurred in the Roman Catholic Orphan Asylum was believed to be due to the poor quality of the milk with which the institution was supplied. The analysis of the milk, made by the officials of the Health Board, showed it to have been skimmed and watered.

Pink Eye.—Numbers of horses in the large stables of various New York car companies have recently been attacked by influenza. It is called "pink eye" by the hostlers. Its symptoms are œdema of the legs, conjunctivitis, Schneider-itis, tonsillitis, and bronchitis. Veterinary surgeons believe that the conjunctivitis may be relieved by steaming the animals' heads. The disease has thus far been of a mild type.

The British Medical Association—The forty-ninth annual meeting of this Association commenced at Ryde on the 9th of August, and lasted four days. Professor Humphry, of Cambridge, President of the Association, was in the chair. Mr. Benjamin Barrow, of Ryde, was unanimously elected President for the ensuing year, and Mr. Humphry, in a few well-chosen words, handed the office over to his successor. Mr. Barrow delivered the customary presidential address.

Mr. Fowler, the General Secretary, read the annual report of the Council, which, among other things, stated that the roll of members now reached 9202, and that the next meeting would be held at Worcester, 1882, being the jubilee year of the Association, and Worcester the town where it was first started by Sir Charles Hastings fifty years previously. Dr. Strange was nominated for the presidency of that year.

Dr. Bristowe delivered the address in Medicine, Mr. Jonathan Hutchinson that in Surgery, and Dr. Sinclair Coghill, of Ventnor, that in Obstetrics.

At the annual dinner of the Association, Dr. J. S. Billings responded to the toast of "the Army of the United States."

Owen County (Ky.) Medical Society.—The physicians of Owen County, Ky., organized in September a County Medical Society, and elected Dr. J. W. Johnson, President, and Dr. R. I. Peck, Secretary.

Vitiated Sea Breezes at Coney Island.—The summer residents of Coney Island, New York, having bitterly complained of the odours emanating from the fat rendering establishments on Barren Island, the Committee of the State Board of Health has visited the premises, and proposes to suppress the nuisance in question.

King's County Lunatic Asylum.—In his annual report upon the condition of the King's County Lunatic Asylum, in Flatbush, L. I., Dr. Shaw, the resident-physician, shows that, according to the statistics of the last two decades (from 1860 to 1880), the percentage of insane persons to the population of the county decreased from thirty-eight to twenty-nine per cent. Dr. Shaw has employed a system of non-restraint, whenever practicable, and reports excellent results from this method. During the year ending July 31, 1881, 428 patients were admitted to the asylum, which now contains 868 inmates. Warden Murray, of the King's County Almshouse, reports that 3255 indigent persons were cared for during the year ending July 31, and that 673 still remain in the institution.

Resignation.—Dr. D. L. Schenck recently resigned the superintendency of the Flatbush Hospital, Brooklyn, N. Y., after occupying that position for seventeen years. Dr. H. O. Plimpton has been appointed temporary superintendent by the Commissioners of Charities and Correction.

Oleomargarine Redivivus.—A so-called "Oleomargarine Bill," in accordance with the requirements of which all oleomargarine exposed for sale was to be plainly marked, passed the New York Legislature, but was vetoed by Governor Cornell.

The New York Night Medical Service has now been in operation about a year. During that time five hundred calls have been made by its corps of physicians. It has been proposed to establish a day medical service which shall be conducted on a similar plan.

Poisoning by Gaultheria (Wintergreen).—Dr. M. L. FICHTNER, of Cranesville, Preston County, West Virginia, sends a report of the following cases of poisoning by oil of wintergreen: Rauhama C. and Malinda C., æt. respectively 14 and 15 years, drank, through mistake, on the 4th of August, 1881, the former about ℥j, and the latter about ℥ij, of the oil of *Gaultheria procumbens*. Both were seized with vertigo, weakness, hot skin, frequent pulse, cold sweats, laboured respiration, and dulness of hearing. In the latter there was also inability to speak, with cramp in epigastrium and convulsions. Warm water and salt were then given as an emetic, and followed by olive oil. In the former case olive oil was continued in half-teaspoonful doses three to four times a day for about ten days, and the patient recovered without any serious inconvenience. In the latter case, bromide of potassium, olive oil, and the decoction of slippery elm bark were used, with cold applications to the head. The patient died in about ten hours after the drinking from congestion of the brain and convulsions. The breath had a pungent odor, and the gaultheria was detected in the perspiration. The patients were treated, at first, by Dr. Daniel Fichtner, afterwards Drs. A. S. and M. L. Fichtner were called.

The Summer Home of the Children's Aid Society, at Bath, Long Island, which was opened on June 18th, has already entertained 2800 poor children from the tenement houses. About 200 children are received, every week, at the home, and are returned to the city, after a week's sojourn at the institution, to be succeeded by an equal number of new-comers.

Literary Notes.—In the *Archives Générales de Medecine* for September, Prof. DUPLAY gives an elaborate "critical review" on the treatment of aneurism by the elastic bandage entirely based on the able paper of Dr. Lewis A. Stimson, of New York, which appeared in the *American Journal of the Medical Sciences* for April last. Dr. Duplay translates and adopts as his own large portions of Dr. Stimson's paper together with his conclusions, but unkindly misspells his name and that of Dr. R. F. Weir, of New York, almost beyond recognition.

The "Atlanta Medical and Surgical Journal" has changed its name to *Atlanta Medical Register*.

G. P. Putnam's Sons announce a "Treatise on the Science and Practice of Medicine," by Dr. A. B. Palmer, Professor of Practice of Medicine in the University of Michigan; and have just published a volume on "Eczema and its Management," based on an analysis of 2500 cases, by Dr. L. Duncan Bulkley, of New York.

—

OBITUARY RECORD.—Died, at Buffalo, on the 28th of September, after a brief illness, aged 70 years, JAMES PLATT WHITE, M.D., Professor of Obstetrics in the University of Buffalo, and formerly Vice-President of the American Medical Association.

Dr. James P. White, a descendant of Peregrine White, one of the "Mayflower" colonists, was born in Austerlitz, Columbia Co., N. Y., March 14, 1811. He received his early education at the Middlebury Academy; his medical studies were commenced at the Fairfield Medical College, where he attended lectures during the years 1831-2-3, and at the Jefferson Medical College, Philadelphia, from which he graduated in 1834. He began professional practice in Buffalo immediately after graduation, and continued in active work almost until his death. Dr. White was one of the founders of the Medical Department of the University of Buffalo, where he occupied the Chair of Obstetrics and Gynæcology, and was in 1850 the first in this country, it is believed, to teach midwifery clinically. He was a-prominent member of the American Medical Association, its Vice-President in 1870, and one of the Vice-Presidents of the International Medical Congress held in Philadelphia, in 1876, and a member of various medical societies. His contributions to medical literature during the last thirty years were numerous and on various subjects, and were mainly published in the *Buffalo Medical and Surgical Journal*; the papers which, however, served the most to establish his reputation were on "Chronic Inversion of the Uterus," published in the *American Journal of the Medical Sciences* in 1858 and 1874. He also was the author of the chapter on "Pregnancy" in Beck's *Medical Jurisprudence*.

Dr. White was a man of strong individuality and wide influence in both public and private life; he was possessed of great executive ability and public spirit, and leaves behind him many warm friends. As a specialist he acquired an extensive and enviable reputation.

—

CORRESPONDENCE.

1300 SPRUCE ST.,
PHILADELPHIA, Oct. 7, 1881.

MR. EDITOR: I have been asked by several of my medical friends for some comments on the case of President Garfield, which was, during its progress, I think, most uncourteously if not unprofessionally appropriated through the newspapers, by some surgeons, as their own. If they had had anything of importance to communicate, I am sure the gentlemen in charge would have given them respectful attention, for access to the White House and to the offices of those gentlemen by mail was not cut off. The case was a public one to members of the profession as citizens only, and doctors not being in possession of all the facts to make intelligent criticism, should have remembered that they were in no position to share "the credit of success or the blame of failure." Now since the death and the official publication of the results of the autopsy, the case has become public, both to professional and laymen, and doubtless its diagnosis, prognosis, and treatment are fair subjects for comment.

From Dr. Frank H. Hamilton's "Military Surgery," New York, 1865, page 338, I make the following extract:—

" In a few cases a ball has been known to pass through the side of the body of one of the vertebra, leaving a round hole or a lateral furrow, *without coming in contact with the spinal marrow or the bloodvessels. It is not probable that we shall be able to diagnosticate such a case clearly during the life of a patient, and if we were able to do so, we do not see what benefit could be derived from any surgical operation.*

In case, however, one of the transverse processes has been broken and sent inwards, although it is not likely to have penetrated the cavity of the abdomen, it may yet give rise to serious results by the *formation of an abscess in the bellies of the psoas muscles, which abscess may eventually make its way along between the fibres towards the groin, or may empty itself into the loose areolar tissue outside of the peritoneum.*"

The italics are mine. Could there possibly have been a more wonderful foreshadowing of the President's case? The fracture of the transverse process is replaced in the case in hand by the fracture of the body, which produced the abscess or channel along the psoas in precisely the same way as described by Dr. Hamilton. The description is perfect. The sinus or channel which was, in the words of the official report, supposed during life to be the track of the bullet, was practically an abscess and sinus caused by the disintegration of a vertebral body through gunshot, precisely as a chronic lumbar and psoas abscess is caused by the chronic disintegration of a vertebral body through disease. How truly Dr. Hamilton sets forth the difficulties of diagnosis, and how absolutely true he is as to surgical interference by operation, having for its object the getting of the missile, which, as the autopsy shows, was lying harmless, compared to the injuries it had inflicted. The diagnosis then was hard; but does it not seem, in the light of our present knowledge, that the deep significance of the nervous symptoms of the President immediately after the shooting, was lost sight of too early in the case? This, if so, was probably the result of the exciting surroundings, and of the fact that the doctors were more occupied in praetical efforts to relieve these symptoms than in speculations as to their cause. They were attributed to injuries or impressions upon nerves of the lumbar plexus, instead of to direct shock to the cord itself. This view seemed to be confirmed by the fact that they promptly subsided under rest and other treatment. That temporary spinal shock does sometimes occur at once after an accident to the column, I will show further on by an actual recent case.

But those pains in the legs, those " tigers' claws," affected *both* sides; what would account for them so well as sudden injury of some kind to the spine? From their bilateral suddenness it is more reasonable to attribute them to direct action upon the centre, than to reflex transfer from the right to the left. The right side I assume exhibited them to a greater degree than the left, but the full force of the impact was received upon the right and was weakened upon the left. If I am not right and the pains were equal on both sides, then there is still stronger reason to refer the phenomena to a central origin.

I have read also, that at first there was hyperæsthesia of the genitals. If so, this, together with the " tigers' claws," pointed strongly to the spine. Some surgeons are sceptical about spinal shock. This summer, in July, Dr. Agnew assisted me in a case that confirms its occurrence.

A boy was shot in the back to the right of the third or fourth dorsal vertebra. He at once had characteristic symptoms in the legs of being wounded in the spine. These soon disappeared. The course of the bullet was not readily made out at first, but the diagnosis was that the column was wounded without injury to the cord, as the symptoms were not continuous. After suppuration set in, the course of the ball was readily traced with a probe, and broken fragments of the vertebral processes were felt. The ball was not felt with a Nélaton or other probe. The patient was etherized. I made a large and deep incision through the muscles in the line of the wound, and removed some clothing and fragments of bone and finally a large bullet, which was lying immediately against the bony bridge of a vertebra. The boy recovered. Whether he will suffer from caries in the future remains to be seen. This boy certainly had spinal shock, without injury to the cord, for there was no remnant of paralysis when he was discharged from the hospital.[1]

But this case is very different from the President's in this, that it was amenable to operation, and we knew about where the ball was. Also here, the ball would have produced great future mischief. In the President's case it did its damage and then hid. If such difficulty occurred in the hunt for it as is stated at the autopsy, imagine the horror of a like attempt on a live man. How long would he have lived? He had better have been killed at a blow.

A surgeon who has *lived* in an accident hospital and receives cases day and night, immediately after injury, gets into the habit of making "snap" diagnoses. It is really not the presumption of ignorance, but it is the quick application of knowledge gained by experience. In nineteen cases out of twenty the "snap" is right; often he who deliberates is lost. Now excuse the egotism, for I have abundant proof of what I say, and I say it for the credit of diagnosis, "snap" though it be. At once, upon reading the accounts of the leg pains and the "tigers' claws," I said to a medical friend, and I have no doubt that many other hospital men said the same thing, "the President is shot in the spinal column." But after the diagnosis was given to the public stating that the direction of the ball was downward and forward, through the liver, and into the anterior wall of the abdomen, I came to the conclusion that in this case the "snap" had failed.

The question of the duty of the consulting surgeons when they first went to Washington has been freely discussed. Should they have reopened and re-examined the wound with probes and fingers? I am assuming that they did not do so, and they were right. A hospital chief, if he has confidence in his residents or assistants, and knows them to be experienced and ready, takes what they say about serious cases which will not tolerate officious disturbance. He recognizes the "snap" if the other symptoms confirm it. For example, the chief visits the hospital on his regular rounds. The resident says, "Doctor, here's a man who was brought in last night shot in the abdomen. He was greatly shocked; I examined him and passed my finger directly into the cavity; I removed some pieces of clothing; I can feel the bullet nowhere under the skin about the whole body; I searched carefully; I have dressed the wound and given some opium; he is now quiet and free from pain." The surgeon looks at the patient, sees that his general symptoms confirm the diagnosis, and that his wounds are carefully dressed. He probably re-examines the body

---

[1] Whilst reading proof of this article, October 18th, this boy walked into my office, having been kindly sent to me, by Dr. W. C. Cox, of the Out-Department of the Hospital. He was perfectly well in every respect.

externally, but if he is a wise man he says practically "hands off, we will await results and act accordingly."

Many a life has been saved by this course; many a one has been lost by deviating from it. I question if one has ever been saved, in the kind of case now under notice, by deviating from it. Now if a surgeon can so treat those who are *under* him, how much more is he bound (unless he sees something positively and absolutely wrong), to receive the statements of his peers, especially when outward appearances seem to confirm them. I question, moreover, whether any more light whatever would have been thrown on the President's case by further exploration at the time when the consulting surgeons made their first visit? By that time, the spinal symptoms had disappeared, or were very much alleviated. Inflammation through swelling of the denser tissues, muscular and fibrous, of the true track of the ball had doubtless closed it. The finger or probes would have passed easily where other fingers and probes had already been, and there would have been almost certainly a positive confirmation of the results of the first examination. When I study the autopsy more closely, I think that this would almost to a certainty have been the case. If I understand the description and the drawing, the ball entered at a place which, if it had had consciousness and an intent to deceive, could not have been better selected in the whole body. It entered "three and a half inches to the right of the vertebral spines," therefore its course began to the right of the psoas mass. Instead of going forward, it traversed the circle of the body transversely, after fracturing the eleventh rib, and went directly on in the direction of a chord of an arc of that circle. It entered the post-peritoneal space and thus penetrated the posterior wall of the abdomen, without opening the peritoneum. It then continued on into the muscular mass, separating the longitudinal fibres, which may have closed behind it. The finger was passed into the wound and also probes. These went readily on in the space mentioned, and the true course was missed. I have no doubt the depending liver, or it may be the kidney, was felt. The wound was one to deceive the very elect. The influence of the inner loin muscles in concealing injuries and diseases of the lumbar vertebra is well recognized. The post-mortem report speaks of the dilated track of the ball, but this dilatation was owing to subsequent changes. I am ignorant of any other explanation of the position taken by fingers and probes, than that I have given.

It is a mistake to suppose the spine escaped attention in the case. Dr. Agnew assures me, that when he operated for the relief of the lumbar abscess, he carefully searched the transverse processes and all of the spine he could feel, and felt nothing wrong. The injury to it was beyond his fingers, and a wise caution here forbade the use of instruments. How truly Dr. Hamilton's remarks are illustrated by this experience. Moreover, by the incisions Dr. Agnew made, which he tells me were carefully planned for drainage, the whole line of the true wound, as well as the mistaken sinus, had full outlet.

The abscess which was found after death, bounded by the liver, the transverse colon, and the transverse meso-colon, for anatomical reasons, was shut off from communication with the wound, and of course was not drained. In the words of the official report, "no communication could be detected between it and the wound." No method of diagnosis occurs to me by which its existence could have been determined during life, unless it had got far enough to cause posterior or anterior bulging.

It was an abscess, arising either from peritoneal inflammation through contiguity or it was a septic deposit.

The case really was one to diagnosticate more by the application of anatomy and physiological and pathological knowledge, than by direct methods. In the light of the autopsy, everything is explained. By the theory of the wound during life, almost nothing.

There were the pains in the limbs and the " tigers' claws." There was most profound depression and a pulse and temperature record which, after the liver theory was abandoned, the accepted wound, at most a severe flesh one, was insufficient to account for. There was the origin of the thoracic duct with its receptaculum chyli right in the line of the wound; hence, the rapid emaciation, and the other nutritive disabilities, further explained by disturbance of the sympathetic trunks and ganglia. There were the radicles of the vena azygos, bathed in the corruption of rotting vertebra, and hence the septicæmia, and there was the abscess and sinus, running toward the groin, a result of the rotting vertebra and not of the ball. What good could it have done to have cut for the bullet after its first mischief? It was then but a small factor in the troubles.

As to the liver, there are recoveries from wounds of it, but they are rare. Between twenty and thirty of such recoveries are reported I think in the surgery of the war. How many even of these were mistakes as to diagnosis? During my last term at the hospital, an old soldier, very peculiarly and deeply jaundiced, fractured his thigh. He told us that the jaundice was an old affair, that he had been shot through the liver in the war, and showed the external scar. He became very sick and died. The liver was most carefully examined, but there was no mark of a wound about it, nor in it. Serious wounds of the liver generally kill promptly by hemorrhage. Hundreds must be killed in this way in battle. On the other hand, recovery may take place and a bullet (strange as it may seem) may become completely encysted in the organ. Dr. Owens, now resident in the Pennsylvania Hospital, has a bullet with the encysting capsule around it which he took from the liver of an old fellow who died in the almshouse from some other cause. It must have laid there for many years.

As to the treatment of the President's case, it was in the light of the autopsy most fortunate. A very valuable life was prolonged beyond all reasonable hope. From a letter I had from Dr. Agnew, dated the 23d of August, 1881, which was confidential then but open now, I know how fully he appreciated the profound gravity of the case, and took an almost hopeless view of it, but still he with his colleagues fought it out nobly. When we come to think of it, it may be a mercy that an exact diagnosis was not made. The temptation to do something more than was done, if it had been made, would have been very great. Outside and inconsiderate pressure would have been clamorous. Whether it would have moved the steady heads in charge, I do not know; but if it had, I am confident the President would have been ready for his grave on the day of the operation. Who can picture the political results that might have followed? Now the perturbing elements have been calmed, and all is peace.

Much has been said about antiseptic treatment in the case. It was practised, I believe, to a very great extent. Its *practice* is grand, except the spray; I heartily agree with the German surgeon who said " fort mit dem spray." Could there be a better commentary on the *unproved theory* of antiseptic surgery than the President's case? Against its theory, or at least the effect of it on many minds, viz., that all sources of contamination producing septic poisoning come from without, I earnestly protest. I have too much respect for Mr. Lister to think that he believes what the extremists among his disciples teach.

The influence of such teaching on the rising generation of physicians and surgeons is bad, in this, that it leads to narrow views and interferes with clear diagnosis. It leads outwardly too much, for contamination comes from within, I believe, more frequently than from without. Was not the decaying vertebra in the President's case enough to account for the septicæmia?

To get all the rats out and then stop the hole with poison and stuffing is a good thing, but to poison and plug the hole and leave the rats in, is a very bad thing. They only undermine and make other holes. A narrow antiseptist looks around the room instead of at the patient, whereas, he should look at both and give due weight to all septic possibilities.

Discussion is now going on as to whether the President's wound was mortal or not. What is mortal? Essentially mortal wounds are extremely limited. A sweep through a certain portion of the medulla oblongata, which is itself a small organ, or a wound opening the aorta, may be instanced as examples. Haller's tripod of life was the heart, the lungs, and the brain. One leg of this tripod gone, the rest falls. The leg must be thoroughly undermined, or else injured in a particular part. Many people get well of wounds of the brain and lungs. Recoveries occur from injuries to the muscular substance of the heart without opening its cavities. Foreign bodies lie imbedded in that substance for years. I saw a large needle taken out of the heart of a negro in the dissecting-room, which must have been there for a very long time, and had nothing to do with his death. Now, setting aside everything else, what was the immediate cause of the President's death? It was from what, in extent of tissue involved, was the smallest serious feature of his injuries. It was the rupture of a traumatic aneurism of the splenic artery! I know of no method in science that would surely locate such an aneurism. If it were located, I know of no measure that would stop its progress. That progress is steadily on to rupture. Anatomy surrounds it with no special sustaining structures. That rupture was essentially fatal, and so with other injuries that might have killed, this one positively did kill.

Such an improbable course as the following was possible in the President's case. The development of the aneurism might have been slower. The bullet was already encysted. The injured vertebra might have cast off its decaying debris, and it, together with the rest of the wound, might have healed. The President might have been pronounced well, and even have resumed his duties. Some day, suddenly, an agonizing cry of pain would have escaped him, and he would have fallen and died as though he were shot a second time! No one would have known the cause until an autopsy revealed the ruptured aneurism. It is but a piece of special pleading to say the wound was not mortal.

WILLIAM HUNT,
Senior Surgeon to the Pennsylvania Hospital.

To Readers and Correspondents.—The Editor will be happy to receive early intelligence of local events of general medical interest, or which it is desirable to bring to the notice of the profession. Local papers containing reports or news items should be marked.

CONTENTS OF NUMBER 468.

DECEMBER, 1881.

CLINICS.

CLINICAL LECTURE.

HOSPITAL NOTES.

MONTHLY ABSTRACT.

ANATOMY AND PHYSIOLOGY.

MATERIA MEDICA AND THERAPEUTICS.

MEDICINE.

MEDICAL NEWS.

THE

MEDICAL NEWS AND ABSTRACT.

VOL. XXXIX. No. 12. DECEMBER, 1881. WHOLE No. 468.

CLINICS.

Clinical Lectures.

ON SOME CATARRHAL AND MUSCULAR DISORDERS OF THE STOMACH.

A CLINICAL LECTURE.

By MORRIS LONGSTRETH, M.D.,

ONE OF THE ATTENDING PHYSICIANS TO THE PENNSYLVANIA HOSPITAL.

GENTLEMEN : In bringing this subject before you it is not so much my purpose to advance any new views of the pathology and treatment of the much-abused organ, the stomach, as it is to give a view of the subject from new aspects. I wish to bring prominently before you certain considerations of the causes and changes in stomach troubles and their requirements for treatment, which, while well known, have been too much put aside and forgotten. While the causes of which we will speak are not the only ones, they are, I think, very much more frequently the source of trouble than is usually acknowledged. These pathological alterations also, while generally spoken of as functional in character, and which exhibit such wide variations of functional disturbance, are yet always of essentially the same type, though exhibiting so widely different grades that their relationship is sometimes with difficulty recognizable, or is even wholly denied.

Let us first arrive at the proper basis for appreciating the points here alluded to, in brief point out the anatomical structure of this organ and the particular relation which its various parts have to its functional activity, both while at work and during periods of rest. The stomach has three coats ; the inner or mucous coat is an arrangement of epithelial cells resting on a basement membrane covering the submucous connective tissue. Numerous gland-tubes are everywhere found, whose office is to secrete the digestive fluid. The submucous connective tissue is a most important part of this coat, and changes in its condition, as we shall see later, bring about most harmful effects on the epithelium and the secreting glands. The next coat is composed of muscular tissue, the bands of which are divided off into compartments, as it were, by more or less broad septa of connective or fibrous tissue. This coat is, I believe, of first-rate importance in the digestive function, much more so than it usually receives credit, and to it I wish especially to call your attention. I believe that in many forms of indigestion it becomes very markedly changed. Let us remember that the bloodvessels which furnish the nutriment for the functional activity of the inner or mucous membrane coat, traverse this layer and the submucous tissue to reach their point of distribution. The peritoneal coat forms the covering of the stomach, but its anatomy and anatomical alterations, though important for certain other stomach diseases, are not of much concern to us in dealing with our present subject.

Let me insist again that the stomach is a mucous membrane organ, specialized, however, as is the rest of the digestive tract, by two factors dependent on its anatomical structure: first, the occurrence of glands supplying the digestive fluid; and second, an abundant and moderately powerful muscular structure in its walls, which is potent in the performance of digestion.

Having, therefore, gentlemen, to deal with a mucous membrane, let us see what forms of disease we should expect, from our knowledge of its structure and functions, to occur as results of deleterious causes acting on it, either from without or within. It is important, also, to call to mind the group of causes which we know are capable of affecting its action. And not the least important of the facts to be remembered are the anatomical and functional relations which this viscus holds to neighbouring organs. In speaking of the anatomical structure of the stomach no allusion was made to its nervous and vascular supplies, or to the arrangement of its lymphatics—all very important factors in its diseased conditions.

Starting, then, with the fact of a mucous membrane, the most important change that can come to it, excluding, of course, morbid new formation and traumatism, is in the amount of mucus which it secretes, whether this is an abatement or an increase from the normal. And with this fluctuation, of course go hand in hand alterations in the amount of the peculiar digestive juices which it is the special function of the stomach to supply.

We know of no morbid influence, and I do not think one can be conceived of, which, acting on a normal stomach, does not at once primarily change the amount of mucus which it secretes. Whether such influences propagate their effects through the nervous system, come from cold, in the sense of catching cold, or through changes in correlated organs, the effects are primarily evidenced by a changed blood supply, and a variation in the amount of this nutritive fluid condition a departure from the normal secretion, both in amount and in quality.

The type of stomach disease is, therefore, of a catarrhal character, and the chief phenomenon of the morbid process, whether we speak of it as inflammation, or a catarrh, or simply a mucous condition, is an alteration of the mucous secretion.

I show you here a man æt. 28, a weaver. The history he gave was that, five months ago, his stomach began feeling badly shortly after each meal, and continuing for some hours after. This feeling of discomfort, and it amounted on some occasions to pain, kept increasing in severity, and seven weeks ago another marked symptom was added, viz., vomiting. The contents of the stomach were rejected about half an hour after eating. He could give no particular account of the appearance of this material, further than that it seemed to be "just the food." About a week ago he was compelled from weakness to stop work. Two days ago, and again yesterday, he says he vomited a good deal of blood, of a fresh character and clotted, and after this felt very weak but not faint.

The amount of food taken during all this time was progressively lessened, and had been previously, and since the commencement of the symptoms, of a coarse character—the rough, ill-prepared food of a common workman boarding house.

Upon examination the man was seen to be pale, not strikingly, if at all, emaciated, but he was very far from showing the rounded fulness of a man of health. He complained of, not headache, as he says, but of a boring feeling through the front part of the head from temple to temple, and through the forehead above the root of the nose. His lips and gums are of a pale pink; the tongue is coated with a thin whitish layer, especially at the back and along the middle portion, reaching about two-thirds to the tip; the sides of the tongue are pale, much paler than other parts of the mucous membrane of the mouth; but mark well, gentlemen, the borders of the tongue, for you will see here something which I believe is of great importance as a sign of the condition of this patient's stomach, as well as perhaps of the intestinal mucous membrane. What do we see? The markings of the teeth. These fluted depressions correspond to the body of the tooth, and the prominent portions to the interstices between the teeth. We see that the intervals between the teeth are, in his case, considerable, and here where he has lost a tooth, we find no fluted depression but a larger projection of the tongue fitting into the interval. We note, too, that his teeth are in good condition.

He complains not of a bad taste in his mouth; though he says he has had a bitter taste at times, especially on waking in the morning; it is now rather a want of taste, and a feeling of cotton-wool or spider webs filling the mouth and fauces. Latterly his food has had no particular taste, and did not excite any relish.

The tendency to vomit since the blood appeared last on yesterday has lessened, but since then he has taken almost nothing, and that of a fluid nature and in very small quantities. However, there has been some nausea, and a little mucus was ejected.

The examination of the abdomen shows no distension, in fact you see it rather flat, and the feeling of it is that of moderate firmness. Percussion gives no especial evidence. You see that this examination has given him no great pain or distress. Let us examine the region of the stomach more particularly. Carefully with the finger tips I pass over the whole upper part of the abdomen. There is no greater sense of resistance or firmness than at other parts of the abdomen, and no especially painful spot to be detected; in fact while the epigastric region is the part where he has had the feeling of discomfort in the past, it has not been confined to this part, and there has been a lesser degree of it at times over other portions. So it is with the sensation. I am now giving him, he feels it most over the region from the umbilicus to the epigastrium and to the borders of the ribs, but there is also discomfort from pressure at other parts. A little nausea is excited by these manipulations, as well as by walking around.

Finally, we note that he has felt no pain at the back, and pressure does not occasion any unpleasant sensation.

The movements of the bowels have been irregular, always tending to sluggishness before the time he dates his present bad feelings; since then usually more closely confined, but this condition he tells you was interrupted by intervals when the movements were loose. So far as he can remember, the loose periods corresponded to occasions of greater pain and discomfort of the stomach. An evacuation of the bowels has occurred spontaneously —forty-eight hours since the vomiting of blood came—and he tells you it was moderately free and about as usual. There was no appearance of blood, no tarry matter in it, and subsequently none has been found. The matter passed was softly solid, varying in colour even in the same movement, but generally light gray, and oftentimes we have found scybalous masses not of great firmness, and these as well as the softer feces were mingled with mucus.

Finally, let me call your attention to the general air of the patient—one who has never had a comfortable lot in life, and is now feeling, as he has been for several months, greatly depressed and despondent. It is well painted on his face. Doubtless from the recent hemorrhage he has been alarmed, but at present dejection is the prevalent tone. This depression comes in the high and low, the rich and the poor, and entirely apart from the accidental cause of alarm which this man has suffered. When the gastric discomfort, sometimes a burning pain, has been most marked, then has he been the most dejected.

Let us now briefly endeavour to determine the cause and the sort of trouble with which we have to deal. This history shows no antecedent acute disease, no intemperance, no excesses of any kind which so frequently lead to stomach maladies. A diet of materials largely difficult of digestion, badly prepared, taken hurriedly, and often at times when tired and exhausted with work. Add to this bad hygienic surroundings both for living and for work. Here are conditions which depressed the patient's strength below the normal, rendering the stomach unequal to performing the function of digestion. The same diet and the same conditions of life are continued, and digestion is each day an incompleted process, and consequently progressively less and less nourishment is derived from the food. Strength for digestion, as well as for work, becomes progressively less. This condition of affairs may continue in a naturally strong man for a considerable time unnoticed, as it doubtless did in this patient, for he, too, was formerly strong.

The next step in the process is, however, taken. A residuum of undigested food, however small, cannot be left in the stomach daily without producing a distinct effect sooner or later. What is this effect? First, on the mucous membrane. The presence of food in the stomach, under normal condition, excites its circulation, and this flow of blood is followed by secretion, and the digestion of the alimentary matters, and the prompt emptying of the organ. Then normally succeeds the ordinary quiet flow of blood, unattended with secretory activity, except a slight flow of mucus.

How is it with the stomach of a strong person when from any circumstance, over-eating, fatigue, nervous emotion, digestion is incomplete or delayed? After an interval, during which there may or may not be symptoms of indigestion, the digestive act recommences, the process is completed, and all is over. At most the evacuation of the bowels on the following day does not occur at the usual hour, or, with some, two movements result. Like the gardener who has not planted and cultivated his crop aright, harvest and seedtime are delayed.

Let this occur habitually in the debilitated. The repeated attempts to recommence digestion of this residuum are as ineffectual as the original effort, and for the same reason. The constant reflow of blood in these attempts leads to change of function, and the continued presence of undigested food acts as an irritant. The flow of blood never ceases, the epithelial and glandular arrangements never have intervals of rest for repair, and the chemistry of digestion is less and less well performed.

The principal product of the mucous membrane activity—over-activity—is, under these circumstances, mucus, and we have arrived at the border land of inflammation. However, gentlemen, we will not give it any name, but be content to understand what has been going on in this man's stomach. This abnormal amount of mucus, present nearly all the time, has another very powerful influence for evil, viz., that the newly swallowed food is immediately immersed in a nearly inactive fluid, and thus surrounded the digestive juices are unable to act on it.

This is a process, therefore, you see, which is constantly promoting itself, and generally pushing forwards from bad to worse. Fortunately, this patient has largely escaped from one feature which so frequently comes in this condition, viz., the fermentation of the stomach contents. He has had no heartburn, no acid eructations, and but little bitter taste in the mouth. The formation of the various fermentation products, many of them of an acid character, develops and tends to render permanent the irritable condition of the mucous membrane, which I have described as bordering on inflammation, more intensely, and certainly more rapidly, than any other fault in digestion.

Now what has been the treatment? Let me say at once, as my remarks will already have shown, that we did not believe from the first that this man was suffering from gastric ulcer. The evidence of ulceration was never very strong, and if once we disbelieve the story of the hemorrhage, or at least discount the amount of blood, the indications of this condition almost disappear. You know how apt the laity are to exaggerate the amount of blood lost, and further than what the man himself told us, no evidence of hemorrhage appeared; no bloody or tarry stools were discovered. Whether ulceration actually occurred, or merely an escape of blood from the overdistended capillaries, no further hemorrhage came, and this, therefore, was not a symptom which had to be combated. The line of treatment which we proposed to follow was not inconsistent, at all events, with a possible ulceration, although perhaps we should have modified it had we been positive of its occurrence and of hemorrhage from that cause.

The man was put to bed, to rest, to quiet him, to quiet his circulation, to save his strength, and this was made absolute for a few days. Then he was gradually allowed to move about, and finally he was ordered exercise in the open air.

The food was entirely fluid—milk or milk and lime-water. Carbonic acid water is likewise useful. Later meat soup; beef tea is not well adapted to this condition. And still later the starchy foods and a little meat were cautiously added to his diet.

For the relief of pain and discomfort of the stomach, he was ordered dilute hydrocyanic acid. A blister, an inch square, was put on the epigastrium; not allowed to remain long; merely to redden the skin; and its position thus frequently changed. This was kept up for several days.

In the course of the week the patient was feeling much better, more cheerful; the sensation through the temples less constant, and not so discomforting; the tongue was cleaner but still coated at the back part, and looked fresher; the swelling not much changed; the bowels acted without assistance, but at long intervals; the upper part of the abdomen felt more comfortable; the vomiting, however, recurred again, but at much less frequent intervals.

The improvement was satisfactory, and was probably largely attributed to rest, the improved methods of feeding, and the better hygienic condition. A return to his former life would certainly have caused a renewal of his symptoms and discomforts. There was as yet no evidence of any essential change in the disturbed action of his mucous membrane. The tongue was still swollen, and furnished the ready index of a turgescence condition of the mucous membrane of the stomach. Is there nothing to be done to relieve or remove this condition beyond time and careful feeding, and these two means are very powerful, nay, essential, if a permanently good effect is to be produced?

Yes, I think there are means to be employed—medicinal agents, which in the large majority of cases are effective in changing the action of the mucous membrane. Without their use, too, time and dieting are ineffective. In making selection of these agents, great difficulty is encountered often in finding the proper ones. This difficulty arises, I think, mostly from the lack of means of distinguishing the exact or even approximate conditions we have to deal with—and by this I mean more especially the grade or stage to which the morbid process has attained. Perhaps, however, this difficulty is not greater than with a similar condition of the respiratory mucous membrane.

One of the most efficient which I have used is calomel, and there is, I believe, nothing new in its use for this purpose. Note, however, gentlemen, the dose in which we administer it to this patient. He is to take the twelfth of a grain, in sugar, every three hours. In this manner we will continue with it until it produces an effect. This effect is often arrived at speedily, but more commonly slowly, and for permanency of result, I think the more slowly the better. It may be continued in this dose for weeks without salivation. The sensations which the patient describes after its use—and here I am speaking of the result in very numerous other cases—are, first, a relief from the feeling that has been present in the stomach; the pain is gone, though often it comes again; the burning, if there has been any, lessens and disappears; the weight or dragging is slowly removed; and a sense of content pervades the usually rather despondent person; and in describing the effect the hands are spread or rubbed over the stomach as expressive of comfort. Nausea and vomiting usually disappear from the first, even after a few doses of the medicine. The temple pain leaves.

Second. The next effect, often not arrived at for a week or ten days, or even longer, is a sensation which is diffused over the abdomen. Some patients describe it as activity of the bowels; others that "something is leaving;" to others it is a griping, as though from diarrhœa; and to others the sensation is almost nil, though they continue to improve.

What changes are observable in the patient apart from his sensations? First, he looks more cheerful; and the colour of the face, often muddy in these cases, clears. Second, the tongue clears off still more and more, or perhaps in the most successful cases entirely. The appetite and taste return or improve, and it is often difficult to restrain the desire for food. The diet, however, must for some time be kept absolutely restricted; nourishment given frequently and in small quantities, and nearly all fluid. Third, the tongue becomes less swollen, and loses the markings of the teeth along its border. The bowels are at first unaffected, but later the movements become more regular. Oftentimes there is what may be looked upon as a critical discharge, an unloading. This fecal matter varies very greatly in character; the element most generally common is mucus, and after this removal of mucus the abdominal sensations are more comfortable. The movements of the bowels previously to this discharge—which does not take place at once, but may be continued through several days—may have been of a diarrhœal character, or at least irregularly so, become at once more natural in time, quantity. and quality. More usually the bowels, during the early stage of the treatment, and indeed before, are constipated. The removal of the accumulated masses, often dry and hard and scybalous, is a great source of relief, and after this digestion is much better performed. and the condition of the stomach improves.

In a word. I may say the result of the medicine given in these small doses, and even smaller ones often suffice, is regulative; if diarrhœa has been present, perhaps occasionally it disappears; if constipation, it is replaced by regularity.

Here is another man, still young, who looks old. Accustomed to hard work, he has now been overtaken with a stomach trouble which prevents labour. The immediate cause of his present trouble—or rather let us say what precipitated an exacerbation of his symptoms—was an apparent attack of intermittent fever. This malady you will not infrequently find does entail a catarrhal condition of the stomach. Why a mild attack of intermittent fever should do so more than other acute diseases, I can but offer this suggestion, viz., that during its continuance, the diet is generally less carefully regulated.

In this man's case I speak guardedly of his having had malaria at all, because I find a condition present in him which may have induced a mild febrile condition simulating intermittent; and then, too, quinine, we have found, did not relieve him. Stomach troubles of the sort this patient has suffered, you will find not infrequently produce pseudo-intermittent attacks.

Look at this man's mouth. There is not a tooth in the lower jaw capable of biting or grinding, and on the upper jaw it is not much better. I have not been able to get from him a satisfactory history of his stomach; he does not seem to be able to tell; but it is self-evident that digestion could not have been well performed, since the first step in its performance, with ordinary diet, was not effected. Food, not masticated, is a fruitful and frightful cause of diseased stomachs.

Whether this man suffered malaria or not is, so far as his stomach is concerned, a matter of small importance to ascertain; for, sooner or later, gradually or suddenly, he was sure, without extreme care, both as to mode of life and diet, to suffer disordered digestion and organic changes in his digestive apparatus.

With this imperfect history I shall not stop at the detail of his symptoms, but merely summarize the probable course of events and speak of the organic alteration with which we have to deal. The unmasticated food created the same inflammatory, or catarrhal, or mucous condition of the stomach as in the previous case. The partly digested pulpy food was forced into the bowel—this man, according to his account, had not suffered from weight, acidity, or vomiting previous to this attack, but had had an irregular diarrhœa.

Why this man's stomach has been able to void its contents, though undigested, promptly, and another man's has not, I am unable to say. Perhaps there was an original difference in the strength (muscular strength) of the two stomachs, and this man is evidently a more powerful man originally than the other. Certain it is, however, that some stomachs have this expulsive power more than others. I have witnessed the effects during life, and every one who is habitually examining stomachs microscopically will see differences in the muscular development in the various specimens.

The prompt expulsion of the undigested food saves the stomach from much damage, or, at least, discomfort, as it has saved this man. As he tells us, he was unconscious of any trouble with his stomach until this attack. Now, however, as you hear from him, as you may see, too, from his face, his stomach has given out. Watch me while I percuss the abdomen, and you can almost hear the evidence of the "giving out." The area of the tympanitic stomach clearness is, you see, greatly increased. We, therefore, have to do with a dilated stomach.

There is no evidence that the pyloric opening is obstructed. There is no tumour to be felt, and I could easily reach it through his thin abdominal walls. The onward flow of his food and of the secretions of the stomach is delayed not by obstruction, narrowing of the outlet, but by deficient expulsive power. We have been washing out the stomach with the siphon, and here I show you the character of the matters that have just been removed. Besides the acid smell, note particularly the amount of mucus, now of course largely diluted with water. You at once see, from the foul, unnatural condition of the cavity of the organ, how nearly impossible it would be for even fluids, like milk, to be digested, and how wholly impossible for a solid, like meat, which this man cannot chew, to be digested,— first, from the failure of the juices, secondly, because, from the dilated condition of the organ, the digestive churning does not take place.

I think you will agree with me when I say this stomach has given out —given out in one of its most essential particulars, viz., its muscular apparatus. There is nothing I can so well compare this stomach to as a heart with valvular disease. In spite of the damaged valve the increasing strength of heart-muscle, hypertrophy, is able to overcome the obstruction to the onward flow of blood, but as soon as the cavity dilates then result symptoms of impeded circulation.

Is there anything we can do for this condition?—and remember what it is we have to deal with—first the catarrhal mucous membrane, second the defective musculature. I don't know how much benefit we can afford this man, but will give you the line of treatment we shall follow, and report the result on a future meeting.

For the mucous condition I have already told what we want to do, but those remedies are hardly in place at this stage, and it is only later that we can avail ourselves of that plan of treatment. I don't think dropping a little pepsin or mineral acid is going to avail much. They would be lost in the sea which we have just removed from this man's stomach. A better plan, perhaps, would be to administer food already partially digested. The antiseptics and non-fermentatives will not be remedial, though they may conduce to the patient's comfort.

The chief condition here is the dilatation, and we will continue to remove the load from the organ by the siphon, and give the enfeebled muscular apparatus the most favourable opportunity to contract and regain its normal tone. Is there any medicinal agent, which, like digitalis for the heart, influences directly the stomach? We do not know of any, but the medicine which, in my hands, has done the most good is nux vomica and its alkaloids. Tincture of nux vomica has long enjoyed a reputation in stomach disorders of various kinds, but how much it will effect in this case I am not able to say.

In other cases where I have had to contend against the food delaying in the stomach, this remedy has proved very serviceable. And in patients suffering from the catarrhal trouble, but in whom no dilatation of the stomach is present, a combination of calomel and extract of nux vomica is exceedingly useful.

Let me now show you a specimen recently removed from a patient who had long suffered from a catarrhal inflammation of nearly the whole length of the digestive tract. This stomach will serve as a diagram, bringing out in an exaggerated manner the changes of which we have been speaking. We find it filled with thick mucus, adhering to this almost destroyed mucous membrane. The submucous connective tissue is very greatly increased. It is from the fibrous change of this portion, through which, you remember, the capillaries run, that the mucous membrane has been destroyed. Its supply of blood has been cut off. Look, too, at the muscular coat, how enormously hypertrophied. Some portions measure a quarter inch in thickness. For the present purpose of our illustration I need only state that this patient did not suffer from symptoms of retained and undigested food—there was no vomiting, no acidity, no heartburn, no eructation of gases. He had a sense of weight, and often burning at the epigastrium, but no other of the ordinary symptoms of dyspepsia. In fact all his food seemed to be hurried through the stomach unchanged, propelled onwards by the increased muscular force of the organ.

Let me sum it up. Stomach disorders, usually accounted functional, as well as others, are essentially catarrhal in their type. The presence of increased quantities of mucus is, in the early stages, one of the chief causes of the failure of digestion. This catarrhal condition, unless promptly checked, leads to organic changes, the most important of which affect first the submucous connective tissue, and secondly the muscular apparatus. The changes in the epithelial structures, of course the initial step in the catarrhal process, are much less important than the others, because complete restoration of the epithelium is more readily effected. The stomach, like the heart, exhibits its most disordered phenomena when the muscular apparatus is defective or begins to fail, and that the improvement or hypertrophy of this structure saves, at least temporarily, much discomfort to the patient.

The essential point in treatment is to change the morbidly catarrhal or mucous action of the stomach, and with the restoration of this action to the normal comes, and by this means alone, an improved quality of digestive fluid. In the presence of the mucus the digestive agents are not able to act. Finally, the addition to the dietary list of pepsin, mineral acids, antiseptics, and anti-ferments, however useful in temporarily assisting digestion, and however comfort-giving to the patient, is not curative.

CLINICAL LECTURE ON THE USE OF SPONGE PRESSURE AS A SURGICAL DRESSING.

Delivered at the Royal Infirmary, Manchester.

By JAMES HARDIE,
Assistant-surgeon to the Infirmary.

GENTLEMEN : A week ago to-day you saw me amputate the leg of a man, aged twenty-five, through the knee-joint, for gangrene, occasioned, as we believed, by embolism from cardiac disease. I dressed the stump in your presence, and I stated that I hoped to be able to-day to make some remarks to you on the special kind of dressing which I then employed. You will be interested to learn that from that time to the present the dressing has not been changed, and not only so, but that there has been no indication for a change of dressing. Not a stain of discharge has been visible; there has been no pain in the stump; the temperature has never been more than one degree above normal; and, in fact, the patient at our daily visit has invariably expressed himself as being quite well. Now, accustomed as you are to see the dressings of an operation changed almost daily, during at least the first week, this brief narrative cannot but be remarkable to you ; and as this is no solitary case of the kind, but one of many, I am desirous of drawing your attention to the lessons which may be learned from it.

It is scarcely necessary that I should justify myself when I say that the ordinary methods of dressing operation cases, whether antiseptic or otherwise, are by no means perfect. To many minds the mention of antiseptic dressings conjures up an infinite amount of trouble and pains and pitfalls. The trouble and pains we might leave out of account, as they soon become a second nature to us, though, for all that, we should be glad to be relieved of some part of them. But, then, every time the dressing is changed the patient is distressed, and there is also a risk of something going wrong. Certainly the handling of the part is not conducive to healing. Quite the reverse, for it may injure recent union. Possibly septic material may gain access to the wound, and the treatment so break down. But still, though everything goes on well, this repeated changing of dressing has to go on too ; and, as I have said, every surgeon admits that this is itself an evil, and the less often he has to do it the better is he pleased.

Let us consider, then, what are the conditions of a wound, say an amputation stump, which require this frequent change of dressing. Dressings are changed because of the amount of discharge which has escaped into them. Whence this discharge ? What does it consist of ? You cannot inflict a wound, however small, on any part of the body without the speedy occurrence of two phenomena —first and immediately the effusion of blood, and second and later the effusion of material for the healing of the wound. Now, this effused blood and so-called inflammatory material constitute the discharge we have to deal with. The former generally early ceases, but as regards the latter, its quantity and quality also depend greatly on the conditions of the part implicated. For instance, you know that in operations on the lip—as for harelip—when the edges have been brought accurately together no great amount of discharge takes place, and union of the wounded surfaces is soon accomplished. Here we have a tissue which is dense and firm, and affording little room for the accommodation of extra-vascular discharge. In the case of a wound under the eye, again, you know that it is followed by a large amount of swelling of the adjoining parts, and this is due to the fact that here the tissue is loose and cellular ; and we find, as a matter of fact, that under ordinary circumstances the healing of a wound in this region is accompanied by the filling up this loose cellular tissue by extra-vascular effusion. This takes place in the case of all wounds in this region to a greater or less extent, but the extent is much less in the case of a clean incised wound than in that of one which is contused or lacerated. If the surgeon has brought the edges of the wound accurately together, and the effusion be large in amount, a further train of phenomena will then probably ensue, which are referable to the tension of the tissues, and which you are all familiar with as acute inflammation. Bearing these cases in mind, then, and reverting to that of the amputation stump, we find that we have an extensive wound through tissues of various degrees of density, some being tough and unyielding and some loosely cellular, while the surfaces of the wound are so uneven that when brought together they afford a multitude of pockets and corners which in ordinary will be filled up by discharge of one kind or another. The wound being an extensive one, and there being considerable bruising of tissue by sawing the bone and ligaturing or twisting the vessels, it is to be expected that the discharges will be somewhat abundant in all cases ; and if the surgeon, forgetful of this, neglect to make due provision for its escape, disastrous consequences will probably ensue. Hence the use of drainage-tubes of one kind or another. But a drainage-tube cannot be looked upon as an innocuous body in a wound. However beneficent its purpose, it is to all intents and purposes a foreign body, and as such must create some degree of irritation, increasing by so much the amount of discharge. A drain, then, is to be regarded as an evil, except so far as it prevents a greater evil.   And here I may remark, somewhat parenthetically, that the present fashion of using drains almost up to the very closing of a wound, the end being clipped off every few days as the latter fills up, although interesting enough, has always appeared to me most inartistic.   Is there nothing better than this mere playing with nature?

We have now to consider the behaviour of those effused products—the blood and the inflammatory discharge—in regard to the healing of the wound.   The blood which remains between the flaps of course first coagulates, and a large proportion of the fluid portion early escapes from the wound.   The clot itself may either break down, and also entirely escape from the interior, as it probably does when it is large, or if small and spread out it may, as it is said, become "organized"—that is to say, it affords a nidus or support for the new interlacing tissue which ultimately unites together the opposed surfaces of the wound between which it lies.   Day by day it loses more of its serum, and becomes more firm, and ultimately, when it has been brought completely under the influence of the tissues, it is probably entirely absorbed.   It is unnecessary for us to consider whether, as some maintain, the clot itself ever contributes actively to the formation of the new connecting material.   This you have doubtless had fully discussed in your pathological studies.   Enough that it is unnecessary, and that it interposes itself as an obstacle to the immediate union of the cut surfaces, and thereby throws on them the necessity of elaborating a larger amount of new growth than would be otherwise required.   As regards the inflammatory material—the serum and plastic · exudation—you will understand that in such parts of the opposed surfaces as are somewhat firm and closely applied to each other, barely more is here thrown out than is actually required for immediate union, while into the loose cellular interspaces, and more particularly into the nooks and crannies of the wound, which have not become occupied by blood, a continuous flow of this discharge goes on, in daily decreasing quantity, until by the shrinking and consolidation of the plastic material, aided by the contraction and compression of the surrounding tissues, this material fills up all these interspaces with firm new growth.   This itself after a time becomes absorbed, but not always readily; and you will commonly find stumps which have recently healed somewhat full or rounded, and not seldom will you find the subcutaneous cellular tissue occupied by solid new material, which not only disappears slowly, but renders the stump incapable of support.   What we find, then, to take place in the healing of wounds is that parts which are closely in apposition unite by immediate adhesion, while those that are separated by an interval, and lack support, unite by the effusion of material from the vessels, a large proportion of which, being fluid, is thrown off as discharge, and that the greater this interval, and the looser the tissue, or, again, the greater the amount of damage done to the part by the operation, the larger is the amount of this discharge, and the longer does it continue.

Now, I do not suppose that any of you will pretend to think that this is a typical mode of healing.   What is a typical mode of healing?   Do we not regard the absence of all discharge and primary adhesion of the wound surfaces, as you sometimes see in small cuts, as the *beau idéal* of the healing process?   Cannot we do something more in our dressing of large wounds that their healing may imitate more closely this *beau idéal?*   This is what, as intelligent beings, we have to aim at.

I have described to you the method which nature adopts to unite wounds which are held together by sutures and dressings as usually applied, and I have insisted especially on the fact that the discharges we are accustomed to see from wounds are due to the exudation of material into the cellular tissue, and into the loose vacant spaces between the surfaces of the wound.   Now, I want you to understand and believe that this discharge is entirely unnecessary for the healing of wounds, and that, were it not for the existence of these loose interspaces which I have mentioned, it would cease to trouble us. This is the point, gentlemen, which it seems to me we have forgotten in our daily surgical life, but forgetting which we have altogether missed the mark to be aimed at in our labours towards perfecting dressings. We have laboured to invent dressings which shall absorb the discharges; what we have to do is to devise dressings which shall render discharges unnecessary. Consider for one moment what it is you desire to do in arranging a stump after amputation. Do you not wish to place the entire wound surface in intimate apposition, and to maintain it so until it has adhered together? If this be so, you can imagine how little likely your ordinary dressings are to carry out your intention. You leave large spaces in the cavity of the wound, particularly at the angle where the bone is situated, and you leave loose connective tissue everywhere, both of which will quickly become occupied by effusion from the vessels. Clearly what we have to do to secure our end is to employ dressings which will exercise a sustained external pressure sufficient not only to bring the opposite surfaces immediately into contact, but also for the time being to obliterate the cellular spaces of the connective tissue, and to prevent the subsequent effusion of blood or inflammatory products. As regards the arrest of hemorrhage in this way, your every-day experience will remind you that it is easily enough accomplished, and we need not therefore pause to consider it. But as regards the prevention of inflammatory exudation by pressure, some theoretical objections will probably occur to you. Remember, however, that we are not dealing with tissues already the seat of inflammatory disturbance, but with tissues in their normal condition, and that we seek to prevent even the first step in the process. That this may be accomplished by means of pressure, in certain cases, is evidenced by the treatment of fractures and sprains by the early use of judiciously applied compresses.[1]

For some years past I have been endeavouring to dress wounds with the end in view which I have enunciated, and, not to take up time with the record of failures, I find now that I have so far succeeded that I am justified in bringing my present method under your notice. I have found, that, by the use of sponge bandaged over the surface of the stump or other part, one is often able to secure perfect union of a wound without discharge and without the need of changing the dressing until the union is complete and sound. Sponge, as you know, is a material which is readily compressible into a very small bulk, and which also possesses a high degree of elasticity or resilience, so that pressure being removed it immediately resumes its former size and shape. Besides this, its highly absorptive properties, which are commonly taken advantage of in surgical practice, are well known to all of you. For these reasons sponge appeared to be a material well adapted for the purpose I had in view, first and chiefly, to exercise a continuous and elastic pressure, and, secondly, to absorb readily any discharge which might perchance escape from the wound. The sponge I have hitherto mainly employed has been the large-celled honeycomb, and the manner in which I used it is briefly as follows. Antiseptic precautions are used throughout. All bleeding points are carefully closed. Frequent sutures are inserted, so as to bring the edges accurately together. No drainage is used. The sponge, having been soaked in carbolic lotion, is squeezed tightly to expel every drop of superfluous moisture. The flaps of the stump are meanwhile carefully pressed together by the surgeon in order to force out any blood which may have collected during previous procedures. And let me urgently draw your attention to this point, since want of thought about it will frequently cause disappointment. However care-

---

[1] Vide Mr. Sampson Gamgee, Fractures of the Limbs; also Mr. R. Dacre Fox, Brit. Med. Journ., vol. ii., 1880.

fully you may close all bleeding points in an amputation, in nine cases out of ten you will find that after closing the wound some further hemorrhage will have taken place. Possibly this may be from the surface of the flaps; very probably it may be from the needle punctures. But be that as it may, to leave this blood in the cavity is to court failure. Diligently compress the flaps together with your fingers, and so squeeze out every drop of blood; then relax not your hold for an instant, but skilfully place the compressed sponge over the surface, and hold it, and as many more sponges as may be required to cover the entire surface, tightly with your fingers, while an assistant secures them in place with a bandage. Sometimes this is rather difficult to do, but by stitching sponges together some assistance may be gained. The bandage having been applied, you may now cover the whole with antiseptic gauze, or with tenax, with a piece of mackintosh over all; these again are secured with another bandage. In many cases it is advantageous to use as a bandage a piece of elastic webbing. This you may do if you choose.

Now, in the case of a wound of moderate size, as in the removal of small tumours or in operating for strangulated hernia, I am almost always satisfied that dressed in this way my care for it is at an end. A few weeks ago I removed a fatty tumour the size of an orange from the shoulder of a woman downstairs. The dressing was not removed until ten days afterwards, when the wound was found perfectly united and dry. So with three cases of hernia I have recently had: one a woman downstairs, and two men in the adjoining ward. In all these cases no further care was needed except the removal of the sutures when the dressing was taken off, ten days afterwards. There are also at the present time two cases of hernia in the men's ward dressed in this way. One was operated on two and the other three days ago. Both are perfectly well, and I advise those of you who are interested to look out for the removal of the dressing, probably on this day week.[1] In the case of large wounds, however, as in an amputation of a fleshy thigh, the case is very different. Here considerable skill is required in the proper application of the dressing, and doubtless in many instances only partial success will be attained. For example, there is a boy downstairs whose thigh I amputated in the lower third thirteen days ago on account of a smash of the leg. From the night of the operation he has been perfectly well. He has never once complained of pain, and, as you see from the chart, his temperature only once reached 100.2°, and has averaged 99°. This entire absence of symptoms caused me to think that on removing the dressing I should find complete union of the wound. On the tenth day, however, the nurse perceived some discharge oozing from the dressings. I therefore removed them, and found some bloody serum trickling from between two of the sutures. At one corner, also, there was some fulness perceptible. On further examination I found that a clot of blood had lodged here, the serum from which had been slowly oozing into the sponges, which, by the way, were wet and heavy. This case is an example of want of skill on my part in the application of the dressing. I do not altogether regret it, as it affords to you a good instance of the readily absorptive property of sponge.

---

[1] One of these men complained on the third day of pain in the region of the wound. This, it was thought, was probably due to flatus; but lest there might be any inflammatory action the dressings were changed. The wound was found perfectly sound, however, and an enema having been administered the uneasiness passed away. In both cases the dressings were removed seven days afterwards. In the case which had not previously been changed, everything was found as it should be—the wound healed, and the surface of the sponge covered with a little dried-up blood. In the other the lower end of the wound was somewhat inflamed; three-fourths of it, however, were perfectly sound.

You will now have an opportunity of seeing for yourselves the result, a week after operation, in another case of extensive wound—in the man, namely, whom I referred to at the beginning of my remarks. Although I should otherwise have left the case alone for some days, that the new tissue might be consolidated, I will take this opportunity of giving you ocular demonstration of how the case has thus far gone on. At present I cannot say with certainty what condition we shall find the stump in any more than any one of you can; but, judging from the general condition of the patient, I can form a pretty safe surmise that there can be nothing very far amiss. [Dressings removed.] You will see, gentlemen, how entirely satisfactory the progress of this case has been. There is not the slightest swelling or semblance of inflammatory action in any part. The flap is closely applied to the bone, showing everywhere the normal contour of the articular surface, the edges of the wound seem united, so that we will remove the stitches, and on the surface of the sponge lying over the wound there is only a little dark-coloured discharge, which has now nearly dried up.

I do not disguise from myself the fact that in this amputation (through the knee-joint) we have not a quantity of vascular tissue to deal with, nor the further fact that in this particular patient the blood pressure in the part is probably less than normal on account of probable plugging of the main arterial trunk. But, on the other hand, we have here a very uneven surface to cover with the flap, and under ordinary circumstances we should probably have had the depressions filled with a quantity of soft new material. And so the case may be regarded from this point of view as somewhat crucial.

I might refer to some other instances in which almost equally satisfactory results have been obtained, especially to two of amputation in the middle of the thigh which I performed elsewhere, and in which the pressure was effected through the medium of finely prepared oakum, not a very satisfactory material, as it lacks the resilience of sponge and soon becomes caked. Not having notes of the cases, however, I shall not draw on my memory for further remark.

Gentlemen, without the great fact of antiseptic surgery, to my mind the greatest achievement which has ever been accomplished in the whole history of the art, all this would be impossible.[1] Without it we pursue a course at best uncertain, and often dangerous, while with this safeguard we go on with secure step, and shall doubtless obtain more and more mastery over those abnormal occurrences which still too frequently impede our path.

Of other instances in which sponge pressure may profitably be had recourse to, I may have something to say on a future occasion.—*Lancet*, Oct. 15, 1881.

Hospital Notes.

Aneurism of the Subclavian and Axillary Artery treated by Galvano-puncture.

C. R., a seaman, aged sixty, was admitted into Mr. RANSFORD'S ward at the Royal Southern Hospital, Liverpool, October 21, 1879. Two years before he fell and injured his left shoulder. Nine weeks before admission he noticed pain for the first time in the left shoulder. About two weeks ago he noticed a swelling for the first time under the clavicle; and that his hand and fingers tingled and

---

[1] Yet possibly this is not the whole truth. It is known (*vide* Dr. Wm. Roberts, "On Spontaneous Generation, and the Doctrine of Contagium Vivum") that septic germs are harmless in the living tissues, and it is thus possible that the careful prevention of useless exudation into a wound may place it in a condition which will enable it to resist their further development even in the absence of antiseptic measures. But in spite of that, the possible collection of discharge through the inadequacy of our dressings will always render the use of antiseptics a desirable precaution.

felt numbed ; his left arm was also colder than the right, and had shooting pains down the arm. These symptoms gradually increased, and the swelling got larger and the arm became weaker. There was no history of syphilis.

On admission, he had a pulsating tumour extending from the left clavicle downwards a distance of four inches. On auscultation, a loud bruit was heard from the clavicle to below the level of the tumour. The left shoulder and arm were œdematous, and colder than the right : and there were shooting pains down the left arm, and over the shoulder-blade numbness and tingling of the fingers. Pulsation extended above the clavicle. The pulse in the left wrist was much quicker and weaker than in the right. Left arm ten inches round ; right nine inches. Ordered iodide of potassium, five grains three times a day, and hypodermic injection of morphia, one-fifth of a grain at night.

Nov. 5th. The tumour seemed to be rapidly increasing in size. Thirty grains of iodide of potassium were given three times a day. In the afternoon two insulated needles connected with the two poles of a constant current battery were introduced into the tumour ; ten cells were employed. The kneedles were kept in for rather more than thirty minutes, whilst the man was under the influence of ether. During the afternoon and evening the pain in the shoulder was about the same as before. Ice applied to the tumour. On the 6th, the pulse was 84, temperature 97°. Pain in the shoulder no less. No apparent change in the size and consistence of the tumour ; pulsation in it and the radial quite as strong. No redness round the needle punctures. No headache. On the 7th he passed a good night after hypodermic injection. Solid feeling around both punctures and tumour, otherwise it appeared the same. Pulsation quite as strong. He went on in this way without much change till the 15th, when two needles were introduced, about three inches in depth ; fifteen cells were used, for about forty-five minutes. Ice omitted. Pulse in the evening 112, temperature 99°. Pulse and temperature remained about the same till the 18th, on which day the pulse was 120, temperature 98.4° ; 19th, pulse 110, temperature 98.4°. On the 20th the pulse was 116, temperature 98.6°. For the last few days there had been great numbness in the hand. Hand and arm swollen and powerless. Red blush over arm. The tumour was in the same condition ; no signs of consolidation. Pain was very severe at the back of the shoulder-blade at night. Evening, pulse 130, temperature normal. Ordered one grain of extract of opium every four hours, as the hypodermic injections caused irritation of the skin at the point of insertion. On the 22d there was puffiness round the shoulder and axilla ; arm still painful. Pulse 120, temperature 99.2°. On the 26th he had severe pain during the night, and this morning at the lower border of pectoralis major. Swelling in axilla extending down the side. Ordered fifteen grains of chloral hydrate and twenty grains of bromide of potassium at bedtime. Arm strapped to the side. Pulse 120, temperature normal.

Dec. 3. Restless during the night, shouted and got out of bed ; quite awake at the time. In the morning pupils were not equal, left smaller than right, neither acted well to light, sight of left eye not so good as right. Pains in arm and shoulder not so severe as usual. Tumour still increasing. Has slight cough. On the 4th the operation was repeated with twenty cells without much hope of doing any good as only negative results had followed the former operations, but the good results obtained by Dr. John Duncan, of Edinburgh, encouraged another trial. For a day or two the tumour felt firmer, but this was only transient, and all melted away again. On the 9th the chloral was increased to twenty-five grains at bedtime, pain was very severe, and without chloral he was very restless. The tumour was gradually increasing. On the 17th the house-surgeon reported that there was no pulsation in the tumour, and he feared rupture of the sac of the aneurism. On examination pulsation was hardly to be felt, the tumour was more diffuse; no pulse could be felt in the left radial; pulsation felt best at the inner side of the tumour, elsewhere hardly to be made out. Ptosis of left eye. Left pupil still contracted more than right. The arm was very œdematous, small gangrenous spots were visible on the back of the hand and knuckles, small slough over spine of scapula, loss of sensation three inches above the elbow. Intercostal spaces filled on expiration, sank in on inspiration. Breath-sounds were heard all over the chest. Left side of chest was very much flattened. Temperature 101.2°, pulse 124. In the afternoon he had a sudden attack of dyspnœa with profuse sweating. This passed off in about an hour. On the 18th he was delirious dur-ing the night; in the morning the breathing was quiet; no delusion; pulse felt again in the left radial; in the evening he had severe pain, and was ordered twenty minims of sedative solution of opium at once; pulse 100. Temperature, morning 96°, evening 100°. On the 19th he passed a fair night; less pain this morning: the skin in axilla red and inflamed; not much change in the tumour since the 17th, beyond that the skin was more distended, and the blood seemed to be finding its way under the skin down the side of the chest; no change in pulse and temperature. On the 20th a bleb formed on the front of the wrist; the hand looked very dusky; the patient appeared brighter. Pulse 100, morning and evening. Temperature: morning 99.4°, evening 101°. On the 24th, the house-surgeon reported that in the morning oozing of bright arterial blood took place from the axilla; parts very sloughy; stopped with a pad of lint steeped in a solution of perchloride of iron, and on moving the patient a large stream of dark blood jutted out from the slough over the scapula; this was also stopped as above, and with tenax. The patient died the next day.

Necropsy, the day after death.—It was noticed that the chest-walls at the upper and outer part were very much pushed in, but there were no signs of any absorp-tion or erosion of the ribs. On carefully dissecting the tumour it was found to involve the whole of the third portion of the subclavian, and the first and second parts of the axillary artery. On dividing it vertically it measured seven inches in diameter in its long axis, and four and a half antero-posteriorly. The anterior portion of the sac was lined with laminated clot, varying in depth from one to two inches; this in one or two places had broken down and formed small abscesses, apparently at the points of puncture; the sac had given way at the lower portion, and communicated with the slough in the axilla. Posteriorly the aneurism ex-tended back to the scapula, and the tissues behind were infiltrated with dark blood, but there did not seem to be any rupture of the sac in this direction, and there was no direct communication with the slough over the scapula. The aorta and the larger vessels were atheromatous, but the other organs of the body seemed as sound as could be expected in an old man of sixty.

Remarks by Mr. RANSFORD.—It was only after many consultations with my colleagues that I decided to try galvano-puncture. The only other alternatives seemed to be to leave him to his fate, or amputation at the shoulder. Dr. John Duncan, in a paper published in the *Edinburgh Medical Journal*, April, 1866, gave fifty cases treated by galvano-puncture, of which twenty-three were cured. These results inclined me very strongly to give it a trial in this case, but I think the lesson it teaches is that in an aneurism of such magnitude galvano-puncture alone is not enough. I should in any similar case be disposed to recom-mend amputation about the shoulder as a preliminary step, and combine it after-wards if necessary with galvano-puncture; or, as in Mr. Heath's plan (see the *Lancet*, Jan. 31, 1880, page 168), the simple introduction of plain steel needles, which were left in some time. This case also illustrates some of the drawbacks so well stated by Dr. Duncan—namely, that, "1st. It is inherently uncertain, liable to cause relapse by the melting of the coagulum, or inflammation by its sudden deposition. 2dly. It is very liable to set up inflammation in the walls and

MONTHLY ABSTRACT.

Anatomy and Physiology.

Influence of the Nerves of the Tympanic Cavity on the Vascularity and Secretion
of its Mucous Membrane.

E. BERTHOLD summarizes the results of a number of experiments as follows: first, that lesions of the trigeminus, both at its trunk and its roots, provoke inflammatory symptoms in the middle ear; but there are differences in the sequels, according to the location of the lesion. The greater intensity of the inflammatory affection occurring after intracranial division may be explained by the prolonged duration of the inflammation. After semilateral division of the medulla oblongata the animals die too quickly to permit the inflammation to reach its height. Still more noteworthy than the difference in the intensity of the phenomena, is the condition of the bulla of the uninjured side. Differing in this respect from intracranial division, there was found as a result of semilateral division of the medulla oblongata almost invariably some secretion in the bulla of the sound side. Inclined though we were at first to regard this disturbance in the lining membrane of the middle ear as a sympathetic one, we still found no reason for the fact that such a sympathetic inflammation never occurred after injury to the trunk of the trigeminus, and we must leave it an open question whether perhaps a crossing of fibres takes place in the medulla, and a part of the trigeminus fibres extends to the middle ear of the other side. The acceptance of the latter assumption would make it self-evident that a lesion confined to one half of the medulla oblongata would affect both ears in the same manner, although in varying degree.

The investigations taught us, moreover, that the sympathetic must be regarded as a vaso-motor, and, according to the extent of our experiments, as an exclusively vaso-constrictor nerve of the entire ear, because a distinct narrowing of the auricular vessels was always observed after irritation of the sympathetic. On the other hand, we obtained negative results respecting the state of the vessels after irritation of the trigeminus as well as after injuries to the sympathetic, trigeminus, and glosso-pharyngeus. Prussak has already called attention to the fact that the constrictor action of the sympathetic, after its irritation, should lead us to suppose a dilatation of the vessels of the ear after paralysis of this nerve; the more so, as we know that division of the sympathetic is followed by filling of the arteries in other parts of the head. However, we fully concur with Prussak that the experiments have not borne out this supposition. Contrary to our expectation, the mucous membrane of the middle ear remained invariably pale, even when the division of the sympathetic had preceded the examination of the drum cavity by several days.

The most surprising result of our investigations, however, was the negative state of the middle-ear vessels both after irritation and after paralysis of the trigeminus, for soon after division of this nerve neither dilatation nor contraction of the middle-ear vessels could be observed. Nor could we, as stated before, observe any visible alteration in the fulness of the vessels by irritating this nerve. Although we could ascribe to the trigeminus neither vaso-constrictor nor vaso-dilator qualities, while division of its trunk or injury to its roots was regularly followed by inflammatory phenomena in the middle ear, it appeared reasonable to acknowledge, in this case, the influence of the neurotomy as a merely trophic one, that is to say, to refer it to the existence of special trophic nerves. If we compare the process in the drum cavity with the so-called trophic keratitis, the phenomena in the drum cavity—protected as it is from injurious atmospheric influences—permit our drawing a more unambiguous conclusion in regard to the existence of these nerves—hitherto always considered doubtful—than the consequences of division of the trigeminus in the eye, which certainly permit of several interpretations. A traumatic otitis after division of the trigeminus could not be thought of, for reasons stated.—*Archives of Otology*, Sept. 1881.

—

Electrical Tetanus.

M. RICHET has found that strong and repeated electrical stimulation will cause, n rabbits and dogs, a tetanus comparable in its results to the traumatic form, and therefore of some practical pathological importance. As a rule rabbits die from asphyxia, and dogs from hyperpyrexia. The asphyxia in the rabbit is due to the arrest of respiration in consequence of the tetanus of the thoracic muscles, and death may be prevented by artificial respiration. Death occurs much more rapidly than in asphyxia from obliteration of the trachea. The latter only kills in three or four minutes, but the electrical tetanus kills by asphyxia in one minute; this rapidity of death is ascribed to the absorption of oxygen and liberation of carbonic acid during the general muscular tetanus. Prolonged applications may, however, exhaust the muscles, so that the contraction of the thorax may cease, and it is even said that respiration may recommence during the passage of the current, probably by the agency of muscles which have not been tetanized. Animals so exhausted cannot be killed by strychnine, if the application of electricity is continued. A rest of a few seconds permits the current to be again effective. In the dogs the electricity employed was not sufficiently powerful to arrest respiration, and death was due to the elevation of temperature. The ascent of the thermometer was extremely rapid, sometimes three-tenths of a degree per minute, so that after the tetanus had lasted for half an hour the lethal temperature of 111° or 112° F. was reached. This pyrexia is due entirely to the muscles, and not to the nervous system. Chloralized dogs, in which reflex action is abolished, present the same elevation of temperature, which occurs, however, a little less rapidly. The proof that the increased body-heat is the cause of death is furnished by the fact that if the animal is kept cool by artificial means, it may bear for more than two hours extremely strong currents, which cause severe tetanus, without dying for some days. The capacity for generating this great temperature under electrization does not disappear even after a prolonged application, and it is not influenced by previous fasting for two or three days. The curve of the rise presents at first a gradual ascent, which becomes more and more rapid, especially after the temperature of 101° is passed. Usually death occurs when a temperature of 112° is attained, but in some cases it reached 112.5° and $113.3.^\circ$ If the temperature did not rise above 110° death did not ensue on the same or the following day; after this point, however, although death may not be immediate, it occurs within twenty-four hours. The electrization does not cause the acceleration of respiration, but this is due to the increased temperature. The thermic dyspnœa commences at 105°. and at 111° the breathing is so frequent that it is hardly possible to count it, and so feeble that scarcely any air enters the thorax. M. Richet believes that these experiments justify the hope that by treating the asphyxia and pyrexia death may be prevented in ordinary tetanus. There is one difference between the facts he observed and traumatic tetanus, which suggests important differences between the two forms—namely, that in the latter the temperature continues to rise after death. This was not noted in their experiments, and it suggests that the cause of the pyrexia, and therefore its treatment, may not be the same in the two sets of cases. Moreover, death may occur in ordinary tetanus from exhaustion, without hyperpyrexia. Recognizing this difference, however, the facts ascertained certainly indicate the importance of keeping down the temperature in those cases in which it exhibits a tendency to rise to the extreme height often attained.—*Lancet*, Sept. 17, 1881.

Materia Medica and Therapeutics.

Action of Berberin.

Berberin has been recommended in Italy as a remedy for enlargement of the spleen consequent on malarial disease; and its mode of action has been carefully studied by Dr. A. Curci, who has made with it a series of experimental, microscopic, and spectroscopic researches. An analysis of his memoir is given in *Lo Sperimentale* for August. He describes first its local and afterwards its general action. The local action of berberin, he says, may be said to consist in irritation and subsequent induration of the tissues. Thus the blood coagulates in the capillaries to which it is applied; the red corpuscles become small, nucleated, granular, and have pale outlines; the muscular fibres lose their distinctness; sometimes the striated fibres become larger and more marked, then lose the transverse striæ, and, the muscular substance coagulating at intervals, special enlargements are produced; the smooth fibres show distinct nuclei and become tortuous. All the tissues are hardened and strongly coloured by berberin; their vital properties are also increased, and there are active proliferation of connective tissue and increase of fibrous tissue. Berberin produces contractions of the intestine, secretion of mucus and of intestinal juices, and tonicity of the tissues. In studying the general effects of berberin, Dr. Curci first tried its effects on healthy animals. In all classes of animals, it produces prostration, muscular relaxation, adynamia, collapse, progressive lowering of temperature, at first increased and afterwards diminished frequency of the heart's action and of respiration, serous diarrhœa, albuminuria, fatty degeneration of the kidneys, and complete anorexia. Hypodermic injections produce these phenomena rapidly, and, if repeated, are followed by death. On the other hand, the administration of berberin by the mouth requires a larger dose for the production of the symptoms; diarrhœa and renal changes are always absent, and death seldom occurs. Towards the end, when sensibility is somewhat diminished, there are tonic and clonic spasm. The temperature is at first lowered, then returns to the normal, and finally falls as death approaches. The vomiting is constant and painful, preceded by contractions; and the vomited matter consists of food and mucus. The abdomen is painful; and the dysentery at last becomes colliquative. The urine is yellow, acid, and albuminous. *Post-mortem* examination only shows diastole of the heart and fatty degeneration of the cortical portion, with hyperæmia of the kidneys. Spectroscopic examination of the blood indicates diminution of its oxidizing and nutrient powers. Berberin reduces the temperature, not through the intervention of the vaso-motor nerves, but by its direct action on the tissues, through which action it also indirectly modifies the blood. With regard to the action of berberin on the spleen, Dr. Curci has found that its administration to animals is followed by an enlargement of that organ. Hence he concludes that, in cases where an enlarged spleen has become reduced under the use of berberin, this has not been due to contraction of the capsule of the spleen, but to the destruction of the malarial miasmatic agent, which is atrophied by berberin in the same way as other histological elements.   Dr. Curci concludes from his experiments that berberin may be found useful: 1, in microscopy, as a means of colouring tissues and rendering them resistant; 2, in the treatment of atonic gastro-intestinal catarrh, of chronic dysentery, of wounds and ulcers (in which it does not cause suppuration, and stimulates the activity of the tissues), and of chronic conjunctivitis.   Its action on the splenic enlargement of malaria is doubtful, and requires to be studied; and it would appear to be an excellent antipyretic, and to be a remedy against the decomposition of hæmoglobin.—*London Med. Record*, Oct. 15, 1881.

—

Influence of Anæsthetics on the Heart, and on the Antagonism of Poisons.

Dr. RINGER has recently published two papers (*Practitioner*, June and July, 1881) which throw considerable light on the action of anæsthetics on the heart, and incidentally on the vexed question of antagonism.   The observations were made with Roy's apparatus, a description of which will be found in Dr. Roy's paper "On the Influences which Modify the Work of the Heart" (*Journ. of Physiol.*, vol. i. p. 452).   Considerable difficulties have hitherto been experienced in working this apparatus, arising chiefly from the inconvenience of having to obtain fresh blood for each experiment.

Dr. Ringer finds that the desiccated defibrinated bullock's blood, imported by Parke, Davis & Co., of Detroit, Michigan, answers the purpose admirably.   It can be readily obtained, as it is frequently used for enemata in cases of gastric ulcer, etc.   For physiological purposes it is dissolved in distilled water, and then diluted with saline, one part of blood-mixture being used to two of salt solution. In each experiment three ounces were used, the same blood being employed in the same series of observations, so that the poison and its antidote were intermixed.

Chloroform acts powerfully on the ventricle of the frog's heart.   Like lactic acid, muscarin, and jaborandi, it lessens both the height and duration of the trace until, finally, the heart is arrested in diastole.   In one experiment, a minim of chloroform nearly stopped the ventricle; and, when the heart had almost ceased beating, the addition of two ten-minim doses of strong solution of ammonia at once restored its action, until the contractions became almost as powerful as at first.   The additions of ten drops of chloroform again stopped the heart.   This shows the powerful paralyzing effect of chloroform, and demonstrates most conclusively the mutual antagonism existing between chloroform and ammonia.

It is clear that chloroform does not arrest the ventricle by stimulating the inhibitory apparatus, for the portion of the heart employed contains no inhibitory nerves.   Chloroform clearly paralyzes the muscular substance of the heart, for it is well known that the muscular tissue will beat rhythmically without the presence of nervous ganglia.   It is evident, therefore, that, did the chloroform paralyze only the ganglia of the ventricle, the ventricle itself would still continue to beat.   Further experiments made with the lower half only of the ventricle render this certain, the ganglionless and nerveless portion being affected in exactly the same way as the whole ventricle.

Atropia does not antagonize the action of chloroform on the ventricle; nor will the previous addition of atropia prevent the action of the chloroform.   Ethidene-dichloride affects the ventricle in exactly the same way as chloroform. Ether affects the heart in a far less degree than either chloroform or ethidene dichloride.   Large doses accelerate the heart's action, and make each beat a little weaker; but the amount of work done is considerably greater, the increased frequency more than compensating for the diminished force of each contraction. Ammonia and ether, like chloroform and ammonia, are mutually antagonistic as regards the whole ventricle. Bromide of ethyl arrests the ventricle, acting on the muscular substance. It is far less powerful than chloroform, but more poisonous than ether.

Iodoform and ammonia are mutually antagonistic, as shown by their action on the ventricle. A fifth of a grain of iodoform nearly stopped the heart, and then ten minims of a one per cent. solution of strong ammonia restored the contractions, which were again arrested by another dose of iodoform. This was repeated on the same heart three successive times.

The importance of these observations cannot be over-estimated, throwing as they do a new light on the whole subject of antagonisms. ROSSBACH (Pfluger's Archiv, Band xxi. Heft 1, p. 1, 1879) contends that drugs are never mutually antagonistic. He maintains that, when a tissue is paralyzed by one poison, it is impossible to stimulate it by another. For instance, whilst atropia, he says antagonizes pilocarpine, pilocarpine cannot antagonize atropia; atropia paralyzes the sweat-apparatus, and pilocarpine is no longer able to stimulate it into action. He admits that after small doses of atropia pilocarpine can produce sweating, and this he explains by assuming that atropia paralyzes first the nerve of the sweat-gland, and later the gland-apparatus itself. After a small dose of atropia the nerve only is paralyzed, and then the pilocarpine can still stimulate the glandular cells; but a large dose of atropia paralyzes the cells also, and then pilocarpine is powerless.

Dr. Ringer's recent experiments demonstrate the fallacy of this argument. The lower half of the ventricle consists of only one substance, muscular tissue, so that the antagonism cannot be due to an action on different structures.—*London Medical Record*, Oct. 15, 1881.

Action and Use of Citrate of Caffein as a Diuretic.

Dr. DAVID BRAKENRIDGE (*Edin. Med. Journ.*, August, 1881) makes the following remarks respecting the action of citrate of caffein as a diuretic. 1. It fails to produce any increase in the amount of the urine in cases in which the renal epithelial cells are diseased—as, *e. g.*, in the early stages of desquamative nephritis —even when vascular and saline diuretics produce a considerable increase. 2. It fails to do so in cases of cardiac dropsy in which, from physiological conditions, we may conclude that the glandular epithelial cells are already doing a maximum amount of work, or are exhausted by transference of work to them from the filtering apparatus. 3. When it acts as a diuretic it increases not only the amount of water passed, but also the amount of urea very markedly, if it have previously been abnormally lowered. 4. Its action is strikingly complementary of that of digitalis; so that, in cases in which both given alone have failed, the two administered together, according to the view suggested, have produced very striking diuretic results. 5. This increase in the amount of the urine may be independent of any increase in the general arterial blood-pressure, sufficient to account for it on any theory of general or local blood-pressure. 6. The combination of digitalis with citrate of caffein causes a striking rise in the amount and percentage of urea, which cannot be explained on any filtration hypothesis. How citrate of caffein stimulates the renal glandular epithelial cells, is still a matter of conjecture. Probably its action is similar to that of jaborandi or pilocarpin on the salivary and sweat glands. In a future paper he hopes to show that the latter substances have a diuretic action like that of caffein. On the other hand, caffein has been observed in exceptional cases to cause both sweating and salivation.

From the foregoing considerations and his whole experience of this drug, Dr. Brakenridge deduces the following practical conclusions regarding the employment of citrate of caffein as a diuretic.   1. In cases in which the renal glandular epithelium is diseased, is already doing a maximum amount of work, or is exhausted, this drug is unsuitable and should not be administered.   2. During recovery from acute desquamative nephritis, when renewal of the renal epithelium has reached a certain point, citrate of caffein, cautiously administered, has appeared to him to have had a decidedly beneficial effect; possibly in such cases it may exert a trophic as well as a secretory stimulant influence.   3. In cases in which the arterial blood-pressure is tolerably normal, citrate of caffein should be given alone, not in combination with a vascular diuretic.   4. In cases of cardiac disease, with absence of compensation, and resulting diminution in the blood-pressure and flow of blood through the kidney, general dropsy, and transference of work in the kidney, from the filtering to the secreting structures, a vascular diuretic, such as digitalis, must be employed in the first place to restore those conditions in the kidney which are essential to the action of citrate of caffein. For this purpose digitalis should be administered for a short period, one to three or four days, before commencing the citrate of caffein.   5. Citrate of caffein, employed in this manner, in conjunction with digitalis, which for obvious reasons, must not be discontinued when the caffein is commenced, is a diuretic of extraordinary power, acts with great rapidity, and is especially valuable in this respect, that it causes a great increase in the elimination of urea (and probably of other solids) as well as of water.   6. It must, however, be remembered that special and powerful stimulation of any gland, especially if it be in a state of malnutrition, may, and usually does, lead, sooner or later, to exhaustion, and must, therefore, be regarded as at best a temporary expedient and of limited duration.   7. For this reason very large doses of citrate of caffein should be avoided.   He has found three grains administered once, twice, or three times daily, according to the circumstances of the cases, amply sufficient for all purposes.   8. Whenever the beneficial effects of the drug have been attained, we should at once endeavour to render them permanent by suitable diet, well selected chalybeate and other tonic remedies, or other remedial measures indicated by the special circumstances of the case.   2. Finally, in cases of very great ascites, in which the blood-pressure in, and the flow of urine through, the kidneys is interfered with by pressure on the kidney and the renal artery and vein, and in which the pressure of the urine within the capsules is increased by pressure on the ureters, neither vascular nor secretory diuretics, alone or combined, can act efficiently until the pressure of the ascitic fluid has been got rid of.   10. The citrate of caffein may be administered either in pill or in solution.—*Lond. Med. Record*, Oct. 15, 1881.

--

Papaya and Papain.

In one of the sessions of the Academy of Sciences in Paris, in August last (*Berliner Klinische Wochenschrift*, Aug. 1881), M. BOUCHUT made some communications regarding the sap of a plant growing in Brasilia, whose botanical name is Carica Papaya, which, according to investigations made by him, with the assistance of Professor Wurtz, possesses distinct digestive and peptonifacient properties.   The sap, which is obtained by incisions made into the bark of the plant, and still more so the essential principle prepared from the same, which has been named papain, if for a certain time left in contact with albuminates, raw meat, fibrin, glue, milk, etc., will enter upon combinations which present all the characteristics of assimilable peptone.   Croupous membranes, ascarides, tapeworm, were changed in a similar manner, even outside the body.

The statements made at that time Bouchut recently revised and enlarged, reporting experiments, which show that this vegetable pepsin exercises its digestive power even upon living tissues. One gramme of a ten per cent. solution of papain, or one gramme of a solution of the sap, in the proportion of 1.5, injected into the brain of an animal, with a Pravaz syringe, proved to have effected a complete peptonic change in the tissue twenty-four hours after the operation. Upon living muscular tissue the same material injected acted in such a manner that, twenty-four hours after, a soft, pulpous, and gelatinous substance is found in the injected locality. Further injections of the same kind were made upon the cervical glands. After three days, which were characterized by great pain and high fever, the injected glands were found to be softened and turned into abscesses, which could be lanced and emptied of their contents.

In one case of cancer of the breast, and in another of scirrhus of the inguinal glands, in the clinic of Professor Pean, in the Hospital St. Louis, softening and disintegration of the diseased parts was induced by treatment with papain. Some of the fluid contained in the softened growth was afterwards subjected to chemical analysis in the chemical laboratory of the medical faculty, by Professor Henning, and proved to be pure peptone with all its characteristics. According to one of the investigations, 47 grammes of the fluid contain 2.91 grammes of albumen, which again contained 0.565 of peptone after being dried at a temperature of 110°. The same result was reached by other investigations, and confirmed by all chemical tests. All the cases like those formerly mentioned were accompanied by great pain and high violent fever.

In conclusion, Bouchut reports an experiment on a living frog. The animal was partially stripped of its integuments, and then completely dipped in a papain solution. After twelve hours, the animal was dead; after twenty-four hours partially digested, and after two days nothing but the skeleton was left.

Vegetable pepsin, consequently, digests living tissue as well as it digests and destroys dead material outside of the body.—*Medical Herald*, Oct. 1881.

—

Hypodermic Injection of Citrate of Iron.

An abstract of an observation made by Dr. CIARAMELLI on the hypodermic injection of iron is given in *Lo Sperimentale* for July. A patient under his care had anæmia of an extreme degree, the affection having lasted several years. For four months he was treated with good food, exercise, pure air, decoction of cinchona, and preparations of iron, without effect. No iron could be detected in the urine; from which Dr. Ciaramelli concluded that the iron salt did not pass beyond the hepatic circulation, but was eliminated with the bile. He then injected daily from two to three grammes of a solution of one gramme of ammonio-citrate of iron in twenty grammes of distilled water. After thirty days the rose tint returned to the patient's face, all the symptoms of severe anæmia being at the same time relieved. On chemical analysis, iron was found abundantly in the urine. Dr. Ciaramelli says that this one case is not enough to serve as the foundation of general principles, but it indicates a line of therapeutic research which may be of great practical value.—*London Med. Record*, Oct. 15, 1881.

—

Hypodermic Injection of Water in the Treatment of Pain.

In the *Gaceta Medica* of Venezuela, Dr. PONTE relates his experiences in several instances in which he employed water hypodermically for the relief of pain. The first case was that of a boy who was suffering from an attack of intercostal neuralgia, so severe as almost to endanger the life of the patient by inter-

ference with respiration. Not having any morphine with him, the author determined to work upon the imagination of the sufferer by injecting pure cold water
over the location of the pain, a procedure which, much to his astonishment, was
followed by permanent relief. Impressed with this fact, Dr. Ponte resolved
upon further experiments. The next case was one of toothache. In order to
eliminate the imaginative element, he informed the patient of the treatment to
be employed, for the execution of which permission was rather reluctantly given.
An injection practised upon the side of the face nearest to the pain was followed
by considerable ardor, but in less than a minute the odontalgia had subsided.
Animated with these results, he employed cold water injections in a variety of
different pains, always with happy issue, even in cases where morphine had been
the drug previously administered. Another patient had been suffering nine years
from intense gastro-intestinal neuralgia, which baffled all remedies. The pain
came on after meals, and its violence was such as to cause her frequently to faint.
When first seen by the writer, she was utterly prostrated. Two injections relieved the pain, and subsequent tonic treatment restored her to perfect health.
Several hundred cases have been treated in the manner described, with good
results. No explanation is given as to the action of the remedy.—*Med. Record,*
Oct. 8, 1881.

Medicine.

On a Peculiar Form of Disease arising from Milk Contamination.

At the meeting of the British Medical Association on August 4th, Mr. R.
BEVERIDGE, M.B., reported that on April 4th, an outbreak of a peculiar form
of disease occurred at Aberdeen, which, from special circumstances, seemed to
be connected with the supply of milk from a particular dairy, on which account
the sanitary local authority intervened, and the supply of milk from that dairy
was stopped. From inquiries made, it appeared that, out of 112 families supplied
with milk from that dairy, 89, comprising 322 individuals, were attacked ; in
most cases, the majority of the members of the families being affected. The bulk
of the cases of the disease were comprised within little more than a week, from
the first to the 8th April, a very few having occurred prior to the first-named
day, and a few appearing after the last-named, but no new families having been
affected after the last date.

Assuming the milk to be the cause, it acted most energetically when used cold
and in quantity, and least so when boiled or used in small quantity. The families
affected were scattered indiscriminately over the town, and seemed to have nothing
in common except the milk. No cases of the same nature occurred in Aberdeen
outside the number using this particular milk, and none occurred elsewhere in
Scotland. In several of those families who, though using this milk, escaped the
disease, peculiar circumstances existed which may have accounted for the immunity they enjoyed. The special symptoms of the disease were a sharp attack
of pyrexia occurring quite suddenly, lasting two or three days, and then subsiding,
leaving great and often dangerous prostration behind. The attack was generally
succeeded, within two or three days, by a second similar one, and in some cases
by a succession of attacks, with complete intermissions between them.

The local symptoms, never specially urgent, were slight sore-throat, with a
feeling of fulness or swelling there, little being seen on looking into the throat,
but a swelling of the deep glands existing at the angle of the jaw. The successive attacks were marked by the involvement of successive glands, on the

same or on opposite sides. In three cases, the disease proved fatal, all these being elderly persons, and in all the immediate cause of death was the extreme prostration following the attack ; death occurring in each case after the lapse of about a week, and several days after all the symptoms had subsided. In one case, a *post-mortem* examination was obtained, which revealed no special lesion connected with the disease, or causing death. The dairy-farm referred to was connected with the Old Mill Reformatory. and was situated about two miles from Aberdeen. The byre was well constructed, large, open from end to end, and contained between forty and fifty cows ; at one end, at such a height as not to interfere with the cows beside it, was a large water-cistern, composed of concrete, and covered with a loose wooden lid. This cistern contained about three hundred gallons of water, was filled twice in the twenty-four hours, and from it was obtained all the water used in the byre and in the dairy. In that dairy were washed almost all the vessels used for conveying milk to the consumers. All those whose milk-vessels were not washed there escaped. When the place was examined by the sanitary inspector, the position of the cistern was at once objected to, and immediately on that, the arrangement of the water-supply was altered. Before this was done, however, a specimen of the water in the cistern was obtained, and found on analysis to be highly contaminated with organic matter, although the water before entering the cistern was extremely pure.

The following were the conclusions at which the author arrived : 1. The milk obtained from the cows was good, but the milk supplied to the consumers was dangerously contaminated ; 2. The contaminated milk was the direct cause of the disease ; 3. The water used in the dairy was dangerously contaminated ; 4. Various circumstances seemed to show that, besides the washing of the milk-vessels with the contaminated water, there had been an intermixture of the water with the milk ; 5. The symptoms seemed to indicate that the disease was produced by a living organic poison introduced into the system by the tonsils and deep lymphatics of the neck. Microscopic examination seemed to show the presence of one particular organism in the water of the cistern, in the milk supplied to consumers, and in the body of the one case where a *post-mortem* examination was obtained ; but the investigations on this point are not sufficiently completed to allow of their being stated in detail. The disease differed from local inflammation in the trifling character of the local lesion, compared with the extreme severity of the constitutional symptoms, in the short duration of the attack, in its periodical recurrence at pretty regular intervals, and in the extreme prostration left behind. From diphtheria it differed in the short duration and periodical recurrence, in the absence of any trace of diphtheritic or false membrane, and in its being absolutely non-contagious.—*Brit. Med. Journ.*, Sept. 24, 1881.

Epithelial Necrosis and Diabetic Coma.

The twenty-eighth volume of the *Deutsches Archiv für Klinische Medicin* contains an article by Prof. EBSTEIN, of Göttingen, on necrosis of the epithelium of the glands in diabetes mellitus, considered with special reference to diabetic coma. He holds that there is not sufficient reason for regarding the presence of acetone in the blood as a *sine quâ non* condition of coma ; although he admits its presence in a certain number of cases, and allows that there may be some connection between it and the symptoms observed.

Having already directed attention to the occurrence of necrosis of the renal epithelium in diabetes (von Ziemssen's *Pathologie und Therapie*, Band ix., 1878), he now expresses his conviction, founded on the observation of a considerable number of cases, that this degeneration plays a prominent part in the etiology of diabetic coma. It is analogous to the necrotic processes occurring in other organs in diabetes, and is met with in two different conditions: 1, in cases where the patient dies with symptoms of diabetic coma, but no coarse anatomical cause of death can be found; 2, in cases where other serious organic changes are found along with the epithelial necrosis. These organic changes—as in acute pneumonia, interstitial hepatitis, and nephritis—may be sufficient to account for death; but still the fatal result may, in the author's opinion, be attributed in some of the cases to the necrosis of the glandular epithelium. This necrosis occurs especially in the kidney, but is also met with in other glands.

In the kidney, the necrosis may affect greater or lesser portions of the organ. In one case, where the patient died of pneumonia, the whole of the epithelium of the cortical portion of the kidney was affected. The necrosis is generally accompanied by an advanced degree of fatty degeneration of the renal epithelium.

On minute examination, the protoplasm is seen to be separated in many places from the tunica propria of the urinary tubules, and to be heaped up in balls and lumps of various sizes, in which the epithelial cells can often be distinctly seen. The epithelium presents either very indistinct nuclei, or none, not even capable of being rendered visible by colouring matter. Along with the dead epithelium, the protoplasm is transferred into simple or fatty detritus. Dr. Ebstein calls the condition of the epithelium necrotic, because it corresponds perfectly to what is met with in other circumstances, where the epithelium is indisputably dead; such as the necrosis of the renal epithelium from ischæmia following infarction or ligation of the renal arteries, or that produced by some poisons, such as the salts of chromic acid.

The necrosis of the glandular epithelium in diabetes is due, in Dr. Ebstein's opinion, much less to anæmia or ischæmia of the organ affected, than to the influence of toxic materials. That the kidneys are most affected, is due to their being the principal emunctories of such matters. In diabetes, these substances are plainly various results of the interference with tissue-change. As far as our knowledge extends, we have to take the following factors into account: 1, the abnormal oscillations of the watery contents of the organism which is the subject of diabetes mellitus; 2, the abundance of sugar in the juices and organs (hyperglycæmia); 3, various substances which appear to be present in abnormal quantities in the blood of diabetic patients, such as acetone, acetic ether, alcohol, etc., as well as oxalic acid; 4, a number of imperfectly known nitrogenous products of decomposition.

The necrotic process in the renal epithelium is of especial importance, inasmuch as it may sometimes produce a sudden arrest of the elimination of toxic substances. Epithelial necrosis thus fills an important gap in the explanation of the sudden occurrence of comatose symptoms in diabetes.

A test of the presence of at least a portion of the products of retrogressive tissue-change, especially those allied to acetic acid, is afforded by the behaviour of diabetic urine with chloride of iron (Gerhardt's test), and by the odour of acetone which the patient exhales. It sometimes happens, in cases where, under the use of a diabetic diet, there is a diminution of the polyuria and glycosuria, that an outbreak of coma occurs, the urine giving the usual reaction with chloride of iron; while in other cases, where the same reaction occurs and the same diet is used, the diabetic symptoms subside, and the patients are better for a certain time. This apparent contradiction is explained by Dr. Ebstein in the following manner. In the cases of the first category, the kidneys retain the power, with the aid of a large amount of urinary water, of completely washing away the products of decomposition, although the necrosed epithelium is no longer capable, when the excretion of water is reduced, of eliminating the waste materials from the body. In such cases, indeed, the comatose symptoms are often seen to disappear when the patient returns to his ordinary diet and drinks abundantly of water, so as to cause a return of the polyuria and glycosuria. In cases of the second category, the renal epithelium is still capable of performing its function, even when the amount of water excreted is diminished.

Necrosis of the glandular epithelium is not confined to the kidneys. Dr. Ebstein has found an analogous change in the cells of the liver in two cases. In one case, there was no interstitial change; in the other, there was interstitial hepatitis, accompanying diabetes mellitus—a combination which he has also observed in two other cases.—*Brit. Med. Journal*, Oct. 22, 1881.

Treatment of Neuralgia and Rheumatism by Electricity and Iodoform.

Dr. Mosso describes, in the *Gaz. Med. di Torino*, 1881, eighteen cases of rheumatism and neuralgia treated by electricity and iodoform. He says that useful effects are often produced by a simple Galffe's apparatus, with a weak induced current, in neuralgia and rheumatism. Sometimes, however, the malady does not yield to electricity; and in such cases he has given iodoform internally with success, sometimes alone, sometimes in combination with quinine, salicylate of soda, or bicarbonate of soda. This treatment gave the best result in neuralgia, but was useless in two cases of traumatic sciatica. The daily quantity was from 5 to 6 decigrammes (about 7¾ to 9 grains), besides what was applied externally; and no inconvenience was produced. In one case in which pure iodoform was applied externally, recovery took place, and iodine was detected in the urine. Dr. Mosso says that iodoform may be given without fear in doses of from 10 to 15 centigrammes several times a day, external friction and other means of promoting the action of the remedy being employed at the same time.—*London Med. Record*, Oct. 15, 1881.

Cerebral Symptoms in Dyspepsia.

M. Leven has reported in *Le Progrès Médicale*, May 28, 1881, one hundred cases which tend to show the existence of cerebral phenomenon whose presence has been heretofore overlooked in dyspepsia. Thus he has seen patients suddenly struck down in the street with true apoplectic attacks which last from ten minutes to a quarter of an hour. Such cases were believed to be epileptic, but M. Leven suggests that they were in reality simply dyspeptic, since the cerebral symptoms entirely disappeared when the digestive troubles had been cured. In dyspepsia the intelligence is unaffected, and there is never any mental disorder. Certain cerebral faculties may be altered, but the *ego* remains intact. This affection of the higher faculties, this weakening of the will, of action, of memory, and of the power of speech, may be readily observed. In some cases the patients are unable to determine upon an act, and they have to make a decided effort to perform what is generally an almost instinctive movement, as for instance to pick up anything that they have just dropped. In such cases the memory is impaired and speech is difficult, more especially after meals. The patients are melancholy, and suffer from cutaneous hyperæsthesia, a point which distinguishes them from the hysterical.—*Practitioner*, Oct. 1881.

A Case of Destruction of the Corpus Striatum without Symptoms.

In the *Deutsche Zeitschrift für Klinische Medizin*, xxvii. p. 520, Honegger narrates the case of a patient aged 56, who had formerly suffered with rheumatism, was admitted to treatment for various symptoms, such as pain in the abdomen, headache, etc. The examination showed chronic nephritis, endarteritis, and hypertrophy of the heart to be present. The patient was not paralyzed in any part of his body, and denied ever having been so. He died of marasmus, and upon post-mortem the following condition was found : In the left corpus striatum a focus of softening extended in to some depth, a similar focus in the thalamus of the size of a lentil, and one of the same size in the upper part of the lenticular body. The whole section of the nucleus candatus, the upper part of the lenticular body and the part of the internal capsule between them were completely destroyed. The centrum ovale was affected for a distance of two cm. around the focus.—*Pacific Medical and Surgical Journal*, Oct., 1881.

—

Left-sided Convulsions followed by Paralysis.

M. D. MACLEOD, M.B. ED., reports the following case in which unilateral convulsions were followed by paralysis and in which an area of local cerebral softening was found after death.

A. A——, aged seventy-three, female, widow, admitted Aug. 9th, 1879, was reported to have had some "fits" about eighteen months before, but no accurate history could be obtained of her case. On admission she was found to be far advanced in senile dementia. She had no idea of her surroundings, nor could she express herself intelligibly. She was very feeble, and could hardly stand, but was able to move her limbs. She could see fairly well, but was deaf. Her lungs, heart, and kidneys were healthy enough. She had a good appetite. Owing to her feeble state she was mostly confined to bed, where she lay quietly. She continued without much change for a year or so, when it was noticed that she did not see so well. Her blindness increased, and, as far as could be judged, was total for months before she died. She had an attack of convulsions at the end of 1880, but it did not last many minutes. On the 19th of April, 1881, she was seized with clonic convulsions confined to her left side. The left side of her face was throughout convulsed; the left eye was spasmodically drawn outwards; her left arm, leg, and the muscles of the left side generally were in a constant state of spasm; the chin was drawn upwards and to the right. The convulsions commenced about 9 P. M., ceased after a short time, commenced again, and continued, but gradually getting weaker, till next morning. On the 20th the convulsions had entirely ceased, and it was seen that she was completely paralyzed along the left side. Her mouth was drawn to the right, her left cheek flapping, and her arm and leg flaccid and powerless. She was unconscious, and continued in a state of coma till 5 P. M. on the 21st, when she died.

The following were the morbid appearances seen in the brain. It is of interest to note, in connection with the blindness in this case, the complete destruction of the angular gyrus of the right hemisphere. The general diseased state of the vessels of the brain, the great atrophy, and the extent of the softening, render a localization of the lesion causing the convulsion difficult; but it is noteworthy that the disease was of the motor area and the tracts connected with it.

Post-mortem appearances.—Head: The scalp was normal; the calvaria was thick, soft, spongy. The dura mater was thickened and tough; the sinuses were full of black clot. On cutting into the dura mater 8 oz. to 10 oz. of cerebro-spinal fluid escaped. The arachnoid was opaque; the vessels of the membranes generally were full of blood. The pia mater was thick and œdematous; it was easily separable from the convolutions except at a spot over the right postero-parietal region, where there was some gelatinous effusion. The arteries of the brain were very atheromatous, markedly so the right middle cerebral; the basilar artery was comparatively healthy. The brain was small (weight 32½ oz. ; right hemisphere 14½ oz., left hemisphere 14 oz., cerebellum and pons 4 oz.). The convolutions were atrophied generally; they were small and much divided by shallow sulci. The cranial nerves were atrophied; the optic nerves, chiasma, and tracts were small and flattened; there was apparently no local atrophy or disease of the right hemisphere. The convolutions of the left hemisphere were small throughout. There was an area of old yellow softening in the left postero-parietal region; this area included the angular gyrus, the posterior portion of the supramarginal gyrus, a small part of the superior parietal lobule just anterior to the parieto-occipital fissure, the upper margin of the first temporal and a very limited portion of the second occipital convolutions. The whole gray matter of this softened area was destroyed, as was the white matter underneath. A band of softening extended inwards and forwards to the posterior part of the thalamus opticus, into which the left optic tract entered, and another line of yellow softening anterior to the other, and separated from it by apparently healthy white substance, was easily traceable to the corpus striatum, the posterior part of which was softened. There was no apparent softening or degeneration in the crura, the medulla, or pons. The convolutional softening corresponded to the area supplied by the branch of the middle cerebral artery running in the horizontal ramus of the Sylvian fissure. This vessel was markedly atheromatous and diminished in calibre. The branch ascending was free of atheroma; the lateral ventricles were dilated; there were gliomatous bodies on the choroid plexus; the cerebellum and pons were soft; the other organs of the body presented no marked abnormality.— *Lancet*, Sept. 17, 1881.

Spinal Lesions from Compressed Air.

The paraplegia which has occasionally been observed in professional divers has been ascribed by M. PAUL BERT to the effect of the compressed air, and he has reproduced it experimentally by subjecting animals to air compressed to seven or eight atmospheres in special apparatus. MM. Blanchard and Regnard have endeavoured to complete these researches by studying the changes in the spinal cord produced by this influence. Some animals (dogs) died soon after the restoration to normal conditions; others lived several days. One of these was attacked with paraplegia, but recovered perfectly. It was ultimately killed, and the spinal cord was found to present numerous foci of hemorrhage and evidence of acute parenchymatous myelitis. There was no sclerosis. The minute hemorrhages existed not only in the gray substance, but were met with in the entire length of the cord; sometimes in the anterior, sometimes in the posterior cornua. The myelitis had the usual characters; hypertrophy and varicosity of the axis-cylinders, and granular masses scattered through the tissue. The change occupied various situations in the white substance, and was in some places of considerable extent. It was least in the lumbar enlargement and was most intense in the dorsal region, where it was so extensive that the recovery of function is difficult to understand.—*Lancet*, Sept. 17, 1881.

Nerve-Stretching in Diseases of the Spinal Cord.

Dr. CARL LANGENBUCH has published, in Nos. 24, 25, 26, and 27 of the *Berl. Klin. Woch.*, his further experiences of the results of nerve-stretching in tabes and other diseases of the spinal cord. He shows that, on account of the long course of tabes, the later stages alone are seen in the post-mortem room, and he also points out that in this disease there are lesions of nerves, as well as of the cord. Sometimes congestion of the nerves, sometimes anæmia, is found. In answer to the question, "Why are the posterior root-zones affected?" he answers that these are the media of communication between centre and periphery, and may be regarded as practically peripheral substance. The columns of Goll connect gray centres with one another, and are only secondarily affected. He regards cold as the great cause of tabes dorsalis.

With regard to the treatment of this and similar diseases, the author observes that even the most useful means—baths, electricity, cautery, etc.—produce only small benefit occasionally; much improvement rarely; recovery never. Such methods act on the end-organs, and thence affect the centres. Nerve-stretching acts directly on the centre; and, although brought forward with caution, it has been abundantly successful. If necrosis of nervous elements have set in, the cure is only partial; but if the disease be taken early, the recovery is complete. Of twenty-eight patients, sixteen suffered from tabes, two from multiple sclerosis, one from lateral sclerosis of both sides, one from lateral sclerosis of one side, one from muscular atrophy, two from tetanus, three from spinal myelomeningitis, one from pemphigus, and one from pruritus. Six of the tabetic patients were dismissed as cured; the others were recent, and were still in bed when the paper was published. The multiple sclerosis was much relieved in both cases. The one-sided lateral sclerosis was entirely cured, and the bilateral case was too recent to be set down in the list of recoveries. The case of muscular atrophy was considerably improved, but was only recently operated on. The tremors were much diminished, but sufficient time had not elapsed for certainty to be attained. Two cases of myelo-meningitis had only just been treated, and the effect was uncertain; in the third there was little, if any, improvement. Both cases of tetanus died; and, lastly, the case of pemphigus and that of pruritus were both entirely cured. During the operation both pulse and respiration undergo considerable but varying changes, and when much alteration was observed, further stretching was not allowed. After the influence of the anæsthetic had passed off the patients had no uneasiness, and expressed themselves, in certain cases, as grateful for the removal of pain. Sensibility was never diminished, but sometimes increased, and there was total removal of the feeling of cold in the extremities. In some cases the one leg felt as if longer than the other, and there was a sensation of being in a strange position. Motility was rapidly restored, and the ataxy removed. Constipation ceased, and involuntary micturition was cured in some cases; and in one case impotence was brought to an end. The sight was improved in cases where it had been affected. The after-results of longer periods have necessarily not been observed as yet; but we have sufficient evidence to lead us to hope for much.

Dr. Langenbuch shows that nerve-stretching has an influence upon the whole nervous system, and in conclusion points out that, in disease of the spinal cord, nerve-stretching is a method of treatment from which, under antiseptic management, nothing is to be feared, and everything may be gained.—*London Med. Record*, Oct. 15, 1881.

Ergot in the Paralysis of Lead Poisoning.

According to Dr. J. A. STITES, in the State of Nevada it may be safely estimated that fifty per cent. of the physician's practice consists of cases of lead-poisoning, the symptoms being in most instances well marked, while in the remainder they are more or less masked. Of the remaining fifty per cent. of practice, the bulk is furnished by accidents and syphilis. The occupation of the male population is mining in silver ore, which is largely associated with lead. Wrist drop is a very frequent symptom, and paralysis of other forms, even hemiplegia and paraplegia, is not an infrequent complication. In the milder manifestations of these symptoms, a cathartic of sulphate of magnesia, followed by iodide of potassium, usually removes them in a few days, enabling the sufferer to resume his work.   The habits of the 'miner render him peculiarly susceptible to attack, and Dr. Stites has found that when his patients abstain from alcoholic stimulants, keep their bowels open, and preserve their appetite by proper living, they are much less apt to suffer from lead-poisoning.

In hemiplegia and paraplegia due to lead-poisoning, Dr. Stites has found ergot in combination with iodide of potassium and nux vomica to expedite recovery. He has tested its efficacy by comparison in the hospital with which he is connected, adopting three varieties of treatment: (1) iodide of potassium alone; (2) electricity with tonics and nux vomica; (3) iodide of potassium and ergot. The latter plan has been attended with the utmost satisfactory results. The following is his standard prescription: ℞. Potassii iodidi, ʒij; ext. ergotæ fluidi, ʒj; ext. nucis vomicæ fluidi, ʒj; tr. cardamomi co., ʒj; syrupi, q. s. ad ʒiv.   Misce.   Sig.—A tablespoonful night and morning.

Usually in a month the power has been restored to the paralyzed parts.   Under other forms of treatment recovery does not usually come under three months. The efficacy of ergot is attributed to the well-known physiological action of ergot on the non-striated muscular fibre.   The dangers which were formerly supposed to be attendant on the prolonged employment of ergot, such as gangrene, etc., are certainly not to be apprehended, according to the author, in the therapeutic employment of the drug.—*Therapeutic Gazette*, Oct. 1881.

Treatment of Empyema.

Dr. W. Wagner of Königshütte, in commenting on a case of empyema successfully treated by operation under antiseptic conditions (*Sammlung Klinische Vorträge*, No. 197), states that the treatment of this affection has now reached a fresh stage; and that, since the introduction of Listerism, an operation, instead of being a mere palliative measure, is to be regarded as justifiable under all circumstances, and, in cases of simple empyema at least, as free from risk.

The surest way, Wagner asserts, of distinguishing an empyema from a simple pleuritic exudation, is to make an exploratory puncture.   This may be done with a disinfected hypodermic syringe and trocar, or, better still, with a larger syringe, such as that used by veterinary surgeons, which holds about five grammes of fluid, and is furnished with a strong and large needle.   The exploratory puncture, however, does not always guard against errors in diagnosis.   In the first place, a case may be met with in which there are two separate and distinct exudations, one a serous, the other a purulent exudation.   Then, again, it may happen, especially in cases of exudation originally serous or sero-purulent, that have become purulent, that the exploratory puncture will give vent to serous fluid in the upper part of the collection and to purulent fluid below.   In a patient lying constantly on his back, this precipitation will take place not to the inferior but to the posterior part of the thoracic cavity, so that serum will be present in front and pus behind.   Dr. Wagner, though acknowledging that cases of this kind are rare, lays it down as a rule that, in every case of pleural exudation in which the general symptoms indicate empyema, several exploratory punctures should be made at different parts of the corresponding thoracic wall, should it happen that at the first or earlier punctures serum and not purulent fluid is withdrawn.

At the present day, no medical man believes in the possibility of the absorption of a purulent pleural exudation.   The so-called "natural cure," in which the pus is discharged through the air-passages, is of rare occurrence, and, when it does occur, is likely to have bad results, and to give rise to phthisis through the contact of the discharge with the lung-tissue, or through its aspiration into the fine bronchial divisions. Spontaneous discharge of an empyema through the thoracic wall cannot be regarded as a favourable termination, as it is often followed by an obstinate fistula.

In a case of well-marked empyema there is, in Wagner's opinion, an almost unconditional indication to operate at as early a date as possible. Unless the affected pleura covering the lung be soft and yielding, and the lung itself be capable of complete re-expansion, the chances of a speedy and good cure will not be favourable. An acute pneumonic infiltration still persisting, whether to a high or low degree, should not prevent early recourse to operative treatment, for with removal of the empyema the pressure on the lung is removed. This organ is thus set free, and as its normal conditions of circulation become re-established, the absorption of the inflammatory exudation is favoured. If the inner wall of the abscess be stiff and unyielding in consequence of thickening of the pulmonary pleura, then cure cannot be effected speedily, and cannot possibly occur at all, unless the resistance of the thoracic wall or that of the tough pulmonary pleura can be overcome. Wagner sums up his remarks on this subject by stating that, when we operate in the early stage of empyema, we meet with the most favorable conditions for the re-expansion of the lung and for the approximation of the walls of the abscess. The older such an abscess, the thicker will be its walls, and the greater difficulty will there be in the obliteration of its cavity. In the application of the above rule, it is, of course, to be understood that the operation be performed under antiseptic conditions. Dr. Wagner is not in favour of treating empyema by simple puncture and aspiration. Such treatment may occasionally prove successful, especially with young children, in which class of patients there is likely to be a rapid re-expansion of the lung after removal of the purulent fluid; but it is attended with this disadvantage, that, as it is almost always impossible thus to remove all the pus, there is likely to remain a small quantity of this secretion, the presence of which invariably causes a relapse of the empyema. The rule is laid down by Wagner that it is not justifiable to try puncture more than once in a case of empyema, and that, if this first attempt do not succeed, the surgeon ought, without delay, to have recourse to incision. The longer an empyema is allowed to run its course, the less favourable become the chances of a cutting operation, and with repetition of simple puncture valuable time is lost.

Though an incision through the thoracic wall low down in the back of the chest may be most favourable for a full discharge during the operation, and in the course of the after treatment, yet, Dr. Wagner holds, this situation can hardly be regarded as being under all circumstances the best in the operation for empyema. The inferior and posterior part of the affected pleural cavity is often obliterated in consequence of pleurisy, and the space may be so contracted through approximation of the elevated diaphragm and the inner wall of the thorax, and also through re-expansion of the lung, that free discharge of pus from the pleural sac is prevented. Dr. Wagner prefers an incision in the fifth or sixth intercostal space, near to the edge of the latissimus dorsi muscle; and in order to promote a free discharge during the after-treatment, he keeps his patient lying on the side, with the pelvis and lower part of the trunk elevated on a firm pillow.

In the cutting operation for empyema, Dr. Wagner recommends the administration of an anæsthetic. With anæsthesia, the surgeon is less likely to be disturbed through restlessness of the patient, and he may, if it be found necessary, proceed without delay to resect a portion of rib. Care, however, must be taken that the movements of the chest on the sound side are not impeded during the operation.

Sudden death, which has occurred in some cases of empyema during operation, cannot, it is stated, be attributed to the anæsthetic. It has been due rather to some disturbance of circulation (thrombosis, cerebral anæmia, embolism of the pulmonary capillaries, pulmonary congestion, or œdema). These instances of sudden death have occurred as frequently during simple thoracentesis without anæsthesia, as in cutting operations for empyema.

The details of the cutting operation are very simple. The surgeon either makes an incision through the skin about two inches in length along the upper margin of a rib, and then slowly divides the muscles until he reaches the pleura, which he opens with a small bistoury ; or, following König's practice, he resects subperiosteally a portion of rib about one inch in length, and then opens the thoracic cavity by incising the posterior layer of periosteum and the pleura. This latter operation should always be performed when the intercostal space is not of sufficient width to admit of the passage of a wide drainage-tube. It is not likely to be attended with any bad result, and in young subjects the resected portion of rib is almost always wholly replaced.

During the flow of pus, which should not be allowed to take place too rapidly, the surgeon should carefully examine the fluid, and also introduce his finger through the opening into the pleural cavity, in order to ascertain the condition of the surrounding wall. He thus endeavours to make out indications for future treatment. If the purulent discharge be free from smell, and do not contain flakes, no injection need be made into the sac ; but if, on the other hand, it be fetid, and be mixed with large and numerous fibrinous masses, then it is necessary to wash out the cavity. Dr. Wagner now uses in such cases a 7 per cent. solution of boracic acid. If the walls of the purulent sac be felt to be thick and rough, and if they be evidently covered by adherent masses of fibrine, then it is necessary to wash out the cavity thoroughly and repeatedly with strong antiseptic solutions, which, in order that chilling may be avoided, should be warmed before they are injected. It is advisable, in dealing with such a condition, to make a second opening into the thoracic cavity.

When the pleural cavity has been opened, relieved of its purulent fluid, and washed out, or, as should always be done in simple cases of pyæmia and with children, has been simply emptied, a piece of drainage-tube of wide calibre, the length of which need not be more than two inches, should be inserted into the wound. Across this tube, near its outer extremity, a needle is thrust. This prevents the tube from falling into the thoracic cavity, whilst two sutures applied to the margins of the external wound and tied around the needle prevent it from being forced outwards. During the operation and immediate dressing, and also during subsequent dressing, Dr. Wagner guards the exposed parts by the carbolic acid spray. The first dressing, by which the whole of the affected side of the chest is covered, and which reaches from the axilla to the pelvis, consists of thick layers of Lister's gauze and of salicylated wadding. The first dressing ought not, it is stated, to be allowed to remain for a longer period than twenty-four hours, even though no secretion has made its way to the surface. The surgeon should then make sure that the drainage-tube remains in position, and that it is patent, and not obstructed by a clot. Retention of pus thus caused is a serious matter in a case of simple empyema, since a continuous and full discharge of the secretion is a necessary condition of a speedy cure. For the same reason, it is held advisable to change the second dressing after a short interval. The thermometer is a sure indicator of retention of pus, but not until this has been established for some hours. During each change of dressing, which, as has been stated, is always done in Dr. Wagner's practice under the spray, the drainage-tube should be removed and thoroughly cleansed, and, if necessary, be shortened before it is replaced. If, during the after-treatment of a primarily simple case of empyema, the pus become fetid and mixed with flakes and shreds of fibrine, the pleural cavity at each change of dressing must be washed out with an antiseptic solution. Dr. Wagner recommends a solution (three to eight per cent.) of boracic acid, or a five per cent. solution of chloride of zinc.

Careful observation of temperature is of the highest importance during the after-treatment of empyema. In a case of simple empyema, the temperature, after an antiseptically performed operation, should from the first be almost normal, unless there be any disease of the lungs or other viscera. An evening temperature of over 101 deg. should always arouse a suspicion that the pus does not flow freely, or that it is no longer in a good condition. A persistence of fever may be caused also by the presence within the pleural sac of fibrinous masses, and, in such case, steps should at once be taken to remove these. In many cases of empyema, these masses exist in abundance, and set up fever by acting as foreign bodies and by becoming decomposed. When the purulent fluid discharged at the time of operation is found to contain fibrinous flakes, and the walls of the cavity can be felt to be roughened and covered by similar deposits, the case can only be treated as one of simple empyema, and an attempt must be made to remove all the material. A portion of rib should be resected, in order that the opening in the thoracic wall may be of sufficient size, and the surgeon should then attempt to remove as much as he is able of these fibrinous masses, by introducing his finger and by washing out the cavity. The injected fluid should be an antiseptic one sufficiently concentrated to disinfect, as far as may be possible, any remaining deposits. The use of such injections should be continued until the purulent discharge becomes free from smell, and is no longer mixed with portions of fibrinous material. The further treatment of complicated empyema, so long as the pus is in good condition, is the same as that of simple empyema.

Dr. Wagner warns against replacing too soon during the after-treatment a thick and short drainage-tube by one of smaller calibre. A weak and narrow tube will more readily become obstructed, and offers less resistance to the tendency of the ribs immediately above and below the wound to come together and obstruct the flow of pus. When there has been no secretion for about eight days, and the temperature has remained during this period quite normal, the drainage-tube may be removed The wound generally heals then very rapidly. If in cases of this kind there occur a reaccumulation of pus, the abscess is usually a small one, and its sac is cut off from the pleural cavity. If the discharge do not cease very soon, it would be advisable, Dr. Wagner states, to brush over its lining membrane a strong solution of chloride of zinc. No injection should be made into this abscess, as the recent adhesions might readily be broken down. — *London Med. Record*, Oct. 15, 1881.

Incision of the Pericardium.

Prof. S. ROSENSTEIN reports the following case in the *Berliner Klinische Wochenschrift*, 5, 1881: On Jan. 16, he examined a boy ten years old. Two weeks before he was taken sick with fever and with gastric symptoms, and since that time he had been short of breath and had a little cough. Careful examination revealed the presence of a very considerable pericardial exudation. Change from lying to sitting made no change in the form or extent of the area of dulness. The boy had no fever, the skin of the thorax was not œdematous. An exploratory puncture with a hypodermic syringe showed pus. The increase of the dyspnœa led Rosenstein to perform puncture with aspiration, by means of which 620 ccm. of purely purulent fluid were withdrawn with the result of immediate and complete euphoria. But on the very next day the pericardial exudation increased, and a left pleuritis developed, so that two days later 1200 ccm. of pleuritic and, again, 120 ccm. of pericardial exudation were removed with the aspirator. The general condition of the patient now growing worse, it was decided, on the eleventh day after admission, to incise the pericardium under antiseptic precautions. This was done, two drains were introduced, and Lister's bandage applied. A magical improvement of the general condition began. Nineteen days after the incision the boy was well, so far as the pericardium was concerned. The pleuritis having meantime become purulent, an incision of the pleura was necessary, but this also healed completely after some weeks. Rosenstein remarks that the case teaches: 1. That purulent pericarditis, like empyema, may run its course without any fever or any œdema of the skin, so that it can only be recognized by exploratory puncture. 2. The fear of myocarditic changes should not hold us back from removing the exudation in suitable cases, because all the symptoms which make such probable can be explained by functional changes in the elasticity and contractility of the heart-muscles. 3. When there is a large collection of fluid in the pericardium, change of the patient's position may have no influence on the height of the area of dulness, so that this criterion cannot be relied upon in differentiating from dilatation of the heart.—*Amer. Journ. of Obstetrics*, Oct. 1881.

Severe Chronic Gastric Catarrh treated by Washing out the Stomach.

Professor RIVA relates, in the *Rivista Ital. di Terapia ed Igiene*, 1881, the case of a man who had suffered for eleven years from gastric catarrh, the disorder becoming steadily worse, until at last he vomited his food mingled with blood. In this condition he was admitted into the hospital at Perugia. He was extremely emaciated, and percussion in the epigastrium showed that the stomach was greatly distended. He suffered while in hospital from extreme weakness, sour eructations, intense thirst, anorexia, vomiting (which was more frequent in the morning than at night), and constipation. The vomited matter was of very offensive odour, frothy and sour; under the microscope it presented digested and undigested fibres of meat, starch-granules, fat-globules, mucus-globules, epithelial cells, and sarcoma. Dr. Riva determined to try the effect of washing out the stomach; and used for the purpose a Nélatou's sound, made rigid by the introduction of a metallic wire; to this was fitted a Kussmaul's pump, and the operation was conducted cautiously, so as not to injure the gastric mucous membrane. The fluid used was a solution of 6 grammes (93 grains) in 1000 grammes (about 35 ounces) of water. After two or three operations, the presence of the tube in the stomach did not cause any attempt at vomiting. As this treatment produced only transient improvement, the quantity of bicarbonate of soda was increased to 10 grammes in 1000 of water. The treatment by bicarbonate of soda having been continued ten days without other marked result than cessation of the vomiting, solution of sulphate of copper (5 grammes in 1000 of water) was injected, and allowed to remain three or four minutes. Under this treatment the patient rapidly improved, and left the hospital a month after admission, having gained 9 kilogrammes (nearly 20 pounds) in weight.—*London Med. Record*, Oct. 15, 1881.

Hydatid Tumour of the Liver in a Young Child.

Hydatid disease of the liver is an affection which attacks young children so infrequently that the following case seems worthy of record.

S. W., a perfectly healthy-looking boy aged four years and a half, came under treatment at the Manchester Southern Hospital on the 22d of September, 1880.

Two days before, while playing with other children, a bigger boy took hold of him round the waist and lifted him from the ground. He ran home crying, and complained of pain about the stomach, and on examining him his mother found a swelling in the abdomen.

When he was admitted to the hospital a bulging prominence was found in the epigastrium, rather to the right of the median line. On palpation a globular tumour could be felt about the size of a small orange; it was smooth, tense, somewhat elastic, but not fluctuating. There was no hydatid fremitus, nor was there any pain or tenderness on pressure. It could be seen and felt to move freely with the respiratory movements. On percussion the dulness over the tumour was found to be continuous with that of the liver. There was no general enlargement of the liver ; in the right mammary line it measured two inches, but slightly to the right of the median line (i. e. in the line of the tumour) three inches and a quarter. The lower margin of the projection was one inch from the umbilicus. There had been no jaundice or other constitutional symptoms. Owing to unwillingness on the part of the boy's parents nothing was done for two months, during which the swelling increased in size, and approached on the surface. On November 15th it was explored by means of the aspirator and a fine needle, and thirteen drachms of fluid were evacuated. The fluid was perfectly clear ; it contained no albumen, but abundance of chlorides, so that, although no echinococci or hooklets could be found under the microscope, there could be no doubt of the hydatid nature of the tumour. There was no urticaria after the tapping, a symptom which is of tolerably frequent occurrence. This sequela has been supposed to be due to an escape of a small quantity of hydatid fluid into the abdominal cavity. If this was the true explanation there certainly ought to have been urticaria in this boy's case. Wishing to insure perfect quiet, chloroform was given, hoping that the small quantity necessary would not be followed by sickness. However, as soon as the needle was withdrawn, violent and repeated retching occurred, so that a drop or two of the fluid could hardly fail to have escaped into the peritoneum. It may be added that in neither of these cases was any blood drawn through the aspirator, as sometimes occurs, on account of the possibility of which event Dr. Murchison advised that the aspirator should not be employed.

In this case the tumour slowly diminished in size, and two months after the aspiration not the slightest fulness could be felt over the region formerly occupied by the cyst.—*Lancet*, Oct. 29, 1881.

Filaria Sanguinis Hominis.

Dr. STEPHEN MACKENZIE recently brought before the London Pathological Society a patient suffering from hæmato-chyluria, in which the filaria were found in the living state. This parasite, like so many similar creatures, presents us with an example of alternation of generations ; or, more correctly speaking, of the need of two hosts for its full development. The minute almost structureless worms found in the blood of the human subject in such vast numbers are the *embryonic* forms of the filaria which requires the mosquito in which to develop into the sexually mature worm. The mosquito feeding on the blood at night, when the filariæ are generally alone to be found, becomes gorged with them. Their growth in the mosquito has been traced by Lewis and Manson, and it is presumed that they are only liberated from the body of their host by its death in the water to which it always finally resorts. The nematoid is thus set free, and possibly undergoes further development ; for the mature worm measures some three inches in length. Its passage into the human body is easily explained ; and the analogy in this respect with the larger nematoid—the guinea-worm—is one which Dr. Vandyke Carter ably illustrated. Once within the human body, the worm lodges in the tissues, but as to its migrations, and, indeed, its ultimate resting-place, but little is known. It would seem, from its discovery in a lymphatic abscess by Bancroft, and in a lymph scrotum by Lewis, to have a peculiar aptitude for selecting the lymph channels for its habitat; a selective power not more remarkable than that which urges the trichina to lodge in muscular tissue. This is further borne out by the fact that its embryos—the filaria sanguinis hominis—are met with in the blood and the urine of the subjects of chyluria and nævoid (or lymphatic) elephantiasis.

Now, although the various discoveries which have been made—at the expense of so much patient research and at such various times that, as Dr. Cobbold remarked at the meeting, they form each distinct "epochs"—have enabled us to form the above complete sketch of the life-history of the parasite, there are lacunæ still to be filled up. Thus knowledge is wanted upon the growth and migration of the parent worm after it has gained entrance into the human body, also as to its duration of life, and particularly as to the question whether it can take on the power of sexual reproduction, and if so, for how long a time. The myriads of filariæ that are probably daily reproduced in the body of such a patient as that under Dr. Mackenzie's care seem to demand such a fact as alternate generations, and also to raise the question as to the time during which the process of reproduction can continue. There is no reason to believe that the embryonic filariæ in the blood can undergo further development within the human body; indeed, analogy, as well as the remarkable discovery of an intermediate host in the mosquito, are opposed to this notion. Again, filariæ have been found in the blood apart from chyluria or any outward manifestation of lymphatic derangement; but this is explicable if it be admitted that the adult worms may lodge in other parts of the body in communication with bloodvessels alone. Conversely, chyluria may exist without filaria, and the case mentioned by Dr. Mackenzie, where the parasite was found in the man's blood in India, but could not be found when he came to England, is explicable on the view that though the parent organism might have perished, or yielded no more embryos, yet the change excited by its presence in the lymphatic channels, and therefore the chyluria, might still have persisted.

The precise mechanism of chyluria still requires to be explained, and until it is elucidated an important part of the subject will remain obscure. The question of the pathology of chyluria was, however, barely touched upon on Tuesday: Dr. Mackenzie limiting himself to the statement of the facts observed in his case; the most important in connection with the urine being that besides having all the chylous characters, it invariably contained more or less blood—that passed by day containing more blood and filaria, that passed by night being more milky; and that filariæ were found in it, especially in connection with blood coagula. The most remarkable feature of the whole case lay in the periodicity shown by the filariæ in their time of appearance in the blood. During the whole period of the man's stay in hospital, the blood had been examined regularly every three hours, with the constant result that, by night, the filariæ abounded and by day were entirely absent. From 9 A.M. to 9 P.M. they were absent; they appeared at the latter hour and increased up to midnight, then decreased till at the first-named hour none were found. These observations entirely confirmed those of Manson, and particular stress was laid upon their nocturnal wanderings and the habits of the mosquito. It is certainly singular that the time selected by the mosquito should coincide with the presence of the parasite in the blood stream, and the connection of these two facts is not the least wonderful chapter in the life-history of the parasite. But whatever the explanation of the periodicity—Dr. Vandyke

Carter pointed out that it was not invariable—a valuable addition to our knowledge of it has been made by Dr. Mackenzie. He found that whereas the time of ingestion of food bears no relation to it, it is otherwise with the time of rest and sleep, for when the patient was up during the night and slept during the day the period of filarial migration was similarly inverted.—*Lancet*, Oct. 22, 1881.

Psoriasis from Borax.

Among the cutaneous eruptions which may result from the administration of drugs, psoriasis has not, according to Dr. W· R. GOWERS (*Lancet*, Sept. 24, 1881), been hitherto included. The following facts, which he narrates, show that an eruption of characteristic psoriasis may result from the internal administration of borax. The facts have been met with in the use of borax in the treatment of obstinate cases of epilepsy, in which bromide fails. The first instance was in the case of a man who had taken borax for nearly two years in doses of first fifteen grains and then a scruple three times daily. An eruption of psoriasis made its appearance on his limbs and trunk, developing to a considerable extent in the course of a few weeks. Five minims of arsenical solution were added to each dose of borax, and the eruption rapidly disappeared. Shortly afterwards Dr. Spencer of Clifton, in mentioning to me a case of epilepsy in which he had given borax with advantage, inquired if I had met with any inconvenience from its use. I told him of this case, in which I thought it possible that the psoriasis was produced by the borax, and he informed me that in his patient the same eruption had just appeared. In this case also the rash rapidly cleared away under the influence of arsenic, and a few weeks later Dr. Spencer wrote to me, "I have not the slightest doubt that the borax caused the psoriasis, or that the arsenic cured it." A third instance has lately come under my notice. The patient was a young man who had suffered from epilepsy since infancy, and was always rendered worse by bromide, so that he was brought to me with the request that bromide might on no account be given. He took borax, first fifteen grains and then a scruple three times a day, with greater benefit than had resulted from any previous treatment, and after eight months an eruption of psoriasis appeared. Arsenic was added, but the result of treatment has not yet been ascertained.

The eruption in these cases occurred on the trunk, arms, and legs, but more on the arms than elsewhere. The face was free. It was located on both the flexor and extensor aspects. The patches varied in size, up to an inch and a half in diameter. Their appearance was quite characteristic, but the scales were not so thick as they sometimes are in ordinary psoriasis. In no case was there a history of syphilis, and in Dr. Spencer's patient syphilis could, with certainty, be excluded.

Gangrenous Eruption in Connection with Chicken-pox and Vaccination.

At the meeting of the Royal Medical and Chirurgical Society on October 25, Mr. JONATHAN HUTCHINSON narrated the details of a case which had been brought before the society two years ago. A child in perfect health was vaccinated with several others from the arm of a healthy infant. None of the other children suffered. In this child nothing unusual happened to the vaccination-vesicles, which ran their course naturally. On the eighth day after vaccination, however, an eruption came out on the body and limbs, which three days later was diagnosed by the vaccinator as variola. Some of the spots had at this time become dusky, and threatened to slough; and afterwards gangrene attacked large numbers of them. Between the eleventh and the twenty-first days, no surgeon saw the child. It died on the latter date; and, an inquest having been held, the coroner requested Mr. Hutchinson to examine the body, and to report on the nature of the disease. The body, which on a former occasion was shown to the society, and of which drawings were again produced, was that of a well-grown healthy child. It was covered with gangrenous sores; the sloughs being black, and in many instances extending into the subcutaneous cellular tissue. Some of them were as large as shillings. There were numerous smaller sores on which no gangrene had occurred. The sores were arranged with tolerable symmetry over the scalp, face, trunk, and limbs; but the hands and feet were exempt. A *post-mortem* examination by Dr. Barlow showed no disease of internal organs. The child had died from exhaustion in connection with the extensive affection of the skin. The author stated that, so far as he knew, this was the first example of a gangrenous eruption following immediately upon vaccination; and that he was inclined to regard it as an instance of the vaccinia exanthem running, in connection with idiosyncrasy, an unusual course. Since the case was first brought before the society in November, 1879, another almost similar one had occurred in Dublin, and had been carefully recorded by Mr. William Stokes. By the kindness of Mr. Stokes, drawings representing the condition of his patient were presented to the meeting. In this instance the patches of gangrene, although larger, were fewer in number and more superficial; and the infant, although for a time in great danger, eventually recovered. The two cases were almost exactly parallel, excepting that in Mr. Stokes's case a much shorter interval between the vaccination and the appearance of the eruption was assigned by the mother. There were, however, great doubts as to her accuracy and truthfulness, since the medical man whom she asserted to have vaccinated the baby said that he certainly had not done it on the day that she alleged. The eruptions affected the same parts in the two children. In both the hands and feet were exempt; and in neither did the vaccination-spots themselves become gangrenous. The author next proceeded to another part of the subject—the attempt to demonstrate that chicken-pox does occasionally assume a gangrenous form, and present conditions very similar to those just described in connection with the vaccinia exanthem. He had, he said, for ten years or more been in the habit of recognizing a gangrenous form of varicella, and several patients suffering from it had come under his care at the Moorfields Hospitals with suppurative iritis. In some cases the disease had proved fatal; but in the majority the patient recovered, with deep scars, and sometimes with great damage to the eyes. In the worst cases, the eruption involved the whole thickness of the skin, and left an abruptly margined, punched-out ulcer. The author quoted from a paper published by Dr. Whitley Stokes, of Dublin, in 1807, in which this malady was, he thought, clearly described. Dr. Whitley Stokes said that it was well known in many parts of Ireland under the name of "the white blisters," "the eating hive," and "the burnt holes." Dr. Whitley Stokes had noticed the resemblance of the disease to chicken-pox, but had attempted to diagnose between them, alleging that, in chicken-pox, the fever always preceded the eruption; and that the pustules always dried quickly. The author of the present paper contended that neither of these distinctions would hold good, and drew attention to the fact that Dr. Whitley Stokes had, like himself, observed that the eruption usually occurred in very healthy children; that at its first stage it was like chicken-pox; that severe inflammation of the eyes sometimes occurred; and that the worst cases ended fatally. The final proof upon which the author relied that the eruption was no other than a modification of varicella was, that he had seen it repeatedly occur to one child in a family whilst several others were going through varicella in its ordinary form. For two examples of this, he had recently been indebted to his friends Dr. Barlow and Dr. David Lees, of the Children's Hospital. Of one of these cases a drawing was shown. The author referred to some wax casts in the Guy's Hospital Museum which, he said, well illustrated the condition which he had been describing. They had been named rupia escharotica; but he could have no hesitation in believing them to be examples of gangrenous varicella. In conclusion, he urged that if the proof were accepted, that, in connection with idiosyncrasy in perfectly healthy children, the eruption of varicella might occasionally assume a severely gangrenous type, there could be but little difficulty in admitting the same possibility as regards the vaccinia exanthem. By the term vaccinia exanthem he intended to designate a general eruption, sometimes erythematous, sometimes lichenoid, and sometimes vesicular, which, although unfrequent, was admitted by all experienced vaccinators to be occasionally seen. It had been especially described by Mr. Ceely, and was referred to by Hebra and others. It was, of course, the analogue of the skin-eruption in variola.—*Brit. Med. Journal*, Oct. 29, 1881.

Surgery.

Operations for Chronic Disease in Phthisical Patients.

At the meeting of the Medical Society of London Mr. BRYANT read the history of a young man who for some years had suffered from disease of the knee-joint, and when he came under Mr. Bryant's care there was evidence of consolidation of both apices of the lungs. The thigh was amputated, the wound healed well, and the chest symptoms improved, while the physical evidence of lung disease diminished. In short, it was a case illustrating, first, the possibility of rapid recovery from a serious operation during the course of phthisis, and, second, the fact that the removal of a chronically diseased joint may be followed by improvement in lung trouble. The case is now by no means isolated, but is one of a series, which have been published from time to time. We may study such a case from two points of view, as showing the influence of general disease upon local conditions, and the influence of local disease upon general affections.

It is not difficult to understand why general constitutional states must influence local disease processes, and it accords with all experience and preconceived ideas that the constitutional effects of pulmonary phthisis may retard, or even prevent altogether, the recovery of a chronically diseased joint. Under such circumstances amputation may be demanded for local conditions quite amenable to milder methods in patients of robuster frame. But the question arises whether the same is true of wounds. Do constitutional states play any part, or any considerable part, in the history of a wound? Hitherto the answer to such a question would have been deemed simple and distinct in the extreme—that they did. But it is now asserted, by some of the more ardent disciples of Professor Lister especially, that our present knowledge of the processes of wound healing, and of the local causes of their failure, has placed us in a position of complete independence of the general systematic condition when called upon to treat a wound. It is asserted that, in every case where certain local conditions are observed, primary union of wounds may be insured. We, at any rate, know that the *vis medicatrix naturæ* is especially exerted and manifest in the healing of injuries of all kinds, and that further knowledge merely adds to the occasions of wonder that so grave and complete injuries can be repaired. It is, however, open to us to say that probably constitutional cachexia, as from phthisis, when very marked, may arrest the healing of a wound. This position seems to be in accord with our present knowledge, and for correction will require demonstration of its error, and not mere assertion. The practical outcome of this is, that, granted amputation to be advisable, there are certain stages of the general disease which admit of the operation, while in others it is inadmissible. Where the lung disease has passed into the third stage, and there are cavities surrounded by large masses of caseous lung tissue, where the pyrexia is marked and constant, and the other organic functions are interfered with, it would be unwise to perform any operation not immediately necessary to save life, as the surgeon's wound might not heal, and, continuing to suppurate, would be a constant drain upon the already enfeebled vital powers. This is the rule as applied to operation for fistula in ano, where it has been found to work well, and where also operating during the more severe stages of the disease in disregard of this rule has proved disastrous.

But it is the other view of such cases as Mr. Bryant's that is the more important, and was more specially raised by him at the Medical Society. This suggests two questions, Whether, and how far, local diseases of bones and joints may cause and·perpetuate phthisical changes in the lungs, and whether, such visceral disease having been lighted up, removal of the diseased bone will ameliorate the condition of the lungs? Although not actually demonstrated as regards man, there is yet every reasonable probability that chronic disease of bones or joints, especially if attended with caseation of inflammatory products, may be the starting point of genuine tuberculosis. But it is by no means so probable that the more common chronic caseating pneumonia of phthisis is due to any similar cause ; and although we cannot assert the negative, and may even be willing to entertain the supposition as one not unlikely to be established as our knowledge becomes more complete, we must at present explain differently the connection between such bone diseases and the common lung changes of pulmonary phthisis. The two affections may be both regarded as expressions of one and the same "dyscrasia," and a man who from an injury gets chronic caseating ostitis and arthritis may be held to be also predisposed to chronic caseating pneumonia from causes inefficient to produce such results in the robust. The pain, the enforced rest, the confinement to the house or to a close room or the ward of a hospital, disturbed sleep, impaired digestion, and especially the prolonged pyrexia, with its necessary increased oxidation and elimination by the lungs, may each and all bear some share in setting up lung mischief. If to this be added suppuration, with the constant drain upon the blood and the unnatural activity of the hæmatopoietic processes, especially in the lymphatic structures, we have a further link in the etiological chain. Should the disease processes in the lungs be once established, it is still more obvious how all these influences must retard if not jeopardize their subsidence. The harmful influence of bone and joint disease both in the causation and continuance of phthisis may thus be granted. And if the above expresses *all* the truth, the indications for treatment are plain—remove at once the offending bone or joint. But if the bone disease be of an infective nature, such a course would be merely closing the stable door after the horse was stolen, if the poison be of a nature to multiply within the body. Amputation of a caseous focus of a general tuberculosis would therefore be useless.

The cases in which this line of practice may be carried out with most hope of success are, then, those in which the pulmonary trouble is distinctly secondary in point of time to the disease of the bone, and where the bone disease is advanced and attended with pain and discharge, while the lung disease is limited in area and early in stage. In proportion as these conditions become altered the indication for treatment gradually shifts, until where the lung condition is primary, very advanced and wide in its area, or is merely a part of a general tuberculosis, and the bone disease is secondary and early and not attended with suppuration, amputation would only be the means of hastening death.—*Lancet*, Oct. 29, 1881.

New Methods of Treating Erectile Tumours.

M. Constantine Paul presented to the French Academy of Medicine, recently, a child whom he had cured of an erectile tumour by vaccinating the growth. M. Paul claimed that he had devised a new method for treating this class of disorders. We are not aware that he claimed for his method of treatment any essential originality. At any rate, vaccination as a method of treating small nævi has long been known to English and American surgery. But M. Paul described a new and peculiar process of performing the operation for vaccination, by means of which he had obtained the specially good results to which he called attention. In vaccinating by the ordinary method it would be quite probable that some part of the tumour's surface would not become affected. In this case the cicatricial tissue resulting from the inflammatory action would be only developed at certain points, leaving the rest of the tumour unaffected. In order to secure uniform inflammatory action throughout the entire surface, therefore, M. Paul covers the tumour with a layer of vaccine lymph, and then through this punctures are made all over the parts desired to be affected.

M. Paul presented a case treated in this way with quite notable success. The patient was a little girl who had had a large erectile tumour on the back of the head. It was situated below the occiput, extending on the right side nearly to the ear. It was, according to M. Paul, at the same time cutaneous and subcutaneous. The vaccination pustule had affected the whole part, and was three months in entirely healing. The skin where the tumour had been was then completely devascularized, but there was some erectile tissue remaining beneath it. This M. Paul believed, from previous experiences, would finally atrophy and disappear.

In a subsequent discussion upon this method of treating erectile tumours, MM. Gosselin and Blot both took the ground that M. Paul's cure was incomplete, and that in all cases where there was any subcutaneous vascularization, vaccination would be nearly futile. It could, however, cure superficial erectile tumours, and in the subcutaneous forms it would at least give a hard, strong covering to the tumour, which would prevent any danger from ulceration or rupturing with hemorrhage.

Commenting upon this procedure, M. E. Ricklin (*Gazette Médicale*) refers to another easy method of treating these tumours, which has been successful in the hands of Dr. Schrumpf. This practitioner treated several cases of bandaging and compression. The tumours were very large, but were situated either on the fore- or upper-arm. By bandaging the extremity from the fingers up, the erectile tissue was made gradually to atrophy and disappear.—*Med. Record*, Nov. 5, 1881.

—

Visceral, especially Renal, Syphilis.

M. Barthélemy reports (*Annales de Derm. et de Syph.* 1881, No. 2, p. 272) five cases of renal disease in connection with syphilis. In the following instance the patient improved under specific treatment A woman, aged 33, who had been infected three years before, was admitted into the St. Louis Hospital, under the care of M. Fournier, in November, 1879. Six months previously she had been under treatment for mucous patches, vertigo, and pain in the head. There was at that time no albumen in the urine, and after three months' treatment the woman went out cured. In October diarrhœa appeared; and at the beginning of November œdema of the lower limbs and genital organs was noticed. On readmission, the face also was puffy. There was intense dyspnœa, and *râles* were audible all over the chest, but there was no dulness, nor pain in the loins. The urine was copious, and contained a large quantity of albumen. The patient subsequently suffered from an iliac abscess, but she gradually recovered under antisyphilitic remedies, and on her discharge from hospital the urine became only slightly cloudy on the addition of nitric acid.—*London Med. Record*, Oct. 15, 1881.

Aspiration of Suppurating Buboes.

In a paper published in the *Annales de Derm. et de Syph.*, 1880, p. 224; and 1881, p. 308, M. LE PILEUR reports nineteen cases of buboes treated by aspiration. Seventeen of the buboes were in the groin; of these, twelve followed soft chancres, six being virulent and six simple abscesses. One was in a syphilitic subject, two were consecutive to scabies, and three were strumous buboes. The remaining two were submaxillary abscesses. In buboes caused by chancre, the author advises that the pus should be inoculated after aspiration, and, if it be found to be virulent, that a solution of nitrate of silver should be injected into the bubo; thus, according to the author, other openings may be prevented. Even if the opening ulcerate, the course is said to be much milder than after the use of the bistoury. M. Le Pileur thinks suppurating adenitis of every kind ought to be treated by aspiration when fluctuation is distinct. The scar is nearly invisible, or at least insignificant. The duration of the affection is shorter than under the ordinary mode of treatment. The nineteen cases gave an average duration of about twenty-four days after aspiration. For the mode of operating, the author refers the reader to his *Etude sur les Adénites Inguinales*, 1874; but, as far as can be gathered from the cases reported, the pus would seem to have been simply drawn off through a trocar, of which the point could be concealed, and a shred of lint placed in the opening and kept there for about twenty-four hours. Poultices were also applied.—*Lond. Med. Record*, Oct. 15, 1881.

Scrotal Calculus.

A unique case of this affection is reported by LIPPOMAN, in the *Wratschebuyja Wedomosti*, 1881, No. 454. The patient, a peasant, sixty-eight years old, stated that fifteen years previously he had suffered from difficulty in passing water, which finally became so aggravated that he consulted a physician, who removed from the scrotum by incision a stone weighing one hundred and twenty grammes. A urethral fistula resulted, through which all the urine passed, at first with ease, but of late with increasing difficulty. On examination a fistula was found just behind the peno-scrotal junction. All endeavours to pass a metallic or an elastic catheter per urethram were futile; only the anterior portion of the pendulous urethra was permeable. The scrotum was as large as a child's head, and was distended by a hard mass. The testicles were dislocated toward the external inguinal apertures, and were very much atrophied. On introducing a catheter into the fistula, it was arrested by a stone. On the following day an incision was carried from the fistula backward along the raphe of the scrotum, and four calculi, weighing in all forty grammes, were removed. They were rough, of a grayish-yellow colour, showed facets, and consisted of phosphates. When placed in apposition they were as large as a goose egg. The cavity left after the operation was cleansed with carbolic acid, drained, and healed kindly, leaving a fistula, through which the patient urinated.' Later he emptied his bladder with the aid of a self-made catheter, consisting of a goose-quill.—*Med. Record*, Nov. 5, 1881.

A Case of Popliteal Aneurism Cured by Means of Esmarch's Bandage and Digital Compression.

E. Z. DERR, M.D., U. S. N., reports the following case: The patient, a strong, robust man, was admitted to the U. S. Naval Hospital, Norfolk, Va., on April 15, 1881. Examination revealed the existence of a large, pulsating tumour in the left popliteal space. The calf of the leg was very much larger than its fellow, and both sensation and motion were very much diminished. Owing to this condition of things, no active surgical interference was resorted to until June 10th, when Esmarch's bandage was applied, and allowed to remain on forty-five minutes. At the end of that time the pain became so intense that it was removed. Pulsation returned after the removal of the bandage, but its force was perceptibly diminished.

On June 16 another application of the bandage was made, and allowed to remain one hour and twenty-five minutes. Pulsation returned on the removal of the bandage, but its force was still further diminished.

On July 9 the bandage was again applied, and allowed to remain one hour. At the same time digital compression was made over the femoral, and continued for six hours after the removal of the bandage. Pulsation returned after the cessation of the pressure, but was greatly diminished, and the tumour was found to be much smaller and firmer.

10th. Digital compression was continued for two hours, causing still further diminution in the size of the tumour.

11th. Compression was continued for three hours to-day, with further good results.

12th. The compression was kept up for five consecutive hours to-day, and on the removal of pressure no pulsation could be detected.

At the present writing—September 9—a hard, fibrous mass, not larger than a walnut, occupies the site of the large, pulsating tumour which previously existed.

The case is reported because it furnished another illustration of the utility of the combined method in the treatment of popliteal aneurism.—*Medical Record*, Oct. 29, 1881.

—

Rupture of the Plantaris Muscle.

In *The New York Medical Journal and Obstetrical Review* for July, 1881, Dr. A. B. JUDSON gives three cases in which he diagnosticated this injury. He remarks that it is seldom found described in systematic works on surgery, although its occurrence is probably not very uncommon. Its most remarkable feature is the trivial nature, or almost entire absence, of an immediate cause. Persons are attacked while quietly walking in the street, stopping suddenly under the impression that they have been shot in the leg. Apart from ecchymosis, which is met with in but a limited number of cases, the only objective signs are œdema and deep-seated induration, and these are by no means constant. If there is an obvious gap in the muscles, with an adjacent muscular tumour, the case is to be considered one of rupture of the muscles, the term *coup de 'fouet* being conveniently used to indicate those cases in which the exact lesion remains undetermined. The diagnosis depends on (1) the suddenness of the attack; (2) the insignificance of the apparent cause: (3) the location of the trouble; (4) the pain, which is absent or slight when the part is at rest, and produced or aggravated by those motions of the limb, active or passive, which disturb the muscles of the calf; and (5) the great disproportion between the objective and subjective symptoms. Recovery is always protracted, and is probably not much facilitated by treatment, which, however, should not be neglected, for the prognosis is sometimes unfavourable, especially when the affected limb is the seat of deep varicose veins, or shows traces of former phlebitis. Local and general remedies should be directed toward the relief of pain. Repair of the injured structures should be promoted by preventing motion or disturbance of the part affected. The condition which seems best adapted to secure this object is that of enforced fixation with the knee moderately flexed and the ankle moderately extended. As recovery progresses, locomotion will be facilitated by a high-heeled shoe, which prevents the foot from being unduly flexed on the leg. Cases of this injury present opportunities for the exercise of judgment in the decision of the question of abandoning further rest and resorting to motion and exercise.

—

Experimental Researches on the Forcible Straining of Genu Valgum.

M. MENARD studies in this paper (*Revue de Chir.*, 10th Sept. 1881) the lesions produced in forcible straining.of the knee on the cadaver, whether with the hands or with the apparatus of Collin. Without entering, he says, upon the clinical side of the question, and without establishing a comparison between this operation and other modes of treatment, some slow and belonging to orthopædic practice, others rapid, such as osteotomy, his object is to clear up the mechanism, and to determine the lesions, of the purely operative proceeding, as constituting one of the elements which permit the question to be decided as to its fitness and uses in surgery. His conclusion is that in rapid straightening of the genu valgum by Delore's method, the operative proceeding carries the knee, not directly outwards but outwards and backwards; at the same time, there is a tendency to bend the tibia inwards on the femur, and to force the extension of the knee. The articulation resists, therefore, not only by its external lateral ligament, but also by those which limit the extension, the posterior ligament and the intra-articular ligaments. This mechanism explains why it is the femur which comes away rather than the articulation. The lesion produced is very generally the stripping of the epiphysis from the inferior extremity of the femur and a large and considerable periosteal attachment, behind and external to the diaphysis. The employment of Collin's apparatus, or of any other similar one, appears to him preferable to manual force. With the hands, somewhat less lesions are produced; the detachment of the epiphysis is accompanied with crushing of the spongy tissue; moreover, the ligaments are apt to be torn away. The results appear to be very analogous in patients from two to six years of age. Beyond that age, it is a question whether the resistance of the femur becomes greater than that of the ligaments. He thinks that even then tearing of the ligaments must be very rare if the operation is well performed. This opinion is indeed only the expression of the results obtained by MM. Farabœuf and Terrillon.—*London Med. Record*, Oct. 15, 1881.

—

A Form of Gonorrhœal Arthritis.

In the *Arch. Gén. de Méd.*, May, 1881, p. 541, MM. DUPLAY and BRUN discuss a form of gonorrhœal arthritis which, according to them, had not before been fully described. This variety of arthritis may come on suddenly, without any known immediate cause, or it may follow slight injury. Most frequently, however, it is preceded by malaise, slight fever, loss of appetite, etc. The first symptom is pain, which comes on with great acuteness. This pain begins, and is always worst, just at the spot where the articular surfaces of the bones touch each other, and is increased at night. Besides this spontaneous pain, acute suffering is caused by pressure above the joint. Swelling soon follows the pain, and it also first appears exactly at the line of junction of the bones which form the joint.

There is little or no effusion into the synovial cavity, the swelling being chiefly due to infiltration of the periarticular tissues. The œdema extends above and below the affected joint, and sometimes there is an obscure kind of fluctuation, leading to a suspicion of abscess. Two cases are mentioned in which incisions were made under this belief. The swelling is not due to effusion into the sheaths of the tendons. In the treatment of this form of arthritis, the most important point is absolute rest of the joint by means of a plaster-of-Paris bandage. The pain then soon disappears, and, in favourable cases, the joint recovers almost entirely. If, however, the joint be not fixed until several days after the onset, more or less stiffness is likely to remain; and if the affection be neglected altogether, ankylosis will probably occur; indeed, this sometimes happens in spite of careful treatment. The wrist and the elbow appear to be the joints most frequently attacked, while the knee, which is frequently the seat of the effusive form (hydrarthrosis) is comparatively seldom involved. However, any joint may suffer, and the authors have seen marked examples of this form of arthritis in the metacarpal, phalangeal, and sterno-clavicular articulations. But whatever joint is attacked, the symptoms are essentially those which have just been described. The paper concludes with notes of six cases (three of the patients being women), illustrating the various points already mentioned; the chief features of this form of joint-affection are the occurrence of pain and swelling, which always begin and remain most marked exactly at the interarticular line, the presence of crackling, and the liability to ankylosis if the joint be not fixed early.—*Lond. Med. Record*, Oct. 15, 1881.

—

Treatment of Floating Bodies in the Knee.

In a recent contribution to the *Rev. de Chir.* (Nos. 5 and 6, 1881) Dr. G. GAUJOT, of the Hôpital du Val-de Grace, states that, since the inquiry of Baron Larrey, in 1861, on the treatment of floating bodies in the knee, direct extraction through a free incision has advanced much in the favour of French surgeons. The subcutaneous operation, though sound in principle, is often attended in practice with certain risks and disadvantages. Penetration of air and blood into the articular cavity cannot always be avoided, and is very likely to result, when through the size of the foreign body it is necessary to cut freely with the tenotomy knife, or when the synovial membrane is much lacerated. This result exposes the patient to the risks of synovitis, which either may be restricted to the plastic form, or may become purulent. Plastic arthritis, in consequence of the functional impairment in which it results, is a serious complication, and purulent arthritis is very often fatal. Another disadvantage attending the subcutaneous operation is the frequent difficulty and, in some instances, the impossibility of effecting extrusion of the floating body through the orifice made in the synovial membrane. Again, during the interval between the first and second stages of the subcutaneous operation, there is always a risk of the foreign body slipping back into the joint, as there is very little tendency for it to contract adhesions to the peri-arthritic cellular tissue. This result is the more likely to occur when the synovial membrane has been freely incised, and when the foreign body has not been moved to any great distance from the opening into the joint.

It is stated in this communication that the death-rate from direct extraction has, during the past fifteen years, been reduced from twenty-two to seven and a half per cent. The author endeavours to prove that this reduction is not solely due to the influence of Listerism. An analysis of fifty-four collected cases in which arthrotomy has been performed since 1863, indicates that a like success to that attained after the use of Lister's method, may be attained by other antiseptic methods, and, indeed, after the use of ordinary dressings. Of twenty-nine cases of floating body treated by arthrotomy, in which Lister's dressing had been applied, two were fatal; whilst of eighteen cases in which ordinary non-antiseptic dressings had been applied, only one had a fatal termination. Such a result, it is pointed out, need not cause surprise if one considers the success that has been attained in ovariotomy and enterotomy by Mr. Kœberle, who does not make use of Lister's dressing.

Articular synovial membranes, when affected by chronic hydrarthrosis, acquire, like other serous membranes that have been exposed to the prolonged contact of morbid products, a certain degree of tolerance that renders them less irritable and less liable to become acutely inflamed. When chronic hydrarthrosis is associated with a floating body within the joint, the tolerance of the synovial membrane is increased through the nature of the original articular affection, since, in changes due to rheumatism, there is much less tendency to suppurative inflammation. In order to insure success after direct extraction of an articular floating body, certain precautions must be taken in order to avoid acute synovitis. Such precautions consist in preventing the free access of air to the interior of the joint; in making a clean and small wound; in avoiding as much as possible irritation of the synovial membrane during the removal of the floating body; and in the exclusion of any septic agent. These evils, M. Gaujot holds, may be guarded against without resorting to any strict antiseptic treatment. In considering the question whether the extraction of an articular floating body can insure a permanent cure, the author states that it is to be remembered that in most cases the foreign body does not constitute in itself the articular lesion. It is very often but an epi-phenomenon superadded to primordial changes of a chronic arthritic character.

The operation usually results in the disappearance of the phenomena due to the presence within the joint of a foreign body, but it does not remove the other results due to antecedent articular changes. There may be a cessation of the characteristic pain and less interference with locomotion, but the symptoms of chronic hydrarthrosis, such as swelling of the joint, crepitus, and a restricted range of articular movements, will too often persist. A decision as to the probability of recurrence should be based rather on the form and composition of the floating body, than on the condition of the joint. The prognosis is favourable in those rare cases in which this body consists of a fragment of bone, or a fibrinous concretion, whilst the indications are just the reverse when it presents one of those many forms which have their common origin in fibro-cartilaginous proliferation of the synovial elements. M. Gaujot states, in concluding, that the operation of direct extraction, though one of very little danger, ought not to be practised save in cases where the functional disturbance is severe, and palliative treatment has already been applied, but without success.—*Lond. Med. Record*, Oct. 15, 1881.

—

Rare Accidents.

In the *Medical Times and Gazette* for October 15th, Mr. CHARLES MCIVHOR GOYDER reports three cases of accidents, which are interesting from the extraordinary character of the injuries. The first case is one of *compound comminuted fracture of the astragalus without fracture of the malleoli*, occurring in a very large and heavy man, and produced by slipping from a pile of chain and falling on his foot from a distance of about two feet. Upon examination, the foot appeared inverted, the external malleolus projected about an inch through a transverse wound over the outer ankle. There was no fracture of the malleoli, but the lower end of the fibula was cleanly divested of all the structures attached to its tip. Upon introducing a finger into the wound, two small chips of bone came away, cancellous in structure and covered in part by a compact layer; a great many smaller fragments were removed from the ankle-joint, when the astragalus was found to be almost completely broken up into comminuted fragments. There was no bleeding, and the foot in other respects was quite natural in appearance. The case was treated antiseptically, and placed upon a back-splint with foot-piece, and two side-splints.

The patient did well for two months, when he got an attack of phlegmonous erysipelas. An abscess formed, which travelled up the sheath of the peronei muscles, and was opened; after which the wound quickly healed, and the patient became an out-patient a month later, his leg and foot being placed in an immovable bandage.

Five years afterwards the injured leg was slightly shorter than the other, but not enough so to make him limp; there was good movement in the ankle-joint, and he can bear the whole weight of his body on his foot.

The second case is one of a *depressed fracture of the malar bone without external wound*, produced in a man while intoxicated, by falling and striking his cheek on the curbstone. When the ecchymosis and swelling were reduced, the malar bone was found to be depressed under the orbit, forcing the eyeball upwards and forwards; there was, however, no interference with sight or with the action of the orbital muscles, and examination showed the fundus to be normal. The man subsequently recovered without any marked deformity.

The third case is an *upward dislocation of the scaphoid bone of the tarsus*, produced by falling a distance of seven or eight feet on the toes and forward part of the right foot. On examining the foot there was a marked prominence in the situation corresponding to the scaphoid bone, wider from side to side than before backwards, with edges well defined, but covered by upraised tendons, etc. The foot was partially extended at the ankle-joint, and its inner border somewhat short. There was a noticeable arching of the sole of the foot, and flexion of the ankle-joint caused great pain. Reduction was easily accomplished under chloroform, and recovery occurred without complications.

Midwifery and Gynæcology.

The Mobility of the Pelvic Articulations.

Dr. KORSCH, of St. Petersburg, contributes to a recent number of the *Zeitschrift für Geburtshülfe und Gynäkologie* an account of an experimental investigation of the above subject. He had dilators so constructed that two opposite parts of the instrument could be separated, and both the extent of their separation, and the force required to effect it, measured. This instrument he applied to different parts of the pelvic cavity, and measured the extent to which its diameters could be altered, and the force required to do it. His experiments were made on the bodies of recently delivered women, of pregnant women, of non-pregnant women, and of men. The following are the conclusions he comes to: 1. Both during pregnancy and in patients suffering from large uterine or ovarian tumours, there is not only yielding of the pelvic articulations, but widening of the pelvic diameters. 2. At the pelvic inlet, the greater widening is of the transverse diameter; at the outlet, of the antero-posterior diameter. 3. To enlarge the pelvic inlet requires nearly double the force needed to widen the outlet. 4. Widening of the transverse diameter of the pelvic inlet is accompanied with shortening of the antero-posterior diameter; but widening of the latter does not alter the former. 5. When the transverse diameter of the brim has been enlarged to the maximum extent, the conjugate may still be slightly lengthened;

but when the maximum increase in length of the conjugate has been attained, the transverse diameter cannot be widened.   6. When the transverse and antero-posterior diameters of the inlet are simultaneously expanded by pressure, the amount of increase in each is not so much as when each is separately expanded. 7. Widening of the pelvic outlet diminishes slightly the conjugate, but leaves unaltered or slightly increases the transverse diameter of the brim.   8. The converse takes place when the inlet is widened.   9. In the majority of the cases the greatest amount of mobility was in the sacro-iliac synchondrosis.   10. In those joints of which the mobility was increased, the quantity of synovial fluid was usually somewhat greater.   11. Lengthening of the antero-posterior diameters depends upon the movement of the sacrum ; that of the transverse diameters upon yielding of the symphysis pubis.   12. Increase in size of the synovial cavity of the pubic articulation leads to a greater mobility of the joint. 13. The number of deliveries has, apparently, no influence on the mobility of the pelvic articulations.—*Med. Times and Gaz.*, Oct. 29, 1881.

A Peculiar Condition of the Cervix Uteri which is found in Certain Cases of Dystocia.

In support of the position taken in his earlier communications, that tonic spasm of the internal os is a more frequent cause of dystocia than the statements of the text-books would lead one to suppose, Dr. ALFRED HOSMER has collected notes of a number of additional cases where this condition of the cervix was found to interfere with labor.   His conclusions are as follows : —

1. Simple elongation of the cervix, even though it be excessive, disables the uterus by perversion of its force, renders spontaneous expulsion improbable, but in connection with artificial delivery does not produce a condition of things to which the term dystocia can be applied with any propriety of significance.

2. Tonic spasm of the internal os may in single labor be developed so early as to imprison the whole fœtus in the cavity of the uterine body, and in a multiple labor its production may be so postponed as to interfere only with the birth of the last child.   Its existence cannot necessarily be referred either to pelvic deformity, to extreme elongation of the cervix, or to the occupation of the cervical cavity by any portion of the unborn child.

Finally, tonic spasm of the internal os has shown a marked tendency to recur in the successive labors of those who have once or even twice survived the danger to which it exposed them, and the patient in whom it occurs for the first time is not necessarily a primipara.—*Boston Med. and Surg. Journ.*, Oct. 20, 1881.

Exfoliative Vaginitis and Membranous Dysmenorrhœa.

It has been a common reproach to gynæcologists that they are too fond of assuming that disorders of the general system, more particularly hysteria and allied nervous symptoms, when met along with uterine disease, are its result. Dr. COHNSTEIN, in a paper on the subject of membranous dysmenorrhœa and exfoliative vaginitis, published in a recent number of the *Archiv für Gynä-kologie*, goes to the other extreme, and, reasoning from a number of cases which he has collected (which collection makes his paper very valuable for purposes of reference), concludes that membranous dysmenorrhœa is not the cause, but the result, of hysteria, or of disorder of the general health.   He points out that in nearly all the cases of his collection the general health was much deteriorated ; that we know of no local treatment which will cure membranous dysmenorrhœa ; that membranes are sometimes passed at the menstrual period without pain ; that in many cases impairment of the general health preceded the painful menstruation. It is very difficult to see in what way hysteria should so modify the functions of the uterus as to make it excrete a membrane each month; and hysteria itself is a thing so difficult to define that it seems hardly possible that proof should be forthcoming of Dr. Cohnstein's theory. But, without going as far as he does, we think he has done good service in calling attention to the facts that nervous and hysterical symptoms going with uterine disease are not of necessity caused by it, and that menstrual pain is modified by the state of the general health in this way—that an amount of pain which a strong, healthy woman would think too trifling to mention, will put a feeble, neurotic individual quite *hors de combat*. In the latter case treatment of the general health may, without modifying the local condition, so improve the patient's power of bearing pain as to remove her from the condition of invalidism.—*Med. Times and Gaz.*, Oct. 8, 1881.

The Origin of Tubo-Ovarian Cysts.

Dr. HENRI BURNIER contributes to the *Zeitschrift für Geburtshülfe und Gynäkologie* a case of the above rare kind, which occurred in the practice of Professor Schroeder. The patient gave a history clearly indicating antecedent peritonitis. When the cyst was removed, it was found that the Fallopian tube, much dilated, opened directly into it, the opening being as big as a shilling (*Markstückgrosse*). Ray-like processes of mucous membrane, continuous with and resembling that of the tube, spread out from the opening over the inner wall of the cyst, some of them meeting at the opposite pole of the cavity. This mucous membrane was everywhere covered with cylindrical epithelium. On examination of the cyst-wall, Graafian follicles could be found, more or less abundantly, in every part of it, except where the tube entered it. The mode in which Dr. Burnier supposes this tumour to have arisen is the following:—First, an attack of peritonitis causing adhesion of the peritoneal surface of the fimbriæ of the tube to the ovary. Then, a Graafian vesicle ripening and coming to the surface at the site of this adhesion. Owing to the greater resistance caused by the inflammatory thickening, this follicle cannot burst, but becomes distended into a cyst (hydrops folliculi). At the same time, the secretion of the Fallopian tube, being retained, dilates the tube (hydrosalpinx). We thus have two collections of fluid, separated by a septum consisting of the wall of the follicle and the fimbriæ of the Fallopian tube. This septum becomes absorbed, and a tubo-ovarian cyst is the result. The adhesion between the tube and the ovary at the site of the dropsical follicle prevents this from projecting from the surface of the ovary, as such follicles are wont to do, and therefore it can only grow by stretching out the healthy tissue of the ovary round it. Hence the presence of Graafian vesicles at every part of its circumference. Dr. Burnier examines the recorded cases of tubo-ovarian cyst. Three of them, he finds, support this theory, and the others contain nothing against it. The theory of Veit, which assumes the coincidence of catarrh of the tube and hydrops folliculi, Dr. Burnier regards as quite compatible with his own view. Richard's theory, that the fimbriæ of the tube embrace the ovary at the time of bursting of the follicle, and that the tubo-ovarian tumour results from the bursting of a dropsical follicle, and effusion of its fluid into the tube, Dr. Burnier regards as untenable—first, because there is not enough evidence that the fimbriæ do embrace the ovary when the follicles break; and, secondly, because it does not account for the presence of cylinder epithelium within the tumour.—*Med. Times and Gaz.*, Oct. 15, 1881.

Incomplete Removal of Ovarian Cysts.

M. TERRIER (*Revue de Chir.*, 10th Aug. 1881) puts the following question : Does the incomplete removal of ovarian cysts, resulting from the existence of extensive solid or vascular adhesions to important organs, give, as has been said, deplorable results, and should it be avoided uniformly, as Kœberlé advises ; or is it, on the other hand, an operation which is acceptable, and even a method counselled sometimes by prudence, and not by necessity (Péan) ? M. Terrier relates some private cases, and examines the recent publication of cases and statistics by Spencer Wells and Péan, with the following results : 1. Incomplete operations ending with the opening of the cysts, suture of the walls to the abdominal wound, and drainage, give very different results, according to the nature of the cystic tumour. 2. When the cyst is unilocular—as serous cysts and dermoid cysts of the broad ligaments are—the results may be excellent, and the cystic cavity ends by being completely filled up. 3. The same result is perhaps possible in certain cysts which are unilocular from a clinical point of view, but which anatomical pathologists class as multilocular cysts. 4. When the cyst is multilocular, and when the cystic walls are clothed with vegetation, the results are very different. The tumour tends constantly to relapse, the abdominal fistula persists, and the interminable suppuration exposes the patient to chronic septicæmia and exhaustion. 5. Finally, it is to be noted, both in the case of young and of multilocular cysts, that there is a possibility of the rapid development of a tumour already pre-existing on the ovary, which has not been touched, and of which the conditions could not be verified at the time of the operation.—*London Med. Record*, Oct. 15, 1881.

Medical Jurisprudence and Toxicology.

Detection of Arsenic in Wall Papers.

Dr. WILLIAM B. HILLS takes exception to the wide publicity given to the nitrate of silver as a test for arsenic in wall-papers. He asserts that it is one of the *least* reliable tests for the purpose mentioned. The cases in which the nitrate of silver test gives fairly reliable results are comparatively few, and are essentially the ones in which arsenite of copper (Scheele's green) or aceto-arsenite of copper (Schweinfûrt green) is used as a pigment, unmixed with other substances. These arsenical compounds are, however, seldom thus used, but are commonly employed in combination with other substances, by which means the green color is modified and various tints are obtained, in which, as a rule, the arsenical green cannot be detected by any physical appearance. Under these circumstances the above test will ordinarily fail to indicate the presence of arsenic, and particularly so if the arsenical green be mixed with organic pigments. Many of these latter, when treated with ammonia, furnish colored liquids, the color varying with the nature of the organic pigments. If nitrate of silver is added to such a liquid, any precipitate produced, whatever its true color may be, will ordinarily assume the color of the liquid. For example : yellow arsenite of silver will usually *appear* red in a red liquid. Obviously no conclusion can be drawn in such cases as to the presence or absence of arsenic. Again, the yellow sulphide of arsenic is sometimes used, and arsenic in such cases cannot be detected by nitrate of silver. The test is also useless in detecting arsenious acid in the aniline colors. Dr. Hill's method of proceeding is as follows : Take a sample three or four inches square, cut into small pieces, moisten with concentrated sulphuric acid, and heat carefully until the paper is thoroughly charred.   Let the charred mass cool, add to it about one fluidounce of water, grind up the black mass so that the water may come in contact with all parts of it; filter and wash.   The arsenic will be found in the filtrate, which is to be examined by Marsh's test.   All chemicals must be free from arsenic.   A paper which, treated carefully in this manner, furnishes no arsenical stain on porcelain, does not contain any appreciable amount of arsenic.—*Louisville Med. News*, Oct. 15, 1881, from *Boston Med. and Surg. Journal.*

Poisoning by Carbolic Acid.

Two cases of poisoning by carbolic acid are reported in abstract in the last number of the *Nordiskt Mediciniskt Arkiv*.   One of them, described by Dr. J. A. Malmgren, is that of a child aged 5½ months, who had an eruption, followed by an ulcer in his groin, which was ordered to be dressed with carbolized oil (8 per cent.). The next day, he had vomiting, which was repeated during the night.   The urine was described by the mother as being "very dark and foul," and the child was very sleepy.   The carbolized oil was removed on the third day; the urine was of a deep coffee-colour, and the child slept almost constantly; the pupils were somewhat contracted; the vomiting continued.   On the fourth day, the patient's condition was about the same; but in the evening the somnolence had ceased, the vomiting was less frequent, and the urine had become much clearer.   The child recovered; but the urine retained a dark colour for a fortnight.   In the second case, related by Dr. Nordenström, a child one year old had a large fluctuating swelling in the left parotid and submaxillary regions; it was opened, and a large quantity of pus discharged.   The part was dressed with cotton-wool saturated with carbolized oil (1 in 10), over which were placed dry cotton-wool and a bandage.   The dressing was changed morning and evening.   About an hour after the application of the dressing, the child had vomiting, which continued through the following day.   The urine was of a dark green colour, and the evacuations were loose.   On the third day, the condition was about the same, and the breathing was impeded.   A mixture of equal parts of camphorated oil and olive oil was now substituted for the carbolized oil; but the child died the next morning.—*Brit. Med. Journal*, Oct. 22, 1881.

Case of Poisoning by Atropia.

The patient, a small, weak, anæmic child, aged 6, took by mistake, between 8 and 9 in the morning, a teaspoonful of a solution of atropia, 0.05 to 10.0, or about 35 milligrammes (a little more than half a grain).   His face soon became flushed, his gait staggering, and his voice hoarse.   An hour later antidotes were administered, including tannic acid, iodide of potassium, and injections of infusion of jaborandi.   Soon the patient exhibited hallucinations, and became delirious.   Seven and a half hours after the dose had been taken, REINL (*Prag. Med. Wochenschr.*, No. 20, 1880) saw the child, who was restless and unconscious and still delirious, the pulse being 140 and respirations 30.   A hypodermic injection was given of 5 centigrammes of morphia (about three-fourths of a grain), and in ten minutes the pulse fell to 100 and the respirations to 20.   The restless movements subsided, and in half an hour the patient slept, the pulse falling quickly to 96, and the respirations to 18.   The following morning, after a good night's rest, the child was quite cheerful, though there remained twitchings of the muscles of the face and extremities which continued three days.   [This case affords no proof that morphia is an antidote to atropia.   Children are curiously insusceptible to the action of belladonna.   Holthouse has recorded the case of a boy, aged 3½ years, who recovered after taking half a grain of atropia; and there have been cases of recovery after taking 0.5, 0.6, 1.0, and 1.5 grains respectively. The injection of an infusion of jaborandi could hardly be expected to do any good. It is true that a hypodermic injection of a one-hundredth part of a grain of atropia will instantly check the perspiration and salivation of jaborandi, but the converse is not the case. Atropia is a much more powerful alkaloid than pilocarpin; and in a case of poisoning by atropia recently recorded by Purjesz, of Buda-Pest, as much as 6½ grains of hydrochlorate of pilocarpin had to be administered hypodermically, before any antidotal properties were observed. It is interesting to note the fall in pulse and respiration after the injection of the morphia. It would appear that, although morphia is not an antidote to atropia, it will retard the restlessness and delirium caused by a poisonous dose of that alkaloid.—*Rep.*]—*London Med. Record*, Oct. 15, 1881.

An Accident with Hydrofluoric Acid.

Fluorine as an element is as yet unknown, it never having been isolated. The reason of this is that it is so destructive to all apparatus used for the purpose. It has been studied in its compounds and reactions, and its atomic weight has been determined indirectly. It is the only element which has no known compound with oxygen. It unites with many other elements as a monatomic acid radical and forms fluorides and also forms quite a number of double salts. Nearly all these compounds affect glass in the presence of moisture. Its hydride is a strong acid like that of chlorine, and is a gas. It dissolves many of the metals to form fluorides, is easily absorbed by water, and hence the liquid acid is obtained by saturating distilled water with the gas. It has little effect upon platinum or lead, and is transported in gutta-percha bottles as it affects neither this nor wax nor paraffine, but its action upon other organic substances is often very energetic. Mr. ROBBINS, Assistant in the Boston Institute of Technology, once attempted to redistil some of this acid as it is formed in these bottles, but neglected to dilute it one-half, as is usually done when it is wished to condense it without a freezing mixture. When heated, the gas began to come over without condensing. It charred the wooden box which surrounded the receiver, and dissolved and volatilized a piece of writing paper which was exposed to it, leaving only a slight film of a gelatinous substance, probably the gum from the sizing of the paper. Concerning the action of this acid upon animal tissues, little is known. Wurtz's dictionary gives the fullest account of it. He says in substance that it corrodes the skin, giving rise to insufferable pain, and produces a deep ulcer which is very difficult to heal; small drops of it being sufficient to produce white and painful blisters. The reporter had not read this, and was not aware of the great severity of the action of this acid, and carelessly used the stump of a match, the wood of which was saturated with the acid above referred to, to remove the lime, etc., from the surface of a piece of porcelain so as to obtain the freest action on the part where it was desired to etch a hole. When he first noticed that it was getting upon his fingers, he washed them and greased them with tallow, and thinking they were sufficiently protected, he went on with his work. For about an hour and a half he had the match in his fingers the greatest part of the time. Just before getting the hole through, he noticed that the ends of his forefinger and thumb were beginning to be unsensitive, and felt a curious sort of dull pain that perhaps might best be described by saying that the fingers "hurt" a little. When through he washed them well, applied dilute ammonia water and washed that off, and then applied bicarbonate of soda, but these measures did not relieve the pain from soon becoming very uncomfortable, and the fingers were dressed in a mixture of linseed oil and lime-water, as it felt more like a burn than anything else. This was done between 11 and 12 A. M. That afternoon the pain gradually increased, and in the evening Dr. Blodgett was consulted.

At this time the ends of the fingers were white and very hard; so hard, indeed, as to dull the scalpel with which he endeavoured to cut away some of the skin. The action was still going on, and as the depth to which it had penetrated could not be determined a dressing of cold cream was applied, and later vaseline was used, but neither seemed to allay the steady increase of the pain which now most nearly resembled the sensation of a burn when held near the fire. The only relief obtained was by the application of cold, and this was only partial, and the only variation in it was from bad to worse, and at last it became the most severe pain imaginable, and it was not till four o'clock the next morning, and with the aid of 110 drops of laudanum, that sufficient relief was obtained for a broken nap. The next day the pain had subsided, and the acid had penetrated quite a distance below the skin, rendering the flesh totally insensible and hard, having abstracted all the water from it. The other fingers were only slightly swollen, and the swelling did not extend back as far as the hand, showing that the blood was not poisoned at all. The course of treatment was to remove the destroyed tissue. This it was thought best not to do with the knife, but poultices alternating with frequent soakings in very hot water were constantly employed, which proved effectual, although slow, in its operation, it being fully twenty days from the time of injury till the slough was all removed. It was very dry and tough, and by no means inclined to separate from the surrounding tissues. In four weeks all dressings to the fingers were abandoned, and he was able to use them a little. Only a small permanent loss of tissue has resulted, but now, after three months, the scars are tender, and the sensation is perhaps permanently destroyed. This agrees with the action of this acid as stated by Wurtz, especially as regards the pain, but he does not mention the very important fact that no pain is felt for some time after contact with the acid, which, in the case reported, was between one and one and a half hour, and by this time the surface has become so hard that it is difficult, if not impossible, to check the action underneath, so that the damage is for the most part done before one finds it out.

The difficulty in healing appears to consist in removing the slough, as it heals very quickly when this is out of the way, and after the first siege of pain, which is a long and severe one, the sore is no more painful than any other of equal size. The author thinks that, should he meet with the same accident again, he should lose no time in washing it off as thoroughly as possible and then apply water-glass. if this were accessible; if not, an alkali should be used, and if possible the part soaked in water as hot as could be borne, and then cold cream applied or some other dressing which will keep the part soft and also exclude the air.

Mr. Robbins also heard of two other persons who have had misfortune with this acid; they were Dr. C. F. Folsom and a Mr. Lodge. The latter had the end of his thumb badly burned. It was three months in healing, and quite a loss of substance resulted. Books on chemistry and teachers of the science should give greater precautions as to the use of this dangerous reagent.—*Boston Med. and Surg. Journ.*, Oct. 27, 1881.

MEDICAL NEWS.

——

To Subscribers.

With this number ends the thirty-ninth year of the "Medical News," and also its publication as a monthly. But two professional periodicals —the "American Journal of the Medical Sciences" and the "Boston Medical and Surgical Journal," are still issued, of those which were in existence at the time of its birth, and during the long period through which it has made its regular monthly visits to its readers, it has witnessed the rise of all the rest of its valued contemporaries, many of which started under flattering auspices only to fulfil a comparatively brief career.

It is with feelings of thankfulness to those whose steady support has enabled it already to outlast a generation that its conductors are able to say that it has not only passed in safety through the numerous financial and political vicissitudes which have wrecked so many promising enter- prises, but that the increasing demands upon it have necessitated at last a change, which has been for some time in contemplation, whereby it will be greatly enlarged in size and converted into a weekly, thus fulfilling more perfectly the mission, which it has always had in view, of convey- ing to the profession early intelligence of all that is of importance to the practitioner. With this object, very extensive and complete arrangements have been made. The editorial staff has been enlarged; assurances of active collaboration have been received from the leading members of the profession throughout the entire country; the services of correspondents have been engaged in every large centre of professional activity through- out the world, and a larger reportorial corps has been organized, so that nothing may be lost, whether in the sphere of clinical observation and experience, original thought, or prompt announcement of improvements and discoveries in the medical sciences wherever originating.

For further details as to the plan of the WEEKLY "NEWS" and its terms to subscribers we refer to the prospectus of the publishers, and to the forthcoming January number itself, which will be shortly issued, and a copy of which will be duly laid before each of our readers. We will only add that a design so extensive, and so much in advance of anything that has hitherto been attempted for the service of the medical public, can only be rendered permanent by commensurate support on the part of the profession—a support very far beyond that hitherto conferred on even the most successful of our medical periodicals. To aid in obtaining this the publishers feel that they can rely upon their old subscribers, not only in view of the friendly association created by prolonged intercourse, but also from the conviction that the wider the circulation of the WEEKLY NEWS, the more perfectly it will be enabled to discharge the functions which it will assume, of a medical newspaper indispensable to all who desire to keep themselves abreast of the progress of medical knowledge.

When the NEWS was started, the population of the United States was less than nineteen millions. We now number fifty millions, with five millions more among our Canadian neighbors—in all fifty-five millions of the most active, intelligent, and progressive race among men. With the wants of such a population to be supplied, the conductors of the WEEKLY NEWS feel that there must be an opportunity for establishing a medical journal on a scale not heretofore attempted, and it will be their earnest effort to fully discharge in every way the very serious responsibilities of the task which they have undertaken.

Ovariotomy under "Modified Listerism."—Dr. GEO. GRANVILLE BANTOCK, in the *Lancet* for Sept. 17, 1881, describes his present method of performing ovariotomy. By the term "Modified Listerism," he means that all the manipulatory details of "Listerism" are followed during the operation, but for the spray, etc., plain water is used instead of what was supposed to be a germicide solution of carbolic acid. The instruments are kept covered in trays with warm water, the hands and sponges are washed with the same, and a spray is made to play *over*, but not *upon* the abdomen. Particular attention is drawn to the mode of using the spray. Previous to October last it was directed upon the abdomen from the right front, so that whenever the parietes were lifted up the cold acid vapour was forced into the cavity from a distance of about four feet. The author thinks that this continuous blast of spray, passing freely as it did over all the parts exposed, produced a very decided cooling effect. The powers of the patient were thus inevitably depressed, and an unnecessary and injurious amount of carbolic acid was thrown upon the peritoneum. Now, following the example of Dr. Keith, the spray producer is placed at a distance of eight or ten feet behind and to the left of the patient, so that the spray passes over, but does not fall upon the field of operation, except in very minute quantity, and without any cooling effect. In this way the peritoneal cavity, in sponging out or looking for bleeding points, is left untainted, and the patient is not chilled. The spray is never used for dressing after the operation, even in drainage cases.

It may be in the recollection of some that at the time of reading of the author's paper before the Royal Medical and Chirurgical Society, it was stated that he had already reduced the carbolic solution to 1 in 100, and intimated that in consequence of the improved results obtained, he should probably dispense altogether with the phenol. After employing this solution in twenty cases, with only two deaths—one from shock and the other from acute uræmia—and with a diminished pyrexia among the recoveries, two ovariotomies were performed and a combined oöphorectomy and hysterectomy with a further dilution of the solutions to 1 in 150. These cases proving still more clearly that the motive was in the right direction, he finally threw aside *all* the acid, and resorted to the pure water metho now followed with apparently equally good results.

Early Experiments in Bovine Inoculation.—It is generally supposed that the attempt to prevent the contagious diseases of animals by prophylactic inoculation, after the manner of vaccination, is entirely a result of the latest development of pathological science. M. Bouley, however, at a recent meeting of the Académie de Médecine, pointed out that this is an error. Ih 1852 a similar attempt was made in Holland. The experiments were designed to confer immunity against the. contagious pleuro-pneumonia, the infectious nature of which, and the protection conferred by an attack, however mild, were pointed out in 1850 by a French Commission appointed at the suggestion of M. J. B. Dumas. The Dutch experiments, however, failed completely, probably in consequence of the mode of inoculation. The place selected was the loose skin below the neck, where the subcutaneous tissue is abundant. When the virus of pleuro-pneumonia is inoculated into such loose cellular tissue, it causes a rapid inflammatory infiltration of such intensity that gangrene and death almost certainly ensue. If, however, the inoculation is made in a situation in which the subcutaneous cellular tissue is dense and scanty, the local effects are slight; the animals escape the immediate results of the inoculation, and acquire the desired immunity. This was recognized a little later by a Dutch observer, Willems de Starrett, who chose the root of the tail as the place of inoculation. Of sixteen oxen inoculated in the throat, twelve died from the local process. Of sixteen others which were inoculated on the tail, all survived; and in all subsequent inoculation in the neck had no effect.—*Lancet*, Oct. 1, 1881.

Hospitals for Contagious Diseases.—The New York Board of Health is about to erect some new hospitals for the reception of contagious diseases upon North Brothers Island, which was granted to the city of New York for the use of the Health Board by the last Legislature. The island is situated in the sound near Port Morris. It has an area of about 13 acres, and is well adapted, both by its size and its isolation, for the sites of the proposed hospitals. One of these, which will be exclusively for smallpox cases, will be erected on the northern shore of the island. It will be of brick, and two stories in height. Other hospitals will be built for patients suffering from typhus fever, diphtheria, and scarlet fever, after the island has been provided with a sea-wall and properly graded. $40,000 have been appropriated for these improvements, but much more will be required. It is hoped that the smallpox hospital will be completed early in the spring of 1882. As soon as the new hospitals are finished, the Riverside Hospital on Blackwell's Island will be abandoned. The Health Board has recently purchased a swift and stanch steam-launch, which is used to convey cases of contagious diseases to the Riverside Hospital, and to carry those who die from such diseases to their burial-place on Hart's Island.

Rules for Authors.—Dr. BILLINGS, in his able, practical, and witty address before the London Congress, laid down the following cardinal rules for authors in the preparation of journal articles, which we heartily endorse :—

1. Have something to say.　2. Say it.　3. Stop as soon as you have said it. 4. Give the paper a proper title.

The Laryngological Congress.—At a meeting of the sub-section for the Diseases of the Throat of the International Medical Congress, the following resolution, moved by Professor Schnitzler, of Vienna, was carried unanimously : "That, opportunity having now been afforded for the first time to laryngology to show its capabilities at an International Medical Congress, and its place amongst the recognized specialties being now fully secured, a repetition of isolated Laryngological Congresses is the less required; and that it is therefore desirable to abandon the plan adopted at the first Laryngological Congress held at Milan last year of holding a second meeting next year at Paris." Although the Section and the

Congress are not the same bodies, and a resolution of one is not binding on the other, it is evident, that, as this resolution was carried by a meeting at which nearly all the leading laryngologists were present, the special Congress is practically merged in the International Medical Congress.—*Lancet*, Sept. 24, 1881.

Health of New York.—The sanitary condition of the city is not so satisfactory at the present time as it was during the months of September and October. During the four weeks ending November 19, there were 2655 deaths. During the same period there were 484 cases of scarlet fever as contrasted with 320 in August and 259 in September. 70 cases of variola were reported, against 75 in August and 46 in September. The number of rubeola cases for the corresponding weeks was 77, instead of 96 and 36, which were the numbers, respectively, for August and September. On the other hand, diphtheria diminished from 355 in August and 276 in September, to 270 during the period in question. The case of supposed typhus fever, reported to have occurred in October, was discovered at the autopsy, conducted under the supervision of one of the Health Commissioners, not to have been a case of that disease. No genuine cases of typhus have been observed in New York since August 27. Nearly all the proprietors of factories at Hunter's point have adopted methods of manufacture which involve a minimum pollution of the atmosphere. The odours emanating from that quarter are consequently much less penetrating and offensive than formerly.

Listerism at Montpellier.—In a clinical lecture, delivered by Prof. DUBREUIL at the St. Eloi Hospital, Montpellier, on a case of amputation (*Gaz. Méd.*, September 17), he observed : " Here we are working with bad surroundings, for we have to complain alike of the faulty construction of our wards, of the unsuitable manner in which they are kept, and of the defective services of the subaltern attendants, who are insufficiently looked after. So that, prior to the adoption of Lister's method, the results of our operations were detestable ; but, thanks be to God and to Lister, all this is now changed, and death after amputation has now become a rare exception, while formerly it was the rule. You observe that I rigorously follow out the precepts of the antiseptic method, for I really cannot understand that mania of some surgeons, who will persist in modifying the precepts of the master, even at the risk of compromising the results. As for me, I follow them out literally, and I declare to you that, in my eyes, the surgeon who at the present time does not adopt the antiseptic method commits an act of criminal folly and odious inhumanity."—*Med. Times and Gaz.*, Oct. 1, 1881.

A Solvent for Quinia Sulphate.—Dr. R. C. KENNER, of Batesville, Ark., recommends (*Louisville Med. News*, Nov. 5, 1881) the solution of quinia in sweet spirit of nitre, in the proportion of twenty grains of the salt to the ounce of the solvent, in cases where there is inability to swallow pills.

The New Manhattan Eye and Ear Hospital, at the corner of Park Avenue and Forty-first Street, was completed on the first of October. It is substantially constructed of red brick with brown-stone trimmings. It has a depth of 100 feet on Forty-first Street, and a frontage of 60 feet on Park Avenue. The walls of the entrance hall, the passages, and the staircase walls are of red brick. The two lower floors are built of brick arches and iron beams, which are covered with ornamental tiling. Out-door patients will be received in the basement and the first story. The second and third stories contain wards and private rooms for the accommodation of patients requiring treatment in the hospital. The capacity of these two floors will be about 80. The fourth floor contains two wards and some private bed-rooms. The kitchen is also located upon the fourth floor. An amphitheatre is situated in the second story, and there is a dining-room on each floor. The engine- and boiler-room, and also the closets, are in a separate building, entirely disconnected from the hospital proper. The buildings will be heated by steam, well lighted with gas, thoroughly ventilated, and provided with three large elevators. There are three broad oaken staircases. The cost of the hospital will be about $120,000.

A Case of Recovery after prolonged Immersion.—Mr. CHAS. POPE gives an account in the *Lancet* for Oct. 1st, of a man who recovered after from twelve to fifteen minutes immersion in water. He was held tightly jammed against a wall by some weight which had capsized his boat, and the reporter attributes his recovery to the fact that this mechanical compression interfered with respiration and thus prevented the filling of the lungs with water.

Deliquescent Salts in Street Watering.—The observations of M Miquel on the constant presence of bacteria—septic, if not pathogenic at all times—in the dust of towns, have recalled attention to the question of the expediency of adding deliquescent salts (if also germicidal, so much the better) to the water used for laying the dust in streets. The idea is not new, the experiment having been made at different times in Glasgow, Paris, and elsewhere, but abandoned for reasons with which we are unacquainted. M. Houzeau, from four years' experience at Rouen, finds that the addition of calcic chloride actually reduces the cost of watering by one-third; for while, under the old system, the operation had to be repeated four times a day, a single watering now sufficed for not less than five or six. The solution employed was the waste liquor from the manufactories of pyroligneous acid, containing, besides calcium chloride, notable quantities of iron and volatile tarry matters also of value as antiseptics. The only reason for its abandonment at Rouen was that improvements in the manufacture of the acid so reduced the strength of the residual liquor that it could no longer be used with advantage commercially. But if the sanitary benefit as well as the comfort of preventing the dispersion of dust were fully realized, no doubt other sources of calcium chloride with the accompanying tar products—as, for example, the manufacture of ammonia from gas liquor—could be found, which would not materially, if at all, increase the cost of street-watering.—*Med. Times and Gaz.*, Oct. 15, 1881.

The Bressa Prize.—The Royal Academy of Science of Turin announces that a prize of 12,000 lire (£480), founded by the late Dr. C. A. Bressa, will be given to the competitor who shall, in the opinion of the Academy, have, during the four years 1879–82, made the most important and useful discovery, or produced the best work, in physical and experimental science, natural history, pure and applied mathematics, chemistry, physiology, or pathology, not excluding geology, history, geography, and statistics. Scientific men and inventors of all nations are invited to compete; the only persons excluded being the members of the Academy.—*British Med. Journal*, Oct. 22, 1881.

OBITUARY RECORD. — At his residence near Philadelphia, on the 31st of October, 1881, WILLIAM FURNESS JENKS, M.D., aged 39 years.

The death of Dr. Jenks finished a life which a few years ago was full of promise. Educated at Harvard, he received his medical degree from the University of Pennsylvania in 1866, and after a term of service as Resident Physician in the Philadelphia Hospital he studied obstetrics and gynæcology in the special schools of Berlin, Vienna, London, and Edinburgh. In 1870 he began the practice of his profession in Philadelphia, and lost no time in finding in dispensary service the opportunity of acquiring a practical knowledge of the sciences which he had so carefully studied, and for three years gave a course of practical obstetrics illustrated by operations on the cadaver. For only a few years, however, was he able to continue his work. In the autumn of 1874, failing health compelled him to pass the winter in Florida. On his return, he made an effort to resume work, but was soon forced to give up, and again seek in a foreign climate the health refused him in his own. From this time his professional labours were over, for he saw that the only hope of prolonging his life was in the entire abandonment of all work. For a few years his search for health was partially successful, and he lived in comparative comfort until last October, when after a short confinement in bed he quietly passed away.

Breaking down almost at the beginning of his professional life, Dr. Jenks left but little behind him by which he could be judged, and the full measure of our loss properly estimated. His exhaustive review of Schrœder,[1] and the paper on "Sarcomatous Growths of the Uterus,"[2] bear, however, sufficient evidence of the extent of his knowledge, and of the close analytical character of his mind. A pupil of Sir James Y. Simpson, he regarded the obstetric forceps as extractors, rather than compressors, and after persistent efforts, succeeded in introducing the Simpson Forceps into Philadelphia obstetric practice. A skilful pathologist, he, at the time of his first illness, was preparing a course of lectures on uterine and ovarian pathology for the College of Physicians. Had he been able to complete this course, it would have been a very valuable contribution to this branch of medical science. It, however, was not to be, and when he died, almost nothing remained to his friends, save the recollection of the brilliancy of his genius, his patient industry, and the sparkling geniality of his manner.

—— At his residence near Dublin, on Oct. 21, ALFRED McCINTOCK, M.D., LL.D., F.R.C.S.I., who is well known in this country as the author of "Clinical Memoirs on the Diseases of Women," and as the editor of Smellie's Midwifery, for the New Sydenham Society.

—— At Paris, October 27, Professor JEAN BAPTISTE BOUILLAUD. Born in 1795, Bouillaud was a young and earnest student when the discovery of auscultation by Laennec gave him the means of making the discovery which will always be connected with his name—the relationship between rheumatism and cardiac disease. He was the author of the word endocarditis, and gave an excellent description of the anatomical changes which accompany that disease. In 1831, he obtained, by open competition, the chair of Clinical Medicine at La Charité, where he was an ardent teacher of the doctrine of Broussais, that all diseases were inflammations, and required treatment by bleeding. In 1842 he was returned to the Assembly by his native town, Angoulême, and after the revolution of '48, he was promoted to the post of Dean of the Medical Faculty. He was a member of the Institute and of the Academy of Sciences.

—— At Glasgow, on the 31st of October, DAVID FOULIS, M.D., aged thirty-five. Dr. Foulis was a rising specialist in diseases of the throat, his wide reputation having been achieved by his performing for the first time in England, the operation for the extirpation of the larynx. Dr. Foulis died of diphtheria contracted from a patient on whom he had performed tracheotomy a few days before.

---

[1] American Journal Med. Sciences, Oct. 1872.
[2] Amer. Supplement to the Obs. Journ. of G. B. and I., Oct. and Nov. 1873.

INDEX.